Interventional Radiology

NOTICE

Medicine is an ever-changing science. As new research and clinical experience broaden our knowledge, changes in treatment and drug therapy are required. The editors and the publisher of this work have checked with sources believed to be reliable in their efforts to provide information that is complete and generally in accord with the standards accepted at the time of publication. However, in view of the possibility of human error or changes in medical sciences, neither the editors nor the publisher nor any other party who has been involved in the preparation or publication of this work warrants that the information contained herein is in every respect accurate or complete. Readers are encouraged to confirm the information contained herein with other sources. For example and in particular, readers are advised to check the product information sheet included in the package of each drug they plan to administer to be certain that the information contained in this book is accurate and that changes have not been made in the recommended dose or in the contraindications for administration. This recommendation is of particular importance in connection with new or infrequently used drugs.

Interventional Radiology

Renan Uflacker, M.D., M.Sc.
HEAD, SECTION OF VASCULAR AND INTERVENTIONAL RADIOLOGY
MED–IMAGEM
Hospital Beneficência Portuguesa
São Paulo, Brazil

Mark H. Wholey, M.D.
CLINICAL PROFESSOR OF RADIOLOGY
University of Pittsburgh School of Medicine
DIRECTOR, DEPARTMENT OF IMAGING AND RADIOLOGICAL SCIENCES
Shadyside Hospital
Pittsburgh, Pennsylvania

McGraw-Hill, Inc.
Health Professions Division

New York St Louis San Francisco Auckland Bogotá Caracas Hamburg
Lisbon London Madrid Mexico Milan Montreal New Delhi Paris San Juan
São Paulo Singapore Sydney Tokyo Toronto

Interventional Radiology

Copyright 1991 by McGraw-Hill, Inc. All rights reserved. Printed in the United States of America. Except as permitted under the United States Copyright Act of 1976, no part of this publication may be reproduced or distributed in any form or by any means, or stored in a data base or retrieval system, without the prior written permission of the publisher.

1234567890   H A L H A L   987654321

ISBN 0-07-065735-1

This book was set in ITC Garamond by Monotype Company, Inc. The editors were Edward Bolger, William Day, and Mariapaz Ramos-Englis; the production supervisor was Richard Ruzycka. The index was prepared by Alexandra Nickerson. The text and cover were designed by Leon Bolognese. Halliday Lithograph Corporation was printer and binder.

Library of Congress Cataloging-in-Publication Data

Uflacker, Renan.
   [Radiologia intervencionista. English]
   Interventional radiology / Renan Uflacker, Mark H. Wholey.
     p. cm.
   Translated and updated ed. of: Radiologia intervencionista.
   Includes bibliographical references and index.
   ISBN 0-07-065735-1
   1. Radiology, Interventional.   I. Wholey, Mark H. (Mark Henry),
   date .   II. Title.
   [DNLM: 1. Angioplasty, Transluminal.   2. Embolization,
Therapeutic.   3. Radiography, Interventional—methods. WN 200
U25r]
RD33.55.U3513   1991
617.4′13059—dc20
DNLM/DLC
for Library of Congress   90-13670
                                                    CIP

To Helena
and to my children,
Andre and Alice
To my parents,
Thank you
RU

To my children
MHW

Contents

CONTRIBUTORS   xvii
PREFACE   xix

Chapter One
Catheterization Techniques / *Renan Uflacker*   1

Introduction   1
Puncture   1
Introducing the Guidewire   3
Catheterization   4
Superselective Catheterization   10
   Exchange catheter technique   10
   Steerable devices (deflecting guidewire)   10
   Coaxial catheters   11
REFERENCES   15

Chapter Two
Embolization Procedures: Techniques and Materials / *Renan Uflacker*   17

Introduction   17
Materials   17
   Short-term embolization materials   17
   Intermediate-term embolization materials   18
   Long-term embolization materials   19
   Other materials   29
Therapeutic Uses   30
   Gastrointestinal bleeding   30
   Intraabdominal extraluminal hemorrhage   30
   Neoplastic bleeding   30
   Bleeding secondary to trauma   30
   Hemoptysis   30
   Pulmonary arteriovenous fistulas   31
   Visceral arteriovenous fistulas   31
   Aneurysms   31
   Arteriovenous malformations   31
Complications of Embolization   31
REFERENCES   43

Chapter Three
Gastrointestinal Bleeding / *Renan Uflacker*   45

General Aspects   45
Upper Gastrointestinal Bleeding   47
Anatomy   47
Angiographic Aspects of Bleeding   47
Difficulties of Interpretation and Treatment   48
Upper Gastrointestinal Bleeding from Mallory-Weiss Tears   49
Gastric Mucosal Bleeding (Gastritis)   49
Gastric Ulcer   51
Duodenal Ulcer   55

Other Situations Associated with Upper Gastrointestinal Bleeding   59
   Infusion of vasopressin   64
   Percutaneous embolization   66
REFERENCES   67
Lower Gastrointestinal Bleeding   68
   Massive intermittent or small-volume chronic bleeding   68
   Massive acute bleeding   68
   Infusion of vasoconstricting agents   68
   Embolization   70
Lower Gastrointestinal Bleeding Related to the Small Intestine   70
   Inflammatory disease   70
   Nonspecific ulcerations (stress, uremic)   70
   Vasculitis   74
   Tumors   74
   Ischemic ulcerations   80
   Arteriovenous malformations   80
   Intestinal varices   82
   Postoperative bleeding   84
Lower Gastrointestinal Bleeding Related to the Colon   84
   Diverticula   84
   Angiodysplasia   86
   Ischemic ulcers   89
   Tumors   90
   Arteriovenous malformations   92
   Stress ulcers (uremic and unspecific)   93
   Inflammatory colonic diseases   93
   Postoperative bleeding   95
   Abscesses   96
   Adenomatous, villous, and hyperplastic polyps   96
   Vasculitis   99
REFERENCES   100
Portal Hypertension and Gastrointestinal Bleeding   101
General Aspects   101
Hyperkinetic Portal Hypertension   103
Extrahepatic Presinusoidal Portal Hypertension   105
   Portal vein obstruction   105
Intrahepatic Presinusoidal Portal Hypertension   110
   Schistosomiasis   110
   Congenital hepatic fibrosis   112
Intrahepatic Portal Hypertension   112
   Hepatic cirrhosis   112
Postsinusoidal Intrahepatic Portal Hypertension   121
   Budd-Chiari syndrome   121
Portosystemic Encephalopathy Caused by a Surgically Created or Spontaneous Shunt   128
Complications from Percutaneous Transhepatic Portography and Embolization
   of Gastroesophageal Varices   133
REFERENCES   134

Chapter Four
Clinical Applications of Embolization   137

Introduction   137
EMBOLIZATION IN THE LIVER *Renan Uflacker*   138
Background   138

Hepatic Artery Aneurysms and Hemobilia   138
Traumatic, Congenital, and Tumoral Arteriovenous Fistulas   144
Hepatic Hemangiomas   147
Bleeding from Hepatic Tumors   149
Metastatic Endocrine Tumors in the Liver   152
Infusion and Embolization of Hepatic Neoplasms   153
Intraarterial Infusion of Chemotherapeutic Agents   153
Hepatic Arterial Embolization   153
Chemoembolization of Hepatic Neoplasms   156
REFERENCES   166

SPLENIC EMBOLIZATION   *Rubens de Souza A. Pinheiro / Renan Uflacker*   167

Partial Splenic Embolization in Hypersplenism   167
   Treatment   168
Splenic Embolization in Cases of Trauma   169
Embolization of Splenic Artery Aneurysms   172
REFERENCES   173

EMBOLIZATION IN THE PANCREAS   *Renan Uflacker*   174

Hemorrhage Secondary to Pancreatitis   174
Functional Pancreatic Tumors   175
REFERENCES   176

RENAL EMBOLIZATION   *Rosa Maria Paolini / Renan Uflacker*   177

Renal Tumors   177
Renal Hematuria of Nontumoral Origin   181
Hypertension of Renal Origin   185
REFERENCES   190

THORACIC EMBOLIZATION   *Renan Uflacker*   192

Pulmonary Arteriovenous Fistulas   192
Postsurgical Thoracic Bleeding   195
Hemoptysis   195
Pulmonary Sequestration   209
REFERENCES   209

EMBOLIZATION IN CASES OF VARICOCELE   *Renan Uflacker*   211

Background   211
Anatomic Considerations   211
Technique   212
Results   215
REFERENCES   215

EMBOLIZATION IN CASES OF BLEEDING FROM PELVIC ORGANS
   Guillherme de Souza Mourão   216

Background   216
Anatomic Considerations   216
Technique   216
Complications   217
REFERENCES   220

EMBOLIZATION IN TRAUMATIC AND ANEURYSMAL LESIONS   *Renan Uflacker*   221

Background   221
Abdominal Organs   221
Pelvic Lesions   222
Lesions of the Extremities   222
Aneurysmal Lesions   222
REFERENCES   226

TUMORAL LESIONS IN SOFT TISSUE AND BONES *Renan Uflacker* 227

Background 227
Technique 227

EMBOLIZATION IN HEMANGIOMAS, ARTERIOVENOUS MALFORMATIONS, AND ARTERIOVENOUS FISTULAS *Renan Uflacker* 233

Classification 233
Hemangiomas 234
Arteriovenous Malformations 236
Arteriovenous Fistulas 238
Angiomatosis 246
Therapeutic Approach 246
Treatment 247
    Observation 247
    Corticosteroids 247
    Radiotherapy 247
    Compression treatment 247
    Sclerosing agents 248
    Embolization 248
REFERENCES 250

EMBOLIZATION OF LESIONS IN THE HEAD AND NECK *Marcio Sampaio / Ronie Leo Piske* 251

Traumatic Arteriovenous Fistulas 251
    Carotid cavernous fistulas 251
    Arteriovenous fistulas of the face, neck, and scalp 260
Angiomatous Lesions 260
    Intracerebral arteriovenous angiomas 260
    Vascular lesions of the face and neck 264
    Vascular tumors 267
    Vascular malformations 267
    Hemolymphangiomas and lymphangiomas 281
    Angiomatoses 284
Dural Arteriovenous Malformations 284
Tumors 289
    Meningiomas 289
    Nasopharyngeal angiofibromas 290
    Paragangliomas 292
    Other tumors 296
    Epistaxis 296
REFERENCES 301

Chapter Five
Interventional Radiology in the Biliary Tract / *Renan Uflacker* 305

Introduction 305
Indications and Contraindications 305
Patient Preparation 306
Materials 306
Technique 307
    External biliary drainage 310
    Internal-external biliary drainage 310
    Internal biliary drainage (endoprosthesis) 322
    Special techniques for biliary drainage 326
    Metastatic disease of the porta hepatis 333
    Pancreatic carcinoma 334

Cholangiocarcinoma 334
Carcinoma of the gallbladder 334
Complications 336
Complications caused by the catheter 336
Complications caused by the technique 344
Results 344
REFERENCES 345

EXTRACTION OF RESIDUAL STONES FROM THE COMMON BILE DUCT *Renan Uflacker* 348

Methodology 348
Indications 349
Stone Size 351
Stone Impaction 352
Results 354
Complications 354
REFERENCES 356

DILATATION OF BENIGN BILIARY STENOSES *Rosa Maria Paolini / Renan Uflacker* 357

Technique 357
Results 357
REFERENCES 359

BRACHYTHERAPY WITH IRIDIUM-192 WIRE IN THE MANAGEMENT OF CHOLANGIOCARCINOMA
 Rosa Maria Paolini 360

Technique 360

BILIARY DUCT RECONSTRUCTION *Renan Uflacker* 362

Technique 362
REFERENCES 367

TREATMENT OF BILIARY STONES *Renan Uflacker* 368

Percutaneous Cholecystostomy 368
Stone Dissolution Agents 370
Oral Bile Salts 370
Topical Agents 370
 Mono-octanoin 371
 Methyl tert-butyl ether 371
Percutaneous Lithotripsy of Biliary Calculi 374
Gallbladder Ablation and Cystic Duct Occlusion 374
Extracorporeal Shock Wave Lithotripsy 376
 Principles 376
 Patient selection 376
 Technique 378
 Results 378
 Conclusions 379
REFERENCES 381

Chapter Six
Angioplasty 383

INTRODUCTION *Renan Uflacker* 383

Indications and Contraindications 383
Techniques, Materials, and Hemodynamics 385
 Basic techniques of angioplasty 385
 Choosing the axillary or femoral approach 390
 Dilatation balloons 390
The Mechanism of Angioplasty 392

Technique for Transluminal Angioplasty of Renal Arteries   394
Mechanisms and Hemodynamics   395
The Dynamics of Flow   399
REFERENCES   400

RENAL HYPERTENSION   *Rosa Maria Paolini*   401

The Pathophysiology of Renal Vascular Disease   401
Frequency   402
The Hemodynamic Effects of Renal Artery Stenosis   402
Renal Artery Stenosis Caused by Atherosclerosis   402
Renal Artery Stenosis Caused by Fibromuscular Dysplasia   402
   Branch involvement   409
Renal Artery Stenosis Caused by Arteritis   409
Measurement of the Stenosis   409
Collateral Circulation   409
Clinical and Laboratory Evaluation of Arterial Hypertension   409
   Etiology   409
   Risk factors   409
   Target-organ involvement   412
   Clinical approach   412
   Laboratory tests   413
REFERENCES   413

RENAL ARTERY PERCUTANEOUS TRANSLUMINAL ANGIOPLASTY (RAPTA)   *Rosa Maria Paolini*   414

Indications and Contraindications   414
Basic Technique   414
RAPTA in Kidney Transplant Cases   415
   Technique   416
REFERENCES   417

ANGIOPLASTY OF THE AORTA AND THE AORTIC BIFURCATION   *Renan Uflacker*   419

REFERENCES   422

ANGIOPLASTY OF THE ILIAC ARTERIES   *Renan Uflacker*   423

Iliac Stenosis   423
Iliac Occlusion   427
Simultaneous Treatment of Iliac and Distal Arteries   429
REFERENCES   432

FEMORAL, POPLITEAL, AND DISTAL BRANCH ANGIOPLASTY   *Renan Uflacker*   433

Femoral Angioplasty   433
Angioplasty of the Popliteal and Distal Branch Arteries   437
REFERENCES   442

ANGIOPLASTY OF OTHER ARTERIES   *Renan Uflacker*   443

Branches of the Thoracic Aorta   443
   Subclavian and brachial arteries   443
   Carotid and vertebral arteries   446
Mesenteric Vessels   446
Hypogastric Arteries   448
REFERENCES   450

VENOUS ANGIOPLASTY *Renan Uflacker* 452

REFERENCES 454

COMPLICATIONS OF ANGIOPLASTY *Renan Uflacker* 455

Reactions associated with arterial puncture 455
Local reactions 456
Hemodynamic problems 460
Reaction to contrast media or medication 460

REFERENCES 461

INTRAVASCULAR STENTS *Julio C. Palmaz* 462

Introduction 462
Types of Vascular Stents 462
  Thermal-memory stents 462
  Spring-loaded stents 462
  Plastic-deformation stents 463
Current Use and Prospective Clinical Application 464
REFERENCES 465

PERCUTANEOUS MECHANICAL RECANALIZATION TECHNIQUES *Mark H. Wholey* 467

Introduction 467
New Recanalization Devices 467
  The Kensey dynamic angioplasty catheter 467
  Atherolytic reperfusion wires 469
  Transluminal extraction catheters 472
Conclusion 478
REFERENCES 478

FIBRINOLYTIC THERAPY FOR PERIPHERAL VASCULAR DISEASE *Mark H. Wholey* 479

Introduction 479
Types of Fibrinolytic Agents 479
Clinical Indications 479
Treatment 481
Conclusions 484
REFERENCES 489

Chapter Seven
Percutaneous Retrieval of Intravascular Foreign Bodies / *Renan Uflacker* 491

Introduction 491
Causes 491
Materials and Results 492
Technical Aspects of Foreign Body Retrieval 492
  Snare technique 492
  Dormia basket 493
  Forceps technique 493
  Modified snare technique 493
  Coaxial (pass-over) technique 496
Difficulties 496
Contraindications 497
Conclusions 497
REFERENCES 500

Chapter Eight
Uroradiologic Procedures 501

PERCUTANEOUS NEPHROSTOMY *João Rubião Hoefel Filho* 500

Introduction 501
Renal Anatomy 502
   Position and location of kidneys 502
   Renal beds, fasciae, and renal spaces 502
   Topographic relationships of the kidney 504
   Renal calices 504
   Renal vascular supply 506
Technical Procedure 508
   General considerations 508
   Opacifying the collecting system 511
   Renal puncture 512
   Diagnostic pyelography 516
   Specific procedures 516
Indications and Contraindications 535
Complications 535
REFERENCES 538

URETERAL PROCEDURES *Renan Uflacker* 540

Urolithiasis 540
Extraction of Ureteral Calculi 540
Dilatation, Ureteral Recanalization, and Stents 542
   Dilatation with a balloon 543
   Dilatation with a catheter 544
   Congenital obstructions 551
REFERENCES 552

PERCUTANEOUS LITHOTRIPSY *Renan Uflacker* 553

Indications for the Procedure 553
Previous Examinations 553
Access 553
Tract Dilatation 556
Nephrostomy and Stones Extraction 557
REFERENCES 558

Chapter Nine
Pulmonary Thromboembolism and Interruption of the Inferior Vena Cava / *Renan Uflacker* 559

Pulmonary Embolism 559
Radiology of the Thorax 559
Pulmonary Scintigraphy 559
Pulmonary Angiography 561
Deep Venous Thrombosis 562
Vena Cava Filters 563
Indications 564
Types of Transvenous Devices 564
Complications 566

New Developments in Filters 569
   Bird's nest filter 569
   Amplatz filter (spider) 569
   Günther filter 571
   Uflacker filter 572
   Simon nitinol filter 572
   Vera tech filter 573
Summary of in Vitro Studies of the Results of Different Filtering Devices 573
Overview 573

PERCUTANEOUS TRANSLUMINAL PULMONARY EMBOLECTOMY 575

   REFERENCES 576

Chapter Ten
Percutaneous Drainage of Abdominal Collections / *Renan Uflacker* 577

Introduction 577
Subphrenic Collections 578
Liver 582
Spleen 594
Kidney 595
Pancreas 597
Intraperitoneal Collections 600
Determining the Access Route 603
Drainage Technique 603
Selection of Materials and Techniques 604
Maintenance of Drainage 604
Conclusion 605
REFERENCES 605

INDEX 607

Contributors

João Rubião Hoefel Filho, M.D.
Assistant Professor of Radiology, School of
Medicine, Pontifícia Universidade Católica;
Chief, Department of Radiology, Hospital
São Lucas, Porto Alegre, Brazil

Guillherme de Souza Mourão, M.D.
Vascular Radiologist, MED-IMAGEM, Hospital
Beneficência Portuguesa, São Paulo, Brazil

Julio C. Palmaz, M.D.
Professor of Radiology;
Head, Section of Vascular and Interventional Radiology,
School of Medicine, University of Texas,
San Antonio, Texas

Rosa Maria Paolini, M.D.
Head, Vascular and Interventional Radiology,
Department of Radiology, Louisiana State
University Medical School, Charity Hospital,
New Orleans, Louisiana

**Rubens de Souza A. Pinheiro, M.D.
(deceased)**
Assistant Professor of Radiology, School of
Medicine, Universidade do Rio de Janeiro;
Associate Professor of Radiology, Universidade
Federal do Rio de Janeiro, Rio de Janeiro, Brazil

Ronie Leo Piske, M.D.
Neurovascular Radiologist, MED-IMAGEM,
Hospital Beneficência Portuguesa,
São Paulo, Brazil

Marcio Sampaio, M.D.
Head, Vascular Radiology and Neuroradiology,
Department of Radiology, Hospital Beneficência
Portuguesa, Rio de Janeiro, Brazil

Renan Uflacker, M.D.
Head, Vascular and Interventional Radiology,
MED-IMAGEM, Hospital Beneficência
Portuguesa, São Paulo, Brazil

Mark H. Wholey, M.D.
Clinical Professor of Radiology,
University of Pittsburgh School of Medicine;
Director, Department of Imaging and
Radiological Sciences, Shadyside Hospital,
Pittsburgh, Pennsylvania

Preface

In 1964, Charles Dotter and Melvin Judkins first described the successful dilatation of a peripheral arterial vessel. They established for radiology a territorial claim to the peripheral circulation. The ground work, however, had been established long before by the Swedish radiologist, Seldinger, who in 1953 described a simple percutaneous method for performing peripheral arteriography. Prior to that time, American radiologists had little or no experience with technical procedures and their training programs were almost entirely based on visual skills. Progress, however, was rapid and diagnostic arteriograms with selective catheterization of essentially every vessel in the body were described. In 1958, the cardiologist, Sones, introduced selective coronary arteriography via a transbrachial arteriotomy. With this single exception, most of the major diagnostic and percutaneous interventional vascular techniques were originally described by radiologists. In 1962, Ricketts and Abrams described their approach to coronary arteriography; alternative techniques were reported by Dotter and Judkins in 1964, Amplatz in 1967, and, finally, Gruntzig in 1977 with his classic description for coaxial balloon angioplasty. Gruntzig's background included experience in both cardiology and radiology.

Although radiologists had inherited the procedure and territorially established themselves, they did not inherit the patient and, over a period of years, they watched the decline of coronary arteriography as a radiologic procedure. Essentially all percutaneous coronary procedures are now under the domain of cardiology. Valuable lessons, however, were learned from this experience, and it spawned the development of a new breed, "the cardiovascular and interventional radiologist." Thus, for the first time radiology has a physician with the ability and interest to admit and treat patients, and accept referrals and consultations equally with vascular surgeons, cardiologists, and general internists. In this role, the radiologist must have a dedicated commitment to patient treatment and the day-to-day care it entails.

The total number of peripheral vascular interventional procedures languishes in comparison to coronary interventions; however, the numbers are deceiving when one considers the overall potential for intervention in the peripheral circulation. For example, an estimated one million people are treated annually for peripheral vascular disease. Of these, 200,000 have undergone a vascular reconstructive procedure. An additional 85,000 are scheduled for amputation, and 150,000 to 200,000 are being medically treated for ischemic ulcerations, pregangrenous conditions, or bypass graft procedures that have failed.

In 1981, less than 3000 percutaneous transluminal angioplasty (PTA) procedures were performed in the peripheral circulation. Similarly, 3000 percutaneous transluminal coronary angioplasty (PTCA) procedures were done. In 1988, the number of PTCA procedures had grown to 285,000, while the number of peripheral PTA procedures had grown to 85,000. Interest in the peripheral circulation, however, has shown a recent dramatic increase. Conceivably, by 1995, the number of peripheral interventional vascular procedures could approach 250,000. Presently, 700,000 diagnostic peripheral arteriograms are done annually. Our experience suggests that 30 to 40 percent of the patients undergoing peripheral arteriography will have an indication for a vascular interventional procedure. If this were extrapolated, approximately 250,000 to 300,000 patients would be eligible candidates each year. This is not the case, however, because unfortunately a large number of these amenable lesions are still being managed surgically.

Of these cases, total occlusions outnumber stenotic disease by a ratio of 3:1. Technically, we have the ability to recanalize even the most lengthy obstruction, with initial success rates approaching 80 percent. However, keeping the vessel patent is another issue. Restenosis rates and total obstructions are still in the 40 to 50 percent range even for relatively short segmental occlusions, and this remains a clinical problem. For these reasons, most of the recent research and development in new device technology is directed to the design of equipment to recanalize total obstructions.

Embolization is now a well-established procedure used to treat trauma, bleeding, tumors, aneurysms, and AV malformations all over the human body. Recent developments in microcatheter construction and occluding balloon technology have made occluding procedures possible in sites never before approached either surgically or by transcatheter technique.

Percutaneous access routes have also been used to treat nonvascular diseases. Techniques for treatment of biliary, gastrointestinal, and genitourinary diseases have been developed and are continually being refined. Percutaneous drainage of fluid collections and relief of obstructions in canalicular compartments of the body have been very successful and are becoming genuine alternatives to surgery in many cases. Percutaneous management of cholelithiasis and choledocholithiasis, while leaving the gallbladder in situ, is gaining more and more acceptance. Considering that approximately 500,000 gallbladders are surgically removed each year, it is reasonable to assume that about 20 to 30 percent of these patients will be eligible for some kind of noninvasive or minimally invasive percutaneous procedure.

Percutaneous interventional procedures may be even more encouraged in the near future, because they typically decrease the length of hospital stay and expenditures compared to the surgical alternatives.

Interventional radiology is an emerging subspecialty that will require a significant increase in both the number of dedicated full-time interventional radiologists and the total number of training programs.

This textbook consists of ten chapters, and although it is heavily weighted to cardiovascular procedures, significant attention is also directed to the nonvascular interventional procedures.

Chapter One is an introduction to catheterization techniques and includes some very basic principles.

Chapter Two is a detailed analysis of the techniques and materials presently being utilized for embolization.

Chapter Three is a comprehensive review of the diagnosis and management of gastrointestinal bleeding by interventional procedures.

Chapter Four is a detailed analysis of the clinical applications of embolization in the thorax, abdominal organs, and the central nervous system.

Chapter Five is dedicated to interventional radiology.

Chapter Six is a technical review of the angioplasty procedure and its therapeutic applications for both simple and complex visceral and peripheral vascular lesions.

Chapter Seven is a review of the percutaneous methods for retrieval of intravascular foreign bodies.

Chapter Eight discusses in detail most of the interventional applications for uroradiologic procedures. This also includes a detailed evaluation of existing approaches to percutaneous lithotripsy.

Chapter Nine details pulmonary thromboembolic disease as well as the numerous percutaneous approaches to inferior vena cava filters.

Finally, Chapter Ten evaluates the percutaneous methods in the management of intra- and extraperitoneal abscesses.

Although the text is not a substitute for practical hands-on experience, it does present current acceptable techniques, recommendations for patient selection, and useful methods that are applicable for both the experienced cardiovascular and interventional radiologist, as well as the beginning resident.

Chapter One

Catheterization Techniques

RENAN UFLACKER

INTRODUCTION

The technique generally used for any type of diagnostic or therapeutic catheterization is that described by Seldinger in 1953 (Fig. 1.1). This technique can be used to introduce a catheter in any artery or peripheral vein.

The arteries most used for vascular catheterization are the femoral, axillary, and brachial. The femoral artery, due to its large caliber and the fact that it is more easily compressed and observed after hemostasis, provides the optimal approach for the majority of procedures. It also allows the patient and examiner to adopt the most comfortable position.

An approach through the axillary artery is second in order of preference because the relatively large dimensions of that vessel lessen the possibility of spasm during catheterization. However, it does entail an uncomfortable and tiresome position for the patient.

Hematomas related to axillary punctures are more difficult to control than hematomas related to femoral punctures and can have more serious consequences since they occur in the presence of the brachial plexus. This route is nonetheless recommended for some types of superselective visceral catheterization and is mandatory in the presence of severe aortoiliac occlusive disease.

Although the brachial route is sometimes preferred for cardiologic procedures, the brachial artery is the least useful for visceral catheterization. Because of the great distance from the point of entrance to the vessel to be catheterized, the natural tortuousness of the arterial system hampers manipulation of the catheter being used and lowers the torque at the tip of the catheter. The brachial artery is subject to spasm and consequent thrombosis and therefore should be approached carefully, using small catheters (4 or 5 French).

Heparinization of the patient is often necessary to prevent thrombosis at the puncture site, and in some cases the use of a systemic vasodilator is indicated.

PUNCTURE

Arterial or venous percutaneous puncture must be done with a thin-walled short beveled needle that has a caliber compatible with the guidewire to be used. It is essential to test the compatibility of the diameters and lengths of the needle, guidewires, and catheters that will be used during the procedure. This simple measure is important to prevent accidents and delays while performing the examination.

Once the approach has been decided on, the Seldinger technique is used for puncture and placement of the catheter (Fig. 1.1).

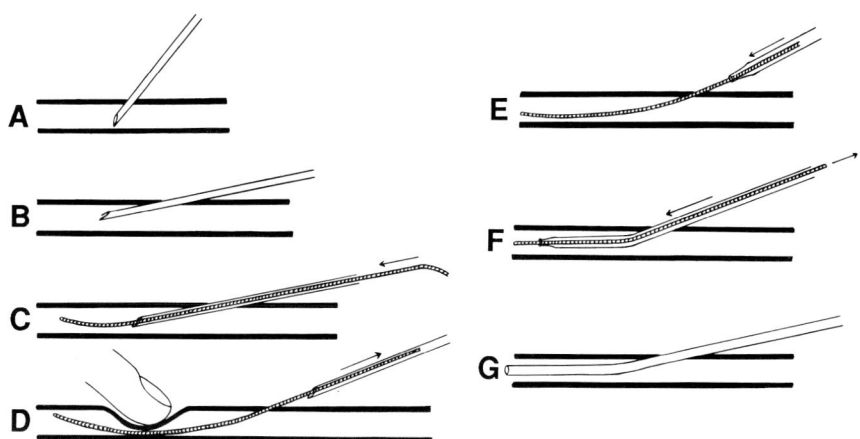

Figure 1.1 Illustration of the Seldinger technique for percutaneous catheterization.
(A) Arterial puncture. (B) Inclination of the needle in the position that is almost parallel to the artery. (C) Introduction of the guidewire in the arterial lumen. (D) Removal of the needle, maintaining the guidewire in the arterial lumen with simultaneous digital compression. (E) Introduction of the catheter over the guidewire. (F) At the same time the catheter is introduced, the guidewire is maintained stationary and removed immediately after. (G) Finally, the catheter is left and manipulated in the vascular lumen without the guidewire.

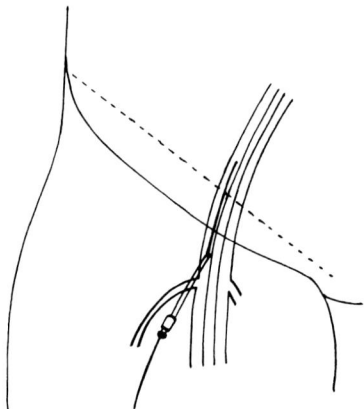

Figure 1.2 Retrograde femoral arterial puncture. This is the standard puncture for access to the aorta and its branches with retrograde introduction (against the flow of the needle and the guidewire). The site of puncture is below the inguinal ligament at the level of the inguinal cutaneous fold (less thickness between the surface of the skin and the vessel wall).

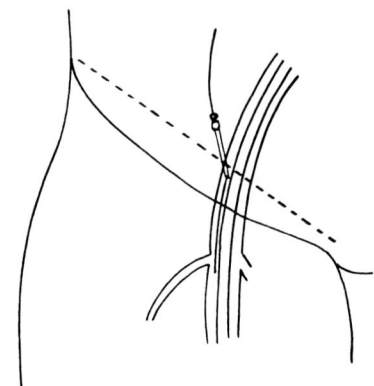

Figure 1.3 Antegrade femoral arterial puncture. This is the puncture used for access to the common femoral artery and other arteries of the leg with antegrade (in the direction of the flow) introduction of the needle and the guidewire. The point of puncture is high, at the level of the inguinal ligament. This puncture is used for femoral popliteal angioplasties and embolization in extremities.

The first step of a successful puncture is careful palpation of the artery to define the site of puncture and vessel entry. Infiltration with local anesthetic is next, usually done with 10 to 15 ml of anesthetic to include the skin, anterior wall of the artery, both areas lateral to the artery, and the area deep to the vessel. This will alleviate any pain and decrease the likelihood of spasm due to puncture or to manipulation of the catheter.

The ideal site for the retrograde puncture of the femoral artery is at or distal to the inguinal crease, below the inguinal ligament (Fig. 1.2). If the puncture is antegrade, for superficial femoral artery access, the entry point is higher, at the inguinal ligament level (Fig. 1.3).

After the artery has been punctured, the mandrel is removed, allowing free blood flow through the needle. A metal guidewire with a flexible tip is introduced. Figure 1.4 shows the dangers of using a long-beveled

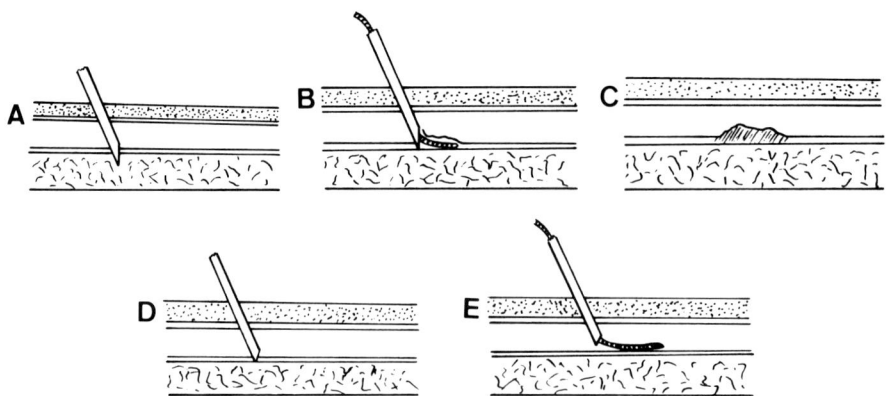

Figure 1.4 Introduction of the guidewire with long- and short-beveled needles.
(A) Arterial puncture with a long-beveled needle situates the needle tip on the posterior wall of the aorta, allowing aspiration of blood with good flow at the same time. (B) Introduction of a guidewire in this situation leads to dissection of the intima. (C) Subintimal dissection causes subintimal hematoma and arterial narrowing. (D) Puncture of the artery with short-beveled needle allows the lumen of the needle to meet the arterial lumen more freely, without attaching itself to the posterior wall of the artery. (E) The introduction of the guidewire is generally free and does not cause lesions to the vascular intima.

needle. Note that the needle tip is positioned in the vessel lumen in such a way that it is as parallel as possible to the axis of the vessel.

INTRODUCING THE GUIDEWIRE

The guidewire should never be forced. Resistance to the guidewire is caused by one of five situations: (1) The artery is tortuous; (2) atheromatous plaque is obstructing the lumen; (3) the guidewire has dissected subintimally; (4) the artery is occluded; (5) the guide tip has entered a collateral artery.

It is difficult for a straight guidewire to negotiate the tortuous artery of a longtime hypertensive patient because there is a large coefficient of friction between the arterial wall and the surface of the guide and its tip (Fig. 1.5). In those cases, a J safety guidewire or a steerable torque-controlled guidewire with a small tip is the best choice.

Among the methods for successfully negotiating tortuous arteries with atheromatous plaques are use of a J-tipped guidewire, a guidewire with a long, flexible segment, and, more recently, a steerable guidewire with torque control distally.

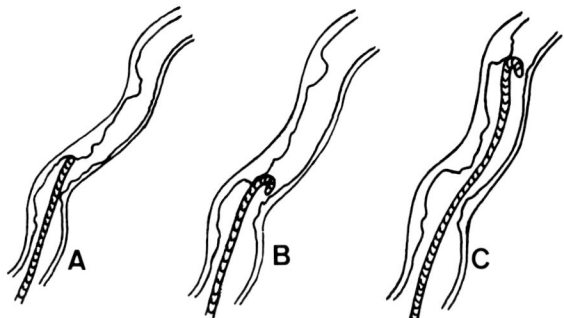

Figure 1.6 Passing an artery with atheromatous plaque with a guidewire.
(A) A straight guidewire cannot pass the obstacles created by atheromatous plaques in the arterial lumen. There is the risk of dissection of the intima and release of the plaques. (B,C) A J guidewire passes the stenoses and intraluminal irregularities quite easily.

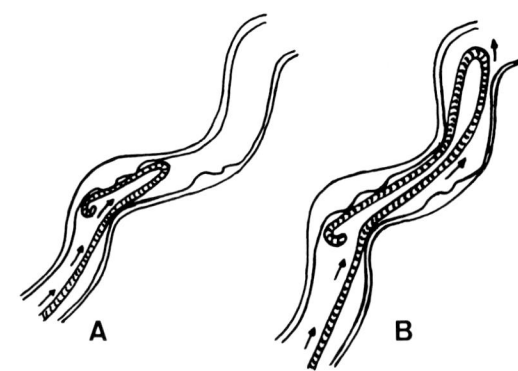

Figure 1.7 Use of the guidewire with a long, flexible tip.
(A,B) The guidewire with a long, flexible J tip tends to curve and uncoil as it is introduced inside the artery.

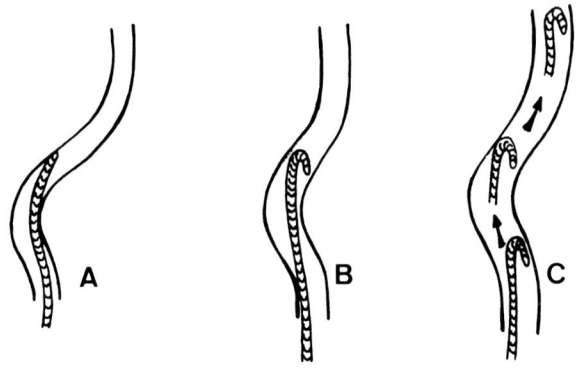

Figure 1.5 Overcoming a tortuous artery with a guidewire.
(A) It is difficult to advance the straight guidewire, because of its straight tip and the friction of its surface with arterial walls, through very tortuous arteries. (B,C) The J guidewire advances easily through a sinuous artery.

Figure 1.6 shows how to negotiate an artery with irregular walls caused by atherosclerosis.

In some tortuous vessels only guidewires with a long, flexible tip will advance the shaft with low friction without linear advance of the tip due to uncoiling within the lumen of the artery. Steerable wires in dimensions from 0.014 to 0.035 in. with 1:1 torque have greatly simplified most catheterization procedures (Fig. 1.7).

The large J tip guidewire (15 mm) is useful to cross plaques and stenosis in atheromatous vessels. A steerable wire may also be used for that purpose (Fig. 1.9). It is more adequate to manipulate within the thoracic aorta with a large J wire (Fig. 1.8).

Bad needle position is an important cause of failure in arterial catheterization. If the needle point is not in the lumen of the artery, but in its posterior wall, the guidewire will be introduced subintimally, causing a dissection or perforation of the intimal layer (Fig. 1.4). Occasionally a slight withdrawal of the needle position will free the tip of the guidewire from the posterior wall of the artery, redirecting the tip into the lumen.

Manipulation of an artery that is occluded near the site of puncture is not indicated unless it is the only vessel available for catheterization or unless it will be used to try to recanalize for angioplasty.

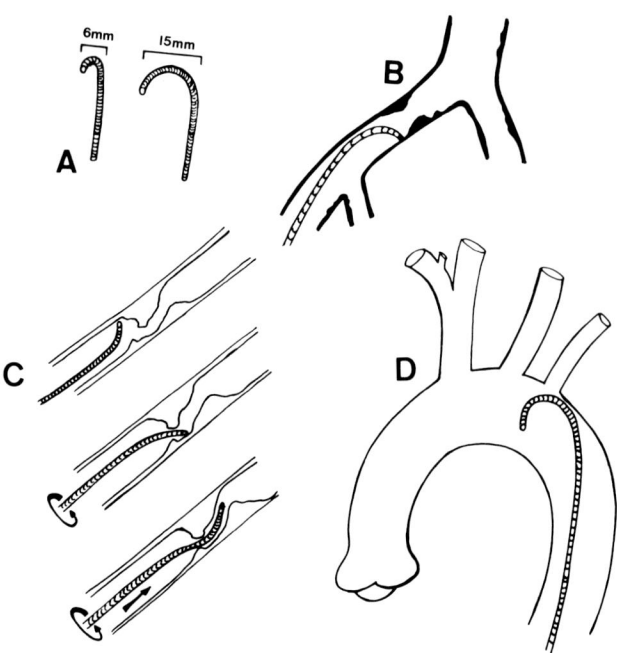

Figure 1.8 Use of the J guidewire.
(A) J guidewire with 6 and 15 mm in diameter at the curved tip. (B) Inadequate use of the large J guidewire. (C) Adequate use of the large J guidewire. (D) Large J tip guidewire used at the thoracic aorta.

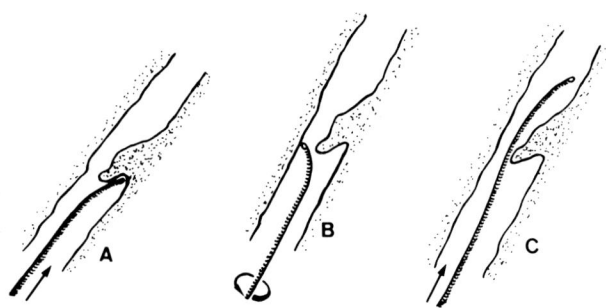

Figure 1.9 Steering the J guidewire.
(A) A steerable J guidewire is used to pass atheromatous arteries. (B) Rotation of the guidewire. (C) Simultaneous advancement during the rotational movement may easily negotiate difficult arteries.

Repositioning the needle at the puncture site is a basic technique when the guidewire persistently enters the vessel that is collateral to the punctured artery (Fig. 1.10). In the case of axillary puncture, the guidewire tends to enter the subscapular artery, lateral thoracic artery, or superior thoracic artery. A 3-mm J steerable guidewire will easily go beyond these collateral arteries in the direction of the subclavian artery, generally after a repositioning of the needle in the caudal position.

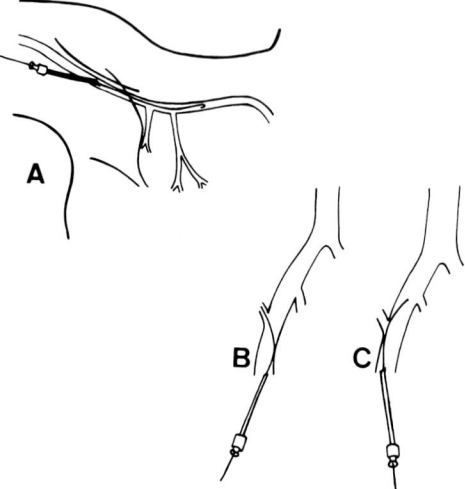

Figure 1.10 Positioning the guidewire in axillary and femoral punctures.
(A) In axillary punctures, it is useful to use a J guidewire to pass the natural anatomic sinuosity and to keep the guidewire from entering collaterals. (B) Femoral puncture with an angulated needle in the medial direction. The tendency is for the guidewire to enter the profound circumflex iliac artery. (C) To avoid this situation, the needle should be angled laterally. The guidewire will steer spontaneously toward the common iliac.

With punctures of the femoral artery, the tendency of the guidewire is to enter the deep, circumflex iliac artery. As shown in Fig. 1.10, a simple lateral redirecting of the needle will prevent the guidewire from entering that artery.

CATHETERIZATION

The catheter can be introduced via the femoral, axillary, or brachial arteries.

Using the axillary route to approach the abdominal aorta, it is more convenient to use the left axillary artery. In young patients, the left subclavian artery forms a rectilinear path, continuous with the descending thoracic aorta, that can be easily reached by the guidewire and the catheter can be introduced through the axillary artery. Maintaining the guide stationary, the catheter is advanced safely toward the abdominal aorta. However, it is convenient to use a preshaped catheter with sufficient torque for manipulation and for selective catheterization of aortic branches.

In older patients, the aorta becomes elongated and tortuous and the left subclavian artery becomes progressively more guided toward the ascending aorta, making the angle with the aortic arch more acute. Because of

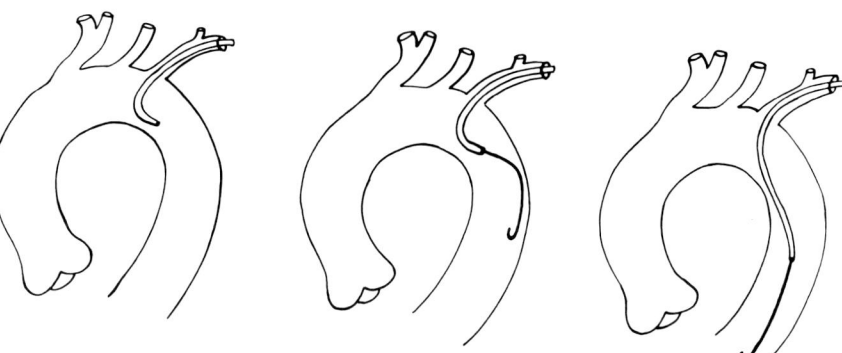

Figure 1.11 Aortic abdominal catheterization through left axillary puncture, using a selective catheter with a simple curve for steering the guidewire toward the abdominal aorta. Once the guidewire is placed in the ascending aorta, the catheter can be advanced, keeping the guidewire stationary. Pigtail-type catheters can be used for the same purpose.

that, successful catheterization of the descending and abdominal aorta is difficult. Different techniques have been described to overcome the problems of left aorta subclavian tortuousness. The simplest is to use a pre-shaped catheter with a closed curve at the tip (Fig. 1.11).

Once the tip of the curve of the catheter has been introduced in the aortic arch, it is steered to the left posterolaterally. Use of rotational fluoroscopy in the left anterior oblique position will also simplify catheterization of the descending aorta. A J guidewire that will tend to go down the descending aorta is then introduced. When the guidewire is well advanced through the descending or abdominal aorta, it is kept stationary and the catheter is advanced down to the desired point. An alternative technique uses a pigtail catheter. Figure 1.11 shows an alternative technique for the left axillary artery approach to the abdominal aorta using a deflecting device or a steerable wire.

Introducing the catheter through the femoral artery generally does not require difficult manipulation, except in cases where it is not easy to advance the guidewire to the iliac artery in patients with arteriopathy, as mentioned before.

Although the catheterization of visceral aortic branches is generally quite simple and quick for an experienced angiographer, there are some general and particular guidelines for success.

One is that the 10 percent rule should generally be observed; that is, the length of the curved tip of the catheter should be at least 10 percent greater than the diameter of the abdominal aorta at the desired level. Observing this affords good stability of the selective catheterization during a contrast injection with high flow and volume, as is the case with the celiac trunk and superior mesenteric arteries. This allows the back of the catheter to be supported on the contralateral aortic wall, maintaining the tip of the catheter in the selected artery. Occasionally, depending on anatomic considerations, aortic tortuousness, and/or the branch that is to be catheterized, it is necessary to use a catheter with a longer or shorter tip.

It is also important to identify fluoroscopically the exact position of the catheter—anterior or posterior. To catheterize the celiac trunk and mesenteric arteries the catheter must be rotated so that its tip is in an anterior direction. If the catheter is rotated clockwise in the inguinal region, the catheter tip will appear to the right of the patient if the tip was posterior and to the left if the tip was anterior. In contrast, counterclockwise rotation will cause the catheter tip to displace itself to the right if anterior and to the left if posterior.

The catheterization of the branches of the abdominal aorta can be done with the catheter tip turned cranially or caudally. If a catheter with a tip slightly larger than the diameter of the aorta is used (Fig. 1.12A), when the guidewire is removed from the catheter, the tip will position itself cranially.

The tip of the catheter can be turned back to its original position and the artery catheterized by simply

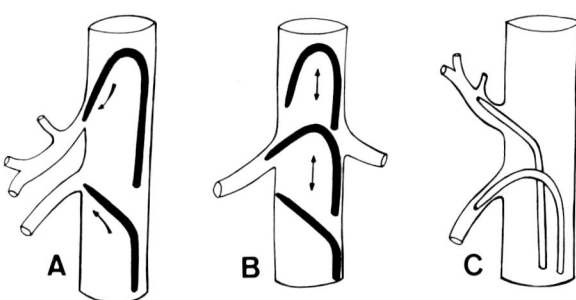

Figure 1.12 Selective catheterization of branches of the abdominal aorta with catheters of different configurations.
(A) The curve of a catheter with a tip that is too long will straighten and open in the aortic lumen. Normally it is not possible to catheterize a branch of the aorta that has a caudal direction without turning the tip of the catheter in the same direction. (B) To turn the catheter tip caudally, the renal artery can usually be used as an anchoring point to reshape the tip of the catheter, using longitudinal movements. It is convenient to remember the 10 percent rule explained in the text. (C) To catheterize an artery in the cranial direction, a catheter with a 30 to 60° curve can be used. To catheterize a vessel in the caudal direction, it is convenient to use a catheter with a 120° curve.

advancing the catheter in such a way that its tip enters the lumen and advances in it. This same orifice can be used to reshape the tip of the catheter or to catheterize an adjacent artery by simply turning the catheter tip downward (Fig. 1.12B). For an aortic branch that goes in the caudal direction, the tip of the catheter must be steered in the same direction. For a branch that goes cranially, the catheter tip must have a more open curve, with a greater radius (Fig. 1.12C). Catheterization of the celiac trunk and the superior mesenteric artery normally requires catheters with longer tips that point downward (Fig. 1.12).

When the catheter tip is too long for the diameter of the aorta, the tip points downward in the direction of the lumen of the aorta, making selective catheterization of the superior mesenteric artery or the celiac trunk impossible. The catheter can be changed for a more appropriate one, or a guidewire can be introduced up to the catheter tip causing a stretching of the extremity of the catheter and steering it against the aortic wall, allowing selective catheterization of the desired branch (Fig. 1.13).

Figure 1.14 shows the basic curves most used in abdominal catheters for selective or superselective visceral catheterization. Each of these catheters has a

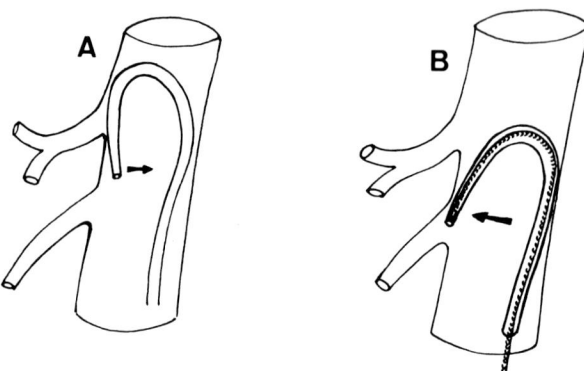

Figure 1.13 A catheter tip that is too long for the diameter of the aorta.
(A) The long tip is turned to the center of the aortic lumen. (B) If a guidewire is introduced in the catheter, the tip of the catheter will steer toward the proximity of the aortic wall and the catheter can then be used for selective catheterization.

specific function and is used most appropriately for specific vessels. There are specific techniques for reshaping the curves of the catheter types shown in the figure once they are placed inside the aorta.

Pigtail-type catheters (Fig. 1.14A) are commonly used

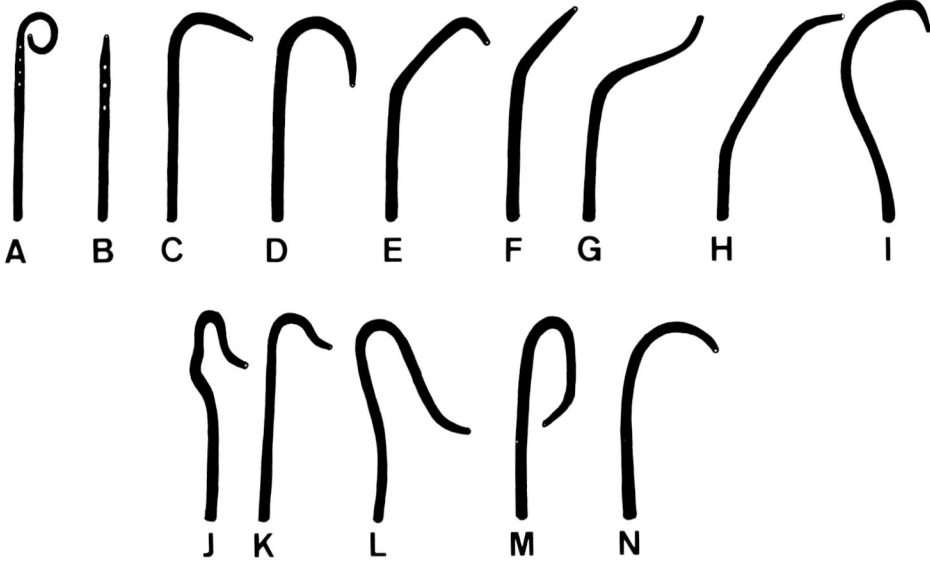

Figure 1.14 Catheters commonly used in the abdominal aorta and for selective visceral catheterization.
(A) Pigtail type. (B) Straight catheters with lateral holes for aortography. (C) Selective catheterization with a simple curve, renal type. (D) Visceral selective catheter with 120 to 180° curve. (E) Visceral selective catheter with a double curve. (F) Multiuse selective catheter with 60° curve. (G) Superselective catheter with a double inverted curve for the left adrenal vein or the left gastric artery. (H) Superselective catheter with a double curve for the gastroduodenal artery and branches of the mesenteric artery. (I) Selective multiuse cobra catheter. (J) Visceral selective catheter (Mikaelsson type, celiac trunk). (K) Shepherd hook visceral selective catheter. (L) Visceral selective catheter or cerebral type (sidewinder). This type is also called a Simmons catheter. (M) Boijsen-type visceral superselective catheter with double curve. When the most distal curve is to the right, it is used in the hepatic artery; when the most distal curve is to the left, it is used in the splenic artery. (N) Visceral selective catheter with a large-radius curve for selective and superselective catheterization.

catheter configurations for thoracic and abdominal aortography. Because of their curved configuration, they have a very stable injection profile during high-flow-rate injections, and are consequently recommended for high-volume, high-flow-rate studies. A risk, however, that does exist with small-diameter pigtail-type catheters is that when they are subjected to high flow rates, there may result a straightening of the tip and opening of the curve. If this occurs, there is the possibility of the catheter being introduced in smaller branches of the abdominal aorta, with all the inherent complications of such an accident, for example, injections of large volumes of contrast in lumbar arteries, as well as the risk of neurologic involvement.

The straight-type catheter with distal and lateral holes is easy to use in angiography. It can be used in the abdominal and thoracic aorta, and can accommodate large flows as long as the internal diameter is wide and the walls are thin. The lateral bores can increase outflow capacity, but high flow capacity is primarily a function of the internal diameter and length of the catheter. Their main deficiencies are the recoil activity and reaction forces that can occur during a contrast injection. Dissection of the intima and plaque fragmentation may occur when straight catheters are used in the diseased abdominal aorta, due to excessive recoil and linear flow in the tip hole.

The selective visceral catheter (Fig. 1.14, C to F) occasionally needs additional manipulation when it is used for selection catheterization, as has already been discussed and presented in Figs. 1.12 and 1.13.

The catheter with a reversed curve (Fig. 1.14G) is useful for superselective catheterization of the left gastric artery, intrahepatic branches of the proper hepatic artery, and especially the left adrenal vein. The use of this catheter is limited because its tip is not appropriate for catheterizing the arterial orifice in the aorta, sliding, instead, along the aortic wall. If a main branch of the aorta or cava is hooked by the tip of the catheter, progression and superselective catheterization of the secondary branches of the arteries are made easier (Fig. 1.15). However, if this is not possible, certain maneuvers can aid in carrying out the catheterization (Fig. 1.15).

The Cobra catheter shown in Fig. 1.14I can be used as a multiuse selective visceral catheter or for superselective catheterization. The best way to use it in superselective catheterization is to employ the Waltman loop technique. Using the bifurcation of the aorta or deep introduction, with or without guidewire, in a visceral artery (generally the superior mesenteric or the renal artery) and pushing the body of the catheter in a cranial direction, a loop is formed that resembles the Simmons catheter (Fig. 1.14L). (Manipulation of the cobra catheter is explained in more detail in the section on superselec-

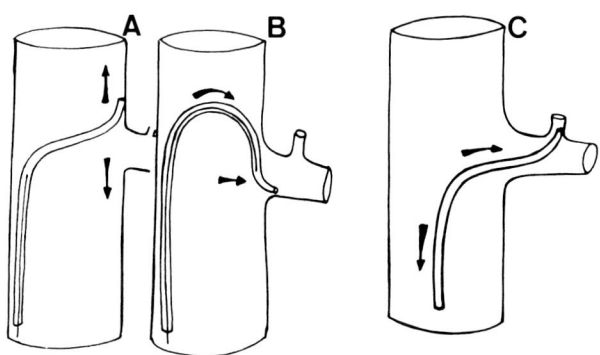

Figure 1.15 Use of the reverse-tipped catheter with a double curve.
(A) The reverse-tip catheter can be moved in the aorta without selectively penetrating any aortic branch. (B) Using a guidewire with a deflector on its tip will give the catheter a shape that can be introduced selectively. (C) Removal of the guidewire with a deflector allows manipulation and superselective catheterization.

tive catheterization.) The catheter with the Mikaelsson (Fig. 1.14J) configuration is generally used for selective visceral catheterization, despite its being designed for injections in the celiac trunk and the superior mesenteric artery, due to its stability during injections with high-volume high-pressure flow. It is frequently possible to catheterize the left gastric artery using a catheter of this type.

Once the tip of the Mikaelsson catheter has been reshaped to its original form inside the aorta, handling it is simple. Nonetheless, some knowledge of the mechanics of the design and experience in its use are required to reshape it with facility. Figure 1.16 shows how to reshape the Mikaelsson catheter.

The shepherd hook catheter is used as a selective visceral catheter, and reshaping its tip is relatively easy. Occasionally, a shepherd hook type catheter is used to catheterize the left gastric artery by anchoring its tip in the celiac trunk, pulling its shaft down and, consequently, raising the tip in the direction of the ostium of the left gastric artery, as in Fig. 1.15.

Simmons catheters can be found in three different sizes with the same shape: types I, II, and III, with progressively larger tips according to the number. Originally, these catheters were used in the aortic arch for catheterization of the carotids in patients with elongated aortic arches. Increasingly, however, they are being used in branches of the abdominal and thoracic aorta. There are four techniques for reshaping Simmons catheters. The original technique included introducing the catheter in the left subclavian artery, with or without a guidewire, and pushing the shaft of the catheter. The distal curve is then reformed in the aortic arch, returning to its

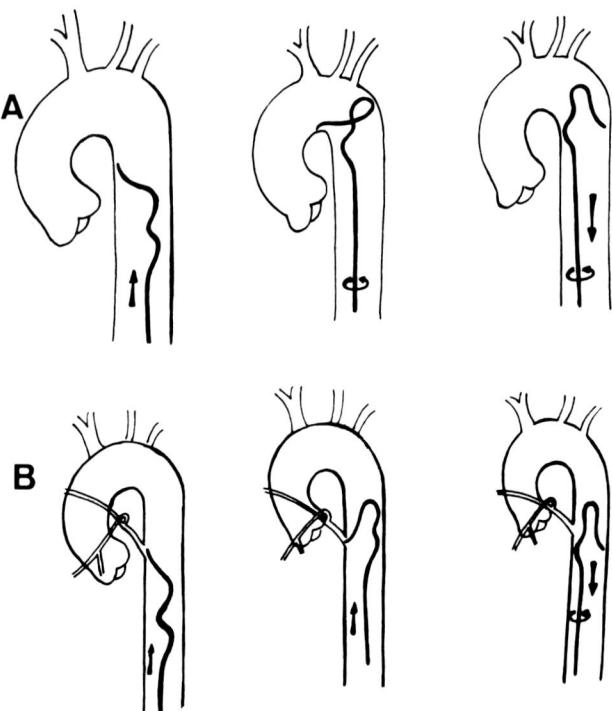

Figure 1.16 To reconfigure the Mikaelsson catheter two techniques are used.
(A) Within the aortic lumen the catheter remains open when advanced. Rotation of the catheter at the arch of the aorta will allow the tip to be reshaped. (B) When pushing the catheter upwards, the tip may enter the intercostobronchial artery and reshape itself as the catheter is pushed and rotated.

original aspect (Fig. 1.17). A variation of that technique is to introduce a large J guidewire, curving it when it reaches the aortic valve, then introducing the catheter over and above the guidewire until the curve of the Simmons catheter has returned to its original configuration (Fig. 1.18). A new technique for reshaping a Simmons catheter is to rotate its shaft clockwise, twisting its curved tip (as can be seen in Fig. 1.19) until it faces the descending aorta, where it tends to reacquire the original shape in the descending aorta or the aortic arch. In such cases, it is helpful to maintain a guidewire inside the catheter, to increase torque and keep the catheter straight.

A final option for reshaping the tip of the Simmons catheter is to use the aortic bifurcation. After aortography, a pigtail-type catheter is pulled down to the bifurcation until the curved tip is lying across the aortic bifurcation (Fig. 1.20). The guidewire is then passed in the contralateral iliac artery as distally as possible, and the pigtail catheter is replaced by the Simmons catheter over the guidewire. Occasionally, it is useful to compress the common contralateral femoral artery to maintain the guide in a fixed position during the introduction of the catheter. Once the catheter has reached the contralateral iliac artery, resting on the aortic bifurcation, the guidewire is removed and the catheter is pushed cranially until its cephalic curve has returned to its original form (Fig. 1.20). Any other type of catheter that makes catheterization of the contralateral iliac artery possible, for example, Waltman's cobra loop, can be used.

An option for selective catheterization of the common hepatic artery or the splenic artery is the hepatosplenic selective catheter designed by Boijsen (Fig. 1.14M). This is a long-tip catheter with a 180° curve and a secondary curve to the right or to the left in the most distal extremity. The Boijsen catheter is easily reshaped by rotating it in the aortic arch as described in Fig. 1.16 or by using a steerable device with a mobile tip (see "Techniques of Superselective Catheterization" below). The open-curve catheter is for general use and has a large-radius curve that advances easily over the guidewire for use in superselective catheterization (Fig. 1.21).

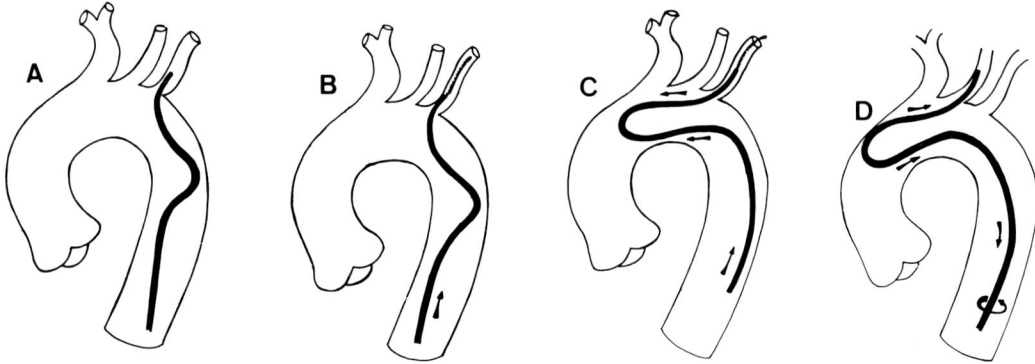

Figure 1.17 Reconfiguration of the Simmons catheter, method 1.
(A) The catheter tip is introduced in the left subclavian artery. (B) A guidewire is introduced in this artery. (C) The catheter, recurved at its tip, is guided cranially. (D) With the guidewire removed, the normal configuration of the catheter can be used for carotid or visceral arteries.

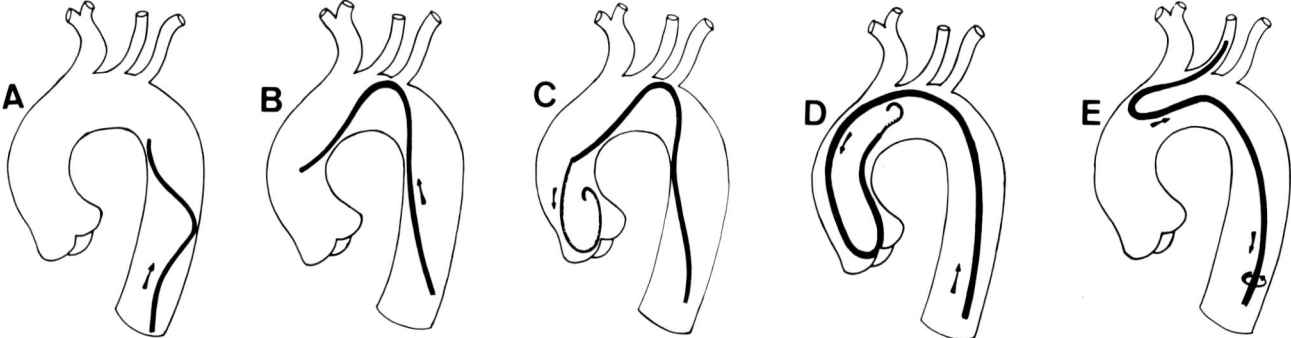

Figure 1.18 Reshaping the Simmons catheter, method 2.
(A,B) Advancing the tip of the catheter up to the ascending aorta, a guidewire is passed up to the aortic valve (C). (D) Once the guidewire is placed against the aortic valve, the catheter is pushed over the guidewire until it has regained its original shape. (E) Once the guidewire is removed, the catheter can be used for superselective catheterization.

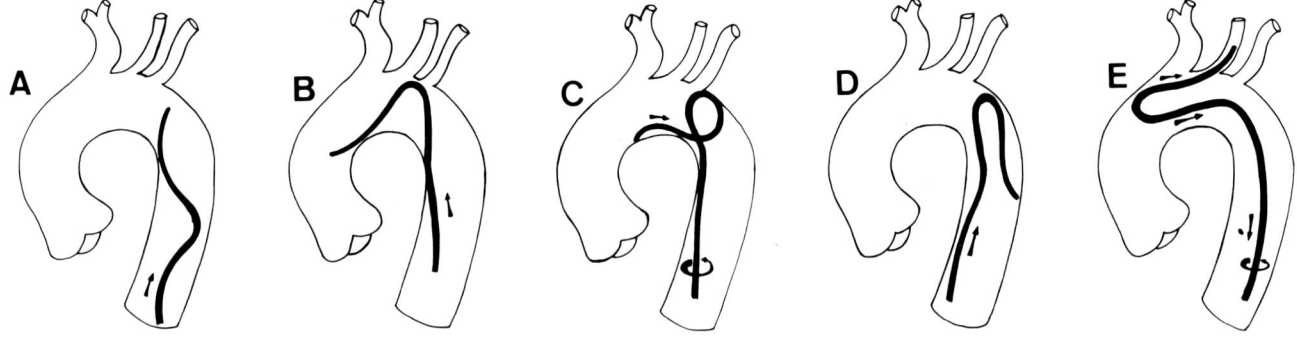

Figure 1.19 Reshaping the Simmons catheter, method 3.
(A) Catheter open in the aorta. (B) Advancing and rotating the catheter in the aortic arch. (C) The catheter is turned over itself until its tip goes to the descending aorta. (D) Once reshaped, the catheter can be used for selective catheterization, as in (E).

Figure 1.20 Reshaping the Simmons catheter, method 4.
(A) Pigtail catheter in the abdominal aorta. (B) Pigtail catheter anchored in the aortic bifurcation. (C) J guidewire introduced in the contralateral iliac artery. (D) The Simmons catheter is exchanged for the pigtail catheter and advanced over the guidewire. (E) The Simmons catheter is advanced over the guidewire up to the contralateral iliac artery. (F) The guidewire is removed and the catheter is pushed cranially, regaining its normal shape. (G) The Simmons catheter, still in the abdominal aorta, is ready to use.

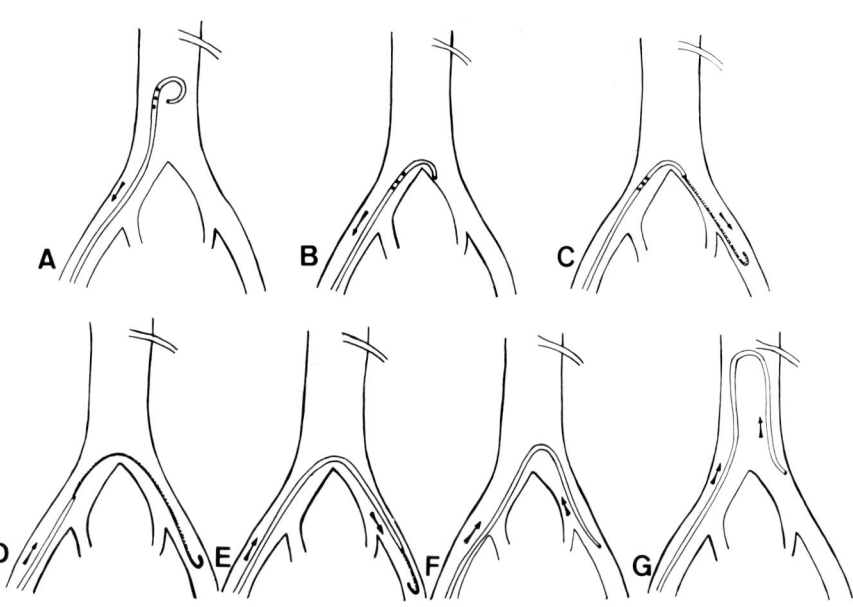

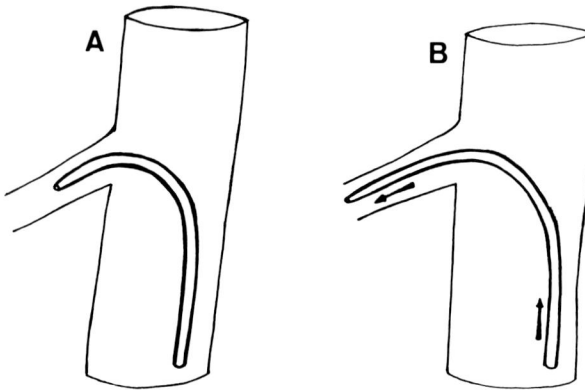

Figure 1.21 (A) An open-curve catheter with a large radius enters more easily and more distally selectively than a catheter with a closed curve. (B) It is sufficient to push the catheter cranially, with or without a guidewire inside it. The catheter, anchored in the artery, will advance deeply.

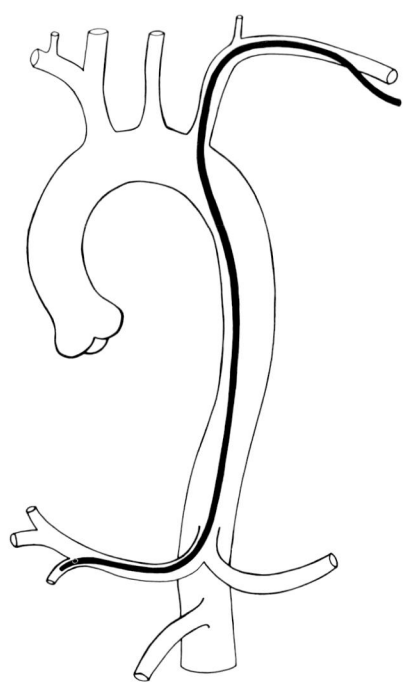

Figure 1.22 Superselective catheterization via left axillary artery, according to Boijsen's description. The craniocaudal position of the celiac trunk and the superior mesenteric artery makes the advance of the catheter into the secondary and tertiary branches easier.

SUPERSELECTIVE CATHETERIZATION

Superselective catheterization was initially developed because of the difficulty of disassociating more complex vascular structures (to avoid superposition) and to facilitate the evaluation of angiographic findings. Superselective catheterization of secondary and tertiary branches of arteries originating from the aorta allows visualization of the vascularization of either a part of or the whole viscera. Superselective catheterization of the branches of the aorta was immediately utilized in therapeutic applications such as embolization, angioplasty, and drug infusion.

An additional advantage of superselectivity in catheterization is that it allows the angiographer to obtain a greater concentration of the contrast medium in the arteries of the target organ and provides better opacification of the venous system.

For diagnostic studies or for pretherapeutic mapping, selective injections in the main vascular trunks should precede superselective catheterization. This measure is necessary because the spasm that frequently accompanies superselective manipulation can simulate arterial or neoplastic disease.

It is to Boijsen that we owe the development of superselective catheterization of abdominal aortic branches via the axillary artery (Figs. 1.10, 1.11, and 1.22).

Exchange Catheter Technique

This is the basic technique for superselective catheterization, using conventional selective catheters and guidewires. Simple progression of the catheter may achieve secondary or tertiary branches superselectively (Fig. 1.21). It is easier, however, to advance the guidewire followed by catheter exchange and manipulation for superselective catheterization (Fig. 1.23). An extra stiff guidewire is very useful for the catheter exchange. Spasm may follow guidewire and catheter manipulation precluding adequate positioning of the system. A vasodilator may be used to relieve spasm.

Steerable Devices (Deflecting Guidewire)

A variety of deflecting and steerable instruments are available. Some are very simple and others are complex to handle and to clean. The Cook deflecting handle is most probably the more useful for vascular catheterization. The Medi-Tech instrument is indicated for nonvascular catheterization (biliary and urinary). Once the artery is identified through a nonselective injection, the catheter and the deflecting instrument are positioned, the tip of the variable stiffness guidewire is positioned, and the catheter is advanced over the guidewire keeping the system still (Fig. 1.24). Rotation of the catheter shaft helps the advancement of the catheter. Intimal dissection and vessel perforation are possible complications of the procedure.

Figure 1.23 Superselective catheterization of the celiac artery, through femoral approach, using a guidewire.
(A) Selective catheter anchored at the celiac trunk. (B) The guidewire is introduced deeply at the hepatic artery. (C) After exchanging catheter, it is advanced over the wire. (D) The catheter is rotated and pulled back until it reaches the gastroduodenal artery. (E) Pushing the catheter upward will make catheterization more selective. (F) To reach tertiary or quaternary branches the catheter is advanced, either over the wire or by itself.

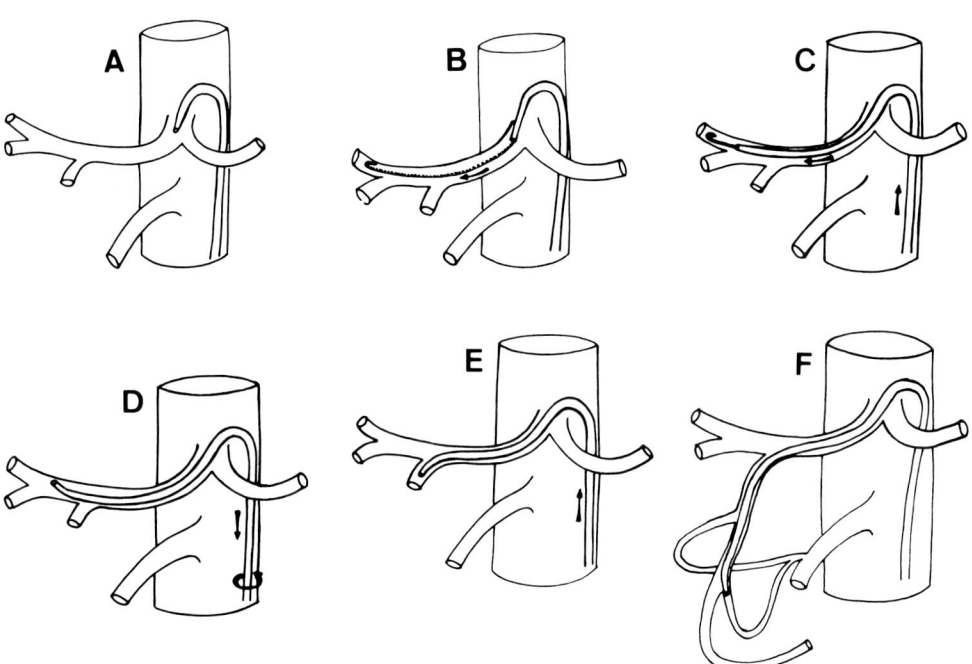

Figure 1.24 Superselective catheterization using the deflector wire.
(A) Catheter in the aorta. (B) Deflector of the catheter tip. (C and D) To select the hepatic artery, the catheter is rotated to the left of the patient. (E) The catheter is positioned at the gastroduodenal artery. (F) To select the splenic artery, the catheter is rotated to the right of the patient.

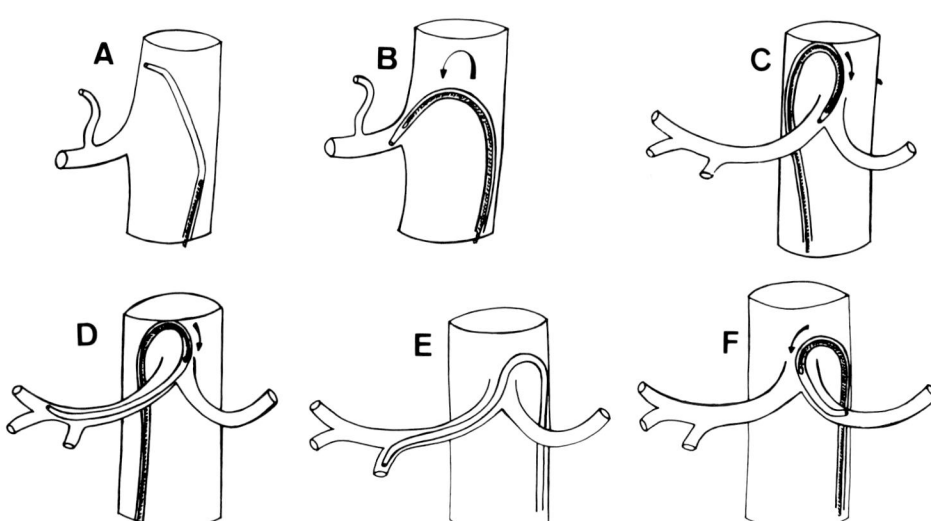

Coaxial Catheters

To use coaxial catheters, it is necessary to have a stable selective catheterization or a superselective catheterization in a secondary branch using any of the techniques described above. Once the No. 6 or No. 5 French catheter guide is in position, the No. 3 French coaxial catheter is introduced with an 0.025- or 0.018-in. guidewire, preferably one with torque control (Fig. 1.25). This coaxial catheter–guidewire set is manipulated until it enters the desired tertiary or quaternary branch. Once the coaxial catheter is placed on target, an injection with small particles or fluids or drug infusion can be done (Fig. 1.25).

The recently introduced 0.038- or 0.035-in. open-ended guidewire with lumen, developed by Sos and collaborators, can be used as a superselective catheter. This guidewire, which combines small size with linear stiffness and flexibility of tip, has been replacing the No. 3 French catheter in the coaxial system for superselective catheterization and embolization with bucrylate and fluid injection. The Sos guidewire is manipulated along with an 0.018-in. steerable guidewire through its lumen. The steerable guidewire has an extremely flexible platinum

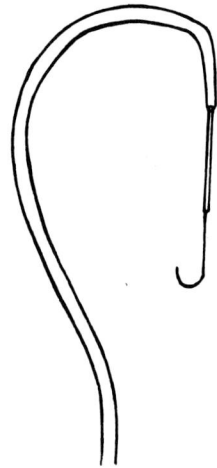

Figure 1.25 Coaxial systems for superselective catheterization according to Waltman. No. 6.5 French cobra catheter and No. 3 French teflon coaxial catheter introduced with 0.018-in. guidewire.

tip, making it highly radiopaque and allowing for the advance of the open-ended guidewire tip up to peripheral vessels. More recently the Tracker catheter has been introduced as a "super" selective catheter for small-vessel arteriography or infusion therapy.

The Cobra-type catheter forming the Waltman loop has proved highly useful in superselective catheterizations, especially if used together with a coaxial catheter guidewire system (Fig. 1.26). The catheter is introduced in the aorta through the femoral artery and its tip is inverted, anchoring it in the renal or superior mesenteric artery. As it is advanced in the femoral artery, the tip enters one of these arteries, and, after a certain point, tends to curve in the free portion of the aorta, forming the loop.

Once the tip is inverted in the cranial caudal direction, it is easy to introduce the catheter in the celiac trunk or the superior mesenteric artery. Continued traction of the catheter provides entrance into the celiac trunk and its branches. Resteering the tip by rotating it and establishing traction of the catheter will lead to superselective catheterization of the left gastric artery and other arteries due to the curve in the cranial direction produced at the catheter tip (Fig. 1.26). Almost any branch of the abdominal aorta can be catheterized selectively or superselectively by the loop technique with the cobra catheter. This technique is especially useful for catheterizing the left gastric artery and the right hepatic artery with anomalous origin in the superior mesenteric artery (Fig. 1.26). Another way of making the loop with the cobra catheter is shown in Fig. 1.27. An option with this method is to advance the cobra catheter through the common contralateral iliac and to continue advancing its body until the tip remains stationary in the hypogastric, contralateral, or external iliac. The shaft of the catheter is then advanced in an upward fashion toward the aorta to form the loop. Once the tip is inverted, by rotating the body of the catheter, the tip can be resteered; then by pulling the body of the catheter, the hypogastric as well as the iliac or femoral artery can be catheterized selectively.

An entirely new generation of small-diameter steerable guidewires (with diameters ranging from 0.010 to 0.035 in.), with highly radiopaque tips has been introduced recently.

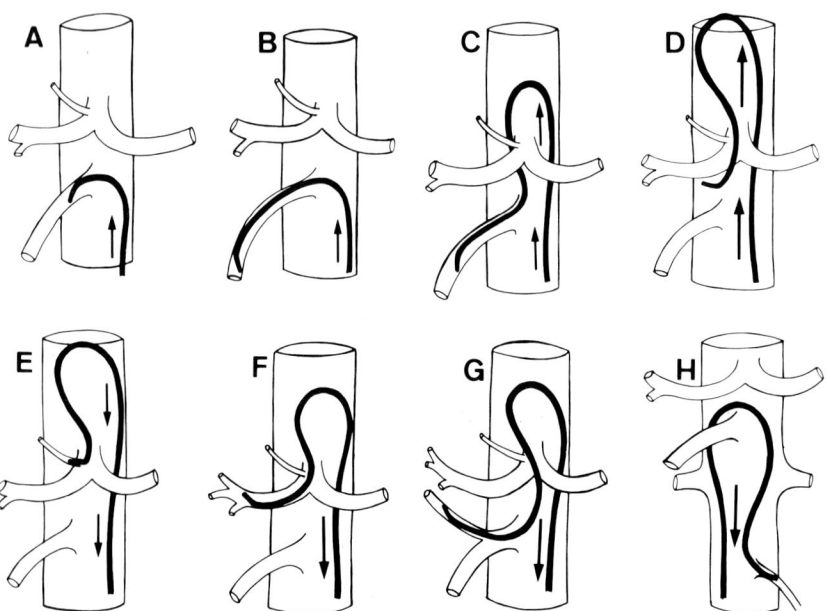

Figure 1.26 Use of the Waltman loop for superselective catheterization.
(A) Cobra catheter introduced in the superior mesenteric artery. (B) Cobra catheter introduced deeply in the superior mesenteric artery. (C) Once the catheter is anchored in the artery, it is advanced cranially, forming a loop. (D) The Waltman loop already shaped. (E) By rotation and traction the tip is steered into the left gastric artery. (F) Hepatic artery. (G) Replaced right hepatic artery. (H) Inferior mesenteric artery.

Figure 1.27 Alternative technique for formation of the Waltman loop with a cobra catheter.
(A,B) Introduction of the catheter in the contralateral iliac artery. (C) Continuous introduction of the shaft of the catheter with a loop formation in the abdominal aorta. (D) The loop is shaped. (E,F,G) Rotation and traction will make it possible to catheterize the hypogastric artery of the same side or to catheterize the common femoral artery and its branches on the opposite side (H).

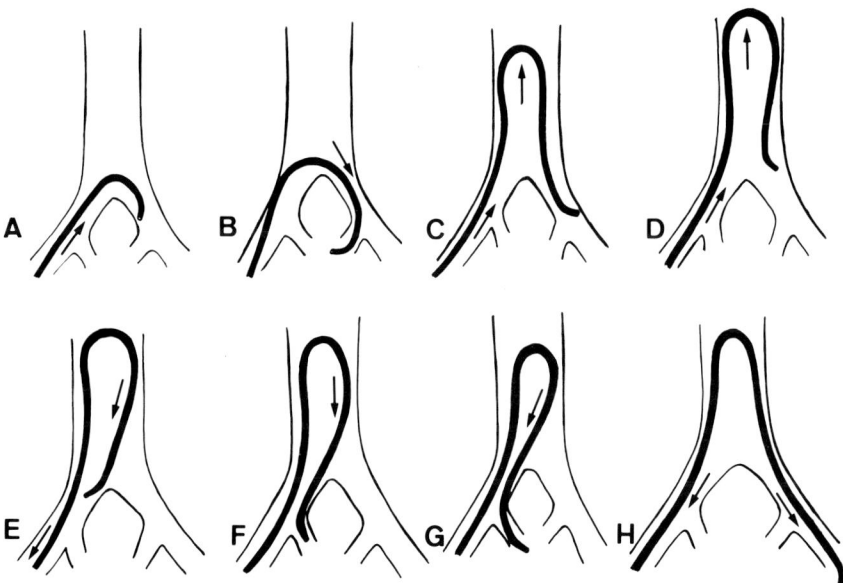

The new generation of superselective catheters allows catheterization of extremely peripheral vessels and delivery of embolic material into small vessels.

Extreme softness of the catheter tip is possible due to introduction of new polymers that combine flexibility and torque control. The 0.5- to 1-mm internal lumens allow particle embolization (250 to 500 μm), and the remarkable suppleness of the last 25 cm removes the risk of arterial spasm. The larger catheters permit routine diagnostic angiography that can be followed by therapeutic selective embolization. A No. 5 to 7 French guiding catheter is required, and a guidewire is usually necessary.

Tiny superselective catheters with a No. 3 French shaft and a tapered distal No. 2.5 French or No. 1.8 French flexible tip, together with a 5 French guiding catheter, are used for chemotherapy (Fig. 1.28). A steel mandrel is used to introduce the extra-supple tip, which has a gold ring for radiopacity. This small catheter may be adapted for use with an occluding detachable balloon for superselective occlusion or aneurysm embolization (Fig. 1.29).

For superselective angiographic studies and embolization with particles up to 500 μm, a No. 4.5 French catheter with a 25-cm flexible tip can be used through a No. 7 French guiding catheter (Fig. 1.30). For superselective embolization with particles up to 250 μm a No. 3 French catheter with an extra-supple 25-cm tip can be used through a No. 5 French guiding catheter (Fig. 1.31).

All this new catheter technology can be used in a system which combines a 2 French flexible catheter with a calibrated leak balloon glued to the tip. The set is introduced through a No. 6 French guiding catheter without a propulsion chamber (Fig. 1.32) and is used for

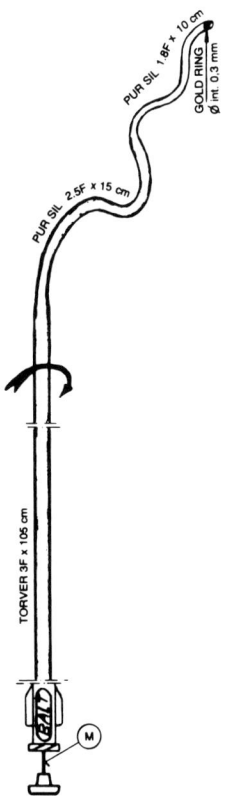

Figure 1.28 Progressively supple No. 3 French–1.8 French catheter for therapeutic drug infusion and bucrylate embolization. These catheters are used for hyperselective catheterization of small vessels in all anatomic locations. Their operation is based on torque control, blood flow, and manual guiding. They are used through a guiding No. 5 French catheter. A gold ring at the tip provides radiopacity. The internal diameter is 0.3 mm.

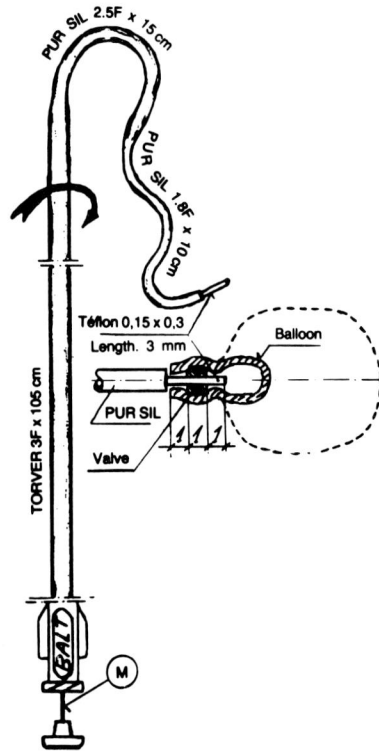

Figure 1.29 Progressively supple No. 3 French–1.8 French catheter, used with detachable balloon. This catheter is adapted to the treatment of intracerebral aneurysms. The balloon is fitted on the teflon tube at the tip of the 1.8 French catheter. The balloon, which is mounted before catheterization, carries the valves at the neck. The system is used through a No. 7 French guiding catheter, and the balloon is detached by withdrawing the catheter. Note the mandrel (M) at the base.

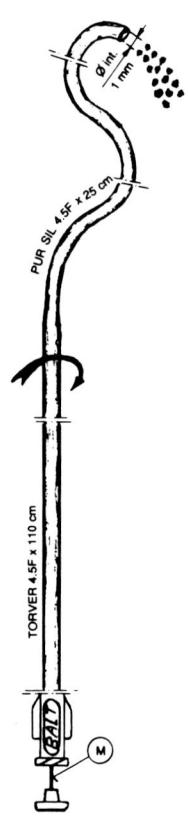

Figure 1.30 Progressively supple No. 4.5 French catheter for particle embolization (up to 500 μm). The very flexible distal catheter allows superselective embolization combining torque control. The internal diameter is 1 mm. A No. 7 French guiding catheter and a steel mandrel (M) are required.

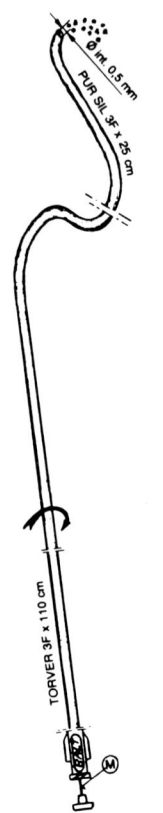

Figure 1.31 Progressively supple No. 3 French catheter for particle embolization (up to 250 μm). The flexible distal No. 3 French catheter allows superselective catheterization combining torque control. The internal diameter is 0.5 mm. A No. 5 French guiding catheter and a steel mandrel (M) are required.

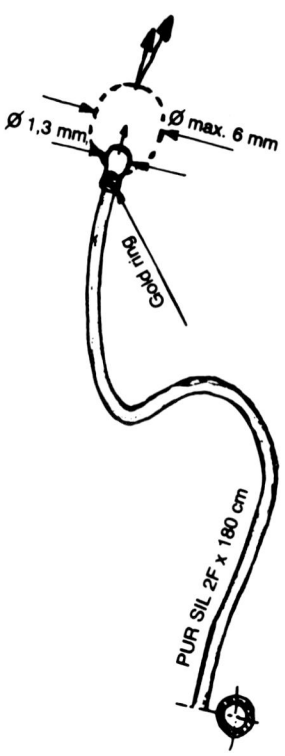

Figure 1.32 Calibrated leak balloon used for selective catheterization of small vessels using blood flow guidance. The gold ring at the tip provides radiopacity.

embolization of arterial venous malformation with bucrylate or histoacryl.

Recently introduced guidewires used to facilitate superselective catheterization with ordinary catheters are also available.

The usefulness of all the materials and techniques for selective and superselective catheterization will be better appreciated in Chap. IV, "Embolotherapy," where the different uses for embolization are presented. However, no matter which types of catheter and guidewire are selected, the most important factor for success is careful, skillful, and experienced angiographic manipulation.

REFERENCES

Almen T. Steering device for selective angiography and some vascular and enzymatic reactions observed in its clinical application. *Acta Radiol*(suppl) 1966;1–260.

Amplatz K. Percutaneous arterial catheterization and its applications. *AJR* 1962;86:265–274.

Ayella RJ. An ideal catheter: The simple curve. *Vasc Surg* 1975;147–150.

Braum S, Abrams HL. A J-shaped catheter for retrograde catheterization of tortuous vessels. *Radiology* 1964;83:436–438.

Beachley MC, Ranninger K. Abdominal aortography from the axillary approach. *AJR* 1973;119:508–511.

Boijsen E. Superselective pancreatic angiography. *Br J Radiol* 1966;39:481–485.

Boijsen E, Judkins MP. A hook tail "closed end" catheter for percutaneous selective cardiography. *Radiology* 1966;87:872–875.

Chuang VP, Soo CS, Carrasco CH. Superselective catheterization technique in hepatic angiography. *AJR* 1983;141:803–809.

Coons HG. Floppy-tipped wire guide for interventional procedures. *AJR* 1985;144:254–255.

Cope C. A new one-catheter torque-guide system for percutaneous exploratory abdominal angiography. *AJR* 1969;92:174–175.

Desilets DT, Hoffman RB, Ruttenberg HD. A new method of percutaneous catheterization. *AJR* 1966;97:519–522.

Dotter CT, Judkins MP, Frische LH. Safety guidespring for percutaneous cardiovascular catheterization. *AJR* 1966;98:957–959.

Driscoll SH, Grollman JH, Ellestedt MH. Single wall arterial puncture with disposable needle. *Radiology* 1974;113:470–472.

Glenn JH. Abdominal aorta catheterization via left axillary. *Radiology* 1975;115:227–228.

Heeney D. Shape your guide wire. *AJR* 1983;141:405–406.

Hawkins IF. A deflector catheter approach to the abdominal aorta. *AJR* 1972;116:196–198.

Judkins MP, Kidd HJ, Frische LH, Dotter CT. Lumen following safety-j-guide for catheterization of tortuous vessels. *Radiology* 1967;88:1127–1130.

Krangure MS, Chow KC, Christensen MA. Accurate and safe puncture of a pulseless femoral artery: An aid in performing iliac artery percutaneous transluminal angioplasty. *Radiology* 1982;144:927–930.

Komaki S. Simplified superselective catheterization of arterial bleeders. *Radiology* 1976;118:727–729.

Levin DC. Catheters for selective arteriography: Additional configuration alternatives. *Radiology* 1983;146:553–555.

Meyerovitz MF, Levin DC, Boxt LM. Superselective catheterization of small-caliber arteries with a new high-visibility steerable guide wire. *AJR* 1985;144:785.

Mikaelsson CG. Polyethylene catheter of new shape for percutaneous selective catheterization. *Acta Radiol* 1965;3:581–591.

Nebesar RA, Pollard JJ. A curved tip guidewire for thoracic and abdominal angiography. *AJR* 1966;97:508–510.

Odman P. The radiopaque polyethylene catheter. *Acta Radiol* 1959;52:52–55.

Rabinov K, Simon M. A new selective catheter with multidirectional controlled tip. *AJR* 1969;92:172–174.

Reuter SR. Superselective pancreatic angiography. *Radiology* 1969;92:74–85.

Rold KD, Smith DC. Guidewire with a J-shaped tip and a tapered movable core. *Radiology* 1983;149:317–318.

Rosch J, Grollman JH. Superselective arteriography in the diagnosis of abdominal pathology: Technical considerations. *Radiology* 1969;92:1008–1013.

Saddekni S, Srur M, Cohn TJ, Rozemblit G, Wetter EB, Sos TA. Antegrade catheterization of the superficial femoral artery. *Radiology* 1985;157:531.

Seldinger SI. Catheter replacement of the needle in percutaneous arteriography: A new technique. *Acta Radiol* 1953;39:368–375.

Sos TA, Cohn DJ, Srur M, Wengrover SI, Saddekni S. New open-ended guide wire/catheter. *Radiology* 1985;154:817.

Sundgren R. Selective angiography of the left gastric artery. *Acta Radiol*(suppl) 1970;1–299.

Vitek JJ. Femoro-cerebral angiography: An analysis of 2000 consecutive examinations with special emphasis on carotid artery catheterization in older patients. *AJR* 1973;118:633–647.

Waltman AC, Coury WR, Athanasoulis C, Baum S. Technique for left gastric artery catheterization. *Radiology* 1973;109:732–734.

Chapter Two

Embolization Procedures: Techniques and Materials

RENAN UFLACKER

INTRODUCTION

There are several methods for partially or totally occluding a vascular compartment. Two of the early uses of this procedure involved the successful embolization of a vertebral angioma, first by Newton and later by Doppman, in 1968. Subsequently, intraarterial infusion of vasoconstrictors such as epinephrine and vasopressin was used to control active gastrointestinal hemorrhage secondary to erosive gastritis or ulcerogenic disease. These early infusion procedures were enthusiastically received, and ultimately the therapeutic potential of the diagnostic arteriogram was recognized. In 1970, Rosch for the first time embolized the left gastric artery to control upper gastrointestinal hemorrhage. Following this, embolization techniques gained significant credibility as a viable alternative to surgical intervention.

At present, interventional embolization is used therapeutically in clinical situations involving trauma; esophageal varices; gastric and duodenal ulcers; arterial pseudoaneurysms; hepatic, renal, and osseous primary and metastatic neoplasms; vascular malformations; varicoceles; significant pulmonary hemorrhage; epistaxis; and lower colonic bleeding.

Currently, there are numerous embolizing and sclerosing agents in clinical use (Table 2.1). Although autologous clot, muscle, fat, fascia lata, and dura matter have been used, the most appropriate particulate material at this time from the standpoints of clinical availability and practical application is hemostatic gelatin (Gelfoam). However, Gelfoam is absorbable, and consequently the occlusion process may result in recanalization after a 3-week interval. For these reasons, the Gelfoam is frequently followed by the application of a Gianturco spiral metal coil. This results in total or permanent occlusion of the vessels, depending on the caliber of the vessel involved. More recently, minicoils have been applied through No. 3 French subselective catheters that pass freely over 0.014-in. steerable coronary artery guidewires. Absolute alcohol has also been utilized to produce permanent occlusion of the vascular bed and all of its extensions. Both detachable and nondetachable balloons can be used as part of the armamentarium for vascular occlusion procedures.

During all these embolization procedures, a superselective catheterization position is most desirable to prevent distal embolization to nontarget organs caused by reflux of the embolization material.

The principal advantage of embolization for acute hemorrhage is that immediate control of the bleeding source is ordinarily achieved. Embolization for control of neoplasm generally results in a reduction in the overall neoplastic mass due to the secondary affects of the infarction, and subsequent surgical resection can be done in a relatively bloodless field.

Before using embolization as a therapeutic procedure, it is important to carefully consider three factors: (1) the natural history of the disease, (2) the appropriate embolization material, and (3) the anatomic peculiarities of the vascular compartment being embolized. A decision must be made regarding whether temporary or permanent embolization is desirable. Frequently, a combination both of techniques and of materials is necessary to achieve effective embolization.

MATERIALS

Embolizing agents can be classified according to duration as short-, intermediate-, or long-term materials. Other classifications are autologous or heterologous, biological or nonbiological, particulated or nonparticulated, and polymerizing or sclerosing. Table 2.1 provides a quick review of types of materials, duration of occlusions, and tissue reactivities described after occlusion.

Short-Term Embolization Materials

A classic example of a short-term embolizing material is the autologous clot, one of the first embolization materials clinically applied. There are several difficulties connected with its use, however. One is that when arterial flow returns in the occluded vessel, lysis takes place

Table 2.1–Materials Used for Vascular Occlusion

Materials	Recanalization	Tissue Reactivity
1. Biological materials		
Autologous clot	6 to 12 h	None
Modified	12 to 24 h	None
Tissues		
Muscle		
Dura mater	Long-term	Moderate
Fascia lata		
2. Absorbable hemostatic materials		
Gelfoam	Days to weeks	
Oxycel (oxidized cellulose)	Days	Moderate
Avitene (microfibrillar collagen)	Days to weeks	
Ethibloc (gel)	Months	
3. Nonabsorbable particulated materials		
PVA (polyvinyl alcohol)	Permanent	Low
Silicone spheres	Permanent	None
Stiff brushes	Permanent	None
Polyesthyrene spheres	Permanent	None
Spiral coils	Permanent	Variable
Detachable balloons	Permanent	Low
4. Fluid polymers		
Bucrylate (isobutyl-2-cyanoacrylate)	Permanent	Controversial
Silicone rubber	Permanent	Low
Polyurethane	Permanent	Severe
5. Tissue sclerosing agents		
Absolute alcohol (99.8 °C)	Permanent	Variable
Ethamolin (ethanolamine oleate)	Permanent	Variable
50% glucose	Long-term	Low
3% Sotradecol	Permanent	Low
6. Catheter with balloons		
Medi-Tech catheter with balloon	Temporary	None
Fogarty (No. 2 or No. 3 French) (coaxial use)	Temporary	None
Wholey occluding balloon catheter	Temporary	None

rapidly. Another is that autologous clot is easily fragmented during embolization, with occasional embolization of a nontarget site. Finally, autologous clots are not a good choice of embolizing agent in patients in whom minimal coagulation can be obtained because of active bleeding disorders or deficiencies in coagulation parameters. The use of ϵ-aminocaproic acid can stabilize the clot and increase the time of lysis from 6 to 12 h to 12 to 24 h. Heating the clot also increases its longevity.

Autologous clot has been obtained by withdrawing, through femoral puncture, 15 to 20 mL of blood and allowing it to coagulate in a sterilized basin for approximately 20 min. Once the clot has formed, it may be serially cut into 2 × 3 mm strips and subsequently placed into a 1- to 3-mL contrast-filled syringe prior to embolization.

Although autologous clot offers low morbidity, because of rapid lysis, it has limited application as an embolizing agent.

Intermediate-Term Embolization Materials

Gelfoam

Surgical Gelfoam has been used for more than two decades as a contact hemostatic. Although a variety of embolizing materials are now available, Gelfoam continues to be a preferred material for clinical embolotherapy because of its availability, low cost, and ease of application through even the smallest of catheter systems.

Gelfoam may be used in particles that vary in size from 1 × 1 mm to 4 × 4 mm strips with 10-mm lengths cut by a conventional blade or scissors (Fig. 2.1). Gelfoam powder is also available for embolization of smaller vessels. The size and configuration of the particles selected depend on the diameter of the catheter used, the type of lesion being treated, and the size of the embolized vessel.

A 1- to 10-mL syringe may be used to introduce the Gelfoam embolic agent, according to the size of the

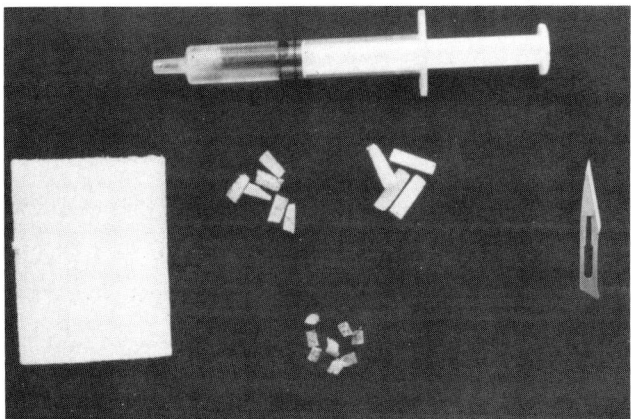

Figure 2.1 Gelfoam used for embolization. The Gelfoam sheet can be cut into small emboli of various sizes that are loaded into syringes full of iodinated contrast to allow fluoroscopic monitoring of the embolization procedure.

particles, the diameter of the catheter, and the flow of the lesion being embolized. Some authors suggest wetting the Gelfoam in a solution of contrast medium combined with broad-spectrum antibiotics.

The Gelfoam particles are back-loaded into the syringe, and the syringe is then filled with a combination of the contrast medium and the antibiotic solution. During injection, the distal aspect of the syringe should be elevated so that the emboli remain close to the outgoing orifice of the syringe at the catheter entrance site. During the embolization procedure, continual evaluation with brief injections of contrast medium allows evaluation of progressive flow reduction. At the first sign of contrast reflux to the parent vessel, the embolization procedure should be terminated. Gelfoam particles ordinarily last, with effective occlusion, for periods varying from 1 to 3 weeks after embolization. A moderate inflammatory reaction may occur during the reabsorption phase, and this may or may not leave a permanent occlusion at the vessel site. Normally, reabsorption of the material is total, and unless infarction has occurred, vessel recanalization will develop. Perivascular fibrotic reaction is a part of the infarction, and frequently when recanalization does occur, intravascular synechia is present. A combination of Gelfoam and vascular sclerosing agents will increase the inflammatory process and produce longer-lasting occlusions. When Gelfoam is used as the sole embolizing agent, the embolization is frequently temporary, and Gelfoam is best applied in situations where intermediate-term occlusion is desired.

Bovine Collagen

Bovine collagen is a fibrillar biological material. In its dehydrated form, when mixed with contrast medium or saline solution, it creates a pasty suspension that is easily injected through small-dimension catheters. Radiopacity can be obtained by the addition of tantalum powder or contrast medium. Bovine collagen acts through the induction of a thrombus by platelet aggregation and fibrin formation.

The distribution of infarction within the tissue is somewhat similar to what occurs when Gelfoam is used. Because the infarction is frequently associated with a periinflammatory process, the use of bovine collagen is not indicated in upper gastrointestinal hemorrhage or in cutaneous vascular malformations adjacent to peripheral nerves.

Oxidized Cellulose

Oxidized cellulose has a cottonlike consistency and functions as a hemostatic surgical agent that acts through platelet aggregation and fibrin deposition. It is mixed with the blood of a patient to stabilize the thrombus. After coagulation, it is cut in particles or strips (like Gelfoam, see Fig. 2.1) and injected through small syringes. Unfortunately, the tendency of this material to occlude the catheter has made its application as an effective emobilizing agent problematic. A intermediate-term occlusion of approximatley 30 days duration occurs. Vasculitis has been described in occluded vessels greater than 1 mm in diameter.

Ethibloc Gel

Ethibloc occlusion material is a radiopaque emulsion with a viscosity approaching that of honey at 37°C. It is precipitated during contact with an ionic solution, resulting in a semisolid substance with a gumlike consistency. The material is available commercially in 7.5-mL bottles in a 60% alcohol solution composed of 210 mg of corn protein, 162 mg of sodium amidotriosate, 145 mg of papaveris oil, and 6 mg of propylenoglycol per mL of alcohol. Precipitation time is increased by the use of 40% glucose, which increases the osmotic effect. Experimental studies have shown that the material will occlude the entire renal arterial circulation, extending into the capillary level, with some filling existing at the renal glomerules. The occlusion lasts several months.

Long-Term Embolization Materials

Gianturco-Anderson-Wallace Coils

Steel coils with attached wool strands can be used for permanent occlusion. Significant evolution of design has improved their safety and allowed better placement techniques. The different types of coils are illustrated in Figs. 2.2 and 2.3.

The first models were constructed out of mechanically

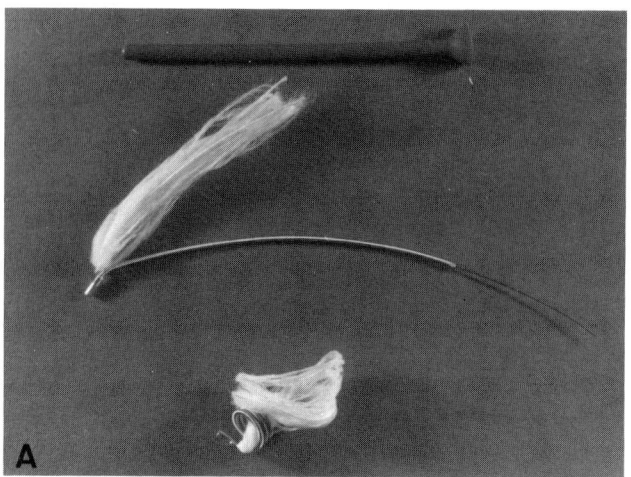
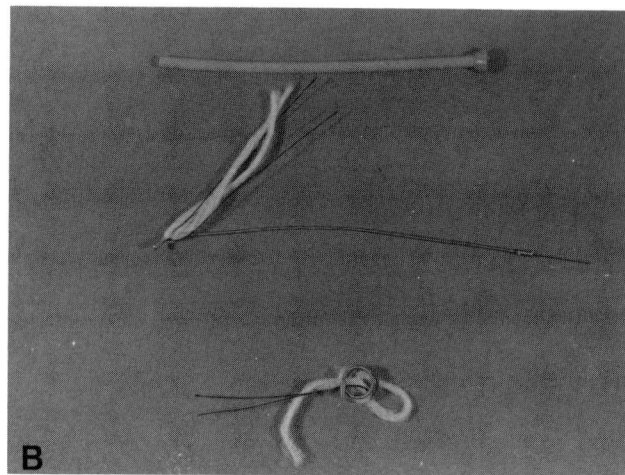

Figure 2.2 Gianturco-Anderson-Wallace coils.
(A) Introducer sheath for the original steel coil with wool tufts. The coil is seen in straightened and functional position. (B) Minicoil composed of 0.021-in. guidewire with dacron tufts. This coil can be introduced by a special No. 5 French teflon catheter. The original coil required a No. 7 or 8 French catheter with a special introducer (see Fig. 2.4).

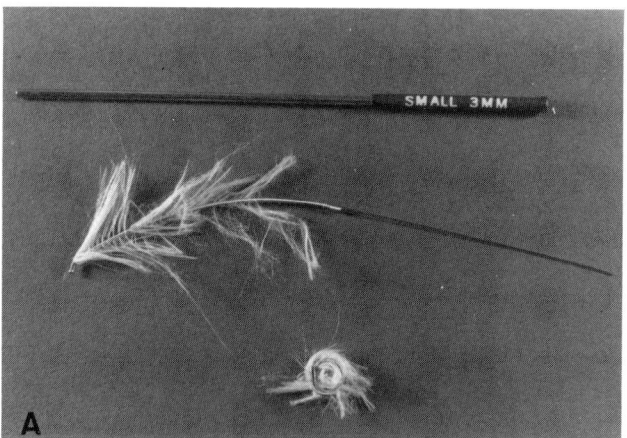
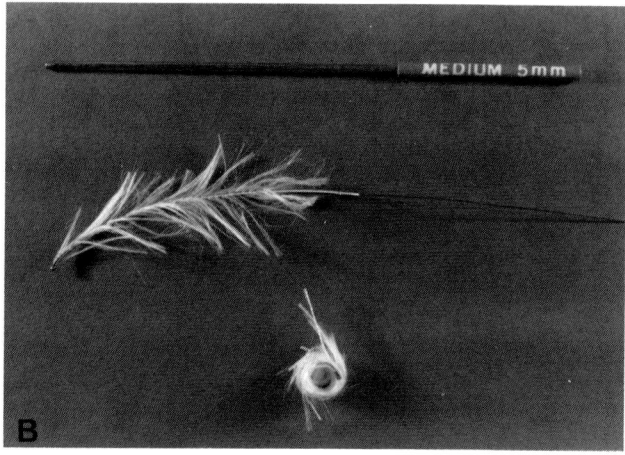
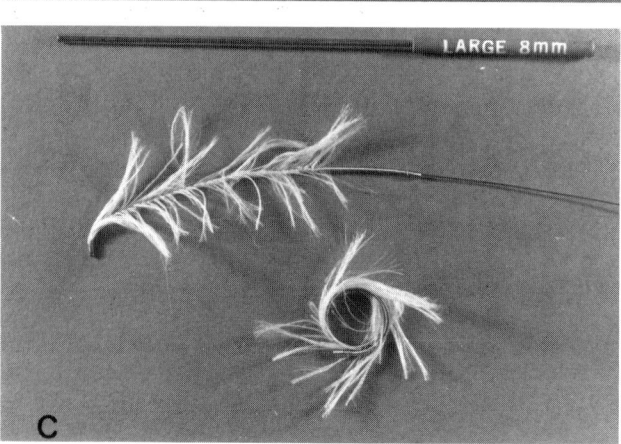

Figure 2.3 New steel coils for embolization. Dacron tufts are distributed along the length of the coil. The coils come preloaded in introducers labeled with the coil diameter. They can be introduced through conventional catheters that take a 0.038-in.-diameter guidewire.
(A) 3-mm-diameter coil. (B) 5-mm-diameter coil. (C) 8-mm-diameter coil.

twisted guidewire segments with a wool strand tied to the tip. The core of the wire had been removed (Fig. 2.2). The coil was introduced through calibrated No. 8 or No. 9 French teflon catheters, and selective catheterization was limited by the size of the catheter (Fig. 2.4). An important improvement in overall coil technology was the development of a minicoil (Fig. 2.2) that could be introduced through a No. 5 French catheter. The minicoil would expand to fit a 3-mm-diameter vessel (Fig. 2.5). A more recent modification, which increased the versatility and simplicity of coil usage, was the creation of 3-, 5-, and 8-mm coils with a dacron cord attachment (Fig. 2.3). These modern coils can be used with conventional angiographic catheters and guidewires (Fig. 2.6). The coils are available in color-coded tubular metal sheaths: black for 3-mm coils, blue for 5-mm coils, and red for 8-mm coils (Fig. 2.3). Recently, "microcoils" with 2-mm diameters have become available for small

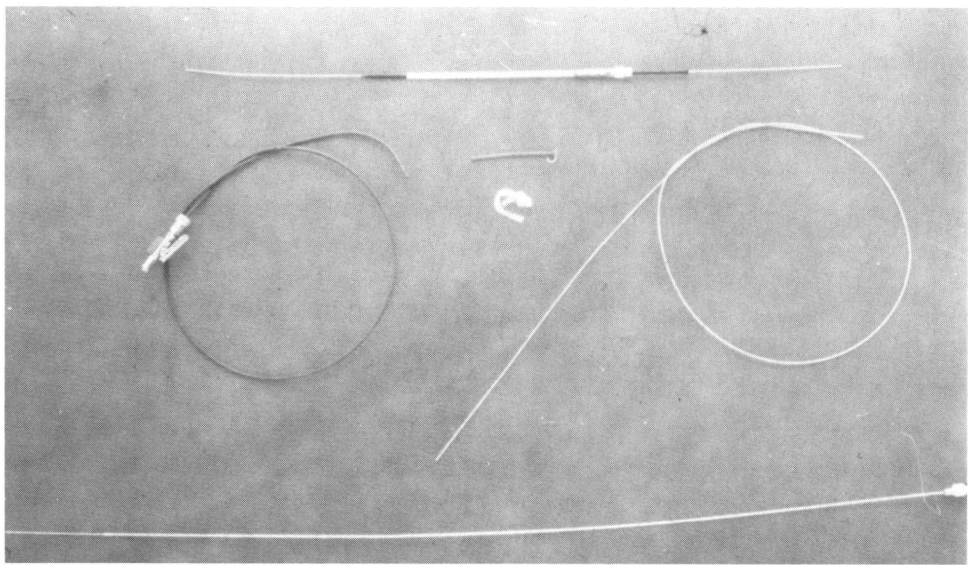

Figure 2.4 Set required to introduce the original Gianturco coils. A No. 8 French Desilet-Hoffman sheath is at the top; a No. 8 French catheter with non-tapered tip is at the left; coils and introducer sheath are shown in center; an 0.42-in.-diameter guidewire is at the right; and the rectifier and stiff introducer with a mobile center are at the bottom.

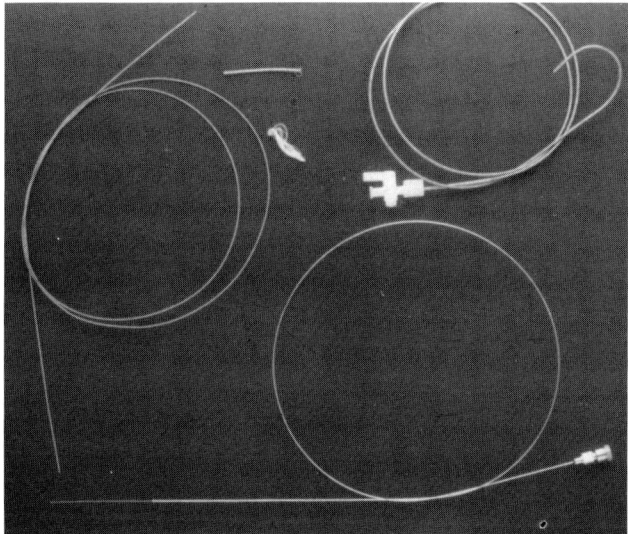

Figure 2.5 Set required to introduce the minicoils. At top left is the special guidewire; the coils and introducer are in the middle; the No. 5 French teflon catheter is at upper right; and the stiff introducer with mobile center is at the bottom.

vessel to be embolized, it will not coil adequately and the maximum occlusive effect will not be obtained. The objective is for the coil to roll and wedge against the arterial wall, forming a solid base for thrombosis.

Vascular occlusion obtained by a coil is frequently permanent, with organization of the thrombus both proximal and distal to the coil. After use of a Gianturco coil, a granulomatous process develops within the arterial wall and periadventitial tissue. It is worth remembering that because the 8-mm coils are positioned in vessels with relatively high flow, they are less thrombogenic and may require an additional coil or supplemental Gelfoam. Because of thrombotic effects around the coil, a brief (5 or 10 min) period of observation is required prior to total occlusion.

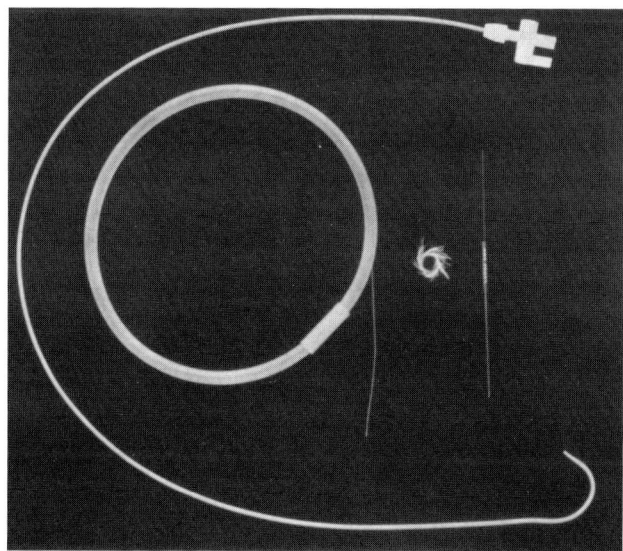

Figure 2.6 The new type of metal coils are introduced with a conventional guidewire and catheter.

vessels. These require 0.021-in. guidewires. Giant coils with diameters of 15 to 18 mm require 0.042-in. guidewires.

With the catheter positioned selectively in the vessel to be occluded, the tube containing the coil with the desired diameter is introduced through the stopcock of the catheter and the coil is advanced 20 or 30 cm inside the catheter with the stiff tip of the guidewire. The sheath is removed, and the coil is then advanced with the flexible tip of the guide until it exits the distal end of the catheter, where the uncoiling is fluoroscopically visible (Fig. 2.7). If the selected coil is too large for the

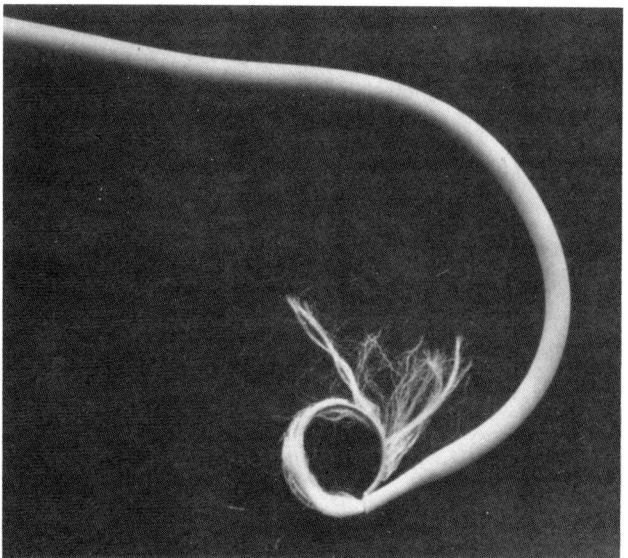

Figure 2.7 8-mm coil resuming its original diameter as soon as it leaves the tip of the catheter.

Embolizations with Gianturco coils are permanent, and although effective, they are always proximal in relation to the capillary vascular bed. Tumoral and AV malformations are frequently inadequately embolized by Gianturco coils because the infarction is only partial. Collateralization occurs and the distal vascular bed remains open. For these reasons, coils are never the primary indication as an embolizing agent for vascular malformations.

Polyvinyl Alcohol (Ivalon)

Polyvinyl alcohol, which is insoluble in water, is semirigid when dry but malleable in the wet state. Polyvinyl alcohol foam (Ivalon) is a hygroscopic material whose wet volume is 20 percent greater than its dry volume (Fig. 2.8). Introduced in the 1960s as a household sponge, it is popularly known by its trade name, Ivalon. In 1975 Tadavarthy published the first paper describing the application of polyvinyl alcohol foam as an embolization material.

When the Ivalon sponge is embedded in live tissue, it causes a mild foreign-body reaction and the cavities of the sponge are rapidly permeated by granulation tissue. Used as an embolization material, Ivalon acts as a mechanical occluder by impaction within the embolized vessel. Although a greater volume of Ivalon is required in comparison to Gelfoam, it produces less perivascular spasm than Gelfoam does.

Occlusion is permanent at the site of particle impaction. The sponge is available in blocks, sheets, or granulated, irregular microspheres with diameters of 149, 250, 420, 590, 1000, and 2000 μm. Homogeneity of the particles is important if systemic shunting through fistulous communications is to be avoided. The material can be made radiopaque by incorporating barium sulfate mixed with a sponge structure. Small strips (1 by 5 mm) of Ivalon, sterilized in ethylene oxide, may be incorporated into a saline solution and introduced in a short connecting tube. The tube is connected to the catheter, and the solution is injected slowly through the syringe.

If the granulated form is used, some modification in the technique may be necessary. To reduce surface tension, the spheres are loaded into a syringe with diluted contrast medium and injected outward and inward into a connecting tube joined to an additional syringe. Eventually the particles will be in suspension in the contrast instead of floating on the surface. The use of a three-way stopcock makes it possible to immediately inject the material into the vascular compartment to be embolized.

Experience is necessary because the Ivalon granules tend to group together and will occasionally occlude the catheter. In most cases, introduction of a guidewire relieves the obstruction. It has been observed that Ivalon particles may be incorporated by the vascular wall and expelled all the way through the skin in some vascular malformations.

Dura Mater

Human lyophilized dura mater has been used for years as a permanent particulate embolizing agent. This material is furnished in small blades and should be cut in 2- by 2- by 2-mm fragments or in 2- by 1- by 10-mm strips. These fragments can be introduced one by one in a 3-mL or 1-mL syringe.

The histologic reactions to the presence of dura mater inside the vascular system are still not adequately known,

Figure 2.8 Polyvinyl alcohol (Ivalon), available in sponge or particulate form.

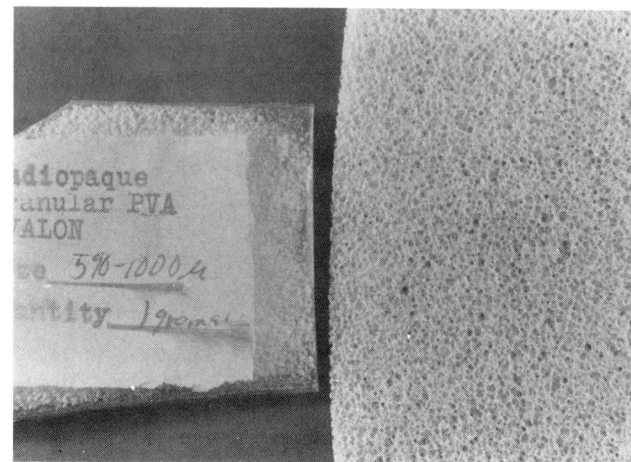

but they seem to be like histologic reactions to an inert material.

Detachable Balloons

In 1974, Serbinenko developed detachable perfusion balloons as aids in superselective angiography and embolization of arterial venous malformations of the central nervous system. Soon thereafter, Debrun improved the system of detachable balloons, developing a concept of calibrated leak balloons in 1975 and 1978.

Methods of vascular occlusion using detachable balloons were developed as alternatives to superselective catheterization involving non-flow-oriented particles. There was need for a flow-oriented occlusive material which would eventually result in permanent occlusion but which would allow the occlusion to be reversed until the material was released at the exact site, thereby eliminating the "all or nothing" phenomenon. Detachable balloons meet these criteria, and are safe for clinical use.

Two types of balloons are available commercially: the latex ones developed by Debrun for neuroradiology and the silicon ones developed by White that are used predominantly in nonneuroradiological embolization.

The latex balloons are mounted on a No. 3 or No. 2 French catheter and tied manually by the interventional radiologist. Their size must be adequate for the dimension of the vessels that are to be occluded (Fig. 2.9). Three catheters are used in a coaxial manner. The balloon is tied to a 110-cm-long No. 2 French teflon catheter that is placed inside a 100-cm-long No. 4 French polyethylene catheter. This set is introduced in the vascular system through a No. 6, 7, 8, or 9 French thin-walled catheter that is 80 or 90 cm long.

Once the introducer is in position and is being carefully watched, the coaxial system with the balloon is advanced through a No. 6 to No. 9 French catheter. When the balloon is properly positioned and inflated, a test injection is done through the introducer catheter to demonstrate the effectiveness of the occlusion. The balloon is introduced to the desired vessel in a flow-oriented manner; that is, the partially inflated balloon is taken to the vessel with greater flow as it is gently pushed by the operator. The balloon is easily visible through fluoroscopy.

A nonionic isosmotic or an iodized oil contrast medium is then used to inflate the balloon. An option for inflation of the balloon is to use liquid silicon, which solidifies permanently after 10 min at 37°C, preventing deflation.

The balloon is detached from the introducer system by advancing the No. 4 French catheter over the No. 2 French teflon catheter. The balloon is left in its place, occluding the artery or arterial venous fistula definitively (Fig. 2.10).

Latex balloons are versatile and can be found in diameters varying from 4 to 20 mm and in several different shapes, e.g., spherical or sausagelike (Fig. 2.9). Detachable silicon balloons can be found in two sizes; one has a 1-mm diameter when empty and a 4-mm diameter when inflated, and one has a 2-mm diameter when empty and an 8- to 9-mm diameter when inflated.

The silicon balloon has a minivalve into which the No. 2 French polyurethane catheter is introduced. When the catheter is removed, the valve closes automatically, preventing deflation of the balloon. Silicon acts as a semipermeable membrane, and it is therefore necessary to utilize radiopaque isosmotic nonionic contrast material to fill the balloon.

To introduce these balloons efficiently, it is necessary to use an expansion chamber that allows for a smooth and progressive introduction of the balloon with the proximal end fixed to the expansion chamber wall to keep the entire system from being pushed through the arterial venous communications. This chamber propels the balloon by means of a saline injection in its interior, producing a flow that draws the balloon and the No. 2 French catheter with it through the introducer catheter.

When the balloon is inflated and vessel occlusion takes place, a test injection is done to demonstrate the position of the balloon in relation to the arterial tree that will be occluded. Permanent occlusion of the embolized artery takes place when the No. 2 French catheter is removed. The balloon is freed by initiating a sudden but smooth traction of the No. 2 French catheter, using a strength of approximately 50 g. If the path is very tortuous, the strength of the traction is dissipated throughout the catheter, and it may become impossible to remove

Figure 2.9 Detachable balloons used with the Debrun technique. The balloons are tied to a white No. 2 French catheter with a rubber string. The black No. 4.5 French catheter is used to release the balloon as it is pushed against the balloon base.
(A) 8-mm-diameter balloon. (B) 10-mm-diameter balloon. (C) 12-mm-diameter balloon.

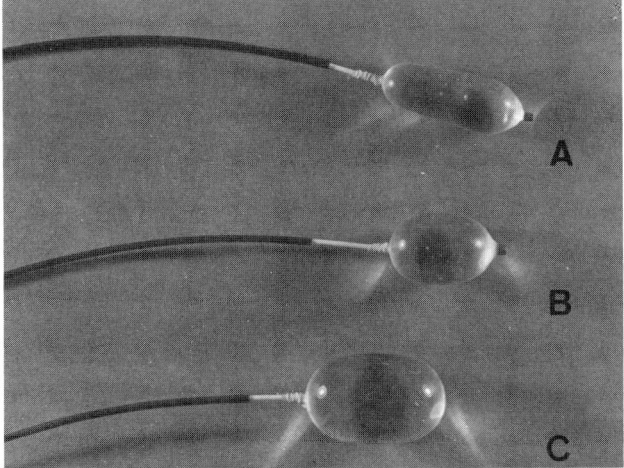

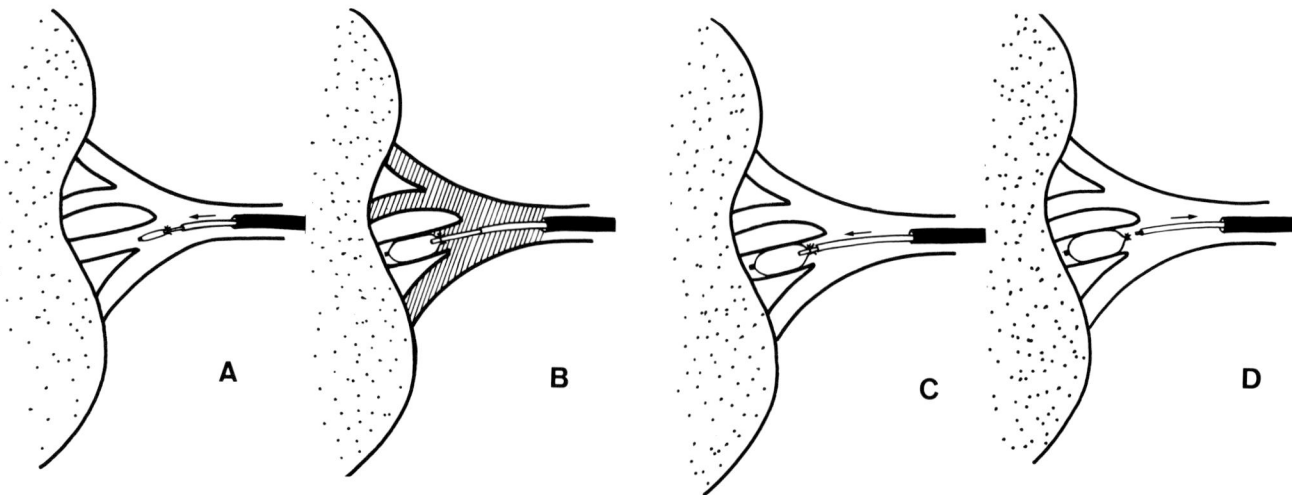

Figure 2.10 Latex balloon placement by the Debrun technique.
(A) The balloon is advanced selectively through a No. 7 or 9 French guiding catheter. (B) The balloon is inflated with angiographic documentation of proper occlusion using a "Y" adapter. (C) The No. 4.5 French catheter is advanced to the base of balloon. (D) The No. 2 French catheter is withdrawn until the balloon is released.

the No. 2 French catheter. In such cases, causing tension in the introducer catheter and the No. 2 catheter simultaneously will generally free the balloon.

If the balloon remains inflated for at least 20 days, the thrombi organize proximally and distally to the site of occlusion and will form an irreversible occlusion.

Histologic studies have not shown significant inflammatory reactions in the arterial wall after prolonged occlusion by the silicon balloon, which testifies to its inert nature.

It is important to reiterate that because the occlusion can be reversed at any time during the procedure, and the balloon can be deflated and removed, changed, or repositioned, detachable balloons are one of the safest and most versatile agents in the interventional arsenal for vascular occlusion.

One potential problem with this procedure is that it is sometimes difficult to inflate and deflate the balloon during positioning maneuvers using the vascular flow, due to the small caliber and tortuosity of the coaxial catheter. Another is that aging of the latex balloon and its elastic valve may occasionally result in premature deflations. The valves of silicon balloons also have a limited life. They can fail if used after 1 year from date of manufacture, causing premature deflation after embolization.

Latex balloons should be prepared the night before the procedure and sterilized with ethylene oxide or with other chemical substances that are noncorrosive for latex, to avoid deterioration of the elastic band and the walls of the balloon.

Isobutyl-2-cyanoacrylate (Bucrylate, IBC)

The cyanoacrylates form a group of rapidly polymerized industrial glues that have been used in various surgical areas including hemostasis and tissue anastomosis. One of the most recent uses of this line of monomers is as an embolizing agent in interventional radiology.

The adhesive property of cyanoacrylates was discovered accidentally during experiments on monomers in 1966. Various cyanoacrylates with different properties are available, but the most commonly used in the biological field is isobutyl-2-cyanoacrylate (IBC).

The polymerization of IBC is obtained through an exothermic reaction that can be initiated by free ionic radicals in the medium. IBC is polymerized in contact with ionic substances or with the endothelium itself. Acid media retard polymerization, and alkaline media slightly accelerate polymerization.

IBC is a low-viscosity material which is quickly polymerized and which can be injected using small-caliber catheters or calibrated leak balloons. IBC is easily rendered radiopaque by mixing it with tantalum power or lipiodated contrast medium (Duroliopaque, Lipiodol) (Fig. 2.11). Tantalum is an inert substance, and its effect on the mixture is limited to a slight increase in viscosity.

The use of IBC is still experimental; however, it is considered the best embolizing agent for the treatment of arterial venous malformations with high flow and medium vascular caliber. Due to the adhesive properties of bucrylate, superselective catheterization is mandatory, and experience is essential to avoid complications.

IBC polymerizes in contact with ionic solutions, and to avoid polymerization 5% glucose must be used to wash the catheter system. The No. 2 French catheter must be pulled immediately after the IBC injection to keep the catheter from sticking to the wall of the vessel or bringing with it fragments of the polymer mass.

When cyanoacrylates are in contact with live tissues, they cause some degree of inflammatory reaction, with

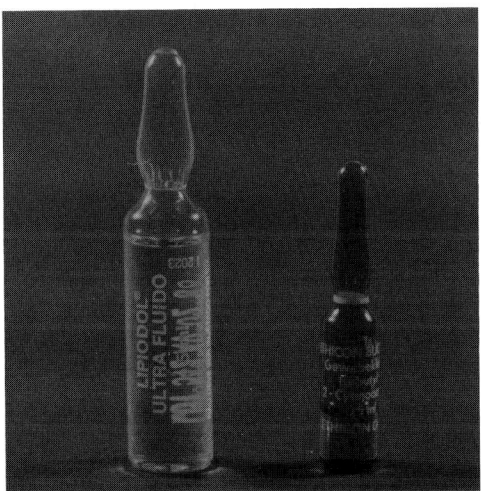

Figure 2.11 A 5-mL vial of Lipiodol and a 0.5-mL vial of bucrylate in dark glass to protect it from light.

polymorphonuclear infiltrate and a granulation appearing between the fifth day and twenty-first day. In experimental studies, a certain degree of absorption of polymers by healthy tissue has been shown. A moderate bacteriostatic effect with the isobutyl monomer has also been identified.

Because cyanoacrylates have caused various adverse effects in the laboratory, some have not been allowed for biological or human use. For example, it has been shown that IBC and the *N*-butyl cyanoacrylates have a mutogenic affect in live beings. And, although there is no documented evidence of carcinogenic effect on human beings caused by any of the cyanoacrylates, the subcutaneous injection of large quantities of methyl metacrylate induced fibrosarcomas in 8 out of 59 rats. In other animals, however, the same substance did not cause the development of any lesion whatsoever.

Embolization with IBC can be used as primary therapy or as a supplement to surgery with resection of vascular malformations. IBC can cause focal parietal vascular necrosis, either because of the heat produced when it is polymerized or because of an unknown physical chemical property, which can cause vascular rupture and localized hemorrhage.

The deposition of IBC in the nidus of the malformation is the most effective way of treating a vascular malformation. The IBC will lead to a progressive thrombosis with occlusion of the nidus and the draining veins (Fig. 2.12).

Bucrylate comes in 0.5-mL low-viscosity sterile ampules (Fig. 2.11), and can be easily mixed with Lipiodol or tantalum to become radiopaque. In a 1:1 bucrylate-Lipiodol solution the polymerization time is about 3.2 s, in a 1:2 ratio it increases to 5 s; and in a 1:3 ratio to 7 s. By increasing the quantity of Lipiodol, the time of polymerization is increased proportionately, allowing the glue (IBC) to reach the circulation at the most peripheral part of the lesion at the capillary or precapillary level (Fig. 2.12).

Once the internal volume of the No. 2 French catheter has been determined, including the volume of the three-way stopcock, superselective catheterization of the artery nourishing the lesion is done with a No. 2 or 3 French catheter or with an open-ended guidewire like that shown in Fig. 1.25.

Using a three-way stopcock, a 1-mL syringe with IBC and Lipiodol is adapted to one way and a 3-mL syringe with 5% glucose is attached on another, and the system is connected to a No. 2 French catheter. The three-way stopcock must be manipulated according to the position of the syringe after the following five steps are carried out:

1. 5% glucose injection in the No. 2 French catheter
2. Injection of IBC (volume equal to or less than that of the No. 2 French catheter)

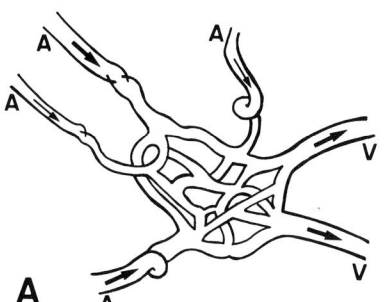 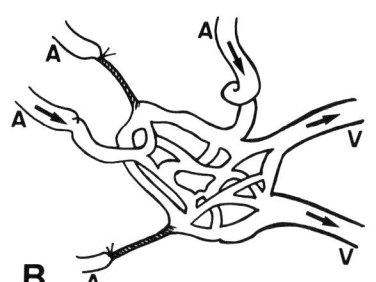 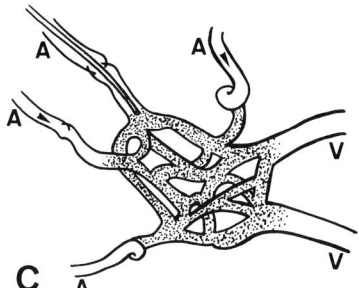

Figure 2.12 Bucrylate embolization of the nidus of an arteriovenous malformation.
(A) Arteriovenous malformation with two large and two smaller supplying arteries. (B) There is an immediate increase in flow through the smaller arteries if there is only surgical ligation of the main arteries. (C) Superselective catheterization and embolization of the nidus can drastically reduce or eliminate total arterial and venous flow.

3. Injection of 5% glucose to take the radiopaque IBC to the vessel that will be occluded
4. Instant removal of the No. 2 French catheter after the outflow of IBC flushed by the glucose solution
5. Postembolization angiographic control

The final objective of embolization with bucrylate is to extend the occlusion to the capillary or precapillary level, causing necrosis or obstruction of the nidus of the angiomatous lesion (Fig. 2.12).

More recently Histoacryl or *N*-butyl cyanoacrylate has been used experimentally and clinically with results similar to those obtained with IBC.

Silicon and Polyesterene Spheres

These efficient embolizing materials cause occlusion of larger vessels if large spheres are used and peripheral occlusion of small vessels if small spheres are used, and produce permanent occlusion of the embolized territory.

Silicon spheres, with diameters ranging from 0.5 to 3 mm, are nonabsorbable and biocompatible, and can be made radiopaque by impregnation with barium sulfate. Silicon spheres are blood-flow-directed. Hundreds of small particles can be introduced in a malformation to diminish the flow and eventually induce thrombosis. At the end of the procedure, larger particles should be used to occlude the main arterial source to the lesion. Although complete occlusion of the lesion is rarely obtained, silicon spheres are an excellent material for palliative treatment of vascular malformations or for use as a presurgical measure. However, because it is difficult to obtain total control over the spheres, they are of limited overall use.

Nylon Brushes (Bristle Brushes)

Nylon bristle brushes, like the brushes used to clean conventional smoking pipes, are made up of a center of braided steel wires with radial nylon spikes. They come in diameters that vary from 4 to 8 mm. The brushes are introduced by No. 7 or 8 French catheters and require selective catheterization for their use. The number of brushes necessary for occlusion depends on the vascular diameter and flow of the embolized artery. There is no trauma to the vascular wall when the brushes are introduced, and at medium term there is minimal inflammatory process involving the three layers of the vessel. The occlusion obtained is permanent and depends on the organization of the thrombus that is formed at the site of the brush. The use and effect obtained by nylon brushes are similar to the Gianturco-Anderson-Wallace coils.

Stainless Steel Spiders

Stainless steel "spiders" were first developed to avoid the passage of embolization material through high-flow large-diameter arterial venous shunts. These spiders act as a filter to prevent passage of Gianturco coils or any other material through their rods, avoiding pulmonary emboli. Later, a large piece of Ivalon was incorporated in their construction so that they would produce definitive occlusion. The new material was called "spiderlon." These spiders are placed percutaneously with No. 7 or 8 French teflon catheters and are available with 10- or 15-mm diameters (Fig. 2.13).

The metal spikes affix themselves firmly to the vascular wall, and in 3 or 4 weeks they are incorporated into the wall. Stainless steel spiders may be used as an initial

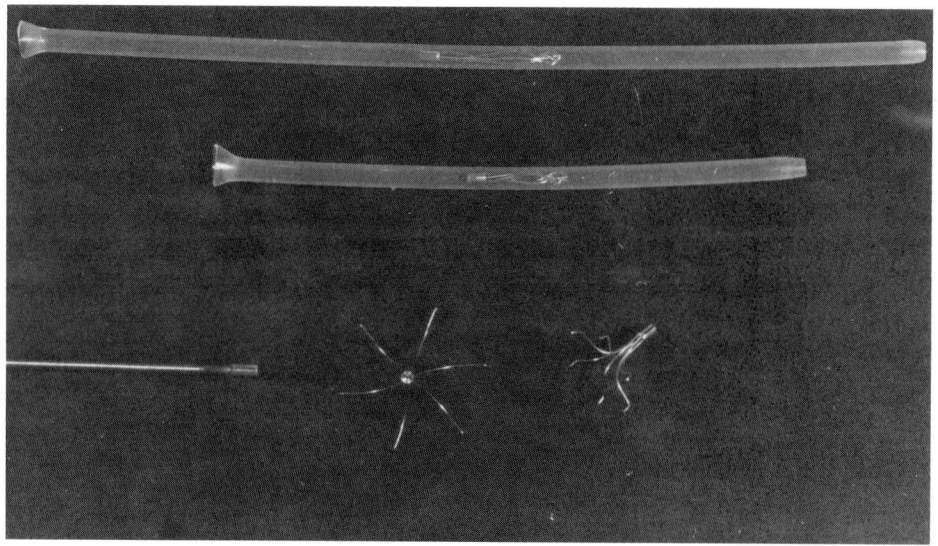

Figure 2.13 Stainless steel spiders. 17- and 9-mm-diameter brushes are loaded into teflon introducers and discharged with the special guidewire shown at left.

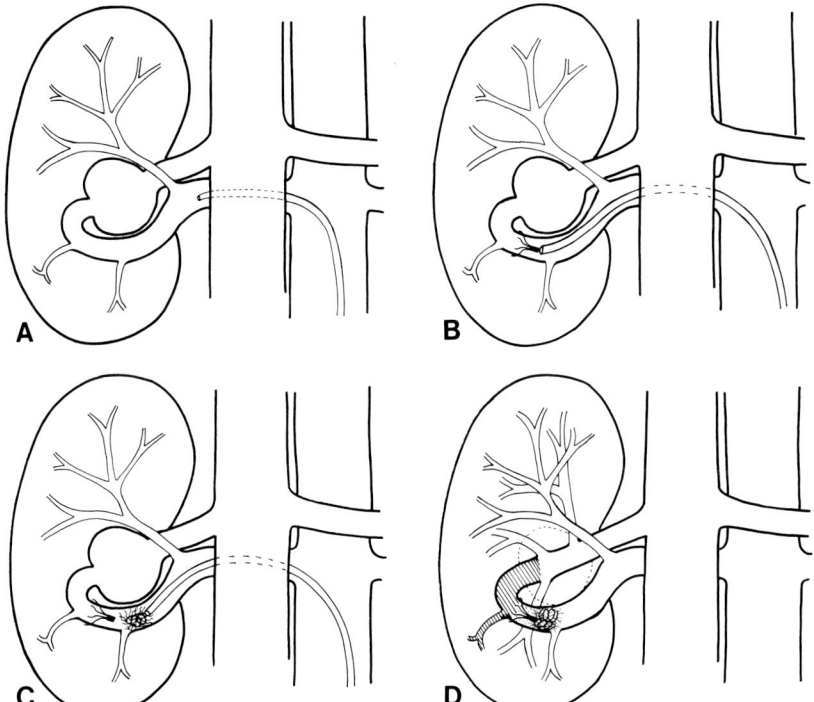

Figure 2.14 Use of spiders in a large-caliber fistula.
(A) A renal arteriovenous fistula with false aneurysm. (B) Superselective placement of spider proximal to false aneurysm. (C) Addition of multiple steel coils whose distal migration is prevented by the spider. (D) Occlusion of the fistula and thrombosis of the false aneurysm. The renal veins draining normal parenchyma can now be identified.

measure (Fig. 2.14) when one foresees a pulmonary or peripheral embolization of an arterial venous fistula the caliber of which is too great for Gianturco coils. Maneuverability is limited due to the high resistance and stiffness of the introducer catheter.

Muscle and Fascia Lata

Muscle and fascia lata are histocompatible biological materials that are removed from the patient, using local anesthesia, prior to that embolization. Autologous muscle was the first material used for embolization of a cavernous carotid fistula described by Brooks in 1930. This technique became popular among neurosurgeons, who used muscle particles to embolize cerebral malformations during surgery.

Both muscle and fascia lata may be obtained through a small incision in the patient's thigh. The materials are difficult to manipulate because they lack opacification and are not easily deformed, and must be used in small fragments when injected by angiographic catheters. Both materials produce permanent occlusion.

Silicon Rubber

Fluid silicon is a biocompatible material that produces permanent occlusion. It is rendered radiopaque with tantalum or barium powder and is introduced through superselective catheterization in much the same way that bucrylate is introduced.

The silicon mixture is made up of a silastic 382R elastomer, a high-viscosity silicon that contains a substance for vulcanization, and fluid medical 360R silicon of lower viscosity that acts as a dilutant of the mixture. The ratio of 382R to 360R ranges from 1:2 to 1:5, depending on the viscosity desired, with 1 g of tantalum powder per mL of mixture.

Two catalyzers are necessary to start vulcanization; Dow Corning Catalyzer M and a disulfiram silicon coagulant. To determine the time needed for polymerization, which varies from 3 to 4 min, in vitro tests are necessary before beginning the injection.

This material can be injected by small coaxial catheters or by a system of balloons occluding the primary artery. There is practically no risk of the catheter or balloon adhering to the silicon, and a real cast of the arterial tree is obtained after injection.

Tissue Sclerosing Agents (Absolute Alcohol, Ethanolamine Oleate, and 50% Glucose)

The main advantage of tissue sclerosing agents over particulate embolizing agents are ease of handling and the fact that they can be injected through thin catheters in superselective and coaxial systems. An additional advantage is that total vascular occlusion occurs after sclerosis. They are inexpensive and universally available (Fig. 2.15). The vascular occlusion obtained with these agents produces obstruction at all levels, from the capillary to the main artery.

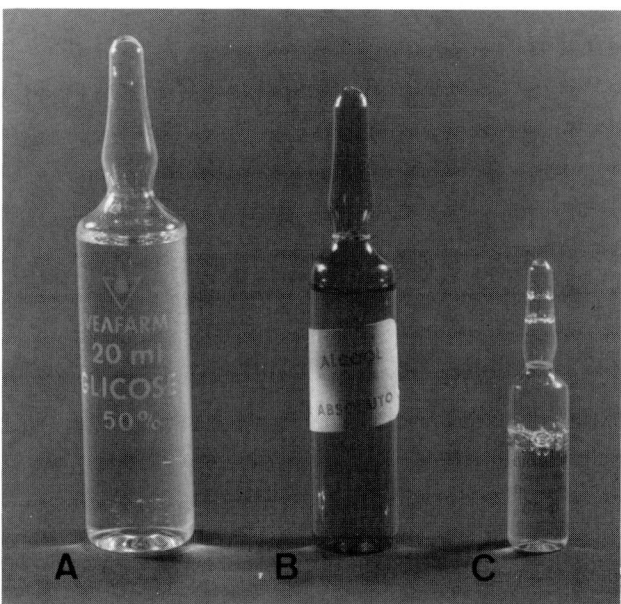

Figure 2.15 Vascular sclerosing agents.
(A) 50% glucose. (B) Absolute alcohol. (C) 2-mL Ethamolin ampule.

Cellular lesions with tissue sclerosing agents result from protein precipitation (sclerosis). In the case of absolute alcohol there is a universal precipitation of blood components and protein denaturation of the vessel wall, with clot formation and dehydration, followed by the sclerosing process itself where the alcohol acts as a histologic fixer. These substances have few systemic effects, and, in the case of alcohol, intoxication levels in the blood are rarely reached.

Some authors suggest the use of a catheter with a balloon to avoid reflux in the aorta and nontarget organs when introducing tissue sclerosing agents. The reflux of absolute alcohol into the aorta can lead to an ischemic lesion of the intestine by vascular obstruction.

The action of 50% glucose is based mainly on its hypertonic action on the blood and the vascular walls of the territory to be occluded.

Absolute alcohol was used initially for renal ablation and later extended to other organs. The injection of absolute alcohol in a vascular territory must be done very carefully, because it will be distributed in all the vessels with blood flow, from the capillary level to the main artery, with deleterious effects in the specific territory catheterized. If absolute alcohol is injected in arteries that irrigate cutaneous surfaces and nervous system tissue, ischemia with necrosis and ulceration will develop in the skin and viscera and there will be devitalization with an important functional deficit in the nervous system. (See "Complications of Embolization" at the end of this chapter.)

Sclerosing agents are especially efficient in venous territories, including varices of the esophagus secondary to portal hypertension, because vascular flow in such vessels is relatively slow, and the vascular wall is more sensitive to sclerosis. Intratumoral injection of absolute ethanol in the liver seems to produce massive tumor necrosis and regression, according to recent reports.

Transarterial Electrocoagulation

Electrocoagulation of blood vessels by application of a direct current via a catheter can produce vascular occlusion. Experimental studies have demonstrated that the size of the clot produced is directly proportional to the quantity and duration of current. The formation of clots and occlusion of the vessel can be secondary to the attraction of platelets to the positive electrode and to the intimal lesion.

An angiographic catheter and a conductor guidewire are used to carry out electrocoagulation.

Electromechanical factors other than the general physiologic mechanisms of coagulation are related to pH alterations, thermal damage, precipitation of proteins and inorganic salts, and diffusion of final toxic products of tissue degradation.

Although electrocoagulation is generally quite efficient, it has never obtained great popularity. Its application is limited to certain centers and to experimental use, and it seems doubtful that it will gain clinical importance in the future.

Catheters with Occlusion Balloons

Catheters with balloons have been available since 1951, but their early use was restricted to experimental diagnostic procedures. The first therapeutic use, for embolectomy, was described by Fogarty in 1963. Later, the technique was employed in the treatment of other intraluminary pathologic conditions and removal of bladder stones. Subsequently, catheters with balloons were developed for interventional angiography to control hemorrhage and for devascularization of neoplastic lesions. They have also been used to occlude either the abdominal aorta or the inferior vena cava. The use of occlusion catheters with balloons as an aid in embolization was introduced by Wholey in 1976.

At present, several catheters having occlusion balloons with diameters ranging from 3 to 40 mm are available for small and large vessels (Fig. 2.16). Balloons with inflated diameters up to 8.5 mm can be introduced percutaneously without a sheath, but the larger ones need sheaths of a size proportional to their deflated diameters.

Occlusion balloons are indicated in acute bleeding due to rupture of large vessels and in temporary occlusion of arteriovenous (AV) fistulas, and are used as protection in procedures involving embolization with particulates or fluids, including absolute alcohol.

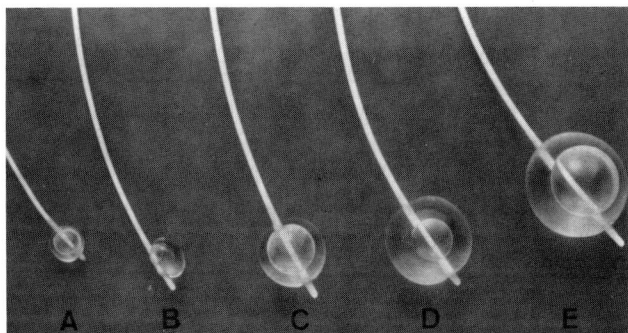

Figure 2.16 Balloon occlusion catheters.
(A) Fogarty catheter. (B) Meditech occlusion catheter with 1.8-cm diameter. (C,D,E) Balloons with progressively larger diameters, up to 4 cm.

Other Materials

Iodinated Contrast Medium

The injection of large quantities of iodinated contrast medium through a wedged catheter will cause, because of its high osmolarity and toxicity, considerable tissue necrosis with ischemia and protein degradation. This effect has been demonstrated experimentally and clinically for ablation of parathyroid adenomas.

The use of a contrast medium heated to a high temperature increases the toxic effect and can be an alternative method for ablation of small organs or segments of organs.

Ferromagnetic Embolization

Particles the size of 0.3 μm of ferropentacarbonyl [$Fe(CO)_5$], which result from the combination of carbon monoxide and iron-producing crystallized microspheres, can be used in a suspension and injected into the vascular system as an embolizing agent. The suspension consists of 0.5 mL of iron microspheres and 40 to 60 mL of heparinized saline solution.

The injection of this suspension, associated with a magnetic field of up to 4000 G (Gauss), almost superselectively directs the iron particles to the target site for embolization, resulting in occlusion of smaller vessels. Unfortunately, the particles may pass through to the venous circulation.

Coil Baffle and Modified Guidewire

After the development of Gianturco coils and vascular occlusion bristle brushes, the need arose for material that would occlude larger vessels, including aneurysms and AV fistulas.

An innovative technique was the production of giant Gianturco coils, 20 cm long, with tufts of dacron threads attached at 3-cm intervals. When introduced, in a vessel of significant caliber, the giant coil winds up causing occlusion in 100 percent of cases. A modified guidewire technique, developed to occlude large AV fistulas, involves the use of 10- to 50-cm-long segments of guidewire with a mobile and flexible core. The form of the guidewire is modified irregularly, angulated, or twisted so the guidewire will wind inside the vessel. The distal tip must be rectolinear in order to anchor onto the vessel walls when introduced.

Coiled Silk Threads

Silk is a material with acceptable biocompatibility and a long history of surgical success. In combination with steel coils or other embolizing materials, the winding of silk thread produces rapid and permanent occlusion in large vessels. This material has been used successfully with arterial venous fistulas and gastric and esophageal varices.

Terbal

Terbal is a new synthetic plastic particulate which is radiopaque, nonreabsorbant, and which is being used experimentally for embolization. Terbal particles are firm and have sharp angles capable of causing an endothelial reaction. The softening temperature of this material is high (120°C), allowing steam sterilization. At this time there is little information available.

Terbal is available in particles of 150-, 250-, 500-, 700-, 1000-, 1400-, and 2000-μm size (Fig. 2.17).

Chemoembolization

The concept of intraarterial chemoembolization introduced by Kato in 1981 has potential. Intraarterial chemoembolization has the direct effect of causing ischemia of the neoplastic lesion by temporary vascular obstruction. In addition, the speed of transit of circulation in the tumoral vascular bed is sharply reduced, increasing the time of contact of the chemotherapeutic drug with neoplastic cells. With an increase in drug concentration, there is likely to be an increase in tissue permeability. The cytotoxic effect is manifest in the tumor lesion and also in the vessel wall. The systemic effect of the chemotherapeutic drug is minimized during primary passage through the organ being infused.

In Kato's system, the chemotherapy agent mitomycin C is placed in 225-μm-diameter microcapsules of ethylcellulose. The technique produced peripheral embolization with gradual and sustained release of the chemotherapeutic agent in the adjacent tissues with practically no systemic effect.

The microcapsules are inert and insoluble in water. Mitomycin C produces an arteritis and a perivascular inflammatory occlusion. More recently, chemoemboli-

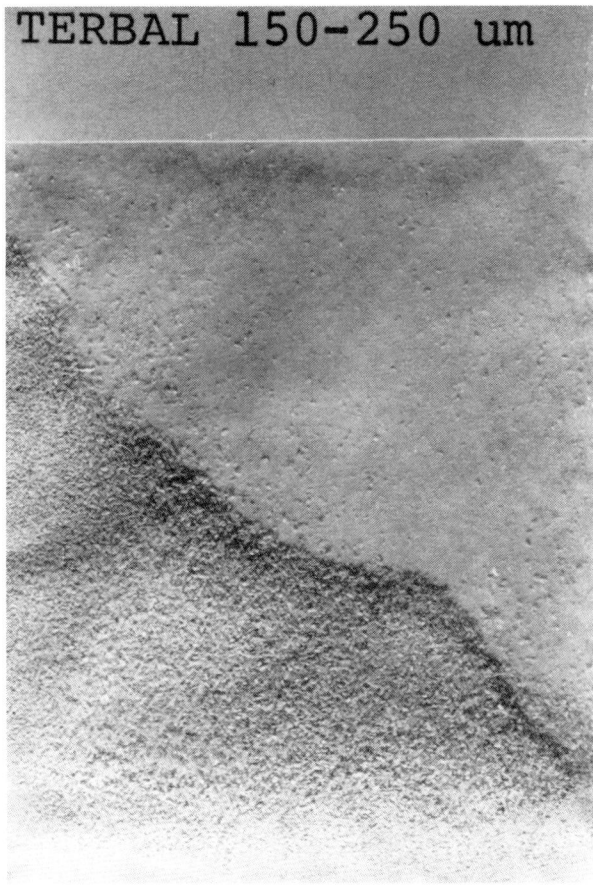

Figure 2.17 Terbal, a new synthetic embolization material. The figure shows 150- to 250-μm particles, but sizes from 150 to 2000 μm are available.

zation has been performed using a suspension of iodinated oil contrast medium and a chemotherapeutic drug.

THERAPEUTIC USES

Gastrointestinal Bleeding

The aspects of infusion of vasoconstrictors compared to embolization are discussed in Chap. 3. At this time, Gelfoam is the most appropriate material for management of gastrointestinal bleeding of arterial or capillary origin. Bleeding of this nature is frequently a self-limiting process. In some cases, only a few particles of Gelfoam placed superselectively will result in excellent control of bleeding with minimal risk.

Acute gastrointestinal bleeding due to esophageal and gastric varices can be adequately controlled with Gelfoam. The addition of a vascular sclerosing agent with the Gelfoam significantly increases the duration of the embolization. Absolute alcohol has also proved satisfactory for the occlusion of esophageal varices. IBC, Gianturco coils, and detachable balloons all play important roles in the proximal and distal occlusion of variceal bleeding.

Intraabdominal Extraluminal Hemorrhage

Intraabdominal hemorrhages in spaces other than hollow viscera have dramatic consequences, especially in patients who suffer from other systemic diseases. One of the sites that bleeds with grave seriousness is the pancreatic bed. In such sites, an absorbable type of embolizing material cannot be used because of the release of pancreatic proteolytic enzymes.

In these situations, permanent occlusion with IBC or small Gianturco-type coils is preferred.

Neoplastic Bleeding

Bleeding within the tissues of the neoplasm requires aggressive interventional control. The use of nonabsorbable material is generally required. Polyvinyl alcohol foam (Ivalon) is generally the particulate material of choice. In certain cases, assuming that the target site is not in close proximity to the peripheral nervous system or adjacent skin, IBC is indicated.

In most cases of lower urinary tract and pelvic bleeding in patients without underlying neoplasm, the use of Gelfoam or Ivalon is satisfactory. Gianturco coils are not indicated for embolization of the internal iliac artery or its branches within the pelvis because this technique would prevent additional embolization if a recurrence of the bleeding developed, which can occur as a result of distal or contralateral collateralization. Embolization of the underlying neoplasm results in infarction with an overall reduction in the size of the mass as well as a significant decrease in the vascular supply. This may result in fewer surgical difficulties during resection with significantly less bleeding at the surgical site.

Bleeding Secondary to Trauma

Embolization may be used as a selective treatment in certain cases of bleeding secondary to trauma. Gelfoam, a frequently used agent, results in effective occlusion (Fig. 2.1). In parenchymal organs, including the kidney and liver, the parenchymal functions must be maintained and hence superselective embolization with Gelfoam and/or Gianturco coals is a satisfactory option (Fig. 2.3). Bucrylate (IBC) and small detachable balloons are also satisfactory options in hepatic bleeding and may be introduced through a system of coaxial catheters (Figs. 2.9 and 2.11).

Hemoptysis

In patients with hemoptysis from underlying inflammatory disorders, the bronchial arteries are frequently hypertrophied and ordinarily present no selective catheterization difficulties. Embolization with Gelfoam, Ivalon, or bucrylate is quite satisfactory. Gelfoam together with a supplemental coil provides permanent occlusion and control of bleeding in approximately 80 percent of patients. When an underlying neoplasm is responsible for the bleeding, smaller-size particles may be necessary so that the proximal vessels can be kept accessible in case a recurrence of bleeding makes reembolization necessary.

Pulmonary Arteriovenous Fistulas

Detachable balloons seem to be most appropriate for the management of arteriovenous fistulas of pulmonary origin. They provide a high degree of selectiveness and steerability, and, because they are flow-oriented, allow evaluation of the effectiveness of the occlusion prior to detachment. Gianturco coils are a secondary option. Their limitation is that the efficacy of occlusion cannot be evaluated prior to final placement.

Visceral Arteriovenous Fistulas

These fistulas are ordinarily postoperative, posttraumatic, or postbiopsy in origin. Detachable balloons and metallic coils are ideal materials for occlusion of visceral arteriovenous lesions. The coils may be used after superselective catheterization is achieved, and the detachable balloon is applied when flow control through the lesion is necessary. The particulate material may be utilized in the smaller arteriovenous fistulas but ordinarily is not applicable in those fistulas with large shunts. In smaller fistulas, Gelfoam or bucrylate may be useful (Fig. 2.14). When temporary occlusion is desirable prior to surgical resection, a nondetachable balloon may be satisfactory for occlusion (Fig. 2.16).

Aneurysms

Both true and false aneurysms generally require both proximal and distal angiographic evaluation prior to embolization. In such cases liquid monomers are useful for intraaneurysmal injection. Coils placed as close as possible to the aneurysmal neck may also result in effective treatment and subsequent thrombosis (Fig. 2.14).

Arteriovenous Malformations

The approach to these lesions is complex, and a protocol involving staged embolization is usually the best option. The use of nonabsorbable particulate material or a bucrylate-type liquid polymer is appropriate. The nidus of the lesion, and not the afferent arteries, must be occluded; otherwise there exists the risk of not treating the lesion adequately and losing access for further embolization. Figure 2.12 shows occlusion of the nidus

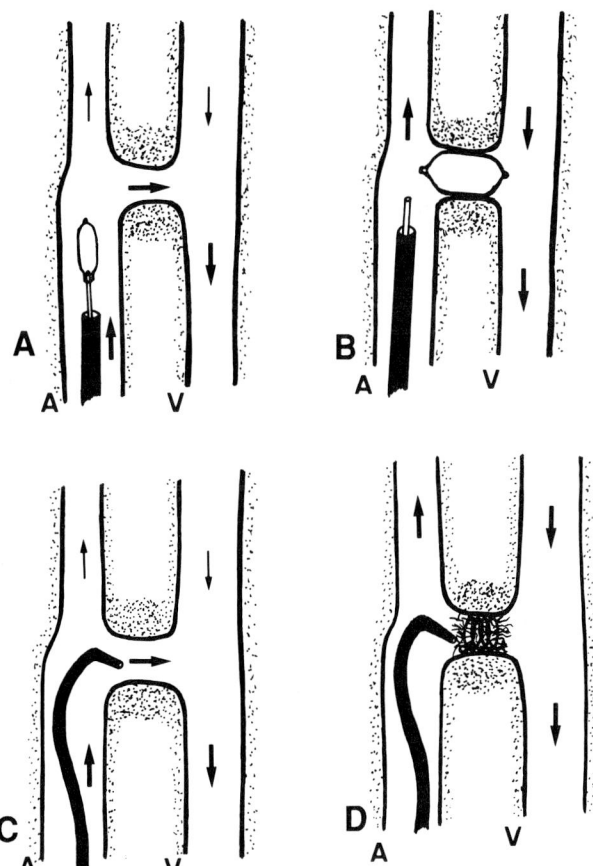

Figure 2.18 (A,B) Use of detachable balloon for occluding AV fistulas. (C,D) use of steel coil for occluding AV fistulas.

of the lesion, maintaining the patentcy of the afferent arteries.

COMPLICATIONS OF EMBOLIZATION

Tissue ischemia with pain, necrosis, and functional alterations is an anticipated complication of embolization, but the most significant complications include reflux of the embolic material and secondary embolization of nontarget organs. Fever may also occur after embolization, with sepsis being a more serious stage of this complication. Gas production within the infarction site is occasionally observed (Fig. 2.19). The presence of pain, fever, and leukocytosis is referred to as the postembolization syndrome. Ordinarily the pain associated with embolization is secondary to the extent of the ischemia, which is greater when there is significant normal tissue adjacent to the neoplasm. Usually, the greater the extent of the neoplasm and the smaller the amount of normal parenchyma present, the less postembolization pain there is.

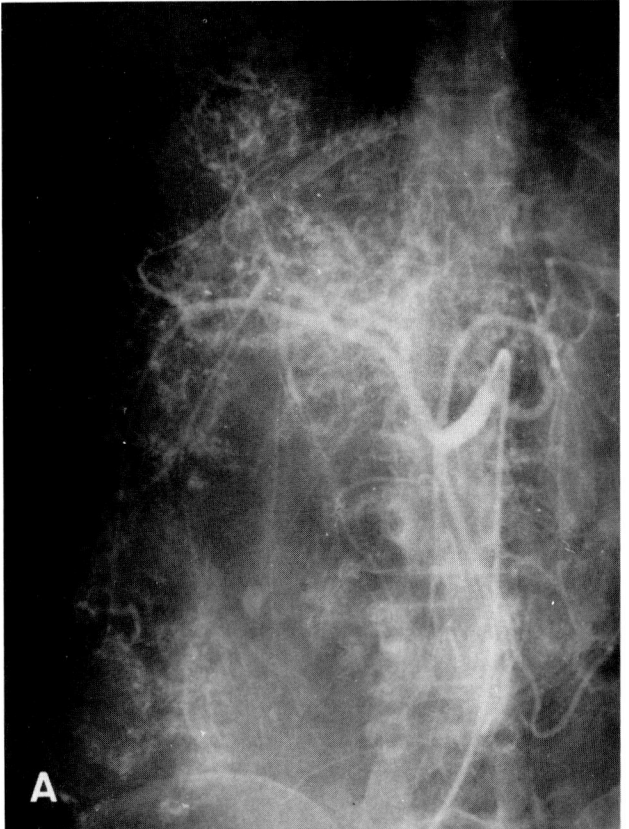
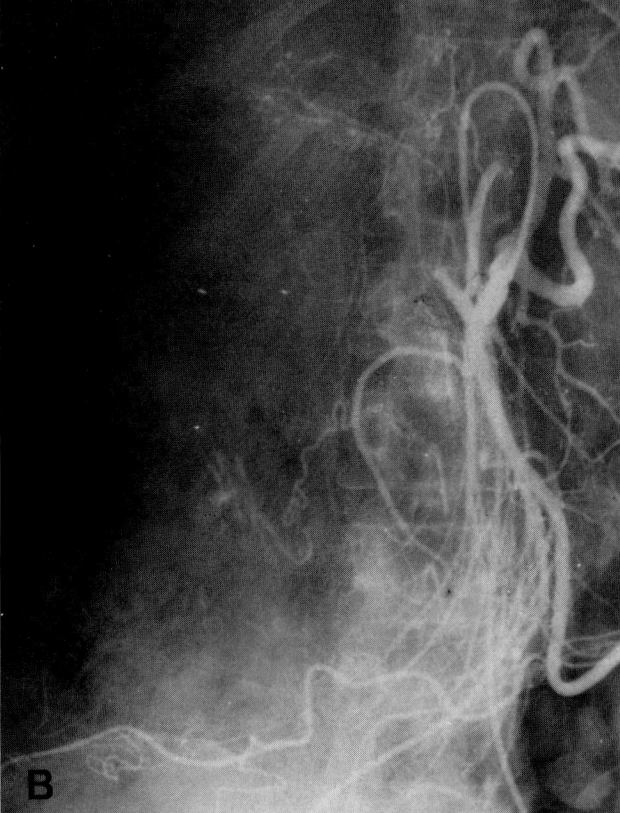

Control of pain during the procedure can ordinarily be accomplished with intravenous analgesics including Fentanyl, morphine, and meperidine. Every 30 min during the procedure, 50 μg of Fentanyl may be given intravenously. Over a 1- to 2-h period, 2 to 10 mg of morphine may also be given intravenously.

Postembolization pain can be quite severe and often requires intensive medication for 24 h. Occasionally pain will last for 3 or 4 days. The extent of pain also varies with the embolizing material. For example, absolute alcohol causes intense pain in the immediate postembolization period, while Gelfoam causes a less intense but more prolonged pain.

The fever that accompanies embolization is apparently related to tissue ischemia and/or the presence of the intravascular foreign body. Fever after the use of Gelfoam is common, as are foreign-body-type reactions. It is essential however, to completely exclude the possibility of the presence of an infectious process.

In most instances, the brief, transient elevation in temperature does not require specific treatment. However, when sepsis is anticipated or exists, extensive antibiotic therapy becomes necessary. This is especially true in cases involving embolization of the spleen or liver. Experimental and clinical studies show that sepsis in these parenchymal organs may be minimized or eliminated by adequate antibiotic coverage and by utiliz-

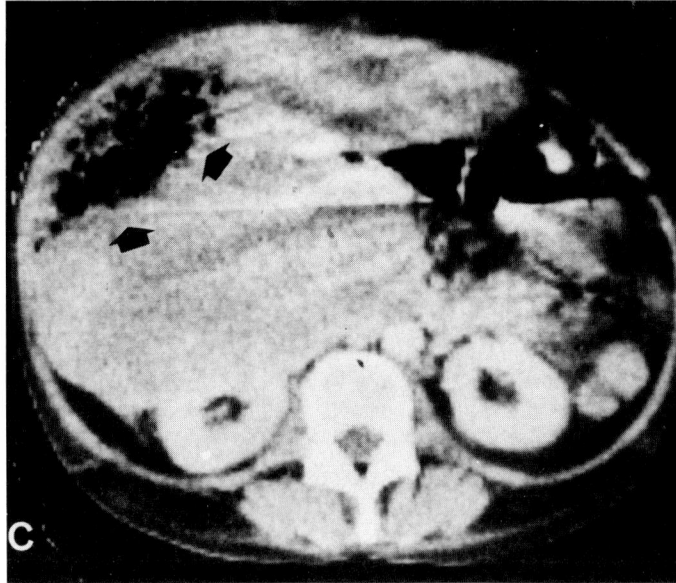

Figure 2.19 Ablation of hepatic metastases from an adrenal primary tumor.
(A) Celiac injection demonstrating hepatomeglay with hypervascular metastases. (B) Celiac injection following ablation with absolute alcohol. Note the arterial devascularization as well as gas in the caudal portion of the liver. (C) Computed tomography (CT) scan demonstrating the collection of gas in the right lobe of the liver.

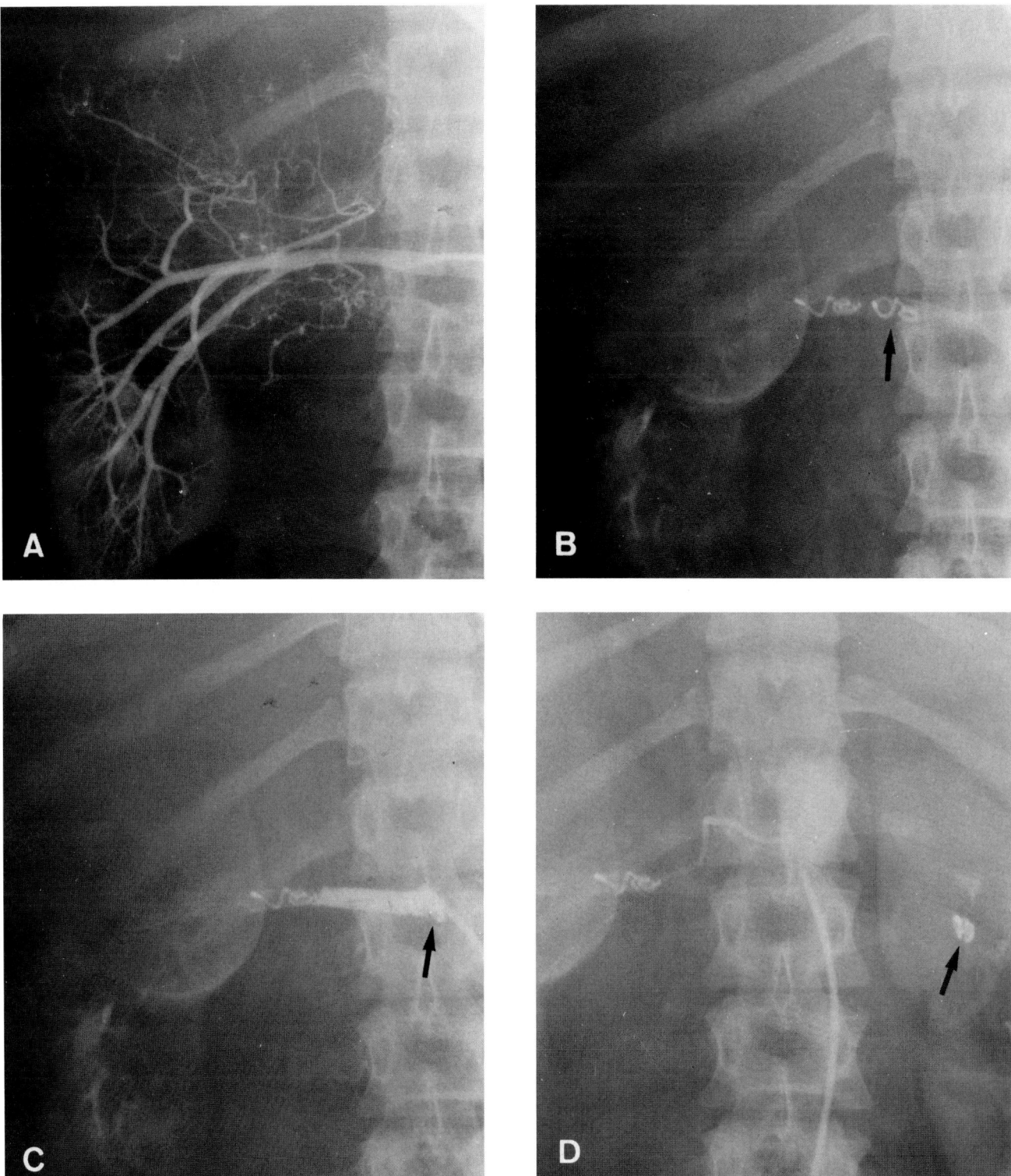

Figure 2.20 Complication occurring during embolization of a right renal adenocarcinoma with Gelfoam and Gianturco coils.

(A) Preembolization angiography. (B) Initial placement of two steel coils. (C) Reflux of the second coil during angiography; it returned to the aortic lumen. (D) Lost coil lodged in the left renal circulation. (This was removed percutaneously with a wire loop technique.)

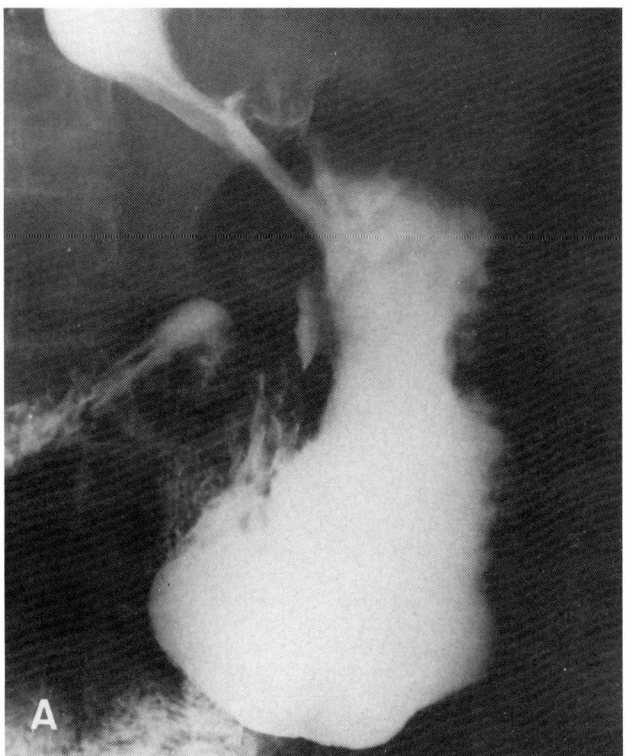 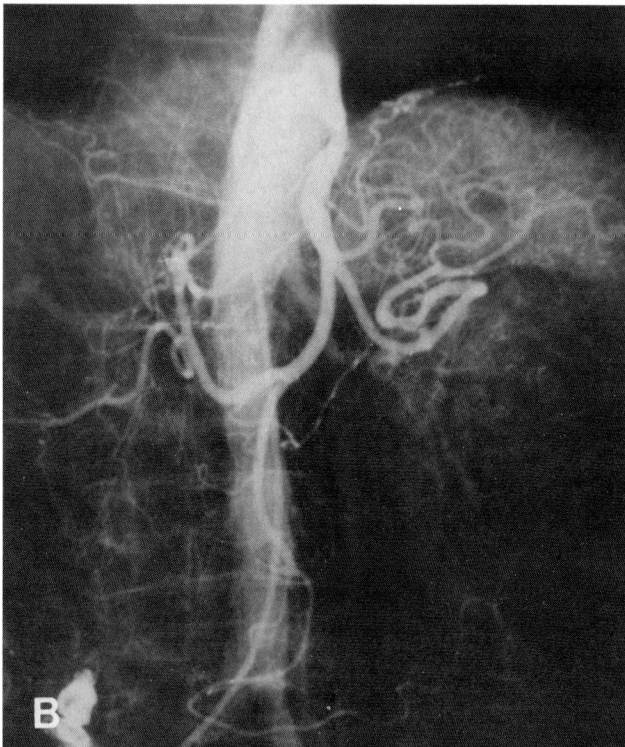

Figure 2.21 Complication during embolization for gastric hemorrhage.
(A) Upper GI study demonstrating a large ulcer on the lesser curve of the stomach which bled shortly after examination.
(B) Celiac axis injection from a femoral approach. Contrast extravasation was not seen at this phase of the angiogram.
(C) Celiac axis catheterization performed from the left axillary approach because of atherosclerotic plaque and the acute angle with the aorta. The celiac trunk was embolized with an 8-mm coil because of inability to catheterize the left gastric artery. While a second coil was being placed, the catheter backed out of the celiac axis, releasing the coil in the aorta. (D) Angiogram following removal of the lost coil by the snare technique.

ing solutions that include antibiotics in the embolizing material suspension. Manipulation of the embolizing material should be minimal; only at the time of injection should it be exposed and then only with the scrupulous application of antiseptic techniques.

Reflux of embolic material into the aorta or into normal adjacent vessels is unusual but can have serious consequences leading to significant ischemia in a normal organ or extremity. Three basic mechanisms may lead to reflux into the aorta.

The first and most common occurs when a small-sized particulate material such as Gelfoam is used. Persistence in introducing the Gelfoam in a partially embolized artery with stagnant flow is the usual cause of reflux, but reflux can also occur if the catheter is dislodged when there is a sudden decompression at the catheter tip as the embolus exits the lumen. Selective contrast injections performed to document or evaluate embolization can also, due to linear velocity at the distal tip of the catheter, displace the embolus causing reflux into the aorta or an adjacent vessel. The phenomenon has also been described during the application of Gianturco steel coils (Fig. 2.20).

When the embolizing agent is greater than the size of the vessel being embolized, a portion of the material may protrude into the aortic lumen. The material may become a source of embolus or eventually displace itself and migrate distally (Fig. 2.21). Occasionally, the percutaneous removal of a Gianturco coil may become necessary (see Chap. 7). Prevention of reflux of particulate or fluid embolizing agents can be accomplished by utilizing diagnostic occlusion balloons. Although the balloon results in some stagnation of flow, the particles can be injected while balloon occlusion is maintained for at least 30 min. In smaller vessels, the catheter can be wedged within the vessel and the embolic material subsequently injected. Another option is the use of coaxial catheters. When occlusion balloons are not utilized for distal embolization, care must be taken to prevent reflux, and when a significant reduction in flow occurs, embolization must proceed cautiously.

Use of absolute alcohol requires special precautions. For example, injecting at high pressure within an occluded arterial system distal to an occlusion balloon may result in the sclerosing fluid being injected in collateral vessels to adjacent organs. This complication has occurred in two of our own cases, one of which involved injection without an occlusion balloon (Fig. 2.22). For

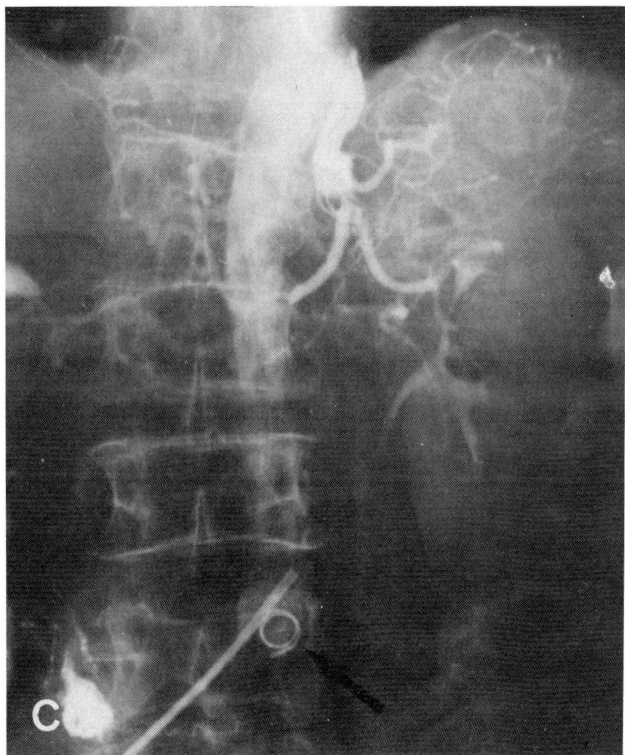
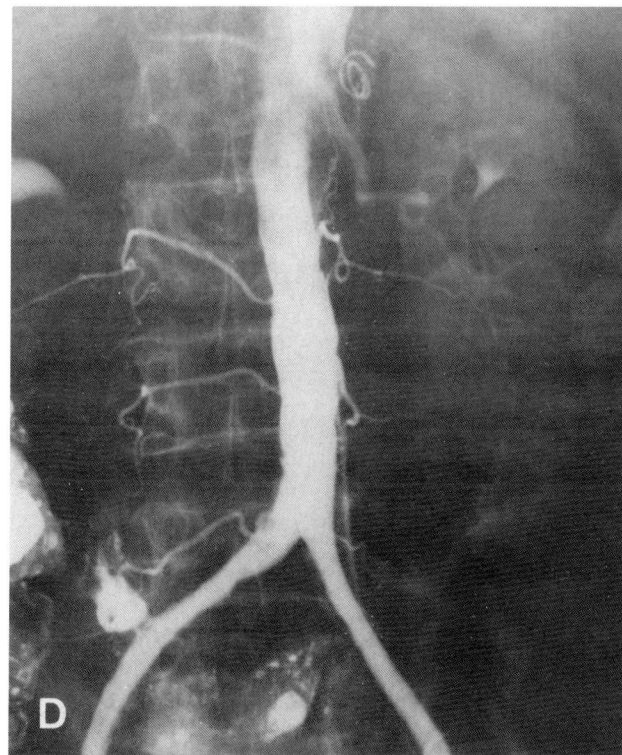

Figure 2.21 *Continued*

Figure 2.22 Complication of left renal tumor embolization using absolute alcohol.
(A) Preembolization angiogram showing tumor involving upper pole of left kidney. Absolute alcohol was injected without the use of a balloon occlusion catheter. (B) Angiogram following embolization. Four days postnephrectomy, an acute abdominal crisis, with necrosis of the colon, occurred. This was probably due to reflux of alcohol into the aorta or passage of alcohol through parasitic circulation.

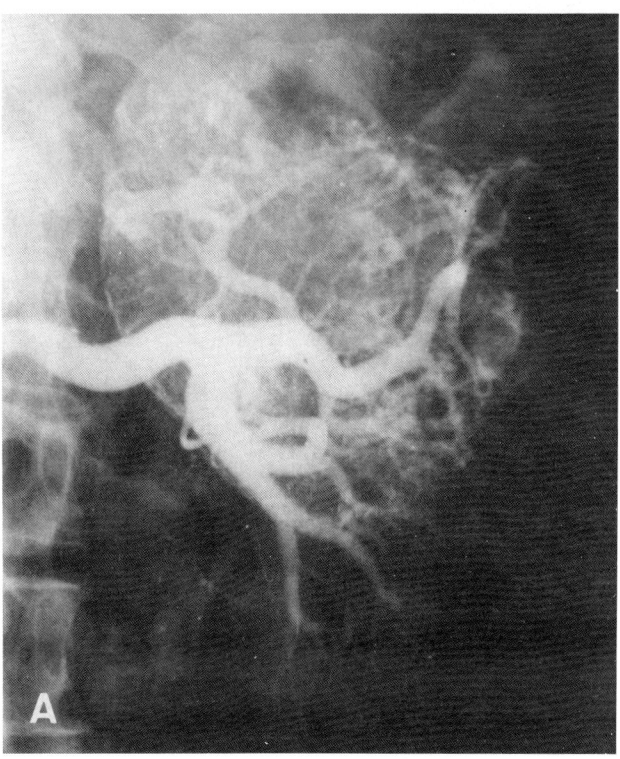
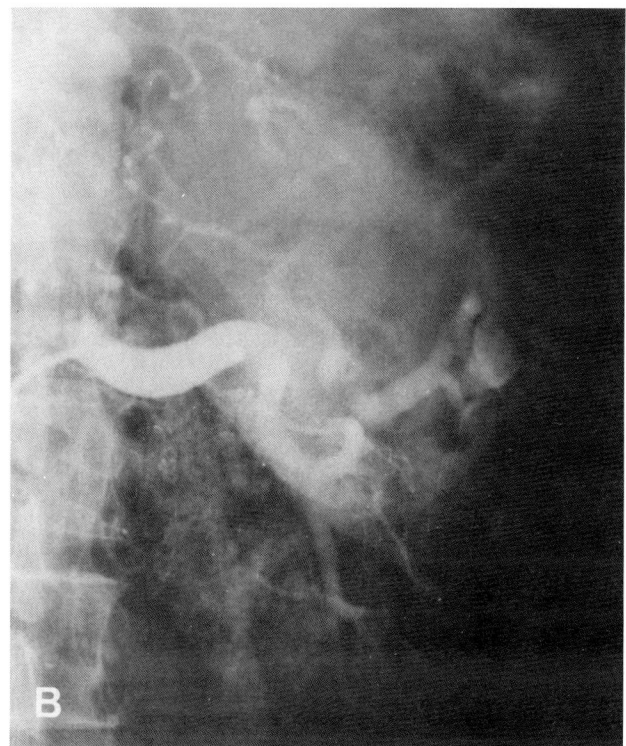

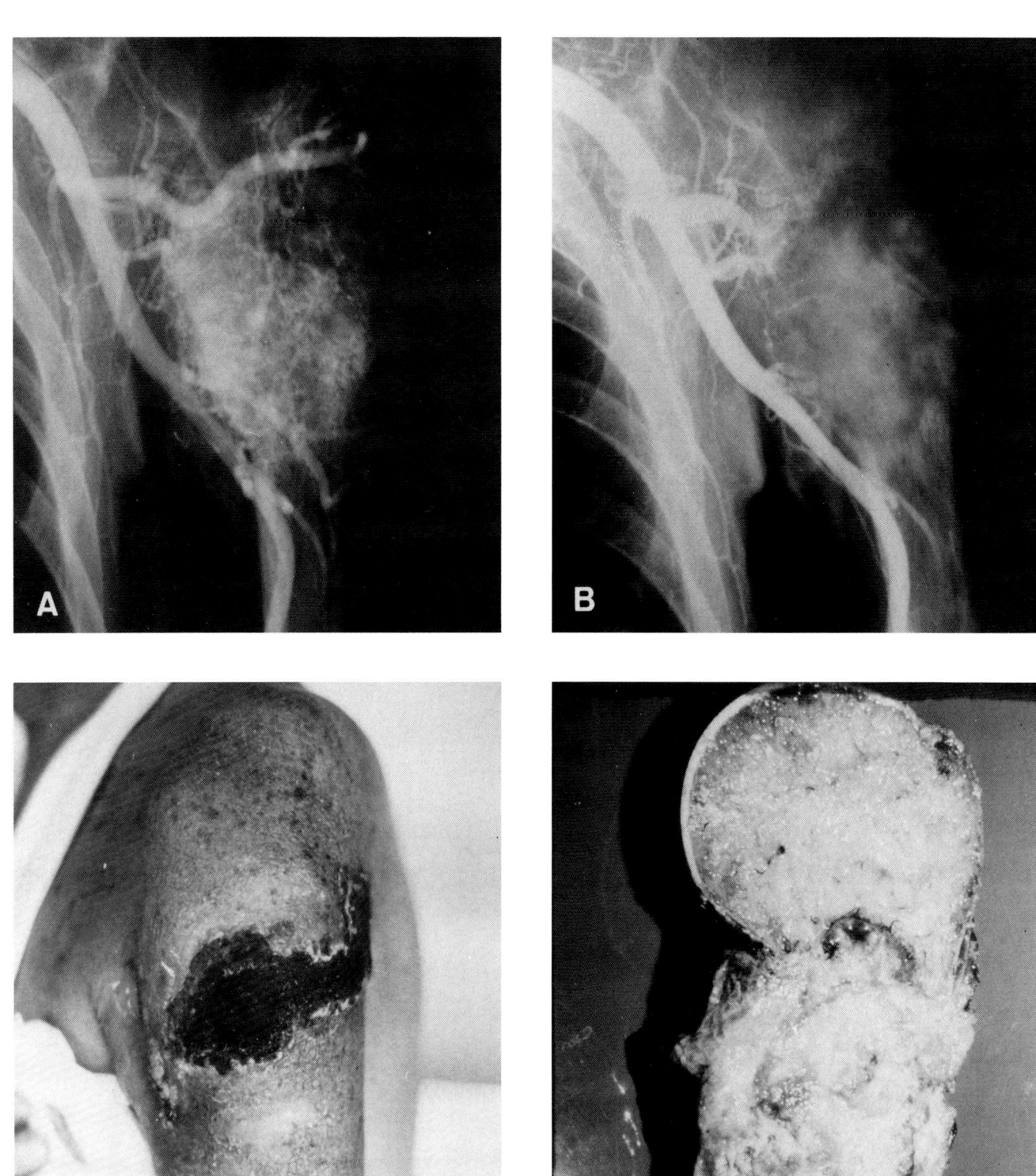

Figure 2.23 Skin necrosis with use of absolute alcohol.
(A) preembolization angiography of metastatic renal cell carcinoma in the left humerus. (B) Devascularization of mass including occlusion of the circumflex humeral arteries. (C) Skin necrosis occurring 2 weeks after alcohol ablation. (D) Pathologic specimen following insertion of a left humeral prosthesis.

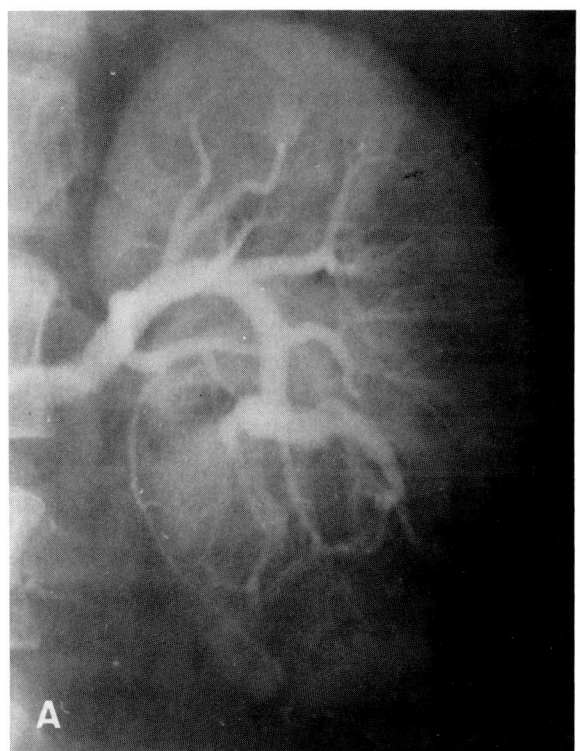
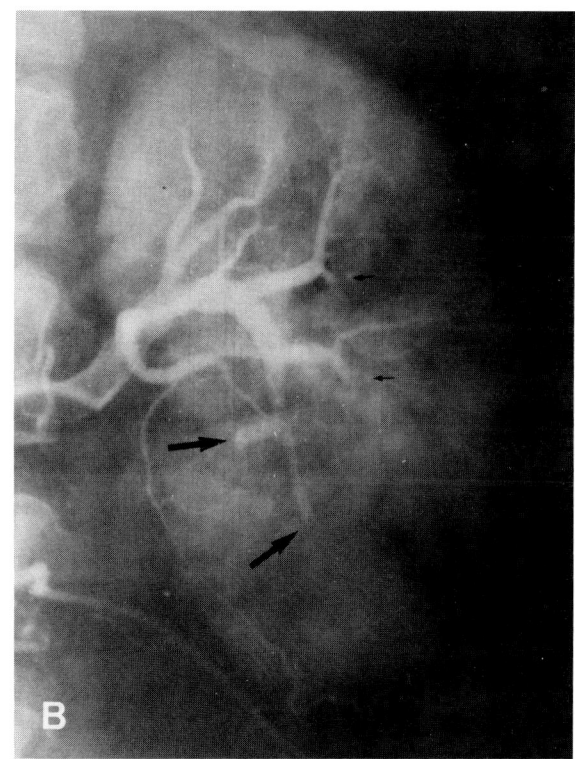
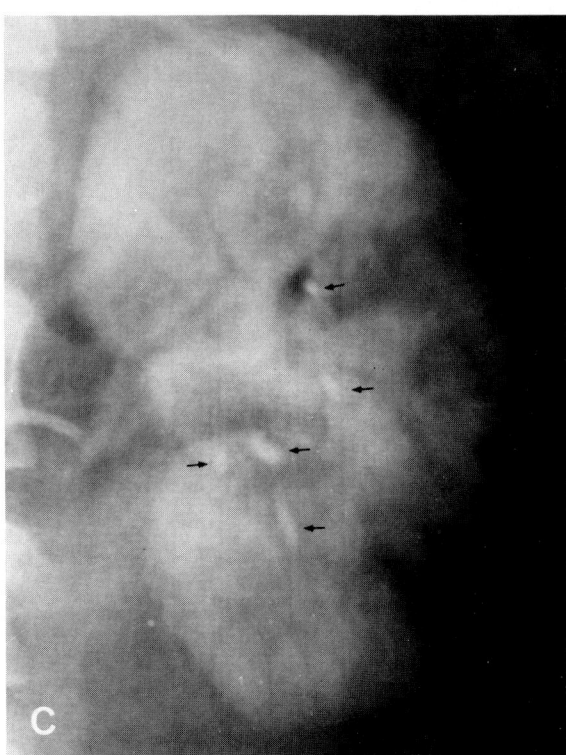

Figure 2.24 Fragmentation of Gelfoam during embolization.
(A) Posttraumatic arteriovenous fistula with false aneurysm in the lower pole of the left kidney. (B) Embolization of arteriovenous fistula (large arrows) and normal arteries (small arrows) by fragmentation of Gelfoam that occurred during introduction through the catheter. (C) Well-opacified Gelfoam fragments.

these reasons, the use of absolute alcohol in vessels that follow a cutaneous distribution carries a significant risk of cutaneous necrosis (Fig. 2.23).

Nonocclusion of a vessel embolized by Gianturco coils can also occur. Occasionally a tuft of teflon threads detaches itself from the coil, and consequently the vessel retains its patentcy. Some of the newer coils, which have smaller diameters and fewer teflon threads, are less thrombogenic than the older ones (Figs. 2.2 and 2.3). In certain situations, proximal occlusion by the coils results in collateral distal circulation with distal reconstitution of the occluded vessel.

One of the most important of the mechanical factors that can lead to complications during embolization is fragmentation of the embolizing particle, with subsequent migration of the fragment to an adjacent vessel. Fragmentation occurs frequently during the utilization of autologous clot and Gelfoam (Fig. 2.24)

An additional mechanical aspect that should be considered in the embolization of aneurysms is the possibility that rupture of the lesion may occur following a sudden increase in pressure during release of the embolization particle. For this reason it may be desirable to release particles without the use of pressure. For example, using metallic coils or balloons will avoid this problem.

Gas-producing organisms with associated sepsis can be detected by conventional methods including ultrasonography and computerized tomographic scanning (Fig. 2.19). Occasionally it is quite difficult to determine the

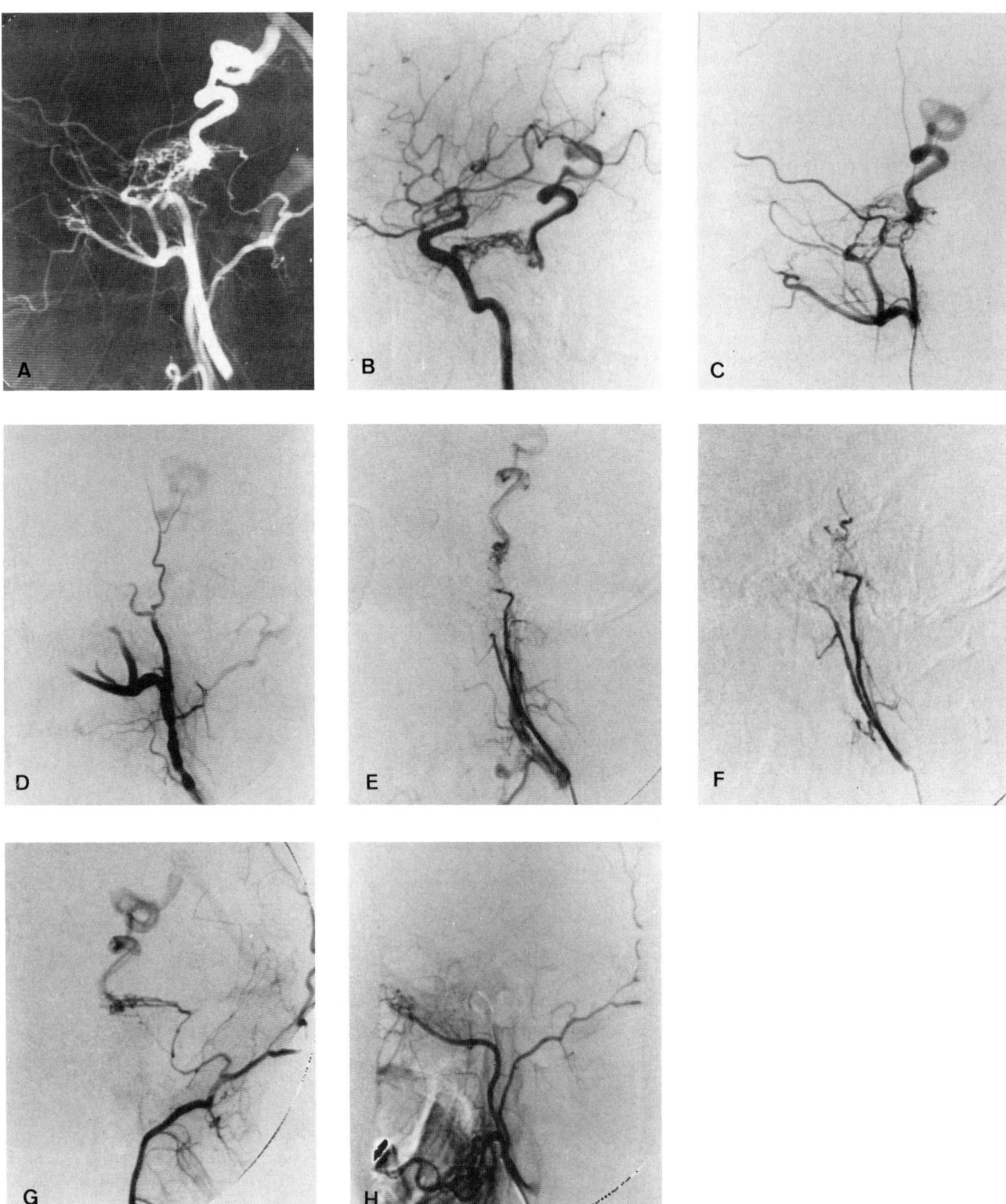

Figure 2.25 Patient with left-sided dural arteriovenous malformation.
(A) External carotid injection demonstrating arterial supply from meningeal and occipital arteries. (B) Internal carotid injection showing supply meningohypophyseal trunk. (C) Middle meningeal artery injection opacifying the lesion. (D) Embolization of middle meningeal artery using Gelfoam. (E) Ascending pharyngeal artery injection opacifying the lesion. (F) Embolization of the ascending pharyngeal artery with bucrylate. (G) Occipital artery injection with a meningeal branch opacifying the lesion. This was embolized with Gelfoam. (H) Final external carotid angiogram following all embolization procedures. Note lack of filling of superficial temporal artery. The internal carotid supply was not embolized. This patient developed motor sequelae of the 7th, 9th, 10th, and 11th cranial nerves which are supplied by the ascending pharyngeal artery. There was some improvement in function after several weeks.

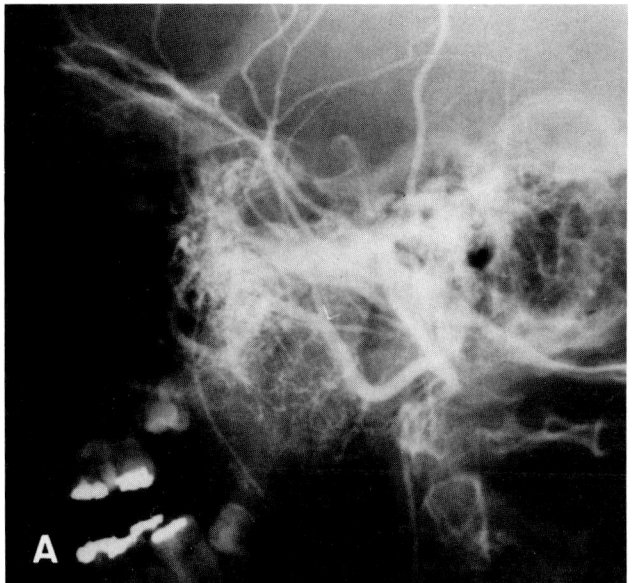 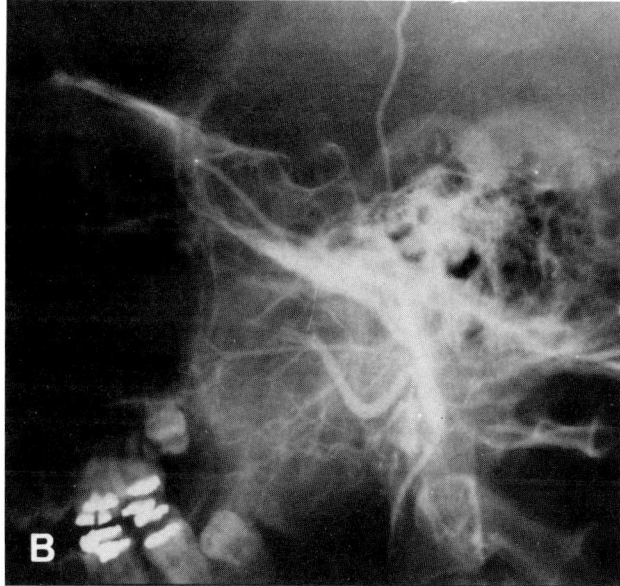

Figure 2.26 Temporary neurologic complication following embolization of an angiofibroma.
(A) Right internal maxillary angiogram demonstrating hypervascular mass in the nasopharynx. (B) Preoperative embolization with Gelfoam. Immediately following embolization, the patient developed a right hemiparesis and dysarthria, which resolved within 30 min. Paradoxically, the neurologic symptoms were that of a left hemispheric event despite the embolization having been done in the right internal maxillary artery.

origin of the gas within the infarcted vessel. Formation of gas within the parenchyma is frequently attributed to the release of oxygen or the presence of carbon dioxide at the embolization site.

The most catastrophic complications occur in neuroradiological interventional procedures in which inadvertent embolization has occurred (Fig. 2.25). Embolization of certain hypervascular lesions in the nasopharynx that are in direct proximity to the base of the skull may cause temporary or permanent neurologic sequelae apparently related to passage of the fragments to the territory of the internal carotid artery (Fig. 2.26). Embolization of the extracranial vessels of the external carotid occasionally results in anastomotic collateralization of the internal carotid or vertebral artery that cannot be identified through conventional angiography. Occasionally successful embolization of a carotid cavernous sinus fistula results in some protrusion of the material into the internal carotid and a release of smaller emboli, with resulting cortical infarcts (Fig. 2.27). Obviously, embolization of AV malformations involves a risk that the material may pass beyond the capillary level and subsequently result in pulmonary emboli. Procedures involving these larger AV communications certainly entail more risks than do procedures involving smaller lesions. With small-sized fistulas between the aorta and the cava, preoperative occlusion may be accomplished with a balloon catheter, but obviously not with coils or other materials that might result in distal embolization through the shunt (Fig. 2.28).

Detachable balloons as large as 20 mm are used in certain large renal AV malformations. Care must always be taken to avoid choosing an embolizing agent that might pass through the fistula and subsequently embolize to the pulmonary circulation (Fig. 2.29). Although pulmonary embolization by smaller particulate material may not produce any major hazard, if foreign bodies are sufficiently large, they must be percutaneously removed (Chap. 7; Fig. 2.29). Inappropriately positioned detachable balloons can be percutaneously deflated using a Chiba needle for direct puncture of the balloon in the abdomen or lungs.

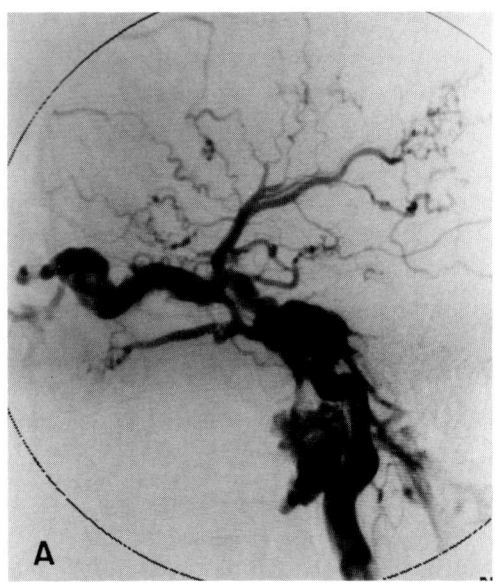
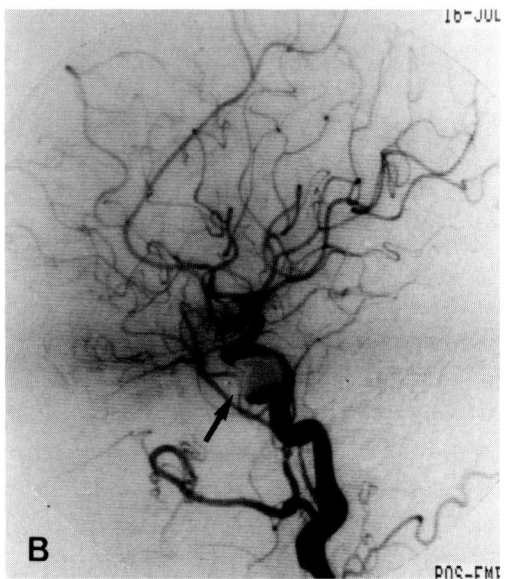
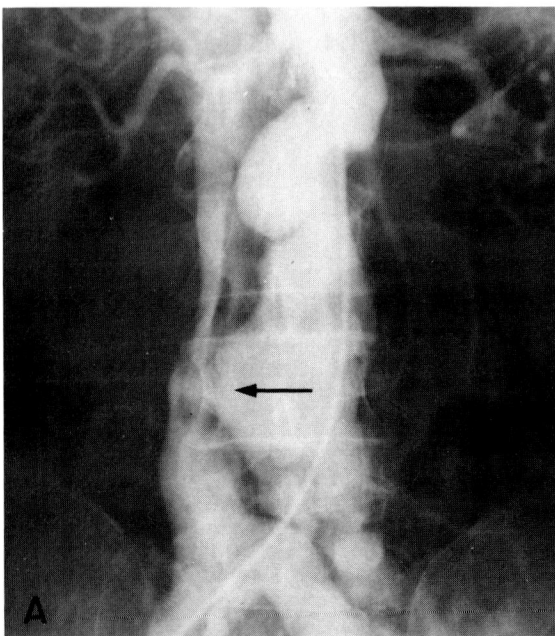

Figure 2.27 A 63-year-old patient with a spontaneous left-sided carotid cavernous fistula.
(A) Internal carotid injection demonstrating massive carotid cavernous fistula with opacification of the cavernous sinus, superior and inferior ophthalmic veins, inferior petrosal sinus, and cortical veins. (B) Embolization of the fistula with a detachable balloon according to Debrun's technique. Note the patent internal carotid artery. Right after embolization there was immediate regression of the proptosis and disappearance of the audible bruit. (C) 15 h following embolization, the patient developed severe headache and vomiting followed by right hemiplegia. A computed tomography scan demonstrated a small cortical infarct. The neurologic symptoms improved after several weeks.

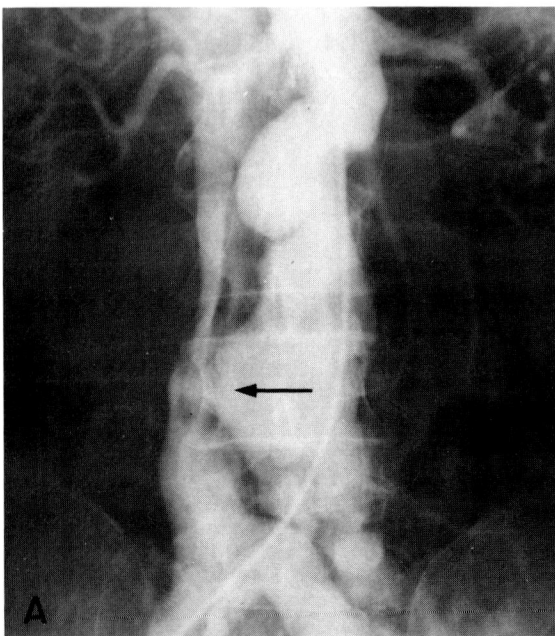
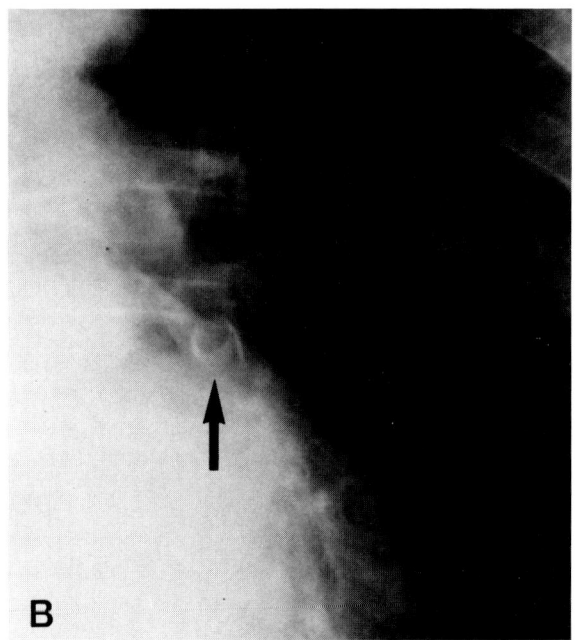

Figure 2.28 High-output congestive heart failure developing because of spontaneous rupture of an abdominal aortic aneurysm into the inferior vena cava.
(A) Aneurysm with spontaneous arteriovenous fistula. (B) An attempt at preoperative embolization using an 8-mm coil resulted in passage of the coil into the venous system and eventually to the left pulmonary artery. This did not cause any symptoms, and the aneurysm was then treated surgically.

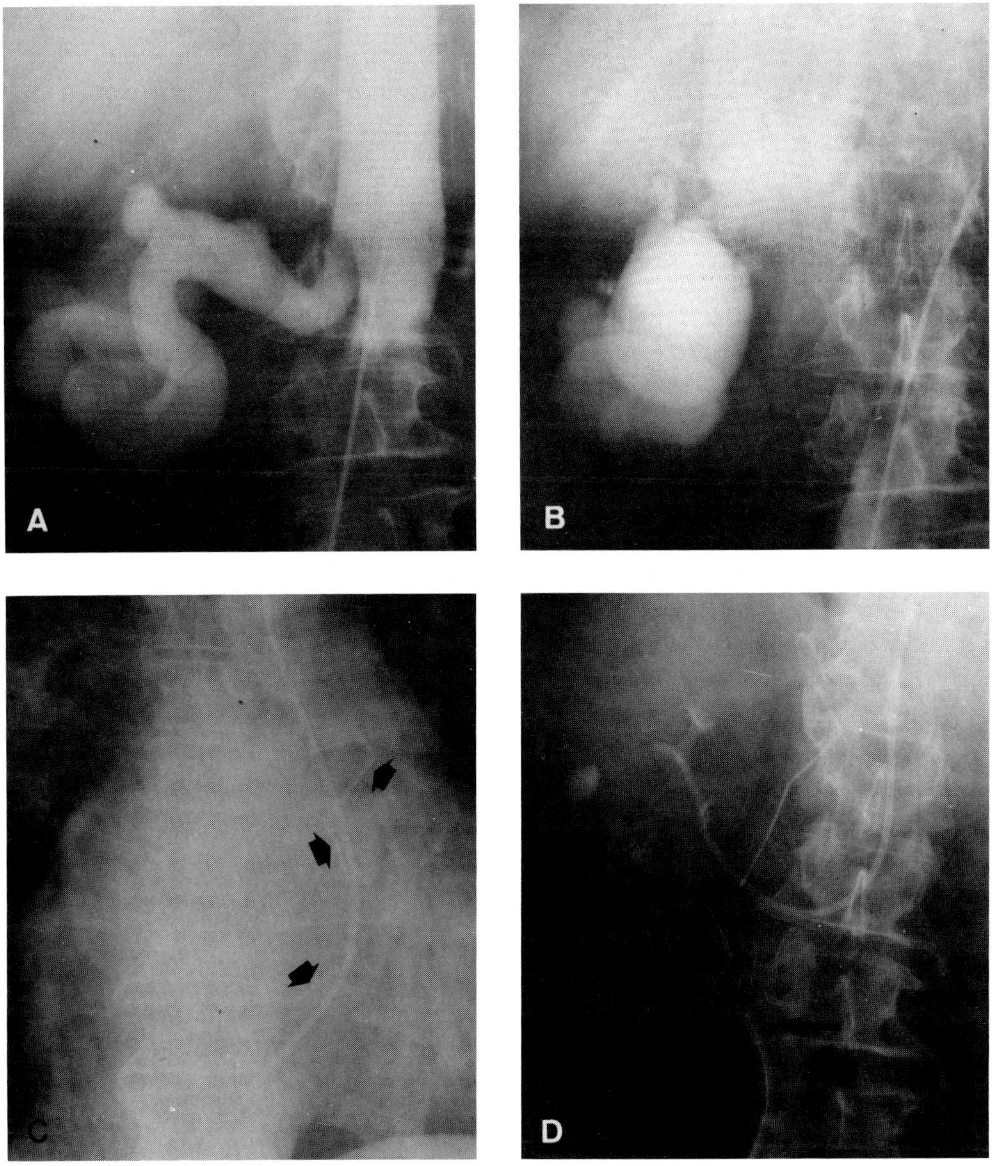

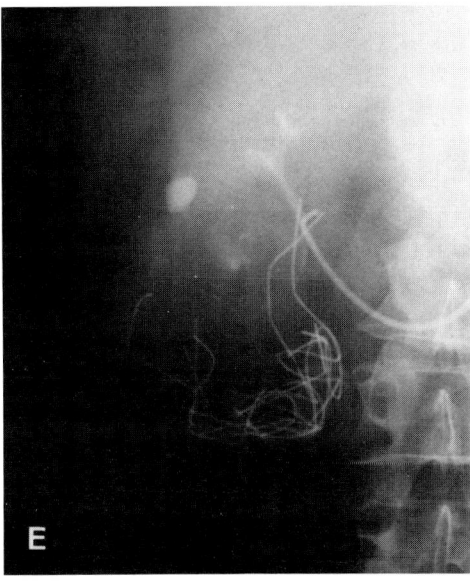

Figure 2.29 Large arteriovenous fistula with false aneurysm in the right kidney, probably due to old penetrating trauma.
(A) Abdominal aortogram demonstrating large renal artery and false aneurysm. (B) Later phase showing venous filling and large-diameter inferior vena cava. (C) Embolization using guidewire fragments. (D) Snare technique (arrow) used to remove guidewire that had been inadvertently passed to the right ventricle. (E) Numerous guidewire fragments forming a metal winding inside the vessel.

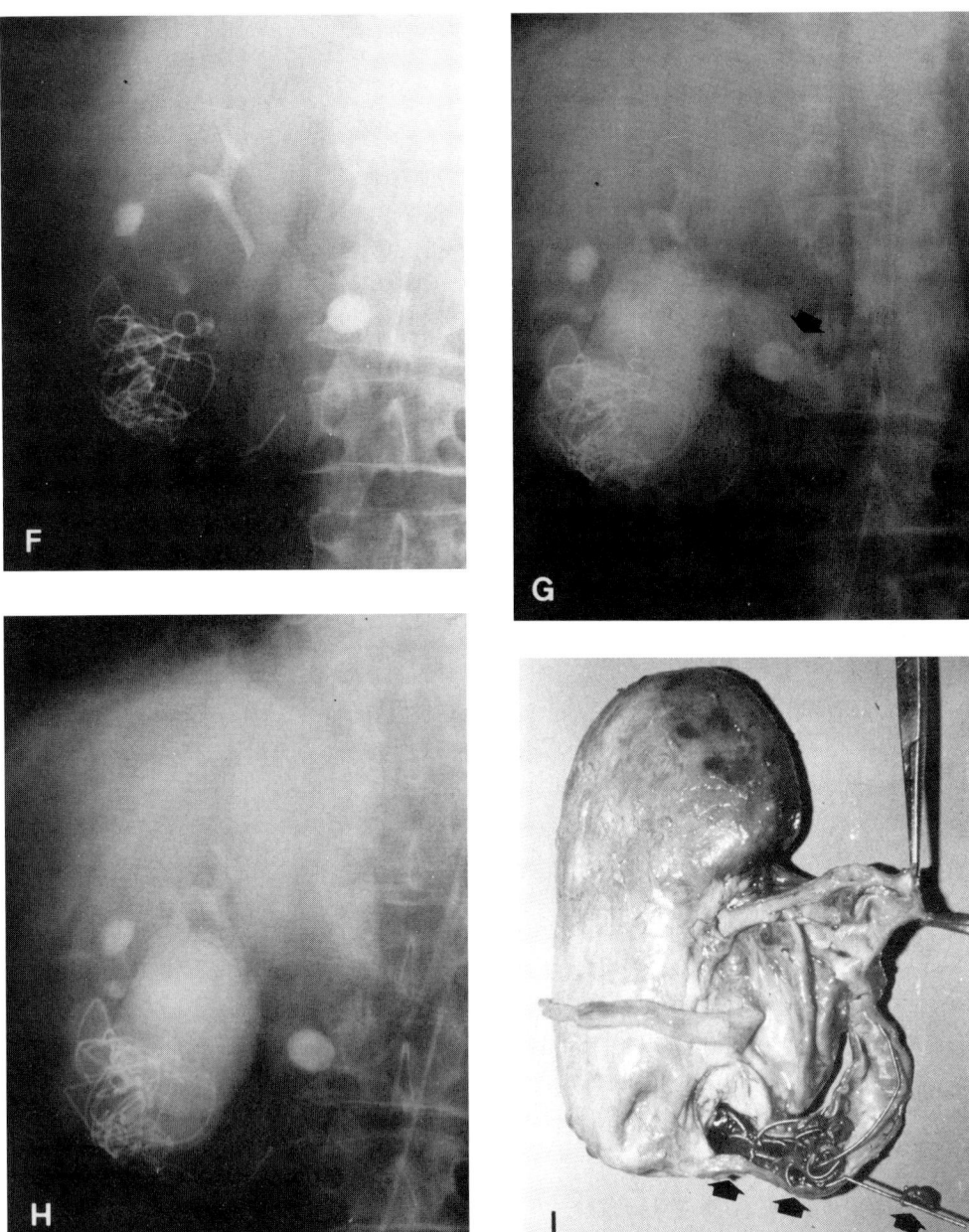

Figure 2.29 *Continued*
(F) Partial migration of metal winding following introduction of steel coils. (G,H) Angiogram showing continued patency of the AV fistula. Note that a 1.8-cm-diameter occluding balloon catheter did not occlude the right renal artery (arrow). (I) Pathologic specimen demonstrating the embolic material and thrombus within the afferent artery of the arteriovenous fistula.

REFERENCES

Anderson JH, Wallace S, Gianturco C, Gerson LP. "Mini" Gianturco steel coils for transcatheter vascular occlusion. *Radiology* 1979;132:301–303.

Athanasoulis CA. Therapeutic applications of angiography. *N Eng J Med* 1980;302:1117–1125.

Barry JW, Bookstein JJ, Alkne JF. Ferromagnetic embolization: Experimental evaluation. *Radiology* 1981;138:341–349.

Buchta KS, Sands J, Rosenkrantz H, Roche WD. Early mechanism of action of arterially infused alcohol U.S.P. in renal devitalization. *Radiology* 1982;145:45–47.

Carrol BA, Walter JF. Gas in embolized tumors: An alternate hypothesis for its origin. *Radiology* 1983;147:441–444.

Castaneda-Zuniga WR, Galliani CA, Rysayr J, Kotula F, Amplatz K. "Spiderlon": New device for simple, fast arterial and venous occlusion. *AJR* 1981;136:627–628.

Castaneda-Zuniga WR, Tadavarthy SM, et al. Nonsurgical closure of large arteriovenous fistulas. *JAMA* 1978;236:2649–2653.

Castaneda-Zuniga WR, Tadavarthy SM, Galliani CA, Laerum F, Schwarten DE, Amplatz K. Experimental venous occlusion with stainless steel spiders. *Radiology* 1981;141:238–242.

Chuang VP, Soo CS, Wallace S. Ivalon embolization in abdominal neoplasms. *AJR* 1981;136:729–733.

Chuang VP, Szwarc RT. The coil baffle in the experimental occlusion of large vascular structures. *Radiology* 1982;143:25–28.

Chuang VP, Wallace S. Chemoembolization: Transcatheter management of neoplasms. *JAMA* 1981;245:1151–1152.

Chuang VP, Wallace S, Gianturco C. A new, improved coil for tapered-tip catheter for arterial occlusion. *Radiology* 1980;135:507–509.

Debrun G, Lacour R, Caron JP et al. Experimental approach to the treatment of carotid-cavernous fistulas with an inflatable and isolated balloon. *Neuroradiology* 1975;9:9–14.

Debrun G, Lacour P, Caron JP, et al. Detachable balloon and calibrated-leak balloon techniques in the treatment of cerebral vascular lesions. *J Neurosurg* 1978;49:635–640.

Di Tullio MV Jr, Rand RW, Frische E. Detachable balloon catheter: Its application in experimental arteriovenous fistulae. *J Neurosurg* 1978;48:717–721.

Doppman JL, Girton M. Adrenal ablation by retrograde venous ethanol injection: An ineffective and dangerous procedure. *Radiology* 1984;150:667–672.

Doppman JL, Popovsky M, Girton M. The use of iodinated contract agents to ablate organs: Experimental studies and histopathology. *Radiology* 1981;138:333–340.

Dotter CT, Goldman ML, Rosch J. Instant selective arterial occlusion with isobutyl-cyanoacrylate. *Radiology* 1975;114:227–230.

Dotter CT, Lucas DS. Acute cor pulmonale: An experimental study utilizing a special cardiac catheter. *Am J Physiol* 1951;164:254–262.

Ekelund L, Jonsson NM, Treugut H. Transcatheter obliteration of the renal artery by ethanol injection: Experimental results. *Cardiovasc Intervent Radiol* 1981;4:1–7.

Ellman BA, Green CE, Eigenbrodt E, Garriot JC, Curry TS III. Renal infarction with absolute ethanol. *Invest Radiol* 1980;15:318–322.

Ellman BA, Parkhill BJ, Curry TS III, Marcus PB, Peters PC. Ablation of renal tumors with absolute ethanol. *Radiology* 1981;141:619–626.

Fellerman H, Dalakos TG, Streeten DH. Remission of Cushing's syndrome after unilateral adrenal phlebography. *Ann Intern Med* 1970;73:585–587.

Finch IJ, Girton M, Doppman JL. Absolute ethanol injection of the adrenal artery: Hypertensive reaction. *Radiology* 1985;154:357–358.

Fogarty TJ, Cranley JJ, Krause FJ, et al. A method for extraction of arterial emboli and thrombi. *Surg Gynecol Obstet* 1963;176:241–244.

Gianturco C, Anderson JH, Wallace S. Mechanical devices for arterial occlusion. *AJR* 1975;124:428.

Gold RE, Blair DC, Finlay JB, Johnston DWB. Transarterial electrocoagulation therapy of pseudoaneurysm in the head of the pancreas. *AJR* 1975;125:422–426.

Goldman ML, Philip PK, Sarrafiazadeh MS, et al. Transcatheter embolization with bucrylate (in 100 patients). *Radiographics* 1982;2:340–375.

Gomes AS, Rysavy JA, Spadaccini CA, Probst P, D'Souza V, Amplatz K. The use of the bristle brush for transcatheter embolization. *Radiology* 1978;129:345–350.

Grace DM, Pitt DF, Gold RE. Vascular embolization and occlusion by angiographic techniques as an aid or alternative to operation. *Surg Gynecol Obstet* 1976;143:469–482.

Greenfield AJ. Transcatheter vessel occlusion: Selection of methods and materials. *Cardiovasc Intervent Radiol* 1981;4:26–32.

Greenfield AJ, Athanasoulis CA, Waltman AC, Le Moure ER. Transcatheter embolization: Prevention of embolic reflux using balloon catheters. *AJR* 1978;131:651–655.

Horton JA, Marano GD, Kerber CW, et al. Polyvinyl alcohol foam -Gelfoam for therapeutic embolization: A synergistic mixture. *AJNR* 1983;4:143–146.

Kadir S, Kaufman SF, Barth KH, White RI. Embolotherapy: Theory materials, technique. In *Selected Techniques in Interventional Radiology*, edited by Kadir S, Kaufman SF, Barth KH, White RI. Saunders, Philadelphia, 1982:24–46.

Kato T, Nemoto R, Mor IH, Takahashi M, Tamakawa Y, Harada M. Arterial chemoembolization with microencapsulated anticancer drug: An approach to selective cancer chemotherapy with sustained effects. *JAMA* 1981;245:1123–1127.

Kauffman GW, Rassweiler J, Richter G, Hauenstein KH, Rohrbach, Friedburg H. Capillary embolization with Ethibloc: New embolization concept tested in dog kidneys. *AJR* 1981;137:1163–1168.

Kim D, Guthaner DF, Walter JF, Pyle R. Embolization of visceral arteriovenous fistulas with a modified steel wire technique. *AJR* 1984;142:1215–1218.

Kricheff II, Madayag M, Braunstein A. Transfemoral catheter embolization of cerebral and posterior fossa arteriovenous malformations. *Radiology* 1972;103:107–111.

Luessenhop AJ, Spence WT. Artificial embolization of cerebral arteries: Report of use in a case of arteriovenous malformation. *JAMA* 1960;172:1153–1155.

Mulligan BD, Espinosa GA. Bowel infarction: Complication of ethanol ablation of renal tumor. *Cardiovasc Intervent Radiol* 1983;6:55–56.

Nakamura K, Tashiro S, Hiraoka T, Ogata K, Ootsuka K. Hepatocellular carcinoma and metastatic cancer detected by iodized oil. *Radiology* 1985;154:15–17.

Ohishi H, Uchida H, Yoshimura H, et al. Hepatocellular carcinoma detected by iodized oil: Use of anticancer agents. *Radiology* 1985;154:25–29.

Pevsner PH. Micro-balloon catheter for superselective angiography and therapeutic occlusion. *AJR* 1977;128:225–230.

Porstmann W, Wierny L, Warnke H, Gerstberger G, Romaniuk PA. Catheter closure of patent ductus arteriosus. *Radiol Clin N Am* 1971;9:203–218.

Serbinenko F. Balloon catheterization and occlusion of major cerebral vessels. *J Neurosurg* 1974;41:125–145.

Spigos DG, Jonasson O, Mozes M, et al. Partial splenic embolization in the treatment of hypersplenism. *AJR* 1979;132:777–782.

Stoesslein F, Ditscherlein G, Romaniuk PA. Experimental studies on new liquid embolization mixtures (Histoacryl-Lipiodol, Histoacryl-Panthopaque). *Cardiovasc Intervent Radiol* 1982;5:264–267.

Tadavarthy SM, Maller JH, Amplatz K. Polyvinyl alcohol foam (Ivalon): A new embolic material. *AJR* 1975;125:609–616.

Thompson WM, Johnsrude IS, Jackson DC, McAlister S, Miller MD, Pizzo SV. Vessel occlusion with transcatheter electrocoagulation: Initial clinical experience. *Radiology* 1979;133:335–340.

Tisnado J, Beachley MC, Cho SR, Amendola M. Peripheral embolization of a stainless steel coil. *AJR* 1979;133:324–326.

Uflacker R. Percutaneous transhepatic obliteration of gastroesophageal varices with absolute alcohol. *Radiology* 1983;146:621–625.

Uflacker R. Radiologia intervencionista: uma especialidade emergente. *Radiol Bras* 1983;16:71–85.

Uflacker R. Transcatheter embolization of arterial aneurysms. *Br J Radiol* 1986;59:317–324.

Uflacker R, Kaemmerer A, Neves C, Picon PD. Management of massive hemoptysis by bronchial artery embolization. *Radiology* 1983;146:627–634.

Uflacker R, Paolini RM, Nobrega M. Ablation of tumor and inflammatory tissue with absolute ethanol. *Acta Radiol (Diagn)* 1986;27:131–138.

Uflacker R, Saadi J. Transcatheter embolization of superior mesenteric arteriovenous fistula. *AJR* 1982;139:1212–1214.

Vinters HV, Galil KA, Lundie MJ, Kaufmann JCE. The histotoxicity of cyanoacrylates: A selective review. *Neuroradiology* 1985;27:279–291.

Vinters HV, Lundie HJ, Kaufmann JCE. Long-term pathological follow-up of cerebral arteriovenous malformations treated by embolization with bucrylate. *N Engl J Med* 1986;314:477–483.

Wallace S, Gianturco C, Anderson JH, et al. Therapeutic vascular occlusion utilizing steel coil technique: Clinical applications. *AJR* 1976;127:381–385.

Weber J, Dociu N, Zabel G. Gas without abscess in renal tumour embolization. *Ann Radiol* 1984;27:305–309.

White RI Jr., Kaufman SL, Barth KH, et al. Embolotherapy with detachable silicone balloons: Technique and clinical results. *Radiology* 1979;131:619–627.

White RI Jr., Strandberg JV, Gross ES, Barth KH. Therapeutic embolization with long-term occluding agents and their effects on embolized tissues. *Radiology* 1977;125:677–687.

Wholey MH. The technology of balloon catheters in interventional angiography. *Radiology* 1977;125:671–676.

Wholey MH, Stockdale R, Hung TK. A percutaneous balloon catheter for the immediate control of hemorrhage. *Radiology* 1970;95:65–71.

Wright KC, Bowers T, Chuang VP, Tsai CC. Experimental evaluation of Ethibloc for nonsurgical nephrectomy. *Radiology* 1982;145:339–342.

Yumoto Y, Jonno K, Tokuyama K, et al. Hepatocellular carcinoma detected by iodized oil. *Radiology* 1985;254:19–24.

Yune HY, Klatte EC, Richmond BD, Rabe FE. Absolute ethanol in thrombotherapy of bleeding esophageal varices. *AJR* 1982;138:1137–1141.

Chapter Three
Gastrointestinal Bleeding

RENAN UFLACKER

GENERAL ASPECTS

Gastrointestinal (GI) bleeding is a relatively common and potentially serious problem, with mortality rates approaching 10 to 20 percent. This is an area of medicine where integration of three disciplines—clinical, surgical, and radiologic specialties—is critical to patient care.

Contrary to what is commonly thought, early diagnosis of GI bleeding does not significantly reduce mortality. This does not mean that early diagnosis is not important but that therapeutic techniques have not developed as quickly as diagnostic techniques have.

When GI bleeding is mentioned in a context of radiologic intervention, it is assumed that the clinical steps of patient maintenance and resuscitation have already been taken.

Managing patients with GI bleeding requires an integrated team approach, which should follow well-defined hospital care policies which concentrate on the problem of bleeding, making use of all available diagnostic and therapeutic resources; all these resources should be centralized in a single specialized intensive care unit. In approximately 75 percent of these patients, GI bleeding can be controlled through conservative clinical treatment. The inclusion of a patient in a specialized protocol for GI bleeding is justified only when bleeding persists after conservative measures have been taken.

The first step in evaluating a patient with upper GI bleeding is to determine whether one is dealing with upper or lower (distal to the ligament of Treitz) bleeding. A nasogastric tube can be introduced. If blood is found in the stomach, upper GI bleeding can be diagnosed with a reasonable degree of certainty. If blood is not found in the stomach, one must consider the possibility of lower GI bleeding.

Hematochezia or melena is generally related to GI bleeding below the ligament of Treitz. However, prolonged upper GI bleeding is frequently associated with melena, and it is not uncommon to see red blood, associated with rapid intestinal transit, in the feces of a patient with upper GI bleeding. The presence of hematemesis suggest upper GI bleeding, though in rare cases hematemesis is caused by lesions distal to the ligament of Treitz (Fig. 3.1).

The patient's clinical history may supply additional information, such as a family history of blood dyscrasia or neoplasm, recent or old trauma, drug intake (aspirin, corticosteroids, anticoagulants), and alcohol abuse. Analysis of the skin surface may be useful when one is looking for signs of chronic hepatitis or a hereditary systemic disease that predisposes a patient to GI bleeding [Peutz-Jegher syndrome, Rendu-Osler-Weber disease, neurofibromatosis, and Ehler-Danlos syndrome (Fig. 3.1)]. Other autoimmune systemic diseases, such as polyarteritis nodosa, may also be accompanied by hematemesis or melena due to the rupture of arterial aneurysms in abdominal organs (Fig. 3.2).

In evaluating bleeding in a patient with cirrhosis or esophageal varices, it is important to remember that bleeding caused by ruptured varices accounts for only 50 percent of such cases. The others may have some degree of gastritis, a peptic ulcer, or esophageal laceration (Mallory-Weiss syndrome).

A history of colon inflammatory disease or melena or hematochezia that occurs immediately after clinical evidence of hypovolemia suggests that the bleeding is of lower intestinal origin. In cases in which it is not possible upon first manifestation of bleeding to identify it as being of upper or lower origin, it is best to assume that the bleeding is of upper GI origin since the incidence of massive hemorrhage is much higher in patients with upper GI bleeding than it is in patients with bleeding distal to the ligament of Treitz.

Many different diagnostic techniques can be used to locate the bleeding site, including angiography, endoscopy, nuclear imaging, barium studies, and exploratory surgery.

The value of angiography as a diagnostic tool lies in its sensitivity (it can identify bleeding as little as 0.5 mL/min) and high specificity regarding location and etiology. Although in recent years upper digestive tract endoscopy has replaced angiography as the technique of choice in cases of upper GI bleeding, angiography remains extremely important as a diagnostic tool for selected patients.

Nuclear imaging is of more value in patients with lower GI bleeding. This technique is highly sensitive in identifying bleeding, although it is less specific in identifying cause or location. The scintiscan is an excellent

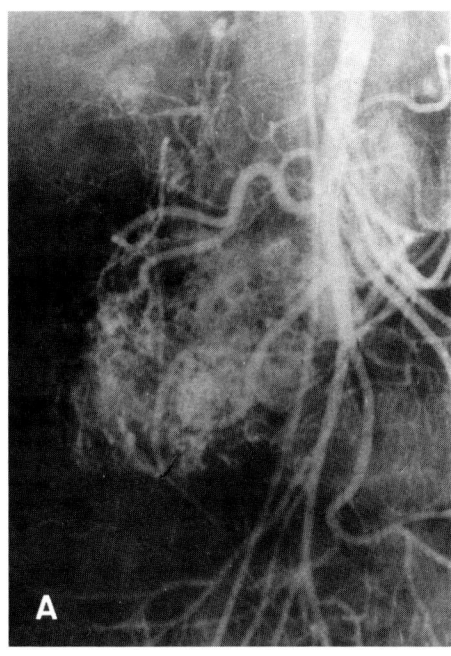
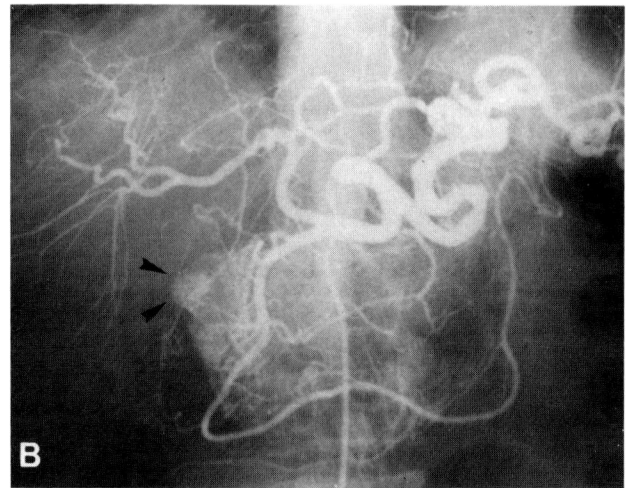
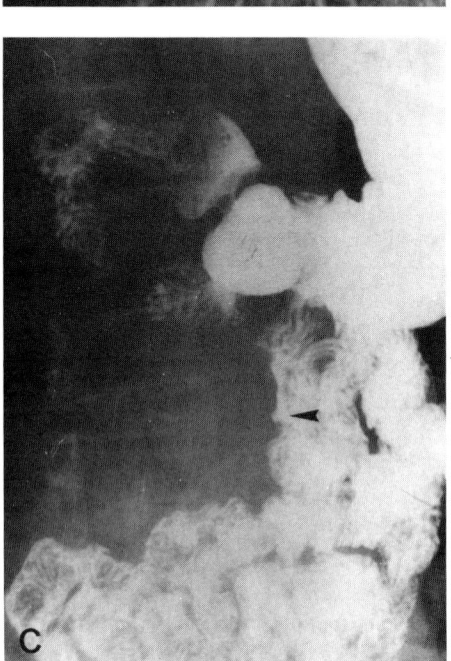
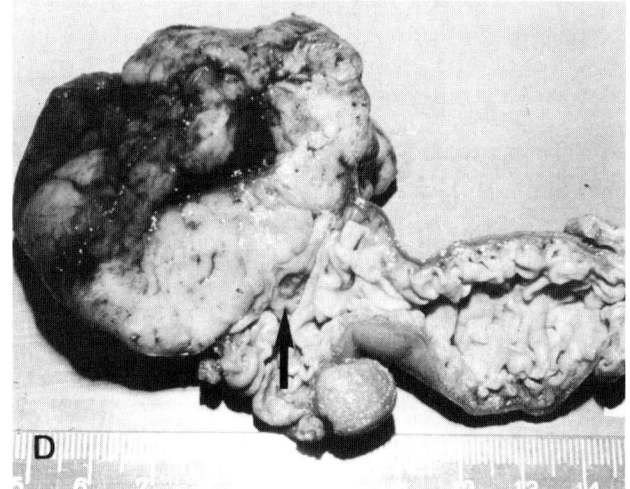

Figure 3.1 A 54-year-old patient with a history of neurofibromatosis since childhood who presented with hematemesis.
(A) Initial phase of superior mesenteric arteriogram demonstrating a large hypervascular neurofibroma. (B) Injection into the celiac axis shows a small neurofibroma on the duodenal wall (arrows). (C) A barium study shows a jejunal loop that is displaced and rigid from ulceration. (D) A surgical specimen of neurofibroma shows extensive hemorrhagic necrosis inside the mass and a small ulcer in the jejunal mucosa (arrow). Note the small satellite fibroma on the other edge of the small intestine. Even though the lesion was located below the ligament of Treitz, hematemesis was the clinical presentation.

means for determining the proper time for angiography. A negative scan suggests no active bleeding, indicating that it is best to postpone angiography. A positive study should encourage immediate angiographic evaluation.

Barium studies are contraindicated in patients with acute upper GI bleeding.

Surgical exploration is a poor method for evaluating GI bleeding because investigation must often be extended to multiple organs. It is contraindicated in patients with chronic liver disease with varices and associated GI bleeding because of the associated unacceptable mortality rates.

When all indications are that GI bleeding originates from a higher location, upper digestive tract endoscopy will pinpoint the location of the bleeding in over 80 percent of cases. Endoscopy performed early in the course of bleeding followed by surgical intervention can lower the mortality rate from 12.5 to 7 percent in patients who are not already debilitated by bleeding. Mortality remains high in surgical patients in whom the precise bleeding point was not known before surgery.

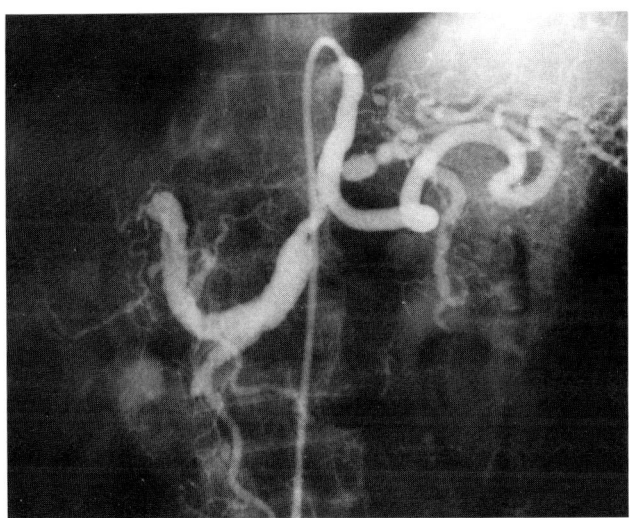

Figure 3.2 A 67-year-old hypertensive patient, with polyarteritis nodosa, including renal lesions seen in the angiogram. There was a prior history of hematemesis and melena. Normal upper endoscopy was obtained. Injection into the celiac axis shows aneurysmal lesions of the left gastric artery and the common and proper hepatic arteries. Note intimal dissection and occlusion at the level of the proper hepatic artery. Hemorrhage in these patients is usually related to aneurysms rupturing into the visceral lumen.

UPPER GASTROINTESTINAL BLEEDING

The clinical protocol and surgical approach in cases of upper GI hemorrhage due to arteriocapillary bleeding are the opposite of those used in treating patients with cirrhosis and bleeding esophageal varices. Early surgery is more effective and arterial embolization procedures are more appropriate in patients with a bleeding peptic ulcer. Most authors agree that early surgery is contraindicated in patients with bleeding varices; procedures such as vasopressin infusion, endoscopic sclerosis, embolization of varices, and placement of an esophageal balloon are more appropriate.

ANATOMY

From an anatomic standpoint, the physician should be familiar with the celiac axis, the superior mesenteric artery and its anastomoses, and the pancreatic and splenic circulation. Figure 3.3 shows a normal celiac axis, as found in over 50 percent of the population. Some common variations exist, such as a left gastric artery originating directly from the aorta and the presence of an anomalous right hepatic artery from which the gastroduodenal artery and its branches may or may not originate. The practitioner must be well acquainted with the anterior and posterior superior pancreaticoduodenal arcades in order to locate and treat duodenal bleeding.

ANGIOGRAPHIC ASPECTS OF BLEEDING

Localized bleeding of arterial origin is identified in the arterial phase of selective arteriography as an accumulation of contrast medium in the bowel lumen. As the angiographic series progresses, contrast medium contin-

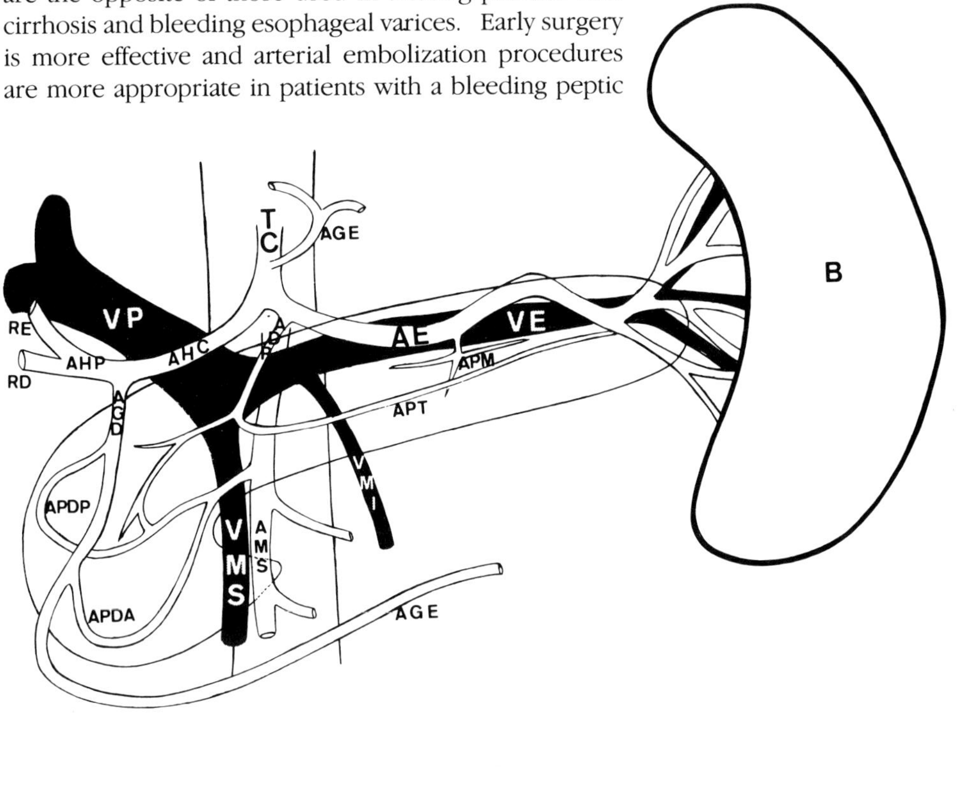

Figure 3.3 Schematic drawing of the vascularization of the celiac axis, with anastomosis of the superior mesenteric artery and the portal vein. B = spleen; VE = splenic vein; VP = portal vein; VMS = superior mesenteric vein; AE = splenic artery; TC = celiac axis; AGE = left gastric artery; ADP = dorsal pancreatic artery; APM = great pancreatic artery; APT = transverse pancreatic artery; AMS = superior mesenteric artery; AHC = common hepatic artery; AHP = proper hepatic artery; AGD = gastroduodenal artery; APDP = superior anterior pancreaticoduodenal arch; RE = left hepatic artery; RD = right hepatic artery.

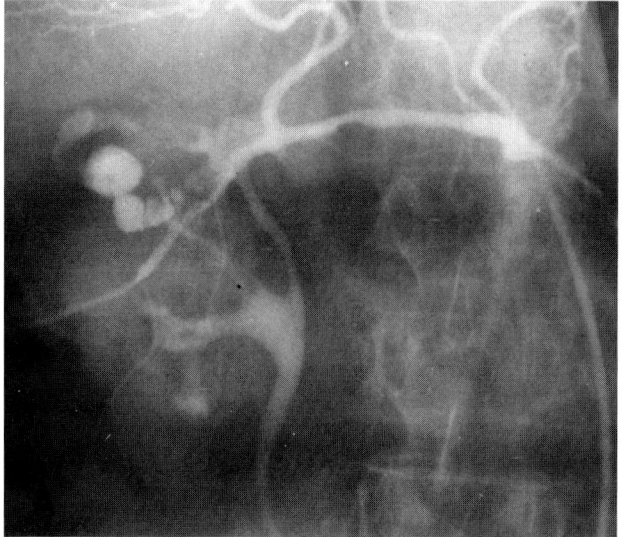

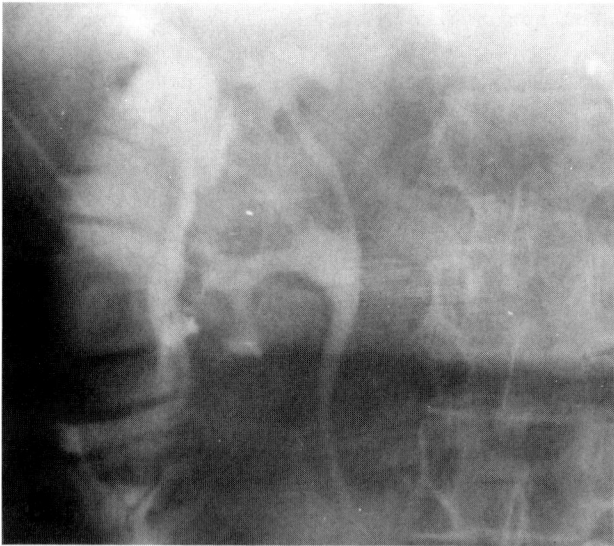

Figure 3.4 A bleeding bulbar ulcer in a 69-year-old patient with hematemesis and abundant melena. Upper gastrointestinal endoscopy did not identify the bleeding site because of the large volume of blood in the stomach.
(A) Final stage of injection into the celiac axis, showing localized contrast extravasation in the bulbar ulcer. (B) A later stage of angiographic injection shows contrast extravasation and duodenal opacification due to extravasation of contrast into the duodenum.

ues to extravasate; this becomes more evident by the end of the series. At this stage, movement of extravasated contrast medium may occur inside the loop of bowel as a result of peristalsis, identifying the point of bleeding (Fig. 3.4). Small amounts of bleeding will form a localized collection, filling an ulcerous or diverticular cavity or remaining around the bleeding site and assuming an amorphous aspect. If there is a large accumulation of clots, extravasated contrast medium may form a small channel through the thrombi, with the appearance of "pseudovein."

Dilution of contrast almost always occurs inside the loop. After a few minutes, the collection of extravasated material is removed by means of peristalsis.

DIFFICULTIES OF INTERPRETATION AND TREATMENT

It is not uncommon for a patient with apparently active GI bleeding to be submitted to angiography and for the exact location of the bleeding not to be shown during the examination. In most patients, blood loss is intermittent, and so extravasation will not be among the angiographic findings if the procedure is carried out between bleeding episodes. The easiest way to identify the time of bleeding and complete the procedure is to observe the aspirate from the nasogastric tube.

Extravasation frequently is not identified by less selective injections. Selective injections must be made into the left gastric, gastroduodenal, splenic, hepatic, and upper mesenteric arteries for the physician to affirm with certainty that there is no active bleeding in the gastroduodenal axis. A previous endoscopy can simplify this routine by locating the lesion before the angiographic procedure does.

Arteriographic study of the wrong territory frequently causes negative results. If the angiographer obtains misleading clinical or endoscopic information, this may result in a false-negative study. For example, patients who bleed as a consequence of a duodenal ulcer, with rapid transit and without hematemesis, present clinically in the same way that patients with lower GI bleeding do. Endoscopy which does not visualize the entire duodenum can worsen this problem. When a bleeding site is not demonstrated in a patient who appears to have lower GI bleeding, upon confirmation of the site, the celiac axis should be studied so that duodenal bleeding is not overlooked.

Arterial anatomic variations can also lead to false-negative results. A left gastric artery originating from the aorta or a middle colic artery originating from the dorsal pancreatic artery may produce false-negative results unless these vessels are sought out.

Gastrointestinal bleeding of venous origin is not usually shown by arterial or venous injection. Bleeding due to gastric or esophageal varices is best detected by means of endoscopy. Arteriography is not indicated as a method of treatment in these cases, which require an approach through the portal vein.

False contrast extravasations are quite common; they result from staining of normal organs or segments of

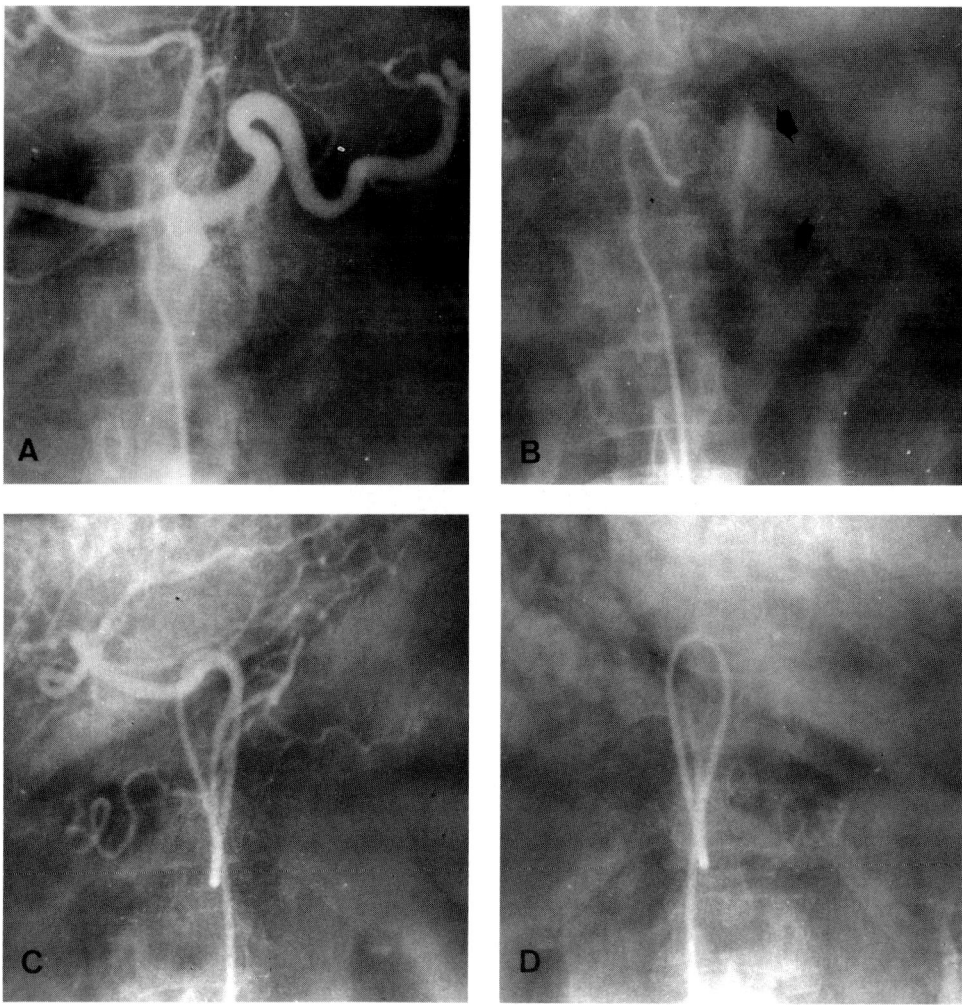

Figure 3.5 False-positive diagnosis of gastric bleeding.
(A) Injection into the celiac axis. No contrast extravasation is seen. (B) Later stage of injection into the celiac axis shows dense opacification of the left adrenal gland, simulating gastric hemorrhage in the lesser curvature (arrows). (C,D) Selective injection into the left gastric artery does not show contrast extravasation or adrenal staining.

organs by contrast medium after selective injection. The most common source of confusion here is staining of one of the adrenal glands by injection into the celiac axis (Fig. 3.5). This occurs through the phrenic arteries and the supply to the upper adrenal gland. Superselective injections may be necessary to demonstrate or exclude this as an angiographic artifact.

UPPER GASTROINTESTINAL BLEEDING FROM MALLORY-WEISS TEARS

Mallory-Weiss tears have been diagnosed increasingly frequently as a recognized cause of GI bleeding, with an incidence as high as 14 percent. The tear occurs during vomiting, and approximately half these patients have a history of alcohol intake during the prior 48 h. At endoscopy, the appearance is that of small tears in the cardia, with active bleeding. Only about 40 percent of Mallory-Weiss patients require blood replacement, and a smaller percentage require more aggressive therapy. This type of lesion, which may be considered as bleeding from the gastric mucosa, can be treated with vasopressin infusion or selective embolization. Selective infusion of vasopressin can control approximately 80 to 90 percent of bleeding; a 16 percent rate of rebleeding has been reported. Treatment by means of embolization of the left gastric artery (Fig. 3.6) produces hemostasis in about 95 percent of patients.

Embolization of the left gastric artery is the treatment of choice for Mallory-Weiss patients. It results in spontaneous healing of the wound and the left gastric artery will recanalize if a temporary embolizing agent is used.

GASTRIC MUCOSAL BLEEDING (GASTRITIS)

The incidence of GI hemorrhages due to acute injury to the gastric mucosa in its different presentations accounts

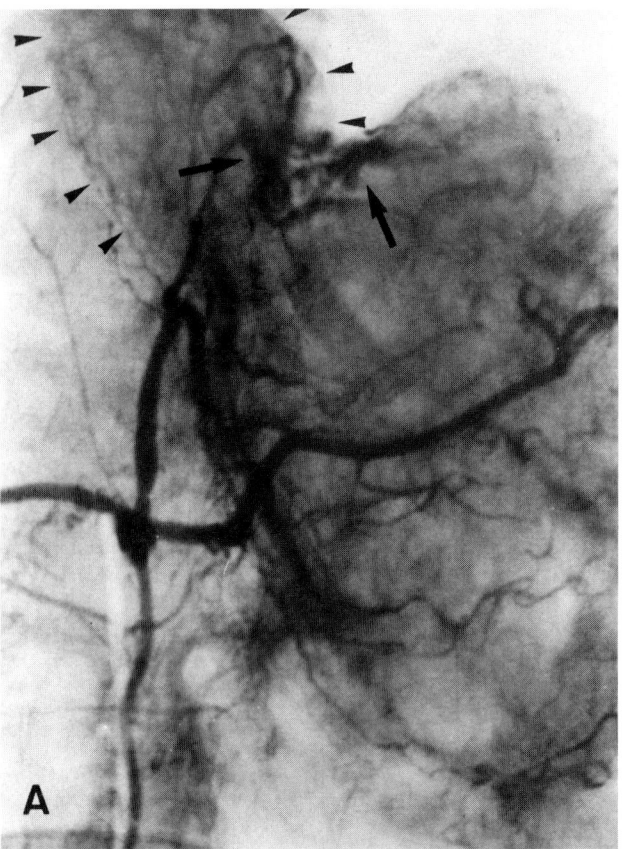
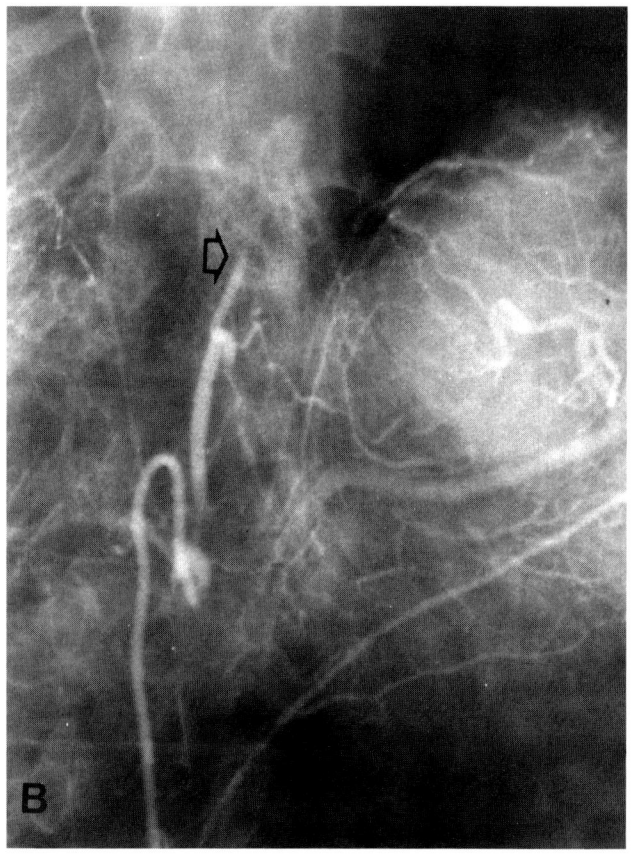

Figure 3.6 Mallory-Weiss syndrome in a patient with vomiting followed by hematemesis.
(A) Selective injection into the left gastric artery shows hiatal herniation (arrowheads) and bleeding in the cardial region (arrows). (B) Control angiography after Gelfoam embolization of the left gastric artery (arrow), with bleeding under control.

for approximately 30 percent of all GI bleeding. Critical patients who now survive for longer periods in intensive care units, frequently have this type of upper GI bleeding. Other presentations include acute gastritis, "stress" ulcer, and Curling's ulcer.

These lesions of the mucosa are superficial erosions that apparently are due to a mucosal ischemic process which breaks down the barrier between the mucosa and the acid content of the stomach, resulting in back-diffusion of hydrogen ions into the submucosa. Predisposing factors include jaundice, sepsis, azotemia, and the use of steroids in about half these cases. Patients with trauma or extensive burns are also at high risk for developing these lesions.

The angiographic presentation is one of diffuse hyperemia of the mucosa. Contrast-medium extravasation is seen infrequently.

Surgical treatment consisting of ligation of a major portion of the gastric vasculature has been advocated, but it is associated with high mortality rates from the primary disease. Most of these patients are recovering from major surgery, have suffered extensive trauma or

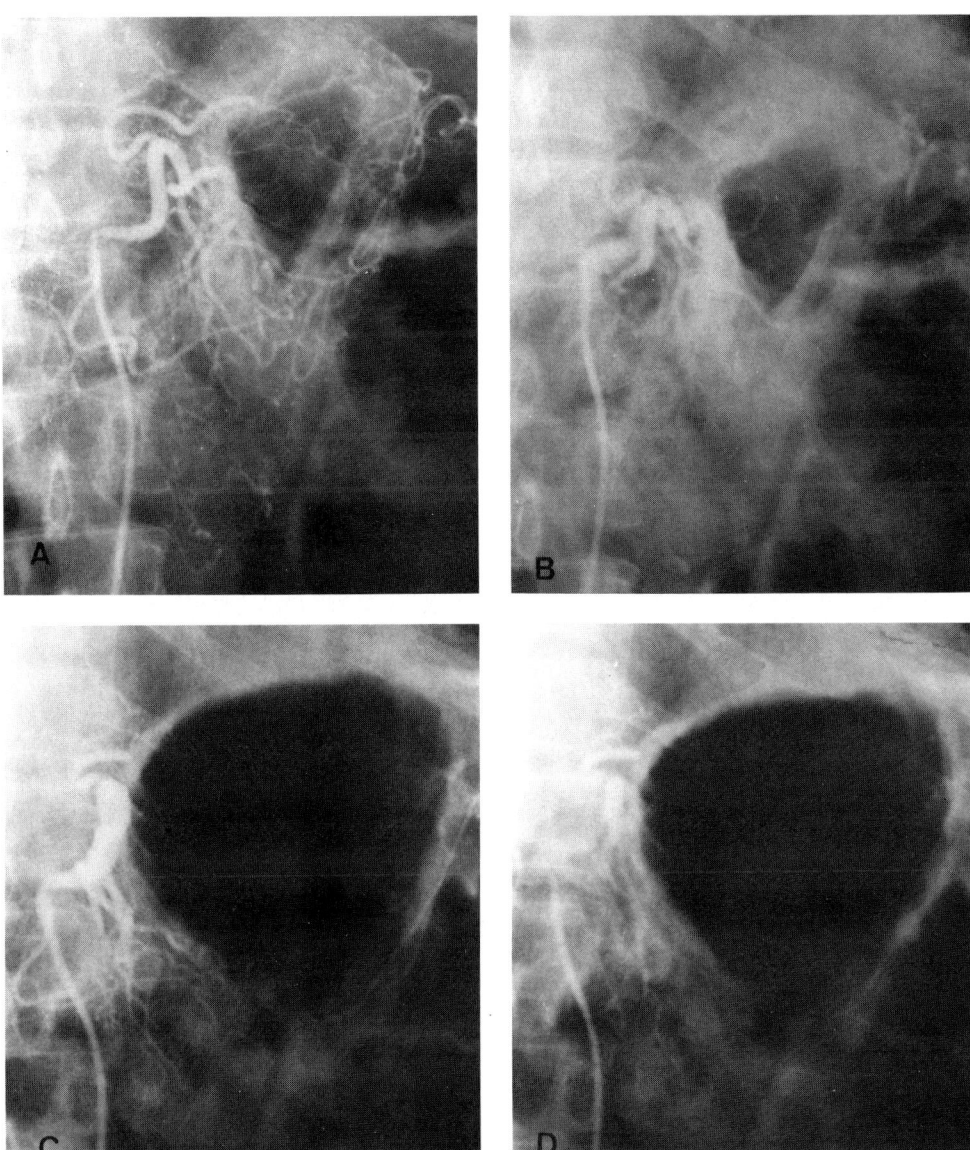

Figure 3.7 Hemorrhagic gastritis in a patient with stroke, gastrostomy, and hematemesis.
(A) Selective injection into the left gastric artery. (B) Later stage of selective injection shows pronounced diffuse thickening of the gastric wall. (C) After Gelfoam embolization of the left gastric artery, occlusion occurred primarily in the arteries of the gastric fundus. (D) A later control shows a significant decrease in wall circulation.

burns, or are recovering from a stroke (Fig. 3.7). The mortality rate from gastric mucosal bleeding in these high-risk patients is approximately 21 percent.

Less invasive and more efficient techniques, such as infusion of a vasoconstricting agent and embolization of the left gastric artery, are preferable in those conditions. Infusion of vasopressin is the therapy of choice in patients in whom the only finding is hyperemia; embolization should be used in patients with active extravasation of contrast medium (Fig. 3.8). These treatment techniques can stop bleeding in approximately 80 percent of patients, although, because of the gravity of the primary disease, the mortality rate is not reduced significantly.

GASTRIC ULCER

Gastroduodenal peptic ulceration is one of the most common causes of upper GI bleeding. The differential diagnosis between a gastric ulcer and a duodenal ulcer is made by means of endoscopy. This distinction is

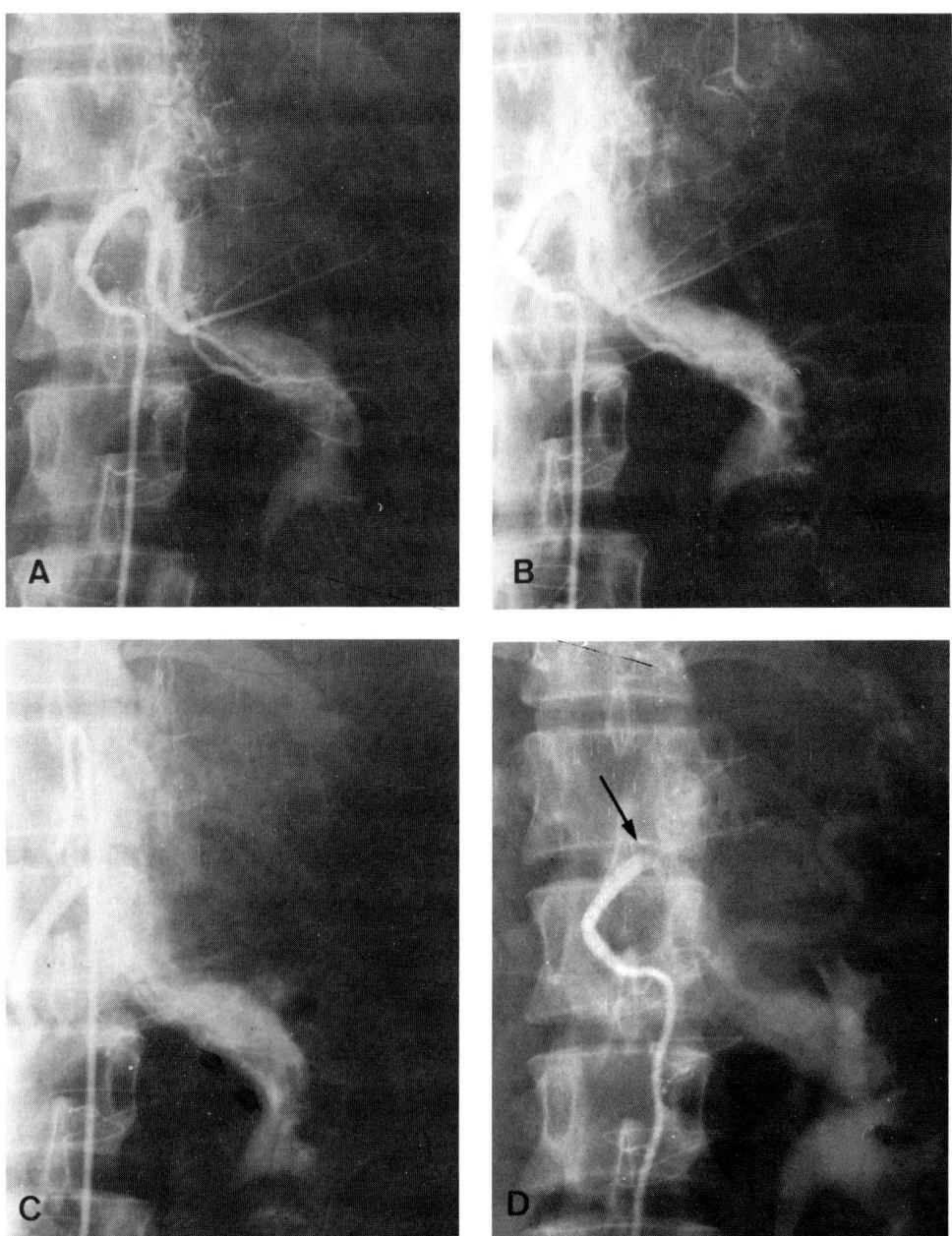

Figure 3.8 A 32-year-old patient with a postoperative perforated gastric ulcer on the lesser curvature.
(A,B) Injection into the left gastric artery shows pronounced thickening of the wall of the lesser curvature caused by localized gastritis. (C) In a later stage of the injection there is intramural extravasation of contrast medium (arrows) without invasion of the gastric lumen. (D) The left gastric artery was embolized with Gelfoam (arrow), and the bleeding was permanently controlled.

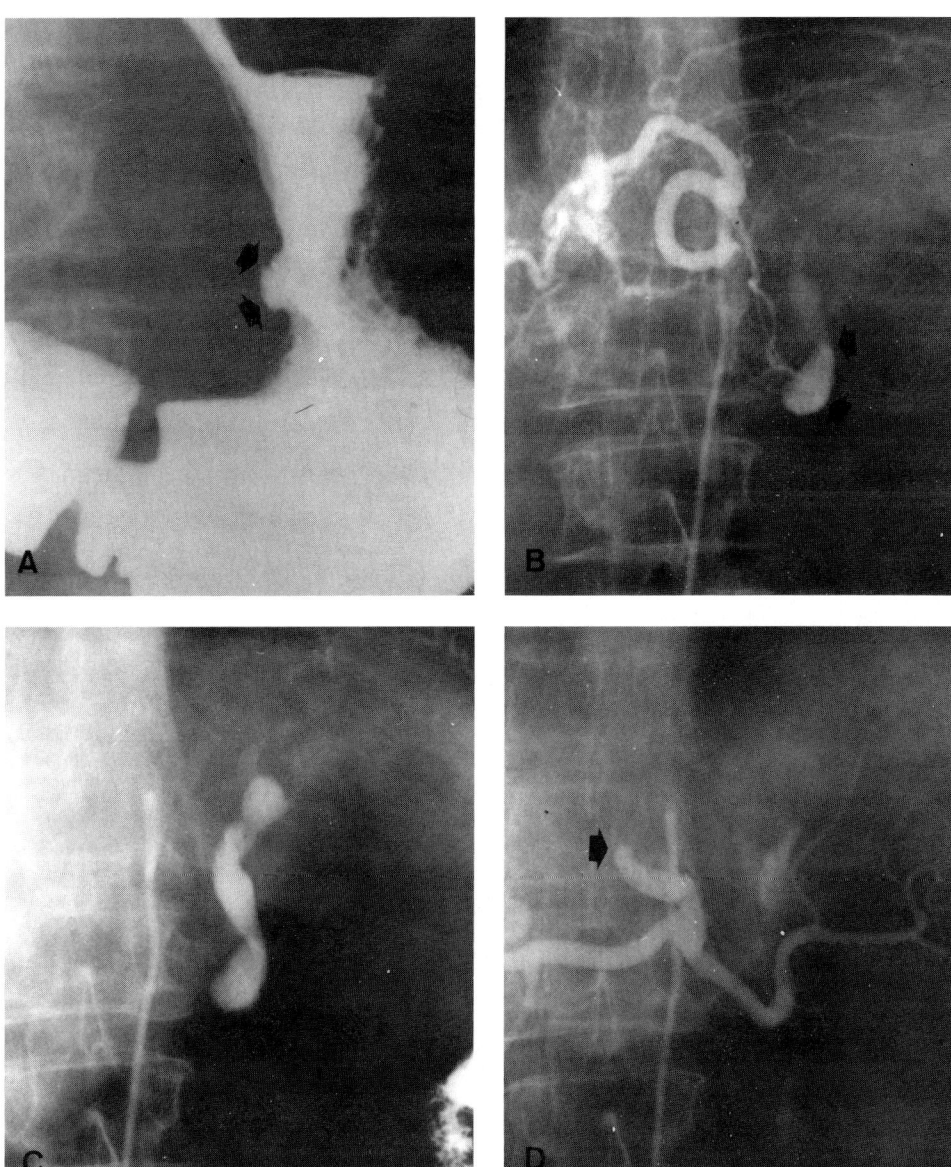

Figure 3.9 (A) A patient with a gastric ulcer in the lesser curvature (arrows) identified during a barium study. The patient was admitted for surgery and had acute bleeding. (B) Selective injection into the left gastric artery showed profuse extravasation of contrast medium into the region of the ulcer (arrows). (C) In a later stage of injection the image of a pseudovein appeared as a result of contrast extravasation among clots in the stomach. (D) Control after embolization with Gelfoam of the left gastric artery (arrow), with bleeding under control. Note the small volume of contrast medium remaining in the gastric lumen. The patient was electively operated on a few days later for treatment of a peptic ulcer.

important, as the angiographic procedure will be shorter and more objective if the artery involved can be identified by prior localization of the lesion. Infusion of vasopressin into the left gastric artery to treat bleeding from ulcers has had a success rate of approximately 60 to 70 percent in some series, although controlled studies have shown a relatively high rebleeding rate without a decrease in mortality. Other centers have had even worse results using vasopressin to treat peptic ulcer disease. These limitations have led to the use of embolization techniques as a preferred method to treat bleeding from gastric ulcers (Fig. 3.9).

In fact, the first use of clinical embolization for the treatment of acute GI bleeding was done by Rosch, who in 1972 successfully treated a bleeding gastric ulcer with transcatheter embolotherapy. Since that time, experience from other centers has shown that embolization is the method of choice in patients with arteriocapillary bleeding.

Gastric ulcers are usually located on the lesser cur-

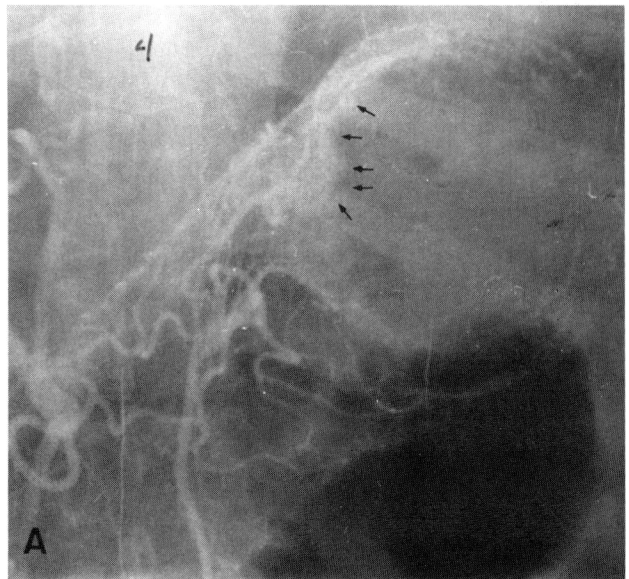

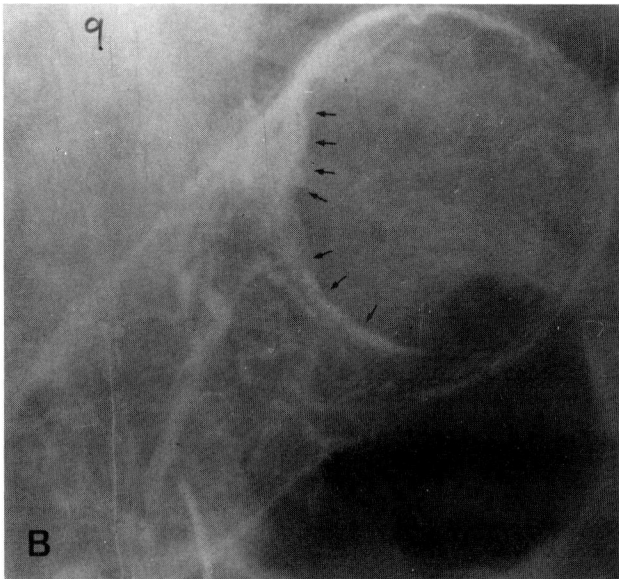

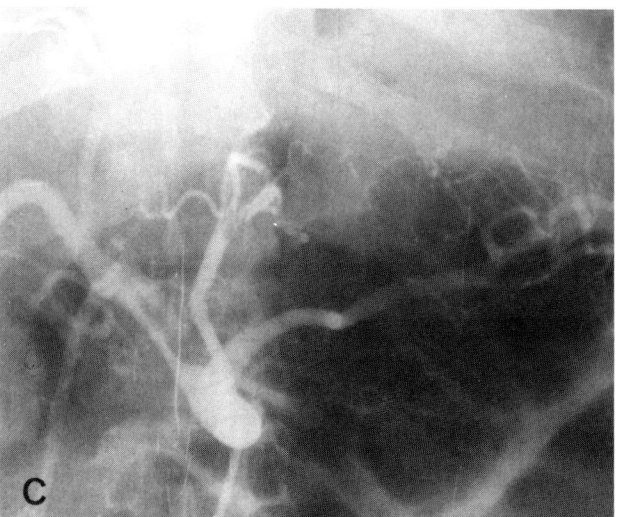

vature, on the anterior and posterior walls (Fig. 3.10), or in the antrum. The artery to be embolized is the left gastric artery (the catheterization technique for this artery was described in Chap. 1, Figs. 1.15 and 1.26). When bleeding occurs on the greater curvature, fed by short gastric arteries, it is often impossible to reach these arteries. Embolization of the splenic artery with one or two Gelfoam pledgets or coils is a valid alternative therapy with a high rate of success (Fig. 3.11). In some cases, embolization of the gastroepiploic artery must be performed.

When embolization is used to treat bleeding in operated stomachs, several problems may arise. Vascular occlusion must be sufficient to stop the bleeding, but it must be limited to preserve gastric wall circulation so that necrosis does not occur. The risk of necrosis rises if a vasoconstricting agent has been used prior to embolization. In critical patients, postoperative bleeding from ulcers in an anastomotic os can be serious; in these patients, embolization can prevent the need for a new surgical procedure (Fig. 3.12). Ulcers on an anastomotic os to the stomach do not respond well to vasopressin. Embolization is the technique of choice in these patients.

Figure 3.10 (A) Gastrointestinal hemorrhage from small ulcers on the upper portion of the lesser curvature. Arrows point at the contrast extravasation. (B) Later stage of injection into the left gastric artery shows diffusion of contrast medium over the mucosa (arrows). (C) Control after Gelfoam embolization of the left gastric artery, with bleeding completely arrested.

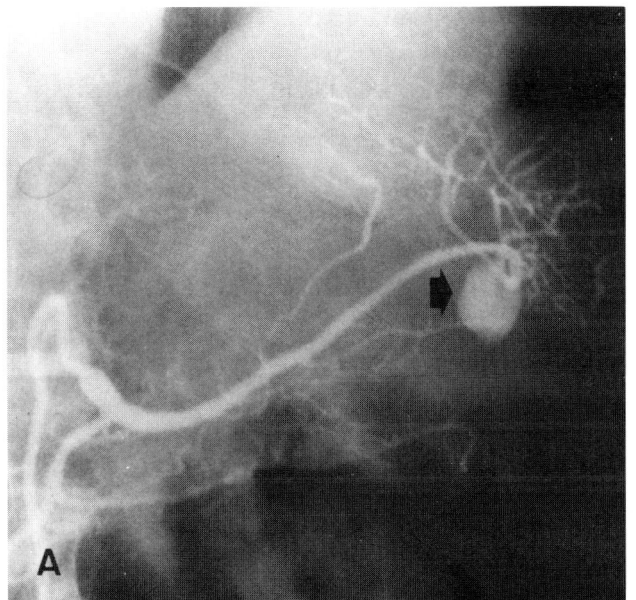

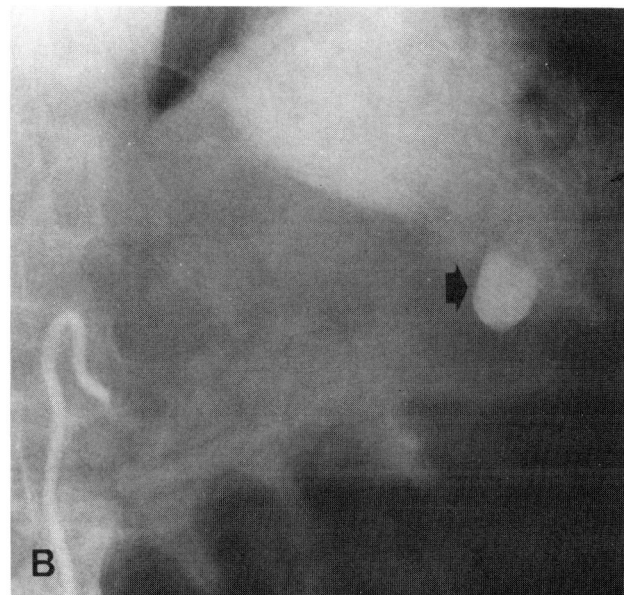

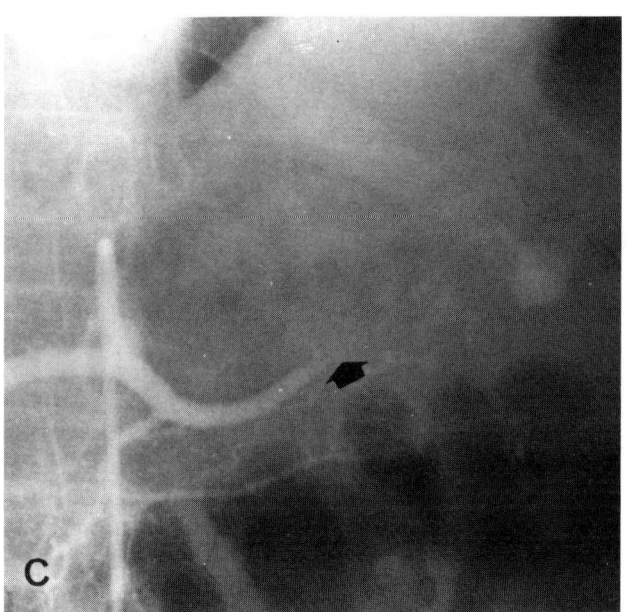

Figure 3.11 (A) Bleeding from an ulcer on the upper portion of the greater curvature of the stomach, vascularized by short gastric arteries; branches of the splenic artery (arrow). (B) Later stage of the arteriogram shows a well-localized collection (arrow). (C) The catheter could not be advanced to the point of bleeding because embolization of the splenic artery had been achieved with two large Gelfoam emboli. The patient stopped bleeding and received elective surgery a few days later.

DUODENAL ULCER

Hemorrhages resulting from duodenal ulcers are usually treated conservatively in patients whose general condition is good. In debilitated or elderly patients, the treatment should be aggressive, depending on the seriousness of the condition. As with bleeding in any ulcer, the angiographic presentation is one of contrast-medium extravasation and pooling, which can spread over the mucosa depending on volume and duodenal peristalsis (Fig. 3.4).

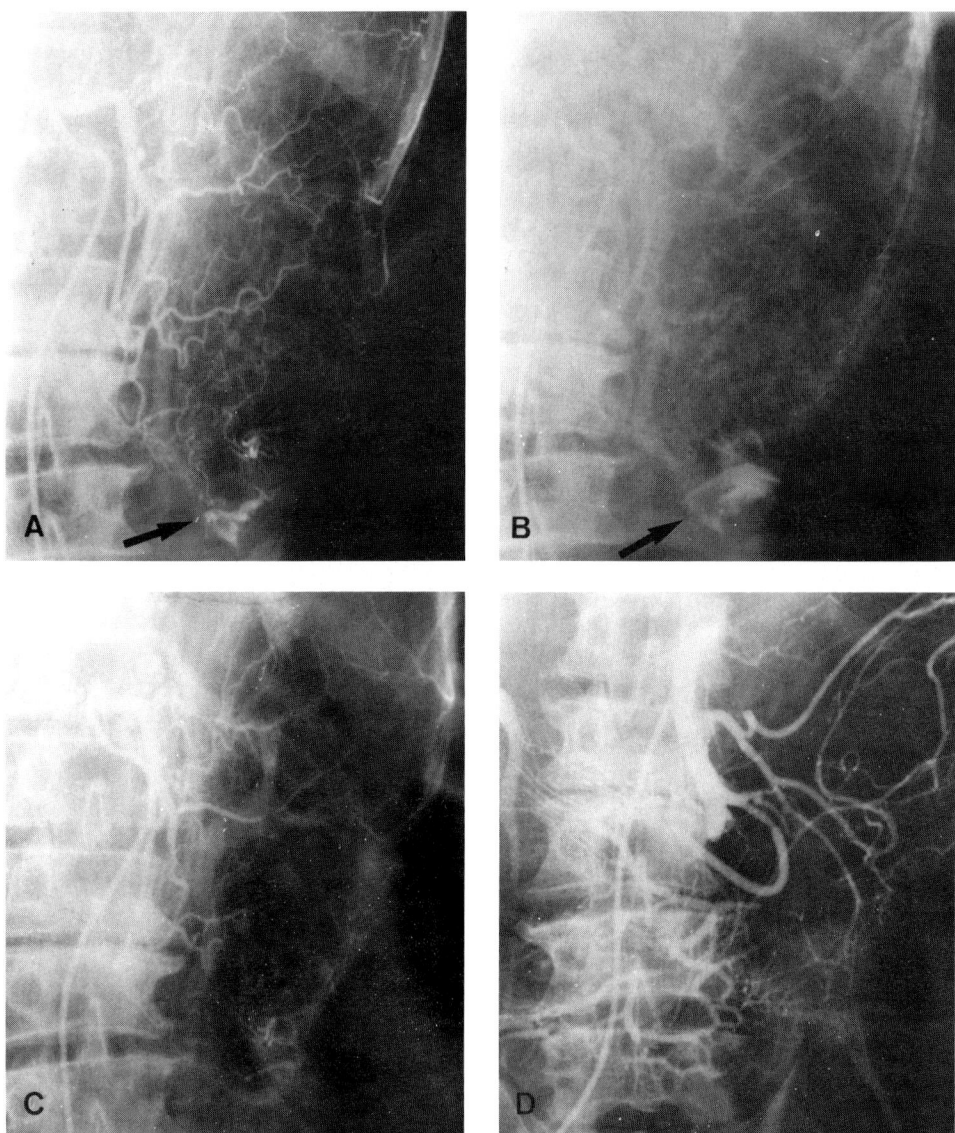

Figure 3.12   A patient in bad general condition in the postoperative period of a duodenopancreatectomy for papillary neoplasm. The patient had presented with hematemesis.
(A) Injection into the left gastric artery shows the site of anastomosis and contrast-medium extravasation in linear ulcerations close to the anastomotic ostium on the gastric wall (arrow). (B) Later stage shows contrast extravasation (arrow). (C) Partial embolization of the left gastric artery was performed with Gelfoam, which controlled bleeding. Embolization was more conservative than it normally would have been because of the risk of necrosis in an already operated stomach. (D) Selective injection into the superior mesenteric artery, showing occlusion from postoperative thrombosis. No bleeding originated from the superior mesenteric artery.

Such bleeding is usually from branches of the gastroduodenal artery or from the main artery itself, depending on the depth of penetration by the ulcer (Fig. 3.13). Treatment of bleeding in the duodenum is complicated by the double vascular supply present (Fig. 3.14).

Embolization of the gastroduodenal artery or its branches is the method of choice for nonsurgical treatment of an acute bleeding duodenal ulcer, with vasopressin infusion playing a secondary role. The results obtained with vasopressin have been inconsistent, indicating a high rate of rebleeding; thus, this technique is generally ineffective when used in clinical patients with upper GI bleeding from a duodenal ulcer. Embolization with Gelfoam pledgets, placed as selectively as possible in the feeding artery, is the most effective method of control (Fig. 3.13).

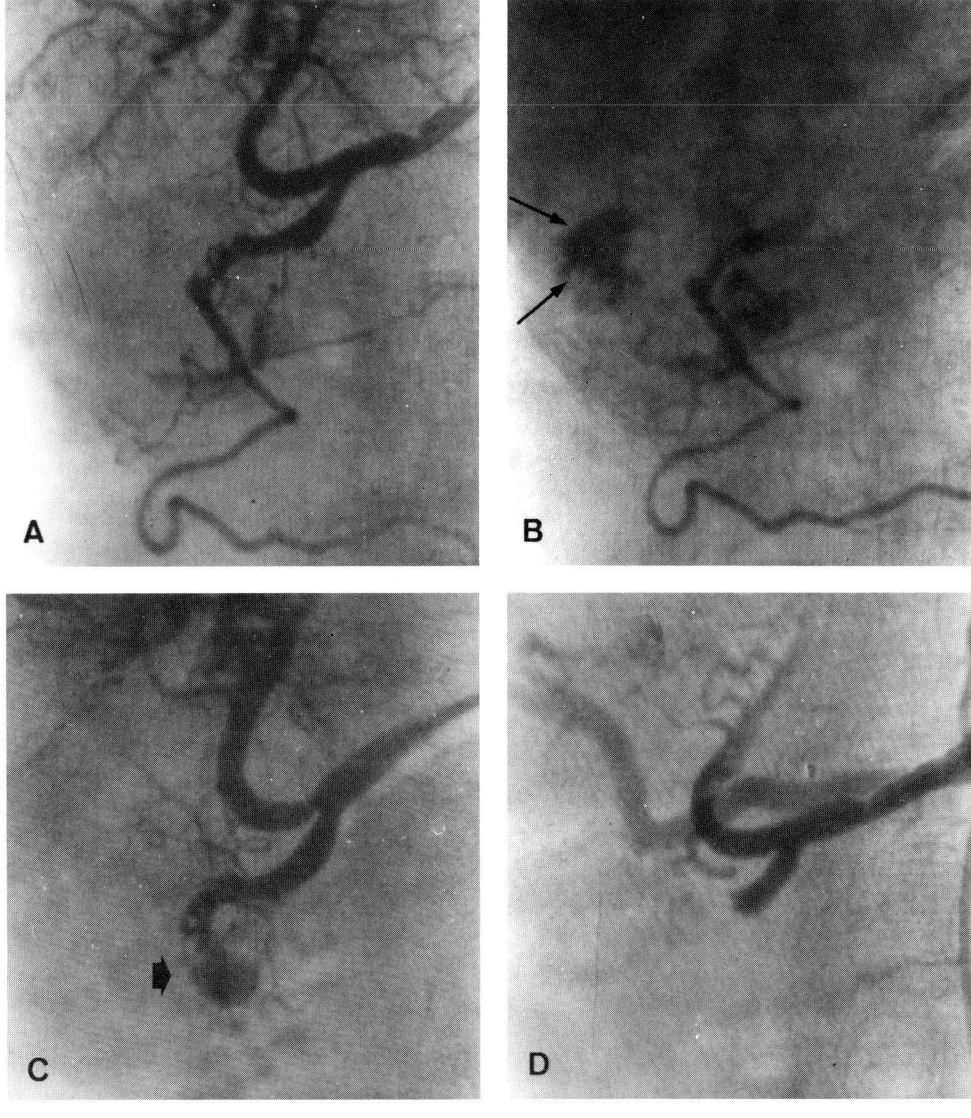

Figure 3.13 Massive upper gastrointestinal bleeding from a duodenal ulcer in an 80-year-old patient.
(A) Selective injection into the hepatic artery shows the beginning of contrast-medium extravasation in branches of the gastroduodenal artery. (B) Later stage of injection shows contrast-medium collection extravasated into the duodenum (arrows). (C) After partial embolization with Gelfoam, contrast-medium extravasation is still present (arrow). (D) Control after final embolization shows that bleeding has stopped because of the occlusion of the gastroduodenal artery and its branches.

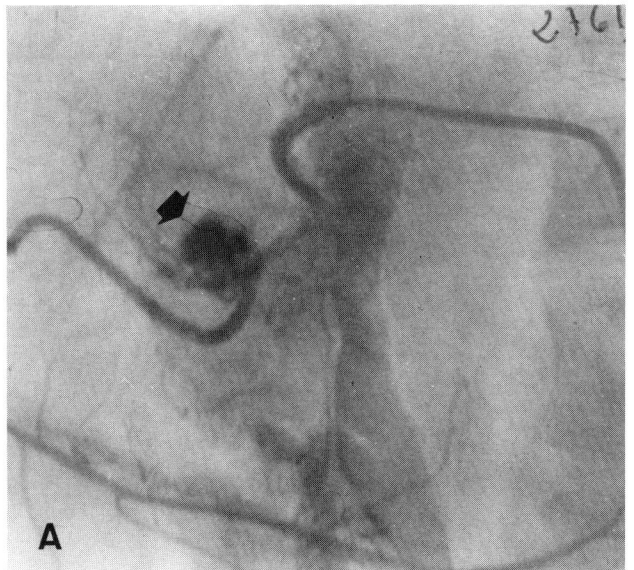
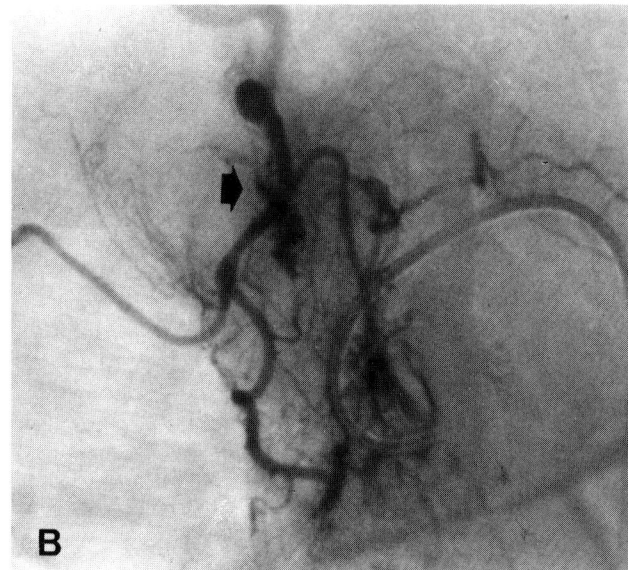
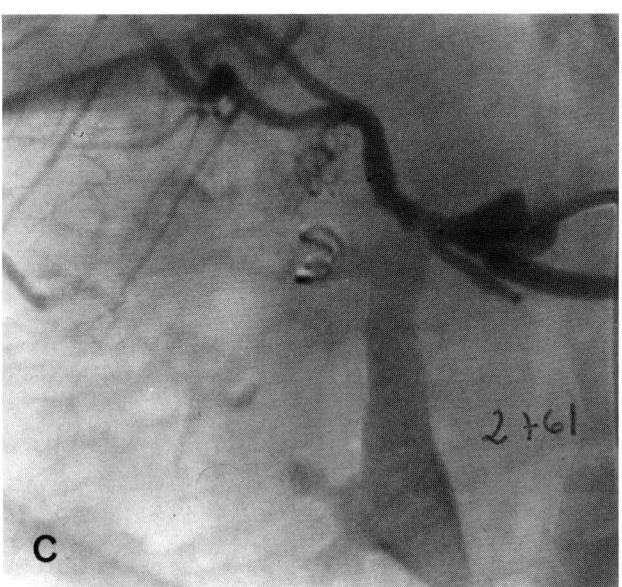

Figure 3.14 Bleeding from a duodenal ulcer discovered by injection into both duodenal circulations.
(A) Injection into the gastroduodenal artery shows extravasation of contrast medium into the duodenum (arrow). (B) Injection into the inferior duodenopancreatic arch, a branch of the superior mesenteric artery, showing the bleeding (arrow). (C) Control in the celiac axis after embolization of both arteries, with bleeding stopped. Gianturco coils and Gelfoam particles were used.

Alternatives to Gelfoam include Gianturco coils, which are used to accomplish a more permanent proximal occlusion (Fig. 3.15), and the use of a fluid, fast-polymerizing embolizing material (bucrylate) that can reach a more distal circulation (Figs. 3.16 and 3.17). Gelfoam has shown good results from an angiographic standpoint in 72 percent of cases, but the clinical rate of success in controlling hemorrhage during a hospital stay is only 44 percent.

There are at least two explanations for this discrepancy. First, hemorrhage from a duodenal ulcer is frequently caused by a large opening in the arterial wall, as opposed to distal arteriolar or intramucosal bleeding in other areas, and consequently is difficult to control. Second, the double circulation in the duodenum, which originates from the celiac axis and the superior mesenteric artery, requires special care, including the occlusion of branches in both arteries, to achieve hemostasis. For these reasons, there has been considerable improvement in the clinical results obtained with embolization when bucrylate has been used to treat duodenal hemorrhage.

A recent study reported that clinical success improved

Figure 3.15 (A,B) Injection into the celiac axis shows active bleeding in the duodenum (arrow) caused by a peptic ulcer. (C) Superselective catheterization of the gastroduodenal artery just before embolization, not showing the low-output bleeding. (D) Control after embolization with Gelfoam and Gianturco coils, showing occlusion of the gastroduodenal artery. Bleeding has stopped.

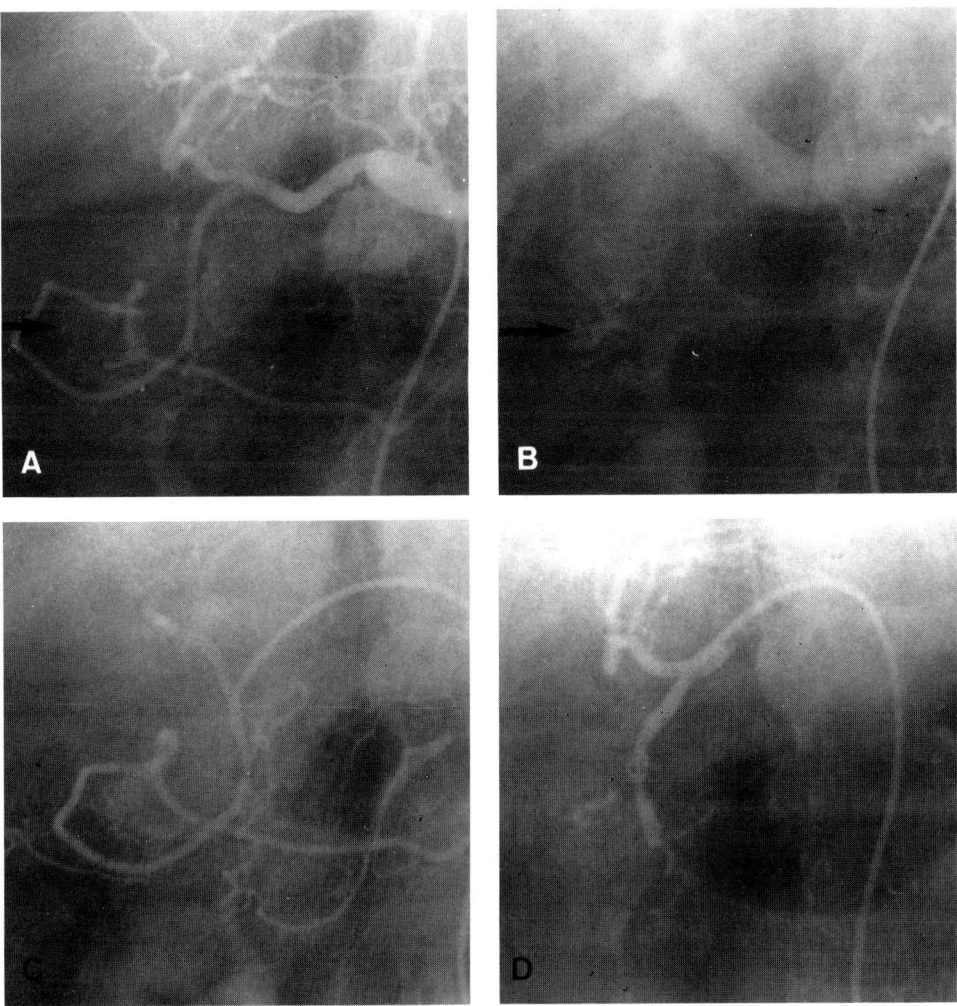

from 33 to 44 percent to 85 percent of cases when bucrylate was used as the embolization agent, and bucrylate is now the method of choice for treating bleeding duodenal ulcers in high-risk patients. Vasopressin has practically been excluded from the treatment armamentarium because of the low level of positive results and the relatively high risk of complications associated with its use.

OTHER SITUATIONS ASSOCIATED WITH UPPER GASTROINTESTINAL BLEEDING

Conditions causing upper GI bleeding other than those already described here are rare, and one must pay careful attention to identify the lesions and select the best method of embolization therapy for each type. The problem caused by the double circulation in the duodenum in regard to the management of bleeding in this area must be mentioned here. Because the direction of flow inside the anastomotic arcades is reversible, when bleeding originates from a branch of these arcades, the hemodynamics becomes very complex. This feature makes the identification of the point of bleeding more difficult and detracts from the results obtained with transcatheter therapy.

Four types of flow artifacts can be identified:

1. Artifact due to contrast injection under pressure
2. Flow reversal caused by catheter-induced spasm
3. Proximal vasoconstriction and changes in flow dynamics caused by vasopressin infusion
4. Collaterals around an embolic occlusion

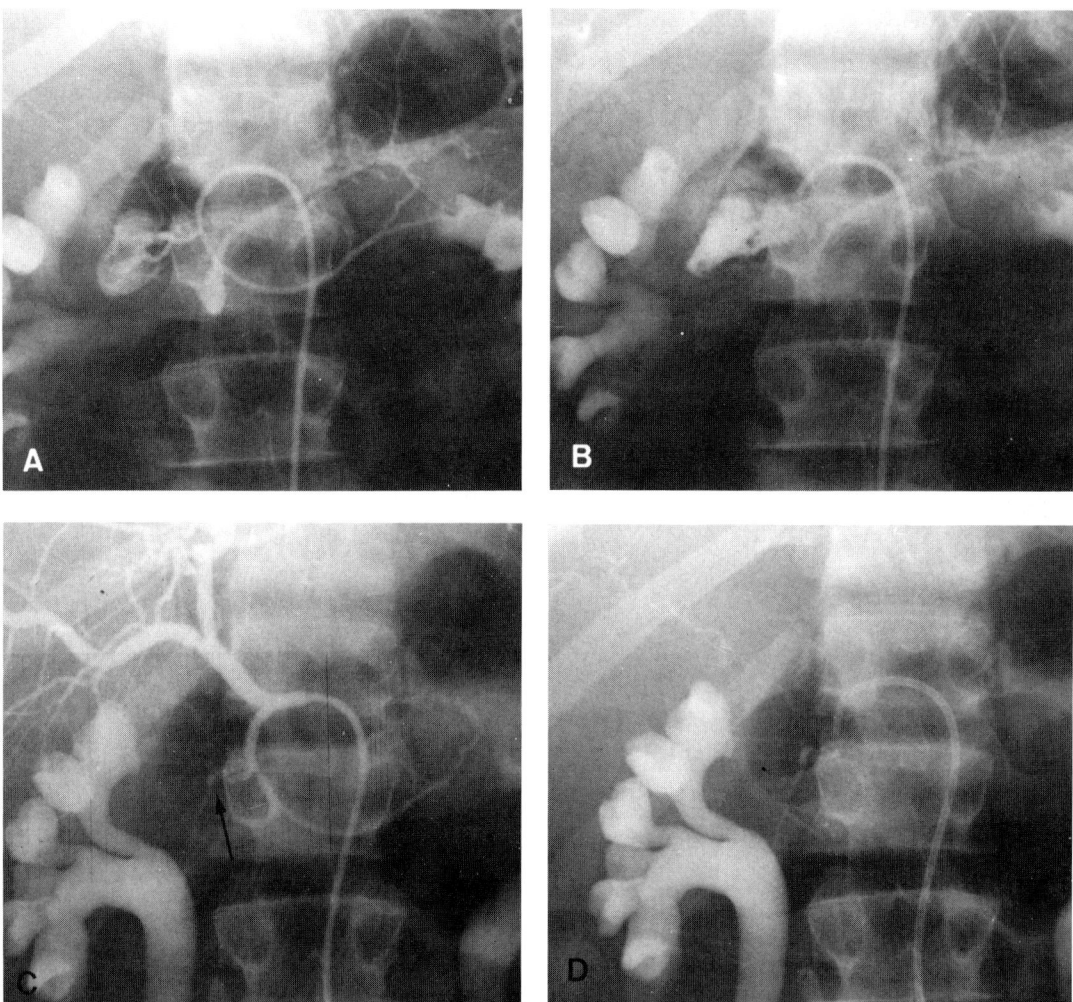

Figure 3.16 (A,B) Duodenal bleeding caused by an ulcer eroding the pancreatic arteries (branches of the dorsal pancreatic artery). (C) Control after embolization with bucrylate, with a view of occlusion in the duodenopancreatic arches (arrow). (D) Plain x-ray showing radiopaque bucrylate in the pancreatic arteries. Bleeding was permanently controlled. Bucrylate is indicated in patients with bleeding of pancreatic origin.

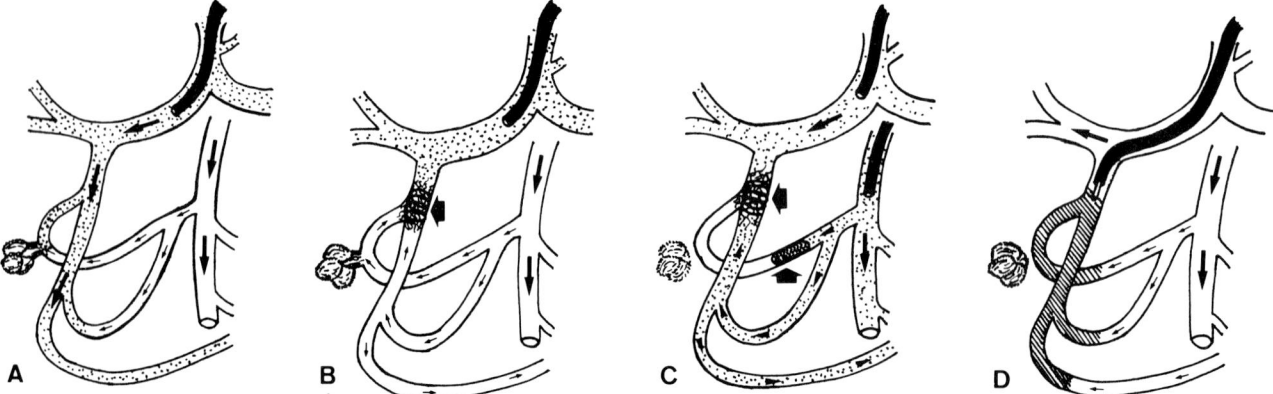

Figure 3.17 Injection of contrast material under pressure into one of the extremities of the vascular arches may exacerbate the flow and erroneously locate origin of bleeding, which actually originates from another artery.
(A) Injection into the hepatic artery shows the main flow (arrows) and contrast-medium extravasation in the superior posterior duodenopancreatic arch. (B) After a relatively central occlusion of the gastroduodenal artery with a coil (thicker arrow), bleeding continues through the lower branches of the vascular arch, which are supplied by the superior mesenteric artery. (C) To control bleeding effectively, it is necessary to superselectively occlude the other portion of the arch (thick arrows). (D) Another way of solving this problem is to use an embolizing fluid such as bucrylate, which will occlude all branches of the duodeno-pancreatic arches, effectively preventing bleeding.

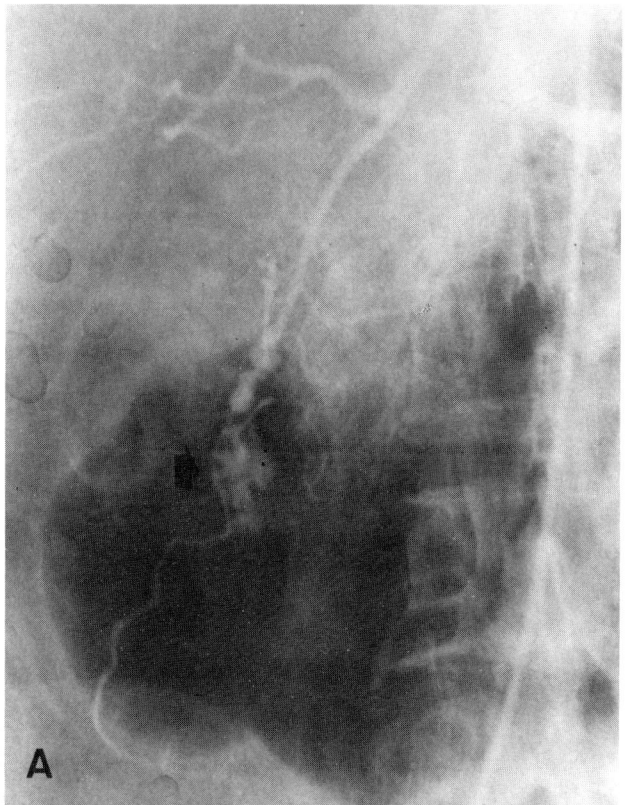 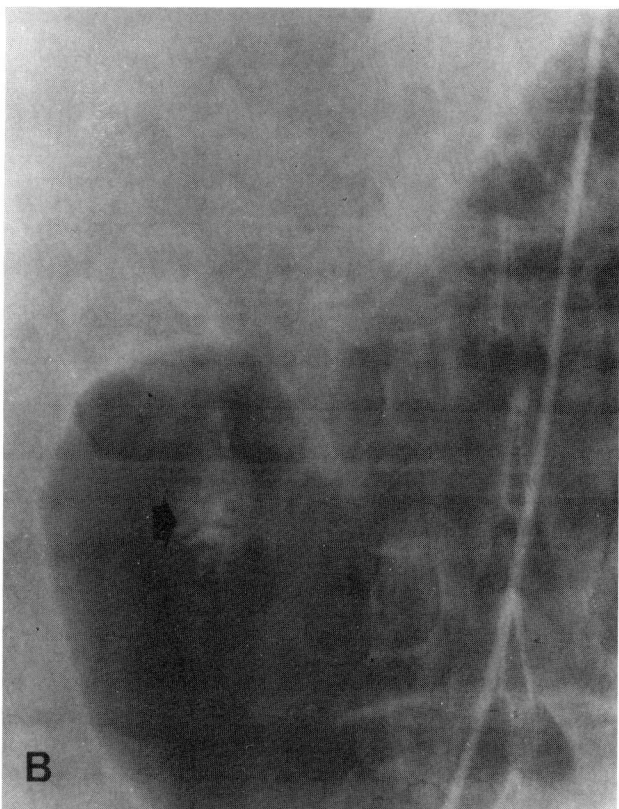

Figure 3.18 A clinical case showing the importance of double embolization in duodenal bleeding because of the doubleness of circulation through the pancreaticoduodenal arches.
(A) Injection into the hepatic artery shows duodenal bleeding after endoscopic papillotomy was performed (arrow). (B) In a later stage of arterial injection, contrast-medium extravasation persists in the duodenal lumen (arrow). (C) Control after embolization with Gelfoam of the gastroduodenal artery; bleeding has apparently been controlled. (D) Injection into the superior mesenteric artery shows that bleeding has persisted through the inferior duodenopancreatic arch. (E) Selective catheterization of the inferior pancreaticoduodenal arch followed by embolization with Gelfoam controlled the bleeding, as seen during control by means of superior mesenteric injection.

The term *vascular arcade* describes an arterial blood supply from two large, independent vessels which may communicate through an ample anastomosis, allowing blood flow in either direction. In the duodenum, the arcades of interest are the superior and inferior pancreaticoduodenal arcades.

Contrast injection under pressure into the common hepatic artery or gastroduodenal artery opacifies the gastroduodenal artery and its branches, usually by inverting the flow in the posterior and anterior superior pancreaticoduodenal branches. This type of injection may reveal bleeding (Fig. 3.17A) during reverse flow; this also applies to injection into the superior mesenteric artery (Fig. 3.14B). Embolization with particulate matter (coil or Gelfoam) which occludes the gastroduodenal artery is not effective in stopping the bleeding permanently (Figs. 3.17B and 3.18, C and D). Superselective embolization of the inferior pancreaticoduodenal arcade is often required, because it occludes the bleeding artery more distally, avoiding retrograde flow (Fig. 3.17D). Figure 3.18 shows the clinical applications of these concepts in particulate embolization.

When vasopressin is infused the same care should be taken. The infusion of a vasoconstricting substance follows the natural distribution of flow, not necessarily reaching the bleeding vessel, whose blood flow may

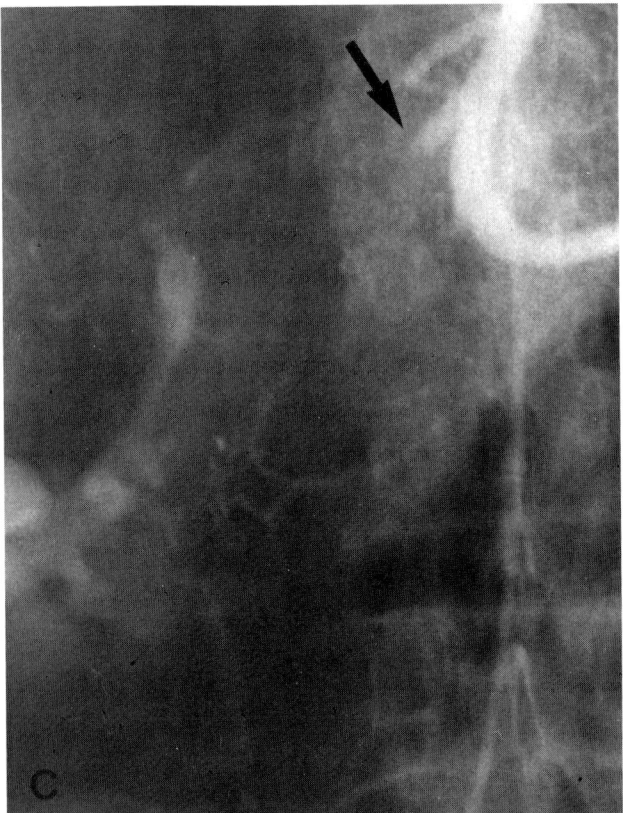

Figure 3.18 *Continued*

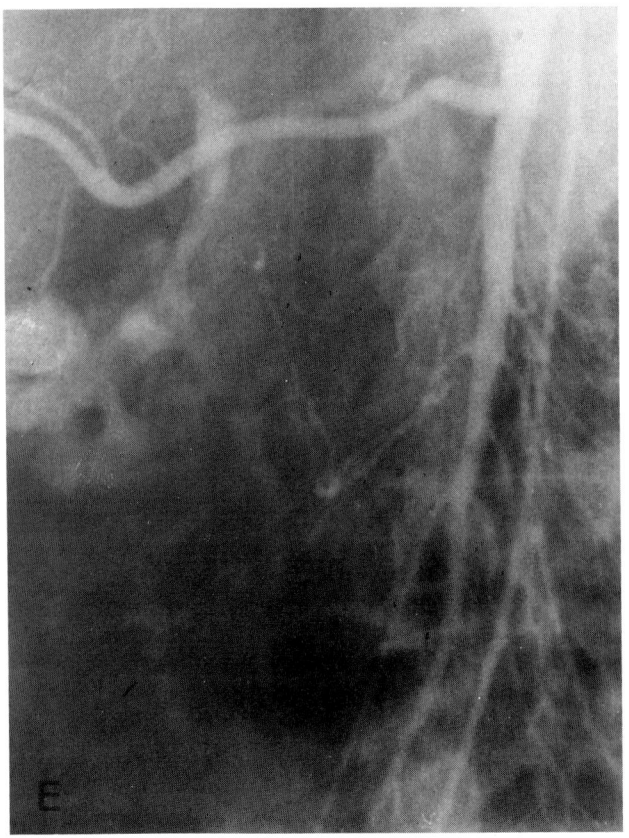

originate from a collateral arcade. Thus bleeding continues in spite of the infusion. One way to overcome this difficulty is to infuse vasopressin into the two main arteries (the celiac and the superior mesenteric).

Most neoplasm bleeding in the stomach is chronic. Certain patients, however, may bleed acutely, requiring treatment by embolization. As a rule these lesions are unresectable because of their size or advanced stage. Furthermore, they do not respond to vasopressin and are better treated with embolotherapy (Fig. 3.19). The lesions may be primary or secondary in the upper GI tract, and their response to embolization may be only temporary while the artery is occluded. The ulcer component of the neoplasm does not heal, and the incidence of bleeding recurrence is quite high.

Hemobilia is not a frequent finding, but when present can be both serious and difficult to diagnose. Hemobilia can cause occult bleeding in patients with closed abdominal trauma as a result of an internal hepatic artery tear with formation of a pseudoaneurysm that communicates into the biliary tree. This condition should be carefully analyzed by means of hepatic angiography.

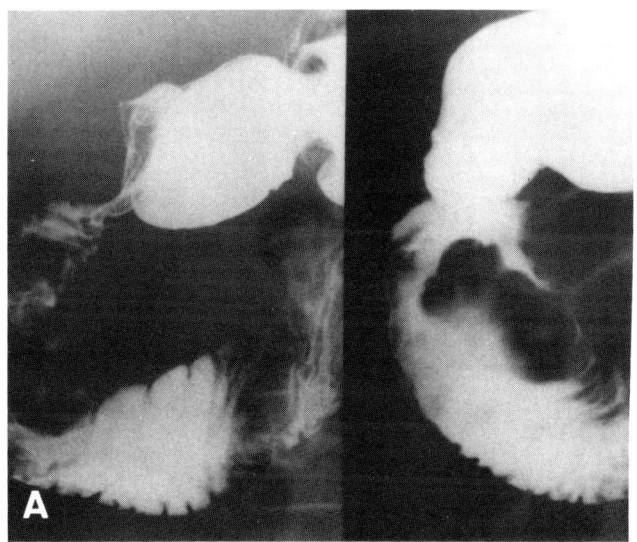
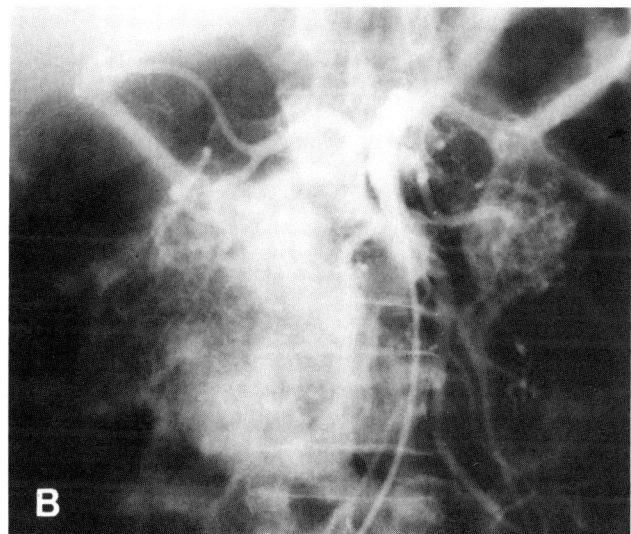
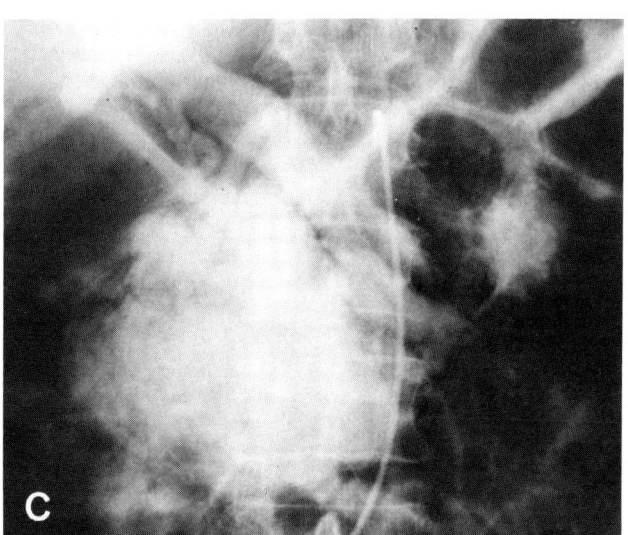
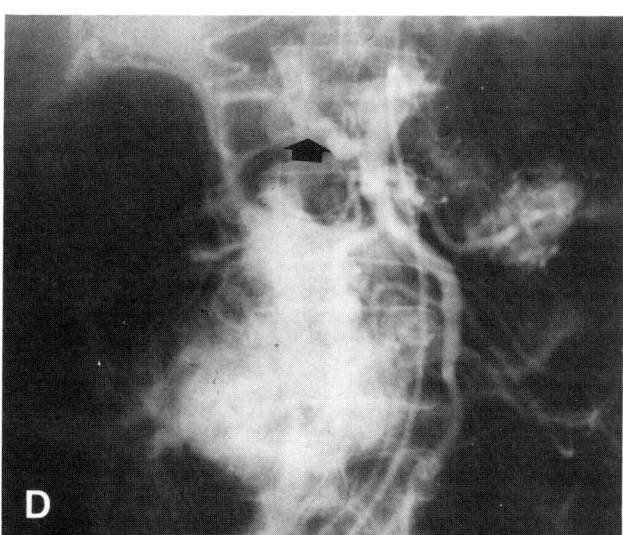
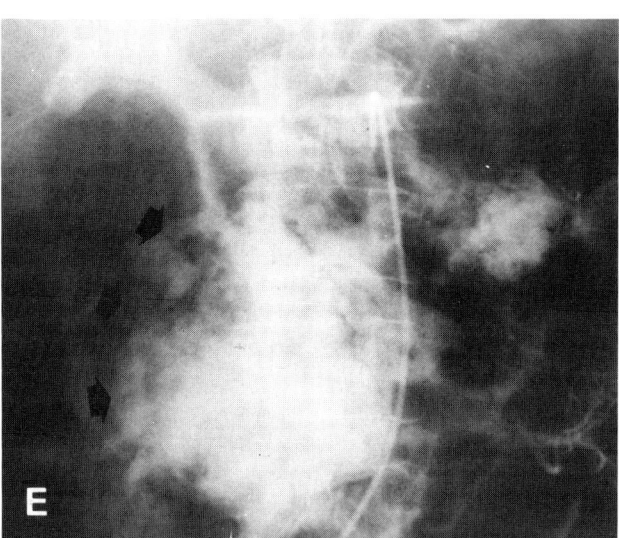

Figure 3.19 A patient with duodenopancreatic metastases of an operated kidney carcinoma, with erosion of the duodenal mucosa and chronic bleeding. There was acute bleeding at examination, although this did not appear in the angiogram.

(A) A barium study of the duodenum shows duodenal infiltration by the tumor mass. (B) Injection into the superior mesenteric shows an abnormal hepatic artery from which the gastroduodenal artery originates, causing dense impregnation of the tumor mass. (C) Later stage of injection shows large, dense impregnation of the tumoral mass and dense venous return. Note a small nodular hypervascular lesion at the root of the mesenterium on the left. (D) Postembolization control of the abnormal hepatic artery and the gastroduodenal artery (arrow). (E) Later stage of injection after embolization shows reduction of contrast impregnation in the duodenal edge of the lesion (arrows). Bleeding was controlled with partial embolization alone. The patient died 6 months after this procedure.

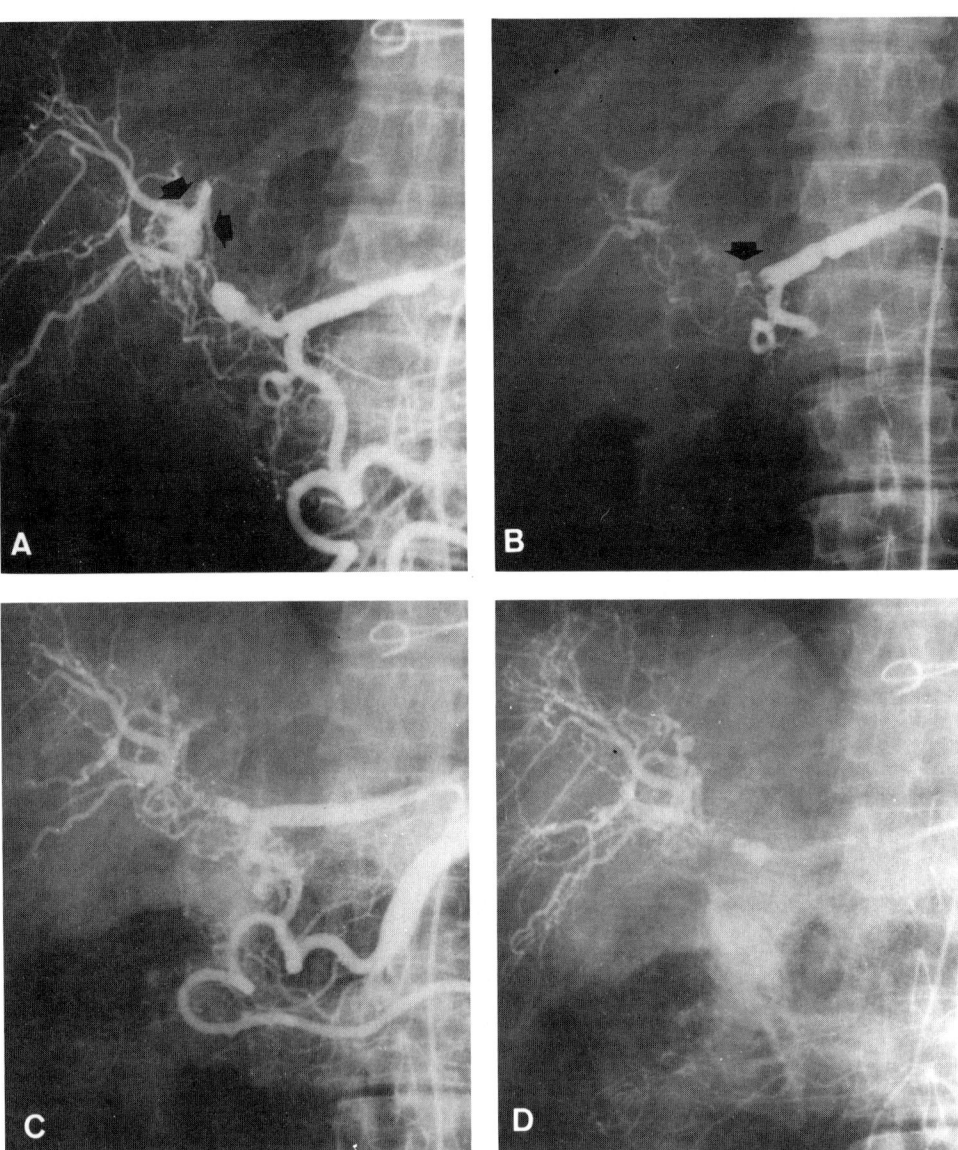

Figure 3.20 This patient with sudden hemobilia received surgery for cholecystectomy and ligation of the hepatic artery. Bleeding recurred.
(A) Injection into the common hepatic artery. Note the partial patency of the proper hepatic artery and fine collateral circulation restoring intrahepatic flow to a certain degree, along with visualization of an intrahepatic aneurysm (arrows). (B) An angiogram after embolization with a Gianturco coil and Gelfoam shows reduction of intrahepatic circulation and only partial refilling of the aneurysm. (C,D) Control angiography 6 months after embolization shows persistence of recanalization of the intrahepatic circulation through fine collaterals, with disappearance of the aneurysm.

Trauma, once the most common cause of hemobilia, has been replaced by hepatic biopsy and percutaneous biliary drainage techniques, which are now the most commonly found causes (Fig. 5.42). Again, the formation of pseudoaneurysms caused by intrahepatic vascular injury is responsible for the bleeding.

Spontaneous hepatic aneurysms and aneurysms of infectious origin (mycotic) are sometimes found. They are usually associated with bacterial endocarditis (Fig. 3.20).

Superselective embolization performed in close proximity to the lesion is the most effective way to treat these patients (Fig. 3.21). Close proximity to the lesion is necessary to avoid the development of collaterals.

Infusion of Vasopressin

Control of nonvariceal upper GI bleeding can be achieved by infusion of vasopressin into the celiac axis, left gastric artery, gastroduodenal artery, or hepatic artery.

Infusion of the left gastric artery is appropriate in patients with bleeding lesions of the cardia and the gastric fundus and body. Pyloroduodenal bleeding can be treated with infusion into the common hepatic artery or the gastroduodenal artery. Infusion into the hepatic artery or splenic artery is used for right gastric artery bleeding and short gastric artery bleeding, respectively.

Infusions of vasopressin into the celiac axis should be avoided because of the low efficacy. Similarly, infusions into the phrenic artery account for occasional

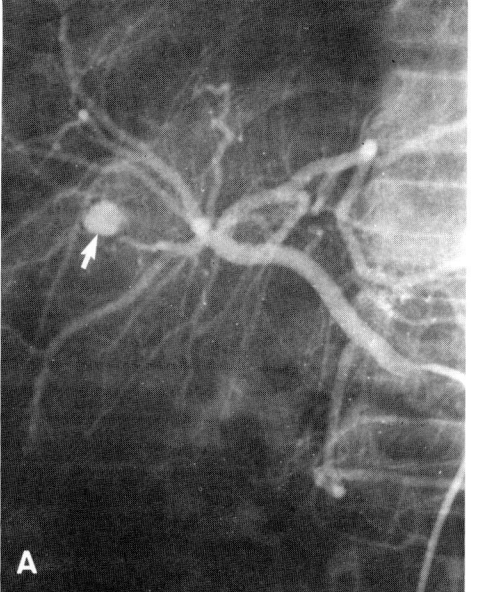
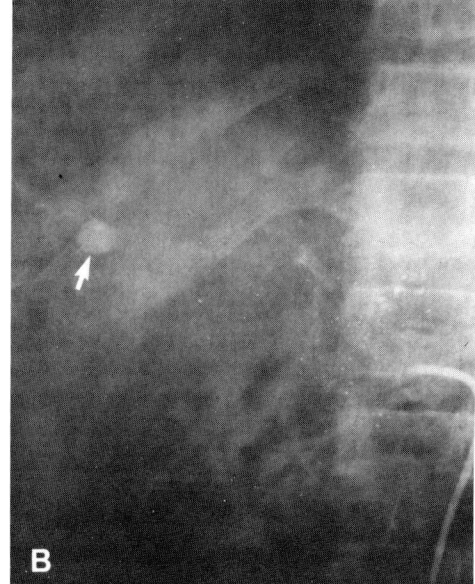
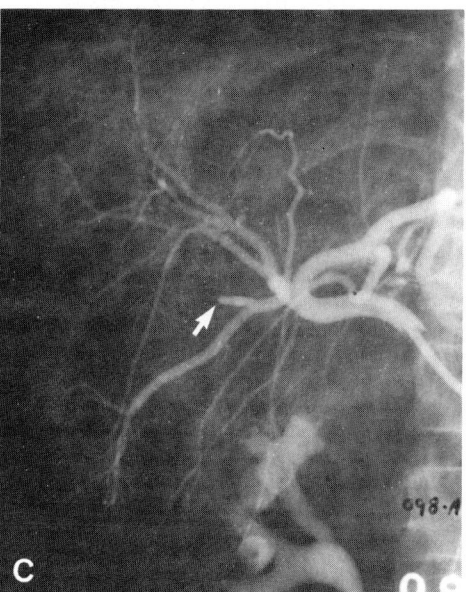

Figure 3.21 A patient with hemobilia after hepatic trauma.
(A,B) Injection into the common hepatic artery shows an intrahepatic pseudoaneurysm (arrow). (C) Angiographic control after superselective occlusion of the artery supplying the lesion (arrow). Bleeding was completely controlled after vessel occlusion.

arrhythmias. Vasopressin is marketed as an oily solution and an aqueous solution. Only the aqueous solution is useful for angiographic therapy. The aqueous solution is supplied in two different concentrations. The 1-mL ampules contain either 10 or 20 vasopressor units. Pitressin doses are calculated in vasopressor units, not milligrams.

The vasopressin solution used for infusion is prepared as 100 IU of vasopressin in 500 mL of normal saline or 5% glucose, yielding a concentration of 0.2 IU/mL. The more concentrated formulation consists of 200 IU of vasopressin in 500 mL of normal saline or 5% glucose, yielding a concentration of 0.4 IU/mL. The injection is made with a continuous arterial infusion pump (an IVAC 530 peristaltic infusion pump) at a velocity of 30 to 60 mL/h, depending on the dose.

Athanasoulis described the following routine for treating GI bleeding with vasopressin infusion:

1. Selective angiogram to demonstrate the bleeding site.
2. Vasopressin infusion at a concentration of 0.2 IU/min for 20 min.
3. Control angiography 20 min after infusion.
4. If no extravasation occurs, the catheter is fixed to the inguinal region with adhesive tape (Micropore), and the patient is then transferred to the intensive care unit (ICU), where the infusion is continued.
5. If extravasation can still be seen, the dose is doubled

to 0.4 IU/min for another 20 min. A new control angiogram is performed after this period.

6. Increasing the vasopressin dose is useless if bleeding has not been controlled. An alternative therapeutic method, such as embolization or surgery, should be considered.

7. If the initial effective dose is 0.2 IU/min the following protocol should be followed:
   –Vasopressin 0.2 IU/min for 24 h
   –Vasopressin 0.1 IU/min for 24 h
   Discontinue if there is no further evidence of GI bleeding.
   If the initial effective dose is 0.4 IU/min, the following protocol should be followed:
   –Vasopressin 0.4 IU/min for 6 to 8 h
   –Vasopressin 0.3 IU/min for 16 h
   –Vasopressin 0.2 IU/min for 16 h
   –Vasopressin 0.1 IU/min for 16 h
   Discontinue if there is no evidence of further GI bleeding.

8. When rebleeding occurs during infusion, it is likely that the selective catheter has been displaced from the infused vessel. The catheter position may be checked with plain x-ray film taken with portable equipment in the ICU, with injection of contrast. If the catheter has been displaced, the patient should be taken back to the angiography laboratory and the catheter should be repositioned or replaced.

Complications due to the use of vasopressin can be minor or major. Major complications are those in which interruption of treatment becomes mandatory. Minor complications can be tolerated or overcome; they are mainly due to the effects of the drug. Minor complications are related to the presence of cardiac arrhythmias, oliguria, hyponatremia, pulmonary edema, and peripheral acrocyanosis. All these are reversible changes that are relatively easy to control.

Major complications include myocardial infarction, severe cardiac arrhythmia, uncontrolled hypertension, intestinal ischemia and infarction, gangrene in the extremities, cerebral edema, femoral thrombosis (at the puncture site), false aneurysm, and sepsis.

Percutaneous Embolization

Embolization should begin at a peripheral site, using small particles of embolizing material to avoid the development of collateral circulation to the area involved. In the digestive tract, however, the particles used should not be so small as to produce capillary occlusion, which can cause mural infarction. The use of Gelfoam powder has been discontinued for this reason.

After a more peripheral occlusion, a more proximal occlusion of the involved vessel can be performed with larger particles, coils, or bucrylate. To prevent tissue infarction, infusion of vasopressin should not be done after embolization. The protocol for embolization to treat GI hemorrhage is as follows:

1. Selective angiogram showing the location of bleeding.
2. An attempt may or may not be made to infuse vasoconstricting drugs.
3. Embolization with small Gelfoam particles (less than 0.5 mm in diameter).
4. Frequent control of the extent of embolization with fluoroscopy.
5. Embolization with large Gelfoam particles (1.0 mm) or coils (optional).
6. Control angiography.
7. Removal of the catheter and inguinal compression.

Embolization for the treatment of GI bleeding should be done with medium-term, absorbable easy-to-handle materials which instantaneously occlude the embolized vessel by adjusting its size to the vascular territory being treated. The material most suitable to these conditions is a gelatin sponge (Gelfoam). In the duodenal area, however, bucrylate is the material of choice in some situations because it achieves a more complete occlusion of collaterals.

Complications of embolization were discussed in Chap. 2.

REFERENCES

Allison DJ, Hemingway AP, Cunningham DA. Angiography in gastrointestinal bleeding. *Lancet* 1982; 3:30.33.

Athanasoulis CA. Upper gastrointestinal bleeding of arteriocapillary origin. In *Interventional Radiology,* edited by Athanasoulis CA, Pfister RC, Greene RE, Roberson GH. Saunders, Philadelphia, 1982:55–89.

Baun S, Athanasoulis CA, Waltman AC, Ring EJ. Angiographic diagnosis and control. *Adv Surg* 1973;7:149–198.

Dantas JC. Arteriografia selectiva no diagnostico das hemorragias digestivas arterials agudas: Revisao da literatura. *Radiol Bras* 1977;10:51–58.

Feldman L, Greenfield AJ, Waltman AC, Noveline RA, Breda AV, Luers P, Athanasoulis CA. Transcatheter vessel occlusions: Angiographic results versus clinical success. *Radiology* 1983;147:1–5.

Gregory PB, Kanuer M, Fogel MR, Andres LL, Rinki MM, Walker JE. Upper gastrointestinal bleeding: Accuracy of clinical diagnosis and prognosis. *Dig Dis Sci* 1981;26:65–69.

Herlinger H. Other diagnostic approaches to upper gastrointestinal bleeding: Utility of contrast radiology. *Dig Dis Sci* 1981;26:76–77.

Kadir S, Athanasoulis CA. Angiographic management of gastrointestinal bleeding with vasopressin. *Fortschr Roentgenstr* 1977;127:111–115.

Larson DE, Farnell MB. Upper gastrointestinal hemorrhage. *Mayo Clin Proc* 1983;58:371–387.

Law DH, Watts HD. Gastrointestinal bleeding. In *Gastrointestinal Disease,* edited by Sleisenger MH, Fardtran JS. Saunders, Philadelphia, 1985:217–240.

Martin EC, Casarella WJ, Schultz RW. Angiographic management of arterial hemorrhage in the upper gastrointestinal tract. In *Interventional Radiology,* edited by Wilins RA, Viamonte M. Blackwell, Oxford, 1982:81–99.

McLean GK, Oleaga JA, Freiman DB, Ring EJ. Angiographic management of bleeding and transcatheter vascular occlusion techniques. In *Interventional Radiology: Principles and Techniques,* edited by Ring EJ, McLean GK. Little, Brown, Boston, 1981:1–117.

Reuter SR, Redman HC, Cho KJ. Gastrointestinal bleeding. In *Gastrointestinal Angiography,* edited by Reuter SR, Redman HC, Cho KJ. Saunders, Philadelphia, 1977:218–268.

Ring EJ, Oleaga JA, Freiman D, Husted JW, Waltman AC, Baum S. Pitfalls in angiographic management of hemorrhage: Hemodynamic considerations. *AJR* 1977;129:1007–1013.

Rosch J, Dotter CT, Rose RW. Selective arterial infusions of vasoconstrictors in acute gastrointestinal bleeding. *Radiology* 1971;99:27–36.

Sedgwick CE, Reale VF. Upper gastrointestinal bleeding: Diagnosis and treatment. *Surg Clin North Am* 1976;56:695–707.

Steer ML, Silen W. Diagnostic procedures in gastrointestinal hemorrhage. N Engl J Med 1983;309:646–650.

Uflacker R, Alves MA, Diehl JC. Gastrointestinal involvement in neurofibromatosis: Angiographic presentation. *Gastrointest Radiol* 1985;10:163–165.

Uflacker R, Amaral NM, Lima S, Wholey MH, Pereira EC, Nobrega M, Tavares T. Angiography in primary myomas of the alimentary tract. *Radiology* 1981;139:361–369.

LOWER GASTROINTESTINAL BLEEDING

Lower GI bleeding by definition originates below the ligament of Treitz in the small or large intestine. It may appear as an exsanguinating hemorrhage or in the form of repetitive bleeding episodes.

Surgical treatment is difficult in these patients. Inspection and palpation are usually negative, and blind surgical excisions are too extensive to be well tolerated by severely debilitated patients. When the origin of bleeding from diverticula in a universal diverticulosis is not known, the only option is to perform a colectomy, which involves morbidity and mortality rates as high as 20 to 50 percent in emergency cases.

It is thus desirable to know the location of the bleeding preoperatively and to use the least invasive interventional technique which can control bleeding. Diagnostic techniques such as scintigraphy and angiography should be used, and therapeutic measures such as vasopressin infusion and percutaneous embolization should be performed. The goal should be to replace an urgent intervention with elective surgery or even to prevent surgery altogether.

The most common cause of lower GI bleeding is diverticulitis, a condition frequently found in elderly patients. Mortality rates from GI bleeding in this age group can be as high as 26 percent, while in younger patients the rate rarely exceeds 13 percent, according to a series published in 1981 that included 136 patients.

In patients with lower GI bleeding, regardless of the nature of the causative lesion, an arteriogram is always performed to localize the bleeding. It is also necessary to obtain temporary or permanent control of the hemorrhage by infusing vasoconstricting agents or performing embolization.

Two main situations may occur in patients with lower GI bleeding: (1) massive intermittent or small-volume chronic repetitive bleeding and (2) massive acute bleeding.

Massive Intermittent or Small-Volume Chronic Bleeding

Included in this group are patients with either several high-volume bleeding episodes or patients with small chronic blood losses who require iron replacement and, occasionally, blood transfusions. A range of intestinal lesions may be associated with these types of bleeding. In these patients a sequence of procedures should be followed to demonstrate the primary cause of bleeding before a more invasive angiographic test is done. Interventional techniques are used less often in this group of patients. Because the site of extravasation cannot be seen, angiography should be used electively in this patient group to search for an anatomic lesion that may bleed. All the splanchnic vessels should be included in the study. Angiodysplasias, malformations, and tumors are the most common causes of this problem.

Massive Acute Bleeding

A few measures should be adopted prior to and during the angiographic procedure to ensure the efficacy of treatment and protect the patient. First, shock should be treated by means of volume replacement. Second, the bleeding level should be determined. Third, the bleeding spot should be identified precisely. Fourth, an attempt should be made to control bleeding through vasopressin infusion or embolization.

Volume replacement, shock treatment, and maintenance of airway patency are priorities. These clinical measures should be done by the team taking care of the patient, with the radiologist serving as a member of the team. A large-gauge venous line for infusion and a Foley catheter for emptying the bladder should be available. To determine the level of bleeding, the measures listed for upper GI bleeding earlier in this chapter should be adopted.

A thorough evaluation of the inferior and superior mesenteric arteries in addition to the celiac axis may be necessary. The inferior mesenteric is injected with a flow rate of 4 mL/s for a volume of 20 mL. The superior mesenteric requires a volume of 40 to 50 mL at a flow rate of 5 to 6 mL/s.

Infusion of Vasoconstricting Agents

To control GI bleeding, a vasoconstricting agent should be injected into the trunk of the bleeding vessel, either the superior mesenteric artery or the inferior mesenteric artery (Fig. 3.22). Superselective injection into the branches of these arteries has not shown additional effectiveness except in cases of ulcer in the gastrojejunal anastomotic ostium.

The infusion procedure is similar to the procedure for upper GI bleeding described earlier in this chapter:

1. Selective angiography is performed to locate the bleeding site.
2. 100 units of vasopressin in 500 mL of normal saline or 5% glucose in a concentration of 0.2 IU/ml is used. Two hundred units of vasopressin in 500 mL of saline will produce a concentration of 0.4 IU/ml.
3. Infusion with a continuous arterial infusion pump at 30 to 60 mL/h is done.
4. Begin tentatively with 0.2 IU/min for 20 min.
5. After 20 min of infusion, control serial angiography is performed to check the effectiveness of the infusion. If bleeding is under control, the infusion is continued in the ICU at 0.2 IU/min for 24 h and then at 0.1 IU/min for another 24 h. The infusion is discontinued if there is no evidence of bleeding.

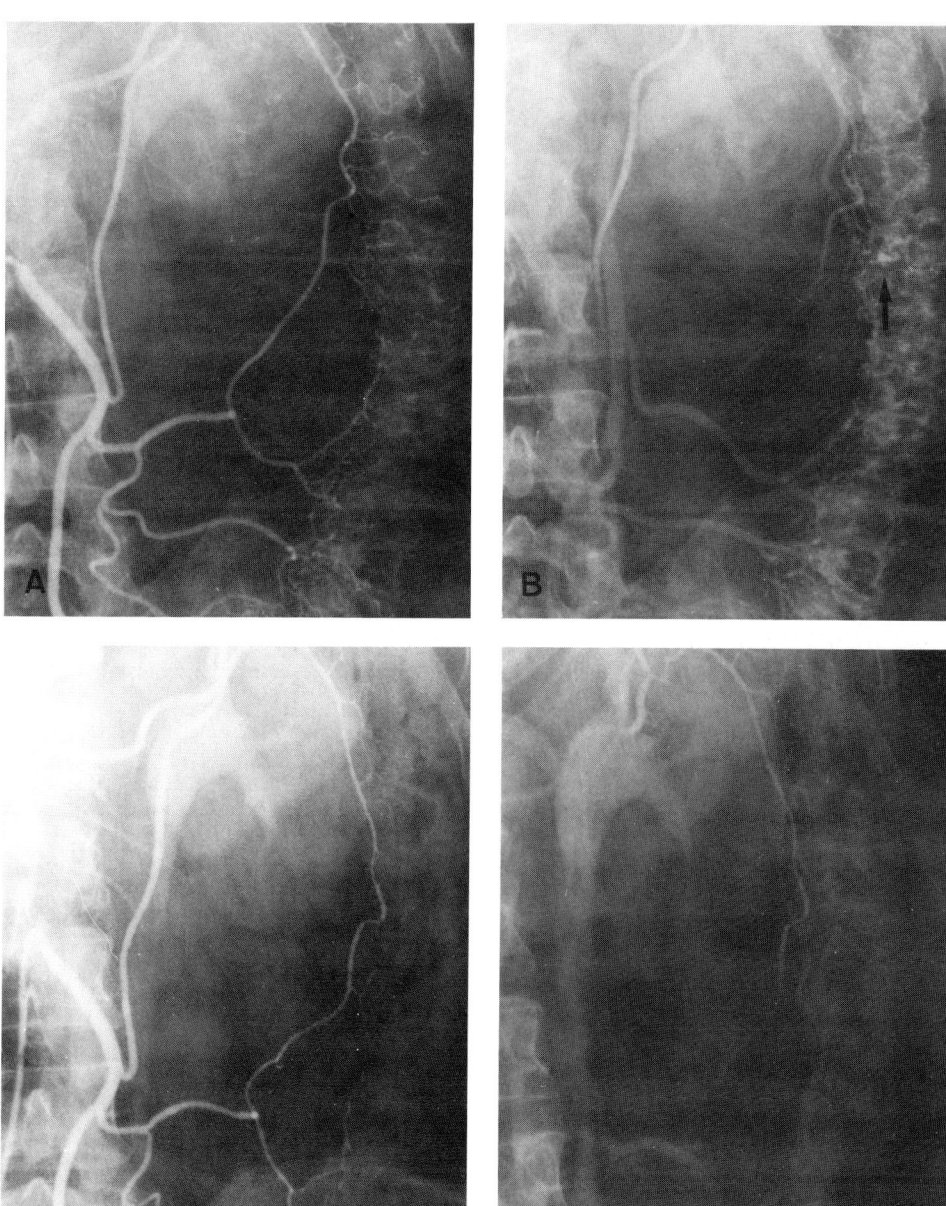

Figure 3.22 A 75-year-old patient who presented with colonic diffuse diverticulosis and lower gastrointestinal bleeding.
(A) Selective injection into the inferior mesenteric artery, early phase. (B) Later phase of injection into the inferior mesenteric artery shows an area of contrast extravasation in the descending colon diverticulum (arrow). (C) A control angiogram 20 min after the infusion of 0.4 IU/min vasopressin shows significant vasoconstriction of straight arteries in the descending colon and sigmoid colon. (D) Later phase shows bleeding control and significant reduction in impregnation of the colon wall. After the infusion was discontinued, bleeding was controlled definitively.

6. If extravasation continues after the first 20 min, the dose should be doubled to 0.4 IU/min for another 20 min. If this is effective, infusion should proceed at the same rate in the ICU for 6 to 8 h and then at 0.3 IU/min for 16 h, 0.2 IU/min for 16 h, and finally 0.1 IU/min for 16 h. The infusion is discontinued if bleeding stops.

If an infusion dose of 0.4 IU has proved to be ineffective, increasing the dose above this level will be useless.

When the right hepatic artery is replaced, the tip of the catheter should be advanced beyond its origin inside the superior mesenteric artery so that a portion of the infusion is not lost into the hepatic circulation.

During the infusion, the patient usually has abdominal pain with cramps, causing the evacuation of blood clots and blood from the intestine; this produces a false impression of increased bleeding activity. Cramps should disappear after 20 to 30 min; if this does not happen, the position of the catheter should be checked and/or the dose should be lowered.

The patient should receive permanent monitoring of

cardiac function and vital signs, since there is a tendency for the development of cardiac arrhythmias and blood pressure elevation.

During infusion, the catheter should remain fixed with Micropore-type adhesive tape onto the skin or should be sutured to the inguinal region. During noninfusion intervals, simple normal saline should be injected through the pump to prevent catheter occlusion.

Development of coronary ischemia is one of the most severe complications caused by vasopressin. It should be promptly recognized.

The physician must be aware that vasopressin has an antidiuretic effect. Thus oliguria should be corrected with a furosemide-type diuretic.

Embolization

Embolization is an alternative to surgery for controlling lower GI bleeding. Even though this technique has been widely used for bleeding lesions of the upper GI tract, it has been almost totally avoided in the treatment of bleeding of the small intestine and colon because of the possibility of inducing serious ischemic infarction.

Many different clinical trials, however, have shown that the incidence of lower bowel ischemic lesions is relatively low and that this method can be highly effective. The prevailing opinion among many authors is that embolization has a high degree of efficacy in achieving both short- and long-term control. This is not, however, a universal concept. Many authors have suggested that embolization should not be used in the mesenteric territory or that it should be used only as an ultimate alternative.

After bleeding has been stopped, the patient is monitored, blood volume is replaced, and electrolyte balance is restored. A waiting period of 3 to 4 days is needed to confirm or exclude the presence of infarction of the bowel loop. Control by means of daily plain abdomen x-rays is recommended to identify signs of irreversible intestinal ischemic damage. Gas appearing on the wall of a loop indicates infarction. Localized dilation, of varying degrees, usually occurs and need merely be observed. When infarction occurs, surgical intervention, directed toward the involved area, should be prompt.

Superselective catheterization of the bleeding segment is necessary in embolizing a mesenteric branch. A guidewire is introduced deep into the distal ileal segments through a diagnostic catheter. The catheter is then advanced on the guidewire. After the guidewire is removed, the catheter is gently pulled till it fits into the bleeding segment and has been identified by test injections. The catheter does not have to be advanced too far into the artery; the introduction of emboli can be done somewhat proximally (Fig. 3.23).

Gelfoam (2 × 2 × 5 mm) or Ivalon emboli are introduced one at a time after the presence of residual bleeding has been documented. When bleeding is under control, the procedure is terminated, and only one injection into the mesenteric trunk is made to document occlusion and the cessation of bleeding. No additional emboli are injected after extravasation has stopped. A more peripheral catheterization may be used when, for example, the bleeding is from the iliocolic artery in a young patient (Fig. 3.24).

Complete occlusion of the bleeding territory is not always necessary; avoiding this procedure can prevent devitalization of the loop wall. In most cases, reducing the blood flow and pressure in the embolized territory is sufficient to allow effective functioning of natural hemostatic mechanisms. Ischemic complications can be minimized by using the lowest possible number of embolic fragments to stop the bleeding.

There are few critical areas, such as the splenic angle of the colon. When the inferior mesenteric artery is occluded, embolization of the middle colic artery will inevitably lead to infarction in the descending colon (Fig. 3.25). This risk is also present when vasopressin infusions are maintained for long periods.

LOWER GASTROINTESTINAL BLEEDING RELATED TO THE SMALL INTESTINE

Inflammatory Disease

Wall hyperemia is the most common finding; in these patients it is associated with arteriovenous shunt and dense opacification of the drainage vein. The clinical example is Crohn's disease. The bleeding can be controlled with intraarterial infusion of vasopressin even when extensive areas are involved.

Nonspecific Ulcerations (Stress, Uremic)

Uremic and transplanted patients develop ulcerative lesions of the small intestine which may bleed profusely. This is superimposed on underlying chronic disease, depleted functions, and systemic arterial hypertension. This combination of factors leads to high morbidity and mortality rates.

These ulcerative lesions should be treated with selective embolization of the branch supplying the bleeding

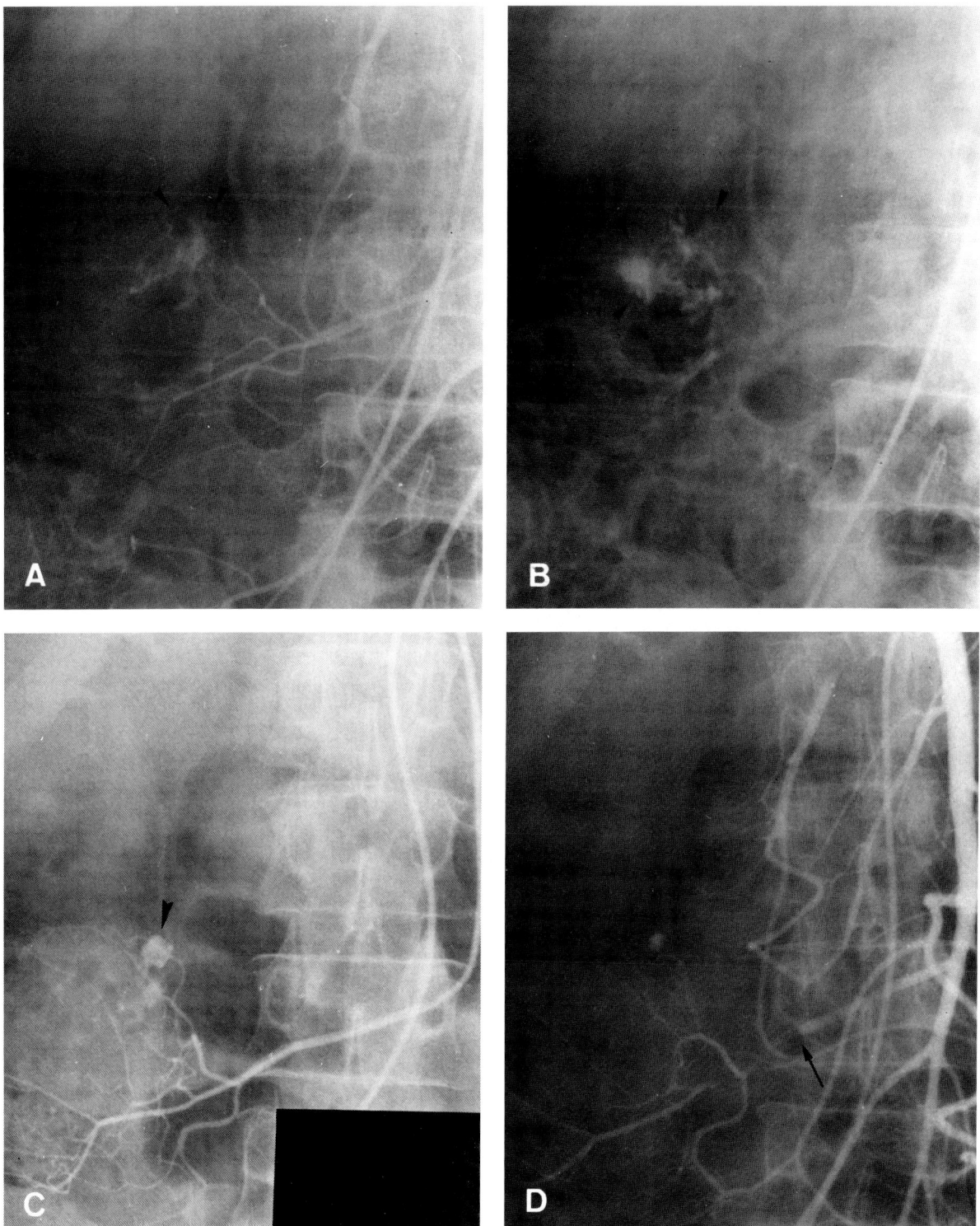

Figure 3.23 A 53-year-old patient with lower gastrointestinal bleeding from a postoperative diverticulum after left hepatectomy for metastasis.
(A) Injection into the superior mesenteric artery shows abundant right colonic bleeding (arrowheads) (B) Later phase of injection shows contrast diffusion into the lumen of the right colon (arrowheads). (C) Superselective injection into the right colic artery, still shows extravasation (arrowhead) into the colonic hepatic angle just before embolization with two Gelfoam emboli. (D) A control angiogram after embolization shows a small amount of residual contrast in the diverticulum, but with bleeding under definitive control.

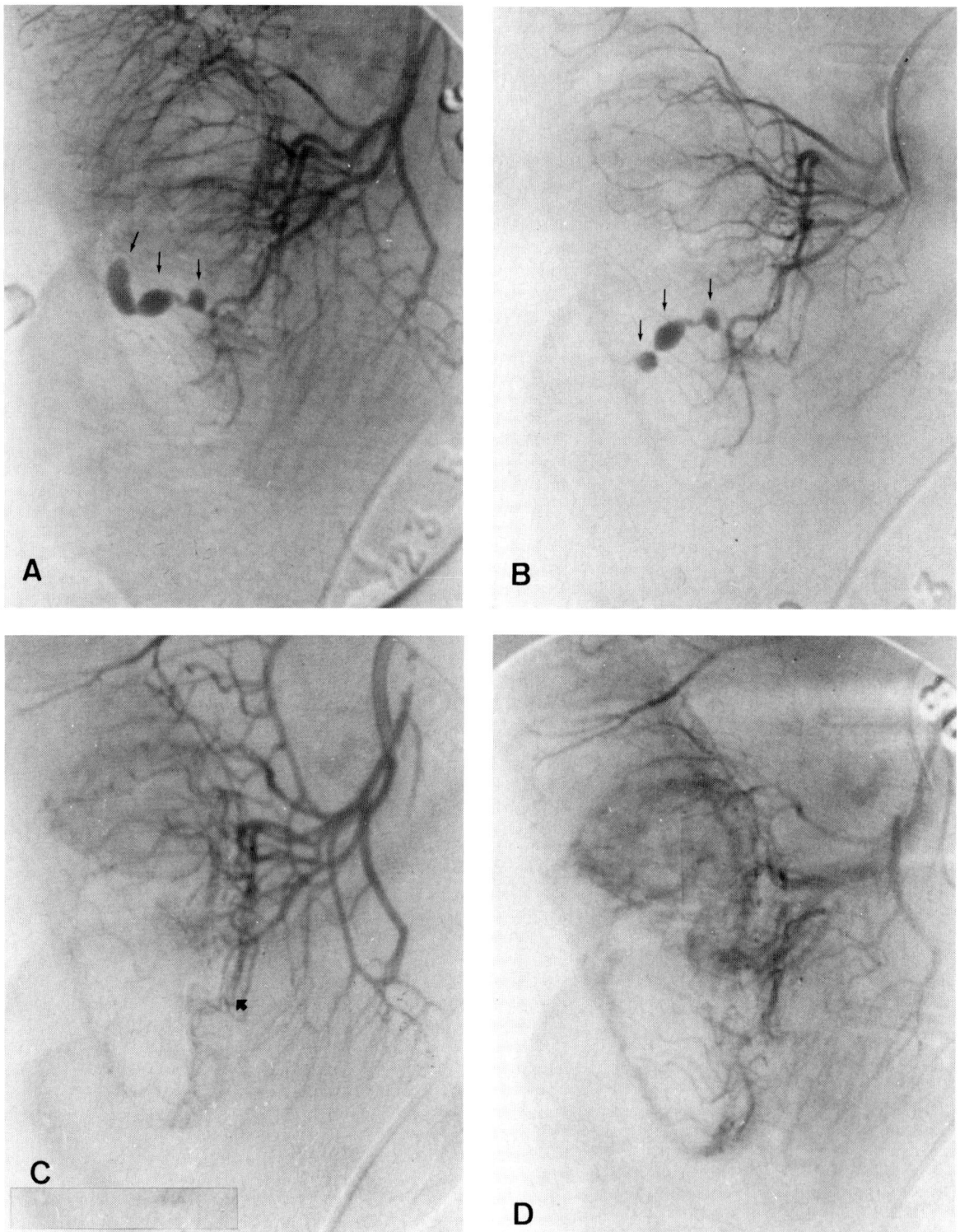

Figure 3.24 A 28-year-old patient with gastrointestinal bleeding after an appendectomy.
(A) Injection at the superior mesenteric artery shows contrast extravasation into the cecum (arrows) originating from the ileocolic artery. (B) Superselective and very peripheral catheterization into the ileocolic artery just before embolization with three Gelfoam pledgets. (C) Postembolization angiogram shows occlusion of the embolized artery and no extravasation of contrast (arrow). (D) Later phase of injection showing inpregnation of the colonic wall and definitive control of the bleeding.

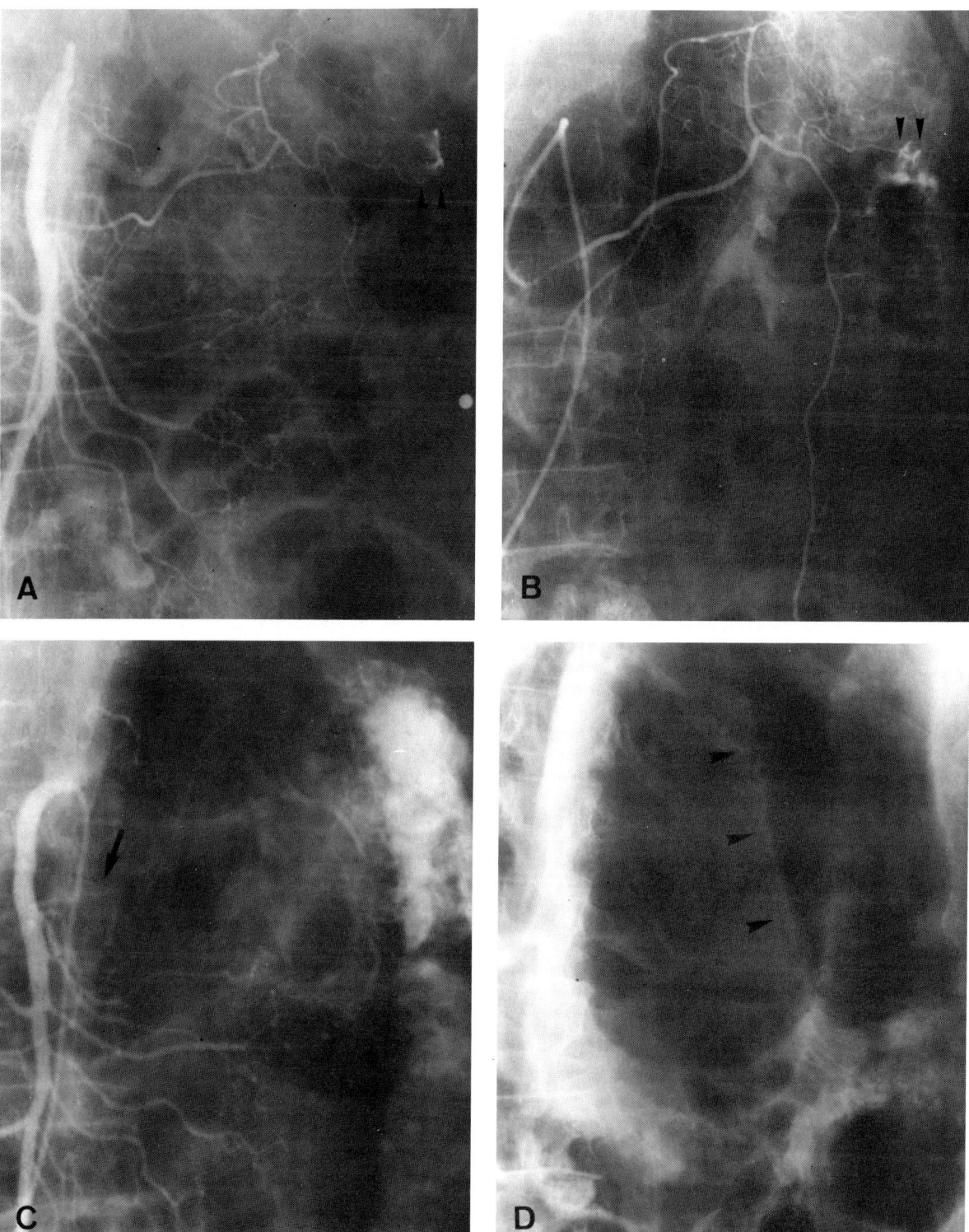

Figure 3.25 A 66-year-old patient with lower gastrointestinal bleeding in hypovolemic shock and unconscious.
(A) Injection into the superior mesenteric artery shows an area of contrast extravasation in the descending colon (arrowheads) through the branches of the middle colic artery. (B) Superselective injection into the middle colic artery shows extravasation into the descending colon just before embolization with Gelfoam. (C) A control angiogram after embolization shows middle colic artery occlusion (arrow) and dense wall impregnation of the colonic splenic angle by contrast medium. (D) As the inferior mesenteric artery was occluded by atheromatosis, infarction of the descending colon developed. Note the air present in the colonic walls (arrowheads) and the significant loop enlargement. Embolization was chosen in agreement with surgeons, since vasopressin was not available at that time and the patient's general condition did not permit surgery. Left hemicolectomy was performed as a semielective procedure 3 days after embolization, with the patient in good general condition.

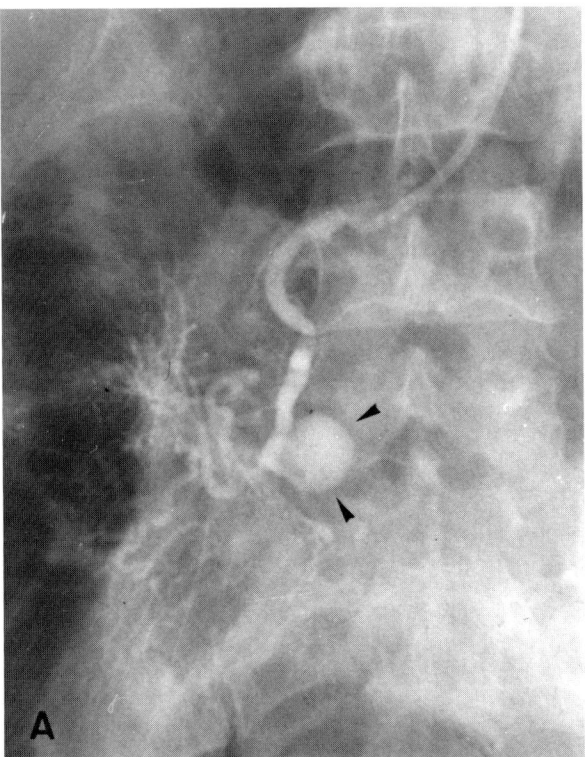 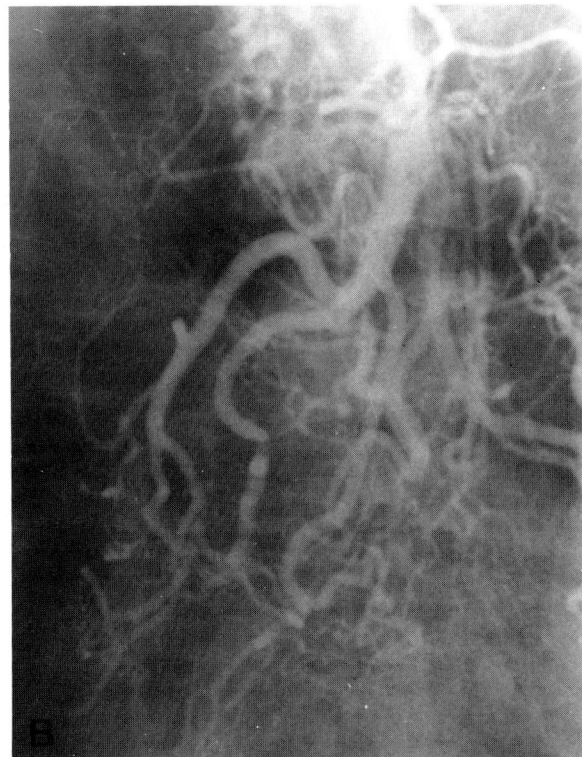

Figure 3.26 An 18-year-old patient, uremic and with lower gastrointestinal bleeding from an ileal ulcer. (A) Superselective injection into the ileal artery, corresponding to abundant bleeding (arrowheads). (B) After embolization with Gelfoam control, showing bleeding arrest. Notice the spasm in some arterial segments.

point (Fig. 3.26). The pathophysiology of such lesions will probably include vascular obstruction with ischemic areas in the mucous membrane (Fig. 3.27).

Vasculitis

Intraluminal bleeding responds well to vasopressin infusion, because the wall musculature contracts. As rupture of a small or large aneurysm is usually the mechanism responsible for bleeding of this type, there is a high possibility of abdominal catastrophe if the bleeding occurs outside the loop, in the mesenteric leaflets. After diagnosis by means of angiography, embolization may be performed and is effective. Most patients, however, should be treated by means of surgical resection. The aneurysmal aspect, as previously mentioned, applies mainly to patients with polyarteritis nodosa. Other types of vasculitis may occur in lymphoproliferative disorders as well as in Wegener's granulomatosis, and the mechanism in these cases is ischemic-type occlusion and ulceration (Fig. 3.28) caused by necrotizing granulomas.

Tumors

From the standpoint of bleeding, leiomyomas are the most important intestinal tumors, even though they are

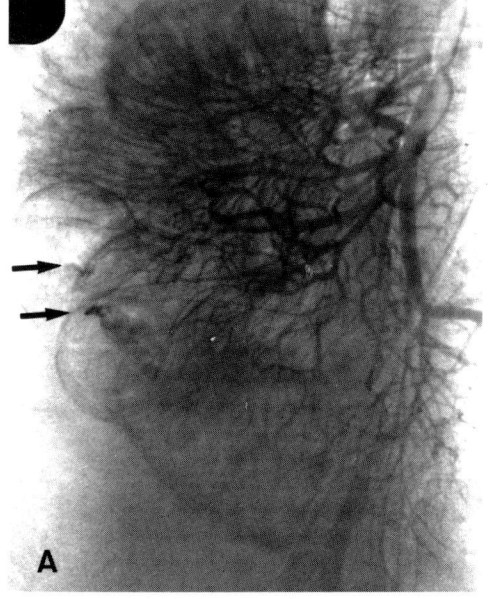
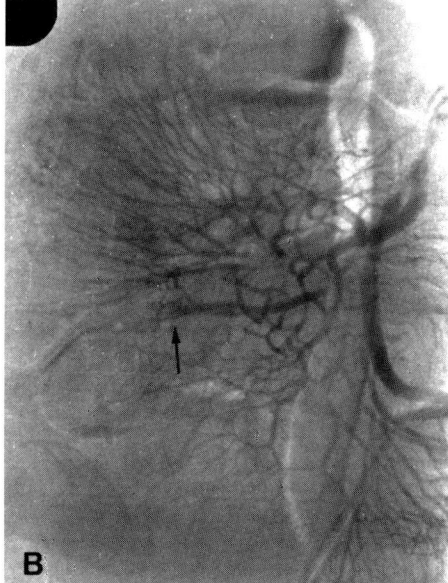
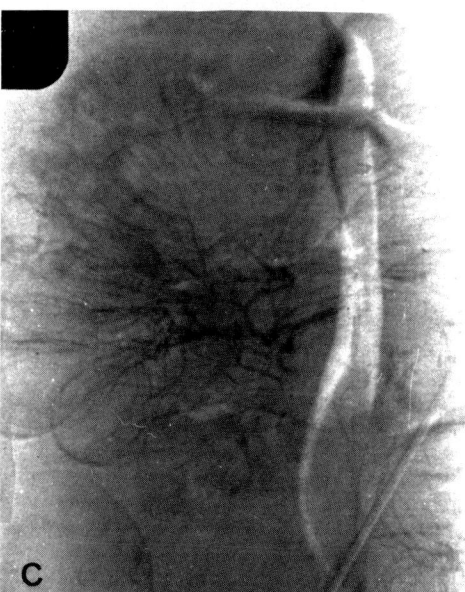

Figure 3.27 A 49-year-old patient with chronic myeloid leukosis for over 6 years during an episode of medullary aplasia and lower gastrointestinal bleeding from ileal ulcerations. (A) Selective injection into ileal arteries shows contrast-medium extravasation (arrows) into the ileal lumen. (B,C) Control after Gelfoam embolization shows bleeding arrest and a small devascularized area in the small intestine (arrow shows occluded artery). Bleeding was controlled, and the patient died 4 months later from pulmonary infection secondary to the immunosuppressive process.

less common than adenomas are. Leiomyosarcomas are next in order of frequency among tumors of the digestive tract.

The clinical presentation of digestive tract myomas, particularly those of the small intestine, is recurrent chronic GI bleeding. Massive bleeding may occasionally occur. These lesions are seldom palpable. Angiography is the technique of choice for diagnosing and locating these tumors.

Angiographic identification of the lesions can be based on a typical and consistent presentation. The findings may include rich vascularization with dense impregnation. A dense drainage vein is usually visualized, suggesting the presence of an arteriovenous (AV) shunt (Fig. 3.29). Arterial invasion is not commonly seen in myomas of the GI tract. The lesions are occasionally hypovascular or present with hypovascular areas. This feature is found more frequently in leiomyosarcomas than in leiomyomas (Fig. 3.30). These lesions usually have well-defined outlines. This contrasts with AV malformations, which

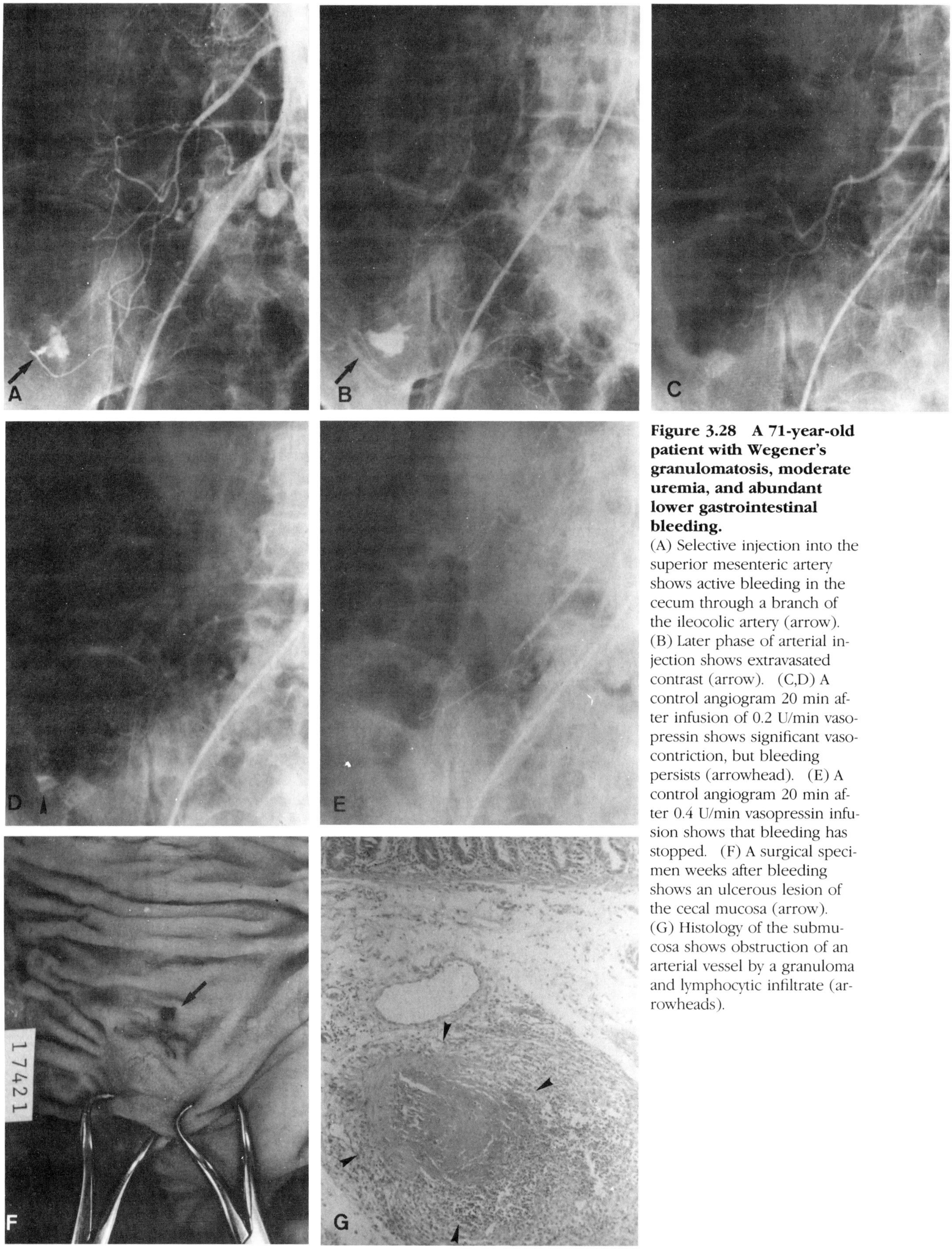

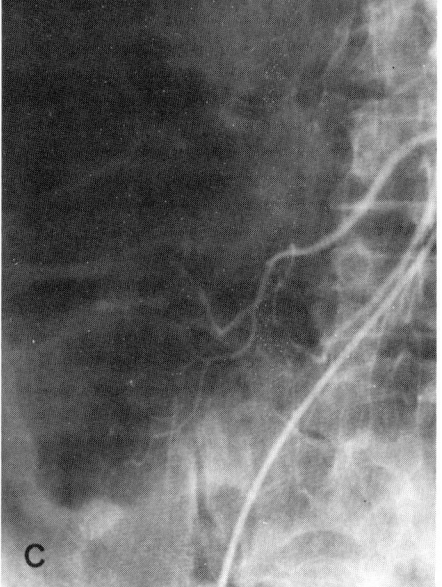

Figure 3.28 A 71-year-old patient with Wegener's granulomatosis, moderate uremia, and abundant lower gastrointestinal bleeding.
(A) Selective injection into the superior mesenteric artery shows active bleeding in the cecum through a branch of the ileocolic artery (arrow). (B) Later phase of arterial injection shows extravasated contrast (arrow). (C,D) A control angiogram 20 min after infusion of 0.2 U/min vasopressin shows significant vasocontriction, but bleeding persists (arrowhead). (E) A control angiogram 20 min after 0.4 U/min vasopressin infusion shows that bleeding has stopped. (F) A surgical specimen weeks after bleeding shows an ulcerous lesion of the cecal mucosa (arrow). (G) Histology of the submucosa shows obstruction of an arterial vessel by a granuloma and lymphocytic infiltrate (arrowheads).

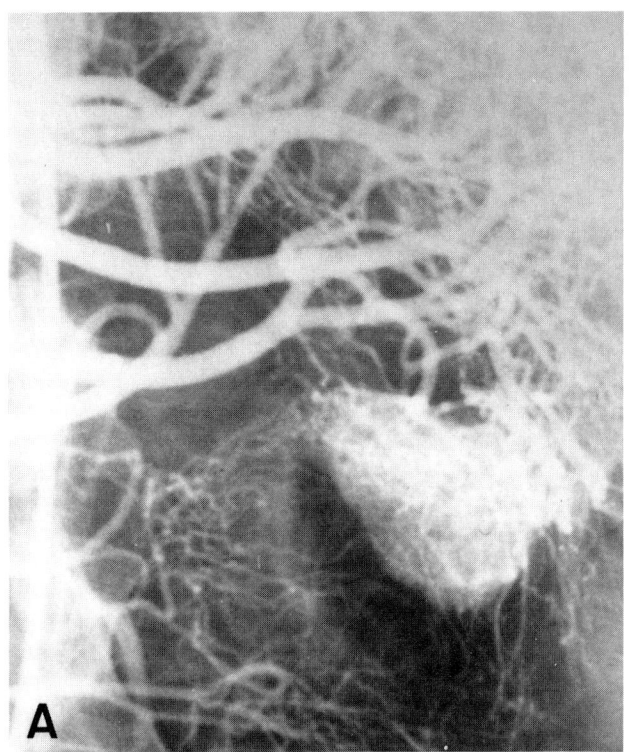

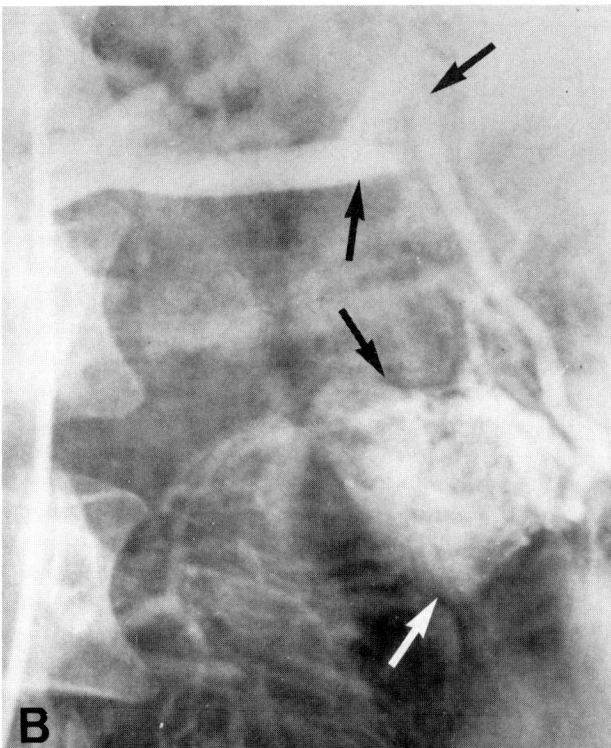

Figure 3.29
(A) A small hypervascular jejunal leiomyoma showing pathological vessels. (B) Later phase of angiogram, with opacification of multiple dense drainage veins (arrows), shows the mass and its outline.

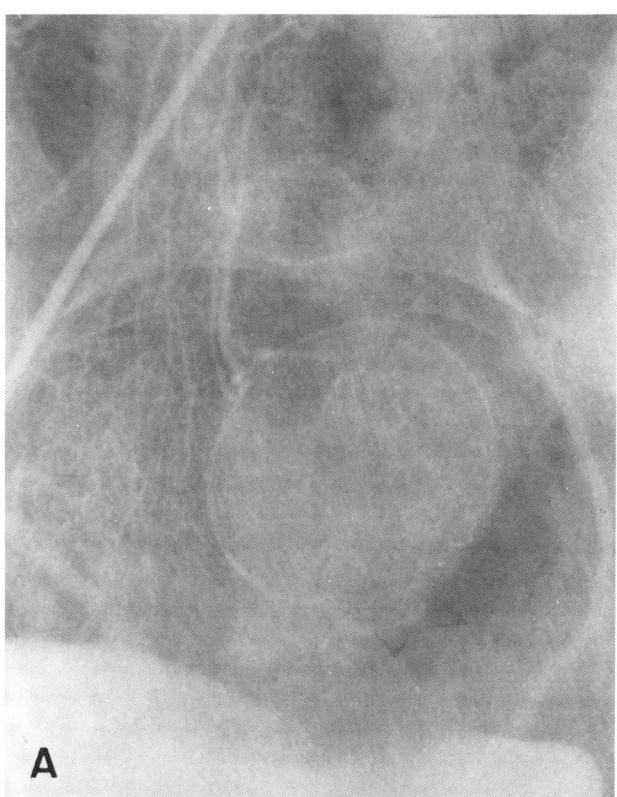

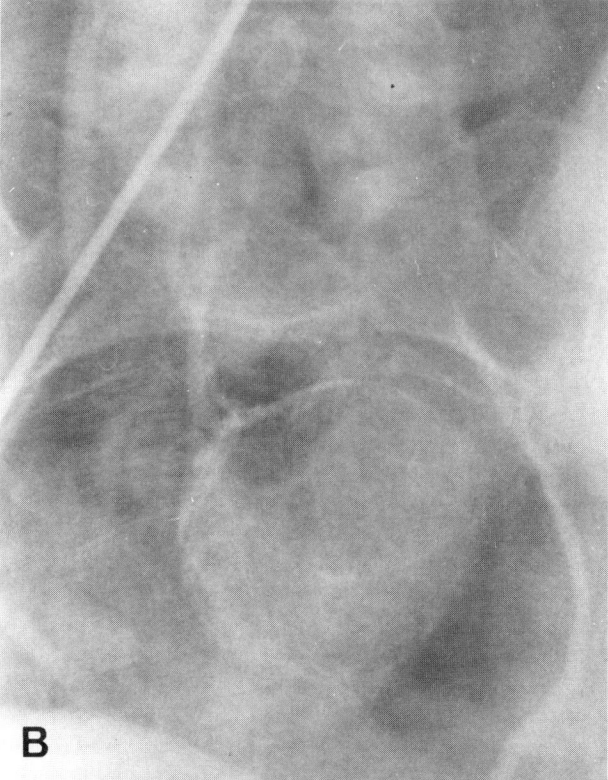

Figure 3.30
(A) A poorly vascularized though well-defined leiomyosarcoma with pathologic vessels and necrotic areas inside the mass. The intraluminal portion of the tumor became ulcerated and bled. (B) Later phase shows moderate venous return. (C) A surgical specimen showing the mass and its relation to a resected loop of the small intestine.

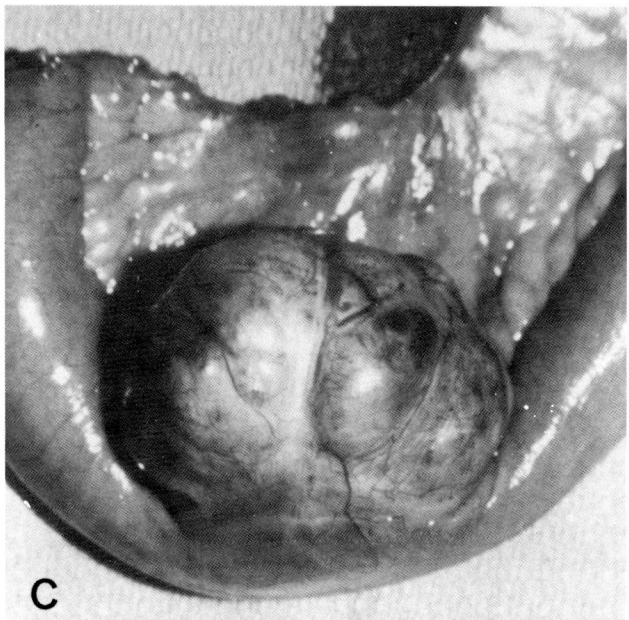

Figure 3.30 *Continued*

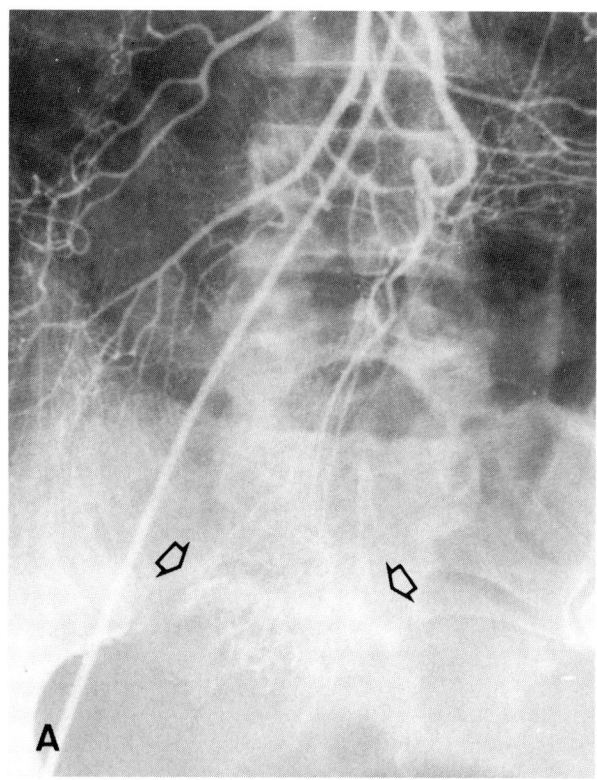

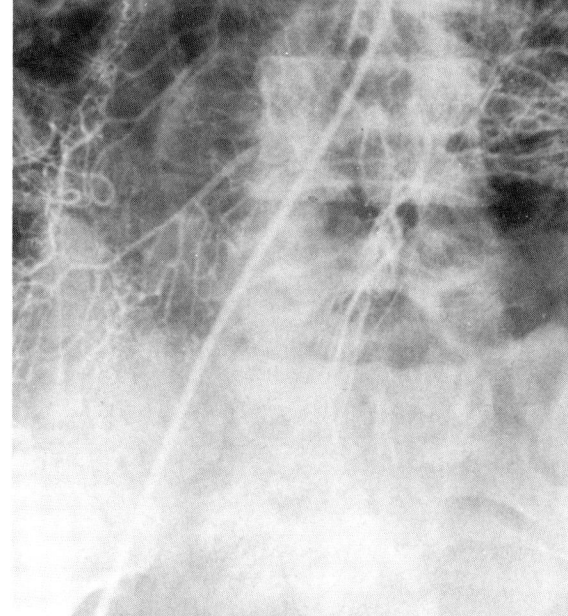

Figure 3.31 A 53-year-old patient with repetitive intestinal hemorrhage for the last 3 years. There was severe bleeding at the time of the study. Jejunal leiomyoma was diagnosed.
(A and B) Injection into the superior mesenteric artery shows a hypervascular lesion with poorly defined borders in the pelvic cavity. Note that the lesion's supplying arteries are stretched jejunal vessels and that the mass protrudes into the pelvis (arrows). (C and D) Injection into the inferior mesenteric artery showing circulation to the lesion through parasitic vessels from adhesions. The lesion adhered to the rectum and uterus. (E) Lateral view of a surgical specimen. (F) With the loop open, a large ulcer of the jejunal mucosa is shown (open arrows).

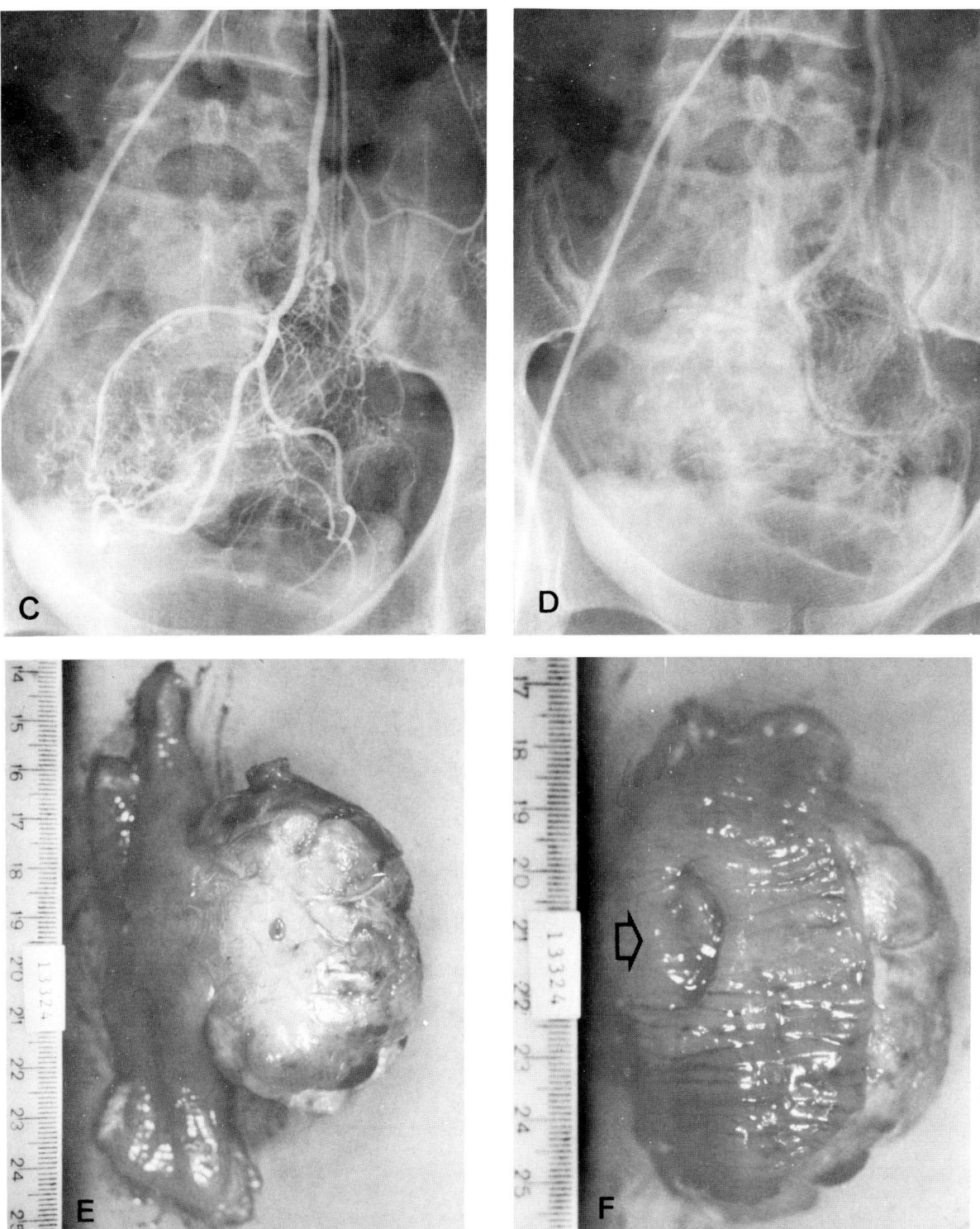

Figure 3.31 *Continued*

should be included in the differential diagnosis (Figs. 3.31 and 3.32).

Bleeding from these lesions does not respond to vasoconstricting agents. If a presurgical therapeutic measure is taken, it should be catheter embolization.

Other tumors of the small intestine may bleed even if they are benign such as polyps, which may or may not be associated with Peutz-Jeghers syndrome.

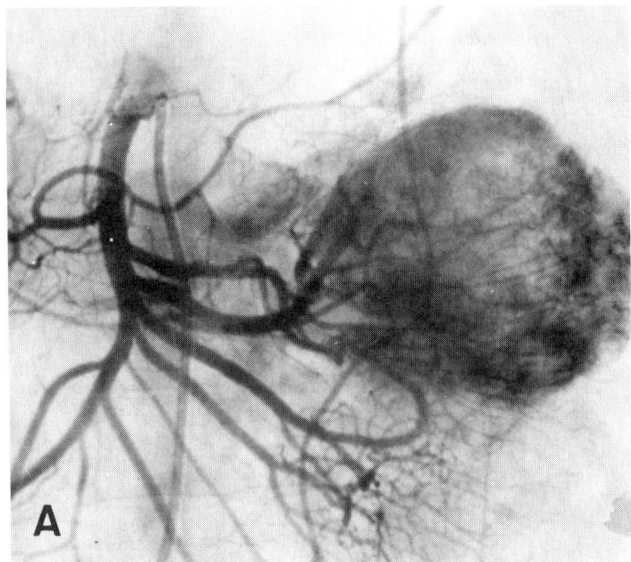

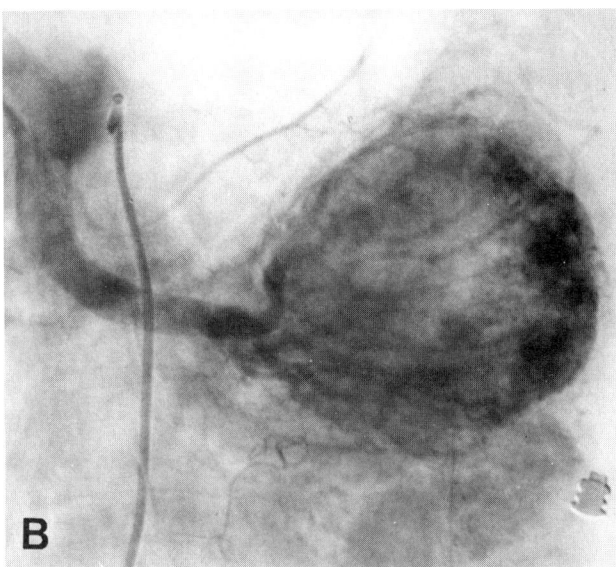

Figure 3.32
(A) Selective injection into the superior mesenteric artery shows a large jejunal leiomyosarcoma. This is a hypervascular lesion with well-defined margins and multiple tumoral vessels inside the mass. (B) Later phase of injection shows dense and somewhat early venous return. A barium study showed significant displacement of jejunal loops.

Ischemic Ulcerations

Ischemic ulcerative lesions of the small intestine as well as those of the colon may have many different etiologies or at least may be related to different chronic primary processes. Therefore, patients with chronic renal failure (uremic), chronic myeloid leukosis, Wegener's granulomatosis, or polymorphous reticulosis may develop ischemic and ulcerated areas which bleed profusely as a result of vascular obstructive lesion, inflammatory response, and lymphocytic infiltration (Figs. 3.27, 3.28, and 3.33). Sepsis can lead to the same type of lesion. Polymorphous reticulosis (also known as lymphomatoid granulomatosis or lethal midline granuloma) may produce nodules or masses resembling metastatic neoplasms (Fig. 3.34). This type of lesion may involve several other organs, particularly in the upper airway, where it may be mistakenly identified as Wegener's granulomatosis. The angiocentric infiltration characteristic of the disease is responsible for the necrotic areas in the intestine due to occlusion of small vessels that may simulate Wegener's necrotizing vasculitis. Although these lesions may respond to vasopressin infusion, the prognosis is extremely guarded.

Arteriovenous Malformations

Several types of vascular malformations in the large intestine have been described. Angiographic observations include impregnating a hypervascular area with poorly defined borders; this area is supplied by an artery larger than the adjacent ones and is drained by a large vein which is opacified early and densely. This is sometimes a discrete finding, with only the larger artery or the early vein being visualized. These are difficult lesions to locate during surgery, since they are of submucosal origin and since the serosa remains normal at the lesion site. Many different superselective catheterization techniques using a No. 3 French catheter or a transoperative methylene blue injection may be used to

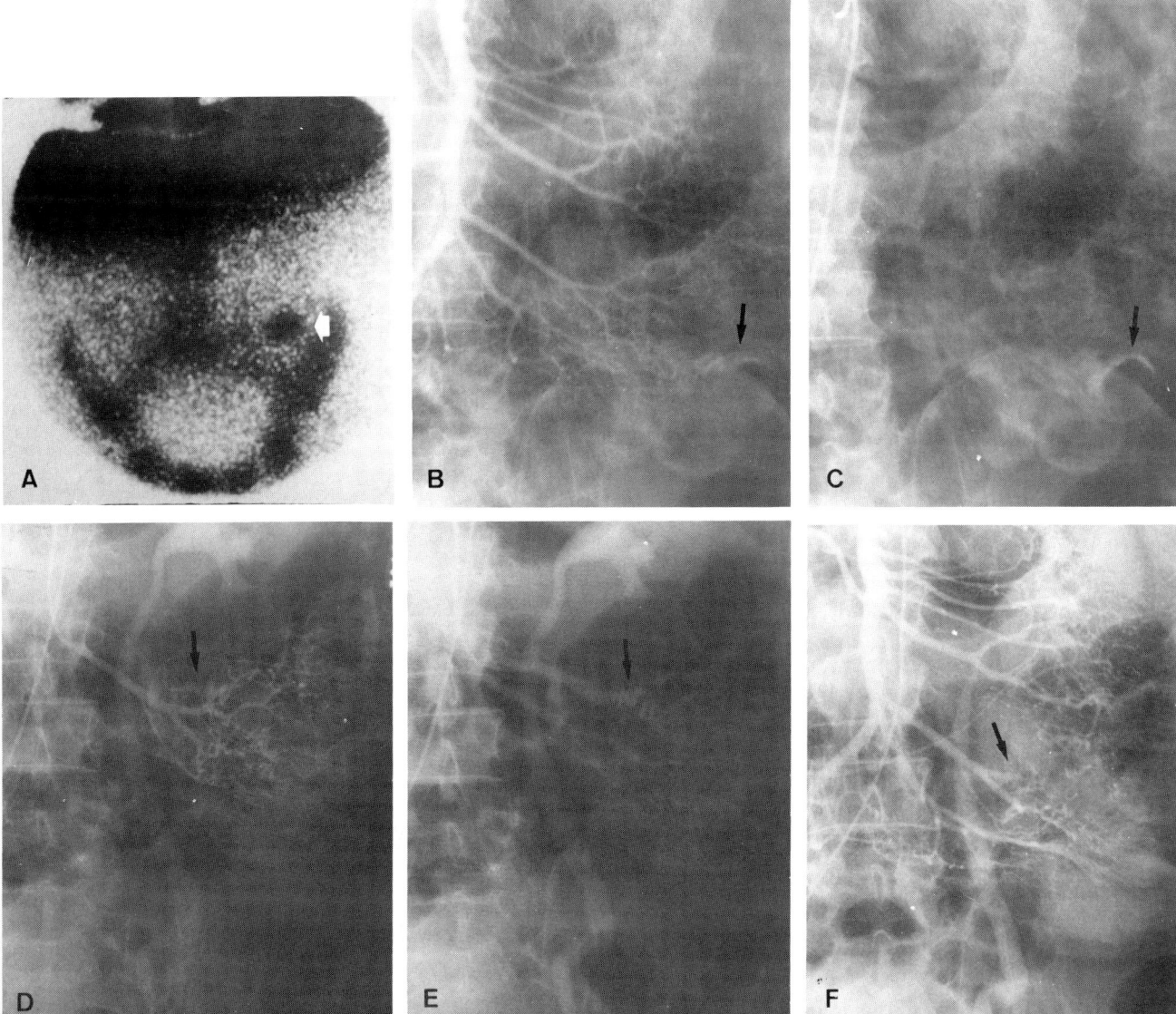

Figure 3.33 A 58-year-old patient with lower gastrointestinal hemorrhage, hematologic changes, and sepsis. (A) Scintiscan with technetium-labeled sulfur colloid shows extravasation of radioactive substance into intestinal lumen, localized in the left iliac fossa, suggesting that bleeding may be in the descending colon (white arrow). (B and C) Arterial and later phase of superior mesenteric injection shows extravasation to the jejunum projected over the left iliac fossa (arrows). (D and E) Superselective injection into the jejunal artery, which is the origin of bleeding (arrows) in another position. (F) Control after superselective embolization with Gelfoam shows occlusion of some peripheral vessels (arrow) and bleeding arrest. This patient underwent surgery, and ischemic signs in the right colon due to a systemic process were found. The patient died 1 month after embolization.

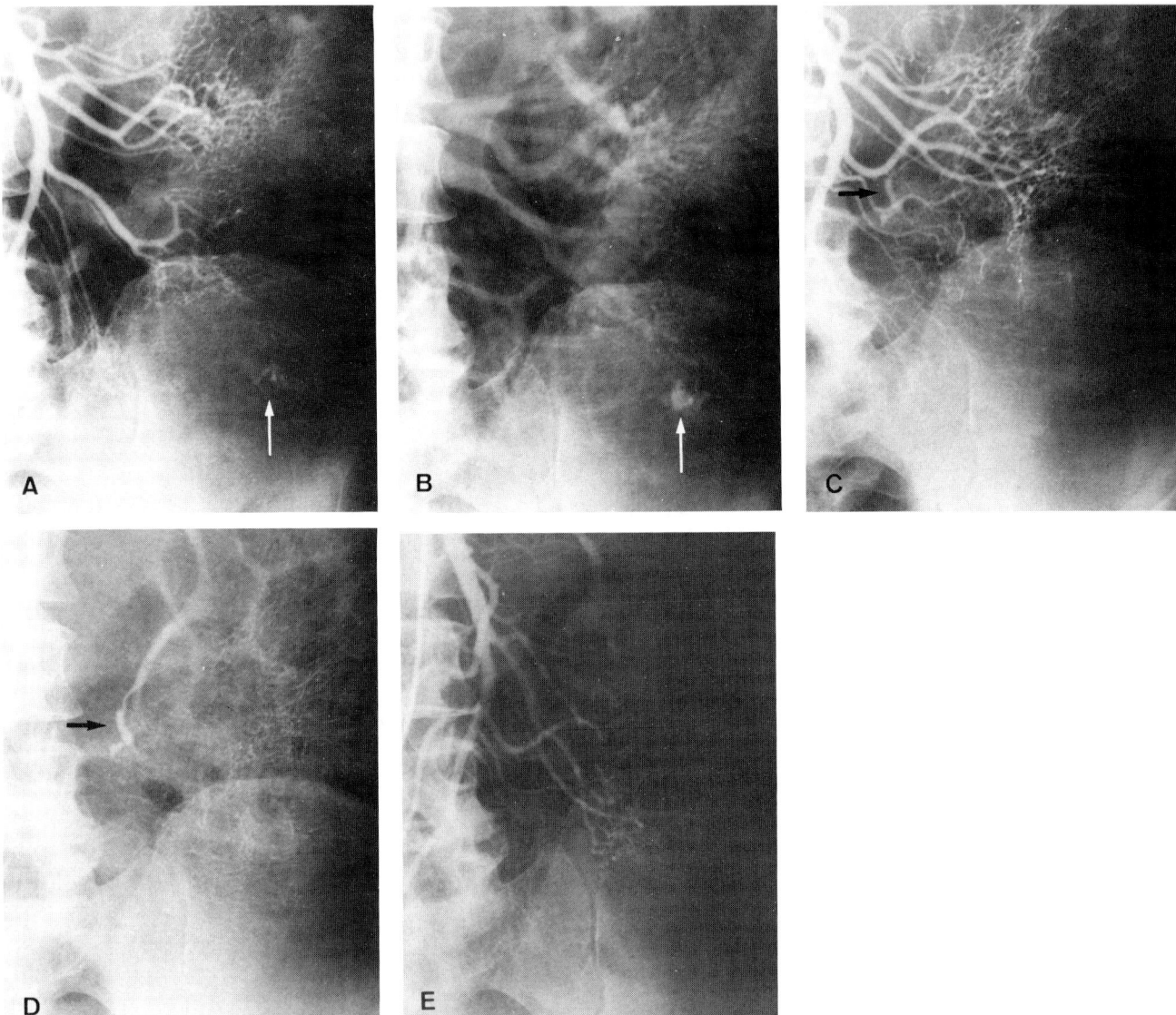

Figure 3.34 A 57-year-old patient who presented with polymorphous reticulosis with involvement of the superior airway, liver, and digestive tract, with lower gastrointestinal bleeding.
(A) Arterial phase of injection into the superior mesenteric artery shows contrast extravasation in the distal jejunum (white arrow). (B) Late phase of injection showing a small collection in the small intestine lumen. (C) After infusion of 0.2 IU/min of vasopressin, extravasation of contrast persisted, now in a different position (black arrow) as a result of movement of loops. (D) Later phase of control angiogram shows a contrast medium collection (arrow) in the intestinal lumen. (E) Control angiogram after the infusion of 0.4 IU/min of vasopressin controlled the bleeding. After vasopressin infusion was discontinued, there was recurrence of bleeding. The patient was operated on and a nodule of polymorphous reticulosis was ressected.

localize the lesion (Fig. 3.35). Embolization of solitary lesions may help stop acute bleeding while the patient is waiting for definitive surgery.

Intestinal Varices

In some patients with portal hypertension, mesenteric varices and varices of both the small intestine and the large bowel wall may develop. These lesions seldom bleed, but treatment is systemic or consists of intraarterial injection of vasopressin to lower the portal pressure (Fig. 3.36). These lesions are occasionally treated with percutaneous transhepatic embolization.

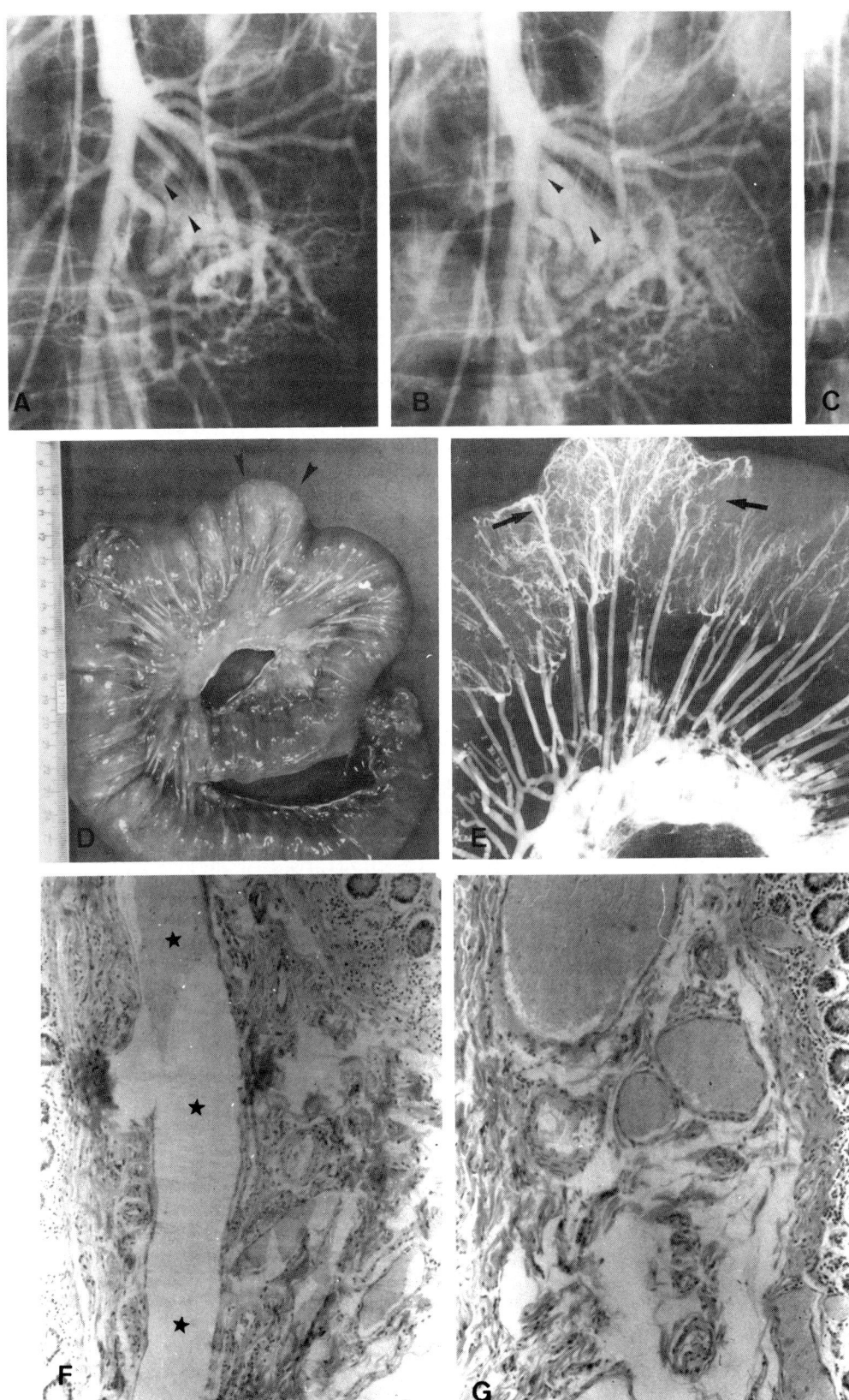

Figure 3.35 A young patient with acute and serious episodes of repetitive lower gastrointestinal bleeding.
(A) Selective injection into the superior mesenteric artery shows a jejunal arteriovenous malformation with dense and early venous return (arrowheads) as well as vein enlargement. (B) Later phase of injection shows higher opacification density of the malformed drainage vein (arrowheads). (C) Venous phase shows persistent opacification of the vein (arrowheads). This patient was operated on, and the lesion was not found. A pyloroplasty and vagectomy was performed to treat a small bulbar ulcer. Bleeding recurred approximately 3 months after the first surgery. (D) During a new surgery, a segment of the jejunum was resected which corresponded to the lesion (arrowheads). (E) Barium injection was performed to locate the malformation (arrows). (F) A histologic section shows a large vessel communicating with the arteriole and venule (stars). (G) A histologic section shows dilated vessels in the submucosa and normal mucosa.

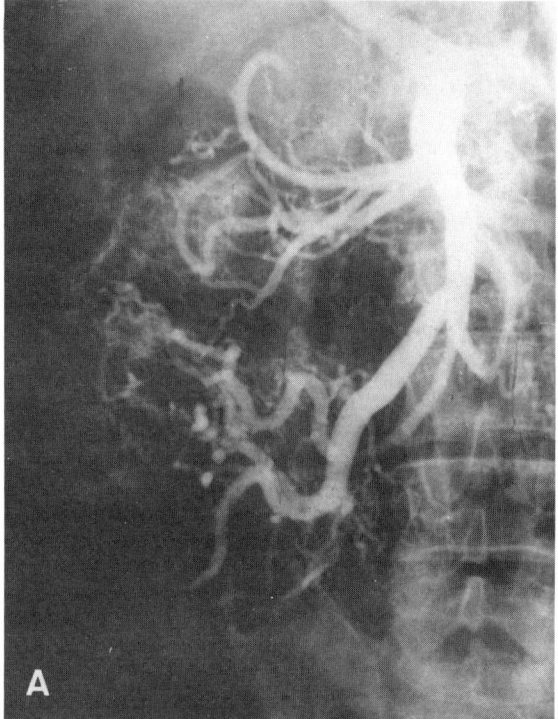
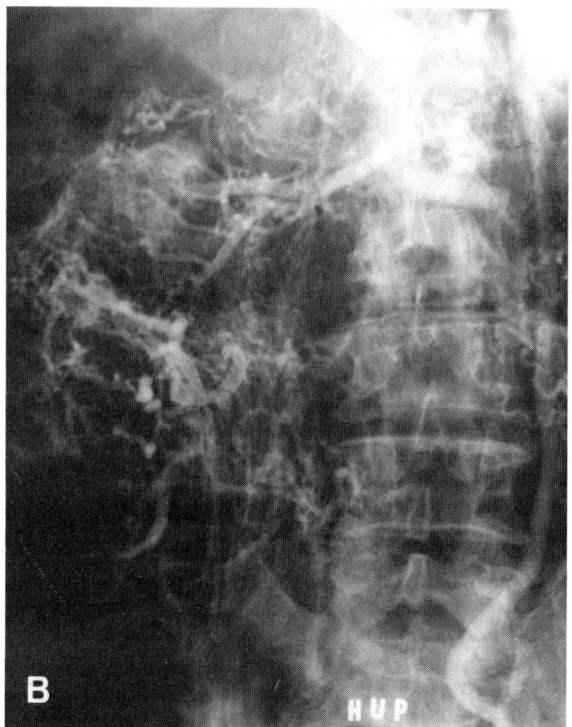
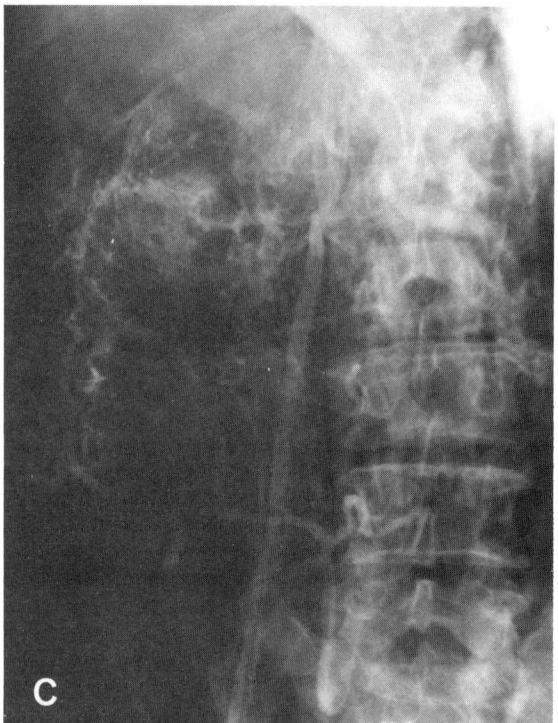

Figure 3.36
(A) A patient with portal hypertension and varices of the right colon with lower bleeding. (B) Note the abundant retroperitoneal circulation. (C) Opacification of the right gonadal vein through retroperitoneal collaterals.

Postoperative Bleeding

Postoperative bleeding in the small intestine is usually associated with enteroenteric or gastroenteric anastomoses due to os ulcerations. The most common location is on gastrojejunal postgastrectomy anastomoses. These lesions respond well to vasopressin infusion. In cases where the bleeding is due to faulty surgical techniques, loose sutures, with abundant bleeding, vasopressin infusion is not adequate (Fig. 3.37).

LOWER GASTROINTESTINAL BLEEDING RELATED TO THE COLON

Diverticula

Colonic diverticula may occur in 25 percent of people from 60 to 70 years of age; approximately 20 to 30 percent of patients bleed during the course of this disease. Although there are many other causes of lower GI bleeding, this is the most frequent cause of colonic hemorrhage. Approximately 80 percent of patients with this condition who are admitted to the hospital recover after clinical treatment, rest, sedation, and blood replacement without needing surgical or other treatment. Angiography for diagnostic and therapeutic purposes should be performed in the 20 percent of patients who do not benefit from these clinical procedures.

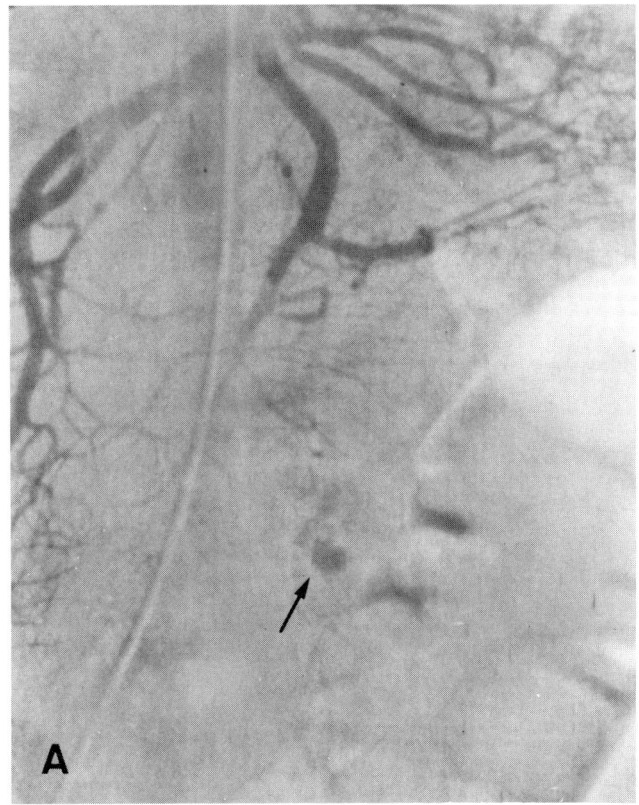 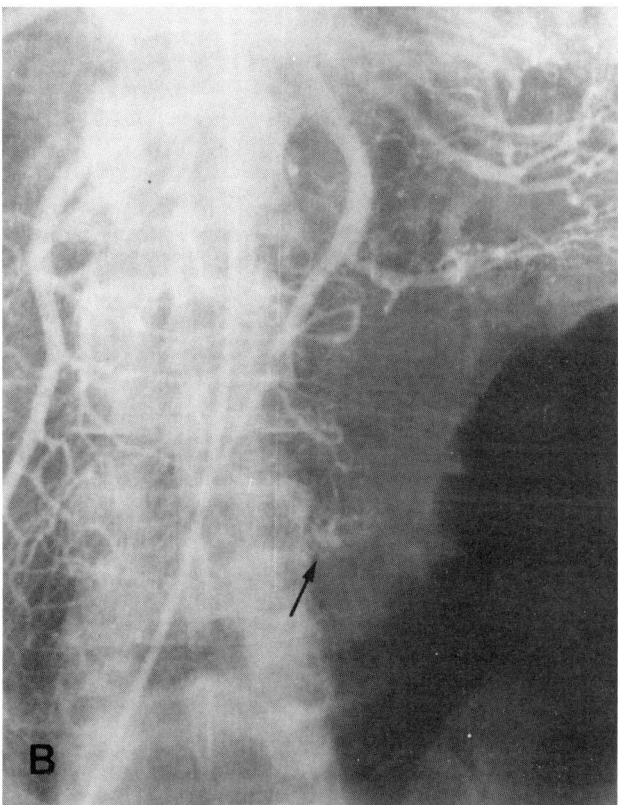

Figure 3.37 A 72-year-old patient with gastrointestinal bleeding after surgical resection of an ulcerated and abscessed leiomyoma in the ileum.
(A) Selective injection into the superior mesenteric artery shows the bleeding site (arrow). A radioisotope study has already identified bleeding. Vasopressin infusion was initiated, starting with a 0.2 IU/min for 20 min, which was ineffective. This was followed by a higher dose of 0.4 IU/min for another 20 min, which was also ineffective because of the use of sodium nitroprussiate to control a hypertensive episode. (B) Control 40 min after treatment still shows extravasation, although it is reduced (arrow). The patient was operated on and had a bad outcome with multiple complications, and died approximately 1 month later.

The location of bleeding is difficult to determine by means of colonoscopy, particularly when the bleeding is acute and profuse. Colonoscopy is best for elective studies of patients with repetitive lower GI bleeding.

Scintigraphy with technetium-labeled sulfur colloid or technetium-labeled red blood cells is highly sensitive in detecting lesions, although its specificity is low in diagnosing the cause of bleeding. This is, however, a procedure that is always used in patients with continuous lower bleeding, since its detection capacity is approximately 0.01 mL/min of blood extravasation. As can be seen in Fig. 3.33, the location is nonspecific, and bleeding, which seems to occur in the descending colon, is actually found in the small intestine, projecting over the left iliac fossa.

Even though diverticula are found predominantly in the descending colon and sigmoid colon, diverticular hemorrhage occurs in the right colon and transverse colon in 75 percent of cases, according to the literature.

The pathogenesis of diverticular bleeding is closely related to the angioarchitecture characteristic of perforating branches. There is no significant diverticulitis in patients with massively bleeding diverticula.

Diverticula are not randomly distributed over the circumference of the colon but originate on lines related to the taeniae coli, which correspond to the larger segments of the vasa recta.

The fibers of colonic wall muscle are separated by connective tissue septa that are obliquely oriented. It is through these spaces that perforating vessels, segments of the serosal vasa recta, penetrate the wall toward the mucous membrane.

A diverticulum is formed by mucosal protrusion into these spaces (Fig. 3.38). The artery, a vas rectus, is positioned on the dorsum of the diverticulum between the serosa and the invaginated mucous membrane of the large intestine. The vas rectus penetrates the colonic wall along the antimesenteric border of the diverticulum, next to its neck and luminal space. A few changes in the vascular wall are found in the vasa recta on the rupture site and the surrounding areas, including intimal

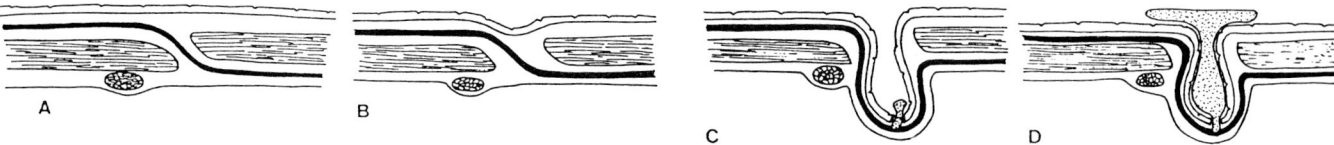

Figure 3.38 Mechanism of diverticular formation in the colon and its anatomic relationship to vasculature.
(A) Intramural penetration in the mesenteric side of the longitudinal muscle fascia by a branch of the vas rectus. The pathway is oblique and passes through connective tissue in a round musculature septum. (B) Mucosal protrusion through a connective septum enlargement, which begins raising the vessel. (C) A transmural diverticular protrusion pointing toward the mesenteric side of the colon. The vas rectus is displaced over the diverticular dome penetrating the submucosa through the antimesenteric side of the colon and the diverticular orifice. Vessel rupture and a small degree of extravasation into the fundus of the diverticular sac are seen in this schematic drawing. (D) As bleeding continues, the diverticulum is filled and blood spreads throughout the mucosa.

thickening, duplication of the inner elastic lamina with lamellar disposition, and thinning of the media. These changes probably result from local repetitive traumatic and inflammatory processes.

Arteries that undergo these changes rupture easily in an eccentric fashion and bleed into the diverticular lumen (Fig. 3.38). Diverticular bleeding from the large intestine results in a round collection of contrast medium, generally small and localized on the colonic lumen, which spreads over the mucosal surface in the late films of an angiography series (Fig. 3.23). Wall "staining" and venous return are not seen during the arteriogram sequence.

Bleeding from diverticula is usually intermittent, and the angiogram is frequently negative because bleeding may have stopped by the time the study is performed. The frequency of angiographic identification of the bleeding site is therefore relatively low. Some authors have suggested the use of a fibrinolytic agent or vasodilator to provoke bleeding when there is a negative angiogram in a patient who is obviously suffering from diverticular hemorrhage. The method is not popular or safe enough, and the problem of false-negative angiograms remains.

As previously mentioned, high morbidity and mortality rates associated with emergency colectomies have contributed to the importance of diagnostic and therapeutic angiography in managing lower GI bleeding.

The standard treatment for lower GI bleeding, particularly when it is of diverticular origin, is vasopressin infusion (0.2 or 0.4 IU/min) into the superior and inferior mesenteric artery, using the protocol described in "Infusion of Vasoconstricting Agents" (Fig. 3.22). This technique can control over 70 percent of patients, with bleeding recurring in about 20 percent. However, approximately half these patients eventually require surgery. Venous infusion of vasopressin through a central catheter is an effective alternative in selected cases.

The use of prolonged infusions of vasopressin to treat diverticular bleeding is associated with a high incidence of bleeding episodes and systemic as well as regional complications. For this reason, a few clinical and experimental studies have been done using selective embolization to treat lower GI bleeding. This alternative has been shown to be effective (Fig. 3.23), but it is associated with a high incidence of predictable complications involving intestinal ischemic lesions (Fig. 3.39) (see "Embolization").

Angiodysplasia

Colonic angiodysplasia is an acquired vascular lesion of the colon which can become a source of chronic or massive intermittent lower GI bleeding. At least in North America, it is considered the second most common cause of lower GI bleeding. This type of lesion is most frequently found in patients above 55 years of age, is not associated with vascular cutaneous lesions or lesions in other organs of the abdomen, and is almost always localized in the cecum or the ascending colon. The lesions have a characteristic angiographic aspect, and diagnosis is essentially angiographic. Cecal angiodysplasia cannot be palpated or examined during surgery; right hemicolectomy, however, has proved to be curative in many patients. The lesion is identified through vascular techniques involving the injection of barium-added gelatin into the surgical specimen and dissection under the microscope.

Cecal angiodysplasia was first described in 1972 by Baum. It is considered to be an acquired lesion.

The pathophysiology of cecal angiodysplasias is not well defined, but the fact that this condition is found mainly in older patients suggests a degenerative process.

Baum has proposed that angiodysplasia is the end result of multiple and chronically repeated subclinical episodes of intestinal ischemia caused by a chronic increase of cecal pressure and enlargement associated with high wall stress. As a result of this high wall

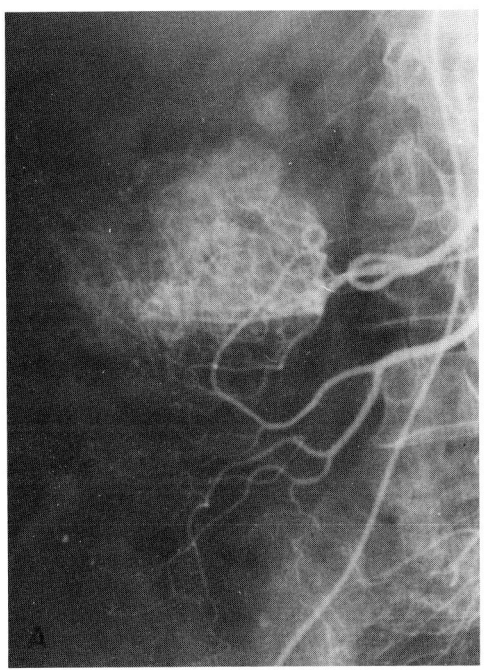 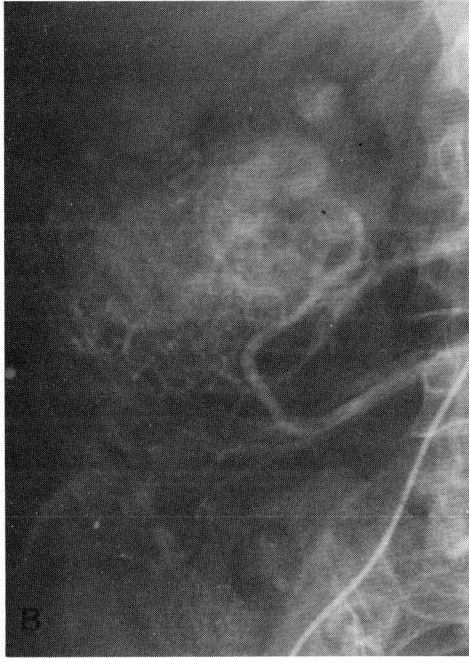

Figure 3.43 Neoplasm of the ascending colon with severe lower gastrointestinal bleeding in a 65-year-old patient.
(A) Injection into the superior mesenteric artery shows a large, moderately vascularized tumoral lesion in the hepatic angle of the colon. Note ill-defined tumoral vessels and borders. It was not possible to embolize the lesion, which did not respond to vasopressin. (B) Later phase of injection shows diffuse impregnation and the abundant venous return of the lesion.

In cases of high-volume tumoral bleeding from an unknown cause, an emergency angiogram is able to demonstrate the lesion (Fig. 3.43) and arrest bleeding by embolizing the supplying arteries. However, this is done only as a preoperative measure or for the palliation of inoperable lesions. Tumoral lesions do not respond well to the use of vasoconstrictors even when they are given by superselective infusion.

Embolization of primary or secondary colonic neoplasms is particularly effective in the rectosigmoid region when only the superior hemorrhoidal arteries are occluded (Fig. 3.44). The low risk involved in this type of embolization is due to the double circulation in the rectal ampule, with anastomosis to the hypogastric vessels.

Myomatous lesions, both benign and malignant, occur less frequently in the colon but can cause abundant hemorrhaging. They are very easy to localize angiographically.

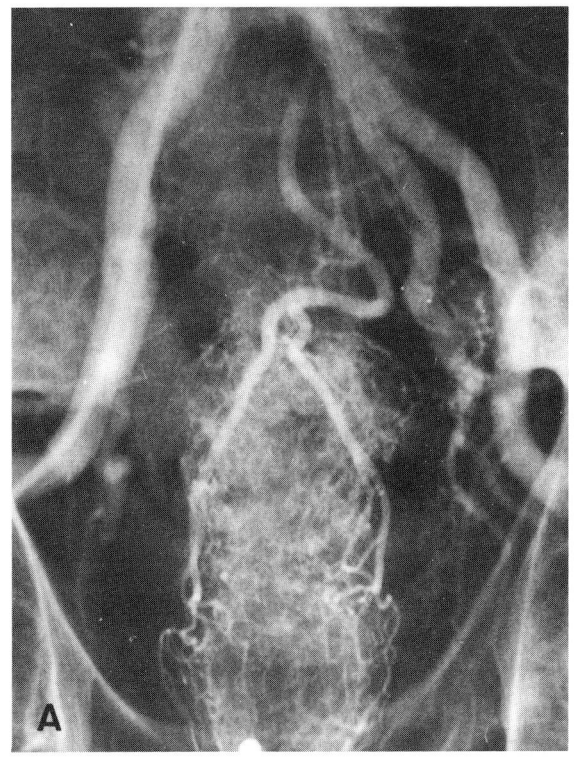

Figure 3.44 A patient with lower gastrointestinal bleeding resulting from rectal invasion by carcinoma of the bladder.
(A) Arterial phase of injection into the inferior mesenteric artery shows dense rectal hypervascularization in the neoplasm. (B) Later phase of injection shows venous return and impregnations localized in the mucosa and submucosa, without unequivocal bleeding. (C) Embolization with Gelfoam was performed, which selectively occluded the superior hemorrhoidal arteries (arrows), with permanent control of bleeding. (D) A barium enema showing infiltrating stenosis of the rectum, with no ulcerated areas.

Figure 3.44 *Continued*

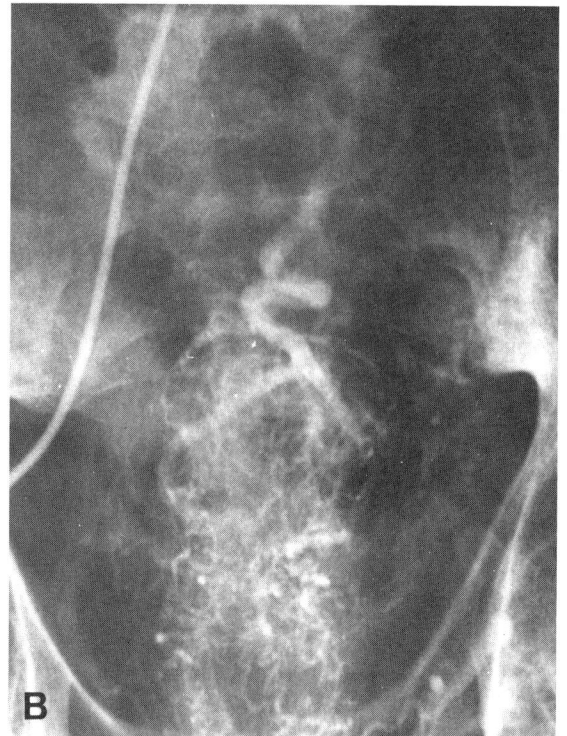
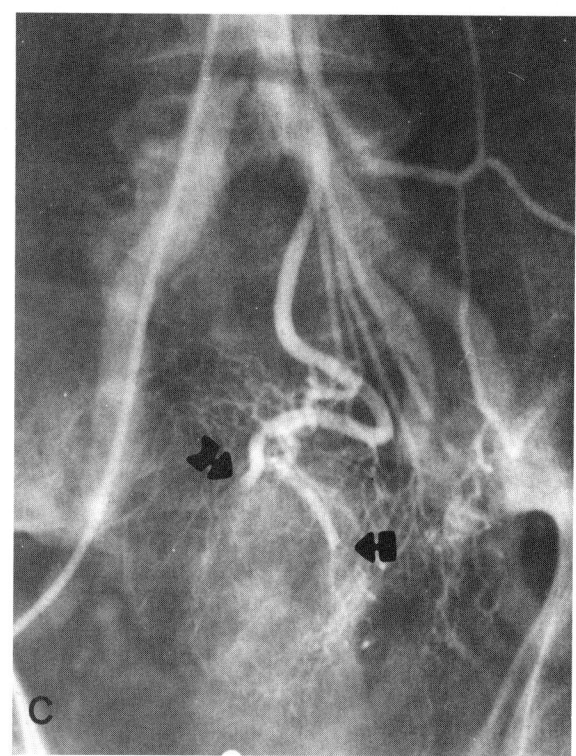
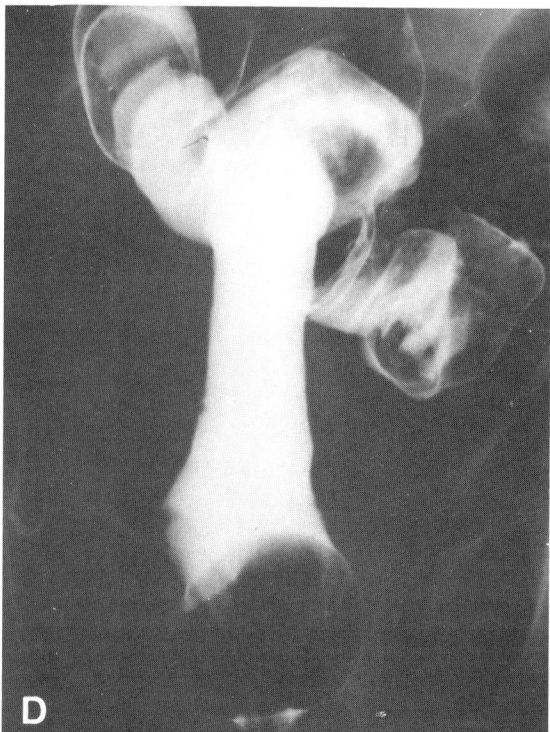

Arteriovenous Malformations

Colonic AV malformations, although not frequently found, can bleed profusely. As opposed to cecal angiodysplasias, these congenital lesions may appear in patients younger than the age group described for colonic angiodysplasias. These congenital lesions are usually larger than acquired ones (Fig. 3.45) and occur randomly in the large intestine. Intestinal AV malformations may be associated with Rendu-Osler-Weber disease and are usually multiple in these patients (Fig. 3.46).

The treatment of choice for these malformations when they cause acute bleeding is usually embolization with Gelfoam and Ivalon. Catheterization should be very selective, and the smallest possible number of emboli should be used. Surgical resection is required in most cases, but there are some areas, such as the rectum, where resection is difficult. Surgical excision is not always possible, and some patients require resections that are too extensive for a benign lesion. The presence of multiple lesions makes surgical treatment more difficult (Fig. 3.38).

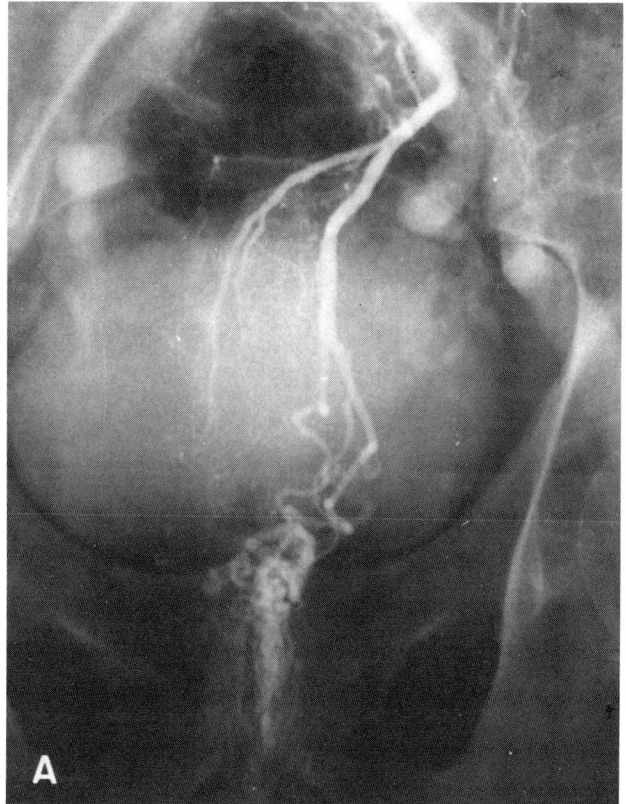 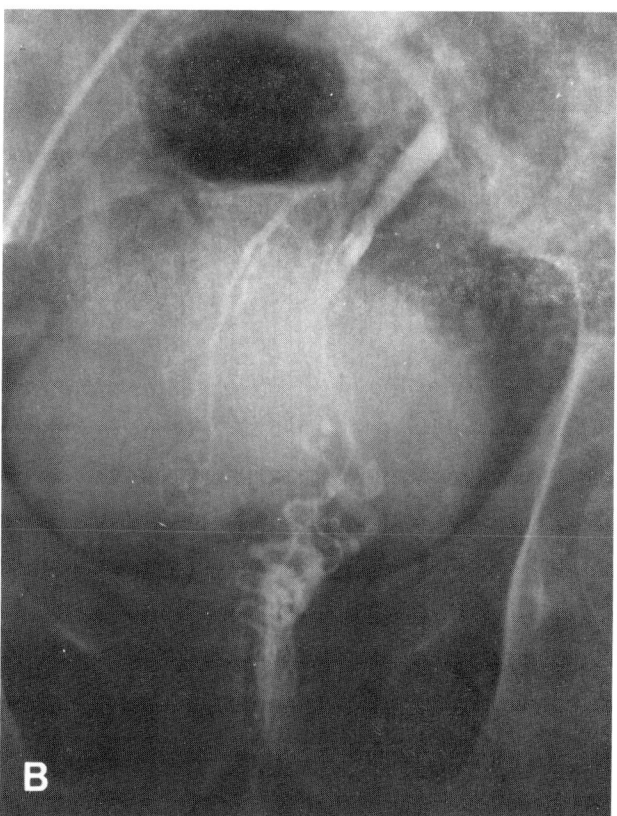

Figure 3.45 A 64-year-old patient who presented with chronic anemia and occult blood in the feces, with repeated negative barium and endoscopic studies, including rectosigmoidoscopy.
(A) Injection into the inferior mesenteric artery shows arteriovenous malformation in the rectum, supplied by the left superior hemorrhoidal artery. Note the vascular entanglement and early venous return as well as the enlarged artery. (B) A later phase clearly shows dense filling of the enlarged vein.

Stress Ulcers (Uremic and Unspecific)

Spontaneous colonic ulcerations or erosions without identifiable cause are attributed to stress. They are found in uremic and/or transplanted and immunosuppressed patients; this may suggest a viral etiology. These lesions can occur anywhere in the colon and may even appear as hemorrhagic proctitis (Fig. 3.47). Their response to vasopressin varies; the safest option is very selective embolization of the lesion (Fig. 3.47).

Inflammatory Colonic Diseases

Local inflammatory diseases with a specific cause and those with more diffuse causes of nonspecific origin may cause copious bleeding into the colon. The first group includes tuberculosis and typhoid fever, which may cause mucosal thickening as a result of an inflammatory process and hypervascularity. The second group includes Crohn's disease and ulcerative rectocolitis. In this group there are characteristic angiographic findings such as mucosal thickening, hypervascularity, and dense and early venous return through submucosal shunts in long segments of the colon.

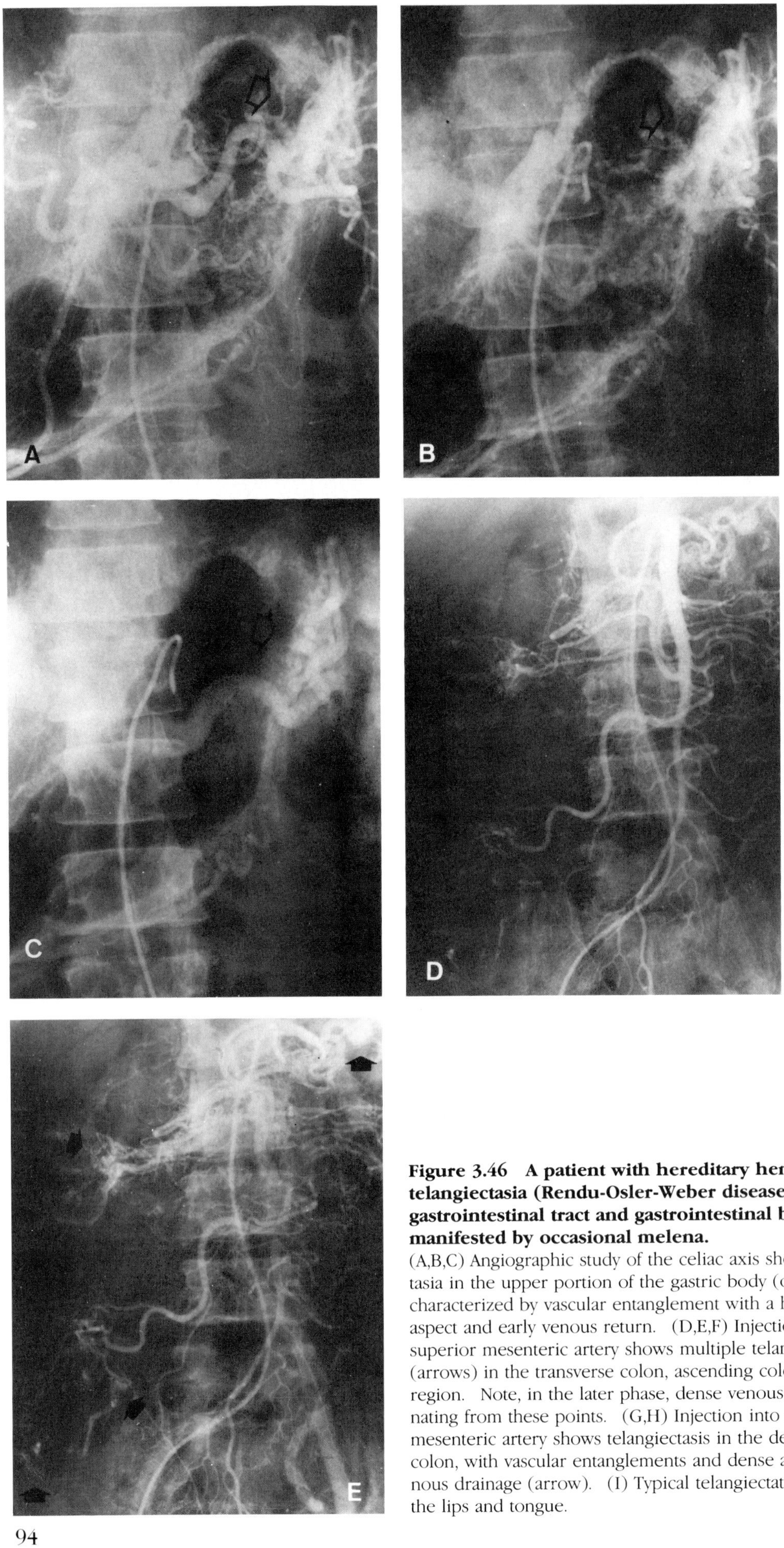

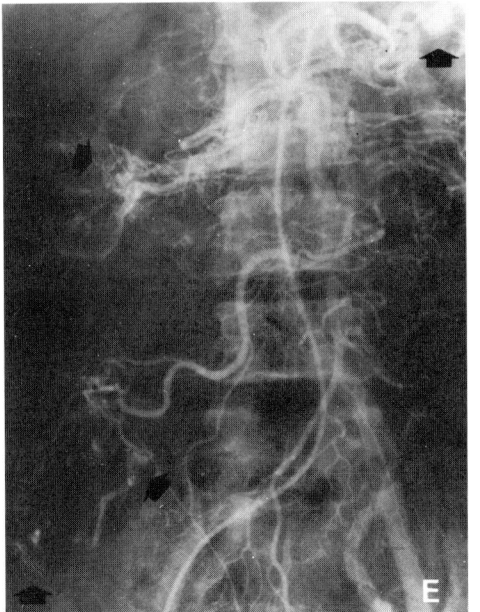

Figure 3.46 A patient with hereditary hemorrhagic telangiectasia (Rendu-Osler-Weber disease) in the gastrointestinal tract and gastrointestinal bleeding manifested by occasional melena.
(A,B,C) Angiographic study of the celiac axis shows telangiectasia in the upper portion of the gastric body (open arrows) characterized by vascular entanglement with a hypervascular aspect and early venous return. (D,E,F) Injection into the superior mesenteric artery shows multiple telangiectasia (arrows) in the transverse colon, ascending colon, and cecal region. Note, in the later phase, dense venous return originating from these points. (G,H) Injection into the inferior mesenteric artery shows telangiectasis in the descending colon, with vascular entanglements and dense and early venous drainage (arrow). (I) Typical telangiectatic lesions of the lips and tongue.

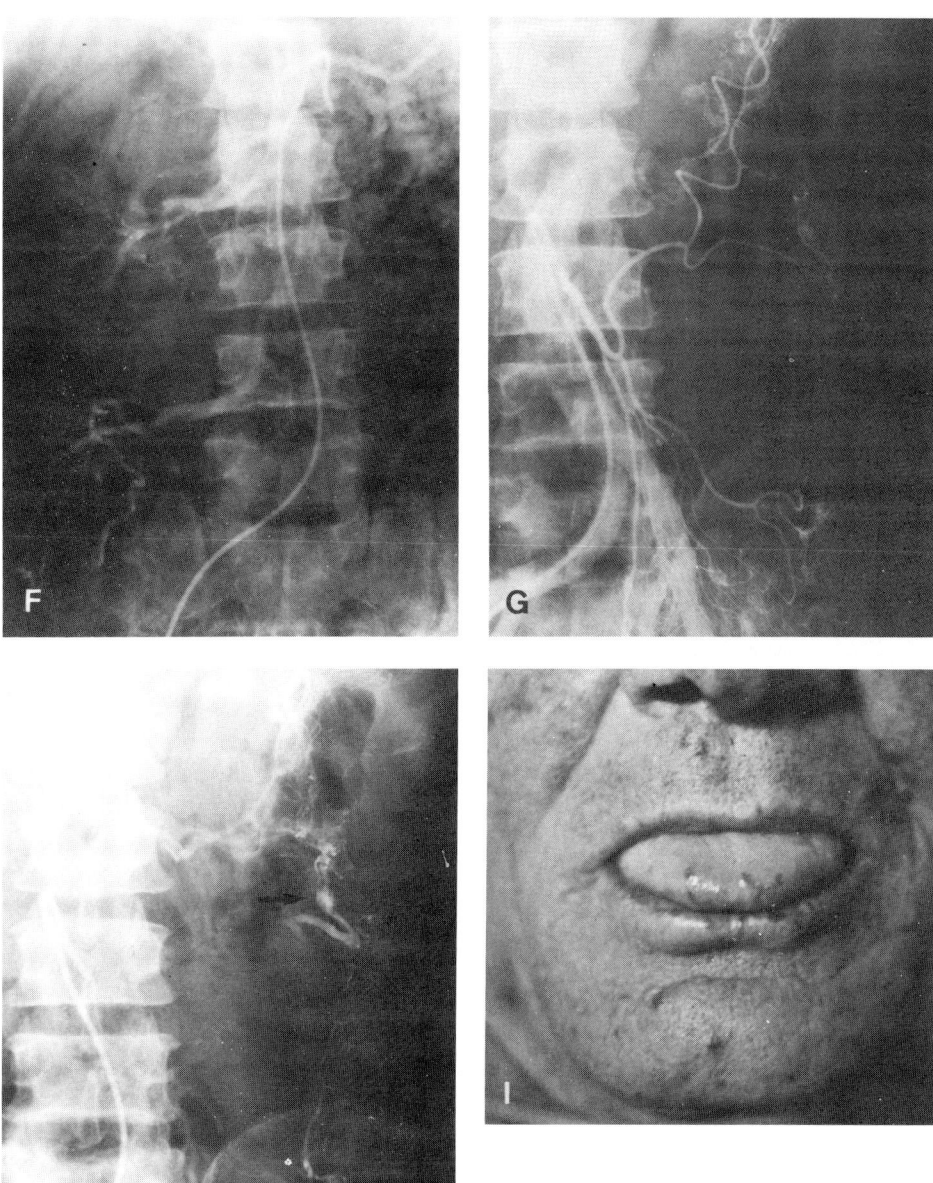

Figure 3.46 *Continued*

All these lesions, when bleeding, usually respond well to the infusion of vasopressin. A specific site of bleeding is seldom identified inside the inflammatory lesion.

Postoperative Bleeding

Bleeding at an appendectomy stump, enteric loop anastomosis (Fig. 3.48), or colostomy, although relatively uncommon, may become serious. These patients usually responded well to vasopressin infusion, with permanent control of bleeding. However, surgical cauterization can destroy the muscle layer of the vessel. The use of vasodilators to control hypertensive episodes may also detract from the beneficial effect of vasopressin. In some cases it is easy to perform superselective catheterization of the involved artery. Embolization is done with only

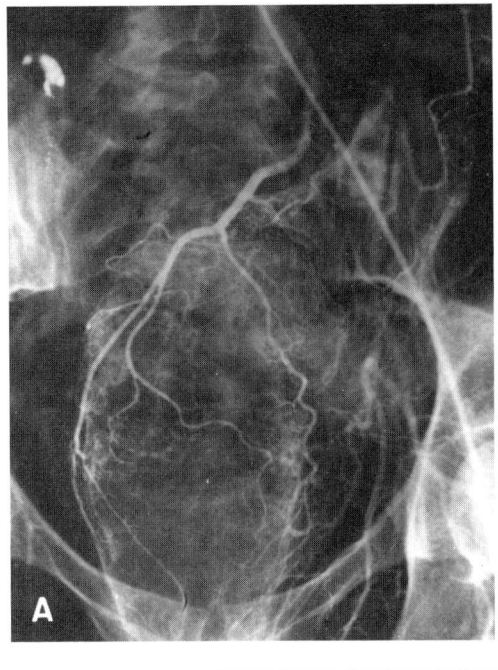
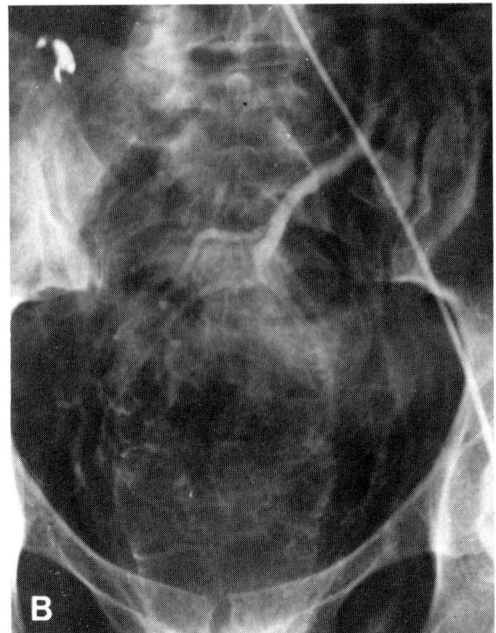
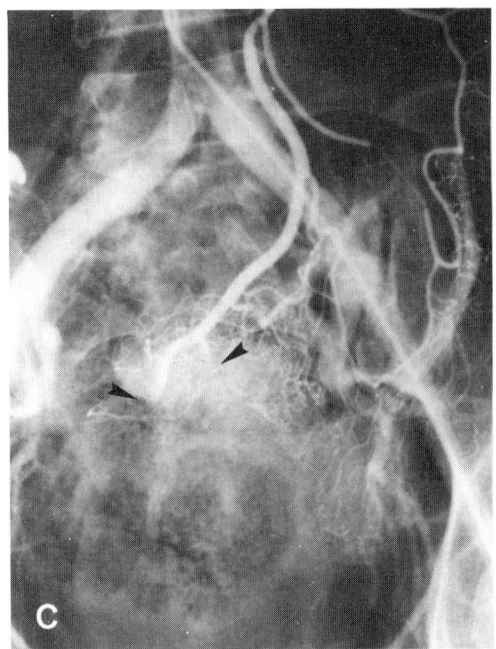

Figure 3.47 A uremic patient with nonspecific proctitis and lower gastrointestinal bleeding.
(A) Diffuse hypervascularity in the rectum. (B) Wall impregnation with normal venous return and some areas of hemorrhagic mucosal suffusion. (C) Control after embolization with Gelfoam of only the superior hemorrhoidal arteries (arrowheads). Note spasm in the sigmoidal arteries.

one fragment of Gelfoam, usually with good results. Bleeding from sigmoidal anastomoses after colostomy closure may also occur, with an indirect sign of bleeding referred to as intermittent arterial filling (Fig. 3.48).

Abscesses

Pericolic abscessed lesions may bleed abundantly as a result of vascular erosion and rupture. These lesions can be intra- or extraluminal. The abscess usually drains spontaneously into the colon. The bleeding can be treated with vasopressin infusion or embolization if access for a catheter is available.

Adenomatous, Villous, and Hyperplastic Polyps

Polyps, which frequently occur in the large intestine, are common sites of intestinal bleeding. Polypoid glandular neoplasms (polyps) can be adenomatous (tubular), pap-

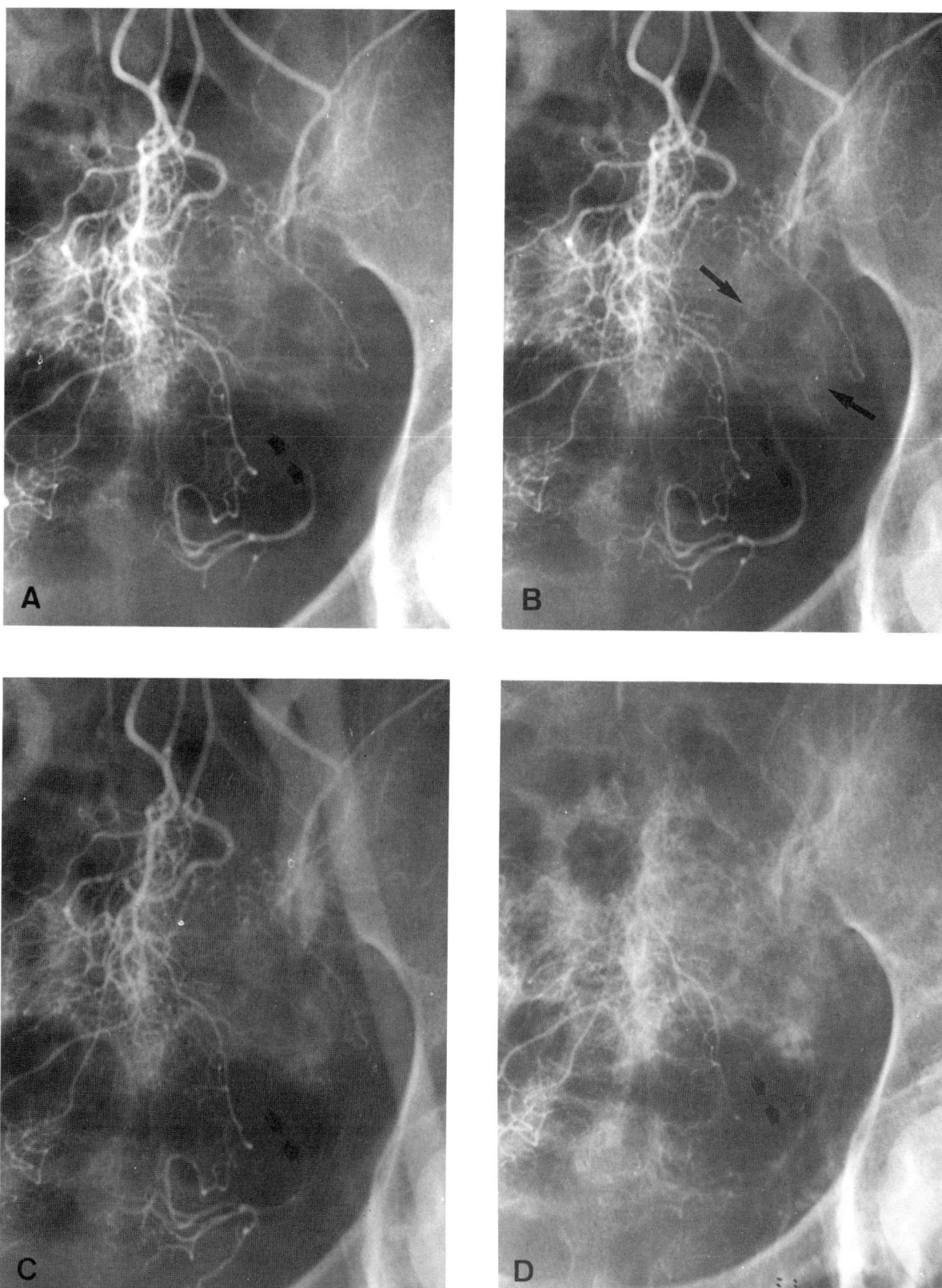

Figure 3.48 Sign of intermittent arterial filling in rectal bleeding at an anastomotic site after colostomy closure.
(A) Artery filling (arrows) near the anastomosis. (B) Artery continues to fill (short arrows). Long arrows show the site of anastomosis. (C) Arterial filling begins to disappear (arrows). (D) The artery previously visualized has disappeared. There is impregnation around the anastomosis but no contrast extravasation.

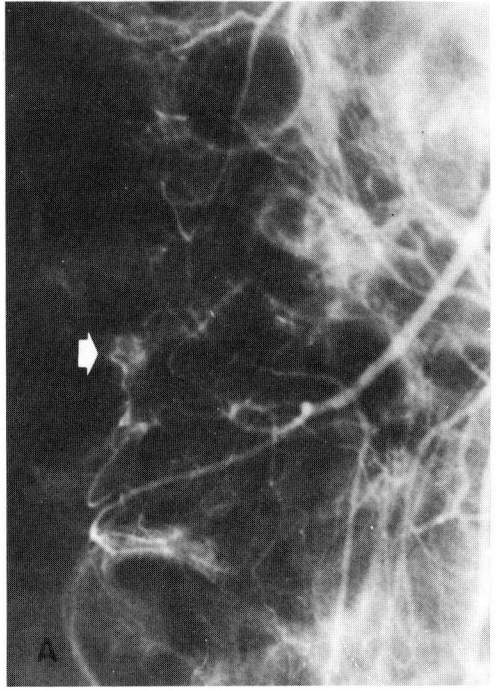
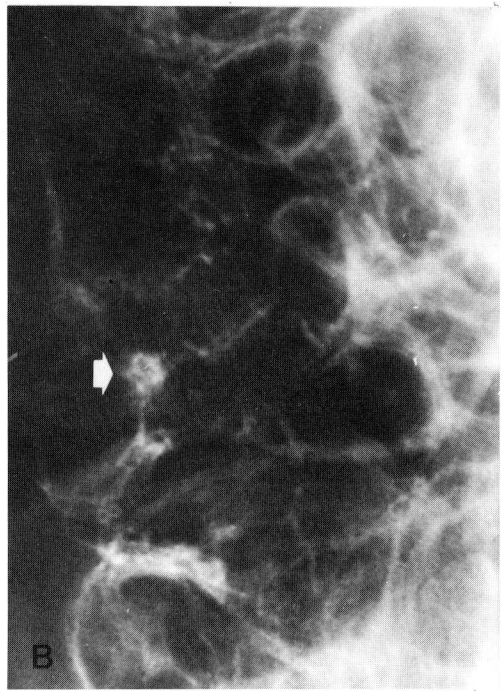
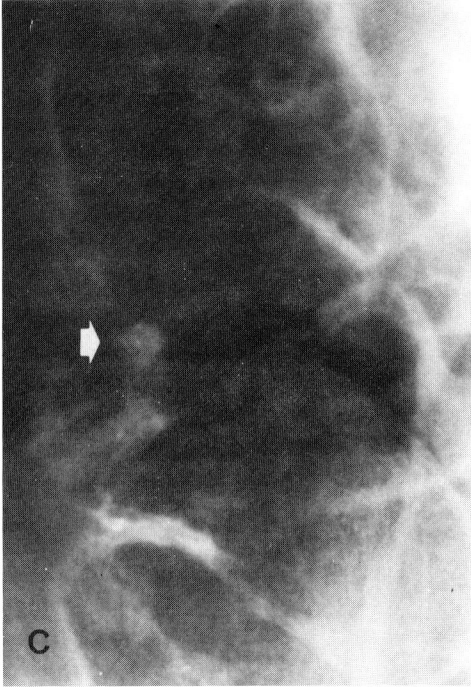

Figure 3.49 A hyperplastic polyp in a young patient causing abundant lower gastrointestinal bleeding.
(A) Arterial phase of superior mesenteric injection shows a localized area of impregnation in the ascending colon (arrow). (B) Later phase shows more significant impregnation of the lesion and absence of early venous filling (arrow). (C) Venous phase shows that this is not a malformation, as there is no increased venous drainage (arrow). (D) Surgical specimen from a right hemicolectomy shows a slightly elevated lesion in relation to the colonic mucosa, covered by hematic crust. (E) Histologic image of the lesion shows normal mucosa in the lower portion of photograph, typical changes in the crypts of the hyperplastic area, and the hematic layer covering the lesion. There are no abnormal vessels in the mucosa or submucosa.

illary (villous), or mixed and may occur anywhere in the digestive tract, particularly in the colon.

Small, flat elevations of the mucosa, so-called hyperplastic or metaplastic polyps, rarely occur. They are formed by enlarged, though normal, glands with excessive mucin secretion but without the potential for malignancy. These lesions may bleed copiously (Fig. 3.49). The best option is intraarterial infusion of vasopressin.

A polyp stump may occasionally bleed after endoscopic removal by means of fulguration. Bleeding of this type can be treated with vasopressin infusion or selective embolization.

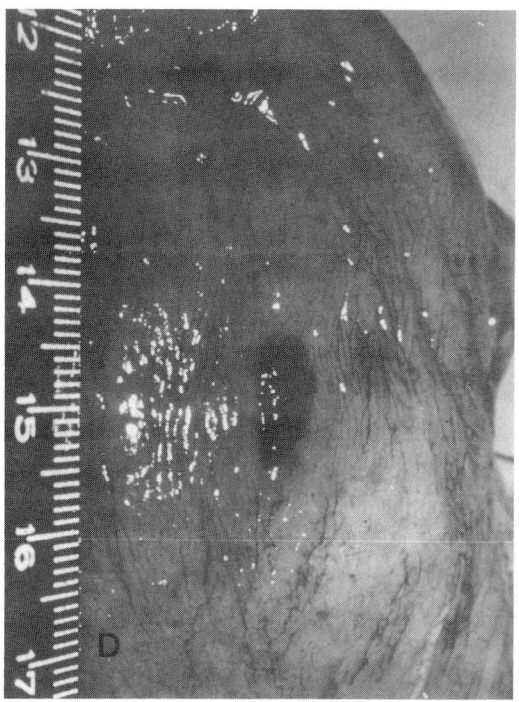 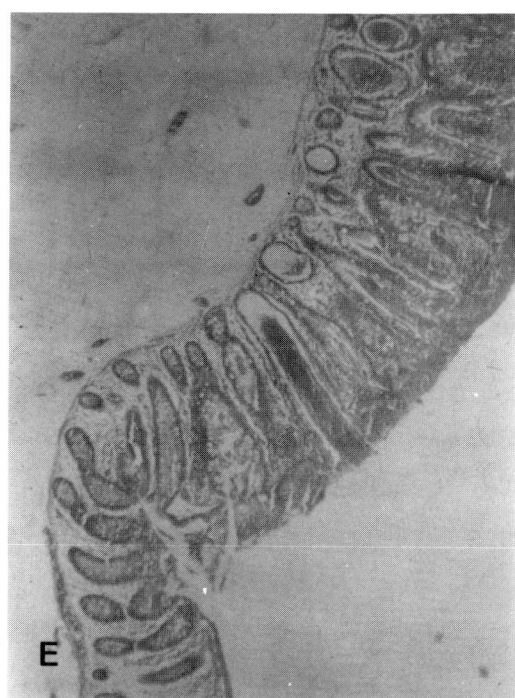

Figure 3.49 *Continued*

Vasculitis

Vasculitis may involve blood vessels in two different ways:

1. From an angiographic standpoint, there may be occlusion or aneurysm formation. Ischemic ulcerations which may bleed can develop with occlusion (Figs. 3.26 and 3.27).
2. When aneurysms are formed, bleeding may be caused by intraluminal rupture of aneurysms (Fig. 3.50). Classical examples of the first type include chronic myeloid leukosis and Wegener's granulomatosis. An example of the second type is polyarteritis nodosa.

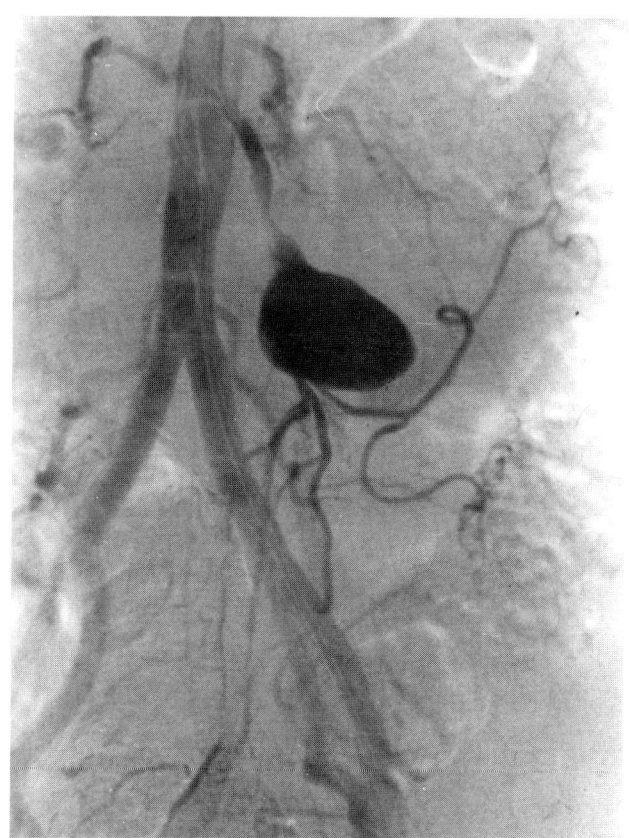

Figure 3.50 Injection into the inferior mesenteric artery of a 32-year-old patient with systemic arterial hypertension who had previously been operated on for a saccular aneurysm in the right common femoral artery. The angiogram shows a large aneurysm in the left colic artery, which was still asymptomatic, but required immediate treatment, as rupture and bleeding rates are very high in these patients.

REFERENCES

Antler AS, Pitchumoni CS, Thomas E, Orangio G, Scanlan BC. Gastrointestinal bleeding in the elderly—morbidity, mortality, and cause. *Am J Surg* 1981;142:271–273.

Athanasoulis CA. Lower gastrointestinal bleeding. In *interventional radiology,* edited by Athanasoulis CA, Pfister RC, Greene RE, Roberson GH. Saunders, Philadelphia, 1982:115–148.

Athanasoulis CA, Baum S, Rosch J, et al. Mesenteric arterial infusions of vasopressin for hemorrhage from colonic diverticulosis. *Am J Surg* 1975;129:212.

Athanasoulis CA, Galdabini JJ, Waltman AC, Noveline RA, Greenfield AJ, Azuleta ML. Angiodysplasia of the colon: A cause of rectal bleeding. *Cardiovasc Radiol* 1978;1:3–13.

Athanasoulis CA, Mondure AC, Greenfield AJ, Ryan JA, Dodson TF. Intraoperative localization of small bowel bleeding sites with combined use of angiographic methods and methylene blue injection. *Surgery* 1980;87:77–84.

Baer JW, Ryan S. Analysis of cecal vasculature in the search for vascular malformations. *AJR* 1976;126:394–405.

Baum S, Athanasoulis CA, Waltman AC. Angiographic diagnosis and control of large bowel bleeding. *Dis Colon Rectum* 1974;17:447–453.

Baum S, Athanasoulis CA, Waltman AC, Galdabini J, Schapiro R, Warshaw A, Ottinger LW. Angiodysplasis of the right colon as a cause of gastrointestinal bleeding. *AJR* 1977;129:789–794.

Baum S, Nusbaum M, Blakemore WS, et al. The preoperative radiographic demonstration of intraabdominal bleeding from undetermined sites by percutaneous selective celiac and superior mesenteric arteriography. *Surgery* 1965;58:797–802.

Baum S, Rosch J, Dotter CT, et al. Selective mesenteric arterial infusions in the management of massive diverticular hemorrhage. *N Engl J Med* 1973;288:1269–1272.

Boijsen E, Reuter SR. Angiography in diagnosis of chronic unexplained melena. *Radiology* 1967;89:413–419.

Boley SJ, Sammartano R, Dams A, Biase A, Kleinhaus S, Sprayregan S. On the nature and etiology of vascular ectasias of the colon: Degenerative lesions of aging. *Gastroenterology* 1977;72:650–660.

Boley SJ, Sprayregan S, Sammartano RJ, Adams A, Kleinhaus S. The pathophysiologic basis for the angiographic signs of vascular ectasias of the colon. *Radiology* 1977;125:615–621.

Bookstein JJ. Angiographic diagnosis and transcatheter therapy of lower gastrointestinal bleeding. In *Interventional Radiology,* edited by Wilkins RA, Viamonte M. Blackwell, London, 1982:111–136.

Cavallezzi JA, Kaufman SL, White RI. Vasopressin control of massive hemorrhage in chronic ulcerative colitis. *AJR* 1976;127:672–675.

Cavett CM, Selby JH, Hamilton JL, Williamson JW. Arteriovenous malformation in chronic gastrointestinal bleeding. *Ann Surg* 1977;185:116–121.

Clark RA, Rosch J. Arteriography in the diagnosis of large bowel bleeding. *Radiology* 1970;94:83–88.

DeRemee RA, Weiland LH, McDonald TJ. Polymorphic reticulosis, lymphomatoid granulomatosis: Two diseases or one? *Mayo Clin Proc* 1978;53:634–640.

Eisenberg H, Laufer I, Skillman JJ. Arteriographic diagnosis and management of suspected colonic diverticular hemorrhage. *Gastroenterology* 1973;64:1091–1100.

Fisse G, Ma CK. Neoplasms. In *Anderson's Pathology,* edited by Kissane JM. Mosby, St. Louis, 1985:1077–1096.

Goudarzi HA, Mason LB. Fatal rectal bleeding due to tuberculosis of the cecum. *JAMA* 1982;247:667–668.

Jackson RS, Cremim BJ. Angiographic demonstration of gastrointestinal bleeding due to aorto-duodenal fistula. *Br J Radiol* 1976;49:966–967.

Koehler PR, Salmon RB. Angiographic localization of unknown acute gastrointestinal bleeding sites. *Radiology* 1967;89:244–249.

Lewi HJE, Goldhill T, Gilmour HM, Buist TAS. Arteriovenous malformations of the intestine. *Surg Gynecol Obstet* 1979;149:712–716.

Massive bleeding from diverticular disease of the colon (editorial). *Lancet* 1963;706.

McDonald TJ, DeRemee RA, Harvison CG, Faeer GW, Devine KD. The protean clinical feature of polymorphic reticulosis (lethal midline granuloma). *Laryngoscope* 1976;86:936–945.

Mellor JA, Chandler GN, Chapman H, Irving HC. Massive gastrointestinal bleeding in Crohn's disease: Successful control by intraarterial vasopressin infusion. *Gut* 1982;23:872–875.

Meyers MA, Alonso DR, Baer JW. Pathogenesis of massively bleeding colonic diverticulosis: New observations. *AJR* 1976;127:901–908.

Meyers MA, Alonso DR, Gray GF, Baer JW. Pathogenesis of bleeding colonic diverticulosis. *Gastroenterology* 1976;71:577–583.

Noer RJ. Hemorrhage as a complication of diverticulitis. *Ann Surg* 1955;141:674–678.

Russell E, LePage JR. Arteriographic bleeding: A new sign. *Radiology* 1975;115:13–16.

Sheedy PF, Fulton RE, Atwell DT. Angiographic evaluation of patients with chronic gastrointestinal bleeding. *AJR* 1975;123:338–347.

Simpson AJ, Previti FW. Technetium sulfur colloid scintigraphy in the detection of lower gastrointestinal tract bleeding. *Surg Gynecol Obstet* 1982;155:33–36.

Taylor FW, Epstein LI. Treatment of massive diverticular hemorrhage. *Arch Surg* 1969;98:505–508.

Uflacker R. Radiologia intervencionista: uma especialidade emergente. *Radiol Bras* 1983;16:71–85.

Uflacker R. Transcatheter embolization for treatment of acute lower gastrointestinal bleeding. *Acta Radiol,* 1987;28:425–430.

Uflacker R, Amaral NM, Lima S, Wholey MH, Pereira EC, Nobrega M, Tavares T. Angiography in primary myomas of the alimentary tract. *Radiology* 1981;139:361–369.

PORTAL HYPERTENSION AND GASTROINTESTINAL BLEEDING

Portal hypertension (PH) accompanied by bleeding esophageal varices obviously can cause upper GI bleeding. However, because of its pathophysiologic peculiarities, clinical and surgical treatment, and specific methods for interventional radiologic therapy, PH is treated here as a distinct category. As in all other cases of GI bleeding, these patients should be treated by a specialized team whose primary interest is GI bleeding in its many different aspects.

As with other forms of GI bleeding, the first step is to define the origin of bleeding. Data from the patient's history related to the existence of chronic liver disease, along with other aspects typical of this condition, should lead one to suspect variceal bleeding.

The initial procedure is upper digestive endoscopy to localize the origin of bleeding. The next step is taking proper action to control the bleeding.

Basically, only endoscopy can safely indicate the etiology of bleeding with certainty and determine whether it is caused by esophageal varices. Identification of varices by itself does not indicate that there actually is bleeding; in fact, only 30 to 50 percent of patients with liver disease present with hemorrhage caused by varices. It is important to identify varices as a source of bleeding, since management will be quite different if the bleeding is of arteriocapillary origin.

In approaching this subject from an interventional radiologist's point of view, one should concentrate on aspects related to angiographic therapy. Of course, there are not universally effective procedures that are accepted without argument in all cases. The approaches discussed here are neither the only correct ones nor necessarily the best ones available.

The recent revival of endoscopic sclerosis as a therapeutic method for patients with esophageal varicose bleeding is of interest in this context. It is an effective alternative which can be jointly adopted or used in a close collaboration between the radiologist and the endoscopist.

GENERAL ASPECTS

Portal hypertension may be caused by increased flow in the portal system, i.e., hyperkinetic PH, or by increased vascular resistance. An arterioportal fistula inside or

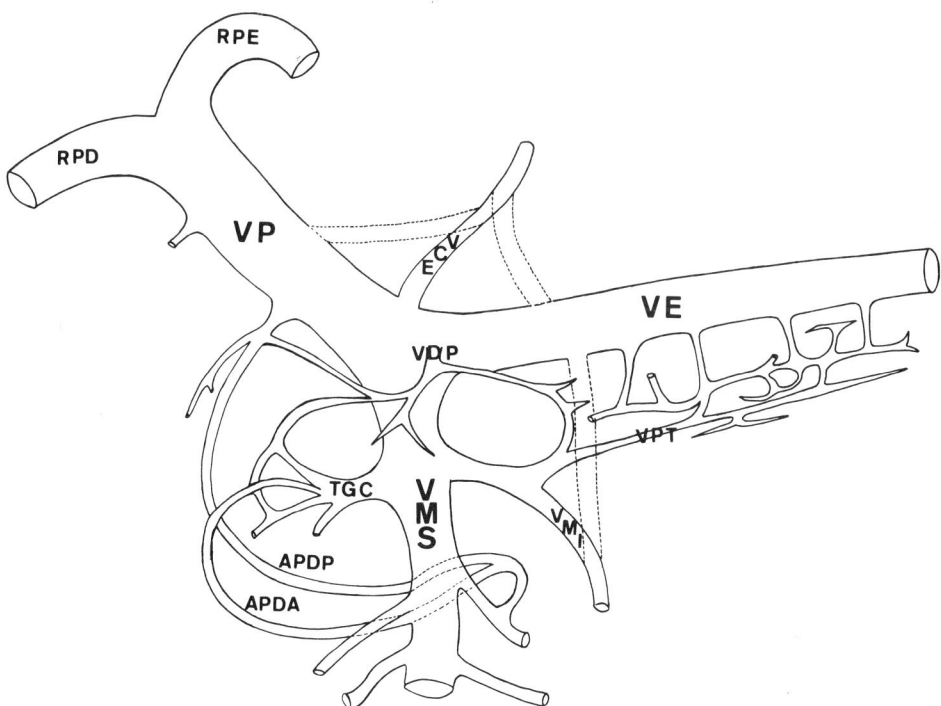

Figure 3.51 Schematic drawing of portal vein system. VP = portal vein; VE = splenic vein; VMS = superior mesenteric vein; RPD = right portal branch; RPE = left portal branch; VMI = inferior mesenteric vein; VCE = gastric coronary vein; VDP = pancreatic dorsal vein; VPT = transverse pancreatic vein; TGC = gastrocolic trunk; APDP = posterior pancreaticoduodenal arch; APDA = anterior pancreaticoduodenal arch.

outside the liver is an example of the first condition; organic lesions of the liver, the portal vein, and the hepatic veins are examples of the second, more common condition.

Whatever the etiology, the result is consistently the same: blood stagnation in the portal system in patients with increased vascular resistance and formation of venous collaterals with blood flow redirected to other sites in patients with all types of PH. The most common site for developed collaterals is the terminal esophagus, which will show varices and frequent bleeding episodes. There are many other functional and hemodynamic changes in the livers of patients with PH which are beyond the objectives of this chapter.

PH due to increased vascular resistance is classified into two groups: (1) presinusoidal extrahepatic or presinusoidal intrahepatic and (2) intrahepatic.

The presinusoidal group is divided into two different types. Presinusoidal extrahepatic PH is caused by obstruction of the portal venous system. This can be related to neonatal sepsis, portal phlebitis, tumor invasion, or diseases associated with increased coagulation.

The presinusoidal intrahepatic form of PH is caused by lesions in the portal space and the hepatic sinusoids. This type of lesion may have many different causes, such as reticuloendothelial system disease, sarcoidosis, congenital hepatic fibrosis, schistosomiasis, and primary biliary cirrhosis. Toxic factors such as inorganic arsenic, copper-containing sprays, and vinyl chloride vapors also can cause these hepatic complications. Lymphocytic infiltration of the sinusoids in patients with Felty's syndrome or chronic malaria can also cause the presinusoidal intrahepatic type of PH.

In all these conditions, an increase in splenic vein flow should be taken into consideration when one evaluates PH patients. Particularly in patients with schistosomiasis, the splenic component of PH is quite significant.

Intrahepatic PH is the most common type worldwide, with cirrhosis as the major cause. Obstruction of portal flow is present at all levels inside the liver. The concept of simple postsinusoidal PH in cirrhosis has been discarded. Obstruction is localized at all portal space levels from the sinusoids to their venous drainage. Budd-Chiari syndrome results in the obstruction of suprahepatic veins. This is therefore a form of intrahepatic PH at the postsinusoidal level. Veno-occlusive disease is also classified as intrahepatic PH.

Diagnostic angiographic procedures play a significant role in the evaluation of all PH patients. Three main conditions should be considered here:

1. Patients with suspected or diagnosed PH who are candidates for a portosystemic shunt
2. Patients without a previous history of chronic alcoholism or hepatitis who bleed from esophageal varices
3. Patients who have been submitted to portosystemic shunt surgery and have complications suggesting the presence of occlusion

Suspected or diagnosed PH in patients who are candidates for a portosystemic shunt is probably the most frequent indication for angiography in this regard. These patients can be divided into two groups: those seen during an upper GI bleeding episode, who are candidates for emergency surgery (an increasingly less common situation), and those who have stopped bleeding and are electively examined before being submitted to surgery. Angiography in these patients provides an accurate measurement of PH; discloses any existing portosystemic collaterals, especially varices; supplies information on the hemodynamic status of portal flow; and rules out the presence of acute-phase arterial bleeding. Clinical and endoscopic evaluation should precede angiography if possible.

There are four major types of angiographic procedures for the evaluation of hepatic blood flow. The first is hepatic venography with manometry. With this procedure, catheterization with hepatic vein occlusion makes it possible to measure transmitted sinusoidal pressure with a water manometer, which represents a static blood column extending from the portal vein through the sinusoids and hepatic venules. This pressure is approximately the same as splenic pulp pressure.

In addition to wedged pressure, free pressures are measured in the hepatic veins and the inferior vena cava. Normal pressures measured by means of catheter wedging vary between 40 and 150 mmH$_2$O. Cirrhotic PH includes two different components: one due to intrahepatic obstruction of portal flow and another which is pressure-transmitted from the inferior vena cava. Therefore, measuring free pressure in the hepatic vein and inferior vena cava is also important. Caval and hepatic venous pressure transmitted through intrahepatic collaterals has an impact on the measurement of wedged sinusoidal pressure. The concept of corrected sinusoidal pressure comes into play when the physician subtracts the free suprahepatic vein value from the sinusoidal figure that has been obtained. This so-called corrected sinusoidal pressure value should be approximately 100 mmH$_2$O as a maximum normal measurement. When the pressure is above this level, one should consider the possibility of PH. In patients with a corrected sinusoidal pressure below 200 mmH$_2$O and acute GI bleeding, the bleeding is probably not of varicose origin.

Injection of 8 mL of contrast medium at 2 mL/s with the catheter wedged into the hepatic vein will homogeneously opacify a group of hundreds of sinusoids drained by hepatic venules and veins in normal subjects. In cirrhotic patients, there is an irregular and nonhomogeneous impregnation pattern, with opacification of portal vein radicles. The more severe the fibrotic sinusoidal process, the greater the opacification of the portal vein in a clearly hepatofugal pattern.

The patency of the hepatic vein and its ostium can be evaluated by means of phlebography and free manometry. This makes it possible to determine the presence or absence of Budd-Chiari syndrome. In patients with advanced cirrhosis the hepatic veins appear to be significantly distorted.

Arterial procedures—the second category—exclude the presence of arterial bleeding during active hemorrhage. The physician evaluates arterial dynamics, the increase in which is proportional to the degree of cirrhosis and reduction of portal flow. These procedures may also determine the existence of a tumoral expanding lesion secondary to liver cirrhosis. When properly used, they can be employed to check the patency of the portal system through an arterial portogram. The arterial route was used in the past for Pitressin infusion to lower portal system pressure and control bleeding from varices. Endovenous infusion of Pitressin, however, can achieve the same kind of bleeding control, leading to a reduction in portal pressure levels similar to what is obtained with intraarterial injections.

Splenoportography and splenic manometry—the third category—are the oldest methods for evaluating the portal system and PH. Even today, splenoportography still supplies most of the information necessary for evaluating PH. Opacification of the portal system and of existing varices and collaterals is usually adequate. In early cases, the splenoportogram appears practically normal, but as liver disease progresses and resistance to portal flow increases, blood velocity inside the portal system decreases and collaterals show hepatofugal flow. In more advanced stages, portal flow becomes hepatofugal and collaterals such as the umbilical vein and portosystemic shunts are open.

Transhepatic percutaneous portography with manometry, sometimes followed by embolization of varices—the fourth category—is the most recent and exciting innovation in portal system evaluation and treatment of its most lethal complication: bleeding from GI varices. Although this technique allows direct access to the portal venous system and offers the possibility of occluding varices during acute bleeding episodes with a high success rate in controlling bleeding, it is not a definitive treatment for bleeding of variceal origin. It is instead the method of choice for controlling acute varicose bleeding which does not respond to the use of Pitressin. Embolization of esophageal varices that is performed electively may control the recurrence of hemorrhage while extending the interval between bleeding episodes. This, however, happens only in some patients, half of whom will bleed again during the 3 months that follow acute or selective embolization by recanalization of varices or the development of collaterals and new varices. Even when one uses powerful vascular sclerosing agents such as absolute alcohol, it is not possible to obtain permanent occlusion of the whole esophageal varicose system. More recently, transhepatic percutaneous portography has been used in association with portal transluminal angioplasty; the results have been excellent.

Some patients without a history of chronic alcoholism or hepatitis occasionally bleed from esophageal varices. These varices are usually diagnosed by means of endoscopy in patients with upper GI bleeding. The cause of PH in these patients is generally intra- or extrahepatic presinusoidal, with portal obstruction or a hepatic lesion caused by schistosomiasis. In endemic regions, such as Brazil, schistosomiasis is the most frequent cause of disease and bleeding in this patient group. Budd-Chiari syndrome also occurs in these patients.

Some patients who receive portosystemic shunt surgery have complications suggesting occlusion. Occasionally the postoperative period of a portosystemic decompression procedure is complicated by occlusion which is manifested by the recurrence of bleeding or the development of ascites. The angiogram in patients with a functioning portosystemic shunt should show side-to-side portocaval, distal or proximal mesocaval, or splenorenal communication. In all these cases except distal splenorenal communication, portal flow tends to reverse itself, with the liver being supplied by an enlarged hepatic artery. The size of the liver tends to be reduced because of a decrease in the input of hepatotrophic factors caused by decreased portal flow. Wedged venous pressure remains within normal limits, and the venogram shows reversed portal flow. In a selective (distal) splenorenal shunt, portal flow is maintained and only blood from the spleen is diverted to the renal vein. In cases of portosystemic shunt occlusion, the patient should be studied from both the arterial side and the venous side.

When there is obstruction, the arterial portogram does not show communication of the portal system with the vena cava or show the occluded portal vein or splenic vein. In some cases, only a stenosed anastomosis is found. When there is thrombosis in the shunt, it is sometimes possible to catheterize the portal venous system through the shunt, using a caval approach. Pressure measurement and shunt disobstruction by means of dilation with an angioplasty balloon catheter has become a frequently used procedure. In a patient whose spleen has been preserved, it is feasible to perform a splenoportogram, which may show the splenorenal anastomosis or its occlusion.

HYPERKINETIC PORTAL HYPERTENSION

Pressure in the portal system is elevated by an increase of flow through an arterioportal fistula or AV communication in an intra- or extrahepatic hypervascular tumoral lesion.

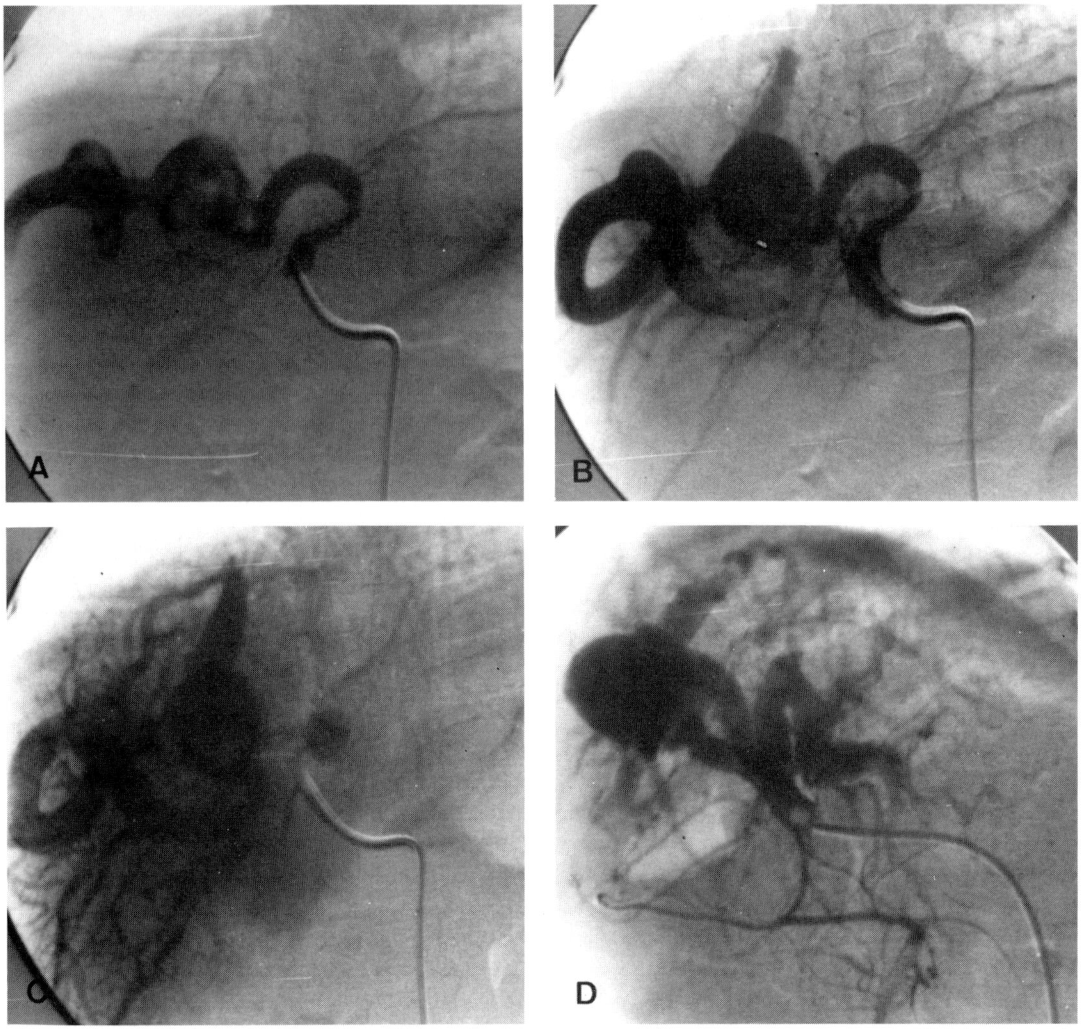

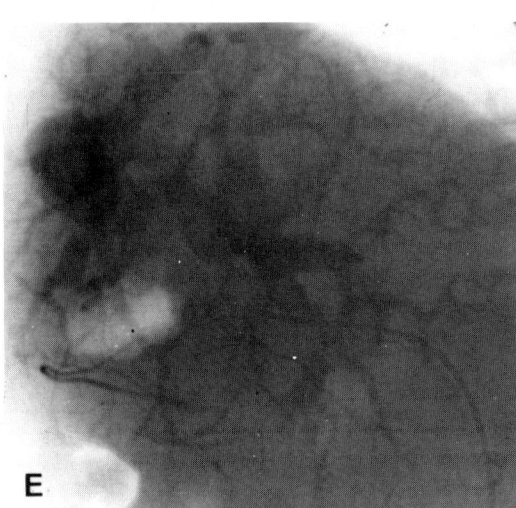

Figure 3.52 A 2½-month-old child with a congenital arteriovenous fistula of the liver causing portal hypertension and bleeding esophageal varices.
(A) Early phase of a hepatic selective arteriogram shows aneurysm dilation and the portal vein starting to be filled from the fistula. (B) Intermediate phase of an anteriogram shows dense filling of the portal vein. (C) Later phase of angiogram shows opacification of the intrahepatic portal system. (D,E) Lateral view of selective hepatic injection shows the fistula. The lesion was treated surgically and totally cured.

Arteriovenous fistulas are rare in the portal circulation. In most cases they are associated with a fistula between the splenic artery and splenic vein or with a fistula in the portal vein. Congenital intrahepatic arterioportal fistula is a very rare condition (Fig. 3.52). Fistulas involving the superior mesenteric artery and vein are even more rare (Fig. 3.53) and can be either congenital or acquired. An intrahepatic tumor mass (hepatoma) or renal tumor metastasis to the pancreas and mesenterium can also cause hyperflow and PH (Fig. 3.19).

The most sensible treatment for this type of lesion is transcatheter embolization, which produces excellent results (Fig. 3.53).

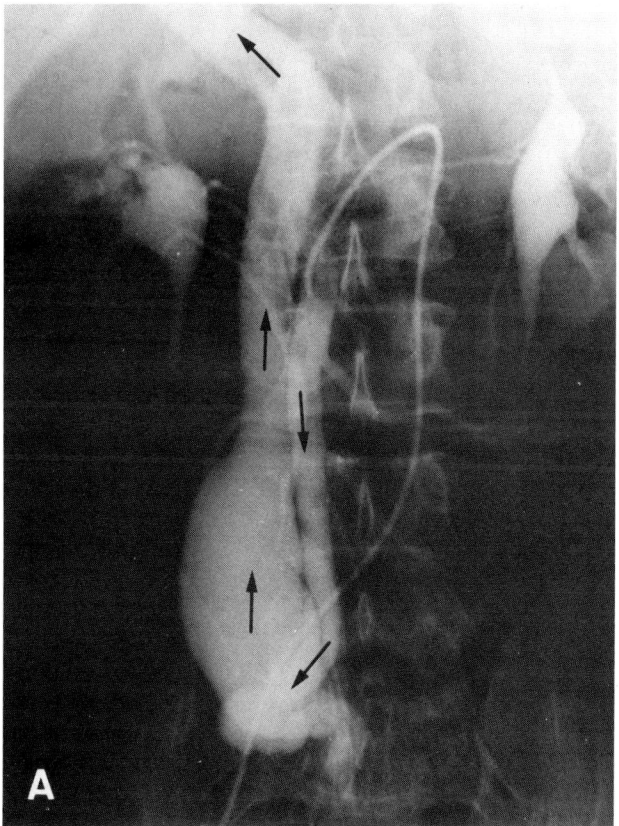
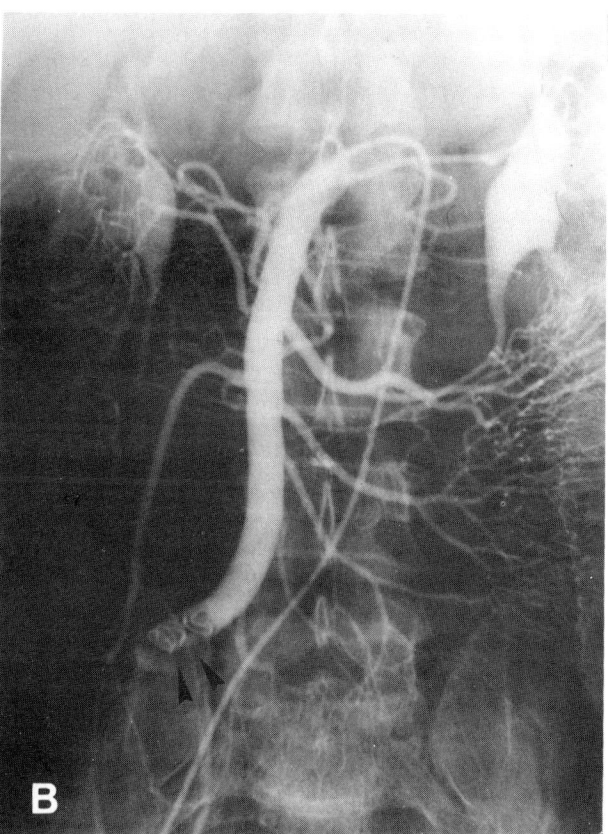

Figure 3.53 (A) Selective angiogram of the superior mesenteric artery. High-output arteriovenous fistula with immediate and dense filling of the superior mesenteric and portal veins. Note dilation in the proximal vein from the aneurysm and poor filling of the intestinal circulation associated with mesenteric angina. (B) Control after embolization with occlusion of the arteriovenous fistula with Gianturco coils and correction of hyperkinetic portal hypertension and intestinal angina pain.

EXTRAHEPATIC PRESINUSOIDAL PORTAL HYPERTENSION

Portal Vein Obstruction

Extrahepatic PH and upper GI bleeding due to obstruction of the portal system occur less frequently than do other types of intrahepatic PH. Many problems may be encountered in these patients in terms of diagnosis and surgical treatment. Portal obstruction is the most common cause of pediatric PH, although according to some authors, 50 percent of these patients are adults (Fig. 3.54). Specific causes of portal system obstruction include infection, trauma, congenital abnormalities, coagulopathies, pancreatic disease, tumoral invasion or compression, retroperitoneal fibrosis, hepatic AV fistula, drugs, hereditary hemorrhagic telangiectasia, and liver biopsy.

Angiographic techniques are valuable in diagnosing obstruction of the portal venous system and in mapping varices and collateral circulation through an arterial or

Figure 3.54 Splenoportogram in a patient with portal hypertension shows gastroesophageal varices due to portal vein thrombosis and cavernomatous change.

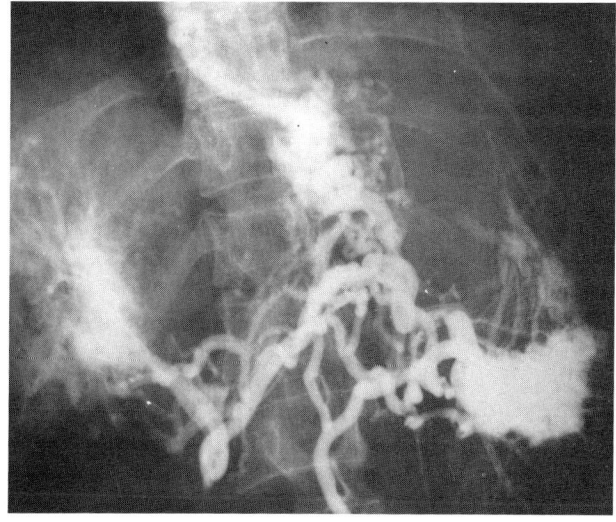

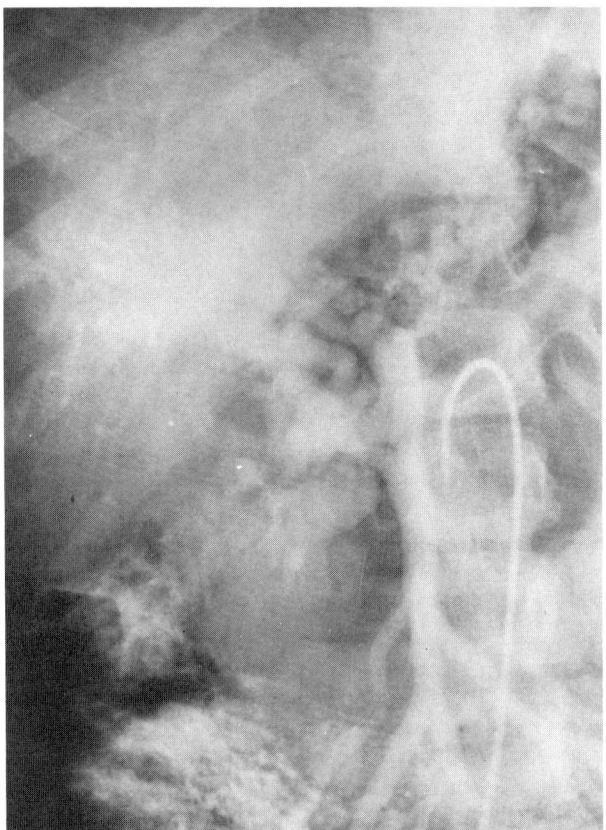

Figure 3.55 **The use of papaverine, 80 mg, as a vasodilator for better visualization of the superior mesenteric vein and portal vein occlusion in a 7-year-old child.**

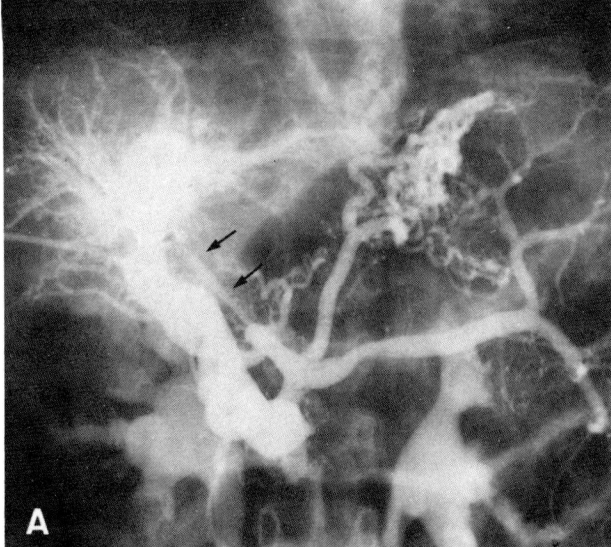

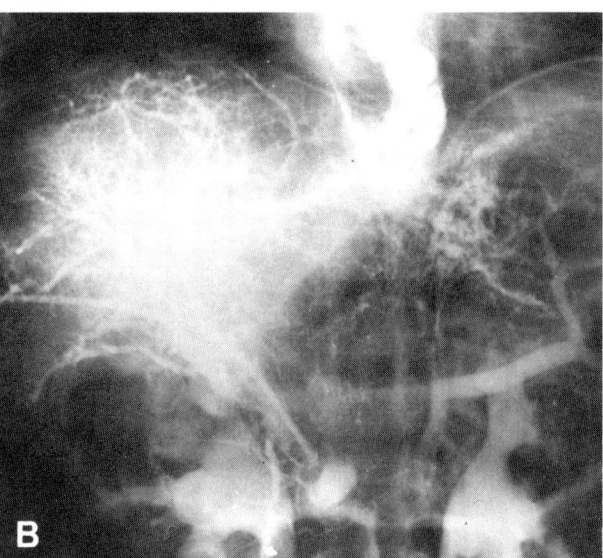

Figure 3.56 **Percutaneous transhepatic portogram (PTP) in a 32-month-old child with portal thrombosis due to postnatal sepsis.**
(A) PTP catheterization of the portal system obtained through innominate venous collaterals in the hepatic hilum. Note the remainder of the portal vein (arrows). Varices could not be selectively catheterized or embolized. (B) Later phase of PTP shows peripheral filling of intrahepatic portal radicles.

phlebographic approach. A diagnosis of portal obstruction can be made by means of hepatic venous pressure measurement, a visceral angiogram with vasodilators, and a splenic and portal venogram (Fig. 3.55). More recently, ultrasound and computed tomography have been used to diagnose obstruction of the portal system.

Until very recently, however, percutaneous transhepatic portography was contraindicated in the presence of portal vein obstruction (Fig. 3.56). A recent report has shown that a percutaneous transhepatic portogram can be performed in most patients who will be treated with embolization (Fig. 3.56). In the same report, transhepatic portal vein angioplasty was mentioned as a possible alternative for treating portal obstruction. Embolization of esophageal varices can be performed in approximately half these patients (Fig. 3.57).

Portal system obstruction is not always clearly seen in the angiogram, and the use of two or more methods

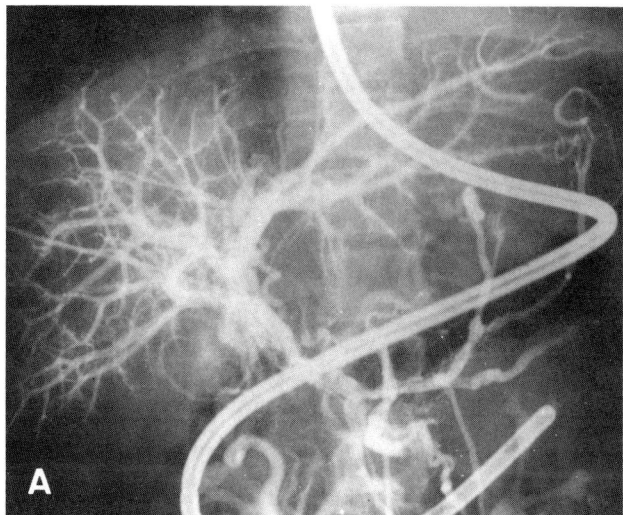

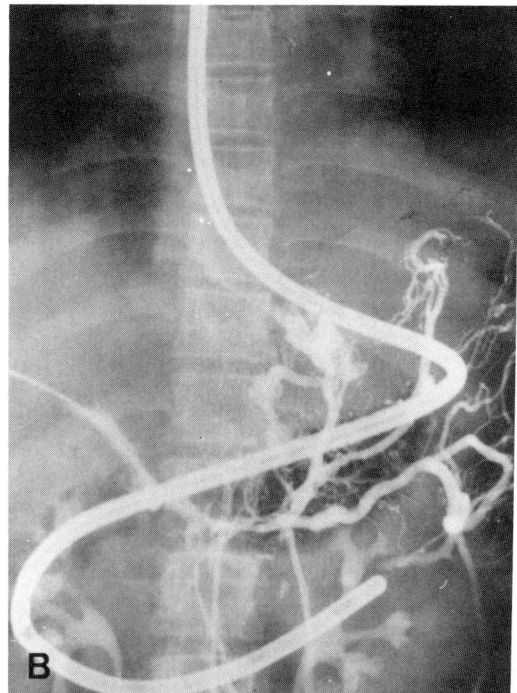

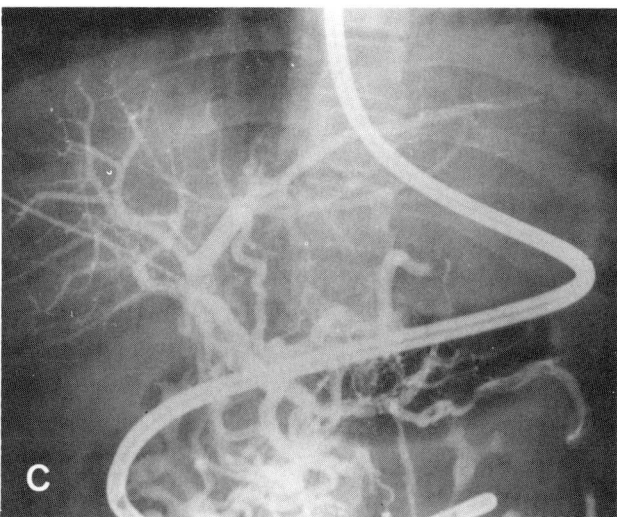

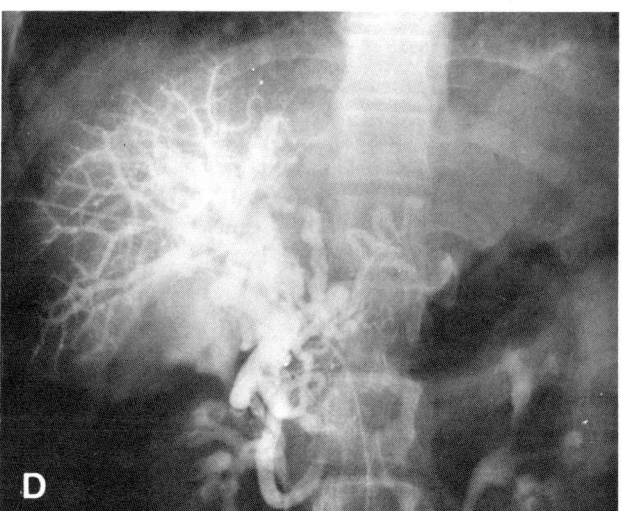

Figure 3.57 Partial occlusion of the portal vein embolization of varices in a patient with a previous splenectomy.
(A) Early phase of a percutaneous transhepatic portogram shows extensive portal vein occlusion and varices. (B) Selective injection with the catheter tip in the ostium of the left gastric vein. (C) Control after Gelfoam embolization without opacification of varices. (D) Follow-up portogram 6 months after embolization shows the evolution of the process and the development of a more extensive thrombosis of the portal system.

may be necessary to show an occlusion. A superior mesenteric arteriogram with a vasodilator (papaverine) and an extended venous phase probably is the best method for detecting portal obstruction (Fig. 3.55). This study, however, must be technically optimal, which is not always possible. Splenoportography is the next best alternative for showing portal obstruction; however, the whole portal venous system is not always visualized because of the formation of hepatofugal flow collaterals and predominant flow shunting to these collateral vessels. A transhepatic portogram can be used to diagnose portal obstruction only when catheterization of the venous system is possible (Figs. 3.58 and 3.59).

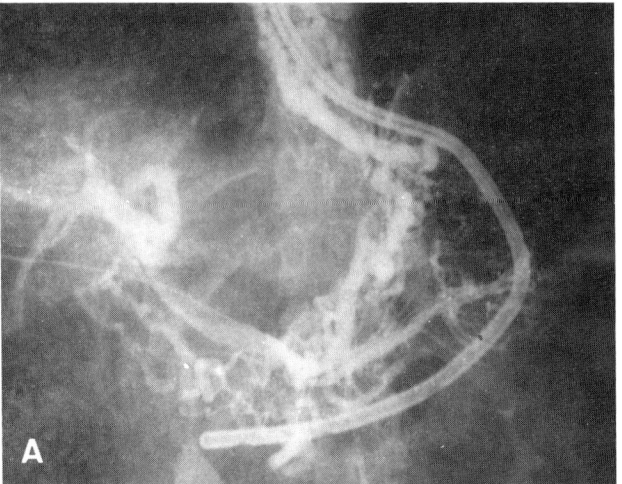
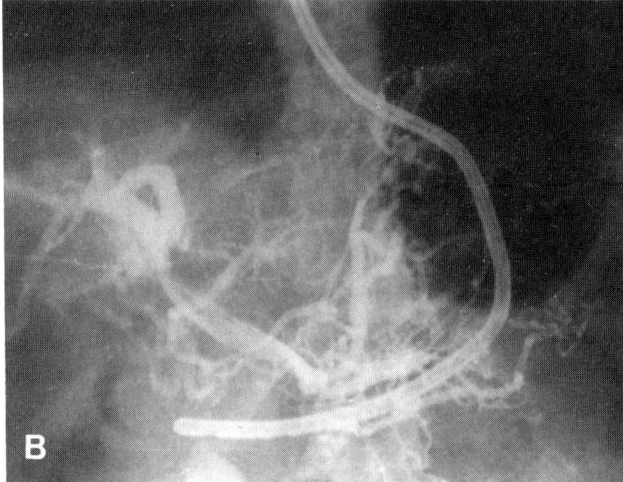

Figure 3.58 Percutaneous transhepatic portogram (PTP) in a 30-year-old patient with alcoholic cirrhosis, acute varicose bleeding, and recent partial thrombosis.
(A) PTP showing varices of the gastric fundus and terminal esophagus. Note the dilated gastric balloon, which does not occlude the varices. Portal pressure was 390 mmH$_2$0. (B) Control PTP after embolization shows occlusion of most parts of the varices, with an increase of portal pressure to 450 mmH$_2$0.

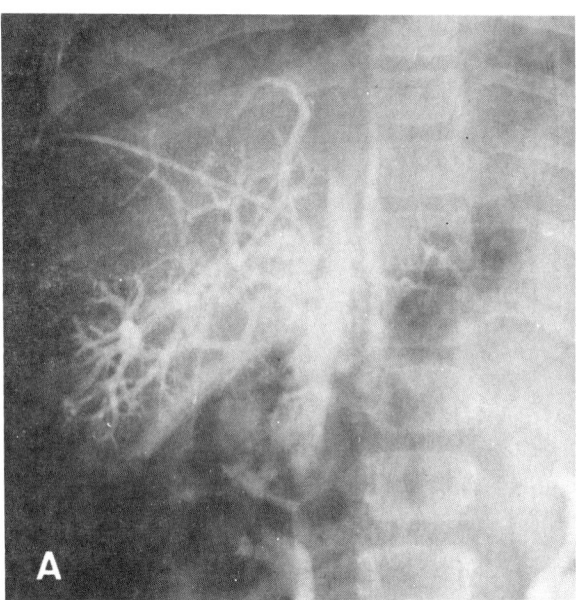
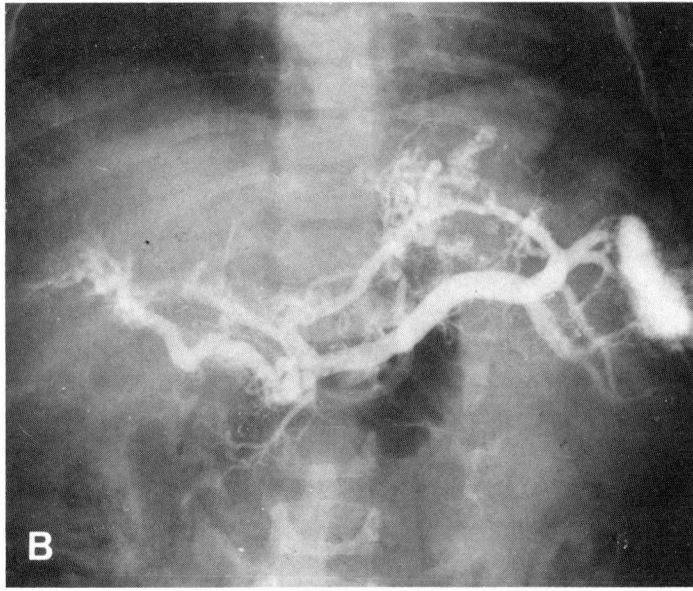

Figure 3.59 (A) Unsuccessful attempt at percutaneous transhepatic portography in a patient with portal thrombosis. The portal vein and collaterals are not identified. (B) Percutaneous splenoportogram showing the portal occlusion site and periportal collateral circulation.

Additional gain may be obtained when the portal system is catheterized, since embolization of esophageal varices can be performed during this procedure (Fig. 3.57). Portal vein dilatation may be attempted in some cases (Fig. 3.60).

Extensive controversies have arisen regarding adequate treatment for bleeding from GI varices secondary to noncirrhotic portal obstruction. Several authors have shown that portosystemic shunting procedures are not effective in these patients. However, more recent reports

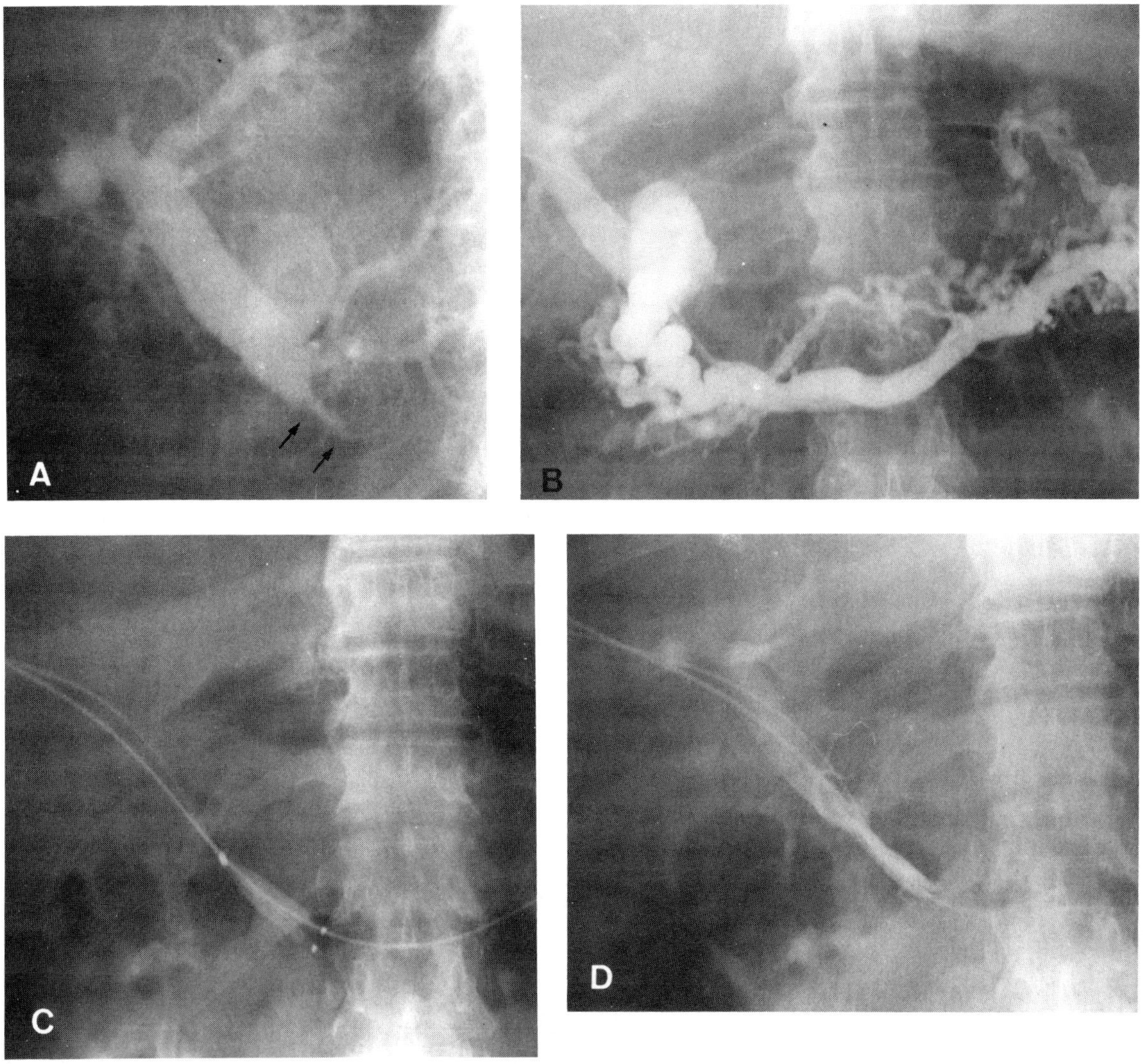

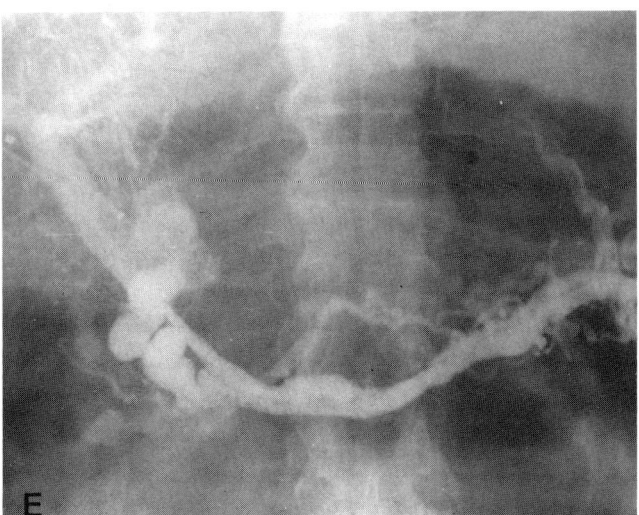

Figure 3.60 (A) A percutaneous transhepatic portogram shows abrupt obstruction of the portal vein and the short and residual lumen of the occluded segment in a patient with chronic pancreatitis (arrows). (B) After catheterization through the occluded segment, the patency of the splenic vein is shown. Notice the multiple collateral veins. (C) Two 6-mm balloon catheters dilating the obstruction. (D,E) Control after dilation of the obstruction showing improvement of the stenosis after angioplasty and reduction of the pressure gradient and varices. (F,G) Two months after the first angioplasty, a new dilation of the stenosis was performed with two 8-mm-diameter balloons. (H) Final control shows significant improvement in the diameter of the stenosis, with the collaterals and gastric varices having disappeared. Pressures did not show a significant gradient. Predilation intrahepatic portal pressure was 28 cmH$_2$0 and splenic pressure was 40 cmH$_2$0 in (A), (B), and (C). Postdilation intrahepatic portal pressure dropped to 23 cmH$_2$0 and splenic pressure was 28 cmH$_2$0 in (D) and (E). After the second dilation, portal pressure was 19 cmH$_2$0 and splenic pressure was 22 cmH$_2$0. There was no significant change in pressures after the second dilation.

Figure 3.60 *Continued*

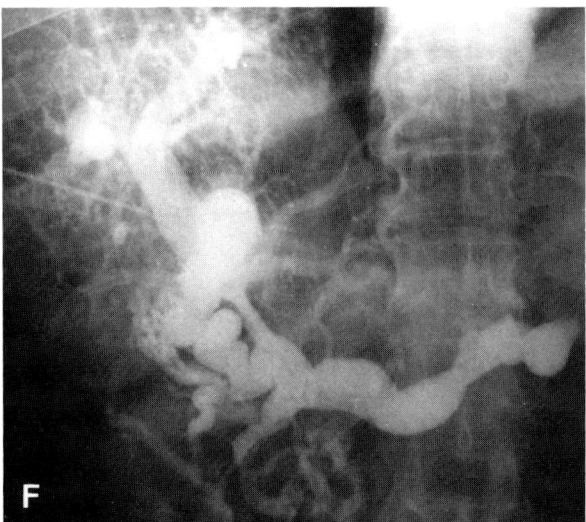

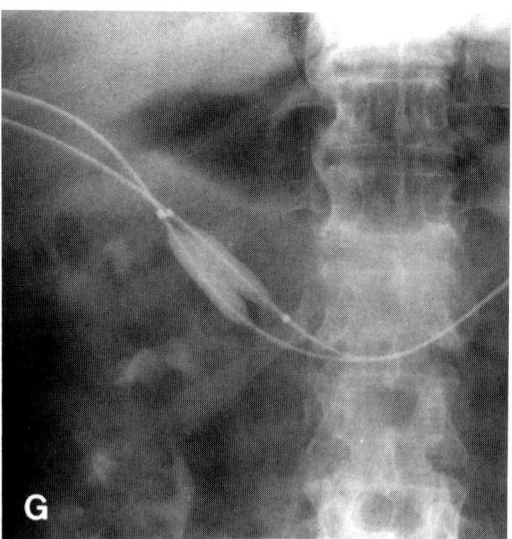

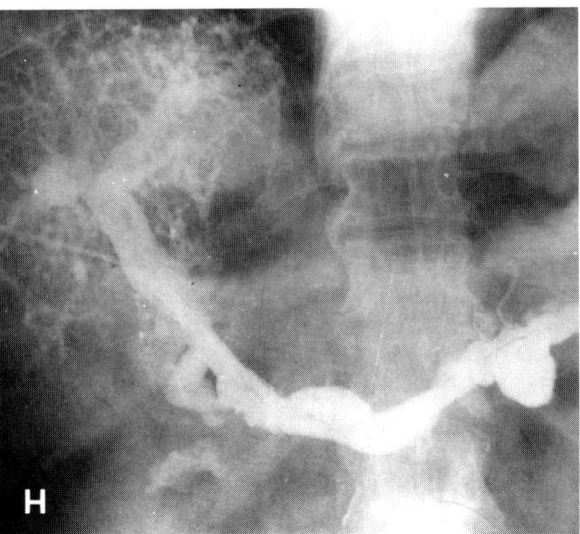

have shown a high incidence of long-term patency and a low rate of occurrence of encephalopathies resulting from shunt procedures or jugular vein interposition. There is undoubtedly a high rate of postsurgical complications in these patients.

Recently developed radiologic and endoscopic techniques have given a new direction to the treatment of patients with recurrent bleeding. Embolization of varices by the transhepatic route in cases of portal system obstruction is possible in 50 percent of adult and pediatric patients. In patients in whom it is possible to catheterize the remainder of the portal vein, angioplasty can be attempted. However, the intrahepatic portal system must be partly patent, and this is not likely to be the case in most children. In patients with portal vein obstruction resulting from pancreatitis, angioplasty can be performed (Fig. 3.60). This seems to be a more physiologic and less traumatic technique than a surgical procedure, but it may be beneficial in only a limited number of patients.

INTRAHEPATIC PRESINUSOIDAL PORTAL HYPERTENSION

Schistosomiasis

Advanced hepatic schistosomiasis is characterized by portal fibrosis and obstruction of branches of the intrahepatic portal vein. A type of presinusoidal PH results from such a lesion and is associated with some or no loss of hepatocellular functions. Hemodynamic study of patients with hepatic schistosomiasis usually reveals PH and normal sinusoidal pressure. In some patients, however, sinusoidal pressure can be as elevated as it is in cirrhotic livers. Increased arterial hepatic circulation has been identified more recently in these patients and is considered to be responsible for increased hepatic sinusoidal pressure.

In hepatosplenic schistosomiasis there is a significant contribution of splenic blood flow to the level of PH. Reductions in portal pressure as high as 40 percent are seen after splenectomy or distal splenorenal shunt is performed in schistosomiasis patients. Splenic artery occlusion with a balloon catheter performed simultaneously with transhepatic portal catheterization with manometry can be helpful in assessing what the effects of splenectomy or a splenorenal shunt will be (Fig. 3.61).

A portal fibrotic process usually evolves slowly but progressively, leading to elevated PH and the development of significant portosystemic collaterals.

Arterial angiographic study shows a typical dilated appearance of the hepatic and splenic arteries, an enlarged spleen, and a reduced liver. A transhepatic portogram or splenoportogram shows a very typical aspect resulting from Symmers' fibrosis. This aspect is

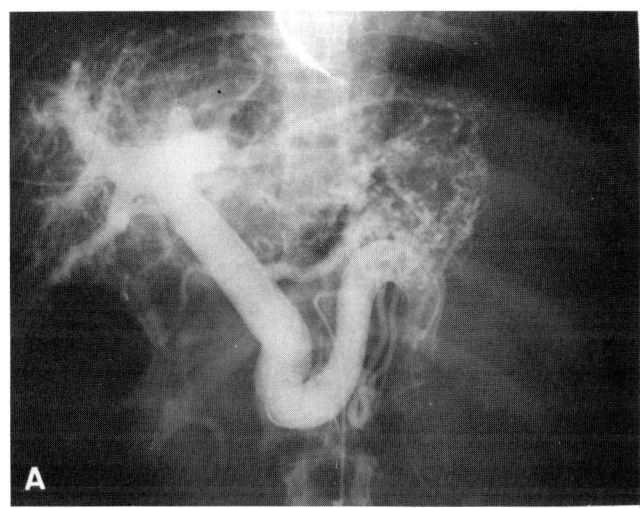

Figure 3.61 A 27-year-old patient with postnecrotic cirrhosis. A splenic selective arteriogram shows an enlarged spleen with increased circulation.
(A) A percutaneous transhepatic portogram shows the portal system. Measured pressure was 390 mmH$_2$0. (B,C) After occlusion of the splenic artery with a balloon, pressure dropped to 355 mmH$_2$0, the portal hypertension splenic component having been removed. (D) Selective injection into the left gastric vein before embolization of varices. (E) Portogram after embolization of varices shows a slight increase in portal pressure to 400 mmH$_2$0.

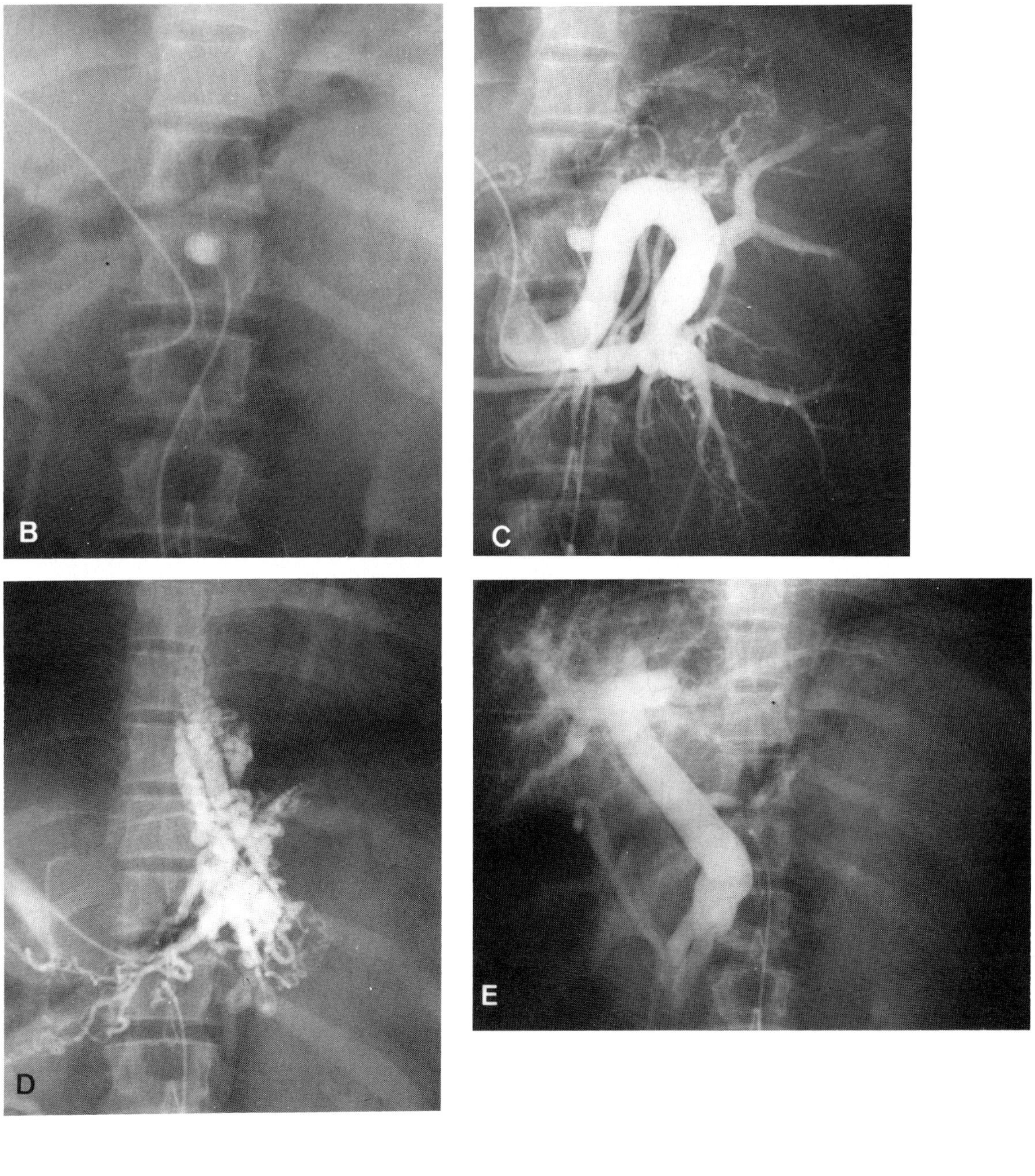

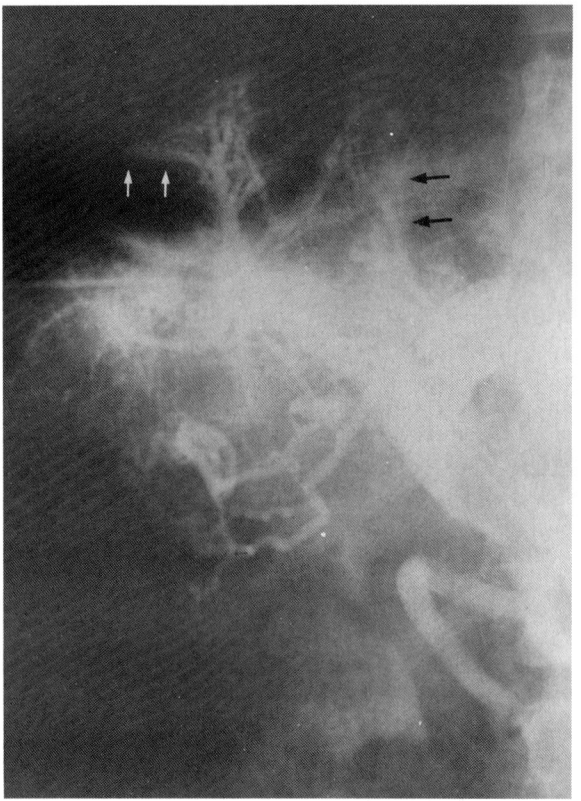

Figure 3.62 A patient with schistosomiasis studied with transhepatic portography shows the Bogliolo sign, i.e., duplication of portal radicles during opacification in the venogram (arrows).

characterized by vascular sheathlike neoformation involving the intrahepatic branches of the portal vein, producing an angiographic image of duplication of the portal radicles (Fig. 3.62). This has been also described as a typical feature in congenital hepatic fibrosis. The fibrotic process is apparently the same, leading to the development of sheathlike venous neovascular circulation.

Congenital Hepatic Fibrosis

Congenital hepatic fibrosis has a typical histologic appearance, with the most important finding being fibrotic tissue deposits in the portal space of liver lobules associated with dysmorphic biliary ducts. These typical aspects are occasionally accompanied by dilatation or compression of the thin walls of interlobular portal branches in the fibrotic area. This disease may cause severe PH with the development of venous collaterals and esophageal varices, sometimes with bleeding. A portal phlebogram of a patient with congenital hepatic fibrosis shows a very typical aspect of duplication of portal intrahepatic branches (Fig. 3.63) that is similar to a phlebographic image of hepatic schistosomiasis. This aspect consists of a vein surrounded by a sheath of venous collateral circulation that develops in the periportal fibrotic tissue. Although this is comparable to Symmers' fibrosis, it occurs only in congenital hepatic fibrosis patients with PH.

INTRAHEPATIC PORTAL HYPERTENSION

Hepatic Cirrhosis

Hepatic cirrhosis of all types is the major cause of intrahepatic PH. Obstruction of portal venous flow occurs at all levels inside the liver. The intrahepatic portal vascular bed is distorted and reduced. Venous radicles of the portal vein and sinusoids are compressed by regenerative nodules. This nodular obstruction has led to the concept of venous drainage obstruction in cirrhosis (postsinusoidal); venous stasis, however, extends from afferent vessels to sinusoids, to the sinusoids themselves, and to the postsinusoidal vessels. Obstruction of portal flow therefore occurs at all levels from the portal space to the hepatic venous drainage.

Figure 3.63 A patient with congenital hepatic fibrosis showing the duplication aspect of portral radicles as a perivascular sheath. This aspect is similar to schistosomiasis.

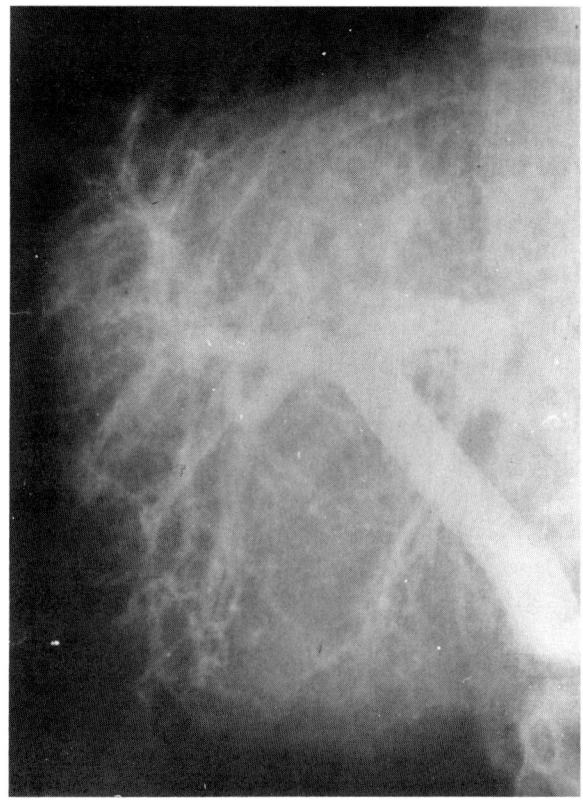

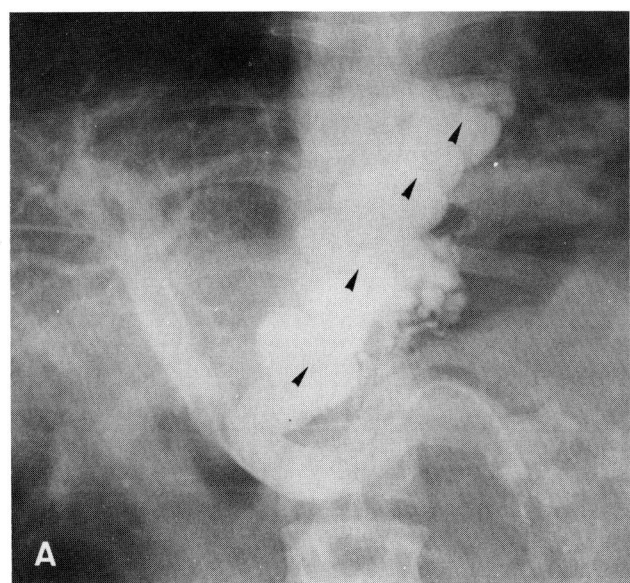
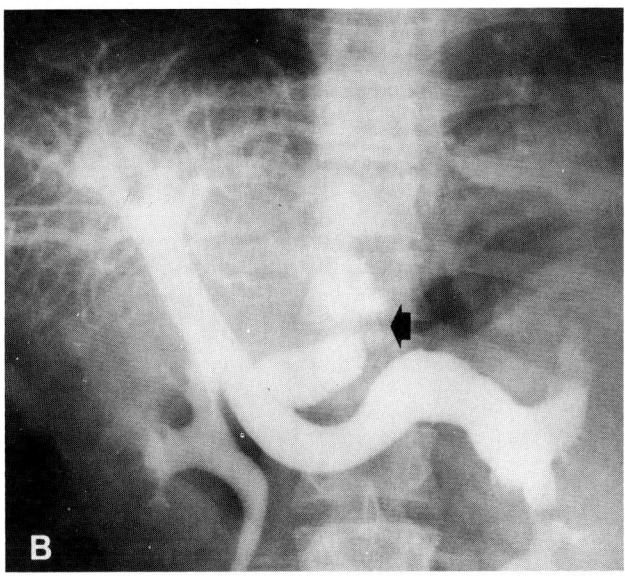

Figure 3.64 A patient with postnecrotic cirrhosis and acute varicose bleeding.
(A) A portogram shows giant varices originating from the left gastric vein, which is larger than the portal vein. Varices were occluded with absolute alcohol and Gelfoam. (B) A control portogram shows occlusion of varices. Portal pressure rose from 310 to 360 mmH$_2$O.

The type of therapeutic procedure used depends on the type of PH. If variceal bleeding is caused by cirrhosis resulting from sinusoidal obstruction, the patient can be treated with vasopressin to lower mesenteric flow and portal venous pressure. Transhepatic occlusion of gastroesophageal varices may be tried if bleeding persists (Fig. 3.64). However, if PH is caused by a high-output AV fistula or by a hypervascular hepatic tumor with AV communication, the best approach is to reduce arterial flow through the fistula or tumor by means of catheter embolization and artery occlusion (Fig. 3.53).

The major problem in patients with sinusoidal blockage is the development of hepatofugal-type collaterals. These collaterals are classified in three main groups:

Group I: veins located in the GI tract, terminal esophagus, gastric fundus, and hemorrhoidal plexus, with varicosity formation
Group II: veins located in the fetal umbilical circulation pathway, with Medusa-head formation (Fig. 3.65)
Group III: veins located in the retroperitoneal GI tract or in adhesions between the intestines and the abdominal wall (Fig. 3.36)

Vasoconstrictors—Pituitrin and later vasopressin—have been used since 1956 in intravenous bolus injections to control varicose bleeding by decreasing portal system flow and pressure. Many different complications, such as myocardial ischemia, hypertension, and arrhythmias, have occurred in spite of success in controlling bleeding. To decrease the number of complications, the concept of selective catheter pharmacoangiography with infusion of vasoconstricting agents into the superior mesenteric artery in doses varying from 0.2 to 0.4 IU/min was developed in 1967. As the incidence of complications apparently was lower, this practice was adopted in some centers until 1974. At that time it was proved that both intraarterial infusion and endovenous infusion of vasopressin have the same effect on portal circulation as they do on systemic hemodynamics and are equally effective in controlling bleeding from varices. The method for transhepatic catheterization of the portal system was introduced in 1971, and in 1974 a paper reported the success of transhepatic catheterization and occlusion of esophageal varices in treating patients with bleeding varices.

Many transhepatic techniques and multiple materials have been utilized to promote occlusion of esophageal varices, including sclerosing agents, autologous clots, Gelfoam, coils, bucrylate, and absolute alcohol.

The first step in treating cirrhotic patients who present with GI bleeding is to check the location and cause through endoscopy and occasionally through angiography. The second step is hemorrhage control by means

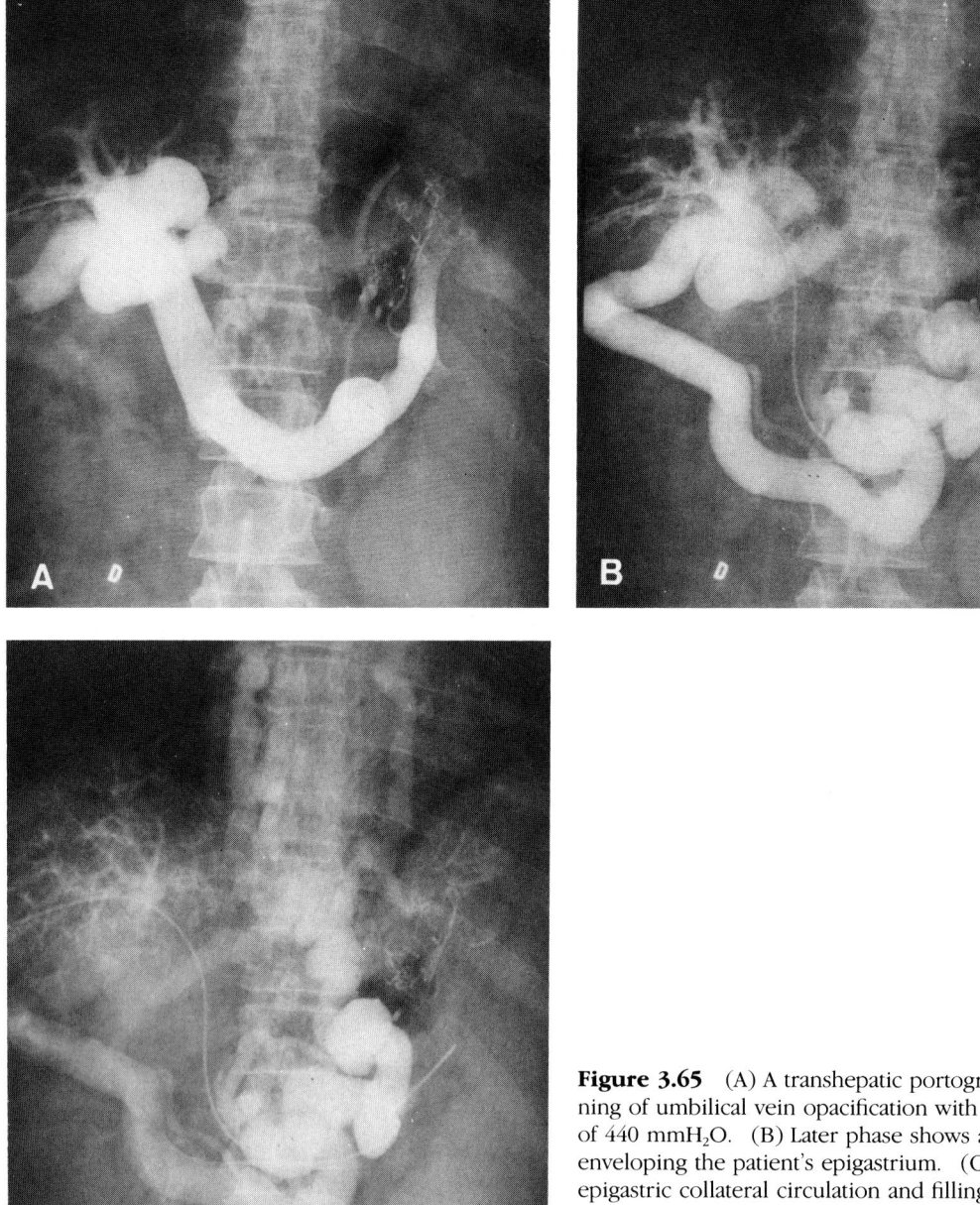

Figure 3.65 (A) A transhepatic portogram shows the beginning of umbilical vein opacification with an average pressure of 440 mmH$_2$O. (B) Later phase shows a large umbilical vein enveloping the patient's epigastrium. (C) Later phase shows epigastric collateral circulation and filling of the internal mammary veins on both sides of the sternum. Pressure after occlusion of varices was 560 mmH$_2$O. The cause of portal hypertension was postnecrotic cirrhosis, and the patient received a splenorenal anastomosis.

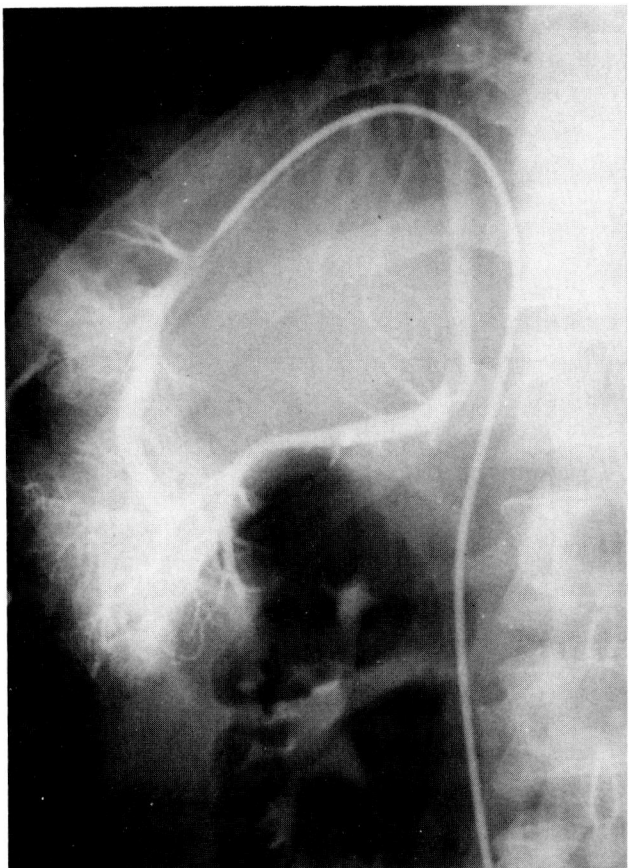

Figure 3.66 Right hepatic phlebogram in a free position in a patient who presented with moderate cirrhosis. Advancing the catheter toward the periphery allows occluded pressure and phlebography to be obtained with an acinogram.

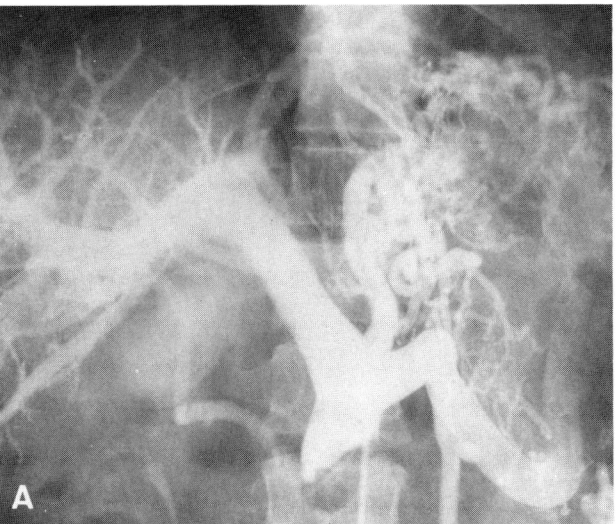

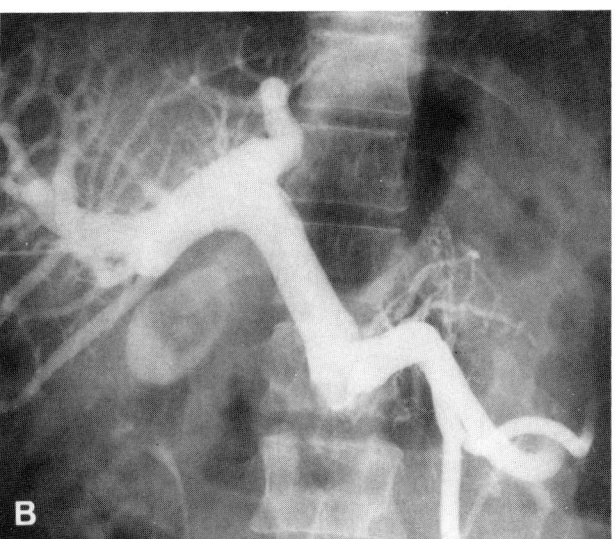

Figure 3.67 (A) A percutaneous transhepatic portogram in a 37-year-old patient with alcoholic cirrhosis and bleeding varices. Note the presence of varices in the gastric fundus and terminal esophagus. Portal pressure was 300 mmH$_2$O. (B) Control angiography after occlusion of varices with absolute alcohol. Pressure increased to 350 mmH$_2$O. Bleeding was controlled, and a splenorenal shunt was performed a few months later.

of endoscopic sclerosis, sometimes before a portosystemic shunt.

Approximately 10 percent of patients with upper GI bleeding bleed from varices. Among the entire population of patients with endoscopically proven esophageal varices, less than 50 percent bleed from these varices during an upper GI bleeding episode.

Emergency arteriography should include injections into the celiac axis and superior mesenteric artery to demonstrate or exclude the presence of arterial bleeding and define the patency of the portal system. If the patient is hemodynamically stable, hepatic venous pressures can be obtained (Fig. 3.66). Depending on the need for evaluation of hepatic lesions, a portal phlebogram can be performed; many significant anatomic aspects may be defined during this procedure (Figs. 3.67 and 3.68).

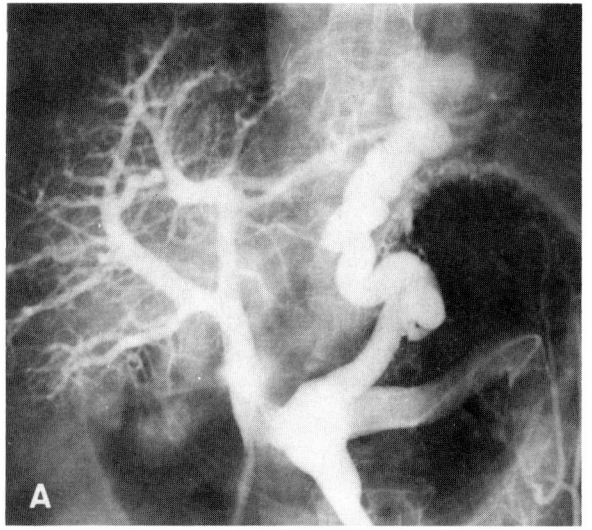
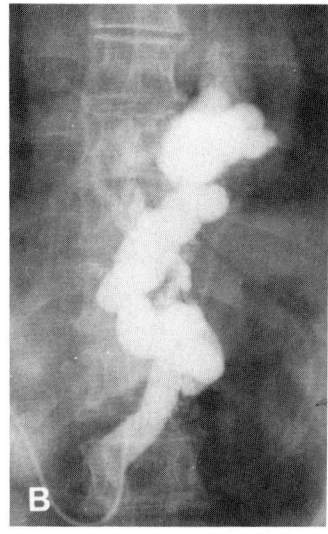
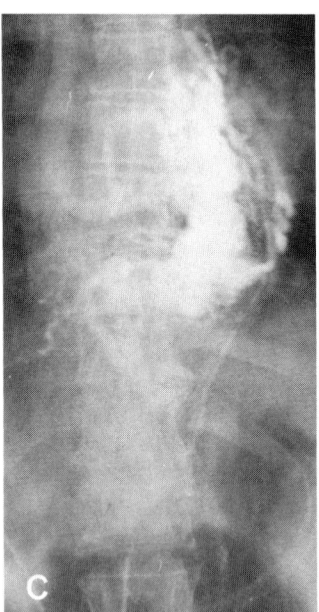
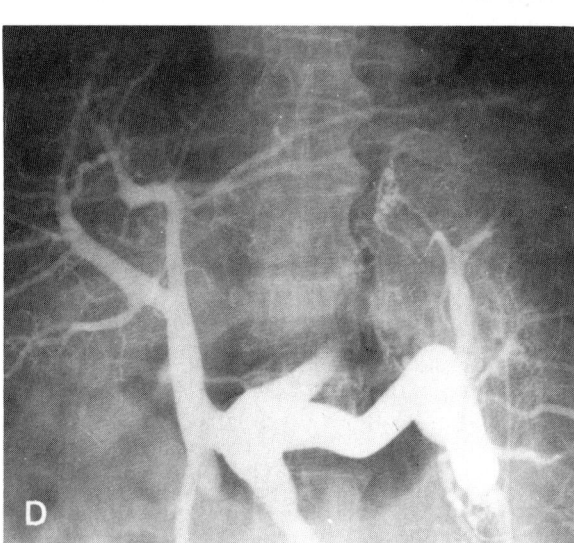

Figure 3.68 A patient with postnecrotic cirrhosis and upper gastrointestinal bleeding from esophageal varices.
(A) A transhepatic portogram shows a patent portal system, a contracted liver, and a large left gastric vein supplying gastroesophageal varices. (B,C) Selective injection into the left gastric vein before occlusion with alcohol and Gelfoam. Note communication of varices with the azygos system. (D) Control after embolization shows occlusion of varices. Bleeding was under control for over 1 year.

In spite of the fact that obliterated gastroesophageal varices may recanalize and despite controversy over reports regarding the effectiveness of transhepatic embolization of varices in the literature, this procedure has been shown to be a significant adjuvant in managing acute varicose bleeding. The results, as expected, are worse in patients in Child's group C. Occasionally no varicose recanalization is evident in the angiogram, and the patient continues to bleed or bleeds again (Fig. 3.69).

Transhepatic embolization of varices may be performed during the acute phase of bleeding as an emergency measure or electively to prevent bleeding recurrence or lengthen the interval between bleeding episodes (Figs. 3.70 and 3.71).

Transhepatic portography is performed through percutaneous transhepatic puncture, under fluoroscopic

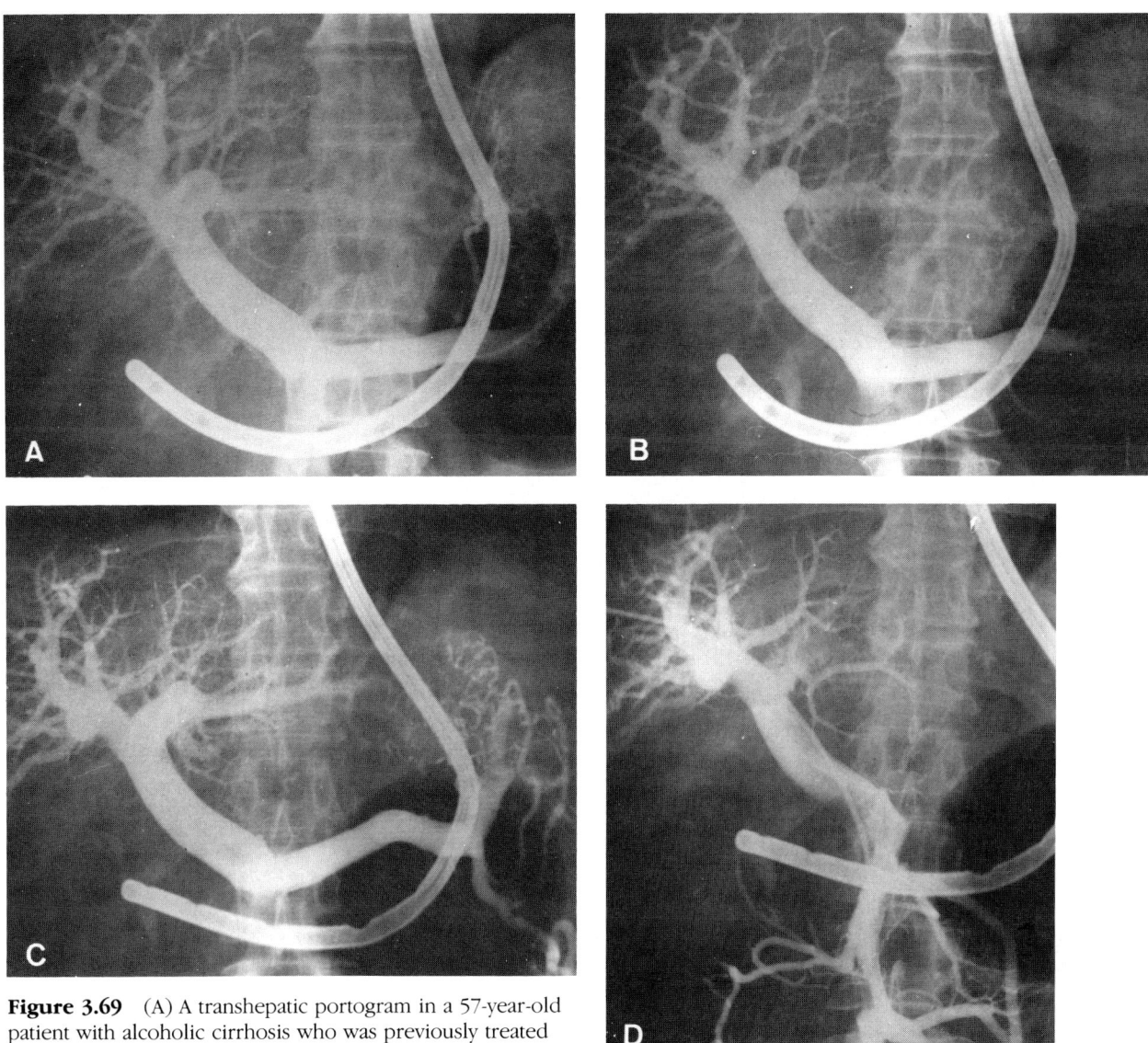

Figure 3.69 (A) A transhepatic portogram in a 57-year-old patient with alcoholic cirrhosis who was previously treated with five sessions of endoscopic sclerosis followed by bleeding. A few varices in the gastric fundus were embolized. The left gastric artery was filled only during selective injection. (B) Control after sclerosis with alcohol of all patent veins supplying the varices. (C,D) Bleeding recurred 10 days after this procedure. A new portogram with injections into the splenic and superior mesenteric veins did not show any varices in spite of clinically active bleeding.

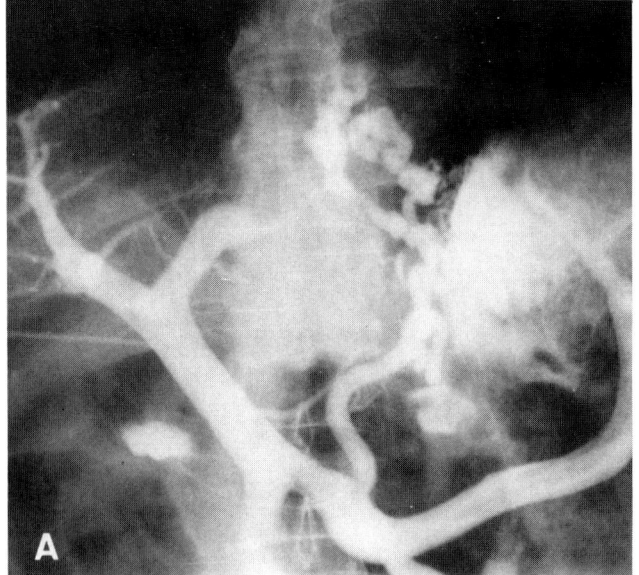
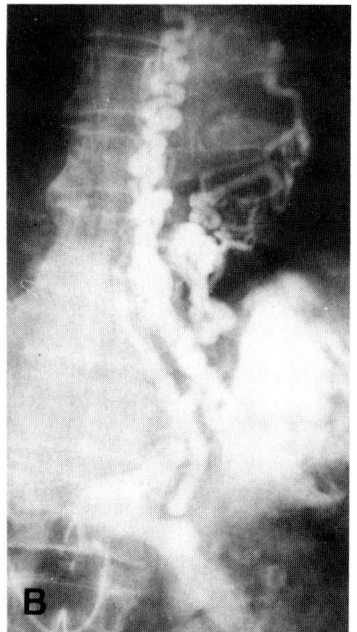
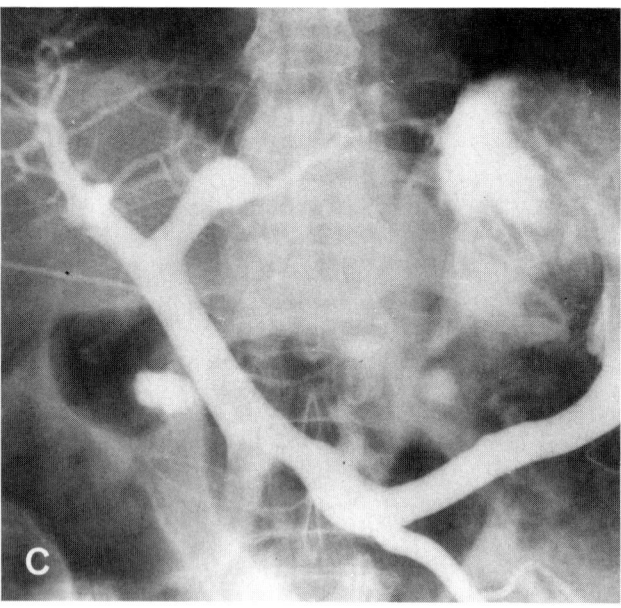

Figure 3.70 A patient with cirrhosis and acute bleeding from varices.
(A) A percutaneous transhepatic portogram showing the portal system and gastroesophageal varices vascularized by the left gastric vein. (B) Selective injection into the left gastric vein. (C) Control after embolization with absolute alcohol and Gelfoam occluded the left gastric vein and varices. Bleeding was under control for only 3 weeks. Note the barium residue in the stomach and duodenum.

guidance, on the right middle axillary line at the 9th and 10th intercostal spaces level. A peripheral portal branch is selected for catheterization and a J tip guidewire is advanced in the main stem of the portal vein, followed by dilatation of the tract and catheter placement. Manometry is performed and a portogram is obtained for varices demonstration.

Once varices have been identified, they are selectively catheterized, and phlebography of the vessels is performed. When adequate catheterization of varices has

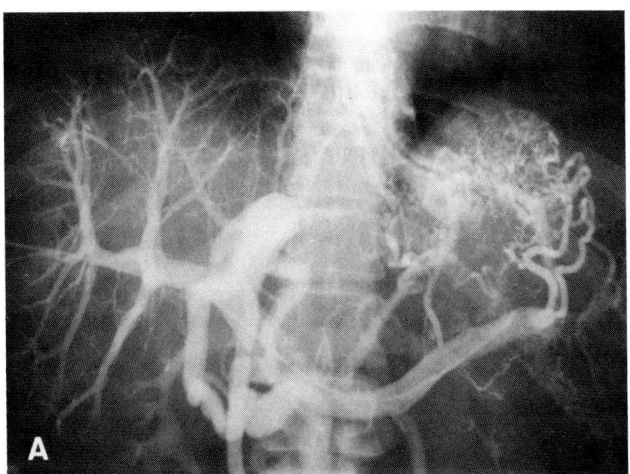

Figure 3.71 A 31-year-old patient with alcoholic cirrhosis, acute bleeding from portal hypertension, and esophageal varices.
(A) A transhepatic portogram shows at least four veins supplying the varicose system. The procedure can be predicted to last for at least 2 h in this situation. (B) Selective injection into the left gastric vein. (C,D) Selective injections into the short gastric veins. (E) After occlusion of varices with absolute alcohol, bleeding was permanently arrested. The preembolization pressure of 590 mmH$_2$O rose to 650 mmH$_2$O after occlusion.

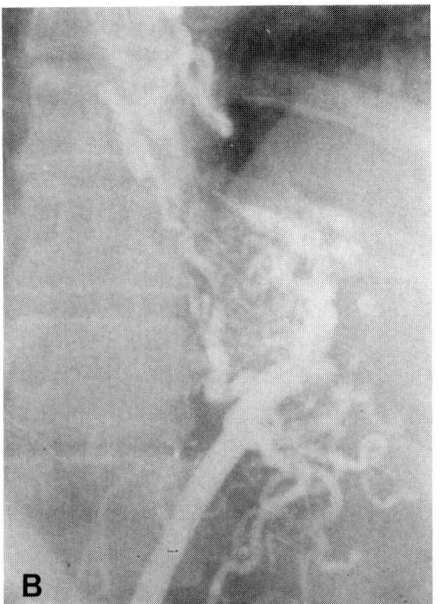
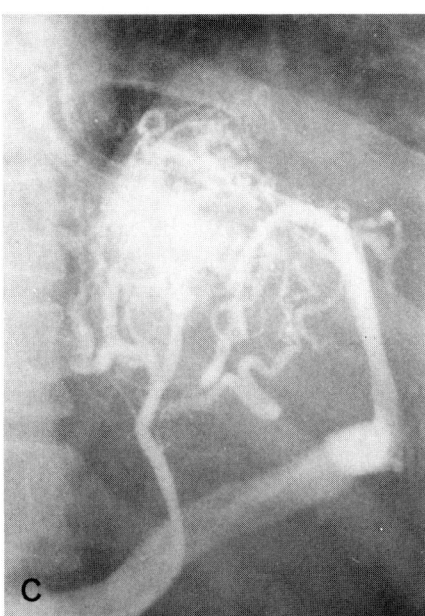
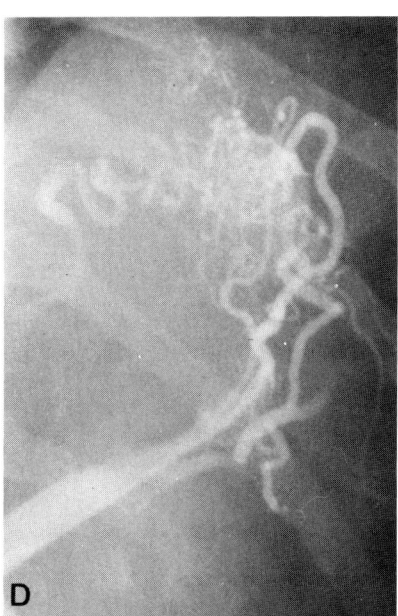
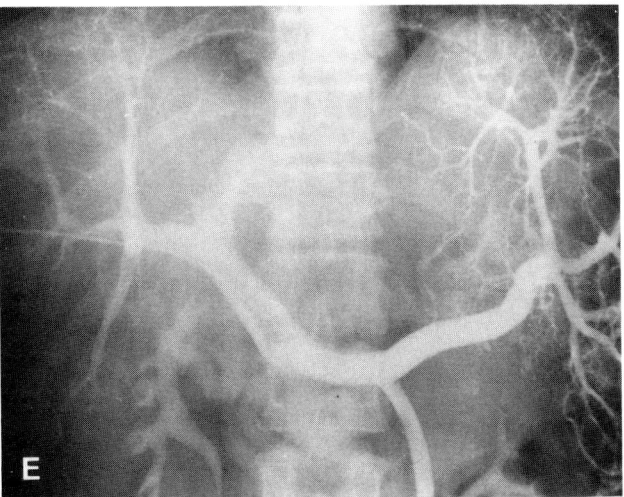

been obtained, obliteration is done with any embolization material. After occlusion of the varices, another portogram is done for control purposes. During removal of the catheter, its pathway through the liver parenchyma is embolized to prevent intraperitoneal bleeding (Fig. 3.72).

Percutaneous transhepatic portography is a valuable complementary method in patients with acute occlusion of proximal splenorenal shunts with varicose bleeding (Fig. 3.73) and in patients with distal splenorenal shunts

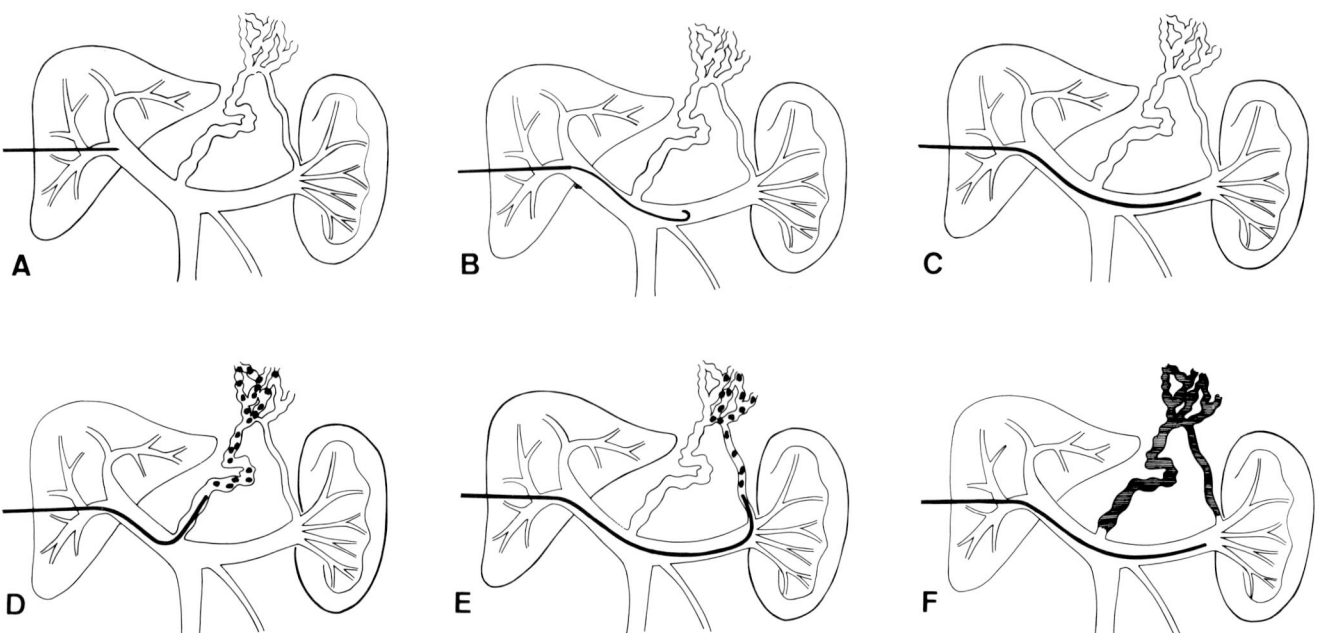

Figure 3.72 A schematic drawing of the embolization technique for gastroesophageal varices through the transhepatic route.
(A) Transhepatic puncture of the portal vein. (B) Catheterization of the portal system initiated with a J-tip flexible guide advanced to the splenic vein. (C) Angiographic catheter placed inside the venous system to perform a scanning portogram of the portal system and its varicose collaterals. (D) Once the varices and left gastric vein have been localized, the vein is selectively catheterized and treated with embolization. (E) Embolization of a short gastric vein. (F) Control portogram after embolization of varices, which appear occluded (in black).

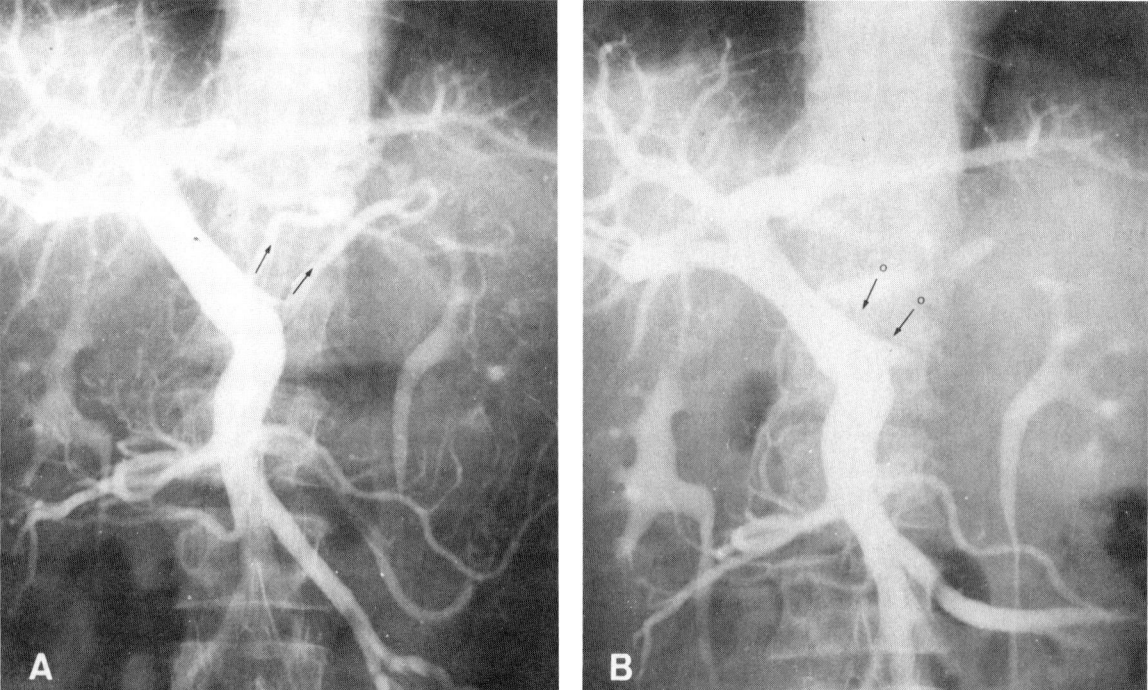

Figure 3.73 A 61-year-old patient with postnecrotic cirrhosis and portal hypertension treated with a proximal splenorenal shunt, which has occluded, with recurrence of bleeding.
(A) A transhepatic portogram shows occlusion of the splenorenal anastomosis and varices. (B) Control after obstruction of varices with Gelfoam emboli shows occlusion of the gastric veins. Bleeding has been permanently controlled.

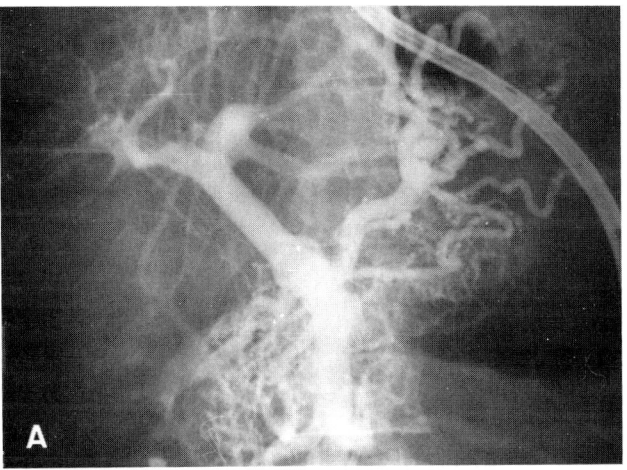
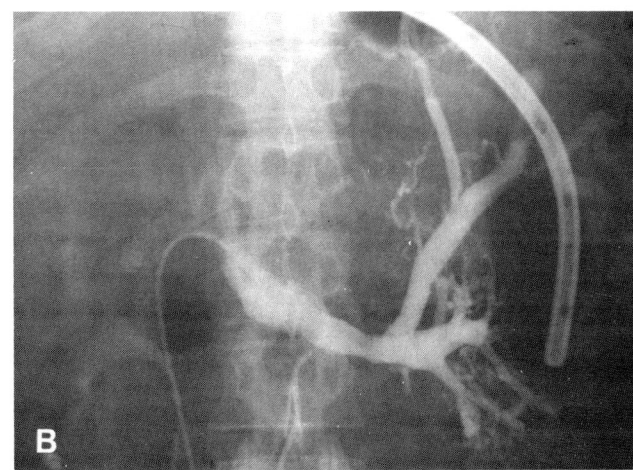
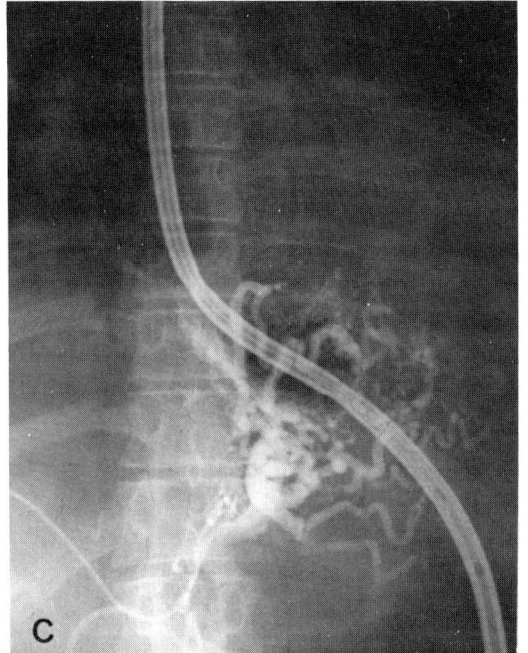
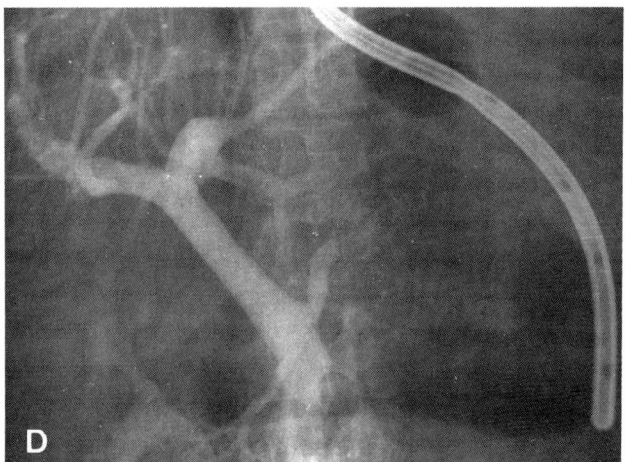

Figure 3.74 A patient with portal hypertension cirrhosis treated by distal splenorenal anastomosis. Rebleeding occurred.
(A) A percutaneous portogram showing varices. (B) Selective injection into the left renal vein shows shunt patency. (C) Selective injection into gastroesophageal varices. (D) Control after embolization of varices. When ligation of the left gastric vein is not done during surgery, the risk of bleeding recurrence persists, as in this patient.

with patency of the left gastric vein and short gastric veins (Fig. 3.74).

Embolization of esophageal varices in our experience is able to control approximately 80 percent of all cases of bleeding from varices. However, in almost half these patients, bleeding recurs during the first 3 months after embolization (Fig. 3.69).

Spontaneous thrombosis of the portal vein related to portal hepatofugal flow and intraportal blood stagnation occurs with relative frequency in patients with liver cirrhosis, particularly patients who have received a therapeutic procedure and then experienced a worsening of hepatic function (Fig. 3.75).

POSTSINUSOIDAL INTRAHEPATIC PORTAL HYPERTENSION

Budd-Chiari Syndrome

Symptomatic obstruction of hepatic venous drainage is rare and may result from constricting pericarditis, ob-

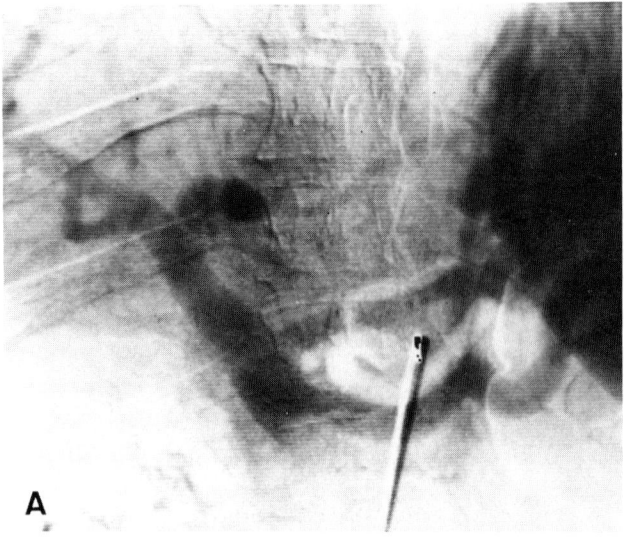
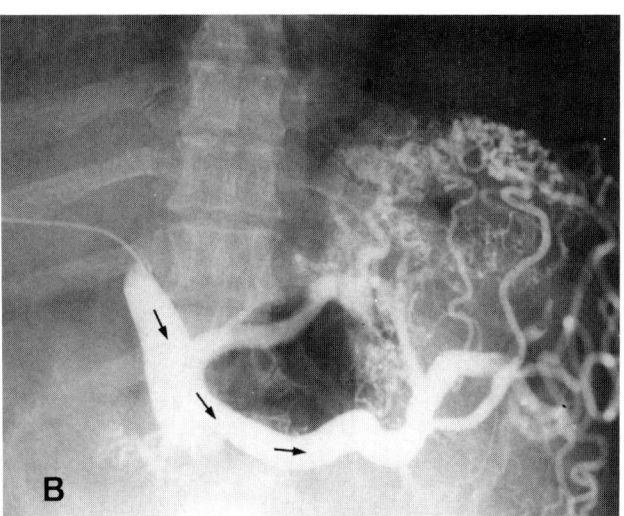
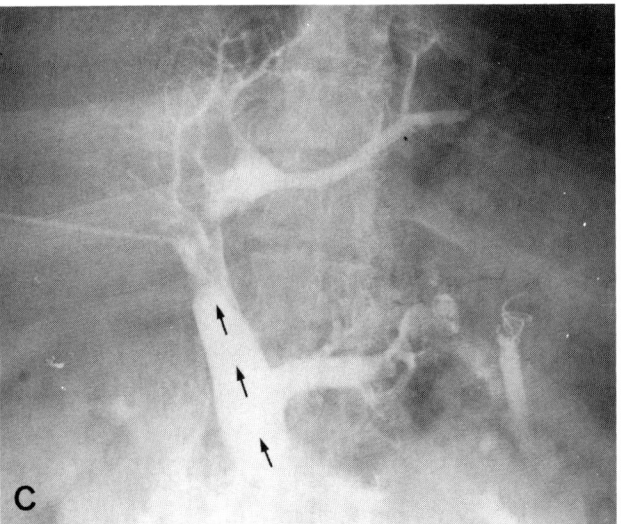

struction of the inferior vena cava, or occlusion of the hepatic veins. This obstruction of hepatic venous drainage may cause ascites, hepatomegaly, hepatic dysfunction, abdominal pain, portal hypertension, and esophageal varices. It is known as Budd-Chiari syndrome.

Obstruction of hepatic veins may be associated with thrombosis, endophlebitis, fibrosis, a hepatic expansive mass (Fig. 3.76), or congenital membranes and diaphragms in the ostium of the hepatic veins or vena cava. The most frequent cause, however, is fibrotic stenosis and/or ostial thrombosis of the hepatic veins. The etiology is firmly established in only about 30 percent of patients. There seems to be a correlation between the occurrence of hepatic vein occlusion and the use of oral contraceptives (Fig. 3.77). Most cases, however, are attributed to the occurrence of primary thrombosis or endophlebitis, resulting in fibrotic obstruction (Fig. 3.78).

Management of patients with Budd-Chiari syndrome is still controversial. Clinical and symptomatic treatment has been the most frequently used form of therapy, although it does not seem to prolong survival. Ascites frequently escapes from clinical control, and 90 to 95 percent of patients die within 2 years after the onset of disease. Surgical treatment is even more controversial because of its high failure rate and is usually oriented toward alleviating hepatic congestion by building a portosystemic anastomosis. Many alternatives have been used, such as surgical correction of caval stenosis, endovenotomy, correction of hepatic vein diaphragms, and transatrial membranotomy. More recently, interventional radiologic techniques have been developed. Balloon membranotomy has been successful in some cases. Transluminal angioplasty has been utilized in two patients with suprahepatic vein diaphragms. In a few more recent cases, transluminal angioplasty has been used to manage

Figure 3.75 A 58-year-old patient who presented with alcoholic cirrhosis.
(A) A digital arterial portogram showing adequate patency of the portal system. The patient was treated with a series of eight endoscopic scleroses, but bleeding recurred. (B) A transhepatic portogram shows varices in the gastric fundus with hepatofugal flow but without filling of the intrahepatic portal circulation (arrows). (C) After embolization of varices, there was partial reversal of portal flow, which now fills the portal radicles of the left lobe and shows thrombi which result from blood stagnation during the hepatofugal flow phase (arrows).

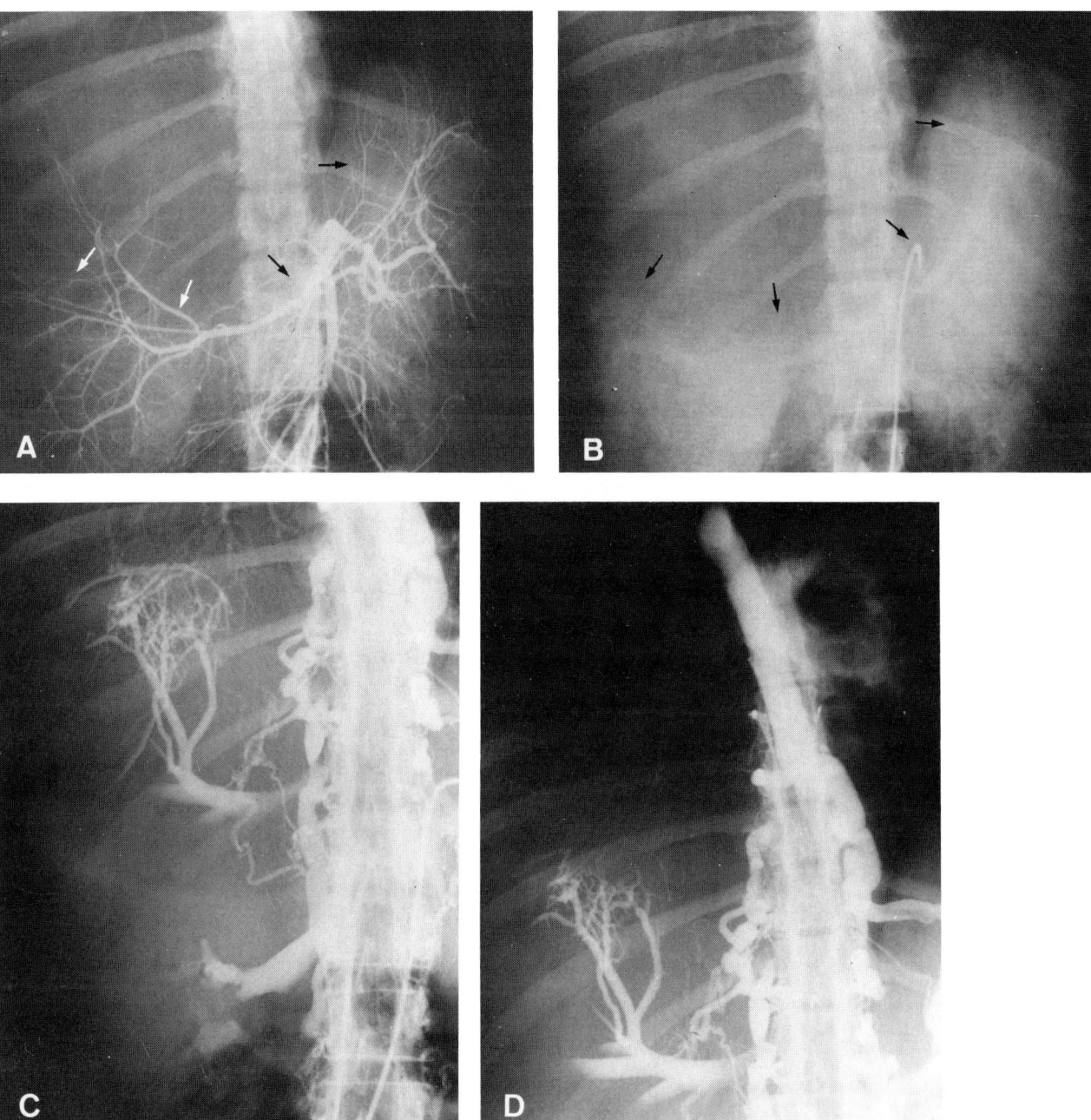

Figure 3.76 A 23-year-old patient with a hepatic hydatid cyst and obstruction of the vena cava and hepatic veins with ascites and Budd-Chiari syndrome.

(A,B) A selective arteriogram of the celiac axis shows a huge avascular expansive hepatic lesion (arrows). (C,D) A cavogram showing caval occlusion and compression of the hepatic veins. Abundant intra- and extrahepatic collateral circulation is identified. (E) Control 18 days after cyst removal. There was clinical improvement and excellent patency of the hepatic veins. (F) A hepatic phlebogram shows the patency of the hepatic veins 3 years after surgery.

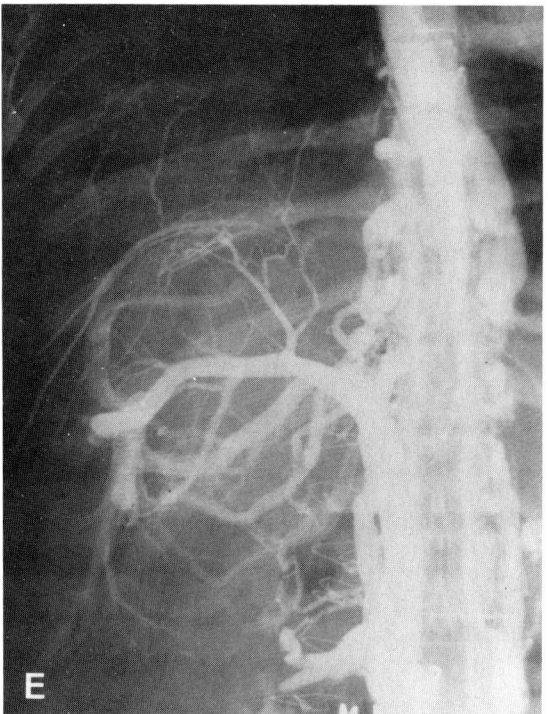
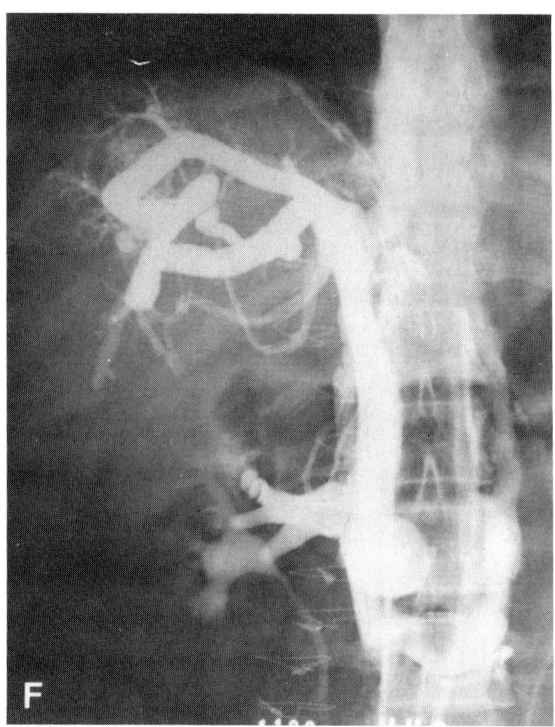

Figure 3.76 *Continued*

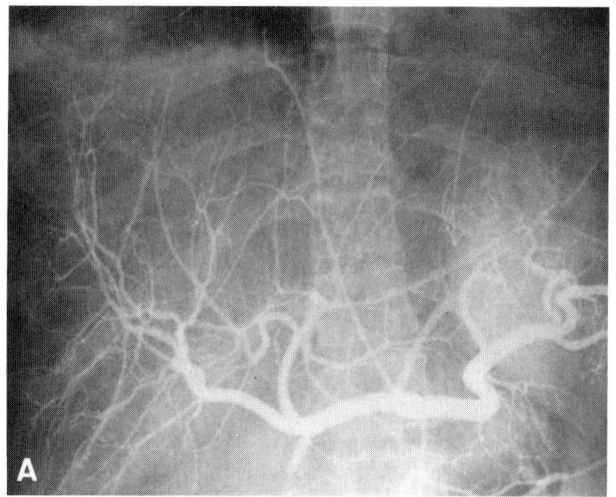
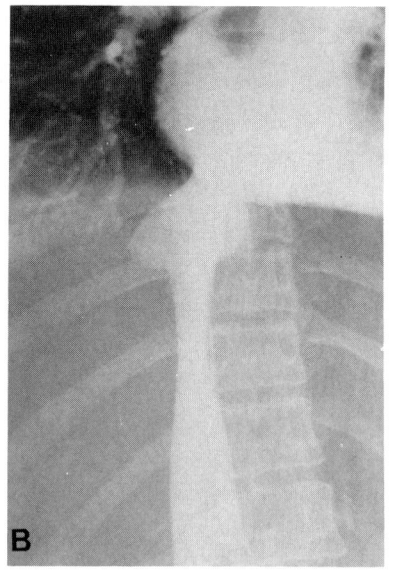
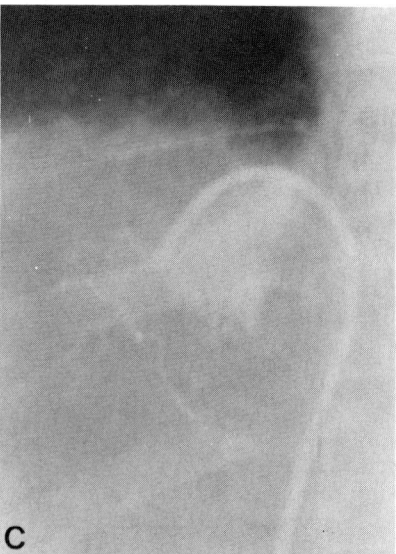

Figure 3.77 A 30-year-old patient with Budd-Chiari syndrome with a history of oral contraceptive use.
(A) A hepatic arteriogram shows artery stretching because of hepatic congestion and volume increase. (B) A cavogram shows constriction of the inferior vena cava and occlusion of the hepatic veins. (C) A selective catheterization trial in the hepatic veins shows right occlusion and poor collateral "spiderweb" circulation.

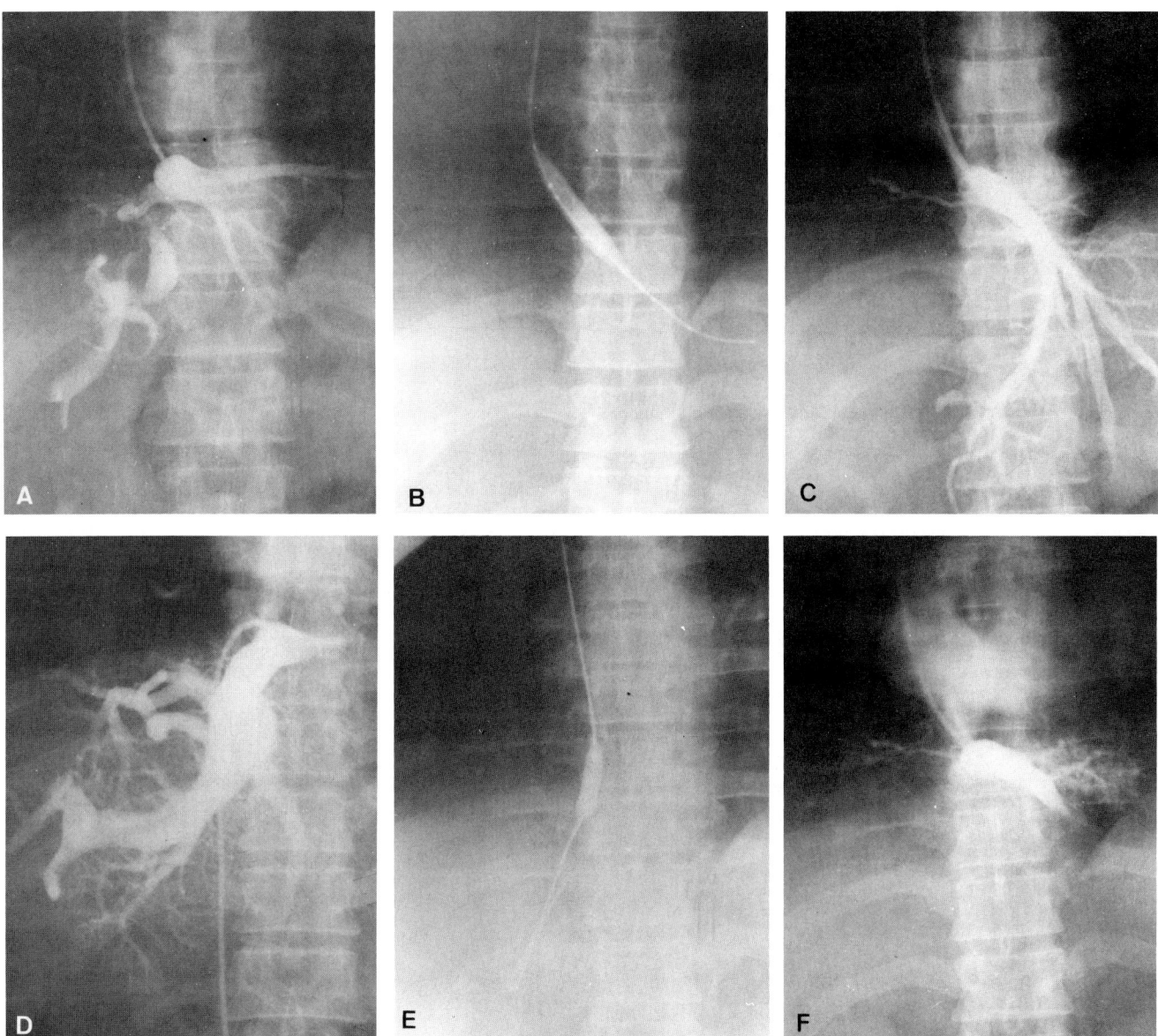

Figure 3.78 A male patient with Budd-Chiari syndrome manifested by uncontrollable ascites which had been leaking for 3 weeks through a diagnostic surgical incision.
(A) A hepatic phlebogram with a wedged catheter in the left hepatic vein. Note the occlusion site (arrow). (B) After diagnostic study, an 8-mm dilation balloon catheter was introduced through the obstruction. (C) Phlebographic control just after dilation shows recanalization at the obstruction site (arrow). Ascitis was clinically cured after dilation with closure of the abdominal incision and reestablishment of the patient's general health. (D) Phlebographic control 2 years after dilation shows recurrence of stenosis and Budd-Chiari symptoms. (E) New dilation was performed with a 6mm balloon. (F) Phlebographic control after dilation shows improvement of stenosis, which was followed by improvement in symptoms.

fibrotic occlusions of suprahepatic veins (Figs. 3.78 and 3.79).

Budd-Chiari syndrome has a pathogenetic aspect associated with many different clinical, angiographic, and histopathologic manifestations. Angiographic methods have been considered the primary means for detecting and confirming the site and extent of this disease. More recently, ultrasound, computed tomography (CT), and magnetic resonance imaging (MRI) have been utilized with good accuracy for diagnosing and evaluating the extension of suprahepatic vein occlusion. In our experience, angiography is of primary importance in detecting Budd-Chiari syndrome but fails to assess the extension of lesions in certain cases.

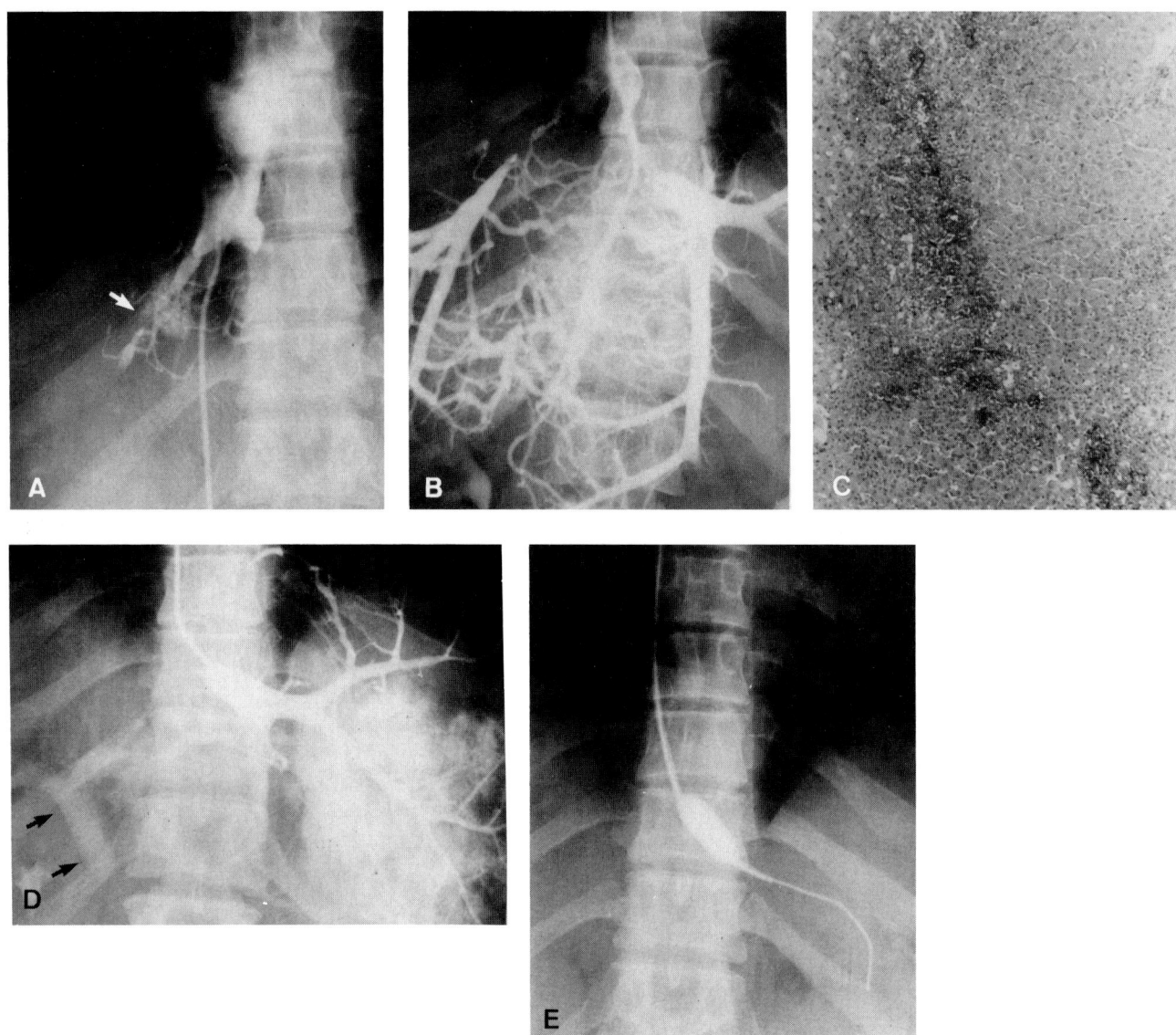

Figure 3.79 A 37-year-old man with abdominal pain, hepatomegaly, and grade II esophageal varices. Budd-Chiari syndrome was confirmed by liver biopsy.

(A) Selective injection into the right hepatic vein shows segmental occlusion (arrows) and collateral circulation in the right lobe. The left hepatic vein is occluded (arrow). (B) Wedged injection into the middle hepatic vein shows a network of hepatic collaterals communicating with the occluded veins. (C) A hepatic histologic image with a severe degree of central congestion, hemorrhage, and necrosis of parenchyma, diagnostic of Budd-Chiari syndrome. (D) Wedged injection into the left hepatic vein shows portal vein occlusion and filling (arrows) (pressure of 490 mmH$_2$O). (E) An 8-mm balloon catheter in the dilation position. (F) A phlebogram obtained just after dilation shows patency of the dilated vein and residual occlusion of the remaining hepatic veins (pressure of 200 mmH$_2$O). (G) A histologic study approximately 1 month after dilation shows improvement of congestion and hemorrhage. A clinical cure with regression of ascites, pain, and hepatomegaly was obtained. (H,I) An ultrasonographic study before (H) and after (I) dilation shows communication of the left hepatic vein with the inferior vena cava (arrows). (J) Scintiscan of the liver shows a significant reduction in peripheral uptake with radionuclide centralization before the procedure. (K) Scintiscan 2 weeks after angioplasty shows improvement of uptake and central localization of radionuclide. (L) Control study 2 months later shows higher peripheral and central uptake. Note the significant improvement in the left lobe. (M) Twelve months after dilation there was recurrence of pain and ascites. Restenosis of the left hepatic vein was identified (pressure of 480 mmH$_2$O). (N) New dilation with a 6-mm balloon and a 4-mm-diameter balloon. (O) Control after left hepatic vein patency (pressure of 170 mmH$_2$O) with regression of symptoms in a 3-year follow-up.

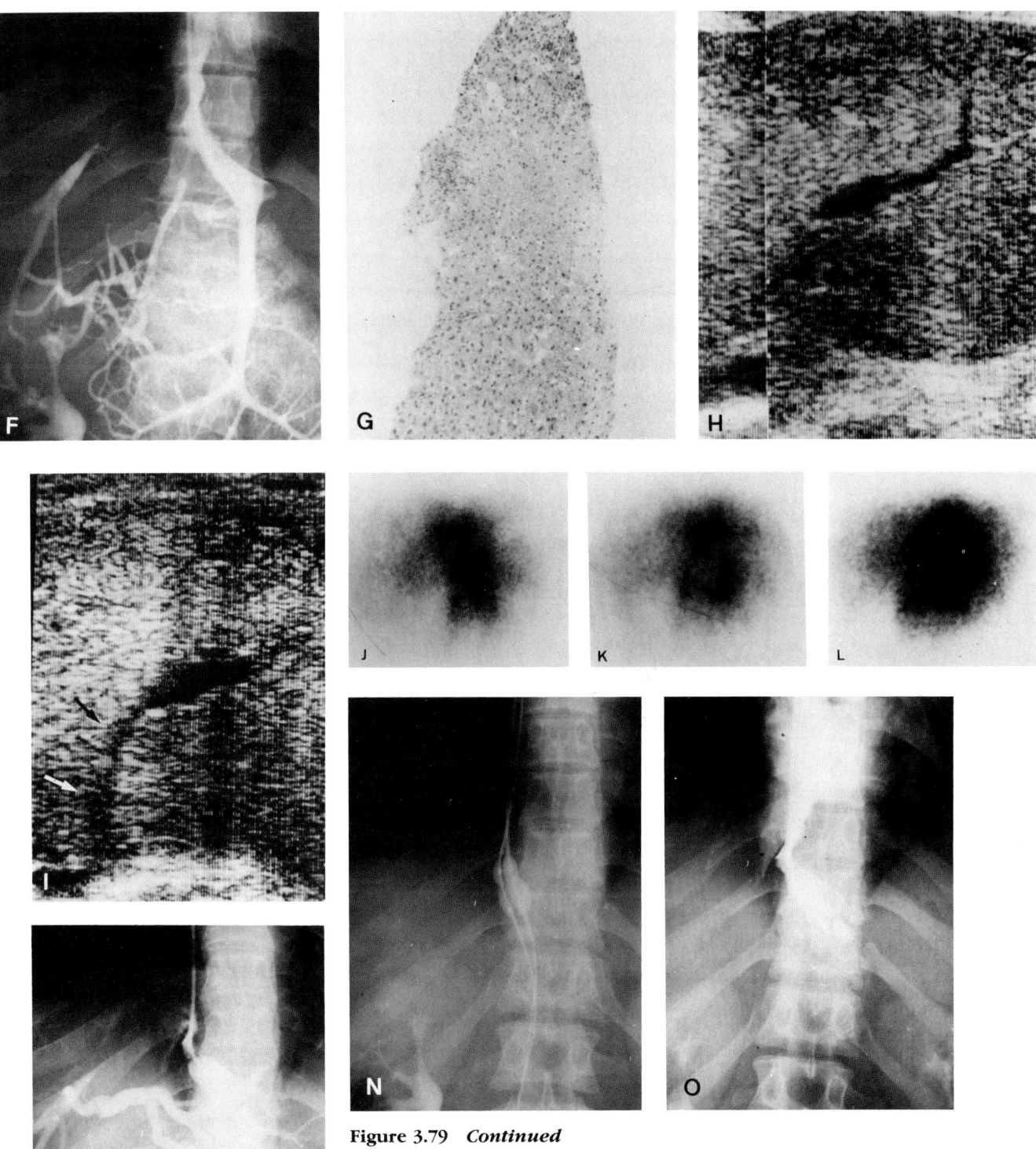

Figure 3.79 *Continued*

Angiographically, Budd-Chiari syndrome is identified by a volume-enlarged liver resulting from edema that causes artery stretching and bulging. In the later phase, parenchymal "staining" is heterogeneous and of high density. Catheterization of hepatic veins may be impossible, although the most frequent finding is evidence of venous occlusion or ostium stenosis and the presence of collateral venous circulation forming what is described as a "spiderweb"—fine collaterals without identification of flow direction. Collaterals of the intrahepatic type are particularly significant, as they make it possible for suprahepatic veins to remain patent in spite of total occlusion of the venous ostium and allow hepatic venous drainage to occur when portal flow is reversed. Although it is theoretically possible for recanalization of a thrombus in the hepatic vein to occur, there has been little evidence of recovery from hepatic venous occlusion after symptoms appear.

It is worthwhile to speculate why transluminal angioplasty with dilatation of only one suprahepatic vein can control all symptoms, as has occurred in our patients who were treated in this manner (Figs. 3.78 and 3.79). Hepatic venous occlusion is encountered with some frequency in postmortem examinations of asymptomatic patients; it seems that in humans a critical level of hepatic venous occlusion must be reached before symptoms of ascites and other symptoms appear. In dogs, occlusion of up to 55 percent of hepatic veins does not produce physiologic changes, although there is a sphincteric mechanism in the ostium of canine hepatic veins which makes it difficult to come to any conclusion regarding human patients. Because of difficulties in managing a severe disease such as this, with its high mortality rate, the use of transluminal dilation seems promising as a treatment option (Figs. 3.78 and 3.79).

Suprahepatic vein angioplasty is a safe procedure, as it is performed inside the hepatic parenchyma, and it may be repeated many times if occlusion recurs. Prolonged survival has been recorded in at least two practically asymptomatic patients, except during periods of occlusion recurrence. Some causes of Budd-Chiari syndrome may be treated surgically, such as the case of a hydatic cyst (Fig. 3.76) or tumor. More recently endovascular stents have been used to treat hepatic venous stenosis and obstructions. They have also been used to create a portal systemic shunt in patients with PH through the jugular-hepatic vein approach.

PORTOSYSTEMIC ENCEPHALOPATHY CAUSED BY A SURGICALLY CREATED OR SPONTANEOUS SHUNT

Portosystemic encephalopathy is a relatively common occurrence in patients who receive nonselective portosystemic anastomoses (52 percent). It occurs less frequently in patients who receive Warren-type selective portosystemic anastomoses (12 percent).

The incidence of postoperative encephalopathy, however, depends on the emphasis given to its investigation by the clinician who treats the patient. Hepatic encephalopathy can be characterized as the occurrence of mental confusion or disorientation episodes detected by a patients' family or the assisting physician. Permanent mental confusion and coma are more advanced stages which usually occur before death from hepatic failure or are related to GI bleeding, electrolytic dysfunction, or the use of drugs, including alcohol. Encephalopathy may be subclinical, characterized by elevated plasma ammonia, electroencephalographic changes, and altered psychometric tests which require sophisticated evaluation.

Deviation of splanchnic blood from the hepatic circulation has been accepted as the major etiologic element in encephalopathy caused by a portosystemic shunt. Portosystemic communication provides access into the systemic circulation to brain toxins that are absorbed by the small intestine, depriving the liver of hepatotrophic substances secreted by splanchnic organs. Reducing pressure in the superior mesenteric artery by creating a shunt also increases intestinal absorption of ammonia, other nitrogen compounds, and d-xylose; all these substances are brain toxins that also promote the development of encephalopathy.

The situation of patients with hepatic encephalopathy caused by a shunt becomes critical when they do not respond to a low-protein or no-protein diet, intestinal antibiotic therapy, and oral lactulose. These patients rapidly develop chronic encephalopathy, dementia, and dependency on their families or the hospital. Coma in these patients can be caused by any precipitating factor, such as infection, protein intake in the diet, drugs, and alcohol. Restoring hepatopetal flow in these patients through surgical obliteration of the portosystemic shunt (surgically created) or by changing a nonselective shunt (proximal splenorenal, portocaval, or mesocaval) to a selective one (distal splenorenal or portal arterialization) has been proposed.

Surgical modification of a portosystemic nonselective shunt into a more selective configuration or its occlusion will cause rehabilitation of mental function with reversal of encephalopathy in most cases. As a major procedure which is performed in severely ill patients whose health and hepatic function are already seriously compromised, surgery has high morbidity and mortality rates when performed in emergency situations. Elective surgery, however, is better tolerated by these patients.

More recently, the use of occlusive interventional radiologic procedures for the management of these nonselective shunts (Fig. 3.80) has been proposed, using

Figure 3.80
(A) After occlusion of a splenorenal anastomosis, a mesenteric caval anastomosis was performed, with interposition of the external jugular vein (arrow), which is seen here catheterized through the inferior vena cava. Encephalopathy developed and was resistant to clinical treatment. (B) Obstruction of the mesenteric caval shunt was performed with a large detachable balloon, which controlled encephalopathy but restored portal hypertension and caused the development of voluminous ascites. (Courtesy of Dr. José Maria B. de Freitas and Dr. Adávio de O. E. Silva.)

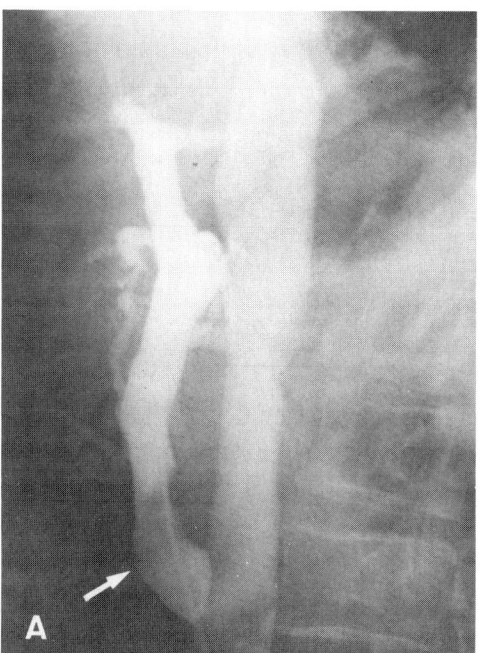
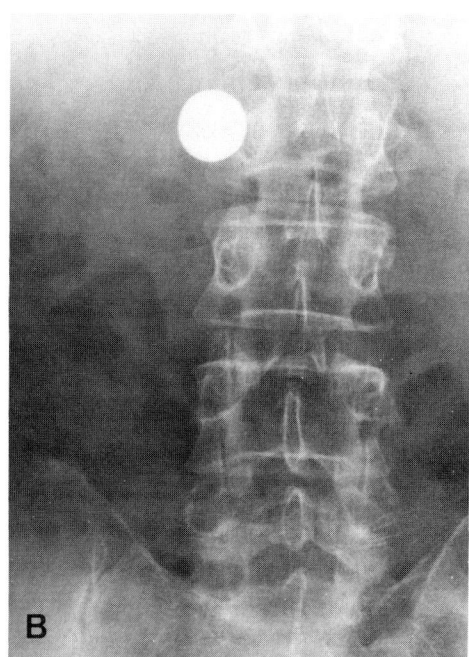

embolization with detachable balloons to achieve definitive control of encephalopathy. However, acute occlusion of a mesocaval shunt leads to severe positive hemodynamic changes such as increased hepatic perfusion by portal blood and negative changes such as the development of ascites. The development of uncontrolled ascites should be avoided, as this condition may cause significant damage to the patient.

There are two additional situations involving patients who develop chronic encephalopathy that is resistant to treatment. The first occurs in patients with a spontaneous portosystemic shunt combined with a small spleen but without hypersplenism; the second occurs in individuals with a spontaneous portosystemic shunt combined with splenomegaly and hypersplenism.

In patients with spontaneous portosystemic communication, chronic encephalopathy, and a small spleen (without hypersplenism), the approach to the portal system should be catheterization by the transhepatic route, with a scanning portogram being performed (Fig. 3.72), along with selective catheterization of the spontaneous portosystemic shunt and embolization with Gianturco coils (Fig. 3.81) or detachable balloons. Portosystemic communications in these patients are generally of the splenorenal type, through the retroperitoneal, phrenic, and adrenal veins, and may become large (Fig. 3.82). Embolization of these communications, although not complete, can significantly reduce the portosystemic flow of blood of splanchnic origin. This will decrease the supply of brain toxins to the systemic circulation and increase hepatopetal flow, which in turn will improve hepatic function. It is important, however, that obstruction of collaterals be performed carefully and only in patients with a certain degree of hepatic functional reserve. These patients must have a portal vascular continent which can withstand a higher volume and pressure of blood.

The most threatening complication in these patients is acute occlusion of the shunt, followed by intraabdominal bleeding resulting from rupture of thin-walled collateral veins in territories which are unable to withstand the new pressure regimen of the portal system (Fig. 3.81). This hemorrhagic complication can be fatal. Besides this complication from bleeding, other aspects should be considered, such as significant changes in hemodynamic systemic patterns which also involve cardiac output and peripheral and pulmonary vascular resistance apart from the development of ascites.

Management of these patients entails a fragile balance of risks; the choices are death from liver failure and the risk of variceal or intraperitoneal hemorrhage. Each case should therefore be judged on its own merits.

In individuals with spontaneous portosystemic communication, chronic encephalopathy, and resistance to treatment who have an enlarged spleen and hypersplenism, it is possible to approach the problem through arterial catheterization and partial splenic embolization.

Patients with PH and hypersplenism have a detectable pressure component in the portal system. This component, which is of splenic origin, is approximately 15 to 20 percent in hepatic cirrhosis and approximately 40 percent in hepatosplenic schistosomiasis. It is reasonable

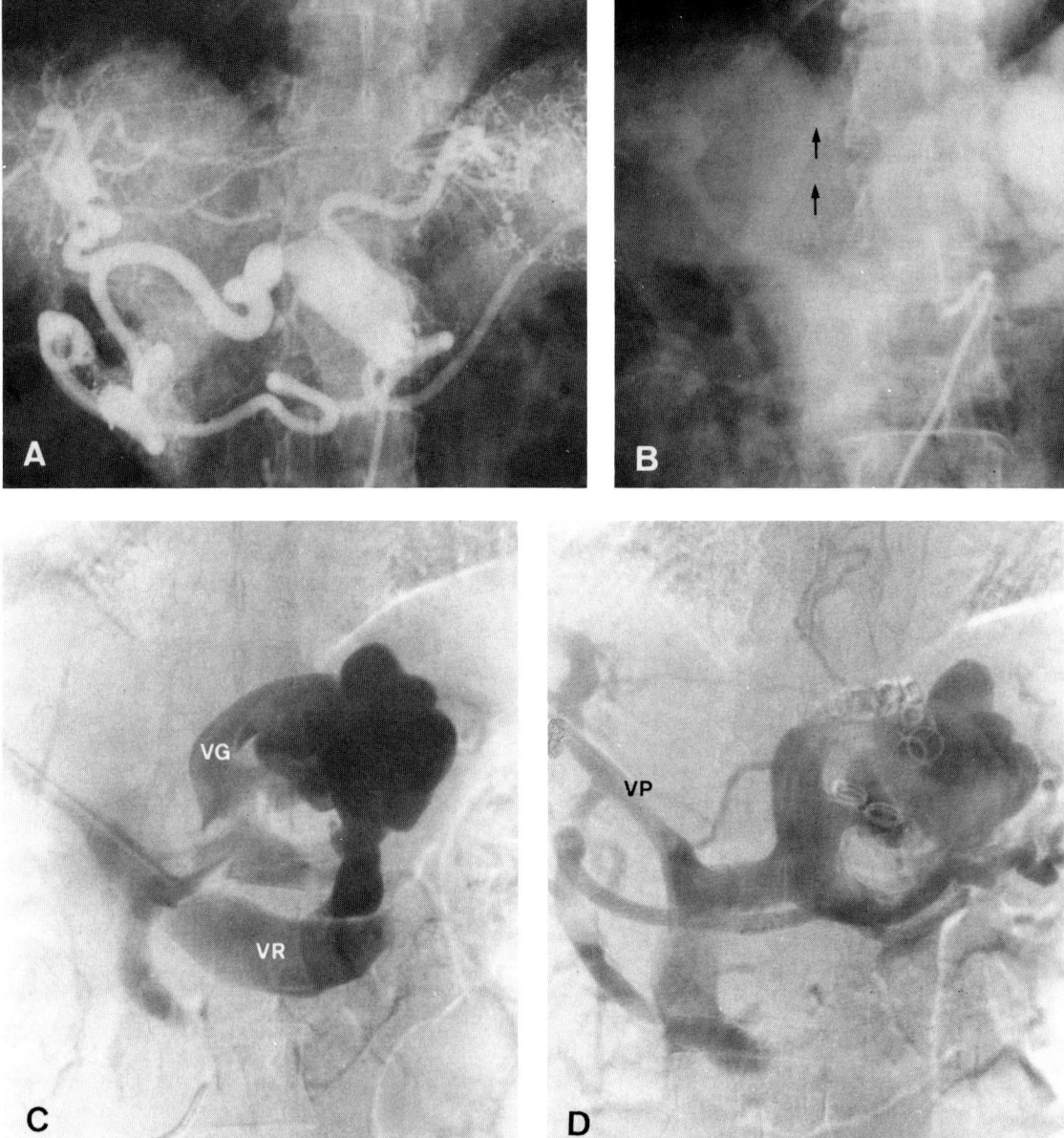

Figure 3.81 A 64-year-old male with hepatic schistosomiasis combined with chronic encephalopathy for 7 years, with three deep coma episodes despite intensive care and a no-protein diet. The patient had already received a splenectomy.

(A) During celiac axis injection, a reduced liver and an aneurysm of the common hepatic artery are seen. (B) In a later phase of arterial injection, venous entanglement of the left gastric vein is seen, with spontaneous shunt to the left renal vein and filling of the inferior vena cava (arrowheads). (C) A percutaneous transhepatic portogram shows hepatofugal flow without portal filling and all blood being drained through the left gastric vein (VG), portosystemic communication with the renal vein (VR), passing through a venous entanglement in the retroperitoneum. (D) After partial occlusion of a spontaneous shunt with Gianturco coils, there was improvement of flow to the portal vein (VP). Although the shunt was successfully occluded, hemodynamic changes made the postprocedure period difficult. Approximately 1 week after embolization was performed, when the patient was already recovering, spontaneous bleeding occurred in the vesicular bed as a result of redistribution and pressure increase in the portal system. Surgical correction of bleeding became necessary. It was ineffective, and the patient died from uncontrollable bleeding during the immediate postoperative period.

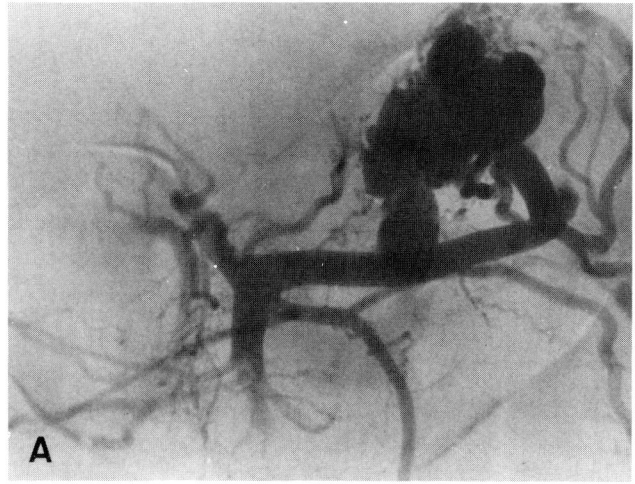
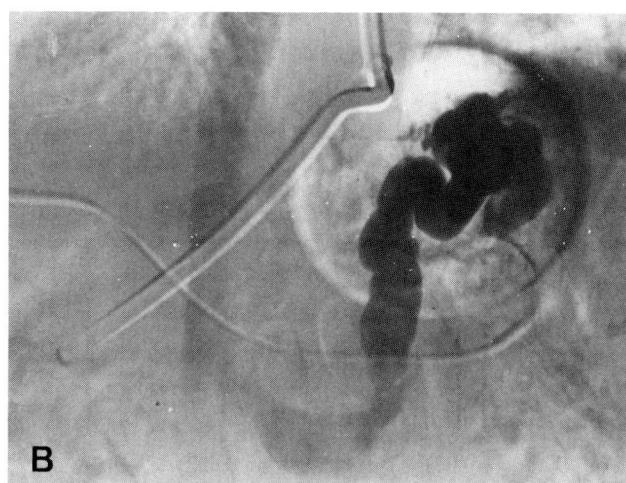
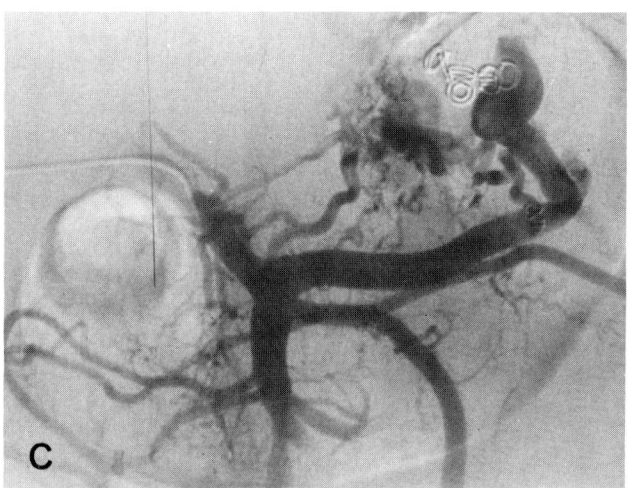
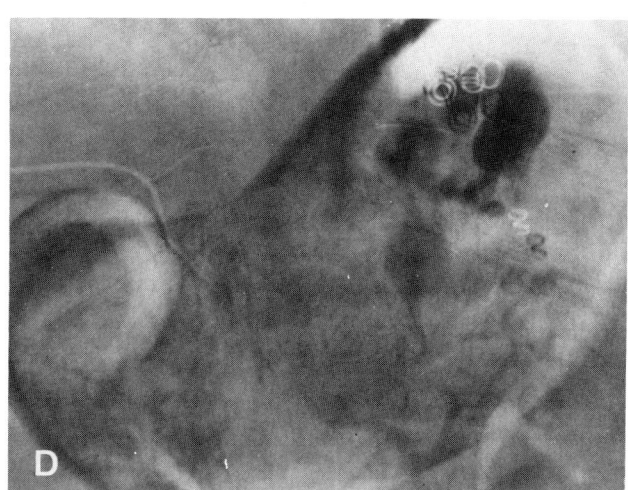

Figure 3.82 A patient with chronic encephalopathy from spontaneous portosystemic shunt and upper gastrointestinal bleeding from gastric varices after endoscopic sclerosis.
(A) A transhepatic portogram shows portal hepatofugal flow and filling of large venous tufts with a spontaneous splenorenal shunt starting from the short gastric vein. (B) Later phase of portogram shows filling of the communication between the renal vein and the inferior vena cava. (C) Occlusion of the spontaneous shunt was achieved with Gianturco coils, which stopped the bleeding and controlled the chronic encephalopathy. (D) Later phase of the injection shown in (C), which showed an absence of significant opacification of the spontaneous shunt.

to assume that if the spleen is partially embolized or its flow is shunted, there will be a reduction in portal system pressure. This reduction is proportional to spleen volume and blood flow (Fig. 3.61).

It is known that severe and persistent leukopenia and thrombocytopenia are found in patients with large splenic volumes and hypersplenism, as these patients are subject to frequent infections and hemorrhagic complications. Besides these aspects, hypoalbuminemia and hepatic functional changes may occur and result in altered enzymatic values. Partial splenic embolization leads to significant improvement of the clinical condition in these patients, with reversal of hypersplenism and recovery of leukocyte and platelet counts to approximately normal levels. However, spleen embolization requires that special care be taken to prevent abscess formation (Chap. 4).

If these patients have a high-output portosystemic shunt related to splenic drainage circulation in addition to a hypersplenic clinical syndrome, the role of spleen blood flow in maintaining the shunt is extremely important (Fig. 3.83). Apart from the clinical benefits of

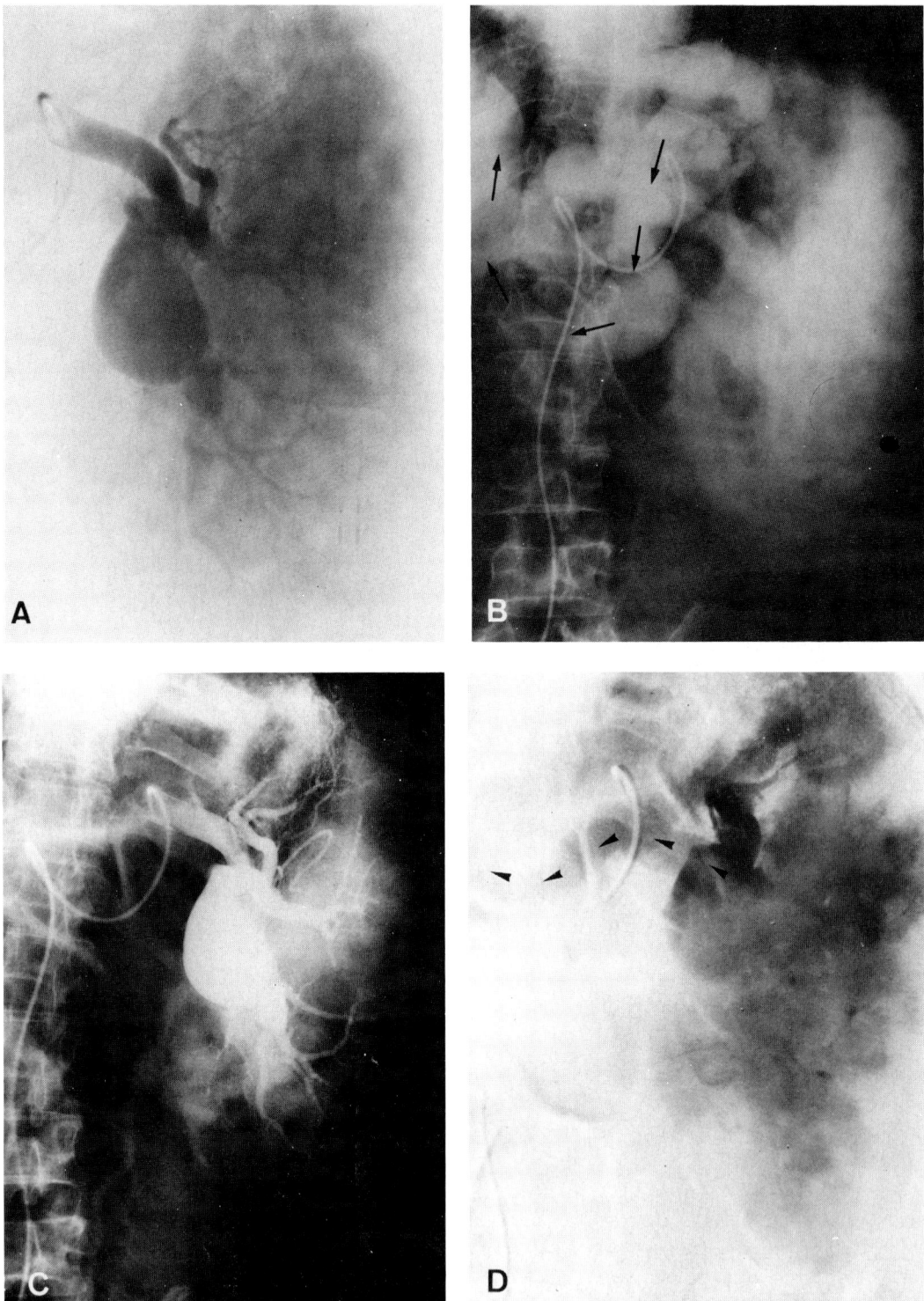

Figure 3.83 A patient with chronic encephalopathy, resistant to clinical treatment and diet, caused by a spontaneous portosystemic shunt to the left renal vein, originating from the short gastric veins and associated with splenic hyperflow due to the hypersplenism.

(A) Splenic selective injection shows an enlarged artery, an arterial saccular aneurysmal lesion, and significant splenomegaly. (B) In the later phase of injection there is opacification of the spontaneous splenorenal shunt (arrows), which was draining into the left renal vein and inferior vena cava. (C) Control angiography after partial spleen embolization shows reduction of arterial flow and parenchymal impregnation. (D) In the later phase there was opacification only of the portal vein (arrowheads) and no opacification of the spontaneous portosystemic shunt. After the procedure, the patient had the so-called postembolization syndrome, with pain, fever, and leukocytosis. The patient, however, had a favorable outcome, with platelet increase and control of encephalopathy during the 1-year follow-up without the use of a special diet.

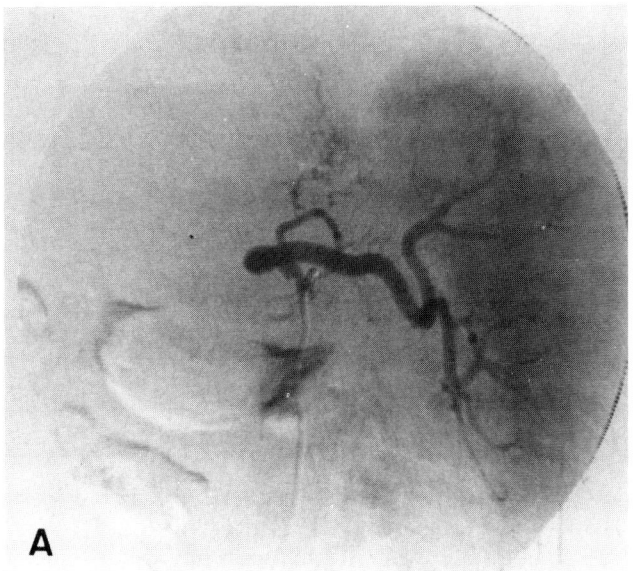
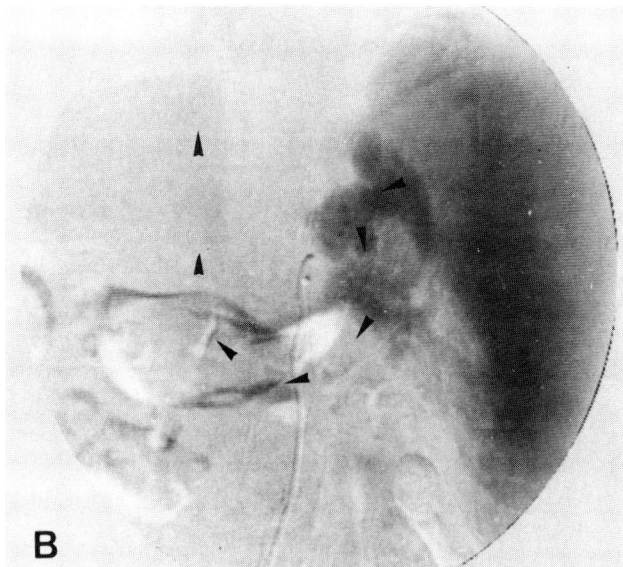
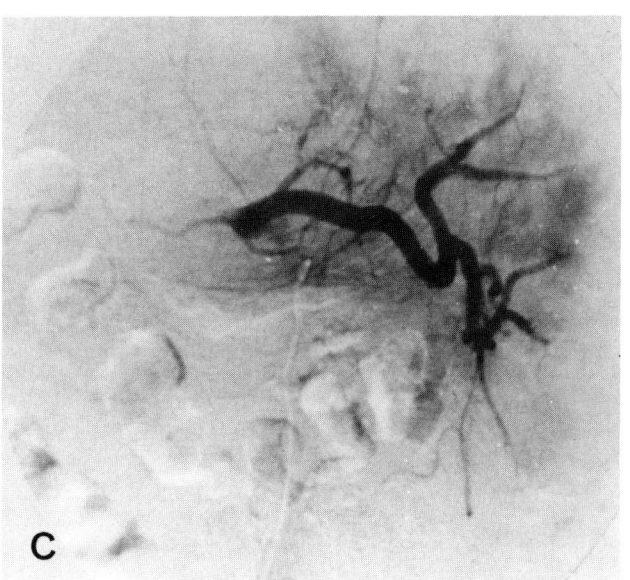
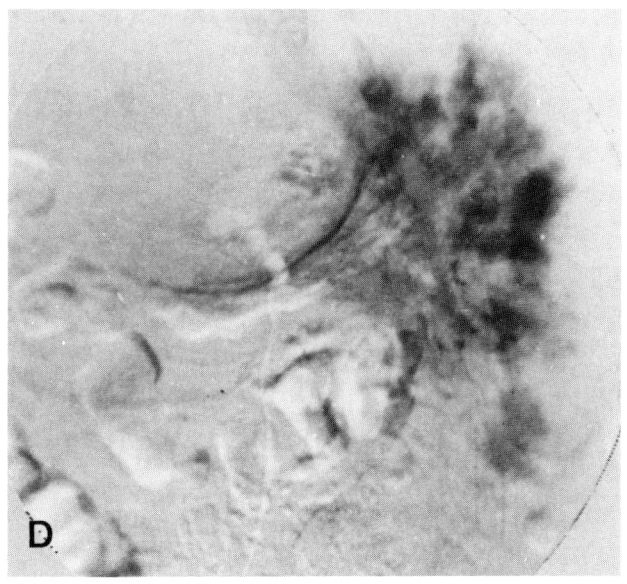

Figure 3.84 A patient with postnecrotic cirrhosis, hypersplenism, and encephalopathy out of clinical control.
(A) Selective injection into the splenic artery shows an enlarged spleen. (B) Later phase shows opacification of the spontaneous portosystemic shunt with filling of the short gastric vein, left renal vein, and inferior vena cava (arrowheads). (C) After partial embolization of the spleen, reduction of splenic perfusion is seen. (D) In the later phase, there is opacification of portions of the splenic parenchyma. The spontaneous shunt can no longer be identified. After the procedure, encephalopathy was controlled without any additional care in a follow-up of approximately 9 months.

managing hypersplenism, partial embolization of the spleen leads to disappearance of or flow reduction in this spontaneous portosystemic shunt by reducing the supply of brain toxins to the systemic circulation (Fig. 3.84). This has occurred in our patients.

COMPLICATIONS FROM PERCUTANEOUS TRANSHEPATIC PORTOGRAPHY AND EMBOLIZATION OF GASTROESOPHAGEAL VARICES

The most serious complication in patients with transhepatic obstruction of esophageal varices is portal vein thrombosis due to blood stagnation occurring inside the vein after the occlusion of collateral branches with hepatofugal flow. This portal vein obstruction can be lethal, but it may pass unnoticed and be identified only in angiographic follow-up studies or by another imaging method. This complication occurs in 2 to 3 percent of patients.

Another frightening complication is intraperitoneal bleeding at the puncture site in the liver. This type of accident occurs with a frequency of about 3 percent in major series. However, the incidence dropped significantly when catheter track embolization following the completion of the procedure became a standard technique.

Other relatively frequent complications include hemorrhagic or ascitic pleural effusion, leakage of ascitic fluid through the puncture site, fever, and hepatic subcapsular hematoma.

Handling of needles and guidewires inside the hepatic parenchyma may lead to the formation of fistulas in different systems. This can cause hemobilia. Accidental puncture of the hepatic arterial system may lead to subcapsular intraperitoneal bleeding or the formation of a pseudoaneurysm (Fig. 3.85).

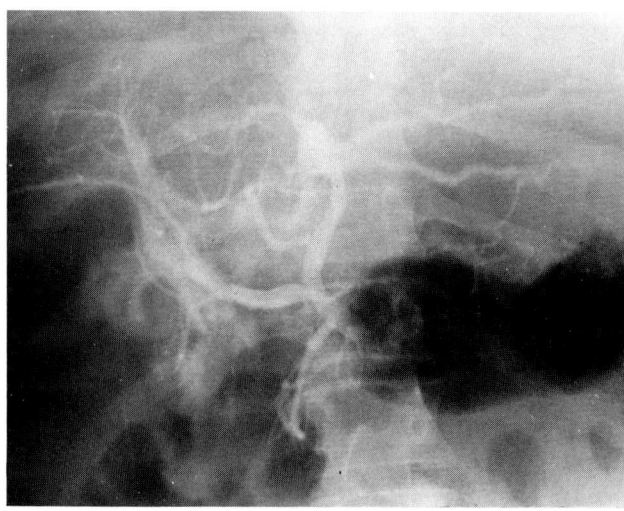

Figure 3.85 A percutaneous transhepatic portogram which resulted in catheterization of the intrahepatic arterial tree. This is a potential cause of intraperitoneal bleeding after this procedure.

REFERENCES

Alvarez F, Bernard O, Brunelle F, Hadchovel P, Odievre M, Alagille D. Portal obstruction in children: I. Clinical investigation and hemorrhage risk. *J. Pediatr* 1983;103:696–702.

Alvarez F, Bernard O, Brunelle F, Hadchovel P, Odievre M, Alagille D. Portal obstruction in children: II. Results of surgical portosystemic shunts. *J Pediatr* 1983;103:703–707.

Alves CAP, Alves AR, Abreu WN, Andrade ZA. Hepatic artery hypertrophy and sinusoidal hypertension in advanced schistosomiasis. *Gastroenterology* 177;72:126–128.

Andrade ZA, Cheever AW. Alterations of the intrahepatic vasculature in hepatosplenic schistosomiasis mansoni. *Am J Trop Med Hyg* 1971;20:425–532.

Azevedo FS, Penas ME, Pinheiro RSA. Embolizacao esplenica parcial. *Radiol Bras* 1983;16:95–99.

Athanasoulis CA. Portal hypertension and bleeding varices. In *Interventional Radiology*, edited by Athanasoulis CA, Greene RE, Pfister RC, Roberson GH. Saunders, Philadelphia, 1982:90–113.

Baert AL, Fevery J, Marchal G, Goddeeris P, Wilms G, Ponette E, Groote J. Early diagnosis of Budd-Chiari syndrome by computed tomography and ultrasonography: Report of five cases. *Gastroenterology* 1983;84:587–595.

Bismuth H, Franco D, Alagille A. Portal diversion for portal hypertension in children. *Ann Surg* 1980;192:18–24.

Bogliolo L. A esplenografia na esquistossomiase mansonica hepatoesplenica, forma de symmers. *Rev Assoc Med Bras* 1957;3:263–269.

Brucharth F. Percutaneous transhepatic portography: I. Technique and application. *AJR* 1979;132:177–182.

Burcharth F, Sorensen TIA, Andersen B. Findings in percutaneous transhepatic portography and variceal bleeding in cirrhosis. *Surg Gynecol Obstet* 1980;150:887–890.

Chandler JG, Fechner RE. Hepatopedal flow restoration in patients intolerant of total portal diversion. *Ann Surg* 1983;197:574–583.

Davis WD, Reichman GR, Storaasli JP. Effect of pituitrin in reducing portal pressure in the human being. *N Engl J Med* 1957;256:108–112.

Deutsch V, Rosenthal T, Adar R, Mozes M. Budd-Chiari syndrome. *AJR* 1972;116:430–439.

Eckauser FE, Appelman HD, Knol JA, Strodel WE, Coran AG, Turcotte JG. Noncirrhotic portal hypertension: Differing patterns of disease in children and adults. *Surgery* 1983;94:721–728.

Fischer JE, Bower RH, Atamian S, Welling R. Comparison of distal and proximal splenorenal shunts. *Ann Surg* 1981;194:531–544.

Hanna SS, Smith RS, Henderson JM, Millikan WJ, Warren WD. Reversal of hepatic encephalopathy after occlusion of total portosystemic shunts. *Am J Surg* 1981;142:285–289.

Hoevels J, Joelsson B. A comparative study of esophageal varices by endoscopy hand percutaneous transhepatic esophageal phlebography. *Gastrointest Radiol* 1979;4:232–329.

Hoevells J, Lunderquist A, Tylen U. Percutaneous transhepatic portography. *Acta Radiol* 1977;19:643–658.

Hunt PS, Korman MG, Hansky J, Parkin WG. An 8 year prospective experience with balloon tamponade in emergency control of bleeding esophageal varices. *Dig Dis Sci* 1982;27:413–416.

Jarhult J, Forsberg L, Lunderquist A. Budd-Chiari syndrome. *Acta Chir Scand* 1984;150:105–108.

Joffe SN. Non-operative management of variceal bleeding. *Br J Surg* 1984;71:85–91.

Johnson WC, Nabseth DC, Widrich WC, Bush HL, O'Hara ET, Robbins AH. Bleeding esophageal varices. *Ann Surg* 1982;195:393–400.

Kallio H, Suorante H, Lempinen M. Hemodynamics after distal splenorenal shunt. *Acta Chir Scand* 1984;150:35–40.

Keller FS, Dotter CT, Rosch J. Percutaneous transhepatic obliteration of gastroesophageal varices: Some technical aspects. *Radiology* 1978;129:327–332.

Koransky JR, Galambos JT, Hersh T, Warren WD. The mortality of bleeding esophageal varices in a private university hospital. *Am J Surg* 1978;136:339–341.

Kreel L, Freston JW, Clain D. Vascular radiology in the Budd-Chiari syndrome. *Br J Radiol* 1967;40:755–759.

Longstreth GF, Newcomer AD, Green PA. Extrahepatic portal hypertension caused by chronic pancreatitis. *Ann Intern Med* 1971;75:903–908.

Lunderquist A, Vang J. Transhepatic catheterization and obliteration of the coronary vein in patients with portal hypertension and esophageal varices. *N Engl J Med* 1974;646–649.

Lunderquist A. Portal vein flow pattern in portal hypertension. *Clin Radiol* 1980;31:395–415.

Lunderquist A, Simert G, Tylen U, Vang J. Follow-up of patients with portal hypertension and esophageal varices treated with percutaneous obliteration of gastric coronary vein. *Radiology* 1977;122:59–63.

Lunderquist A, Borjesson B, Owman T, Bengmark S. Isobutyl 2-cyanoacrylate (bucrylate) in obliteration of gastric coronary vein and esophageal varices. *AJR* 1978;130–136.

Murphy FB, Steinberg HV, Shires GT, Martin LG, Bernardino ME. The Budd-Chiari syndrome: A review. *AJR* 1986;147:9–15.

Norlinger BM, Nordlinger DF, Fulenwider JT, Millikan WJ, Sones PJ, Kutner M, Steele R, Bain R, Warren WD. Angiography in portal hypertension: Clinical significance in surgery. *Am J Surg* 1980;139:132–141.

Nusbaum M, Baum S, Sakiyalal P, et al. Pharmacologic control of portal hypertension. *Surgery* 1976;62:299–304.

Odievre M, Chaumont P, Montagne J, Alagille D. Anomalies of the intrahepatic portal venous systems in congenital hepatic fibrosis. *Radiology* 1977;122:427–430.

Orloff MJ, Johansen KH. Treatment of Budd-Chiari syndrome by side-to-side portocaval shunt: Experimental and clinical results. *Ann Surg* 1978;188:494–512.

Ou QJ, Hermann RE. The role of hepatic veins in liver operations. *Surgery* 1984;95:381–391.

Parker RGF. Occlusion of the hepatic veins in man. *Medicine (Baltimore)* 1959;38:369–402.

Passariello R, Thau A, Rossi P, Lombardi M, Simonetti G, Stipa S. Control of gastroesophageal bleeding varices by percutaneous transhepatic portography. *Surg Gynecol Obstet* 1980;150:155–160.

Pereiras R, Viamonte M Jr, Russell E, LePage J, White P, Hutson D. New techniques for interruption of gastroesophageal venous blood flow. *Radiology* 1977;124:313–323.

Potts JR, Henderson JM, Millikan WJ, Sones P, Warren WD. Restoration of portal venous perfusion and reversal of encephalopathy by balloon occlusion of portal systemic shunt. *Gastroenterology* 1984;87:208–212.

Reuter SR, Redman HC. Cirrhosis and portal hypertension. In *Gastrointestinal Angiography,* edited by Reuter SR, Redman HC. Saunders, Philadelphia, 1979:219–261.

Scott J, Dick R, Long RG, Sherlock S. Percutaneous transhepatic obliteration of gastroesophageal varices. *Lancet* 1976;2:53–55.

Shaldon S, Sherlock S. The use of vasopressin in the control of bleeding from esophageal varices. *Lancet* 1960;2:222–224.

Sherlock S. Portal circulation and portal hypertension. *Gut* 1978;19:70–83.

Smith-Laing G, Camilo ME, Dick R, Sherlock S. Percutaneous transhepatic portography in the assessment of portal hypertension. *Gastroenterology* 1980;78:197–205.

Smith-Laing G, Scott J, Long RG, Dick R, Sherlock S. Role of percutaneous transhepatic obliteration of varices in the management of hemorrhage from gastroesophageal varices. *Gastroenterology* 1981;80:1031–1036.

Spigos DG, Jonasson O, Mozes M, Capek V. Partial splenic embolization in the treatment of hypersplenism. *AJR* 1979;132:777–782.

Tavill AS, Wood EJ, Kreel L, Jones EA, Gregory M, Sherlock S. The Budd-Chiari syndrome: Correlation between hepatic scintigraphy and the clinical radiological and pathological findings in nineteen cases of hepatic venous outflow obstruction. *Gastroenterology* 1975;68:509–518.

Terblanch J, Northover JMA, Bornman P, et al. A prospective management of patients after esophageal variceal bleeding. *Surg Gynecol Obstet* 1979;148:323–328.

Thompson EN, Sherlock S. The etiology of portal vein thrombosis with particular reference to the role of infection and exchange transfusion. *Q J Med* 1964;132:465–480.

Tylen U, Simert G, Vang J. Hemodynamic changes after distal splenorenal shunt studied by sequential angiography. *Radiology* 1976;121:585–589.

Uflacker R. Radiologia intervencionaista: Uma especialidade emergente. *Radiol Bras* 1983;16:71–78.

Uflacker R, Lima S. Percutaneous transhepatic portography for obliteration of gastroesophageal varices in partial and total vein occlusion. *Radiology* 1980;137:325–330.

Uflacker R, Alves MA, Cantisani GG, Souza HP, Wagner J, Moraes LF. Treatment of portal vein obstruction by percutaneous transhepatic angioplasty. *Gastroenterology* 1985;88:176–180.

Uflacker R. Percutaneous transhepatic obliteration of gastroesophageal varices using absolute alcohol. *Radiology* 1983;146:621–625.

Uflacker R, Saadi J. Transcatheter embolization of superior mesenteric arteriovenous fistula. *AJR* 1982;139:1212–1214.

Uflacker R, Francisconi CF, Rodriguez MP, Amaral NM. Percutaneous transluminal angioplasty of the hepatic veins for treatment of Budd-Chiari syndrome. *Radiology* 1984;153:641–642.

Uflacker R, Silva AO, Albuquerque LAC, Piske RL, Mourão GS. Chronic portosystemic encephalopathy: Embolization of portosystemic shunts. *Radiology* 1987;165:721–725.

Viamonte M Jr, Lepage J, Lunderquist A, Pereiras R, Russell E, Viamonte M, Camacho M. Selective catheterization of the portal vein and its tributaries. *Radiology* 1975;114:457–460.

Viamonte M. Radiologie des obstructions des veines viscerales. *J Radiol Eletrol* 1976;57:853–863.

Viamonte M, Pereiras R, Russell E, Lepage J, Meier WL. Pitfalls in transhepatic portography. *Radiology* 1977;124:325–329.

Viamonte M, Pereiras R, Russell E, Lepage J, Hutson D. Transhepatic obliteration of gastroesophageal varices: Results in acute and non-acute bleeders. *AJR* 1977;129:237–241.

Warren ND, Millikan WJ, Henderson JM, Wright L, Kutner M, Smith RB, Fulenwider JT, Salan AA, Galambos JT. Ten years portal hypertensive surgery at Emory: Results and new perspectives. *Ann Surg* 1982;195:530–542.

Warren WD, Milikan WJ Jr, Smith RB, Rypins EF, Henderson JM, Salam AA, Hersh T, Galambos JT, Faraj BA. Non-cirrhotic portal vein thrombosis. *Ann Surg* 1980;192:341–349.

Weeb LJ, Sherlock S. The etiology, presentation, and natural history of extra-hepatic portal venous obstruction. *Q J Med* 1979;192:627–639.

Widrich WC, Robbis AH, Nabseth DC, Johnson WC, Goldstein SA. Pitfalls of transhepatic portal venography and therapeutic coronary vein occlusion. *AJR* 1978;131:637–643.

Wiechel KL. Tekniken vid perkutan transhepatisk portapunkton (PTP). *Nord Med* 1971;86:912.

Chapter Four
Clinical Applications of Embolization

INTRODUCTION

Embolization is most frequently performed to control bleeding of traumatic origin, an inflammatory process, or a neoplasm. In other situations embolization is used to alter the function of an organ or vascular territory, for instance, by controlling the development of a neoplasm. In still others, the objective is to correct a vascular malformation with or without arteriovenous fistula, if possible, without altering the function of the affected organ. Occlusive techniques predominate because vasoconstrictive agents are not effective in most situations occurring outside the GI tract, due to the size of the vessels involved, trauma to the arterial wall, association with an inflammatory process, and the presence of tumor vessels in the lesion.

One application of embolization therapy that is not directly related to those discussed in Chapters 1, 2, and 3 is the treatment of visceral neoplasm as a form of lesion therapy (either palliative or definitive), without attempting to treat any of its occasional complications, such as bleeding.

The selection of embolization techniques depends on the type of vessel and lesion to be treated (various methods used for embolization are described in Chap. 2). In general, however, the following principles hold.

For embolization of a small peripheral hepatic lesion a particulate material, such as Gelfoam or Ivalon, may be used in small volume.

When dealing with a ruptured aneurysm of the splenic artery, a more proximal, definitive embolization will be performed, with larger-size material, such as a detachable balloon or Gianturco coils.

If the site to be embolized is an organ which may bleed and digest the embolic material (for example, as the pancreas digests Gelfoam), a cyanocrylate-type polymer should be used.

The individual aspects specific to each situation will be described in the following sections.

Embolization in the Liver

RENAN UFLAKER

BACKGROUND

It has been estimated that under normal circumstances, the hepatic artery supplies the liver with 25 percent of its blood and around 50 percent of its oxygen. The portal vein supplies the liver with the other 75 percent of its blood and 50 percent of its oxygen. When the arterial supply is discontinued, the oxygen demand is adequately met by portal blood, due both to an increase in total portal venous flow as a result of absence of competition over the common vascular bed by the two systems at the hepatic sinusoidal level and to an increase in extraction of portal blood.

Another important hemodynamic aspect of intrahepatic circulation is the existence of collateral exuberance through phrenic and intercostal arteries, the gallbladder vascular bed, the gastrohepatic and falciform ligaments, the duodenopancreatic arches, and the interlobular anastomoses, which precipitates the recanalization of intrahepatic circulation practically immediately when hepatic artery occlusion takes place at any more proximal level (Fig. 3.20). This recanalization through the collaterals led to total failure of hepatic devascularization procedures by surgical hepatic artery ligation at any of its levels (Fig. 4.1). Even though a degree of ischemia and necrosis may be identified in intrahepatic neoplastic lesions after surgical ligation, the fact that flow is reestablished through the collaterals allows the viability of most of the existing tumor tissue (Fig. 4.1).

A few aspects of hepatic embolization well established in the literature should be mentioned here. Hepatic necrosis after arterial occlusion is a rare condition in humans, provided that the portal vein remains patent. Embolization in abnormal hepatic territory should be superselective and peripheral enough to prevent ischemia and infarction of normal surrounding tissue. However, hepatic arterial occlusion cannot be "too peripheral"; if it reaches the sinusoids, the natural shunts between the artery and the portal vein will be occluded and infarction will occur. "Micro" sized particles or fluids, such as absolute alcohol and polymers, should not be used diffusely in the liver, as they may cause extensive infarction of normal tissue. Only superselective use, and in isolated lesions, is advisable.

Small 2- by 1-, 2- by 2-, or 2- by 3-mm particles should be used in small bleeding vessels or hepatic tumors. Aneurysms and lacerations should be treated with larger particles. Infection of embolized hepatic parenchyma can be prevented by adequate antibiotic coverage. Oxygen supplementation should be used to increase the supply of oxygen to the liver. Reduction in food intake for 48 h after the procedure is also advised.

Hepatic embolization generally should not be performed if hepatofugal flow is present in the portal system or if the portal vein is occluded. However, limited embolization of hepatic neoplasm with arteriovenous fistula, even when portal hepatofugal flow is present, is admissible since shunt occlusion will invert the portal flow to its usual direction or at least will reduce pressure in the venous system, improving hepatic function.

Because canine portal blood is not sterile, experimental studies with hepatic embolization in dogs have resulted in a high rate of complication due to abscess. In humans, the risk of abscess is quite low, although this complication has been described.

HEPATIC ARTERY ANEURYSMS AND HEMOBILIA

Aneurysms of the hepatic artery may be detected as masses or by bleeding inside the biliary tree. When the aneurysm is of intrahepatic type, hemobilia is more likely to happen. Severe intraperitoneal bleeding may be the first sign of an extrahepatic aneurysm. The most common causes of hepatic artery aneurysm or pseudoaneurysm are trauma (blunt, penetrating, biopsy, or surgical), infection (mycotic aneurysm) (Fig. 4.2), arteriosclerosis (Fig. 3.20), and collagenous disease with vascular involvement (Ehlers-Danlos syndrome). In the past, the most common cause of hepatic artery aneurysm was infection (Fig. 4.2); presently, however, the most frequent cause is trauma, with formation of pseudoaneurysms and

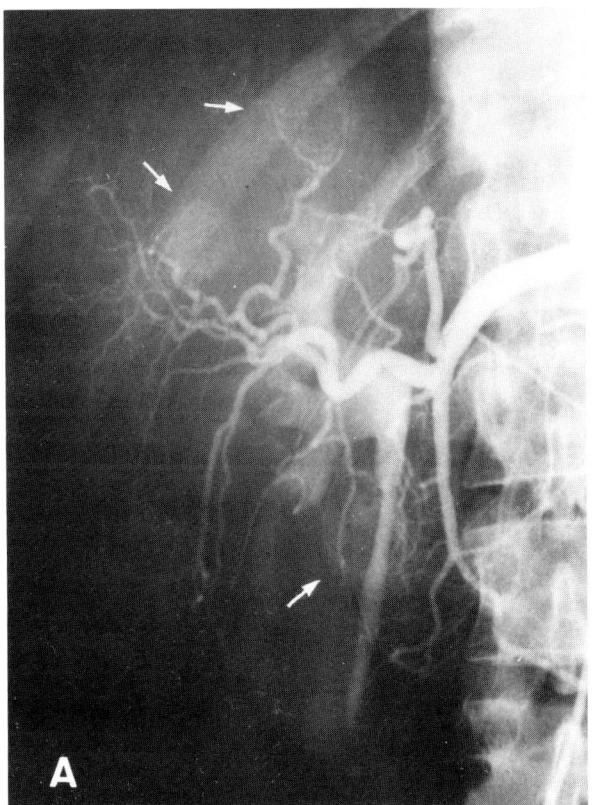
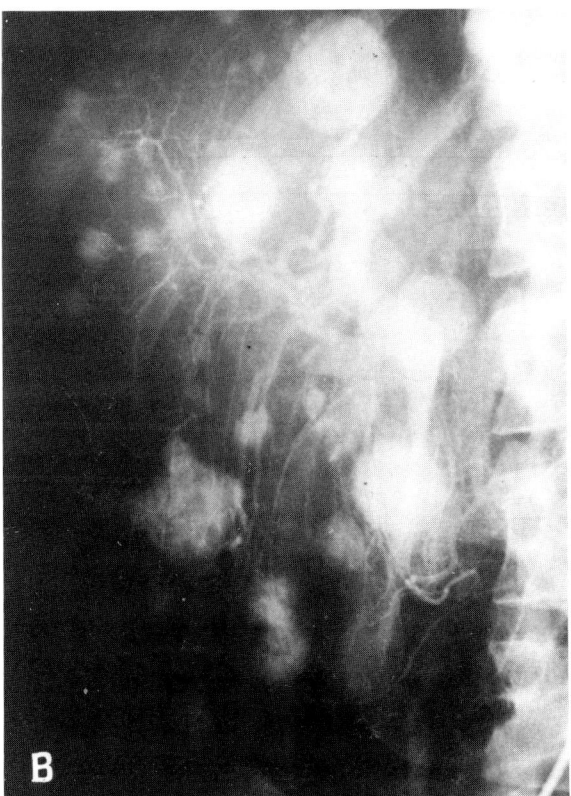
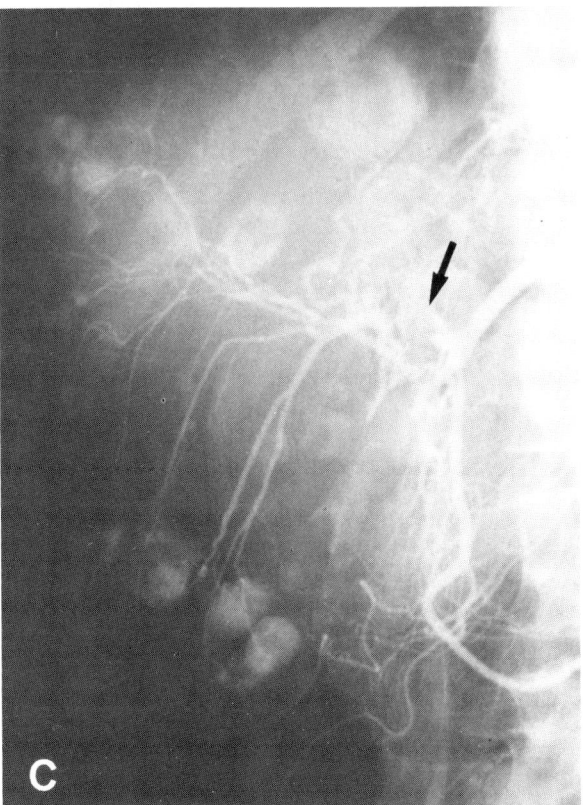

Figure 4.1 (A) Early arterial phase of injection into the celiac axis, showing the beginning of impregnation of hepatic nodules (arrows). (B) Early later phase of injection into the celiac axis, showing several hypervascular metastatic nodules of the carcinoid tumor. (C) Control angiogram after surgical ligation of the proper hepatic artery (arrow), showing abundant collateralization, with recanalization of intrahepatic circulation. Notice that even though the metastatic nodules have not shrunk, they are displaying signs of cavitation with necrosis.

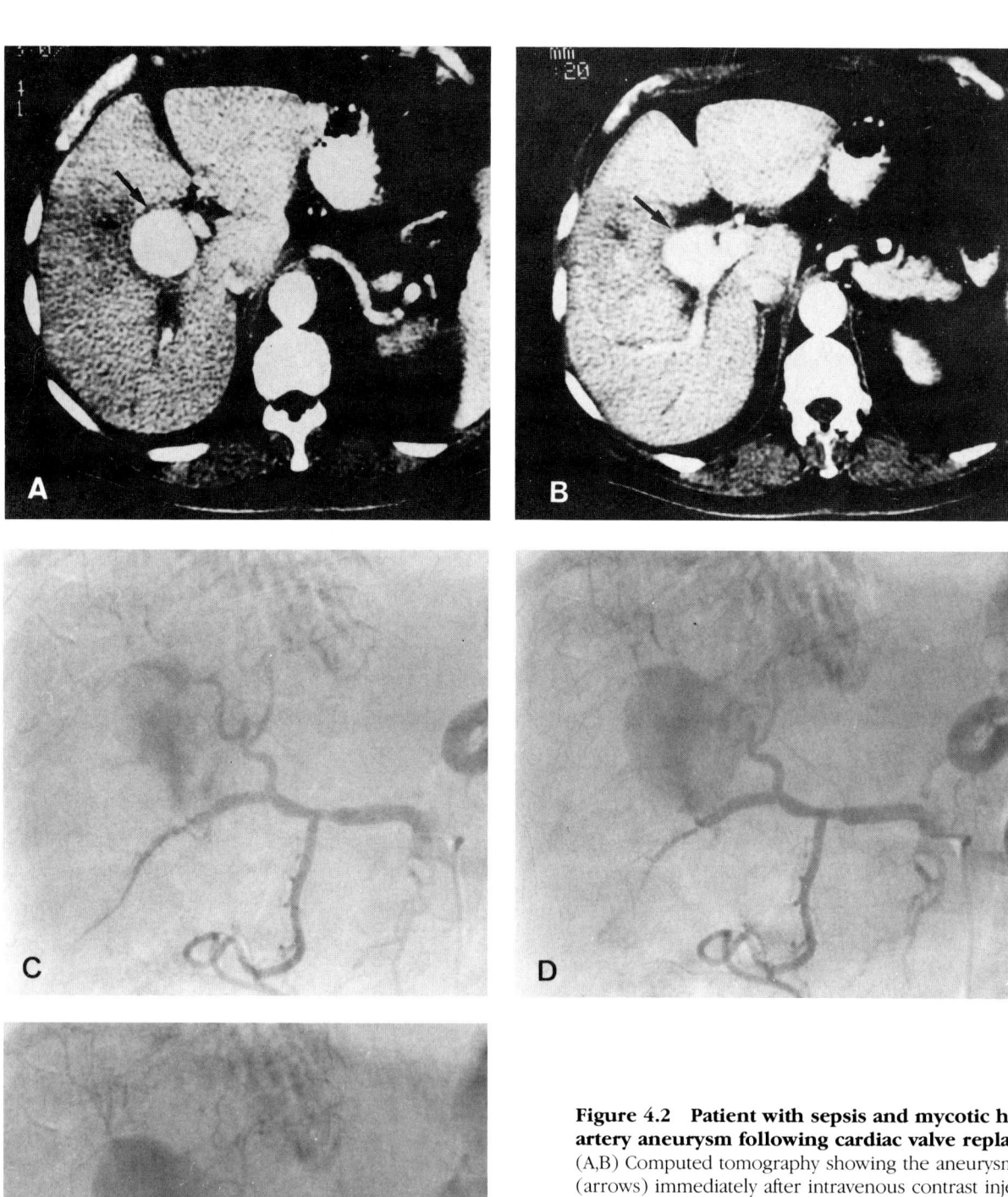

Figure 4.2 Patient with sepsis and mycotic hepatic artery aneurysm following cardiac valve replacement. (A,B) Computed tomography showing the aneurysm cavity (arrows) immediately after intravenous contrast injection. (C,D,E) Different stages of an hepatic selective angiogram showing the progressive filling of the pseudoaneurysm cavity with localized rupture of the right hepatic artery. (F) Later phase of injection into superior mesenteric artery, showing portal vein compression on the portion of the artery near the bifurcation, by the pseudoaneurysm. (G) Control angiogram showing arterial and pseudoaneurysm occlusion after embolization of right hepatic artery performed with two Gianturco coils (arrow). (H) Computed tomogram 4 days after embolization showing thrombosed aneurysm with residual contrast inside. A computed tomograph 3 months after embolization showed complete resolution of the aneurysm.

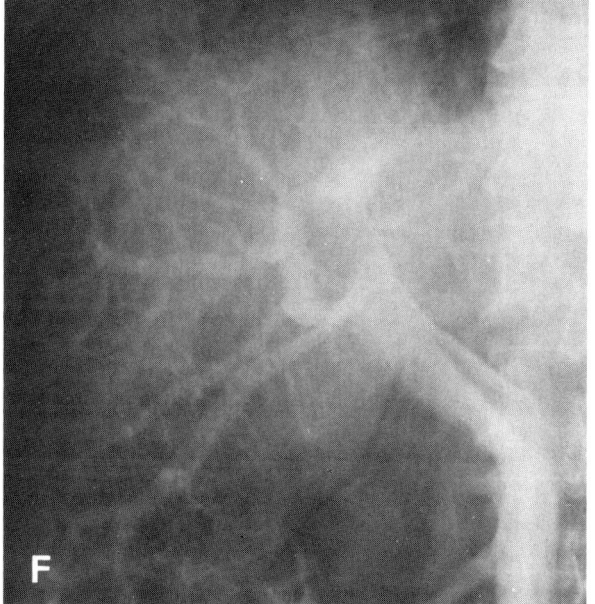
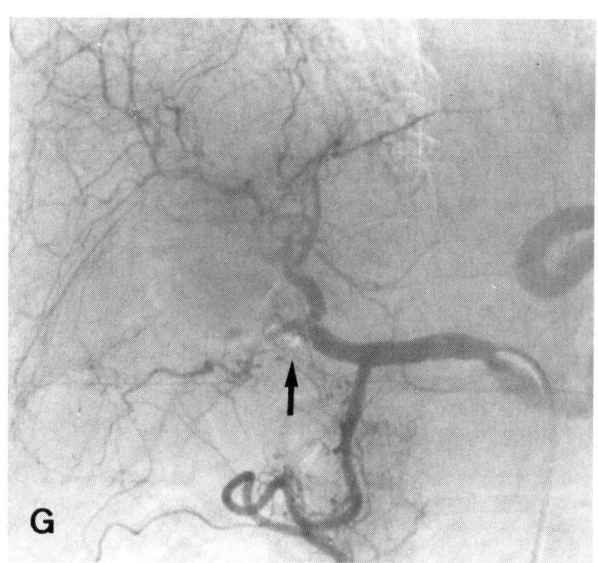
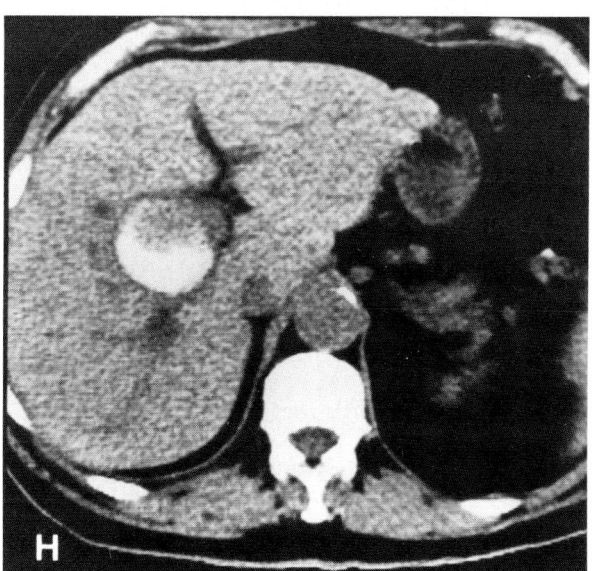

Figure 4.2 *Continued*

hemobilia (Fig. 4.3). Computed tomography and ultrasonography are valuable tools for identifying these lesions (Fig. 4.2). The classic therapy has been ligation of the hepatic artery, but surgical reconstruction of the artery was occasionally performed in cases of extrahepatic aneurysm. Pre- and postsurgical mortality was around 75 percent before embolization started being used. With or without surgery, the mortality rate has been reduced by 30 percent, according to recent studies. Aneurysms that remain unruptured may cause pain and jaundice.

Today embolization is the most widely accepted therapeutic method for treating hepatic artery aneurysms. The techniques used include filling the cavity of the lesion with Gianturco coils or a plastic polymer and closure of the artery feeding the aneurysmatic lesion, in any of its presentations. The treatment of choice for hemobilia is superselective embolization of the arterial branch supplying the lesion (Figs. 3.20 and 3.21). When the lesion cannot be reached through arterial catheterization, direct percutaneous transhepatic puncture of the lesion, with direct embolization of the aneurysmatic cavity, may be performed (Fig. 4.3).

An alternative for controlling hematobilia is prolonged plugging of the artery with a detachable balloon or a Fogarty-type occlusion balloon catheter (Fig. 4.4).

All hepatic artery aneurysms should be treated whether or not bleeding is present because the chance of acute rupture in these cases is quite high and is associated with a high mortality rate.

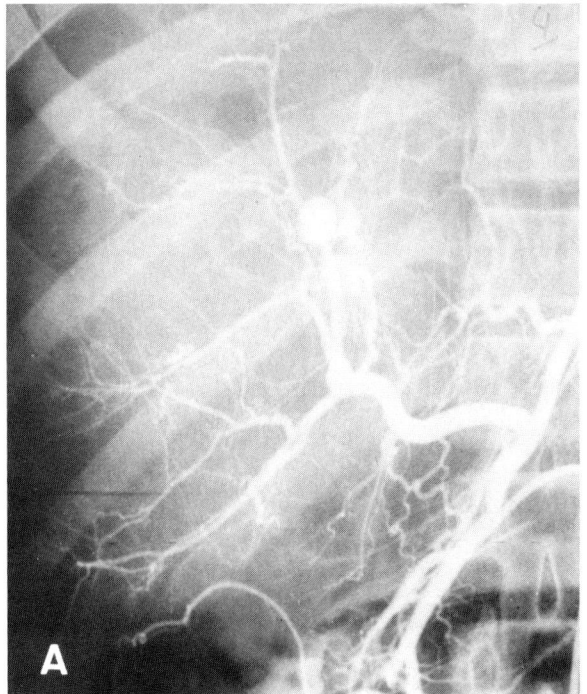
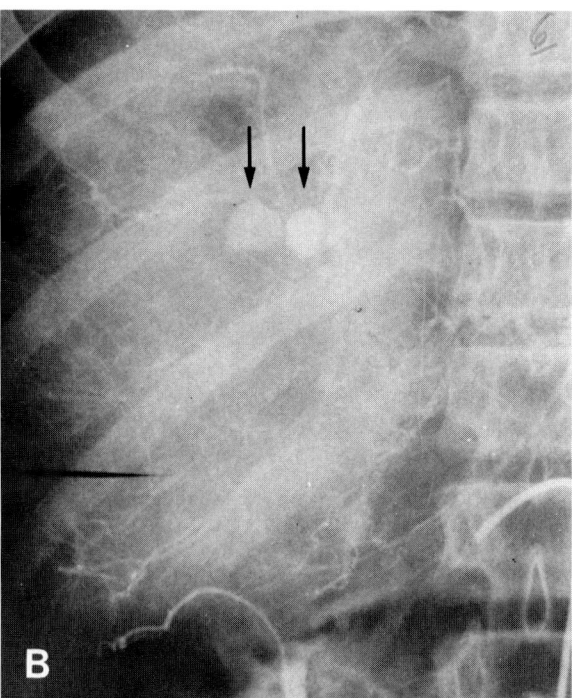
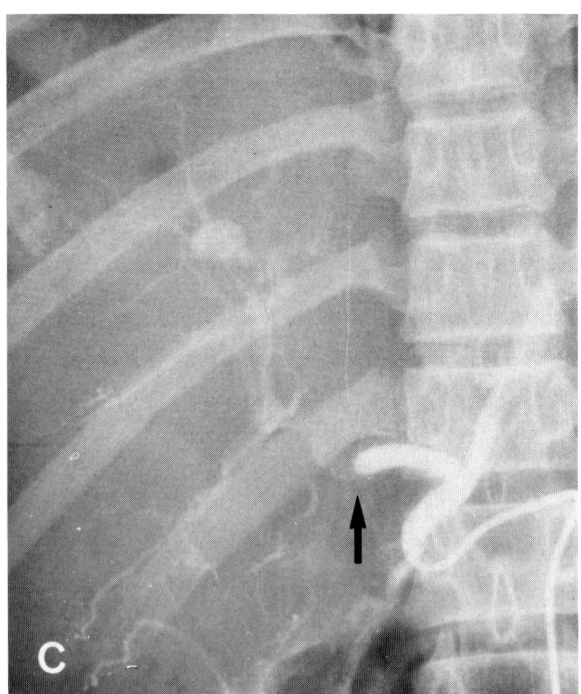

Figure 4.3 Liver pseudoaneurysm of traumatic origin, with severe hemobilia, treated by direct percutaneous puncture and embolization. Gelfoam embolization permanently occluded the cavity and cured the hemobilia.

(A,B) Contrast collection inside the liver (arrows) after injection into common hepatic artery. (C) After multiple selective catheterization attempts, dissection of the proper hepatic artery occurred (arrow), which prevented intravascular embolization. (D) Direct percutaneous puncture of aneurysm cavity with contrast injection. (E) Injection of additional contrast has resulted in biliary tree opacification, showing the communication. Embolization with Gelfoam pledgets was successfully performed through the percutaneous puncture.

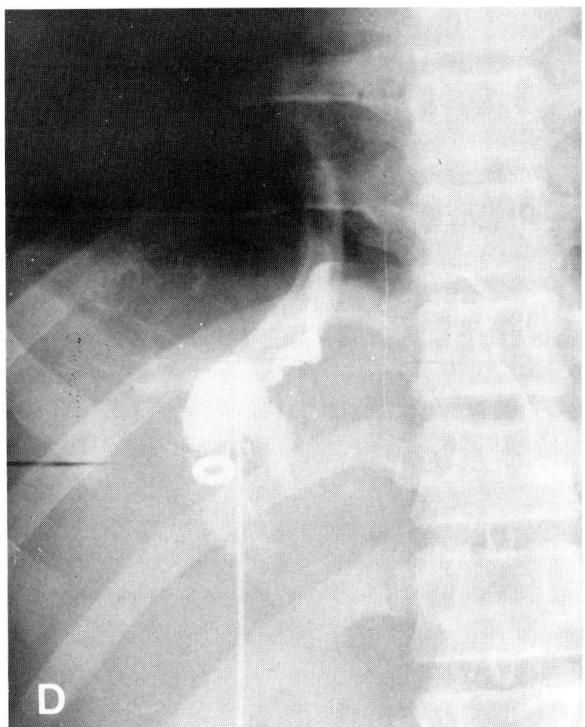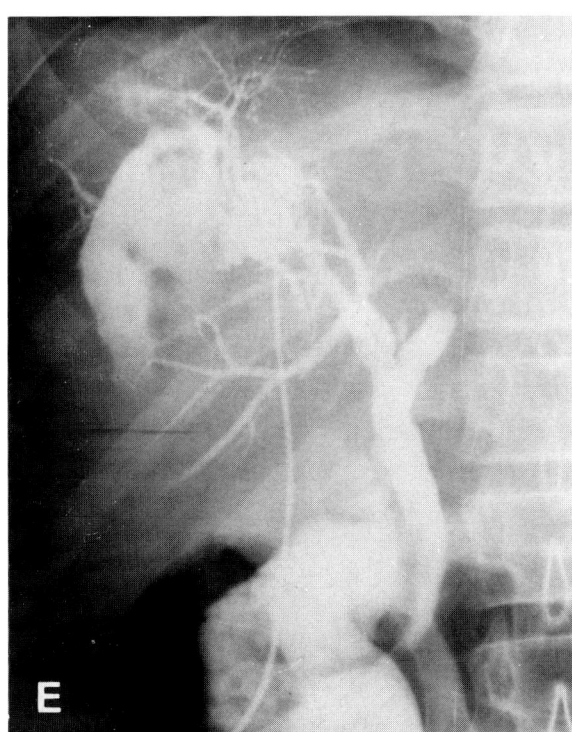

Figure 4.3 *Continued*

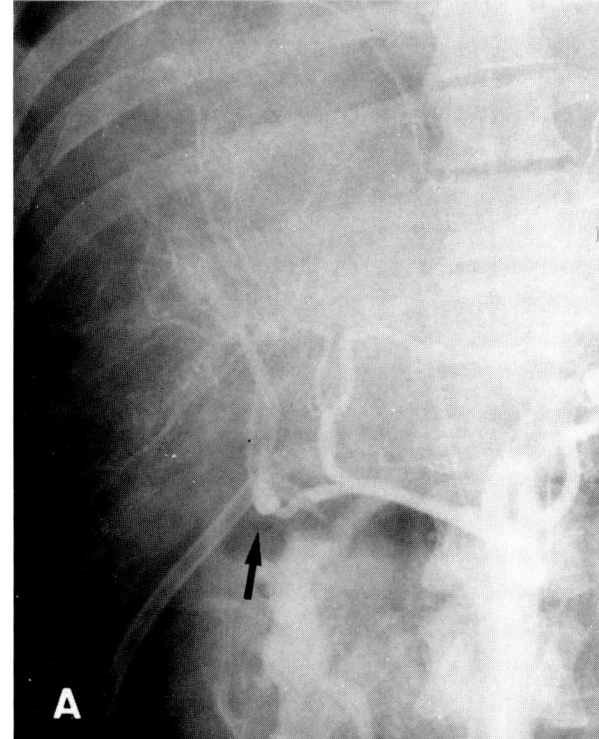

Figure 4.4 (A) Patient with hemobilia due to trauma during surgery for pseudoaneurysm formation on the site of cholecystectomy (arrow). (B) Cholangiogram through T tube showing the biliary tree filled with blood and contrast medium. (C) The proper hepatic artery was occluded with a No. 2 French Fogarty-type balloon catheter, coaxially introduced through the angiographic catheter. Bleeding was permanently controlled.

Figure 4.4 *Continued*

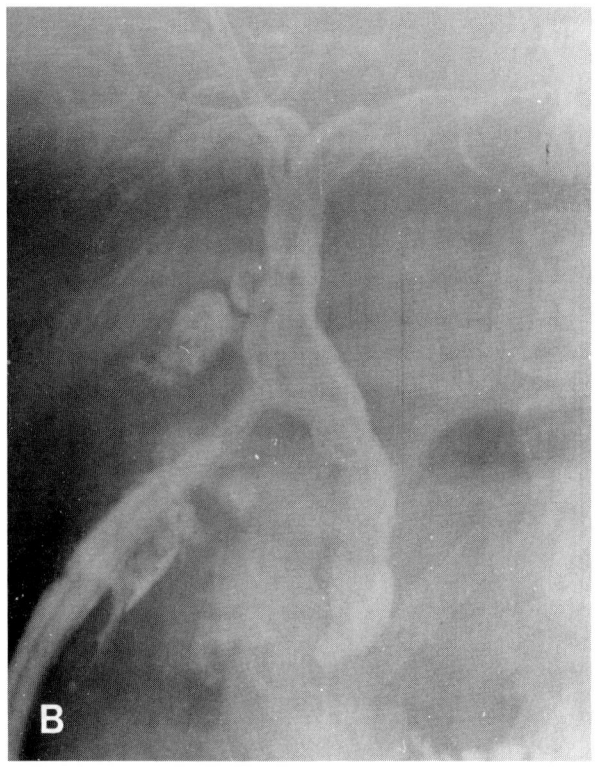

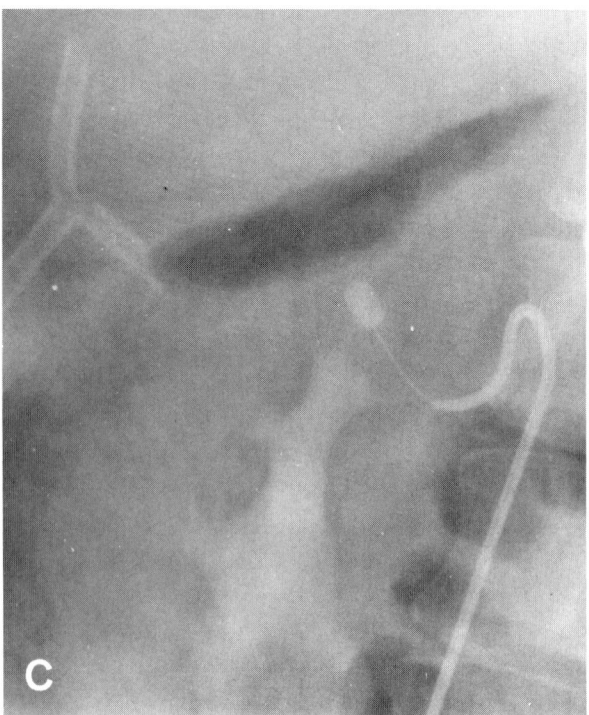

TRAUMATIC, CONGENITAL, AND TUMORAL ARTERIOVENOUS FISTULAS

The type and size of the hepatic AV fistula determine the embolization material to be utilized. For fistulas up to 8 mm, detachable balloons may be used; in larger fistulas, a combination of materials is desirable.

Traumatic AV fistulas are the result of puncture, trauma, or surgical biopsy. Definitive occlusion can usually be achieved by embolization with a Gianturco coil (Fig. 4.5).

Congenital hepatic AV fistulas usually have a high output, causing severe portal hypertension (Fig. 3.52). In small children, congenital heart failure often occurs also. Embolization is the treatment of choice for these lesions.

Tumoral AV fistulas are associated with the presence of a hypervascular neoplastic lesion, usually hepatic carcinoma, which promotes a high-output communication between the hepatic artery and the portal vein, causing reversal of portal venous flow and severe portal hypertension with collateral circulation and esophageal

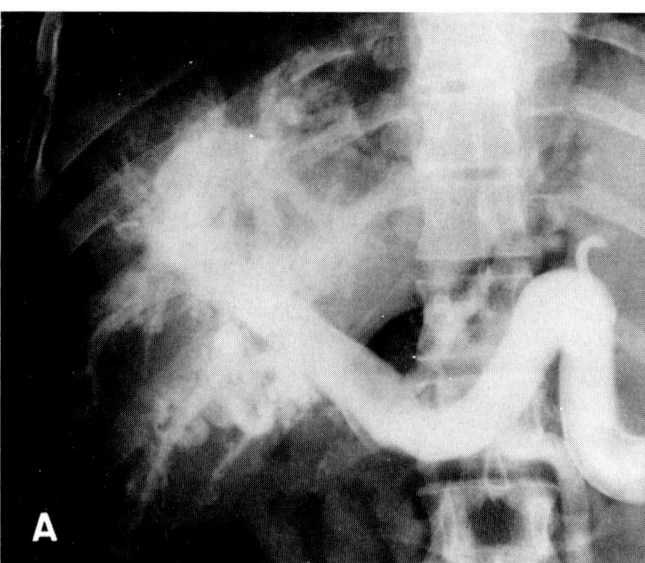

Figure 4.5 Patient with hepatic schistosomiasis and portal hypertension after selective Warren-type shunt and wedge-shaped hepatic biopsy.
(A) Preoperative splenoportogram showing large-sized portal vein and changes in portal intrahepatic radicles. (B,C,D) Selective injection into the left gastric artery showing arterioportal fistula (arrow) on the anterior border of the liver causing portal vein opacification and portal pressure increase. Notice the presence of ascites. (E) Superselective embolization of left hepatic artery was performed with a Gianturco coil (arrow). The control angiogram showed the fistula closed.

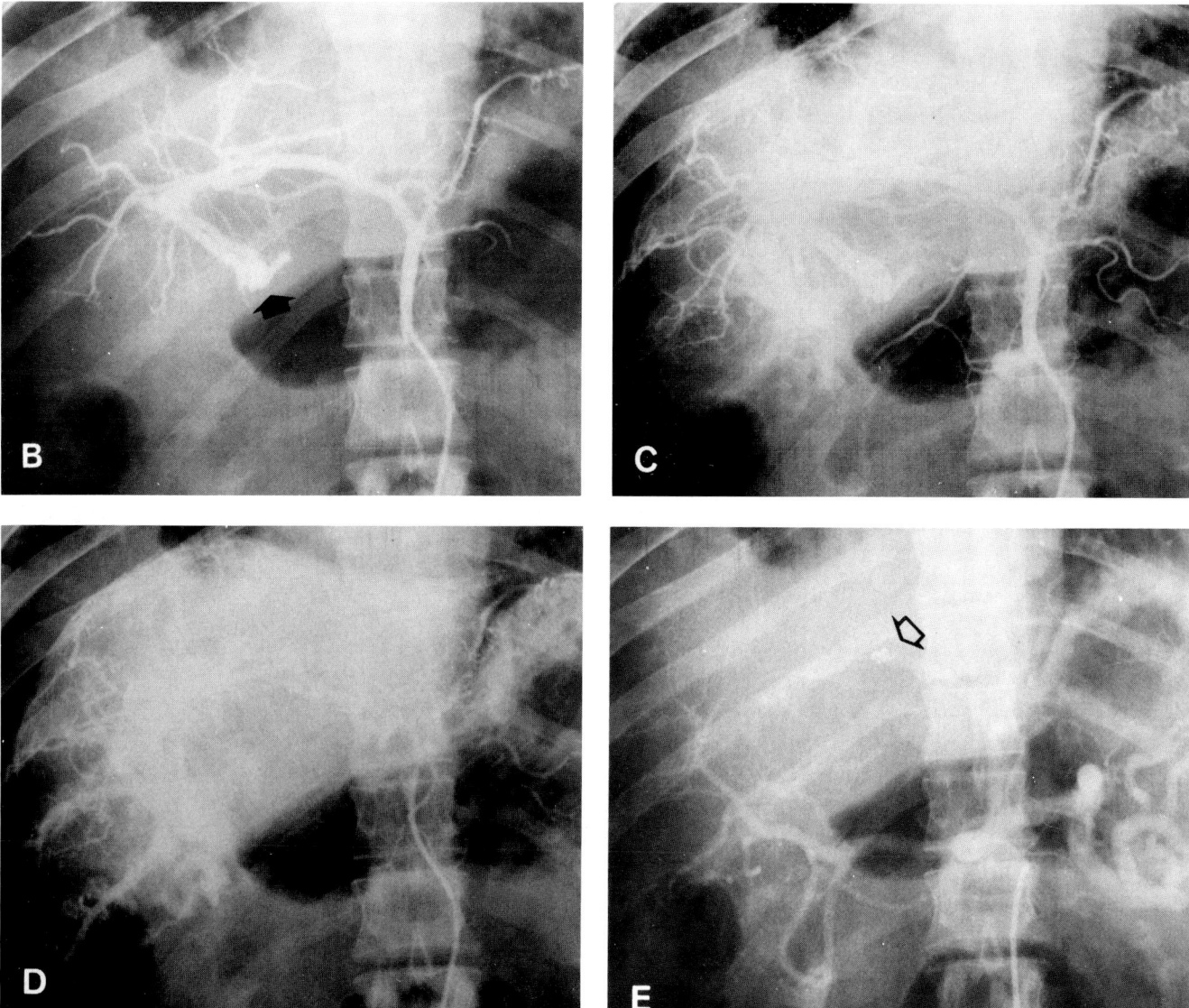

Figure 4.5 *Continued*

varices (Fig. 4.6). The lesion may be highly aggressive, frequently invading the portal vein. In these cases, in addition to hepatofugal flow in the portal vein, there is reduced luminal capacity to accommodate the portal system blood. Segmental, selective embolization of the artery most involved in the AV shunt should adequately control this problem (Fig. 4.7), in some cases providing portal flow reversal (Fig. 4.6). The arterial system should be preserved insofar as possible, because there is a high probability of hepatic necrosis followed by death if embolization beyond what is absolutely necessary is performed. In any case, the prognosis for patients with tumoral AV fistulas is very poor, with expected survival of only a few months.

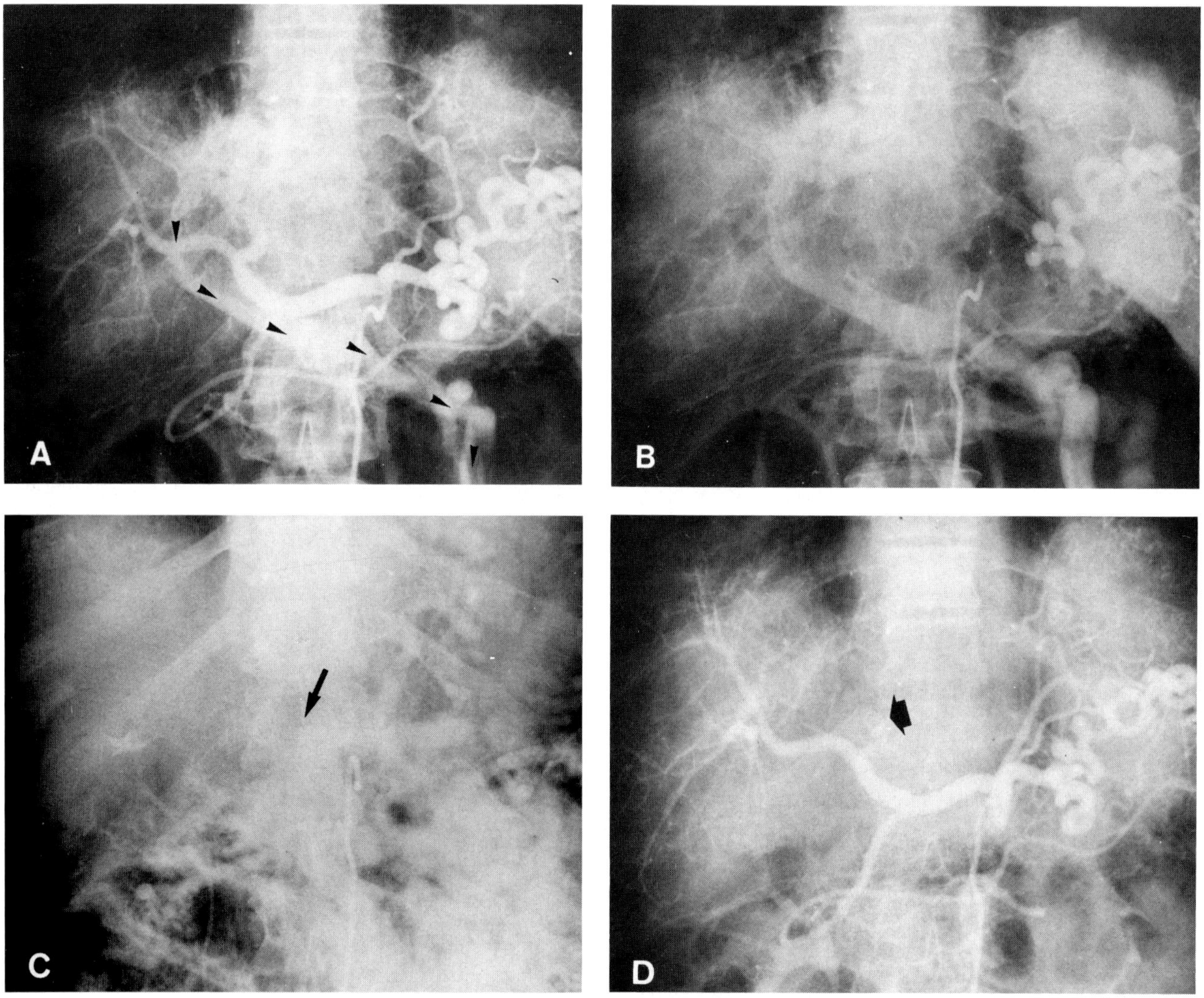

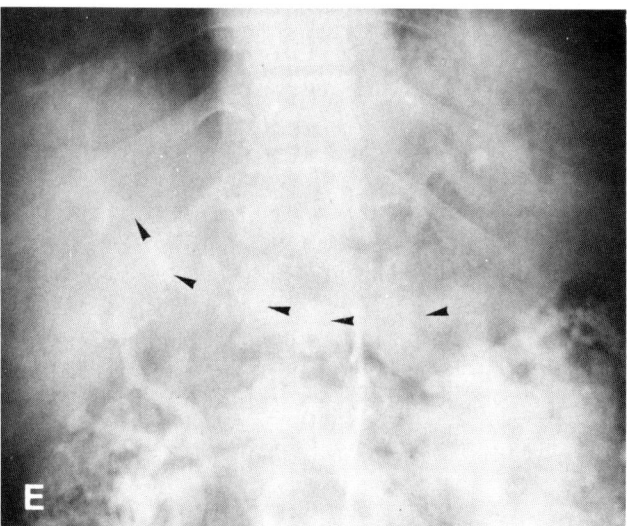

Figure 4.6 A 36-year-old patient with postnecrotic liver cirrhosis. A murmur has developed in the right hypochondrium, and there are clear signs of portal hypertension, with development of large-diameter portal-type circulation in the anterior portion of the abdomen.

(A,B) Injection in the celiac axis has shown a hypervascular tumor in the left hepatic lobe, with massive arterioportal shunt and inverted portal vein flow (arrowheads), as a result of partial portal occlusion for tumor invasion. (C) Later phase of injection into the superior mesenteric artery using papaverine (80 mg), showing portal vein "occlusion" (arrow) by hepatofugal flow. (D) Following superselective embolization of the left hepatic artery with Gelfoam and one Gianturco coil (arrow), the arteriovenous fistula has disappeared. (E) Injection into superior mesenteric artery after embolization showing portal flow reversal to hepatopetal flow (arrowheads), in spite of partial portal vein invasion. Portal-type circulation immediately disappeared from the abdominal wall, resulting in improvement in the patient's general condition, and the patient survived almost 6 months.

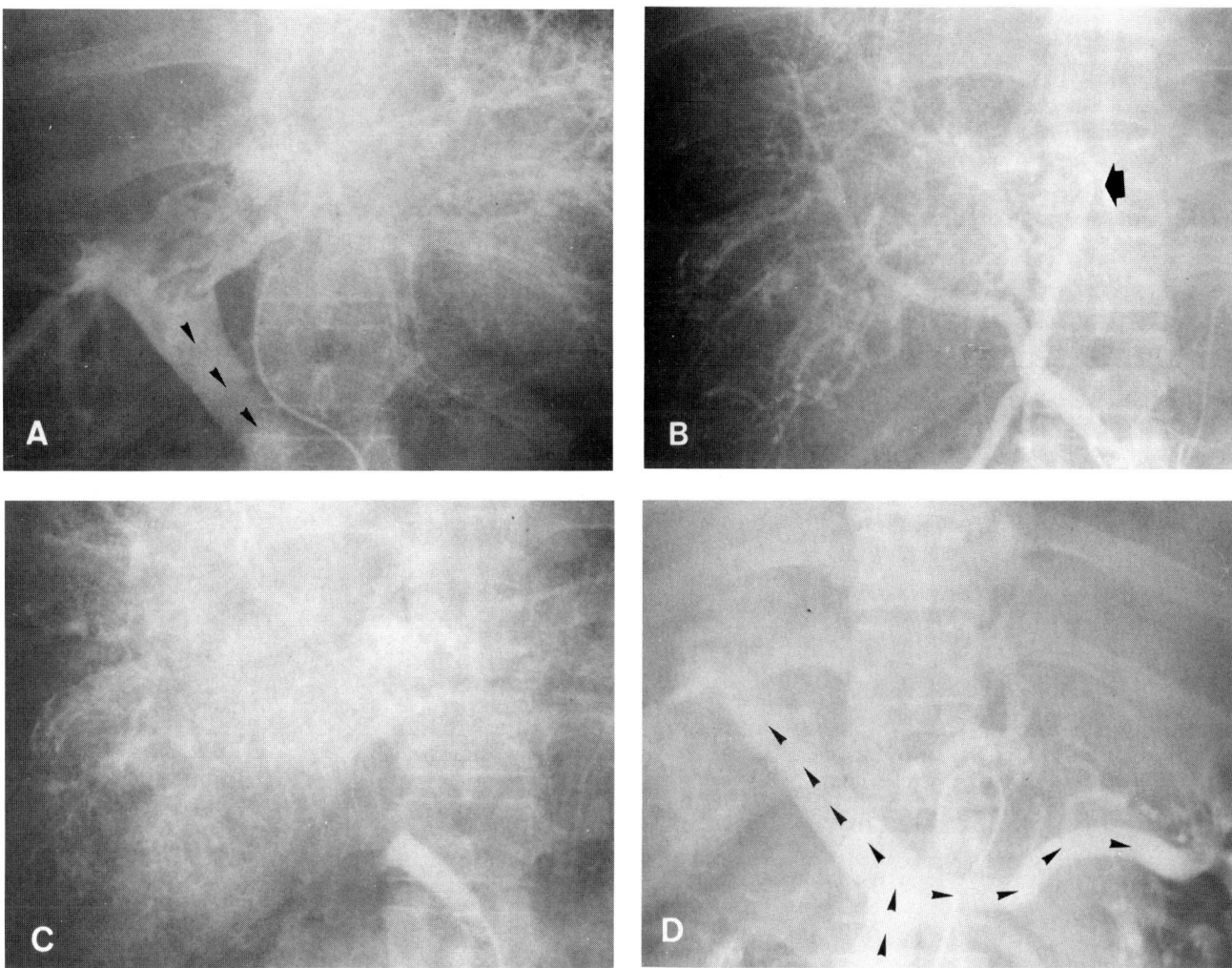

Figure 4.7 (A) Patient with postnecrotic cirrhosis and hepatoma with portal vein invasion and arterioportal shunt with hepatofugal flow (arrow). (B,C) Following embolization of the left hepatic artery with a Gianturco coil (arrow), occlusion of arteriovenous shunt has occurred. Notice a small dissection of the common hepatic artery. (D) Later phase of superior mesenteric injection showing portal vein flow reversal (arrow) and splenic vein inversion (arrow).

HEPATIC HEMANGIOMAS

Hepatic cavernous hemangiomas are congenital lesions, which may remain silent for long periods of time, without clinical manifestation, before they are accidentally identified by ultrasonographic study or CT. Asymptomatic cases do not, of course, require any surgical or radiologic treatment. Interventional techniques are justified only in cases of uncontrollably growing lesions, which may cause damage due to a mass effect, with displacement of adjacent organs; pain due to hepatic capsular distention (Fig. 4.8); or untreatable pain as a consequence of smaller hemangiomatous lesions (Fig. 4.9).

Embolization in such cases should be as selective as possible; the embolizing material may be Gelfoam or any type of material of higher durability, such as Ivalon. With larger lesions, embolization results in a decrease in total flow volume. In most cases, this decrease occurs immediately after the procedure is performed, making embolization useful as a presurgical measure for diminishing blood loss and facilitating transoperative reposition.

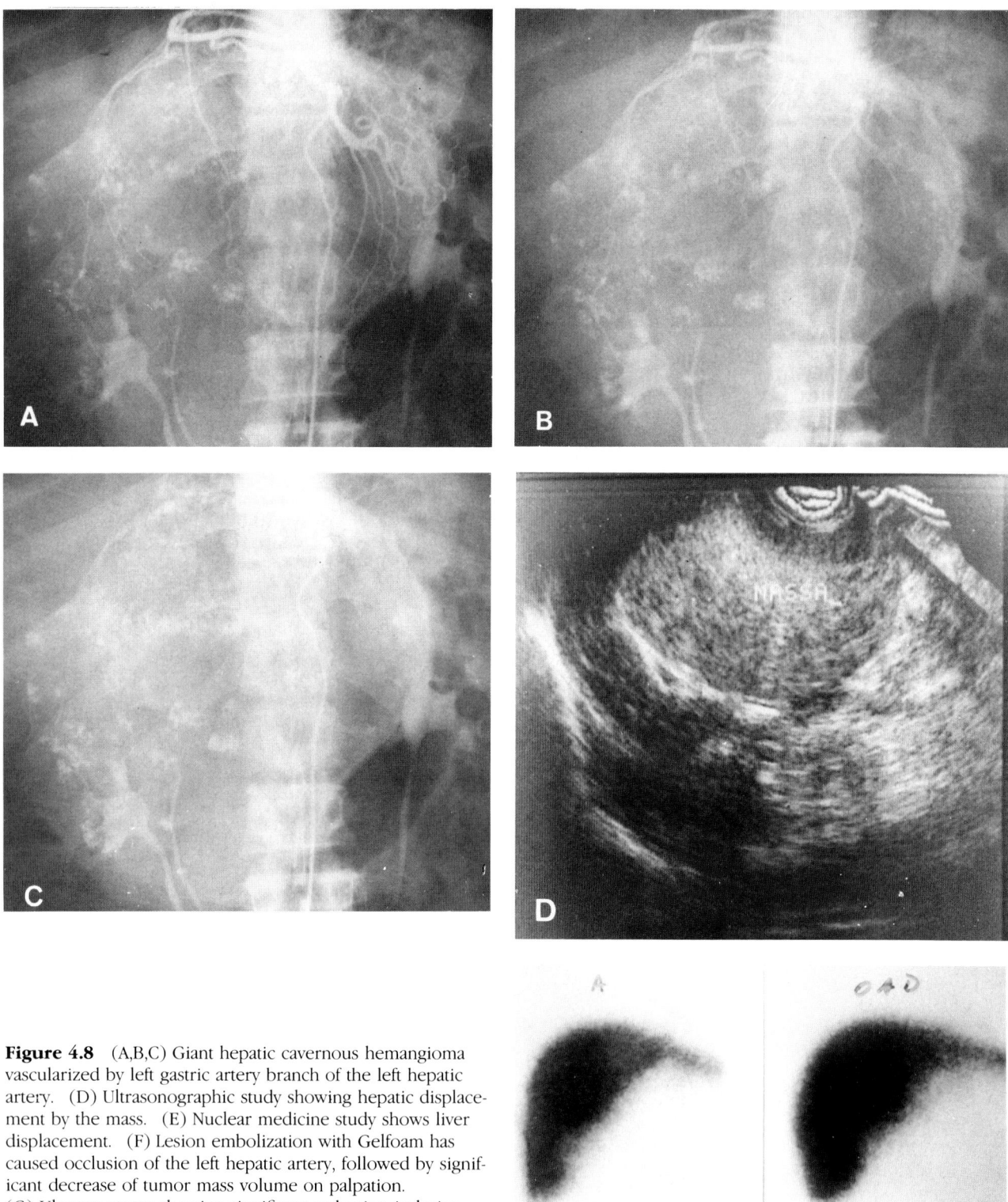

Figure 4.8 (A,B,C) Giant hepatic cavernous hemangioma vascularized by left gastric artery branch of the left hepatic artery. (D) Ultrasonographic study showing hepatic displacement by the mass. (E) Nuclear medicine study shows liver displacement. (F) Lesion embolization with Gelfoam has caused occlusion of the left hepatic artery, followed by significant decrease of tumor mass volume on palpation. (G) Ultrasonogram showing significant reduction in lesion volume. This remained unchanged during a 3-year follow-up.

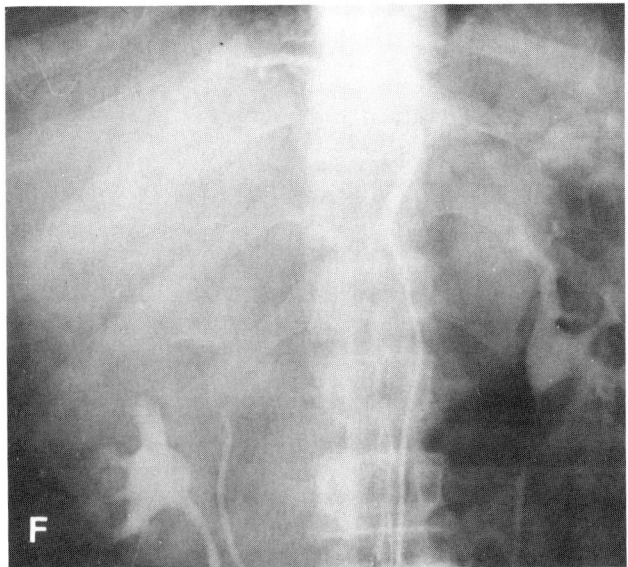

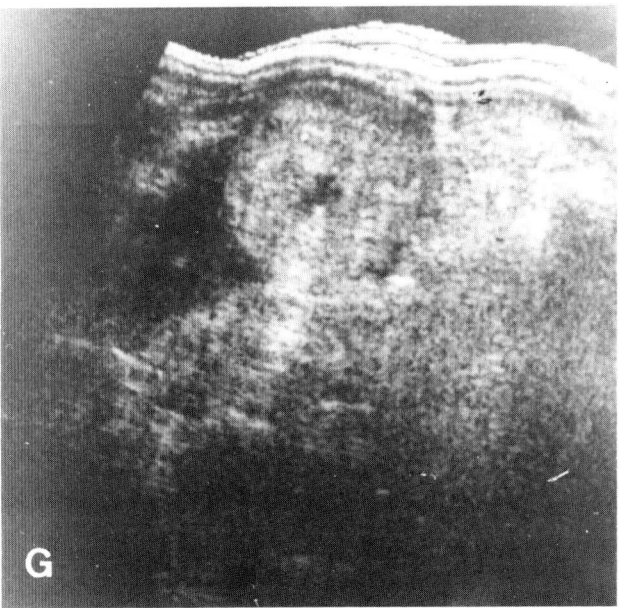

Figure 4.8 *Continued*

In cases of childhood liver hemangioendotheliomas, which are benign tumors, massive shunts may cause congestive heart failure and severe hepatomegaly. Gelfoam, which may cause systemic embolism, should not be used in these cases. Detachable balloons, or Gianturco coils, which are able to occlude the fistulas permanently, are the materials of choice. The tumor itself spontaneously recedes with age.

BLEEDING FROM HEPATIC TUMORS

Spontaneous rupture of hepatic tumor is a rare cause of intraperitoneal bleeding. [As of 1979, only 191 cases of such ruptures, out of 2526 cases of liver cell carcinoma (a 7.5 percent incidence) have been described in the literature.] Traditional treatment has usually been surgical, including hepatectomy, hepatic packing with Gelfoam, and hepatic artery ligation. The most successful method is hepatic artery ligation. Although hepatic artery embolization would seem to be an obvious treatment, it has not been frequently used.

Other hepatic lesions or systemic diseases, including liver cell adenoma, hepatic cavernous hemangioma, and polyarteritis nodosa aneurysms, have been associated with spontaneous liver rupture.

Severe abdominal pain and free blood in the peritoneal cavity may be the first manifestation of chronic liver disease. When a diagnosis is not made until surgical inspection, the prognosis is poor. Survival in cases of hepatoma is limited from a few days to 6 months following treatment.

According to the literature, hepatic artery ligation followed by partial hepatectomy during a "second-look" operation is the best management protocol considering the surgical limitations due to complications and the possibility of hepatic failure. However, in severely ill patients, with advanced cirrhosis and a ruptured tumor, the surgical trauma can be as deleterious as the bleeding itself, and in these cases, transcatheter embolization is an attractive, if more conservative, alternative. After embolization and percutaneous occlusion have improved the acute phase, partial hepatectomy may be effective in certain patients. Catheterization should be superselective, occluding only the tumoral area involved.

However, even if one is able to achieve bleeding control through emergency intervention, and even if the immediate response is excellent, the prognosis may be poor (see Fig. 4.10). Surgical ligation of the hepatic artery may be temporarily effective, but it will prevent any future use of therapeutic catheterization.

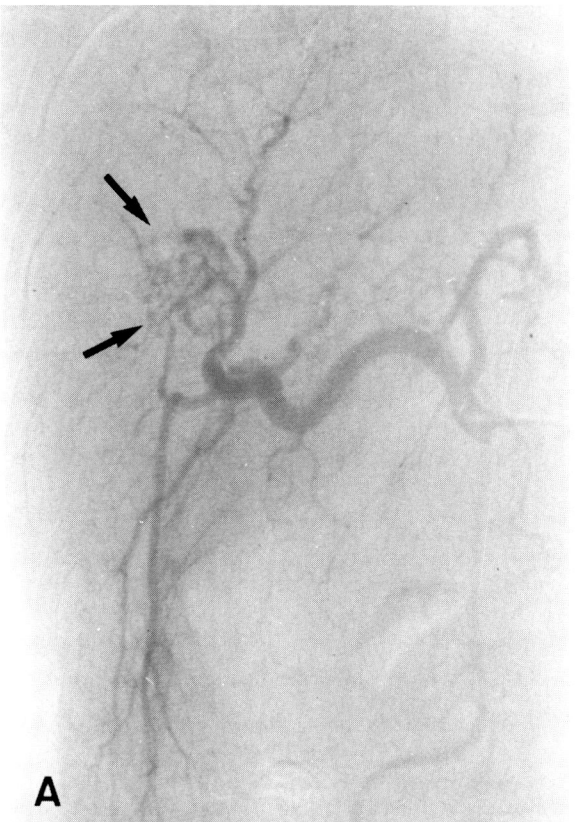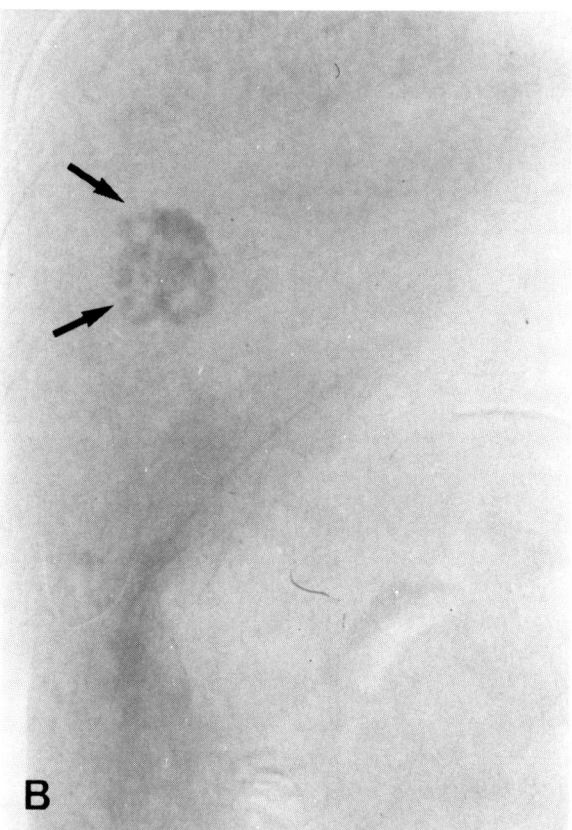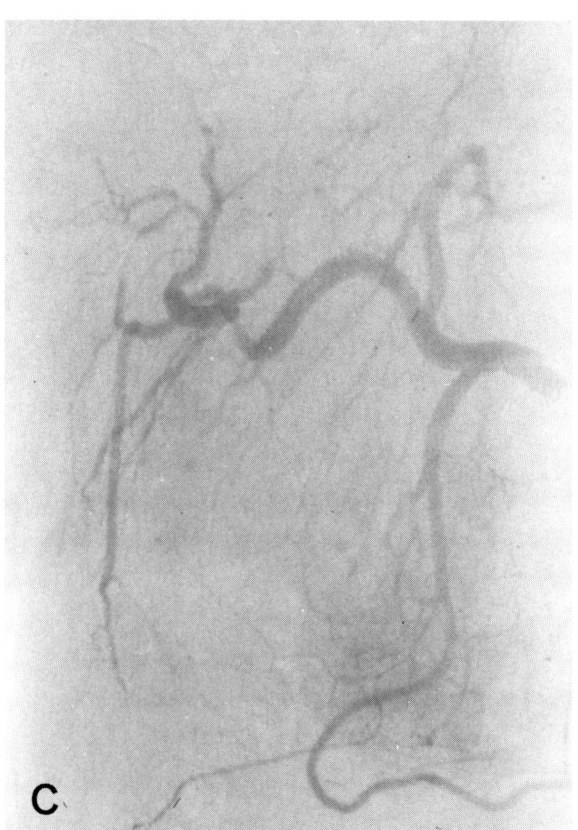

Figure 4.9 A 45-year-old patient with pain in the right hypochondrium related to the presence of a small-sized cavernous hemangioma.
(A,B) Selective injection into the proper hepatic artery showing the hemangiomatous lesion (arrow). (C) Following embolization with Lipiodol-impregnated Gelfoam, the lesion was occluded, with significant improvement of symptoms after moderate postembolization syndrome pain.

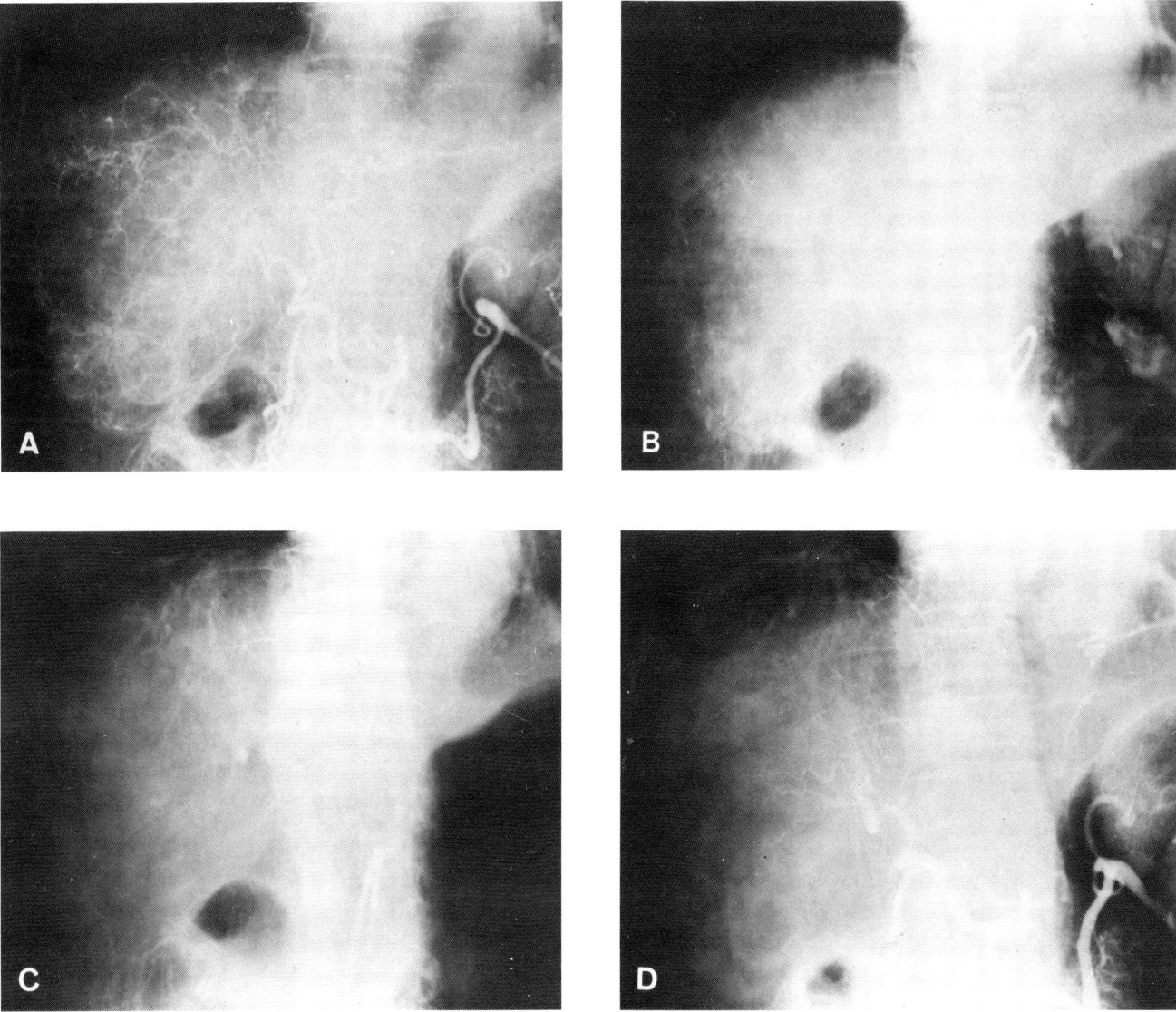

Figure 4.10 Postnecrotic cirrhosis in an 80-year-old patient with shock and acute abdominal pain. Surgery did not control bleeding on the surface of the liver.

(A,B) Angiogram showing the presence of hepatoma with spontaneous subcapsular hematoma without contrast medium extravasation. (C) Later phase of injection into the superior mesenteric artery showing portal vein patency; however, the portal vein is being medially pushed by the expanding lesion.

(D) Control angiogram following embolization with Gelfoam, which controlled bleeding. Results were good for the first 5 days following embolization, but soon irreversible encephalopathy developed, and the patient died 8 days after the procedure was performed.

METASTATIC ENDOCRINE TUMORS IN THE LIVER

Malignant pancreatic or intestinal endocrine tumors generally metastasize in the liver because of the natural filtration performed by the organ through the portal circulation. These metastases are usually larger in size than the primary lesion, so a larger percentage of the tumoral volume, and hence higher hormonal activity, is found in the liver. Endocrine tumoral lesions, even when malignant and metastatic, usually grow slowly as compared to other tumors, allowing for long survival periods. During those periods, the patients are usually subject to extreme discomfort caused by endocrine disease activity. The symptoms presented will depend on the nature and origin of the dominant hormone in the tumor. Symptoms may include diarrhea, skin lesions, bronchial spasms, heat flashes with skin flushing, heart failure, and changes in arterial pressure. In advanced stages, the cumulative effects of hepatomegaly will predominate, with pain, dyspnea, discomfort, and portal and caval obstruction. Palliative treatment is extremely important, although the prognosis must be cautious because dissemination may cause discomfort so excessive that the patient's life becomes totally unbearable.

Curative forms of treatment may be tried prior to embolization. When metastasis is limited to one hepatic lobe, partial hepatectomy may be curative. The use of tumor metabolite antagonists, specific chemotherapy (either local or systemic), and embolization are probably the most effective forms of treatment. Hepatic artery ligation today is considered ineffective for treating these hepatic lesions, for the reasons given at the beginning of this chapter (see Fig. 4.1).

The favorable reputation that embolization has for the treatment of hepatic metastatic endocrine lesions is justified. It involves minimal aggression to the patient and has a high rate of effectiveness, especially when compared to surgical procedures that may demand a laparotomy, general anesthesia, and ligations or resections in patients who appear hemodynamically unstable and are subject to cardiovascular and respiratory collapses.

Hepatic artery ligation will prevent any other devascularization procedure by catheter or local infusion of chemotherapeutic agents. When the main artery is kept open, embolization may be repeated as many times as necessary. Subsequent embolization may also be performed through the collaterals or through recanalized arteries with new metastatic deposits, but with increased difficulty.

The choice of embolization as a treatment for hepatic metastasis is usually made independently of whether or not resection of the primary tumor is involved. It may be indicated in cases in which chemotherapy did not obtain the desired results and in those in which there has been recurrence after partial hepatectomy.

Depending upon the type of tumor, a pharmacologic antagonist of the hormone being produced may be required to prevent fluctuations in hormone production and distribution both during the embolic procedure and, if tumor necrosis develops, following embolization. The carcinoid syndrome is the most significant example of an acute hormonal release accompanied by severe vasoactive phenomena. In these and similar cases, substances such as cyproheptadine and p-chlorophenylalanine are used before and after embolization and the prophylactic use of antibiotics is generally required. As with all embolization procedures, one should make sure that the portal vein is patent, and determine which hepatic arteries are present, taking into account anatomic variations.

The embolization material used will vary according to availability, experience of involved personnel, and type of lesion. In all cases, however, long-duration, small-sized material, which may be peripherally lodged inside or on the periphery of the metastatic lesions, must be used. This material may be used in conjunction with larger, medium-duration particles (Gelfoam or collagen). The two basic materials for long-duration or permanent particles are 150-μm Ivalon and lyophilized dura mater.

Occlusion of the main artery with a coil is not advisable unless redistribution of intrahepatic flow is being sought in order to make the procedure easier. The Gianturco coil will produce a permanent, very proximal, occlusion, which acts as a surgical arterial ligation.

In cases of hormone-producing hepatic metastatic lesions, embolization should be as extensive as possible, in order to render hormone production as inactive as possible. It is generally accepted that the great advantage offered by embolization in the treatment of these metastatic lesions is that in most cases the procedure produces significant regression of hepatic metastases while controlling the clinical syndrome (Fig. 4.11). Hepatomegaly is usually reduced, which may later be followed by ultrasonography or computed tomography.

This technique may also be used in case of carcinoid syndrome and metastatic manifestations of endocrine pancreatic tumors, such as insulinomas, vipomas, gastrinomas, somatostatinomas, and other, less frequently encountered, ones.

Contraindications for this procedure are jaundice, significantly reduced hepatic function, portal vein occlusion, and sepsis.

Complications include occlusion of nontarget organs, causing ischemia and pain, and nausea and vomiting. Other effects of embolization are decreased hepatic function, abscess formation, and sepsis. The presence of gas in the liver parenchyma is frequent, but is not necessarily caused by an infectious process (Fig. 2.18).

All hepatic embolizations involve a risk of gallbladder

necrosis, and ischemia of this organ is probably the main factor responsible for the postembolization pain syndrome. There are special techniques available for preventing occlusion of the arterial bed of the gallbladder.

INFUSION AND EMBOLIZATION OF HEPATIC NEOPLASMS

In Western countries, metastatic hepatic neoplasms are much more frequent than primary hepatic tumors, although the latter are relatively frequent in some regions of Africa and the Far East. The presence of primary hepatic tumors (also called hepatomas or hepatocarcinomas) is more commonly related to liver cirrhosis of posthepatitis B etiology. Today, the relationship between hepatitis B virus and the development of hepatocarcinoma has been unequivocally established: the presence of a primary hepatic lesion is related to loss in hepatic function due to concomitant postnecrotic cirrhosis.

Once hepatoma has been discovered, survival time without treatment is around 2 to 6 months. The average survival time for patients with hepatic metastases is 6 to 12 months, depending on the histologic type of the lesion. In these patients, however, metastases rule over the course of the disease and survival time. The average survival of patients with untreated hepatic metastases of colon carcinoma is 150 days; of stomach carcinoma, 60; and of pancreatic carcinoma, 50.

Metastatic colon carcinomas, and primary liver lesions that are single and limited to one hepatic segment, are better treated by surgical resection, provided that a few specific criteria are met. It is rare, however, that these criteria are met; in addition, partial hepatectomy may be associated with high morbidity and mortality rates. For these reasons, interventional radiologic techniques have become the treatment of choice in most cases. Traditionally, two transcatheter treatment modalities have been advocated: intraarterial drug infusion and embolization. More recently, chemoembolization procedures that combine the advantages of both methods have been used.

INTRAARTERIAL INFUSION OF CHEMOTHERAPEUTIC AGENTS

This technique has been used for about 20 years. Over the years, countless changes in the procedure have been introduced. Wallace and Chuang, for example, advocated the use of superselective catheterization in all cases, with the introduction of high drug concentrations at short time intervals (2 h to 5 days), infusion cycles repeated every 4 to 6 weeks, and hepatic flow redistribution in the presence of multiple hepatic arteries.

In many cases, because of the existence of two or more hepatic arteries, it is necessary to redistribute hepatic arterial flow in such a way that arterial irrigation of both the liver and of the tumor lesion is performed through a single artery. In these cases, the arterial occlusion should be proximal, in order to allow the development of intrahepatic collaterals between the different segments. This type of occlusion is performed with Gianturco coils following superselective catheterization of the target artery.

Both femoral and axillary approaches may be used. For short infusions, up to 24 h, the femoral approach is advised; for infusions up to 5 days' duration, the axillary route is preferred because it does not interfere with the patient's mobility. The catheter should be fixed onto the skin with a micropore-type adhesive tape or sutured with anchorage stitches. The catheter tip should be well positioned in either the common hepatic artery or the recommended subselective vessel.

Heparinization with 10,000 to 20,000 IU is advisable to prevent thrombotic complications.

In order to monitor arterial position and patency, catheter position should be evaluated daily, with plain abdominal x-rays or using small contrast injections.

Some authors recommend that the infusion catheters be put into place by transsurgical gastroduodenal and proper hepatic artery catheterization. This technique allows the catheter to remain in place in the artery to be infused for long time periods, with minimal interference with the patient's mobility. However, the surgical procedure required for its implementation is subject to all the obvious limitations found with cancer patients. Simultaneous portal vein infusion has been suggested by some authors. The most frequent complications of this technique are occlusion of the infused artery, occlusion of the punctured artery in the periphery, and formation of arterial aneurysms. Infusion of chemotherapeutic agents into hollow visceral arteries may cause mucosal ulcerations with bleeding. Cholecystitis and pancreatitis may also occur.

According to the literature, the treatment protocols proposed show partial response in 55 percent of cases and full response in 12 percent, with prolonged survival from 7 to 14 months. (Response is determined by angiography, ultrasonography, or computed tomography.)

HEPATIC ARTERIAL EMBOLIZATION

As mentioned earlier, the portal vein supplies the liver with 75 to 80 percent of its blood volume and 50 percent of its oxygen. Two other important facts to remember when considering hepatic arterial embolization are (1) 90 to 95 percent of the blood flow feeding neoplasms,

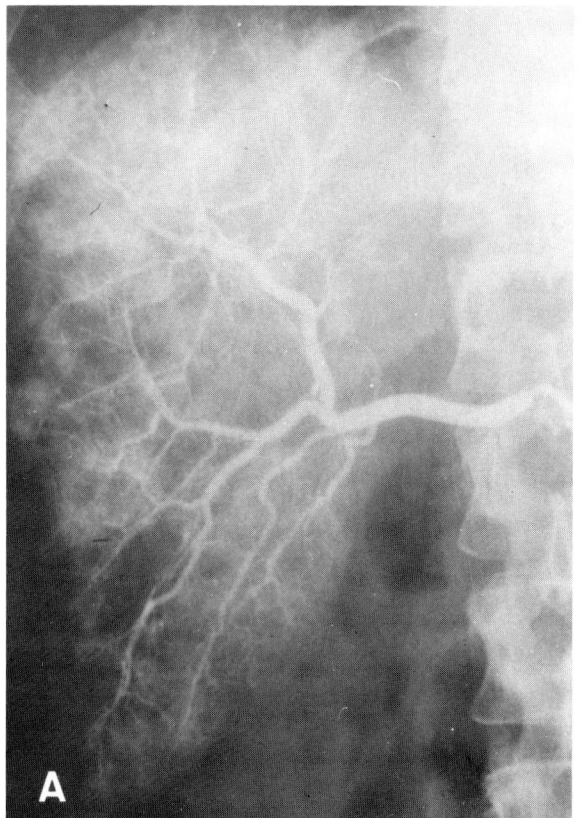
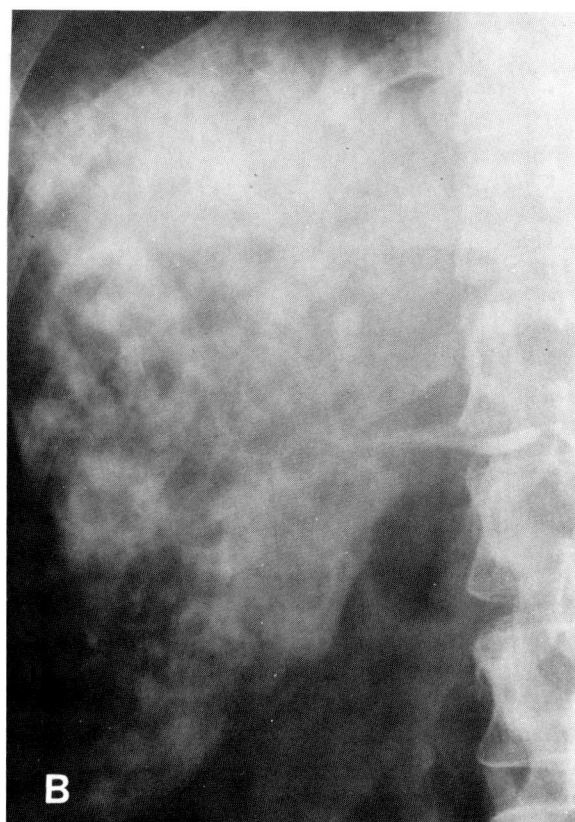
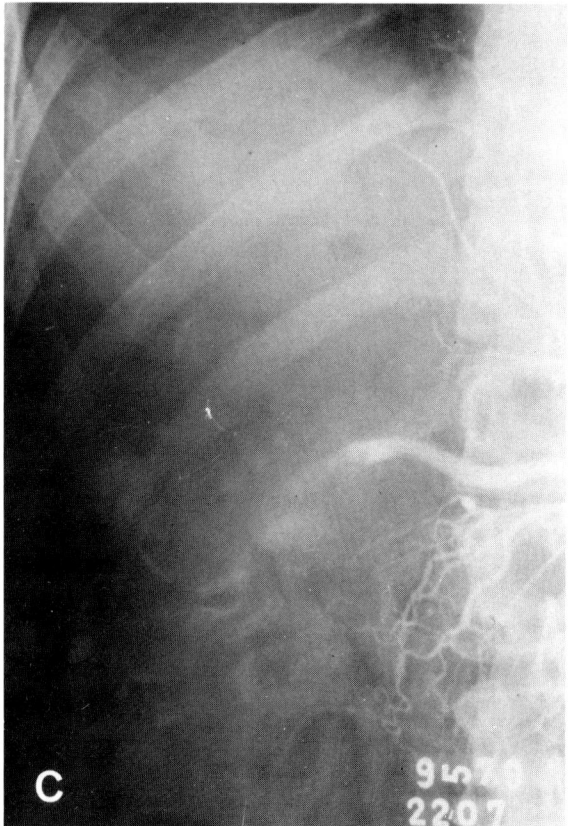

Figure 4.11 Patient with pancreatic (vasoactive intestinal polypeptide-producing tumor, causing untreatable diarrhea (pancreatic cholera) due to hepatic metastases (Werner-Morrison syndrome).
(A,B) Proper hepatic selective angiogram showing metastatic liver with countless moderately hypervascular nodules.
(C) Control angiogram after embolization with Gelfoam, showing hepatic circulation occlusion. Diarrhea was under control for about 1 year. (D,E) New hepatic angiogram taken after recurrence of diarrhea, showing intrahepatic circulation recanalization with multiple hepatic nodules. (F) New embolization with Gelfoam and one Gianturco coil was performed to obtain a more central occlusion. A 2-year follow-up showed continued control of the diarrhea-causing syndrome.

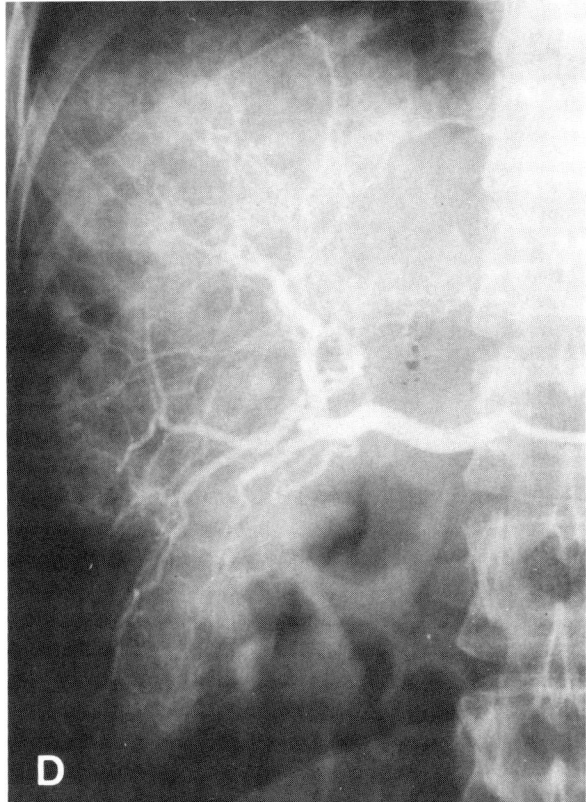
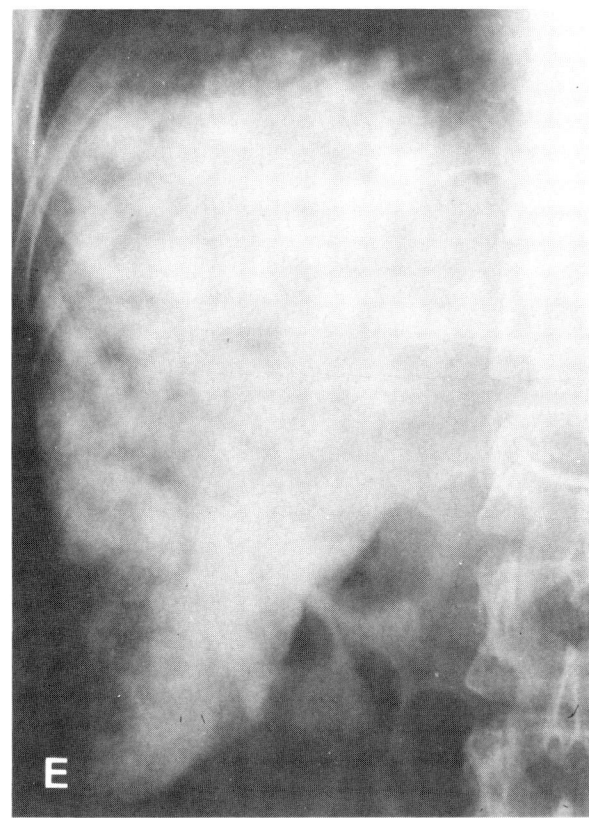

Figure 4.11 *Continued*

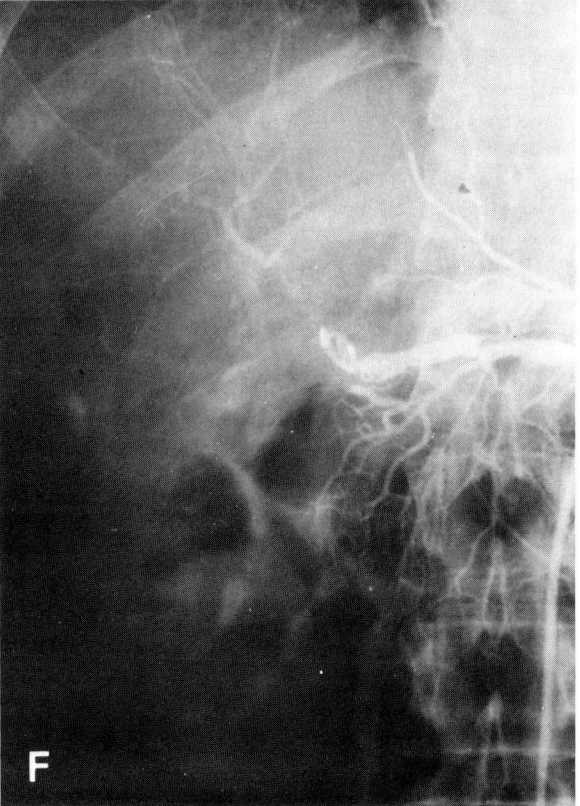

both primary and secondary, is arterial, and (2) 10 percent of the liver is enough to maintain life.

Portal patency is a necessity if hepatic embolization is to be performed. It is established by angiographic opacification using 45- to 60-mL contrast injection into the superior mesenteric or celiac arteries. Late-phase films must be obtained to demonstrate opacification of the portal vein.

Liver embolization is not indicated if the tumoral lesion involves over 70 percent of hepatic volume, due to the risk of acute liver failure after vascular occlusion.

Hepatic arterial embolization for treating tumor lesions is best performed through peripheral vascular occlusion with particulate embolic material of the Gelfoam type; small Ivalon particles are also appropriate.

In some cases, simultaneous proximal occlusion of the artery with a Gianturco coil is indicated in order to decrease distal bed recanalization (Fig. 4.12). Proximal occlusion, however, will prevent subsequent access if additional embolization becomes necessary. Absolute alcohol is generally contraindicated for hepatic tumor lesion ablation (Fig. 2.18). It may, however, be used in single isolated lesions and with superselective catheter-

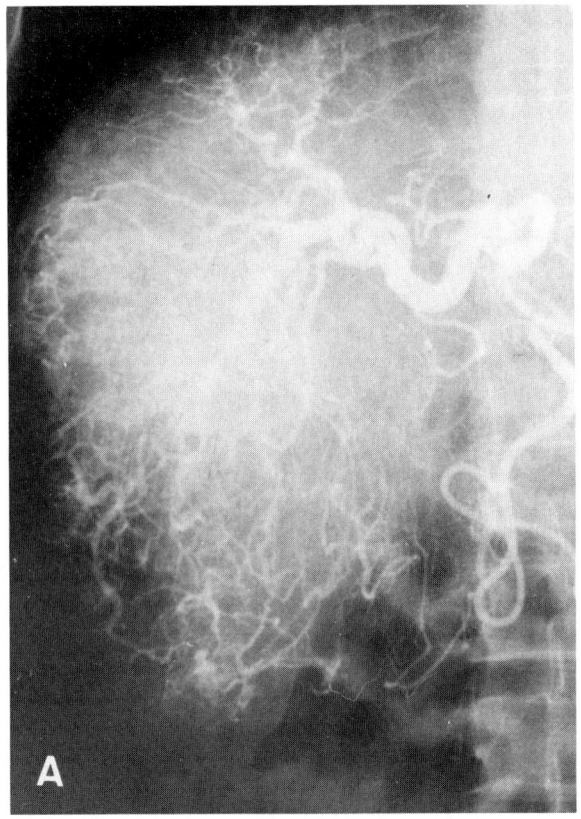
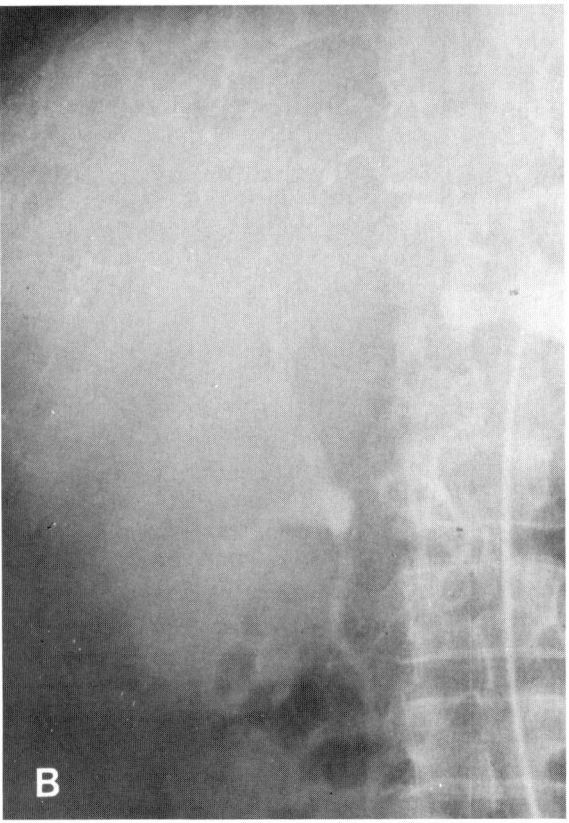

ization. Nonselective injection of ethanol will cause diffuse sinusoidal lesions in normal liver tissue (see Figs. 4.13 to 4.15).

CHEMOEMBOLIZATION OF HEPATIC NEOPLASMS

Chemoembolization is a combination of intraarterial infusion of a chemotherapeutic agent and the introduction of an embolizing agent for occlusion of the neoplastic vascular supply. This relatively recent technique was introduced by Kato in 1981. Its considerable potential will continue to be developed and experimentally studied over the next few years.

In addition to producing ischemia in the tumoral vascular bed, chemoembolization significantly reduces flow, thereby extending the time of contact of the chemotherapeutic drug with the neoplasm, increasing the pharmacologic concentration of the drug, and causing changes in vascular permeability and patency. The cytotoxic effect occurs on the vascular wall, apart from the tumor mass, causing capillary occlusion.

The original idea was to utilize methylcellulose microcapsules with enclosed mitomycin C aliquots, which, while producing peripheral embolization, would slowly and uniformly release the chemotherapeutic agents into adjacent tissue, with marked reduction of systemic effects. Mitomycin produces a perivascular inflammatory process and arteritis; the microcapsules are inert. (See Figs. 4.16 to 4.21.)

Figure 4.12 48-year-old patient with postnecrotic cirrhosis and right liver lobe hepatoma.
(A) Angiogram showing hypervascular lesion in right hepatic lobe, with pathologic vessels. The portal vein is patent.
(B) Control angiogram after embolization with Gelfoam particles and Gianturco coils, showing total occlusion of the lesion. The patient survived for almost 2 years, which is exceptional in cases of primary hepatic tumor.

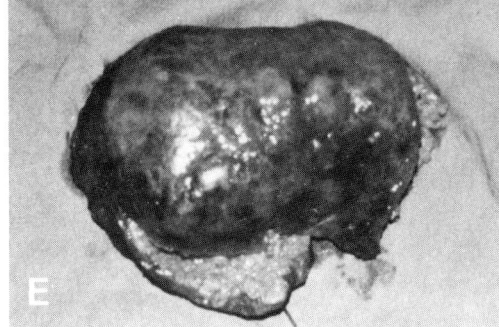

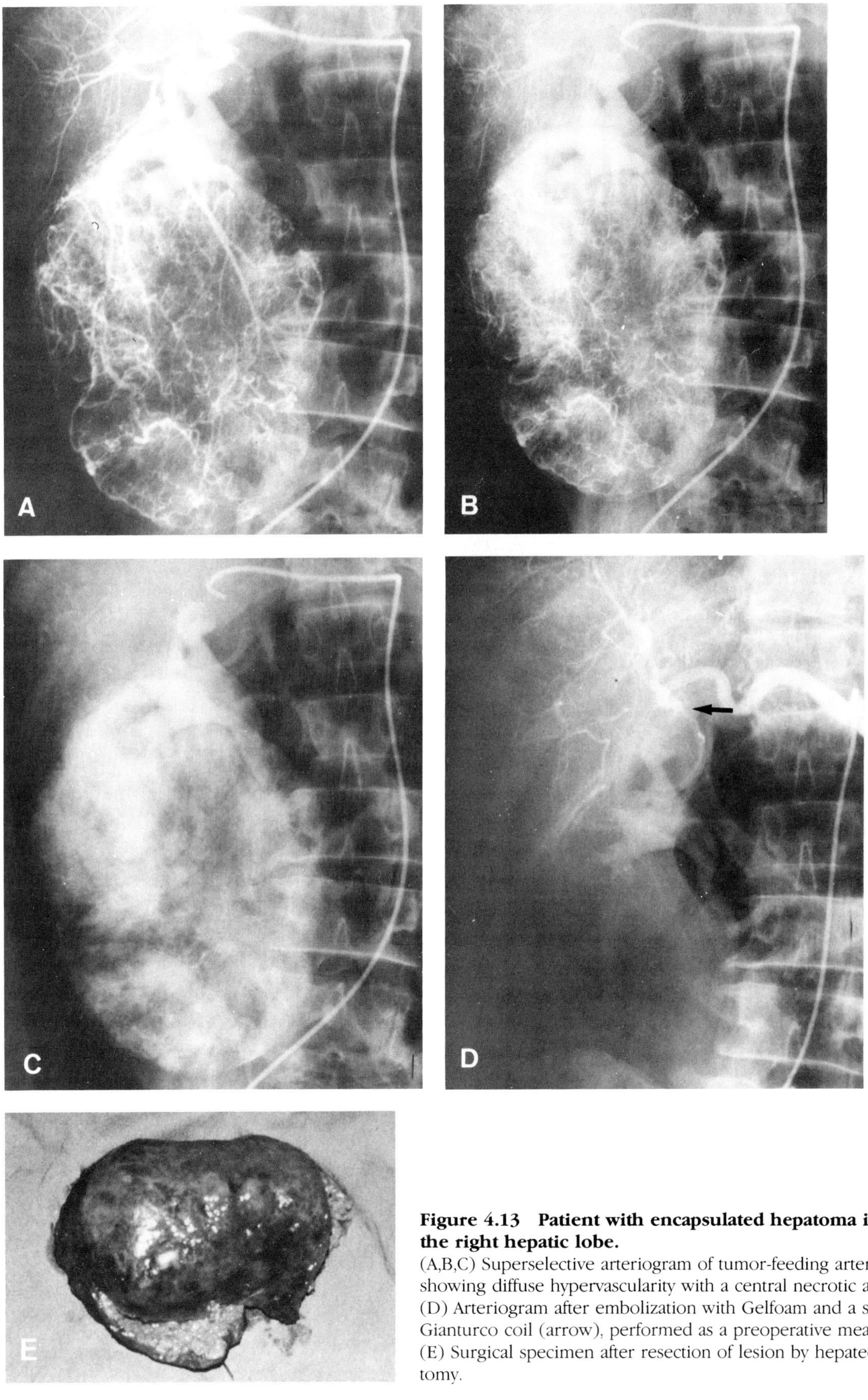

Figure 4.13 Patient with encapsulated hepatoma in the right hepatic lobe.
(A,B,C) Superselective arteriogram of tumor-feeding artery, showing diffuse hypervascularity with a central necrotic area. (D) Arteriogram after embolization with Gelfoam and a small Gianturco coil (arrow), performed as a preoperative measure. (E) Surgical specimen after resection of lesion by hepatectomy.

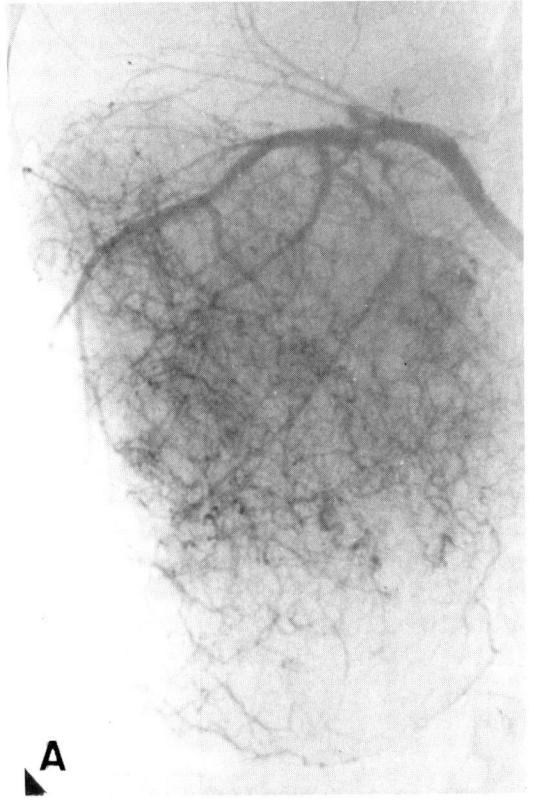
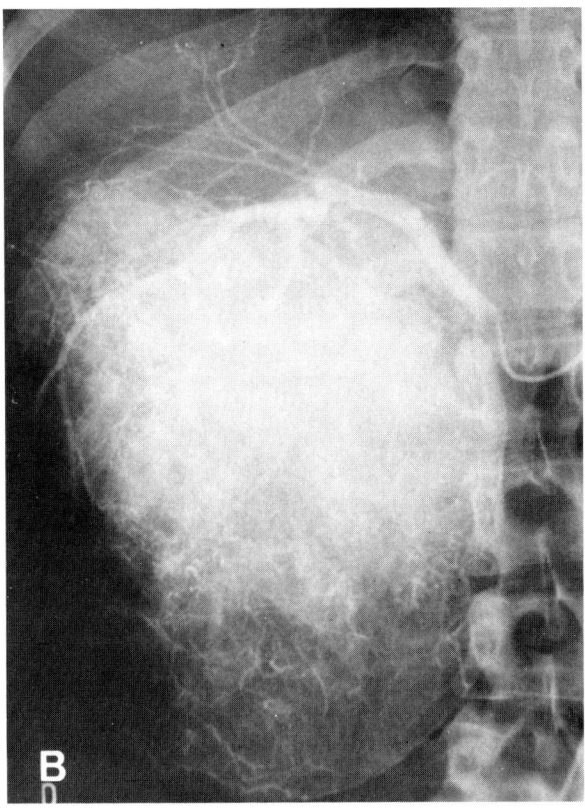
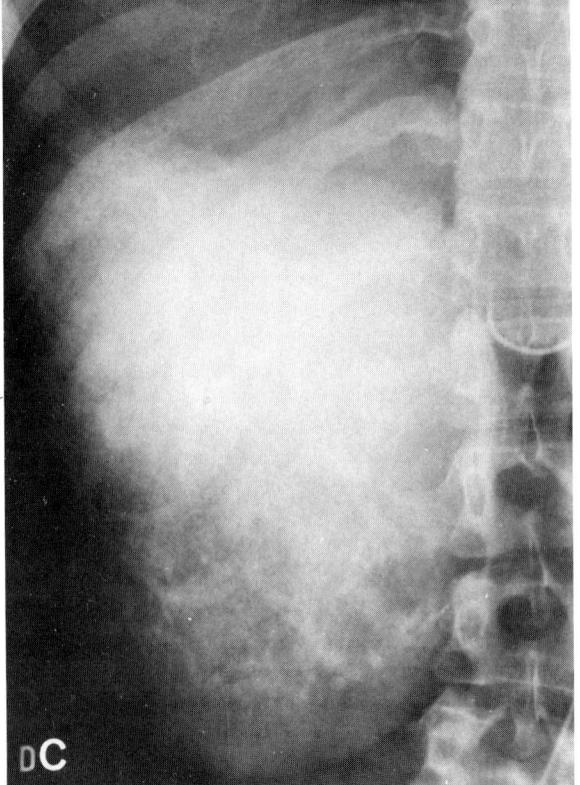

Figure 4.14 23-year-old patient, not using any contraceptive pill, with hepatic mass, abdominal pain, and abdominal distension.
(A,B,C) Hepatic selective arteriogram showing expansive hypervascular lesion with tumoral vessels, densely impregnated in the later phase. (D) Computed tomogram showing the homogeneous mass inside the right liver lobe. The distance from A to B is 15 cm. (E,F) Control angiogram after superselective embolization with small Gelfoam particles, showing significant devascularization of the mass, with main right lobe arteries preserved. (G) Computed tomographic study 3 weeks following embolization, showing large areas of tumoral necrosis and reduction in mass size. Symptoms have disappeared. An aspiration biopsy puncture showed liver cell adenoma, a finding that was confirmed by analysis of the surgical specimen after right hepatectomy.

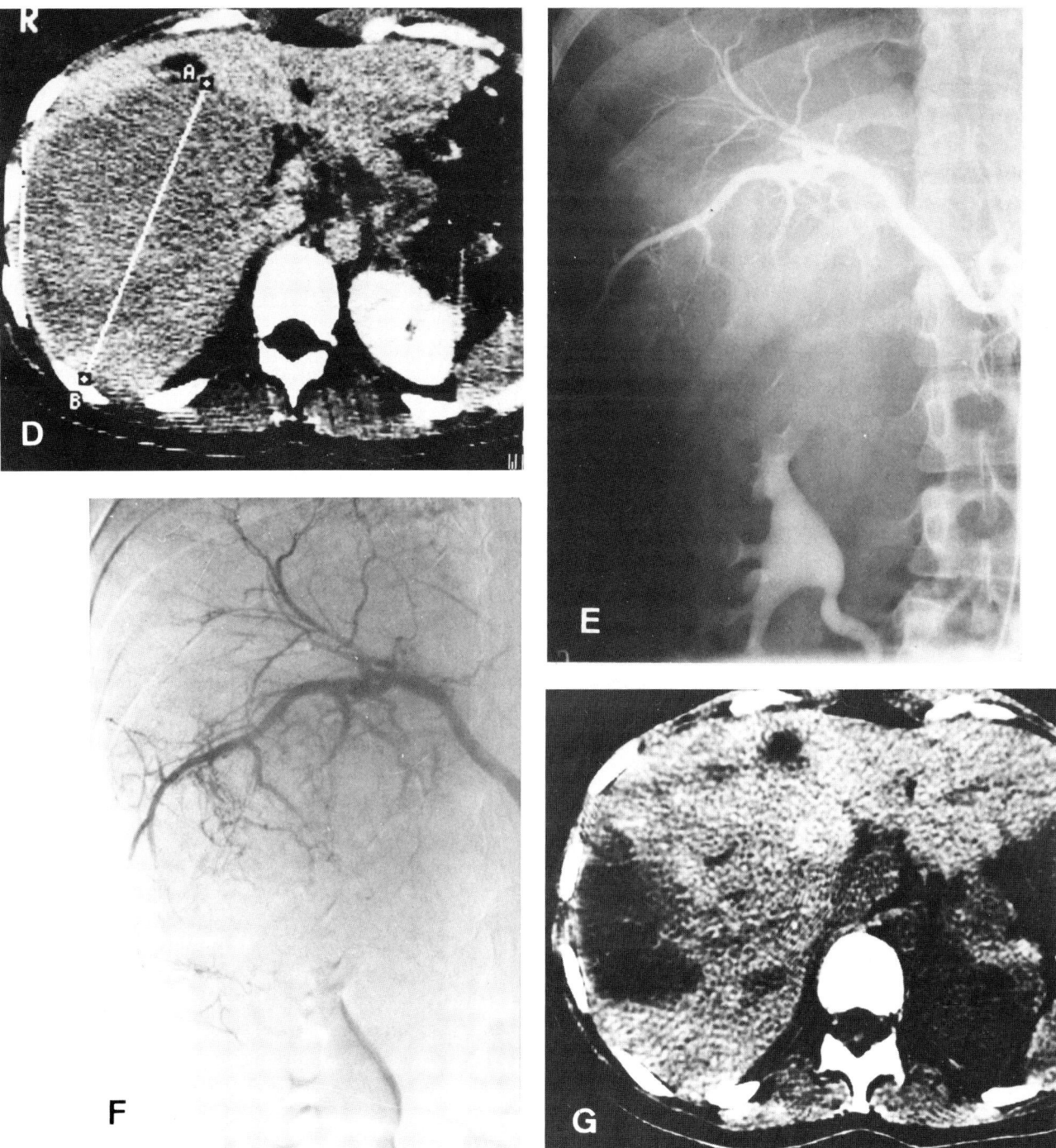

Figure 4.14 *Continued*

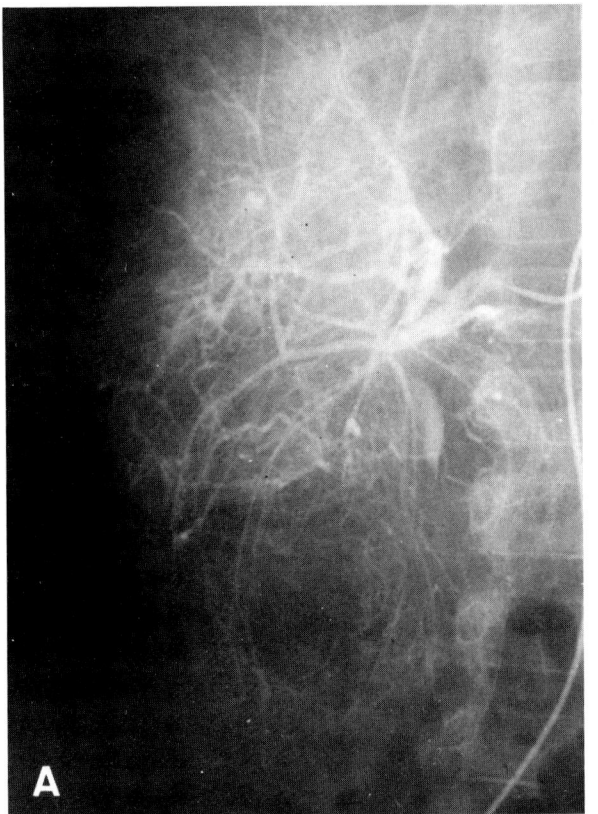
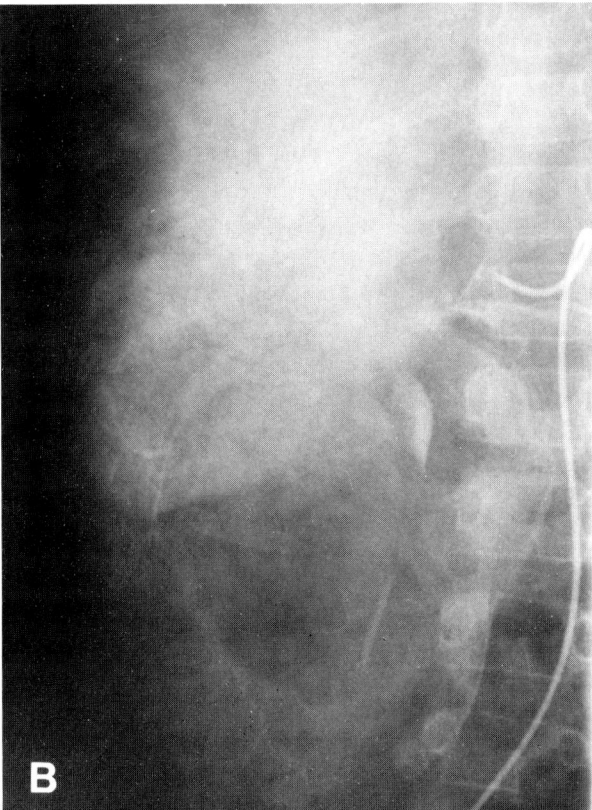
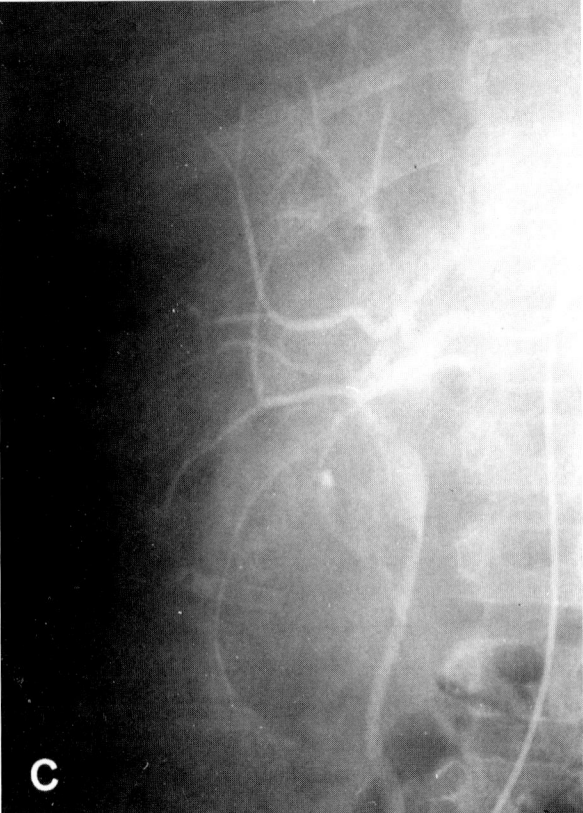

Figure 4.15 12-year-old patient with hepatic hemangiosarcoma presenting with abdominal pain, hepatomegaly, and ascites. The tumor is unresectable.
(A,B) Hepatic selective angiogram showing a multinodular diffuse tumoral lesion in the right liver lobe. (C) Control hepatic angiogram following peripheral embolization with Gelfoam.

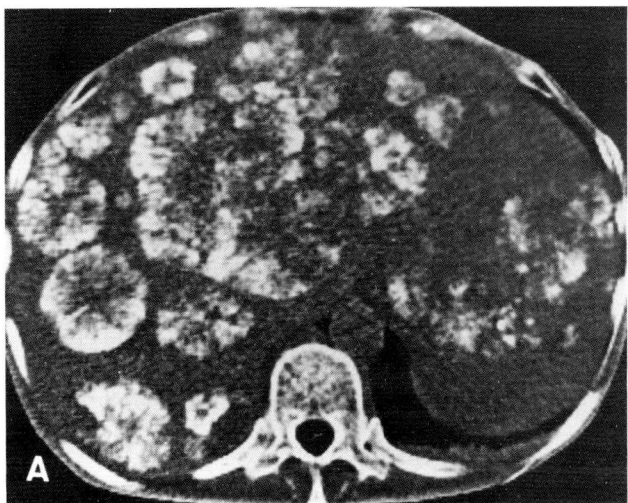
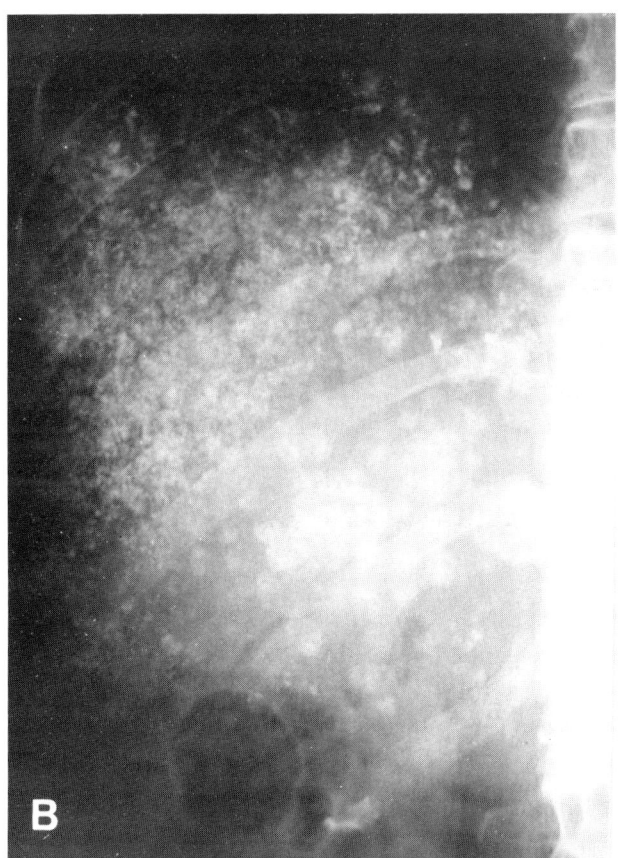

Figure 4.16 58-year-old patient with diffuse hepatoma in both liver lobes.
(A) Example of selective impregnation of hypervascular hepatic lesions (hepatoma) with Lipiodol–mitomycin C suspension. (B) Plain liver x-ray after injection of the suspension, showing impregnation of the hepatic lesions. The patient survived for only 6 months in spite of significant regression in volume of liver lesions after chemoembolization (not shown).

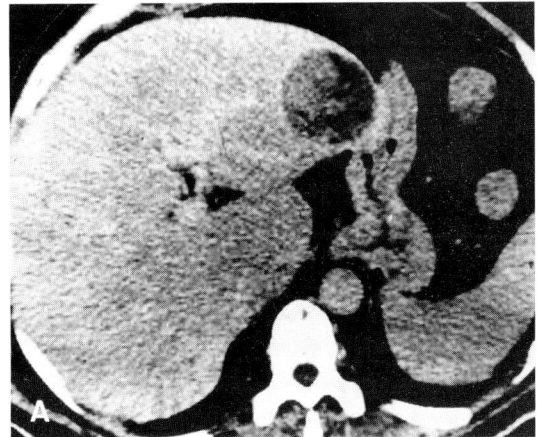
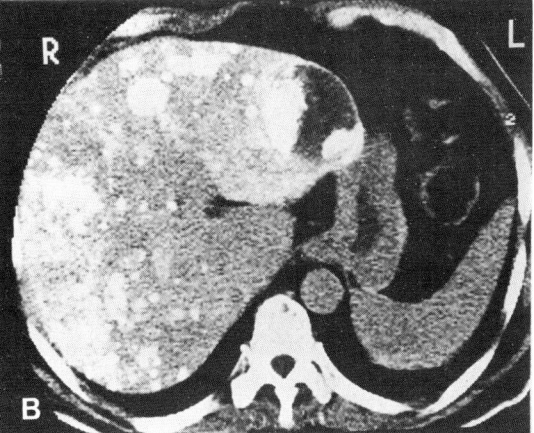

Figure 4.17 (A) 71-year-old-hepatoma patient, with lesion apparently restricted to the left lobe with necrotic area. (B) Computed tomography view after injection of Lipiodol–mitomycin C solution, showing impregnation of left and right lobe lesions. Note the partial impregnation of the larger left lobe lesion. Survival was only 4 months following diagnosis.

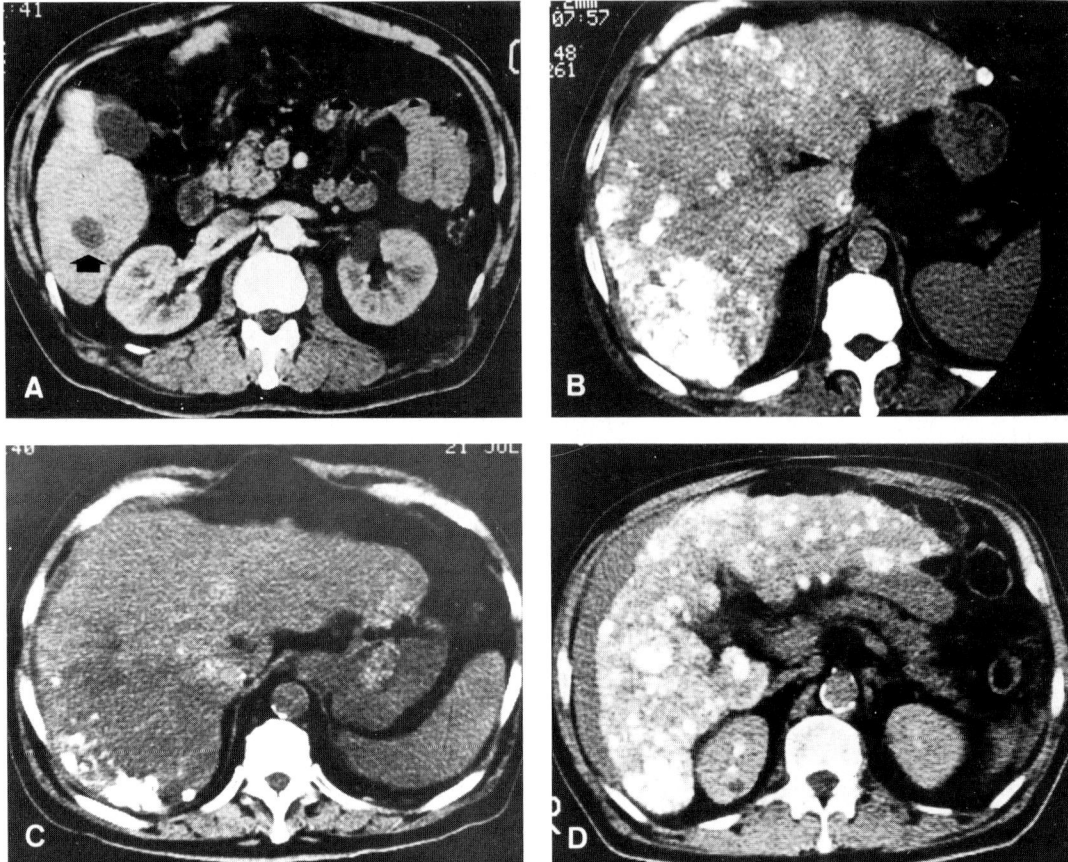

Figure 4.18 Patient with cirrhosis and hepatoma.
(A) Computed tomogram showing only one nodule in right liver lobe (arrow). (B) Computed tomogram after injection of Lipiodol–mitomycin C mixture, showing impregnation of several other hepatic nodules. (C) Control tomogram 2 months after the first chemoembolization, showing reduction of liver size, with Lipiodol residue in right liver lobe lesion. (D) Computed tomogram taken after second chemoembolization [1 month after control tomogram (C)], showing increased number of lesions and presence of ascites. The hepatic tumor became nonresponsive to treatment, and the patient died 1½ months after a final chemoembolization procedure, approximately 7 months after diagnosis.

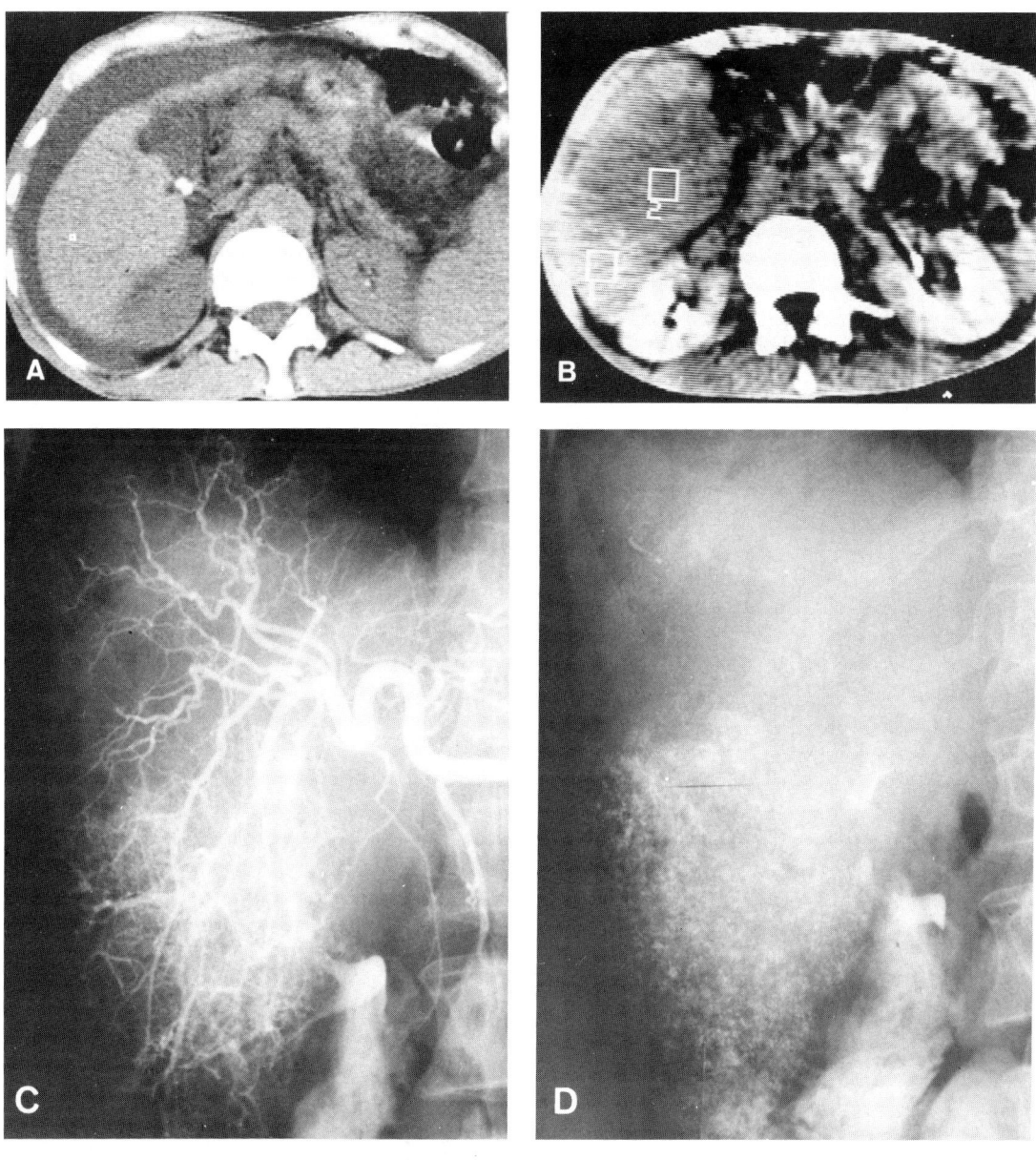

Figure 4.19 65-year-old patient with cirrhosis and hepatoma.

(A) Computed tomogram showing ascites due to noncompensated cirrhosis and homogeneous parenchyma. (B) Computer tomogram performed 1 year later, showing expansive lesion in right liver lobe (square marked 2). (C) Selective hepatic arteriogram showing hypervascular lesion and pathologic circulation in right hepatic lobe. (D) Plain liver x-ray showing selective impregnation of tumoral lesion after chemoembolization with Lipiodol and Mitomycin C. (E) Computed tomogram study, 6 months after diagnosis, showing lesion impregnation on the right side of the liver. The general condition of the patient is good.

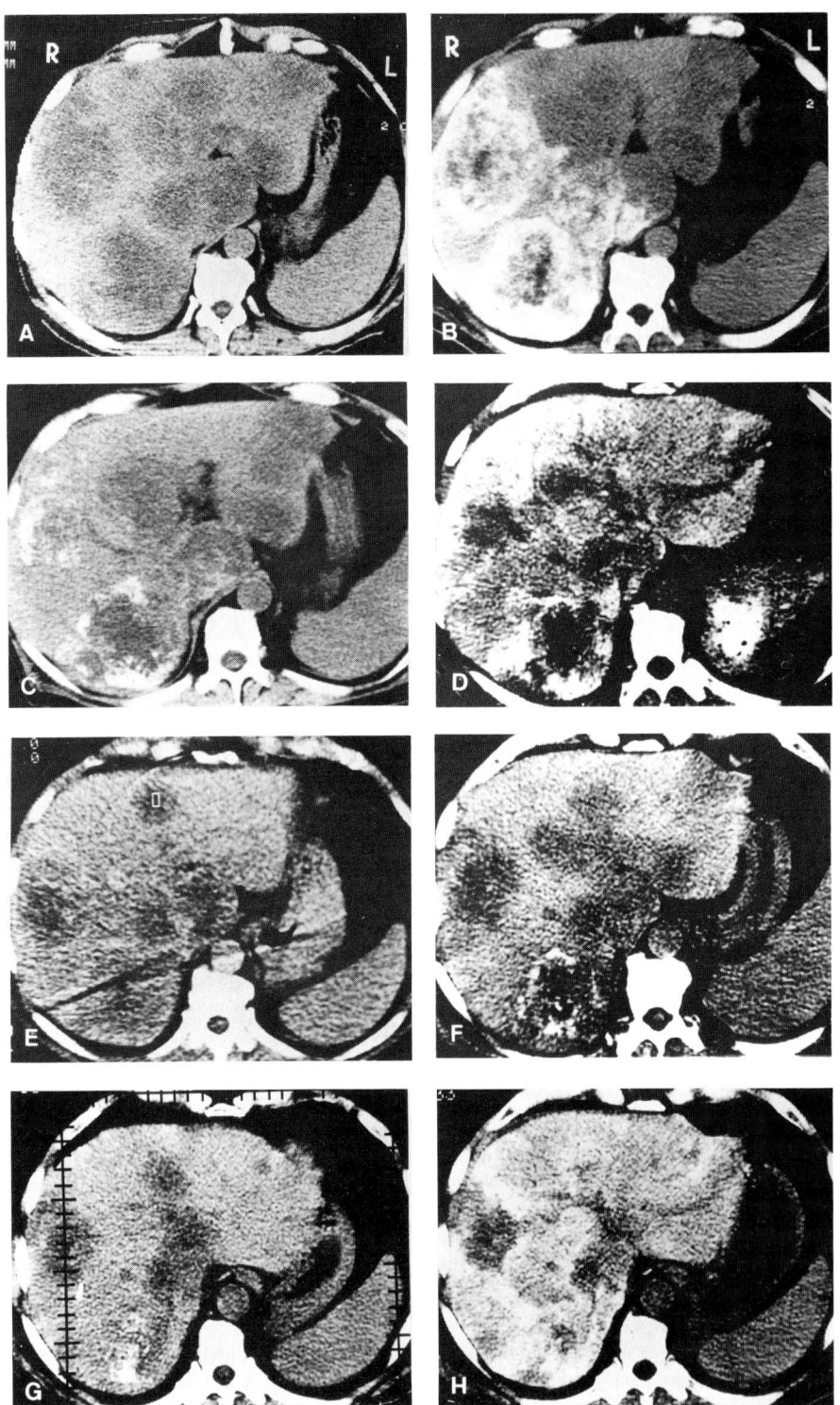

Figure 4.20 65-year-old patient with hepatic metastases of colon adenocarcinoma.
(A) Extensive hepatomegaly due to multiple metastatic nodules and poor general condition. (B) Control tomogram taken immediately after first chemoembolization, which, due to vascular anatomic problems, was inadvertently restricted to the right lobe. (C) Control tomogram taken about 1 month after (B), showing a slight reduction in the right lobe lesions and a slight increase on the left. (D) A second chemoembolization procedure was performed, covering both hepatic lobes. (E,F) Control tomogram, and new chemoembolization, respectively, about 1 month after (D). (G,H) Control tomogram, and new chemoembolization procedure, around 1 month after (F). Note the reduction in hepatic volume as compared to (A) and the decrease in number of nodules. There has been significant clinical improvement, and functional values are normal.

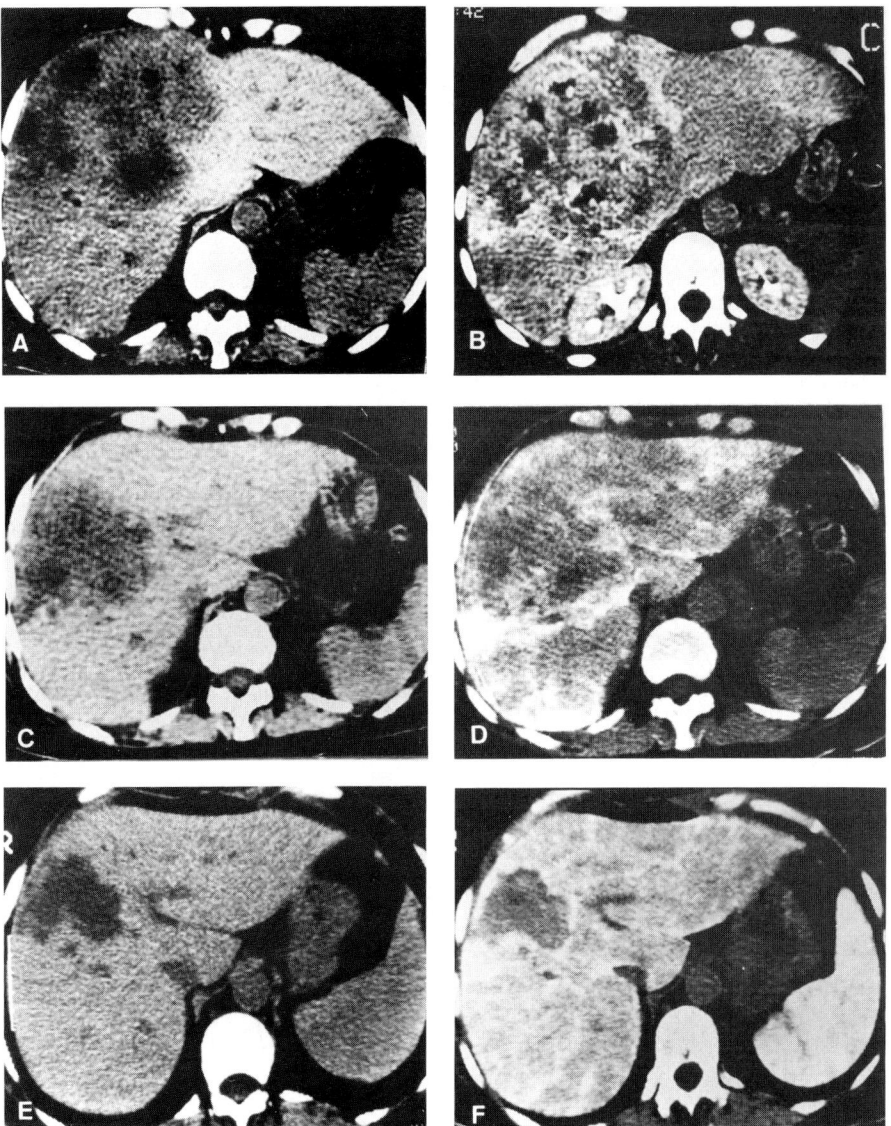

Figure 4.21 54-year-old patient with breast carcinoma and large-volume hepatic metastases.
(A) Computed tomography showing metastatic liver.
(B) Control tomogram taken immediately after Lipiodol–mitomycin-C chemoembolization. (C) Control tomogram about 1 month after first chemoembolization. There has been a significant response to treatment, with over 50 percent regression in lesion size and hepatic volume. (D) Control tomogram taken immediately after a second chemoembolization application. (E) Control tomogram taken 5 months after the third chemoembolization procedure, showing an almost 80 percent reduction in metastatic mass size. (F) Control tomogram after the fourth chemoembolization procedure, showing further reduction in tumor size. Response to treatment continued to be positive 36 months after diagnosis.

REFERENCES

Ackerman NB. The blood supply of experimental liver metastases: IV. Changes in vascularity with increasing tumor growth. *Surgery* 1974;75:589–596.

Allison DJ, Jordan H, Hennessy O. Therapeutic embolization of the hepatic artery: A review of 75 procedures. *Lancet* 1985; March: 595–599.

Bengmark S, Rorengren K. Angiographic study of the collateral circulation to the liver after hepatic artery ligation in man. *Am J Surg* 1970;119:620–625.

Bookstein J, Cho KJ, Davis GB, Dail D. Arterioportal communication: Observations and hypotheses concerning transsinusoidal and transvasal types. *Radiology* 1982;142:581–591.

Carrasco CH, Chuang VP, Wallace S. Apudomas metastatic to the liver: Treatment by hepatic artery embolization. *Radiology* 1983;149:79–83. Case Records of the MGH: Case 19-1980. *N Engl J Med* 1980;20:1132–1140.

Cho KJ, Rauter SR, Schmidt R. Effects of experimental hepatic artery embolization on hepatic function. *AJR* 1976;127:563–567.

Chuang VP, Wallace S. Hepatic artery embolization in the treatment of hepatic neoplasms. *Radiology* 1981;140:51–58.

Chuang VP, Wallace S, Carrasco H, Charnsangavy C. Embolization as a therapeutic modality. *Cancer Bull* 1984;36:15–20.

Clouse ME, Lee RGL, Duszlak EJ, et al. Peripheral hepatic artery embolization for primary and secondary hepatic neoplasms. *Radiology* 1983;147:407–411.

Ekelund L, Stigsson L, Sjogreen HO. Transcatheter arterial embolization of normal livers and experimental hepatic tumors in the rat. *Acta Radiol* 1977;18:641–651.

Furui S, Otomo K, Itai Y, Iio M. Hepatocellular carcinoma treated by transcatheter arterial embolization: Progress evaluated by computed tomography. *Radiology* 1984;150:773–778.

Grace DM, Pitt DF, Gold RE. Vascular embolization and occlusion by angiographic techniques as an aid or alternative to operation. *Surg Gynecol Obstet* 1976;143:469–482.

Healey JE. Vascular patterns in human metastatic liver tumors. *Surg Gynecol Obstet* 165;120:1187–1193.

Heimbach DM, Ferguston GS, Harley JD. Treatment of traumatic hemobilia with angiographic embolization. *J Trauma* 1978;18:221–224.

Kato T, Nemoto R, Mori H et al. Arterial chemoembolization with microencapsulated anticancer drug. *JAMA* 1981;245:1123–1127.

Kerlan RK, Bank WO, Hoddick WK et al. Occlusion of a hepatic artery to portal vein fistula with bucrylate. *Cardiovasc Intervent Radiol* 1983;6:138–140.

Kobayashi H, Hidaka H, Kajiya V et al. Occlusion of a hepatic artery to portal vein fistula with bucrylate. *Cardiovasc Intervent Radiol* 1983;6:138–140.

Koehler RE, Korobkin M, Lewis F. Arteriographic demonstration of collateral artery supply to the liver after hepatic artery ligation. *Radiology* 1975;117:49–54.

Kuroda C, Iwasaki M, Tanaka T, et al. Gallbladder infarction following hepatic transcatheter arterial embolization. *Radiology* 1983;149:85–89.

Madding GF, Kennedy PA. Hepatic artery ligation. *Surg Clin North Am* 172;52:719–728.

Mathisen DJ, Athanasoulis CA, Malt RA. Preservation of arterial flow to the liver. *Ann Surg* 1982;196:400–410.

Matsui O, Kawamura I, Takashima T. Occurrence of an intrahepatic porto-arterial shunt after hepatic artery embolization with Gelfoam powder in rats and rabbits. *Acta Radiol* (Diagn) 1986;27:119–122.

McDermott WV, Paris AL, Clouse ME, Meissner WA. Dearterialization of the liver for metastatic cancer. *Ann Surg* 1978;187:39–46.

Nagasue N, Inokuchi K, Kobayashi M, Saku M. Hepatoportal arteriovenous fistula in primary carcinoma of the liver. *Surg Gynecol Obstet* 1977;145:504–508.

Nakamura H, Tanaka T, Hori S, et al. Transcatheter embolization of hepatocellular carcinoma: Assessment of efficacy in cases of resection following embolization. *Radiology* 1983;147:401–405.

Nakao N, Miura K, Takahashi H, et al. Hepatocellular carcinoma: Combined hepatic, arterial and portal venous embolization. *Radiology* 1986;161:303–307.

Nouchi T, Nishimura M, Maeda M. Transcatheter arterial embolization of ruptured hepatocellular carcinoma associated with liver cirrhosis. *Dig Dis Sci* 1984;29:1137–1141.

Ohnishi K, Tsuchiya S, Nakayama T, et al. Arterial chemoembolization of hepatocellular carcinoma with Mitomycin-C microcapsules. *Radiology* 1984;152:51–55.

Okuda K, Jinnouchi S, Nagasaki Y, et al. Angiographic demonstration of growth of hepatocellular carcinoma in the hepatic vein and inferior vena cava. *Radiology* 1977;124:33–36.

Onodera H, Oikawa M, Abe M, Goto Y. Gallbladder necrosis after transcatheter hepatic arterial embolization: A technique to avoid this complication. *Radiology* 1984;152:209–210.

Sarr MG, Kaufman SL, Zuidema GD, Cameron JL. Management of hemobilia associated with transhepatic internal biliary drainage catheters. *Surgery* 1984;95:603–607.

Stagg RJ, Lewis BJ, Friedman MA, Ignoffo RJ, Hohn DC. Hepatic arterial chemotherapy for colorectal cancer metastatic to the liver. *Ann Intern Med* 1984;100:736–743.

Stridbeck H, Ekelund L, Jonsson N. Segmental hepatic arterial occlusion with absolute ethanol in domestic swine. *Acta Radiol* 1984;25:331–335.

Takayasu K, Moriyama N, Muramatsu Y, et al. Splenic infarction: A complication of transcatheter hepatic arterial embolization for liver malignancies. *Radiology* 1984;151:371–375.

Tegtmeyer CJ, Bezirdijian DR, Ferguson WW, Hess CE. Transcatheter embolic control of iatrogenic hematobilia. *Cardiovasc Intervent Radiol* 1981;4:88–92.

Uflacker R, Paolini RM, Nobrega M. Ablation of tumor and inflammatory tissue with absolute ethanol. *Acta Radiol* (Diagn) 1986;27:131–138.

Yamada R, Sato M, Kawabata M, et al. Hepatic artery embolization in 120 patients with unresectable hepatoma. *Radiology* 1983;148:397–401.

Wallace S, Chuang VP. Transcatheter management of hepatic neoplasms. In *Interventional Radiology,* edited by Wilkins RA, Viamonte M. Blackwell, Oxford, 1982:177–187.

Wright RD. The blood supply of newly developed epithelial tissue in the liver. *J Pathol Bacteriol* 1937;45:405–414.

Splenic Embolization

Rubens de Souza A. Pinheiro
Renan Uflacker

PARTIAL SPLENIC EMBOLIZATION IN HYPERSPLENISM

The spleen is a brittle, highly vascularized organ located in the left hypochondriac region and protected by the rib cage. It is fed by the splenic artery, which emerges from the celiac axis distally to the origin of the left gastric artery. The initial segment of the splenic artery may be directed toward the left side, the right side, or ventrally. It is rarely a straight branch of the aorta or of the superior mesenteric artery, and it generally follows a slightly tortuous, dorsally inclined course until reaching the splenic hilum. In elderly patients, particularly those with splenomegaly and portal hypertension, the splenic artery has a considerably enlarged lumen and its course is markedly tortuous.

From the splenic artery originate branches which take part in vascularization of the stomach (short gastric arteries, toward the greater curvature) and pancreas. The dorsal pancreatic artery emerges from the proximal portion of the splenic artery in 40 percent of all individuals; one of its main ramifications is the transverse pancreatic artery, which runs toward the tail of the pancreas. Many fine pancreatic branches originate from the splenic axis, the pancreatica magna being the most important. The pancreatic caudal artery originates at the distal portion of the splenic artery. A rich network of anastomoses connects the several components of the pancreatic vascularization network.

The angiographic demonstration of these vessels is subject to varying hemodynamic factors, which determine the flow of the contrast medium bolus injected. The intraparenchymal course of splenic arterial vessels is variable: primary dichotomy occurs near the hilum, and the upper and lower branches give origin to tributaries with progressively smaller diameter toward the periphery. The presence of polar branches is quite common, and the upper polar branch should not be mistaken for the accessory left gastric artery.

Intrasplenic blood transit is complex: experimental evidence supports a microcirculatory "open type" bed, in which blood coming from follicular arteries flows between red pulp cords, returning to the intravascular compartment through large venous endothelial openings. Formed blood elements pass through without any morphostructural deformation.

The splenic veins converge toward the splenoportal venous axis, appearing considerably distended in cases of congestive splenomegaly. Numerous venous collaterals establish a connection between intrasplenic circulation and the azygos system, through capsular perforating branches.

The radiologist's contribution to the treatment of splenomegaly and hypersplenism effectively began with the work of Spigos in 1979. Standardization of partial embolization procedures has drastically reduced complications, the prevalence of which had given rise to doubts whether such procedures would ever be practical.

A large body of cumulative data now exists regarding the embolization treatment of hypersplenism related to immunosuppressive states. Indications gradually began to increase as the method was applied in palliative treatment of splenomegaly and hypersplenism related to chronic liver disease and portal hypertension. In such situations, the significance of hypersplenism within the patient's overall clinical picture is less important, and the main objective of partial splenic embolization is to alleviate the discomfort caused by the abdominal mass, while improving liver cell function (presumably by improving arterial perfusion).

Hypersplenism is characterized by sequestration of formed blood elements inside the spleen, accompanied by splenomegaly and medullar hyperplasia. Portal hypertension is a consequence not only of anatomic or hemodynamic restrictions to venous blood flow in the visceral bed, but also of hyperdynamic conditions, which are affected to a considerable extent by enlargement of the splenic territory. Splenectomy, the classic surgical treatment, is associated with high morbidity rates, even when performed by experienced hands. The surgery itself is technically difficult, especially when the spleen is enlarged, and pre- and postoperative difficulties are well documented in the literature. In addition, splenectomy fails to alleviate portal hypertension, and absence of a vital organ compromises the immune system.

When partial splenic embolization (PSE) is indicated, careful consideration should be given to the disease's underlying etiology, particularly with regard to the patient's life expectancy. Those expected to survive for only a short time (e.g., uncompensated cirrhotic patients, immunosuppressed patients without adequate clinical support) are not good candidates for PSE. The procedure is appropriate for patients in whom the alleviation of symptoms offered by PSE may result in significant improvement, usually those who have a good hepatic reserve.

The natural history of the disease must also be taken into account. Elimination or control of those factors which may worsen the patient's general condition, as well as careful management of the basic course of the disease, are critical for the success of PSE. A few indispensable measures are health and dietary reeducation, drug therapy for schistosomiasis, correction of hydroelectric imbalance, and treatment of the consequences of hepatocellular dysfunction (ascites, hypoproteinemia, hepatorenal syndrome, etc.).

Finally, the clinical environment must be carefully controlled, with good coordination among all members of the health team. It is crucial that patients understand and accept the reasons for therapeutic actions and cooperate during all treatment stages. A common cause of failure, for example, is interruption of long-term follow-up when patients drop out because of lack of proper guidance or because of resistance to the treatment regimen.

PSE is regarded as a reliable and safe alternative to classic splenectomy. It reduces spleen volume, controls hypersplenism, and improves hepatic arterial perfusion. PSE is a palliative measure, one that is part of a multidisciplinary therapeutic plan.

Treatment

Preembolization

After the patient is admitted to the hospital, laboratory and clinical investigation should include the following:

Liver and renal function stabilization.
Complete hemogram, including reticulocyte and platelet counts and coagulation study.
Measurement of serum electrolytes, enzymes (SGOT, SGPT, GGT), protein, bilirubin (total and fractions), urea, and creatinine level.
Abdominal anatomic and functional evaluation. (We use conventional radiology, ultrasonography, and hepatosplenic scintigraphy.)

In addition, respiratory physiotherapy may be necessary to improve pulmonary ventilation, particularly of the lower lobes.

These tests establish the overall abdominal anatomy, including the sizes of solid organs and epigastric vessels. The presence and magnitude of ascites and of collateral circulation, and any coexisting lesions (cholelithiasis, pancreatitis, neoplasm, etc.), are carefully listed. The degree of hepatic perfusion can be measured with reasonable accuracy by studying the radioisotope uptake ratio by the spleen and the liver.

It has been observed that the post-PSE period is more difficult in patients with ascites and low levels of serum albumin. Therefore, protein supply should be at least increased, if not normalized, and ascitic volume reduced to a minimum. Volume replacement is not necessary; administration of albumin or fresh human plasma is preferred.

The patient should receive 1.2×10 IU of procaine penicillin 6 h before PSE is started. Administration of anxiolytics or sedatives is not indispensable as premedication.

Embolization

Access is obtained through femoral artery puncture, using Seldinger's technique, under strict aseptic conditions. Preformed Cobra visceral-type (No. 5 French) catheters are utilized; contrast medium injection flow should not exceed 10 mL/s. Superselective catheterization is indispensable; the catheter tip should be positioned near the hilum of the splenic artery, beyond the emergence point of pancreatic vessels. In view of splenic artery tortuosity, a few maneuvers are required, for example, the formation of a Waltman loop for antegrade catheterization, and finer and more flexible catheters and guides should be available for passing bends.

The angiographic study will document splenic vascular anatomy, the type of parenchymal opacification, venous return, and any anatomic variations in circulation. If the study reveals expansive lesions, lack of splenic parenchymal impregnation, occlusion of the splenoportal venous axis, or redirectioning of visceral venous flow, continuation of the procedure is contraindicated. These, however, are not frequently encountered. Errors can occur when a lymphoma patient is embolized, particularly if the condition is clinically occult when PSE is performed. The splenogram is not homogeneous in patients with hypersplenism, compensated postnecrotic cirrhosis, and portal hypertension.

Contrast medium (preembolization) should be injected at a rate of 6 to 10 mL/s for 4 to 5 s. Not more than 50 mL of contrast medium is required, even for patients with voluminous splenomegalies (lower spleen border located below the iliac crest, and internal border to the right of the abdominal midline). The intensity of opacification will be inversely proportional to splenic volume.

For studying massive splenomegaly, x-rays are exposed in a sequence of two films per second for 3 s with a delay of 3 s from the beginning of contrast injection. Late films should be obtained at the 12th, 16th, 20th, and 25th seconds. For smaller spleens, contrast medium volume, flow rate of injection, and film sequence should be adjusted accordingly.

The embolizing mixture consists of 2 mL of dry particles (Gelfoam, cut down to 2- by 2- by 2-mm sizes after manual compression of the plate supplied with commercially available packages), 8 to 10 mL of an antibiotic solution (80 mg gentamycin, 5 × 10 IU of crystalline penicillin G, and 40 mL of saline solution). This mixture is made radiopaque by adding 1 part of contrast medium for each 2 parts of embolizing solution.

After the mixture has been homogenized by vigorously agitating the syringe, the embolization itself is performed. The mixture must be introduced slowly, and it is recommended that a metallic nozzle be adapted to the syringe, so as to obtain higher resistance, and that the syringe be put in a vertical position (with the nozzle up) during injection. This allows the embolizing material to float immediately. Embolization is manually performed, and its several stages should be sequentially monitored by arteriography (10-mL contrast medium injection for 1 s, with exposure of 1 film per second for 3 s).

Quantification of the extent of embolization is based on empirical criteria. Measurement of the embolized area is not advisable. Besides being difficult to perform during examination, it requires the utilization of complex mathematical formulas. A practical method that has produced satisfactory results for us consists of completing the procedure when occlusion of fifth-order arterial branches, which corresponds to 30 to 40 percent embolization of peripheral parenchyma, is attained. One should wait at least 15 min after the embolizing particles have been injected before performing control angiography. Radiographic studies performed before that will not reflect the true extent of embolization. Presumably there is an initial period of emboli "accommodation" inside the spleen, during which the particles are gradually distributed by inflowing arterial blood (Fig. 4.22, A and B). No angiographic evidence of arterial "spasm" is seen during embolization.

The final control angiogram should display splenic venous drainage patency (Fig. 4.22, C and D) If all recommended procedures have been meticulously followed, embolization should not occur in any other territory. In patients who have undergone intestinal arteriography (injection into the superior mesenteric artery) after splenic embolization, venous blood reflux into the distal splenic vein is sometimes seen.

Postembolization

Pain is the most frequent and constant symptom. During the first 72 h we inject an analgesic solution (meperidine, 100 mg; dipyrone, 2 mL; distilled water, 10 mL q.s.p) every 4 h. Individual responses dictate whether to maintain treatment, substitute oral analgesic medication, or interrupt therapy. The pain is usually intense, radiating to the whole abdomen and to the left shoulder. Abdominal distension and restricted diaphragmatic mobility will accentuate the patient's discomfort, and may be minimized by physiotherapy.

Administration of fluids and electrolytes is particularly important during the first 6 to 8 h, when the patient should not ingest food. After that, food intake is usually resumed, although patients with persistent vomiting should remain without food for a longer period.

During the initial postembolization period, fever will sometimes exceed the 38°C threshold. For the first 7 days after embolization, prophylactic antibiotic therapy is recommended.

Some practitioners have reduced the duration of antibiotic therapy, and a few have eliminated it. Although no complications were observed in those cases, the validity of this approach has not been adequately demonstrated, and we recommend following the conventional protocol.

The initial postembolization syndrome, which is satisfactorily tolerated by most patients, lasts from 7 to 10 days. In some patients, an increase in abdominal circumference and spleen size is seen during the first 15 days. Leukocytosis is also common. On average, the clinical condition stabilizes around the fifteenth day and hospital stay does not exceed 3 weeks. There are, however, exceptions.

After the thirtieth day, spleen size starts to diminish rapidly. Patients are significantly improved (both subjectively and objectively) and resume their normal activities. Their laboratory counts return to normal or stabilize at subnormal levels that are better than those obtained before the procedure (Fig. 4.23).

SPLENIC EMBOLIZATION IN CASES OF TRAUMA

Spleen rupture is a relatively common occurrence in cases of blunt and penetrating abdominal trauma, and the most frequent indication for splenectomy is trauma. Less commonly, transoperative splenectomy is performed after accidental surgical lesion of the spleen. The hematologic and immunologic effects of asplenism following splenectomy have only recently been defined.

The first evidence signaling the importance of the spleen in resisting infection was published in 1919: splenectomized rats were identified as being more susceptible to infection and having shorter survival than controls. This signal was ignored until the 1950s, when it was demonstrated that a group of young children submitted to splenectomy for trauma were more suscep-

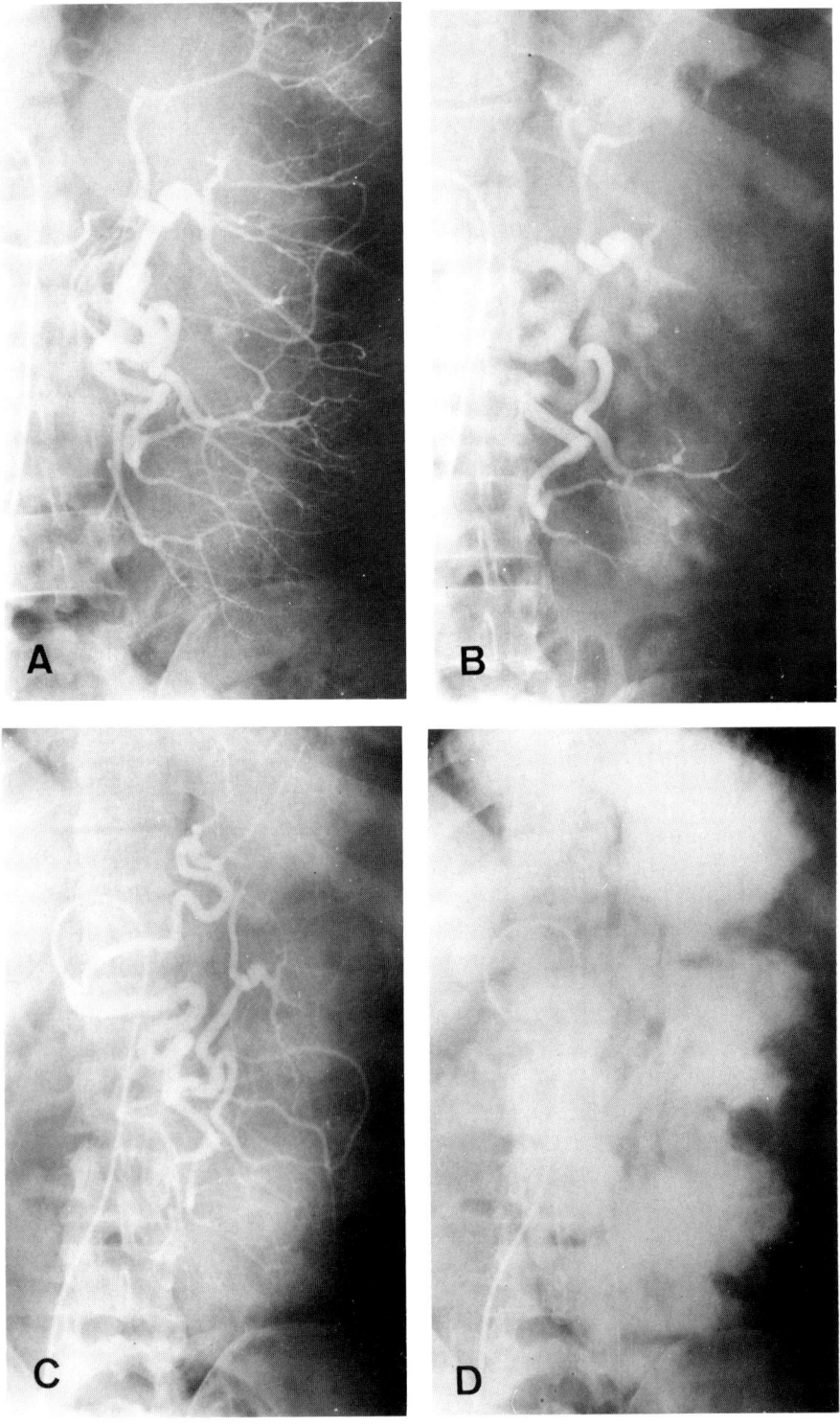

Figure 4.22 Representative stages of partial splenic embolization in two different patients.
(A,B) Intrasplenic vascularization before and after PSE. Figure B documents the end of PSE; notice the apparently "excessive" embolization. (Study after 15 min showed opacification of a larger area of the parenchyma and obstruction of fifth-order branches.) (C,D) Final stages of PSE in portal hypertension patient. Note occlusion of fifth-order branches and venous drainage patency with esophageal gastric varices.

tible to frequent infection and/or death due to sepsis than unsplenectomized children. Similar findings were later described for older children and adults.

Changes in the immune system caused by splenectomy are age-dependent, being most significant during the first year of life. IgM levels fall drastically, remaining low for at least 1 year. IgG levels remain unchanged while IgA levels are elevated. Tuftsin levels drop, which in turn decreases phagocytosis by neutrophils. For all these reasons, there is decreased capacity for opsonization and phagocytosis of encapsulated microorganisms.

There are several alternatives to emergency splenectomy. Conservative treatment may be an option preoperatively, when imaging diagnosis of the splenic rup-

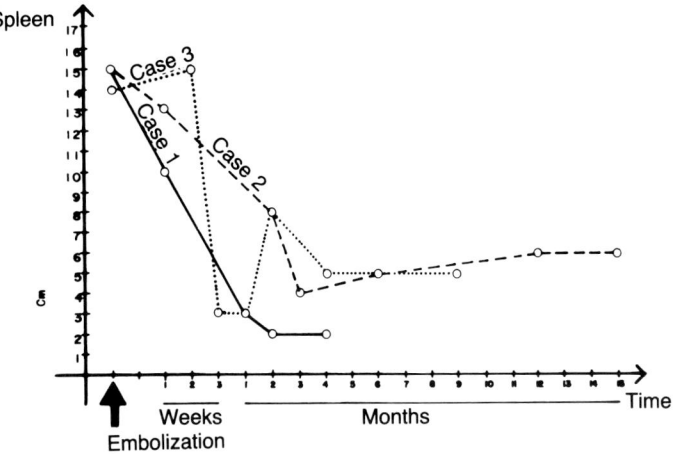

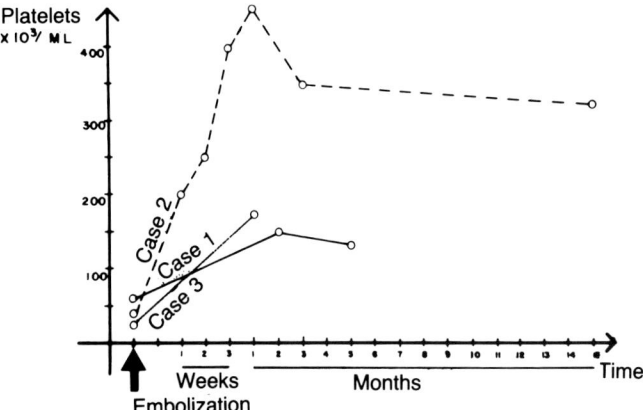

Figure 4.23 Examples of individual variations in platelet counts and in splenomegaly regression following partial splenic embolization.

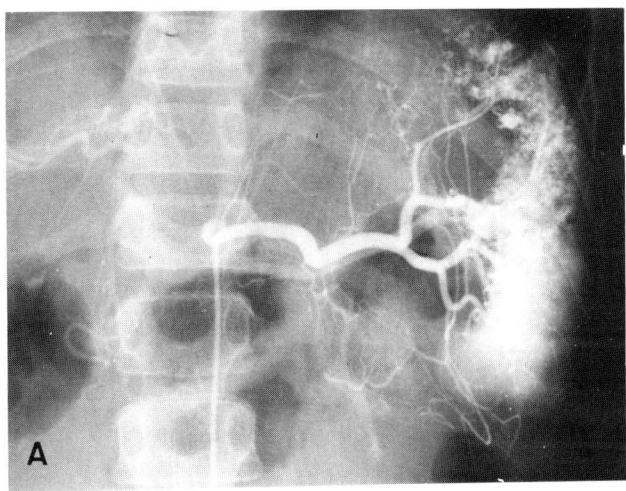

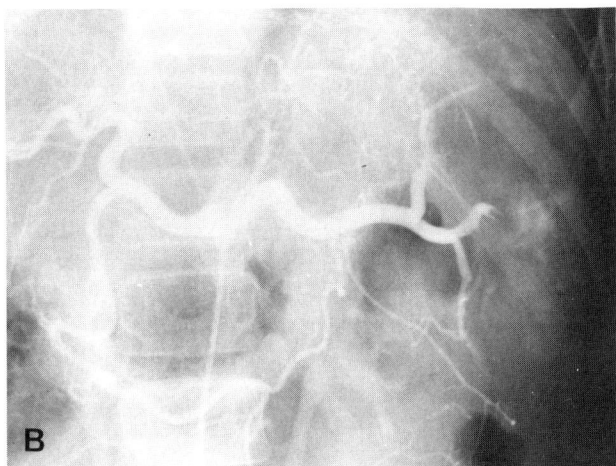

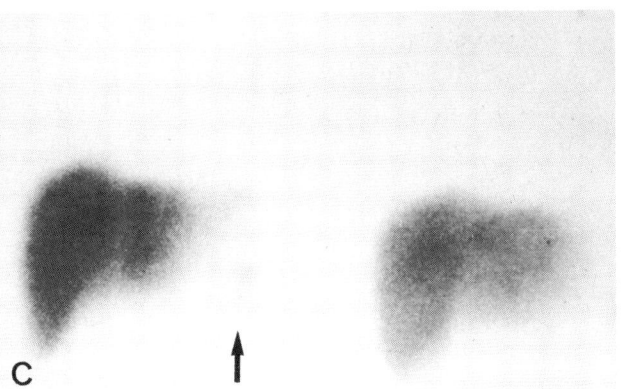

Figure 4.24 Blunt abdominal trauma in 8-year-old child, with spleen laceration and free blood in the peritoneum.
(A) Angiogram of celiac axis showing splenic upper pole laceration, and early venous filling. (B) Control angiogram following spleen embolization with Gelfoam. Bleeding control was achieved, and the clinical condition improved without further surgery being necessary. (C) Hepatosplenic control scintigram 2 months following embolization showing radioisotope uptake by splenic lower pole (arrow).

ture shows stable evolution of the lesion, and even intraoperatively, when capsule rupture is present but bleeding has stopped and a stable clot is plugging the laceration. A number of papers have been published showing the excellent results obtained with conservative surgical and nonsurgical treatment (observation) in children. Surgical alternatives include arterial ligation, splenorraphy, partial splenectomy, splenectomy with autogenous transplant, and spleen embolizaiton or occlusion with balloon of the splenic artery.

The full potential of interventional radiology in cases of traumatic damage to the spleen has not yet been explored. However, splenic embolization for control of bleeding is highly effective, and, being partial, preserves a sufficient amount of parenchyma to prevent infectious complications (Fig. 4.24).

To obtain an effective embolization, ablation of about two-thirds of spleen volume should be performed with fragments of Gelfoam-type resorbable material. The antibiotic therapy protocol described above should be followed in these cases.

Occlusion of the splenic artery with a Gianturco coil or a detachable balloon may also be effective, but the risk always exists that collateral circulation will develop and that bleeding will persist.

Follow-up of spleen viability should be performed through nuclear imaging (Fig. 4.24).

EMBOLIZATION OF SPLENIC ARTERY ANEURYSMS

Around 10 percent of all aneurysms of the splenic artery rupture, causing shock and death. According to many authors surgery is indicated when an aneurysm is identified in the splenic artery, even without bleeding or symptoms of rupture.

In 1978, the wiring technique for occlusion of splenic artery aneurysms was described; the procedure met with reasonable success. Later, it was verified that in many cases, the simple occlusion of the splenic artery with a Gianturco coil or detachable balloon is enough to occlude the aneurysm, thus controlling bleeding (Fig. 4.25). An alternative is temporary occlusion of the splenic artery by balloon catheter, performed as a preoperative measure.

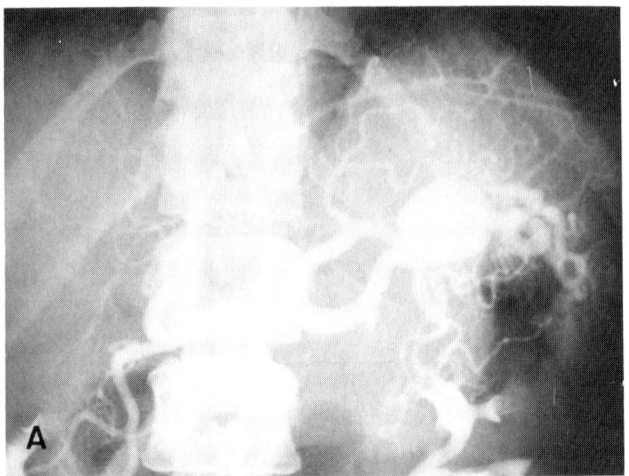

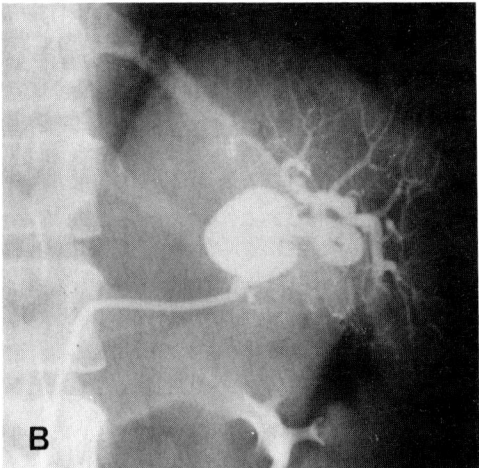

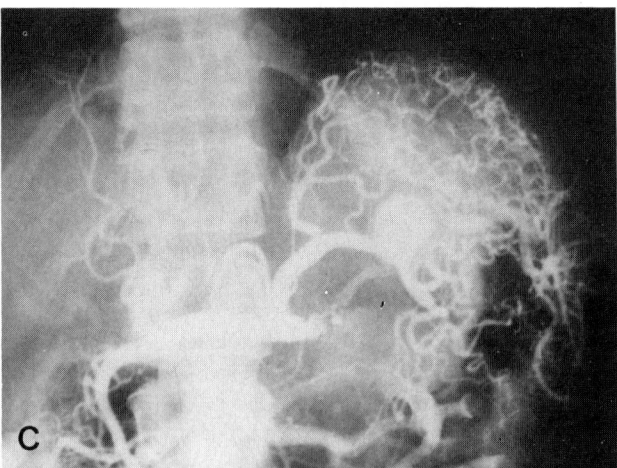

Figure 4.25 61-year-old patient with retroperitoneal spontaneous hemorrhage.
(A) Injection into the celiac axis showing a 5-cm-diameter aneurysm in the splenic artery, without evidence of bleeding. (B) Superselective injection into the splenic artery. (C) Post-embolization control angiogram showing splenic artery occlusion, residual filling of aneurysm with contrast, and development of collateral circulation through the left gastric artery. Bleeding was controlled, and later on, during surgery, the aneurysm was found thrombosed and distal arterial ligation was performed.

REFERENCES

Allison DJ, Fletcher DR, Gordon-Smith EC. Therapeutic arterial embolization of the spleen: A new cause of free intraperitoneal gas. *Clin Radiol* 1981;32:617–621.

Alwmark A, Bengmark S, Gullstrand P, Joelsson B, Lunderquist A, Owman T. Evaluation of splenic embolization in patients with portal hypertension and hypersplenism. *Ann Surg* 1982;196:518–524.

Azevedo FS, Penas ME, Pinheiro RSA. Embolizacao esplenica parcial. *Radiol Brasil* 1983;16:95–99.

Castaneda-Zuniga WR, Hammerschmidt DE, Sanchez R, Amplatz K. Nonsurgical splenectomy. *AJR* 1977;129:805–811.

Chuang VP, Reuter SR. Selective arterial embolization for the control of traumatic splenic bleeding. *Invest Radiol* 1975;10:18–24.

Chuang VP, Reuter SR. Experimental diminution of splenic function by selective embolization of the splenic artery. *Surg Gynecol Obstet* 1975;140:715–720.

Cooper MJ, Williamson RCN. Splenectomy: Indications, hazards and alternatives. *Br J Surg* 1984;71:173–180.

Ferguson A. Hazards of hyposplenism. *Br Med J* 1982;285:1375–1376.

Gerlock AJ, MacDonell RC Jr, Muhletaler CA, Parris WCW, Johnson HK, Tallent MB, Richie RE, Kendall RI. Partial splenic embolization for hypersplenism in renal transplantation. *AJR* 1982;138:451–456.

Goldman ML, Philip PK, Sarrafizadeh MS, Sarfeh IJ, Salan AA, Galambos JT, Powers SR, Balint JA. Intra-arterial tissue adhesive for medical splenectomy in humans. *Radiology* 1981;140:341–349.

Guilford WB, Scatliff JH. Transcatheter embolization of the spleen for control of splenic hemorrhage and "in-situ" splenectomy: An experimental study using silicone spheres. *Radiology* 1976;119:549–553.

Kakkasseril JS, Stewart D, Cox JA, Gelfand M. Changing treatment of pediatric splenic trauma. *Arch Surg* 1982;117:758–759.

Kumpe DA, Rumack CM, Pretorius DH, Stoecker TJ, Stellin GP. Partial splenic embolization in children with hypersplenism. *Radiology* 1985;155:357–362.

Levy JM, Wasserman P, Pitha N. Presplenectomy transcatheter occlusion of the splenic artery. *Arch Surg* 1979;114:198–199.

Levy JM, Wasserman PI, Weiland DE. Nonsupurative gas formation in the spleen after transcatheter infarction. *Radiology* 1981;139:375–376.

Maddison F. Embolic therapy of hypersplenism. *Invest Radiol* 1973;8:280–281.

Mazer M, Smith CW, Martin VN. Distal splenic artery embolization with a flow-directed balloon catheter. *Radiology* 1985;154:245.

Mineau DE, Miller FJ Jr, Lee RG, Nakashima EN, Nelson JA. Experimental transcatheter splenectomy using absolute ethanol. *Radiology* 1982;142:355–359.

Pinheiro RSA, Azevedo FS, Palma JK. Radiologia intervencionista em hipertensao porta. *Radiol Brasil* 1986;19:63–65.

Probst P, Castaneda-Zuniga WR, Gomes AS, Yonehiro EG, Delaney JP, Amplatz K. Nonsurgical treatment of splenic artery aneurysms. *Radiology* 1978;128:619–623.

Spigos DG, Jonasson O, Felix E, Capek V. Transcatheter therapeutic embolization of hypersplenism. *Invest Radiol* 1977;12:418.

Spigos DG, Jonasson O, Mozes M, Capek J. Partial splenic embolization in the treatment of hypersplenism. *AJR* 1979;132:777–782.

Spigos DG, Tan WS, Mozes MF, Pringle K, Jossifides I. Splenic embolization. *Cardiovasc Intervent Radiol* 1980;3:282–288.

Thanopoulos BD, Frimas CA. Partial splenic embolization in the management of hypersplenism secondary to Gaucher disease. *J Pediatr* 1982;101:740–743.

Trajanowski JQ, Harriet TJ, Athanasoulis CA, Greenfield AJ. Hepatic and splenic infarction: Complications of therapeutic transcatheter embolization. *Am J Surg* 1980;139:272–277.

Uflacker R. Transcatheter embolization of arterial aneurysm. *Br J Radiol* 1986;59:317–324.

Vujic I, Lauver JW. Severe complications from partial splenic embolization in patients with liver failure. *Br J Radiol* 1981;54:492–495.

Yoshioda H, Kuroda C, Hori S, et al. Splenic embolization for hypersplenism using steel coils. *AJR* 1985;144:269–274.

White JJ, Goldman ML, Lepow M. Correction of hypersplenism without splenectomy. *J Pediatr Surg* 1981;167:967.

Wholey MH, Stockdale R, Hung TK. A percutaneous balloon catheter for the immediate control of hemorrhage. *Radiology* 1970;95:65–71.

Wholey MH. The technology of balloon catheters in interventional angiography. *Radiology* 1977;125:671–676.

Wholey MH, Chamorro HA, Rao G, Chapman W. Splenic infarction and spontaneous rupture of the spleen after therapeutic embolization. *Cardiovasc Radiol* 1978;1:249–253.

Wright KC, Anderson JH, Gianturco C, Wallace S, Chuang VP. Partial splenic embolization using polyvinyl alcohol foam, dextran, polystyrene, or silicone. *Radiology* 1982;142:351–354.

Embolization in the Pancreas

RENAN UFLACKER

HEMORRHAGE SECONDARY TO PANCREATITIS

False aneurysms in the pancreatic and peripancreatic arteries are well-defined complications of chronic and necrotizing pancreatitis, due to vascular wall digestion by the proteolytic enzymes produced in the pancreas. The most important enzyme in this process is trypsin. These pseudoaneurysms may be the cause of severe digestive-tract and intraperitoneal bleeding that is difficult to control either clinically or surgically.

Although pancreatitis-related pseudoaneurysms are relatively uncommon, they were found in 10 percent of a series of 72 patients.

True splenic artery aneurysms may be fortuitously found, or related to pancreatic cystic tumor.

Digestive bleeding from rupture of a pseudoaneurysm into the pancreatic or biliary ducts or into a pancreatic pseudocyst into the duodenum is rare. Even more rare is intraperitoneal bleeding from such pseudoaneurysms. Patients presenting with digestive bleeding due to a ruptured pancreatic pseudoaneurysm have a 47 percent mortality rate if treated surgically.

Embolization by catheter and electrocoagulation can be used to control bleeding in cases of pseudoaneurysm due to pancreatitis or trauma. However, depending upon the embolization technique used, the procedure may cause rupture of the aneurysm, which will complicate the course of the disease.

A large number of peripancreatic pseudoaneurysms are located in the splenic artery, though other arteries may also be involved. Due to the high risk and low effectiveness of surgical procedures, angiography is a major tool in the diagnosis and treatment of these cases (Fig. 4.26). Angiography or embolization may cause spontaneous rupture of the fragile aneurysm wall if injection of emboli leads to a sudden increase of pressure inside the aneurysm. Significant pressure increase can occur if the fluid volume is too rapidly injected into the aneurysm; this force will be transmitted to the aneurysm wall, often causing rupture.

The use of Gelfoam as an embolizing material in cases of peripancreatic pseudoaneurysms is not advisable for two reasons. First, they are rapidly digested by the pancreatic fluids, which decreases occlusion time. Second, injection of Gelfoam particles will cause sudden

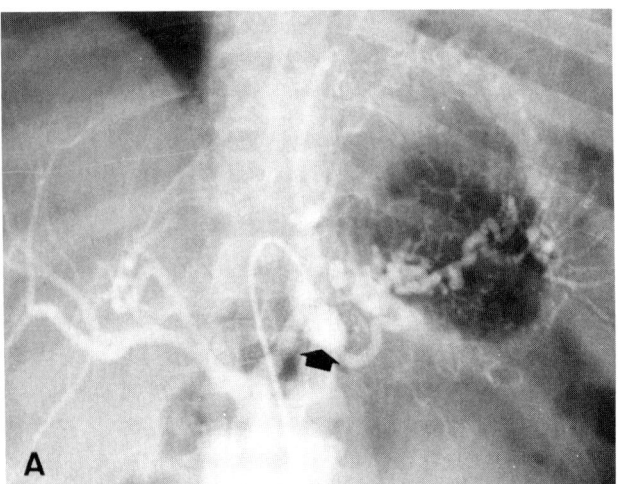 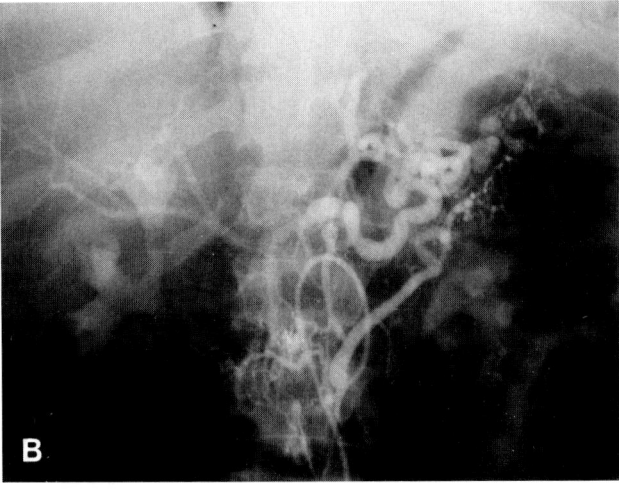

Figure 4.26 44-year-old alcoholic patient, with necrohemorrhagic pancreatitis. The patient was previously operated on, and the epiploic retrocavity drained into the epigastrium, causing profuse and repetitive bleeding. (A) Injection into the celiac axis showing a pseudoaneurysm in the proximal splenic artery (arrow). The distal splenic artery is occluded; gastric fundus collaterals to the splenic hilum are visualized. Embolization with two Gianturco coils was performed at the splenic artery origin. (B) Control angiogram 2 weeks following embolization performed by catheterization of a collateral branch originating from the superior mesenteric artery. The celiac axis is occluded, and the splenic artery, being also patent, no longer displays the pseudoaneurysm seen in (A). Bleeding stayed under control during a 5-year follow-up.

pressure variations inside the aneurysm. An embolization system utilizing low-pressure emboli introduction is more desirable. Gianturco coils, detachable balloons, or bucrylate are probably the best options, since they cause no significant pressure variations, not even when large volumes of fluid are used for introducing the emboli or glue (Fig. 4.26). Moreover, it is not necessary to occlude the pseudoaneurysm cavity itself. Obstruction of the afferent artery alone is successful in treating most lesions.

It should be recalled that the principles described here are also valid for treating pancreatic bleeding due to trauma and in postsurgical conditions. In such cases, bucrylate has proved to be the most effective of the embolizing materials, used with the coaxial system described in Chap. 2.

FUNCTIONAL PANCREATIC TUMORS

Endocrine pancreatic tumors (apudomas) are relatively rare, although over a period of a few years a busy angiography center may see a reasonable number of patients with hyperinsulinism and other endocrine syndromes.

A few recent reports indicate that it is possible to control hormone production by insulinomas through superselective embolization of the pancreatic vessels feeding the lesion. Control of hormone production is similar to that obtained in patients with hepatic metastases of endocrine tumors. In some cases it may be necessary to repeat embolization after a few months. A properly embolized insulinoma will show a clinical and laboratory response equal to the response observed after total

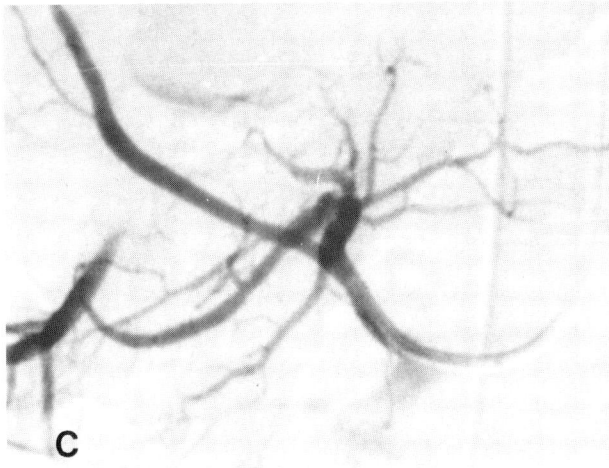
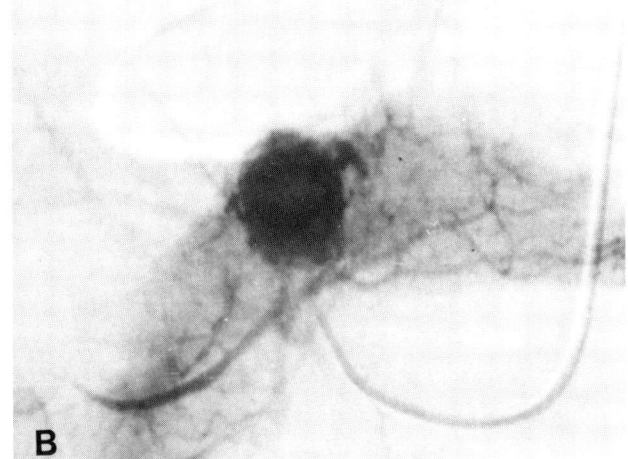
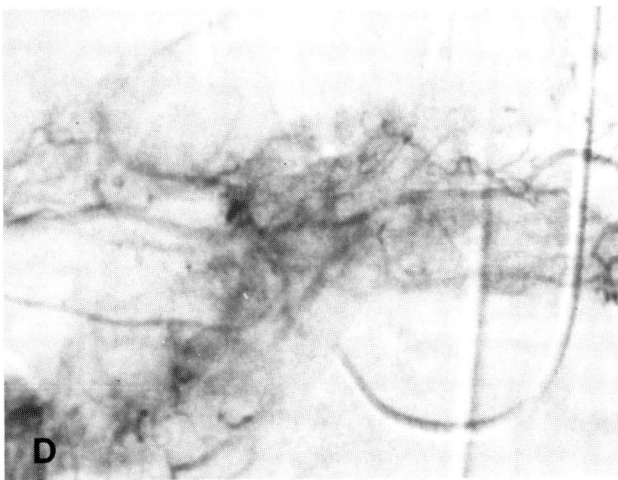

Figure 4.27 45-year-old patient with hyperinsulinism (360 μU/mL) and hypoglycemia (plasma glucose as low as 17 mg/dl) who had undergone several coma episodes and exhibited behavioral changes.
(A) Selective injection into the dorsal pancreatic artery arising from the superior mesenteric artery. Notice the insulinoma staining. (B) Late arterial phase showing the dense impregnation of the adenoma between the head and body of the pancreas. (C) After embolization with 150-μm Ivalon particles, the lesion has been devascularized; no contrast impregnation is yet evident. (D) Later arterial phase showing no insulinoma staining after embolization. Eight hours after embolization, glucose levels had risen to 205 mg/dL and insulin had dropped to 11.5 μU/mL. The hyperglycemia gradually tapered off, reaching normal levels within a week.

surgical tumor resection. A few hours after embolization the patient will present with hyperglycemia and low insulin levels due to suppression of normal pancreatic functions. To control high glucose levels a low-glucose diet, and even insulin therapy, may be necessary. Hyperglycemia lasts for 5 to 7 days, and gradually tapers off to normal levels.

Long-term follow-up data on patients with insulinoma treated by embolization is lacking, but the existing data indicate that such treatment is highly effective (Fig. 4.27).

REFERENCES

Eckhauser FE, Stanley JC, Zelenock GB, et al. Gastroduodenal and pancreaticoduodenal artery aneurysms: A complication of pancreatitis causing spontaneous gastrointestinal hemorrhage. *Surgery* 1980;88:335–344.

Harper PC, Gamelli RL, Kaye MD. Recurrent hemorrhage into the pancreatic duct from a splenic artery aneurysm. *Gastroenterology* 1984;87:417–420.

Lima JR, Jaques P, Mandell V. Aneurysm rupture secondary to transcatheter embolization. *AJR* 1979;132:553–556.

Milavelle R, Venables CW. Chronic pancreatitis as a cause of gastrointestinal bleeding. *Gut* 1982;23:250–255.

Miyake T, Sakai M, Ueda S, et al. Arteriopancreatic duct fistula in juvenile pancreatitis: A cause of massive gastrointestinal hemorrhage. *Dig Dis Scienc* 1981;26:760–764.

Moore TJ, Peterson LM, Harrington DP, Smith RJ. Successful arterial embolization of an insulinoma. *JAMA* 1982;248:1353–1355.

Ranson JHC. Surgical treatment of acute pancreatitis. *Dig Dis Sci* 1980;25:453–459.

Schecter LM, Gordon HE, Passaro E. Massive hemorrhage from the celiac axis in pancreatitis. *Am J Surg* 1974;128:301–305.

Starling JR, Crummy AB. Hemosuccus pancreaticus secondary to rupture splenic artery aneurysm. *Dig Dis Sci* 1979;24:726–729.

Stroud WH, Cullom JW, Anderson MC. Hemorrhagic complications of severe pancreatitis. *Surgery* 1981;90:657–665.

Uflacker R. Transcatheter embolization of arterial aneurysms. *Br J Radiol* 1986;59:317–324.

Uflacker R, Diehl JC. Successful embolization of a bleeding splenic artery pseudoaneurysm secondary to necrotizing pancreatitis. *Gastrointest Radiol* 1982;7:379–382.

White AF, Baum S, Buranasiri S. Aneurysms secondary to pancreatitis. *AJR* 1976;127:393–396.

Renal Embolization

Rosa Maria Paolini
Renan Uflacker

RENAL TUMORS

Renal tumors, particularly hypernephromas, which account for 75 percent of all renal tumors, are well vascularized, and preoperative embolization of such tumors has been extensively used for the last 10 years to facilitate surgical removal of the mass. Many surgeons will not perform a nephrectomy without first carrying out embolization. Some evidence exists that this procedure also increases immunity and decreases metastases.

The hypernephromas can be diagnosed using ultrasonography, CT, and intravenous pyelography. Angiography is no longer performed merely for diagnostic purpose, but rather for mapping out and displaying the vasculature. In order to reveal any metastatic thrombi the vascular study should include analysis of the inferior vena cava and renal vein.

To avoid the risk of tubular injury to the contralateral kidney that may result from injection of a large volume of contrast medium, embolization is not performed simultaneously with the diagnostic examination.

Absolute alcohol, Gelfoam, and Ivalon are all used in the embolization of renal tumors. The technique for using Gelfoam or Ivalon, which is a time-consuming but safe procedure, is the same as already described for other lesions, the catheter being introduced deeply into the renal artery to avoid reflux of any particles into the aorta and/or contralateral renal artery. An occlusion balloon catheter is sometimes used, although this is not mandatory.

More recently, absolute alcohol has become the material of choice for use as an occluding agent. It acts by injuring the vascular endothelium while causing cell vacuolization and thrombosis. Evidence of gas formation inside the tumor is provided by postembolization ultrasonography when echogenic areas are seen within the lesion (Fig. 4.28). Absolute alcohol should be used carefully. The renal artery may be catheterized with an occlusion balloon catheter in order to prevent reflux of ethanol into the aorta and/or the contralateral renal artery, which can lead to irreversible damage to nontarget organs. The use of an occlusion balloon catheter does not, however, prevent (and may even facilitate) the alcohol's passing into the left colic artery circulation, through parasitic circulation between the tumor and the left colon, every time the injection pressure exceeds the arterial pressure in the collateral vascular bed.

The alcohol is injected at a rate of 2 to 4 mL/s, the amount that will cause definite injury to the tumor. Fifteen milliliters is usually enough to cause a good occlusion, although if the tumor is very large, more may be necessary. The maximum dose of absolute alcohol, which was established on the basis of experimental gas chromatography studies, is 0.5 mL per kilogram of body weight. Higher doses may cause alcohol intoxication and even alcoholic coma. When a good occlusion is not obtained with the maximum dose, embolization is completed using Gelfoam or Gianturco coils (Figs. 4.29 and 4.30).

The occlusion balloon is deflated after injection of the alcohol in order to control the degree of embolization. Embolization is considered complete when the intrarenal branches are occluded and the contrast medium stagnates in the renal artery and the intrarenal branches. No thrombi or Gelfoam particles should remain in the main renal artery.

Surgery is carried out from 3 to 7 days following the embolization, when all symptoms of the postembolization syndrome, such as back pain, nausea, and fever, have disappeared and when no collateral circulation has yet been formed. When Gelfoam is used, no recanalization of thrombi will take place during this period.

Pain during and after tumor occlusion is in direct proportion to the extent of normal renal tissue infarcted in addition to the tumor embolization.

The use of absolute alcohol may cause damage to the contralateral kidney and left colon necrosis due to reflux of the absolute alcohol in the aorta. These complications are however, rare.

Alcohol allows a much faster procedure than Gelfoam does and offers longer-lasting occlusive effects. With alcohol, the damaged arterial segments do not recanalize or recover, although formation of new vessels may occur. With Gelfoam, recanalization of thrombi is seen within 30 days. Absolute alcohol is therefore now almost exclusively used for palliative treatment of hypervascular renal tumors. Sarcomas and Wilms' tumors have also been successfully embolized.

Palliative embolization is performed in those cases when the tumor is irresectable and the intent is to improve the patient's symptoms. Some authors maintain that embolization alone can increase a person's immune resistance; this remains unproved.

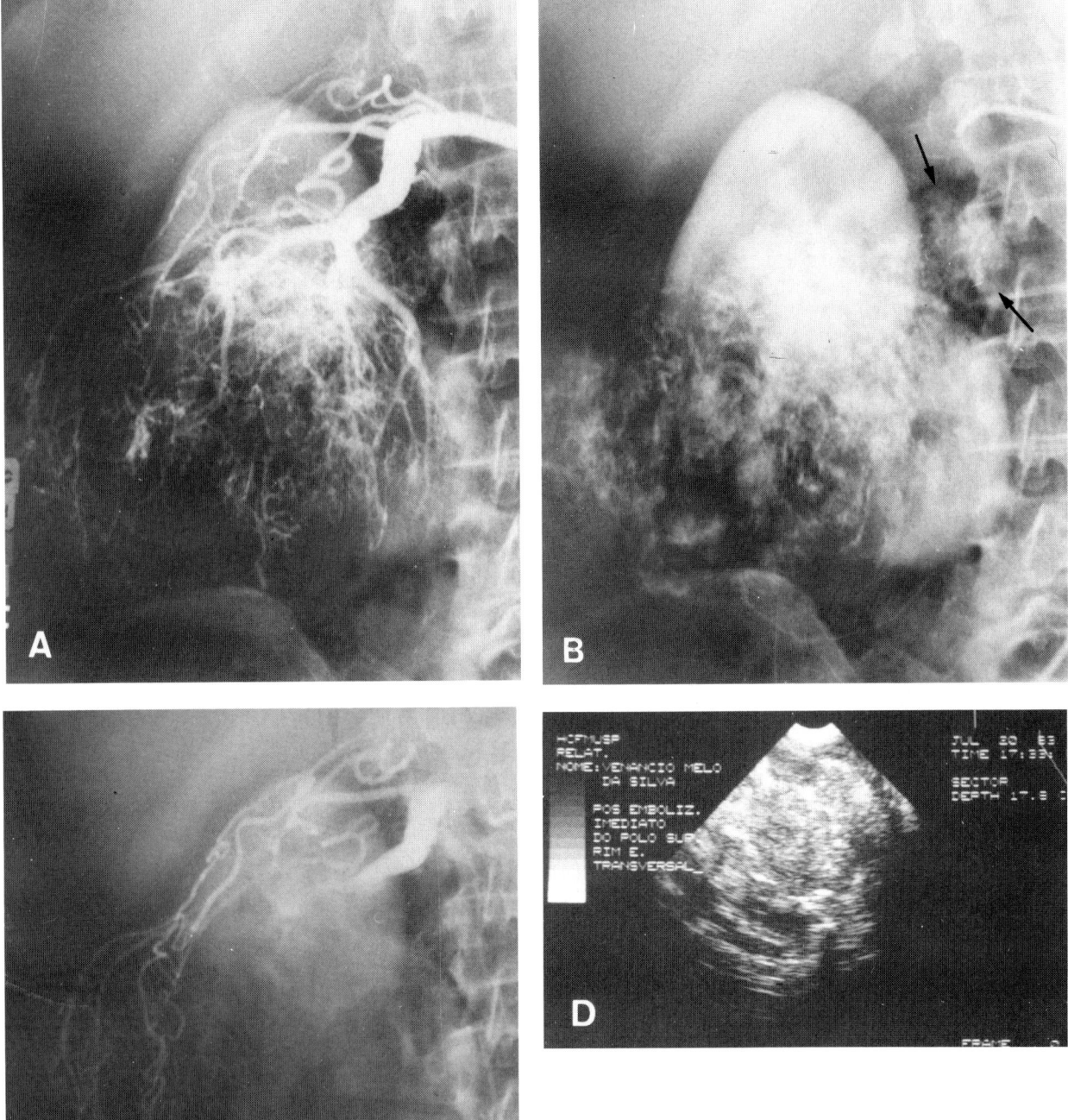

Figure 4.28 (A) Patient with extensive, densely vascularized renal cell carcinoma on the right. (B) Later phase showing impregnation of the lesion and tumor extension into the renal vein (arrows). (C) Control after occlusion of venous circulation with absolute alcohol without using an occlusion balloon. Note the continued patency of capsular arteries, which have not been occluded. (D) Ultrasonographic image showing gas inside the necrotic mass. The lesion was easily dissected without excessive bleeding.

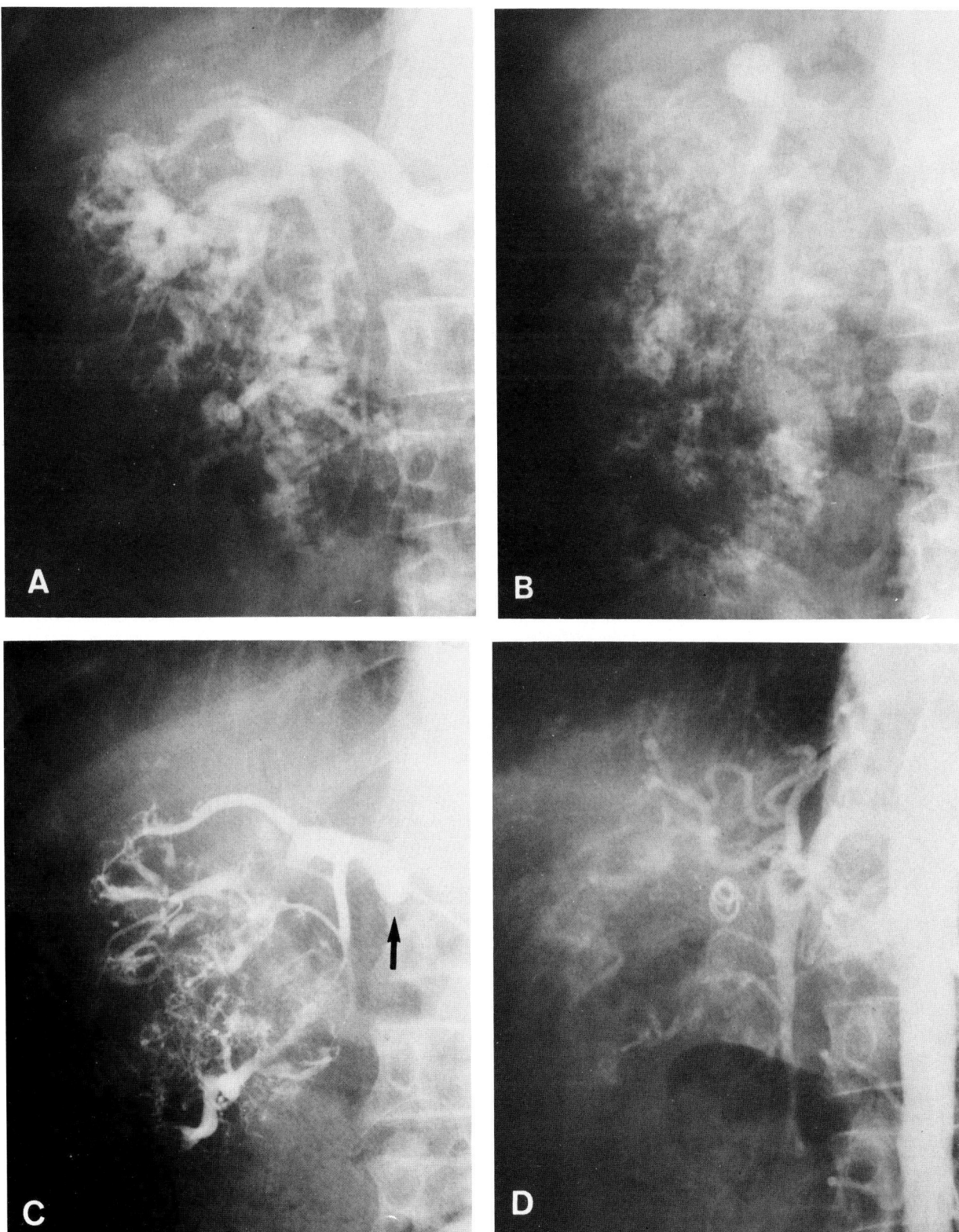

Figure 4.29 (A) Large renal hypervascular tumor mass with high-output arteriovenous fistula. (B) Later stage of the arterial injection showing the tumor's diffuse impregnation. (C) Embolization made with absolute alcohol occluding the main artery with balloon (arrow). (D) Absolute alcohol–balloon embolization was not enough to occlude the AV fistula. Control angiogram showing occluded main artery and Gianturco coils closing the fistula. The mass was removed by surgery.

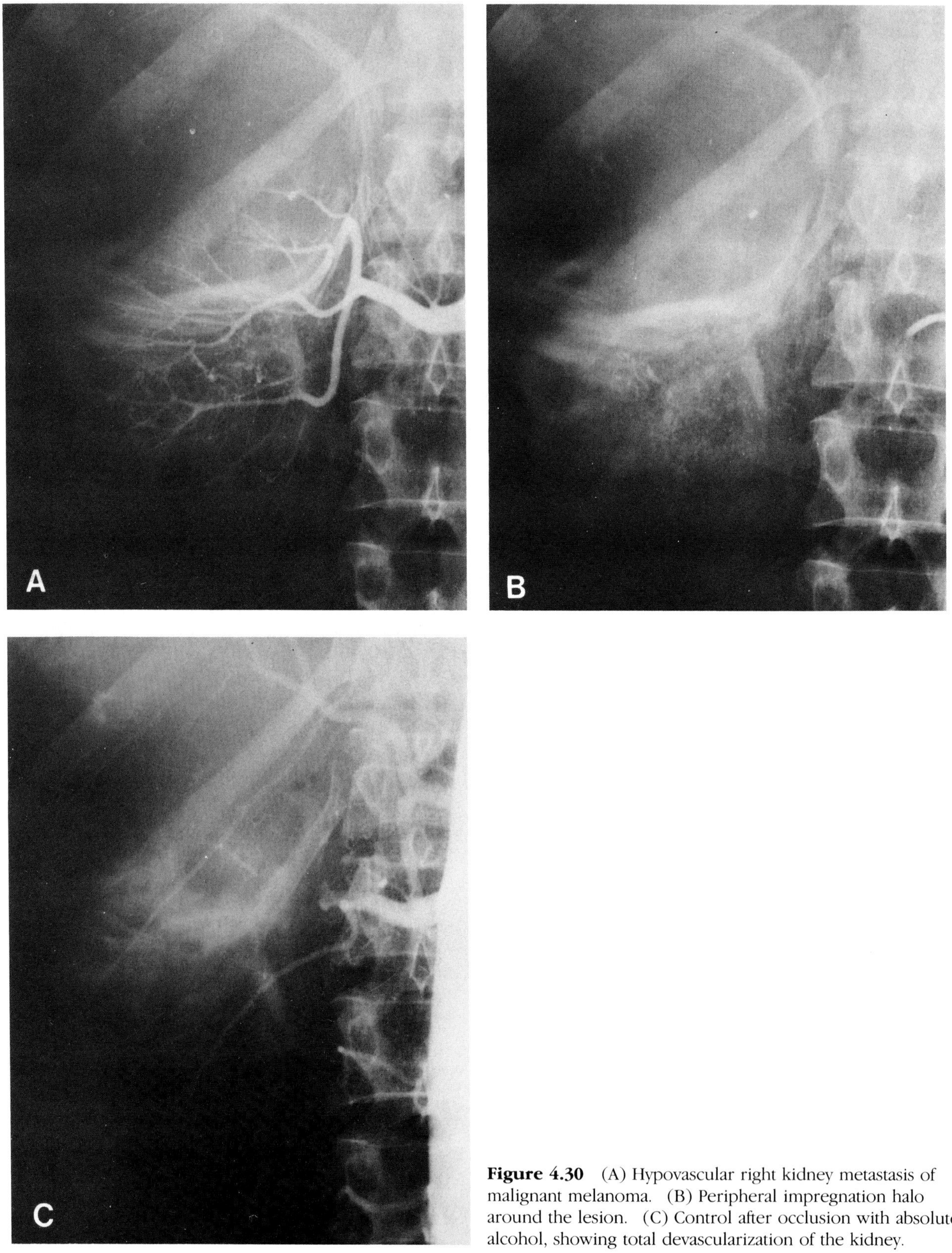

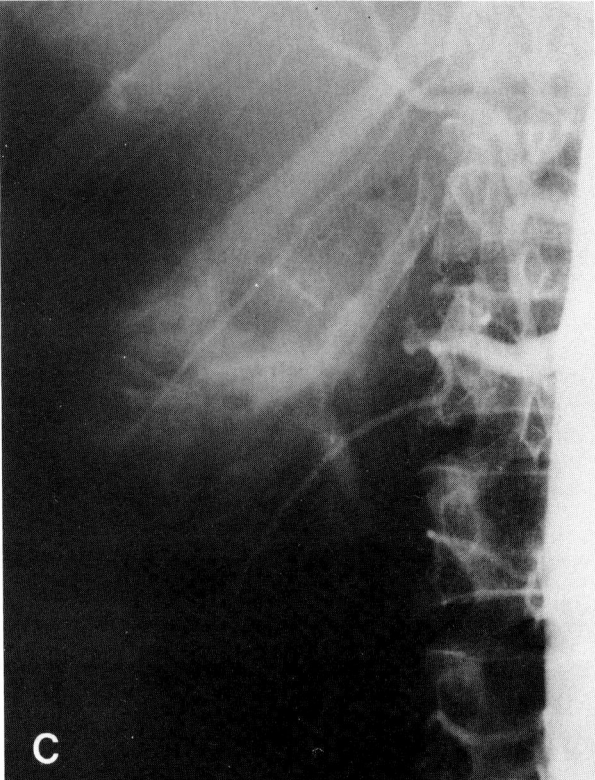

Figure 4.30 (A) Hypovascular right kidney metastasis of malignant melanoma. (B) Peripheral impregnation halo around the lesion. (C) Control after occlusion with absolute alcohol, showing total devascularization of the kidney.

RENAL HEMATURIA OF NONTUMORAL ORIGIN

Hematuria of nontumoral origin can be secondary to a contusion caused by penetrating trauma, diagnostic needle biopsy, or open or percutaneous surgical procedures (e.g., nephrostomy or percutaneous lithotripsy), or due to spontaneous rupture of an aneurysm or renal vascular malformation.

As attested to in the literature, renal trauma with AV fistula and/or a pseudoaneurysm with massive or persistent bleeding frequently requires partial or total nephrectomy to control bleeding. Alternative procedures tried in an attempt to preserve more of the renal parenchyma and function include fistula excision, endofistulorraphy, ligation of renal branch arteries, and occlusion of venous channels.

The therapeutic approach to renal trauma, however, is generally conservative. The patient is kept under observation, and only a few cases eventually require further treatment.

Therapeutic embolization offers an attractive and elegant nonsurgical alternative, with maximum conservation of renal parenchyma and function. The potential of therapeutic embolization has been increasingly recognized as the number of invasive percutaneous and surgical procedures has grown (Figs. 4.31 and 4.32).

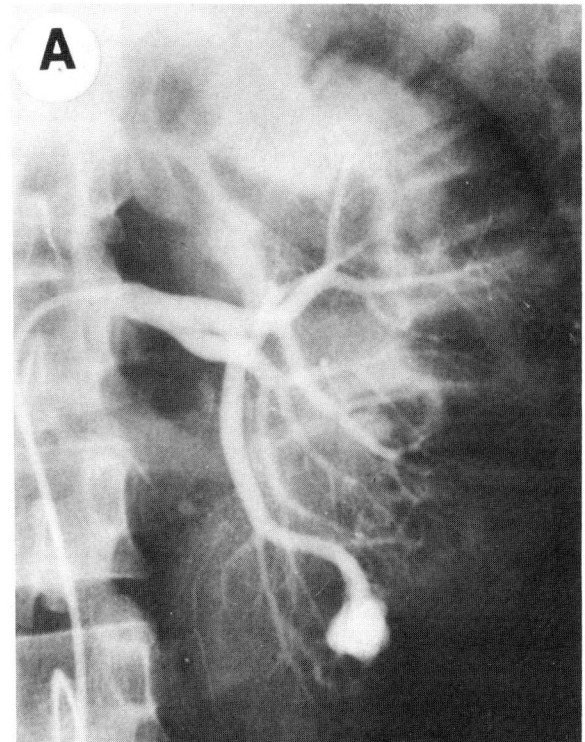

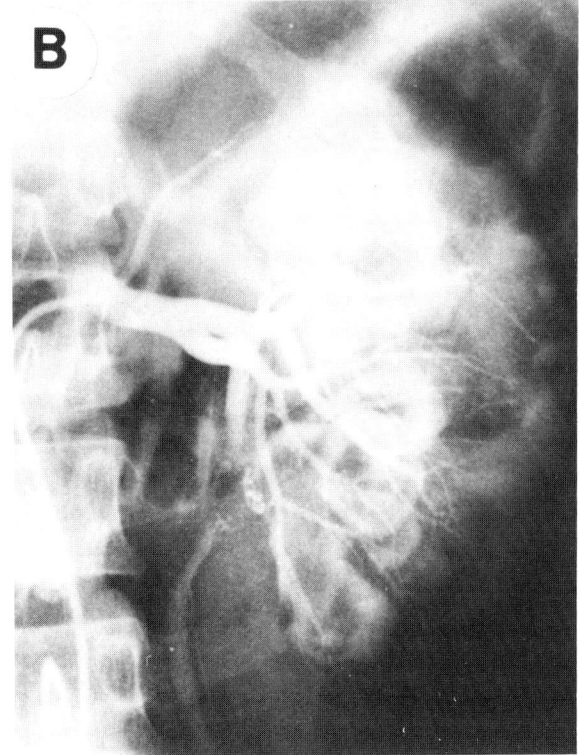

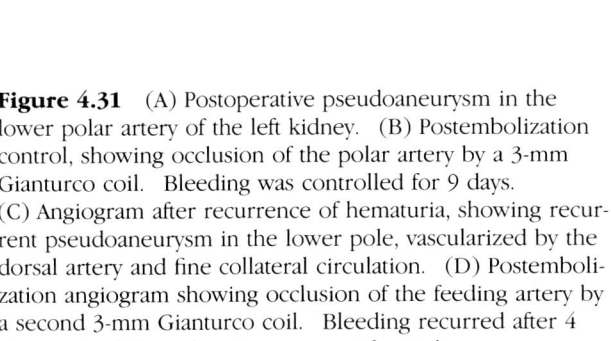

Figure 4.31 (A) Postoperative pseudoaneurysm in the lower polar artery of the left kidney. (B) Postembolization control, showing occlusion of the polar artery by a 3-mm Gianturco coil. Bleeding was controlled for 9 days.
(C) Angiogram after recurrence of hematuria, showing recurrent pseudoaneurysm in the lower pole, vascularized by the dorsal artery and fine collateral circulation. (D) Postembolization angiogram showing occlusion of the feeding artery by a second 3-mm Gianturco coil. Bleeding recurred after 4 days, and a left nephrectomy was performed.

Figure 4.31 *Continued*

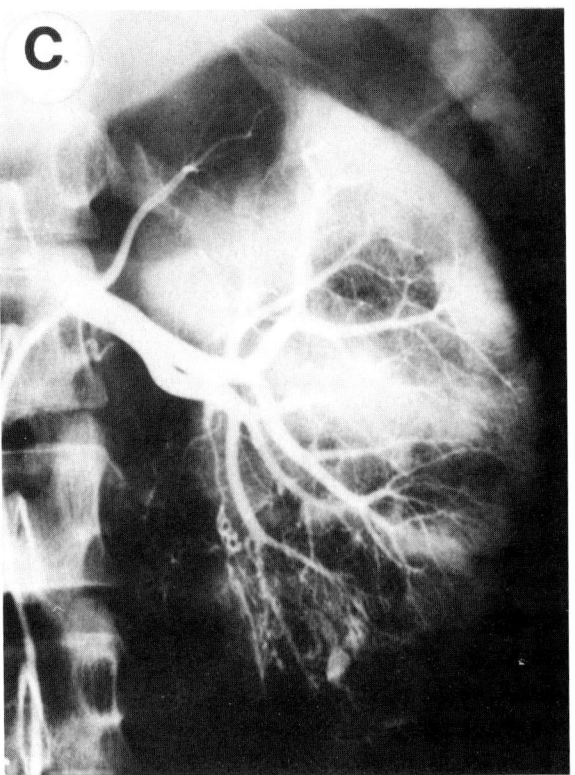

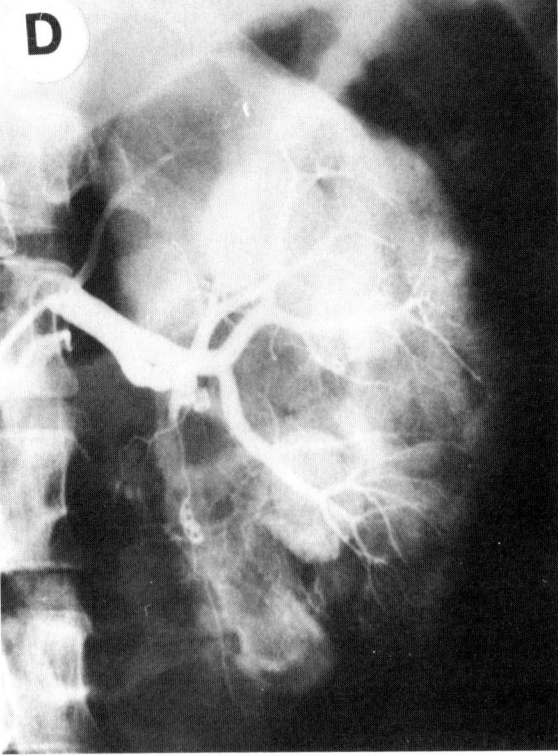

During the last few years, renal embolization for controlling both traumatic and postsurgical hematuria has become so widely accepted clinically that it is now the method of choice for such cases.

In a recent series of 21 cases transcatheter embolization was effective in immediate control of hematuria in 98 percent of patients, even though bleeding recurred in 4 of the 21 (19 percent), requiring new catheterization.

Catheterization and embolization should be very selective in all cases; otherwise ablation of the renal parenchyma will be too extensive. This is of the utmost importance, since the objective of transcatheter occlusion is to preserve the kidney. It is important to utilize a type of occluding material that does not break during introduction (Fig. 2.23). For example, one autologous clot may be enough to temporarily occlude the target renal artery branch and thus to control hematuria, but it is easily broken during injection and may reach a larger number of vessels than intended. Of the range of materials that have been used in embolization of renal hemorrhages, only muscle, dura mater, detachable balloons, and Gianturco coils will not break while being introduced. Of these four, current preference is for balloons and Gianturco coils (Figs. 4.33 and 4.34), which are more easily handled and were effective in the majority of cases in a recently published series.

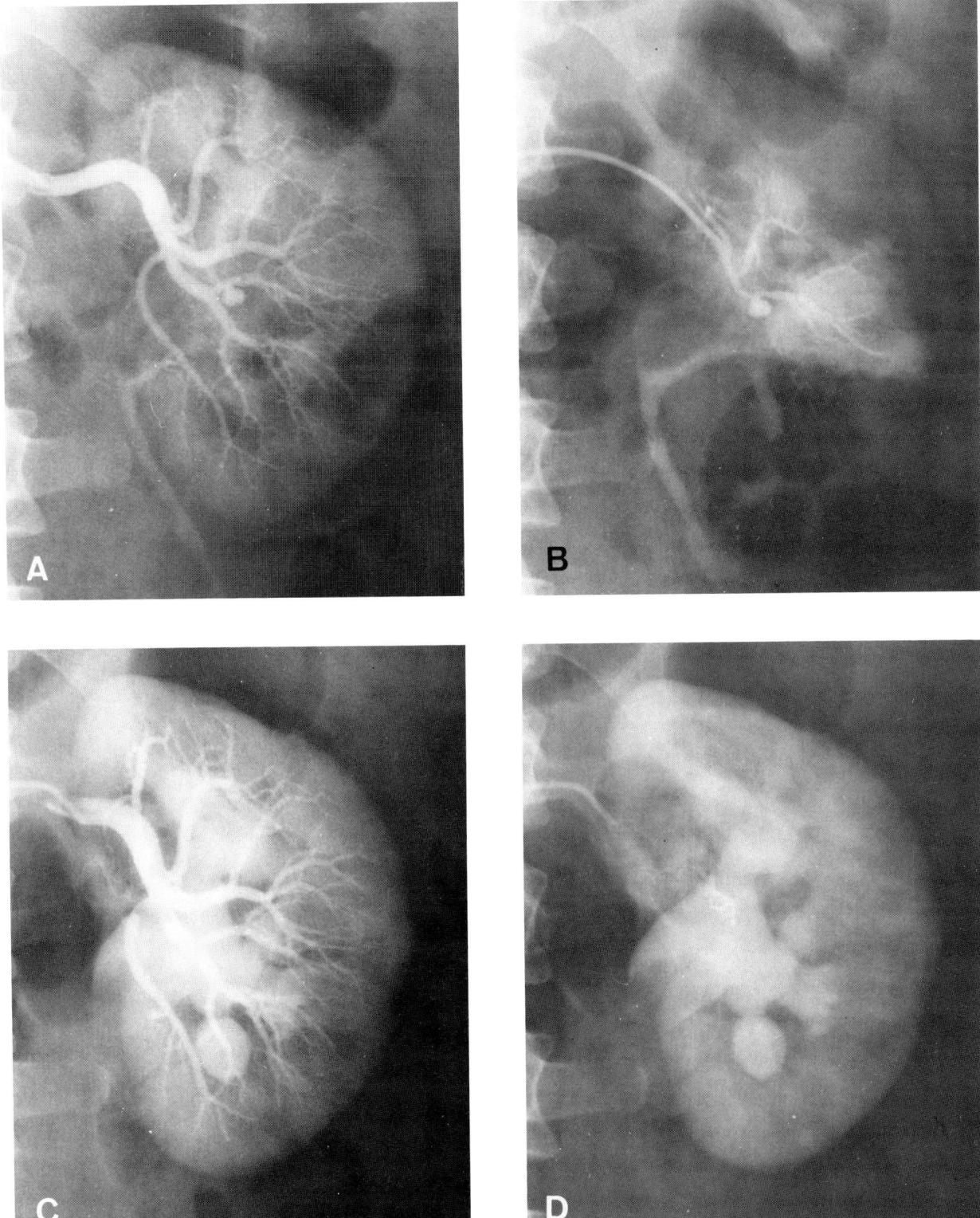

Figure 4.32 35-year-old patient who had surgery for stone removal and percutaneous lithotripsy 20 days earlier, with massive hematuria occurring during the last 7 days.
(A) Selective left renal angiogram showing a small pseudoaneurysm of the renal dorsal arterial branch. (B) Superselective injection into the involved artery showing the lesion. (C,D) Postembolization control angiogram. Embolization with a 3-mm Gianturco coil has completely occluded the vessel and stopped all bleeding. Note that there was no significant loss of renal parenchyma during the nephrographic impregnation stage.

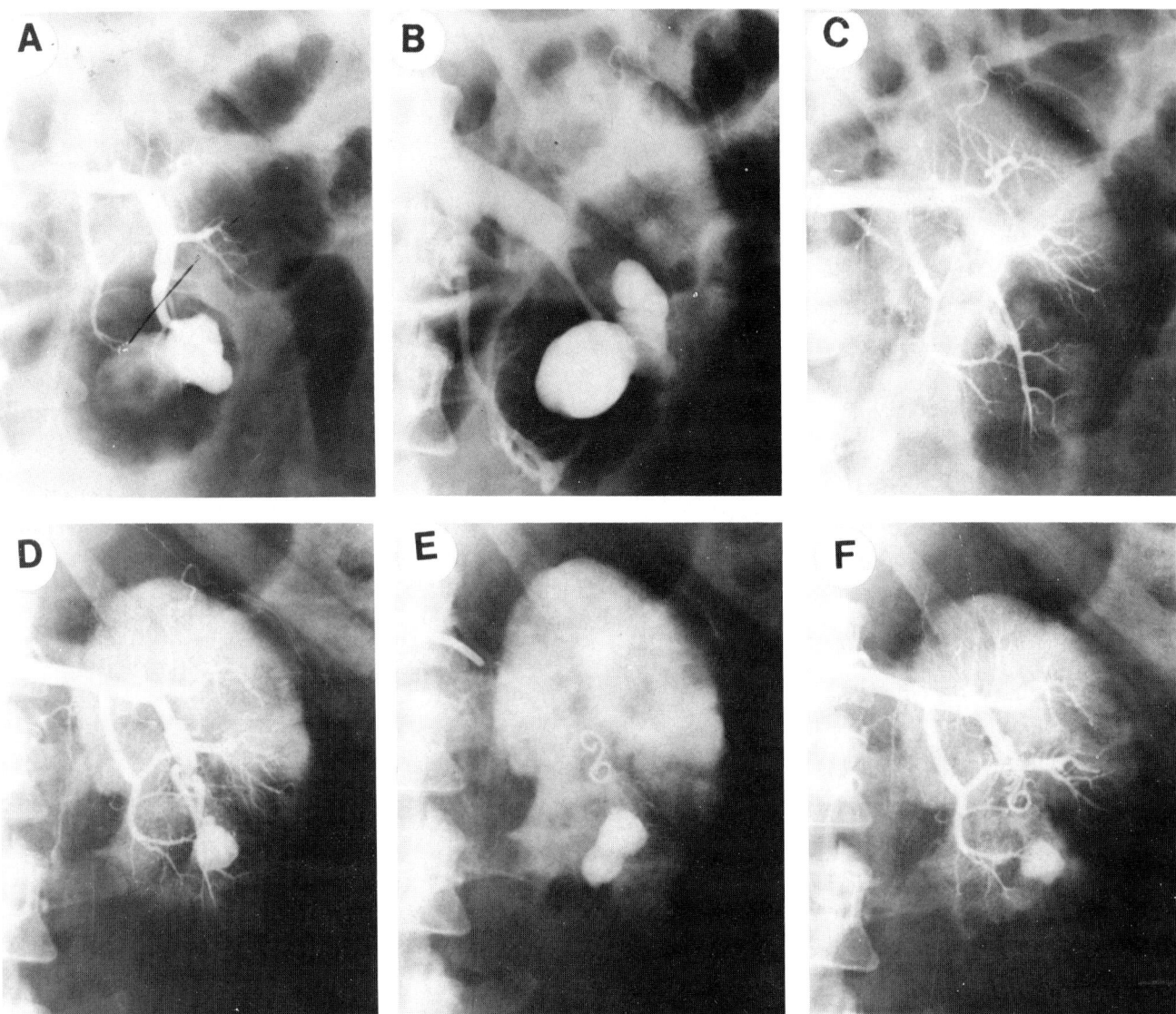

Figure 4.33 Massive hematuria and arteriovenous fistula with pseudoaneurysm following nephrolithotomy.
(A,B) Selective renal angiogram showing a large pseudoaneurysm and massive AV fistula in the lower pole of the left kidney. (C) Control angiogram after embolization of branch artery with a Gianturco coil, preventing opacification of the pseudoaneurysm. Hematuria was controlled, but bleeding recurred after 13 days. (D,E) New angiogram showing recanalization of the pseudoaneurysm through collateral circulation. (F) New angiographic study after embolization with a second Gianturco coil showing occlusion of collaterals and of pseudoaneurysm. Note the residual contrast inside the aneurysm cavity. Hematuria has been permanently controlled.

In more serious cases of trauma with laceration and in kidney transplant patients, the embolization alternative is undoubtedly the best option, as it prevents surgical intervention in these high-risk patients (Figs. 4.35 and 4.36).

In cases of hematuria due to spontaneous rupture of a renal artery aneurysm, careful selective embolization with Gianturco coils, with occlusion of the aneurysm cavity (Fig. 4.37), is effective, allowing for maximal recovery of functioning renal parenchyma. This is particularly important when there is only one kidney (Figs. 4.37 and 4.38).

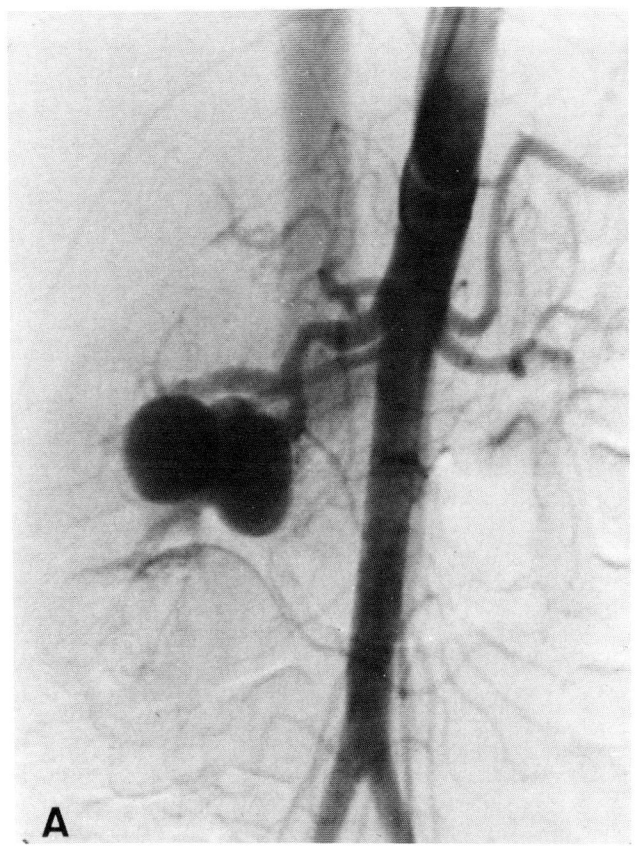
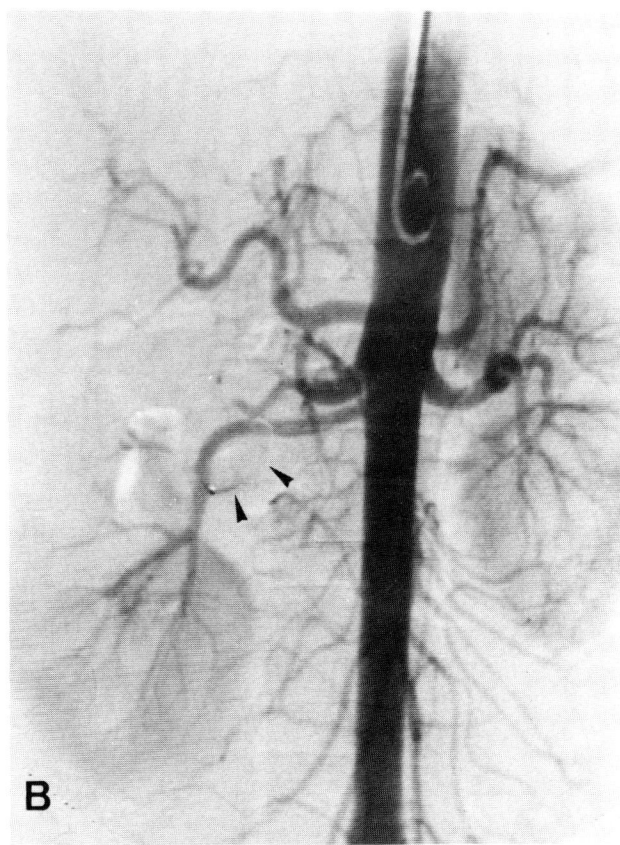
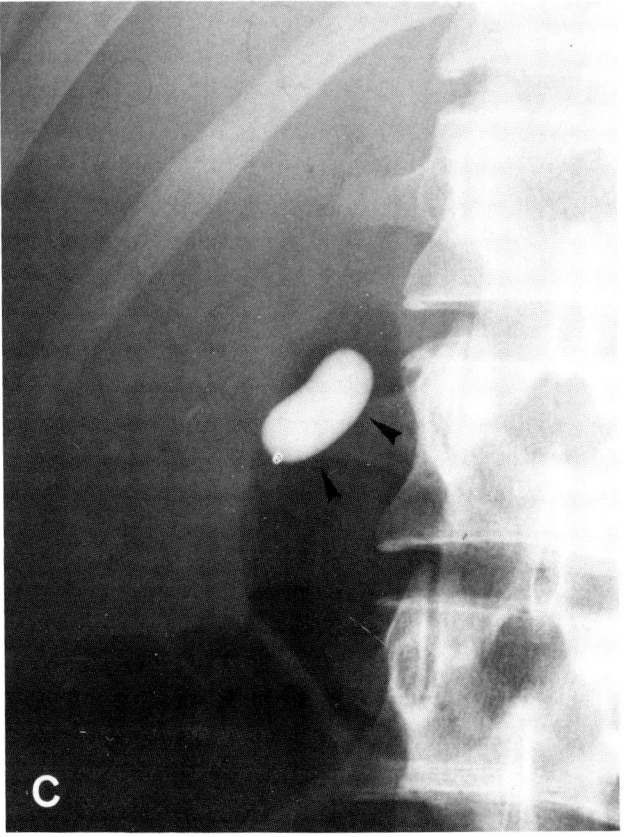

Figure 4.34 15-year-old patient with previous renal needle biopsy followed by hematuria and hypertension for 1 year.
(A) Aortogram showing two pseudoaneurysms with massive arteriovenous fistula on left kidney. Notice the rapid filling of interior vena cava. (B) Control angiogram after embolization of the AV fistula with detachable latex balloon (arrowheads) through left axillary route. Notice occlusion of the involved artery by the AV fistula. (C) Plain abdominal x-ray showing detachable balloon inside the renal artery (arrowheads) filled with nonionic contrast (iopamidol).

HYPERTENSION OF RENAL ORIGIN

To date there is little clinical experience with management of renal hypertension through embolization procedures. However, embolization can be used in two situations for treating the renal causes of systemic hypertension: (1) in cases of segmental arterial stenoses where percutaneous angioplasty cannot be performed, and (2) when the kidney or a segment of the kidney is compromised by a nephrosclerotic type of parenchymatous lesion or renin-producing chronic pyelonephritis. In both cases, the

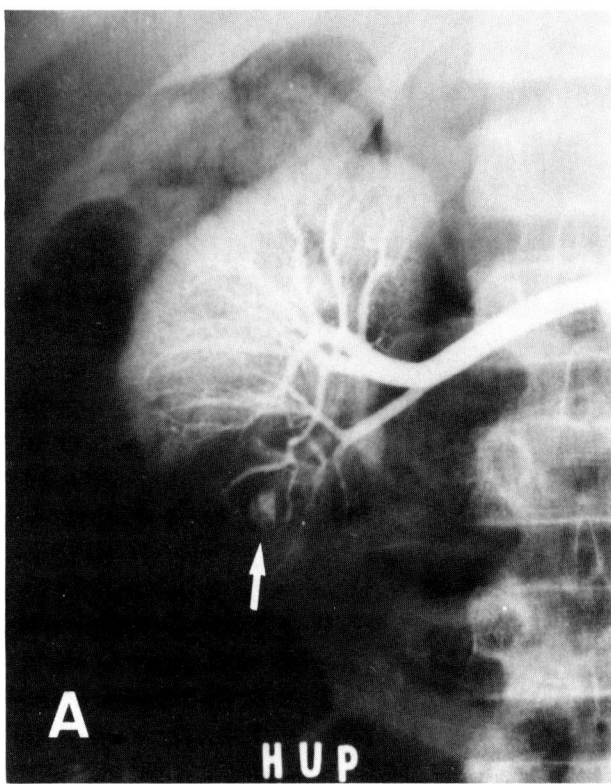
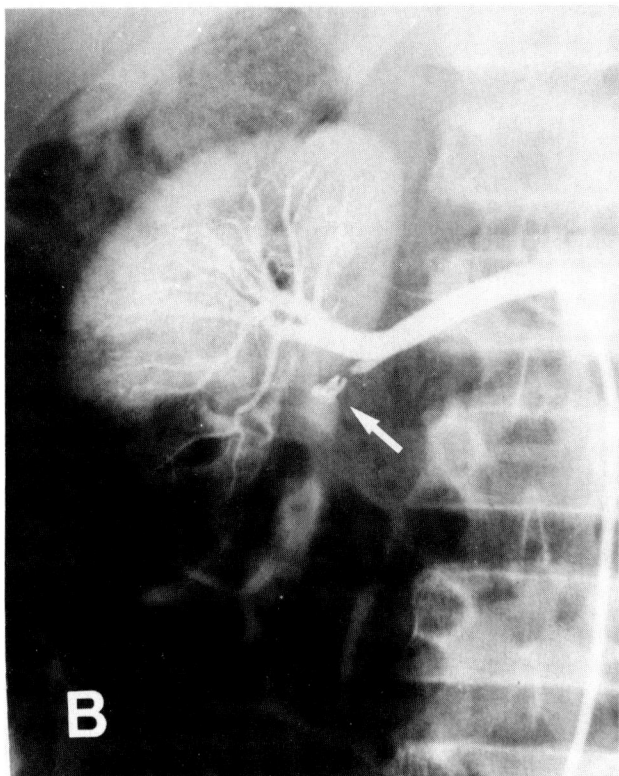

Figure 4.35 (A) Posttraumatic pseudoaneurysm (arrow) with massive hematuria and a cutaneous fistula after surgical drainage of perirenal hematoma. Also evident is a small AV fistula in the lower pole of the kidney. (B) Angiogram following embolization showing occlusion of lower polar artery by 3-mm-diameter Gianturco coil (arrow). Hematuria was permanently controlled after embolization, and the cutaneous fistula closed after 5 days.

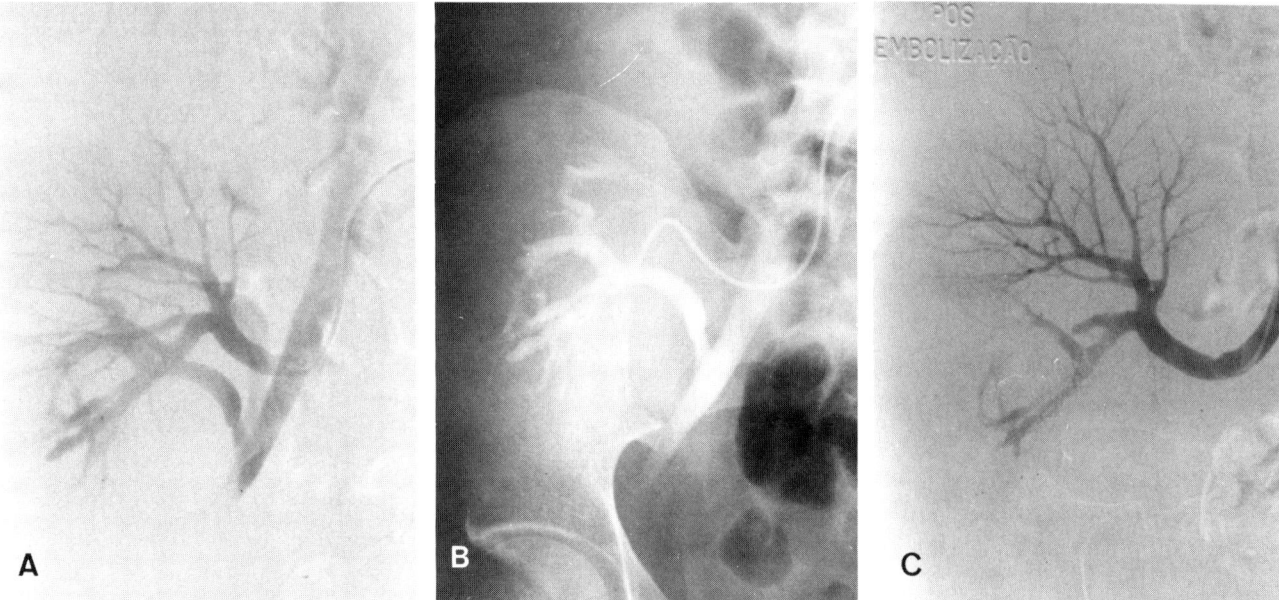

Figure 4.36 Kidney-transplant patient 40 days after operation, with rejection symptoms and perirenal abscess, who received transoperative puncture biopsy during abscess drainage.
(A) High-output AV fistula with high-intensity hematuria.
(B) Superselective catheterization of the involved artery.
(C) Control after embolization with 3-mm Gianturco coils and two Gelfoam particles showing AV fistula closure and hematuria under control. The kidney was eventually rejected and removed about 4 months after the procedure.

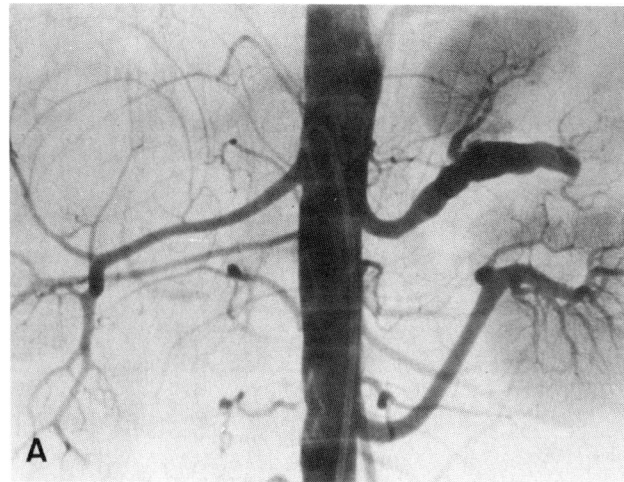
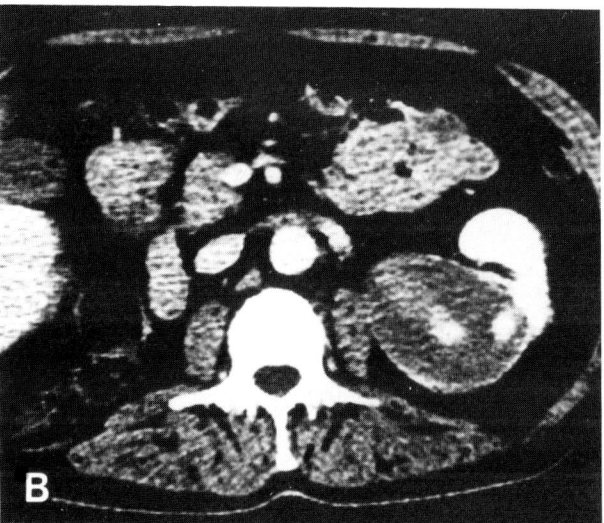
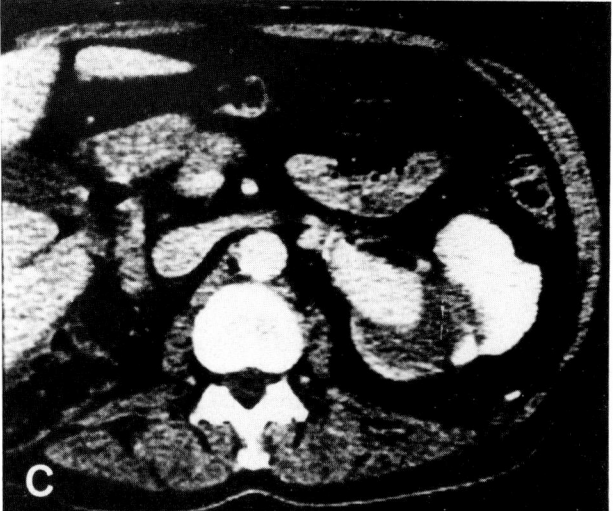
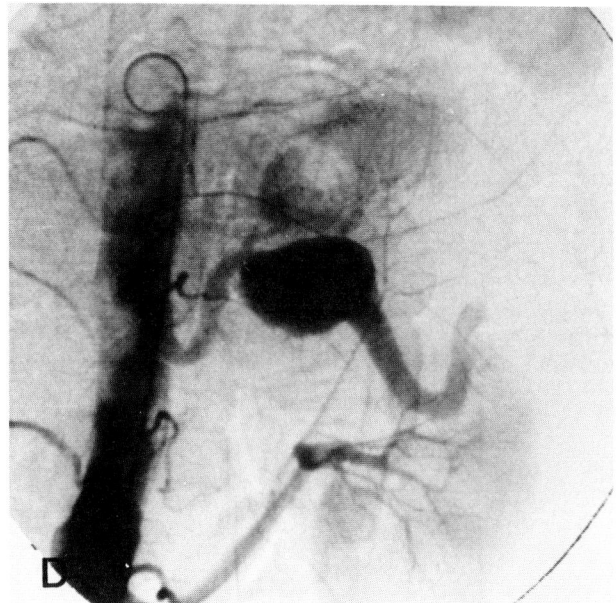

Figure 4.37 58-year-old patient who had right nephrectomy 7 years earlier, for renal tuberculosis. Left intrarenal aneurysm with acute massive hematuria has evolved.

(A) Aortogram showing right kidney with arterial displacement due to tuberculosis and hydronephrosis. Aneurysmatic changes may already be seen in the left renal artery. (B,C) CT scan 7 years after the image in (A) showing axial slice of aneurysm, with opacified lumen and parietal thrombus. (D,E) Digital and conventional angiographic studies showing enlargement of the lumen of aneurysm. (F) Aneurysmal lumen was selectively catheterized, followed by embolization with multiple Gianturco coils and Gelfoam particles and by closure of the ostium with an occlusion balloon catheter. (G,H) Postembolization control angiogram showing occlusion of aneurysm and the remaining renal parenchyma being fed by lower polar renal artery. About one-third of the parenchyma of the single kidney remains. Renal function was maintained within normal limits, and hematuria has been under total control for 6 years.

occlusion of the involved artery should control renin production by suppressing the function of that segment.

The potential for effective use of embolization is increased and the procedure is easier when the involved portion of the kidney is vascularized by an artery independent of the main renal artery (polar artery) (Fig. 4.39).

As the technique of peripheral angioplasty continues to improve, incorporating miniaturized catheters and balloons, it is becoming possible to perform angioplasty in segmental renal branches in more and more cases.

Figure 4.37 *Continued*

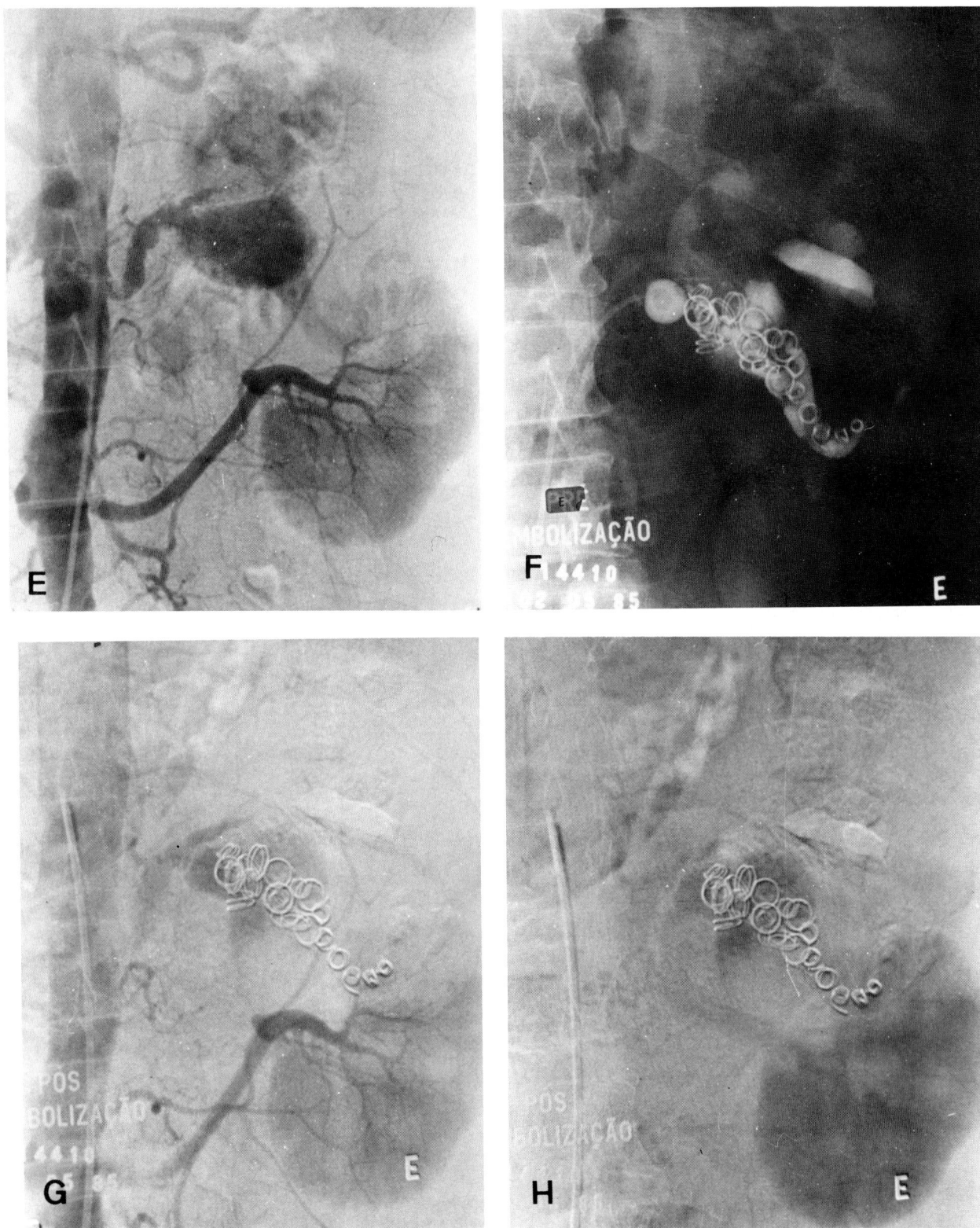

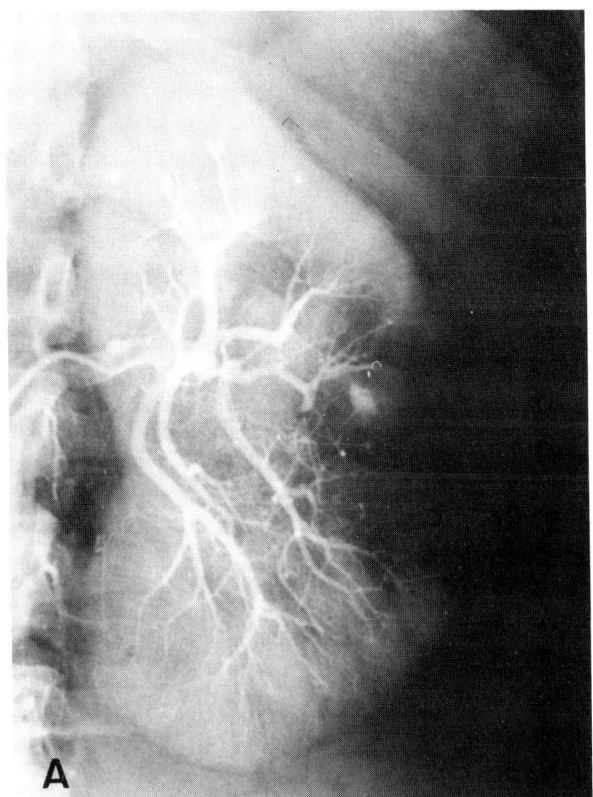
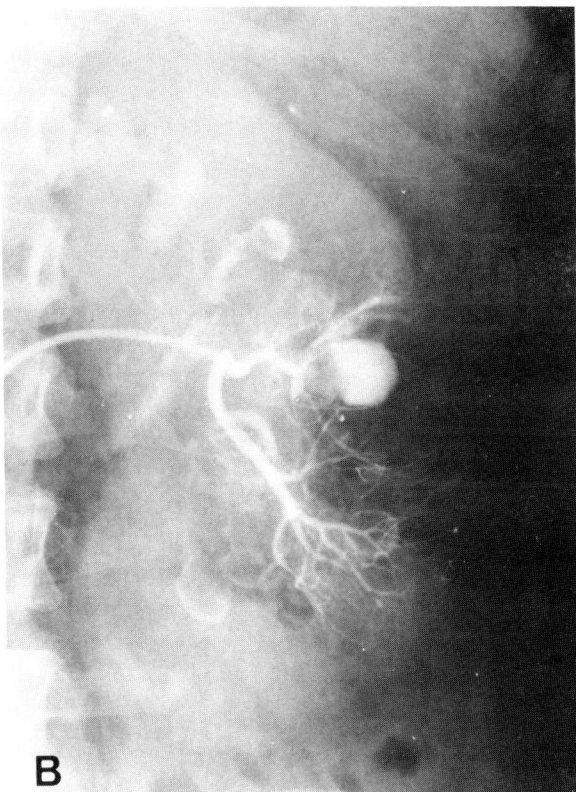
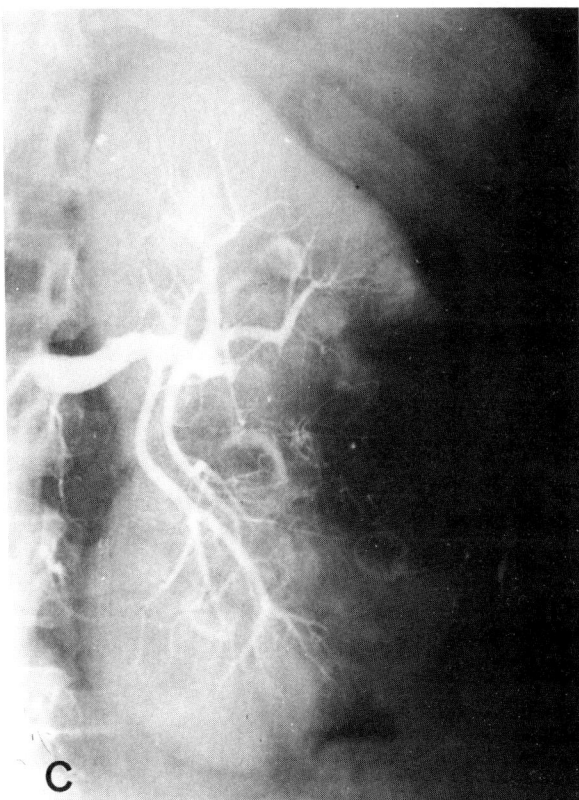

Figure 4.38 Massive hematuria in single kidney following nephrolithotomy.
(A,B) Selective and superselective angiograms showing a filling defect in the nephrogram and pseudoaneurysm formation. (C) Control angiogram after superselective embolization, with 3-mm coil Gianturco, showing occlusion of the involved artery and of the pseudoaneurysm. Bleeding gradually stopped, and renal function remained normal. A perirenal abscess was drained about 2 weeks following embolization, and the patient is still asymptomatic.

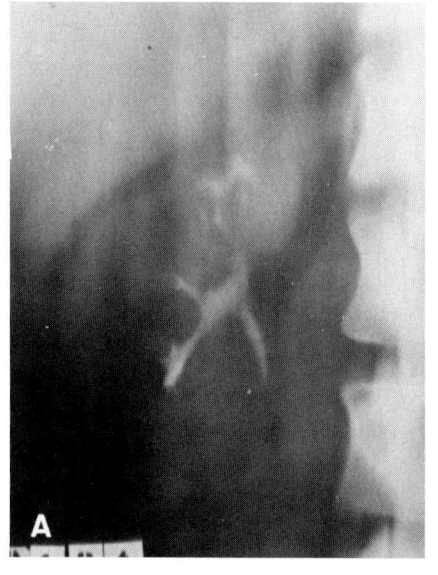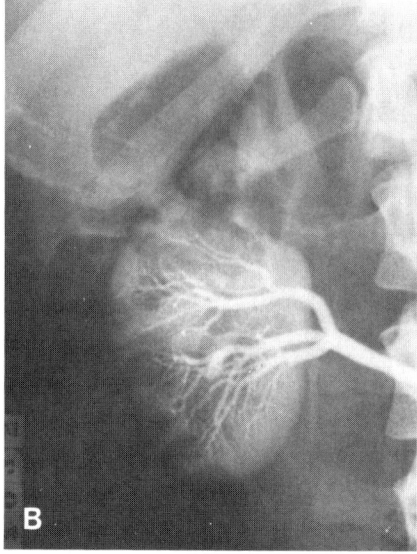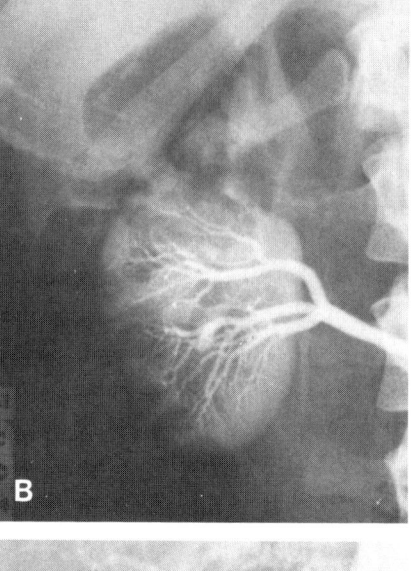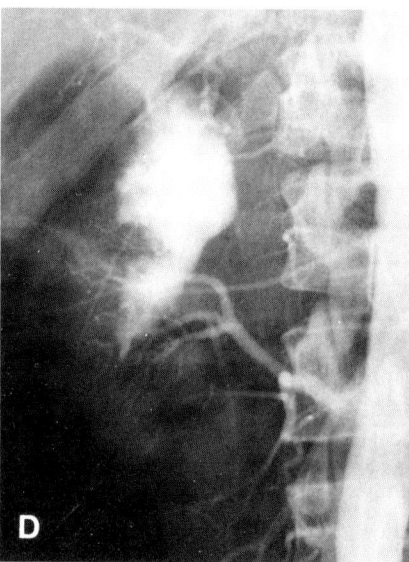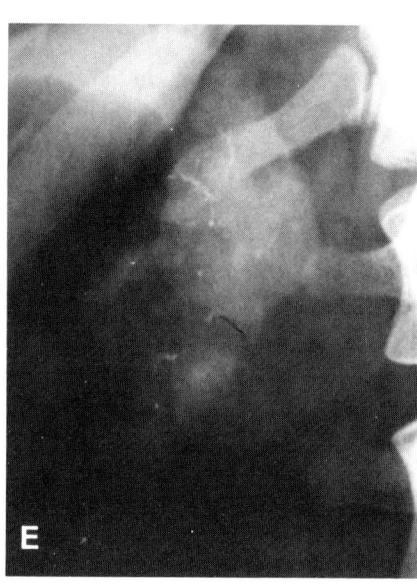

Figure 4.39 Embolization of a pyelonephrotic sequela in a patient with arterial hypertension of renal origin.
(A) Nephrotomogram showing scarring and irregularities on the right upper renal pole. (B,C) Selective arteriogram of right kidney upper polar artery showing vascular lesions consistent with chronic pyelonephrotic lesion. The main artery appears normal. (D) Control after embolization with Gelfoam soaked in Lipiodol, showing arterial occlusion. (E) Right kidney x-ray showing radiopaque material in the right upper pole occluding the arterial vessels. Permanent control of hypertension has been achieved.

REFERENCES

RENAL TUMORS

Cox GG, Lew KR, Price HI, et al. Colonic infarction following ethanol embolization of renal cell carcinoma. *Radiology* 1982;145:343–344.

Ellman BA, Green CE, Eigenbrodt E, et al. Renal infarction with absolute alcohol. *Invest Radiol* 1980;15:318–321.

Ellman BA, Perkhill BJ, Curry TS, et al. Ablation of renal tumors with absolute ethanol: A new technique. *Radiology* 1981;141:619–621.

Paolini RM. Embolization of the renal artery in dogs using alcohol (99.8°C). In *Interventional Radiology*, edited by Oliva P, Viega-Pires JA. Excerpta Medica, Amsterdam, 1982:15–18.

Uflacker R, Paolini RM, Nobrega M. Ablation of tumor and inflammatory tissue with absolute ethanol. *Acta Radiol (Diagn)* 1986;27:131–138.

Wallace S, Chuang VP, Swanson DA, et al. Embolization of renal carcinoma: Experience with 100 patients. *Radiology* 1981;138:563–567.

RENAL HEMATURIA OF NONTUMORAL ORIGIN; HYPERTENSION OF RENAL ORIGINS

Almgard LE, Fernstrom I. Embolic occlusion of an intrarenal aneurysm: A case report. *Br J Urol* 1973;45:485–486.

Andersson I. Renal artery lesions after pyelolithotomy: A potential cause of renovascular hypertension. *Acta Radiol* 1976;17:685–695.

Barbaric ZL, Cutcliff WB. Control of renal arterial bleeding after percutaneous biopsy. *Urology* 1976;8:108–111.

Bookstein JJ, Goldstein HM. Successful management of postbiopsy arteriovenous fistula with selective artery embolization. *Radiology* 1973;109:535–536.

Castaneda-Zuniga WR, Tadavarthy SM, Murphy W, Beranei KI, Amplatz K. Nonsurgical closure of large arteriovenous fistulas. *JAMA* 1976;236:2649–2650.

Chang J, Katzen BT, Sullivan KP. Transcatheter Gelfoam embolization of posttraumatic bleeding pseudoaneurysm. *AJR* 1978;131:645–650.

Charron J, Belanger R, Vauclair R, Leger C, Razavi A. Renal artery aneurysm. *Urology* 1975;5:1–11.

Cho KJ, Stanley JC. Nonneoplastic congenital and acquired renal arteriovenous malformations and fistulas. *Radiology* 1978;129:333–343.

Chuang VP, Reuter SR, Walter J, Foley WD, Bookstein JJ. Control of renal hemorrhage by selective arterial embolization. *AJR* 1975;125:300–306.

Cohen AM, Fisher MF, Voon VS. Total therapeutic embolization of the kidney for hypertension in a child with a mycotic aneurysm. *Cardiovasc Intervent Radiol* 1983;6:121–124.

Cosgrove MD, Mendez R, Morrow JW. Branch artery ligation for renal arteriovenous fistula. *J Urol* 1973;110:632–638.

D'Souza VJ, Glass TA, Velasquez G, et al. Nonsurgical treatment of childhood hypertension: Embolization of an intrarenal aneurysm. *Cardiovasc Intervent Radiol* 1984;7:229–231.

Ehrlich RM. Renal arteriovenous fistula treated by endofistulorrhaphy. *Arch Surg* 1975;110:1195–1198.

Goldman ML, Fellner SK, Parrott TS. Transcatheter embolization of renal arteriovenous fistula. *Urology* 1975;6:386–390.

Grace DM, Pitt DF, Gold RE. Vascular embolization and occlusion by angiographic techniques as an aid or alternative to operation. *Surg Gynecol Obstet* 1976;143:469–475.

Kadir S, Marchall FF, White Jr. RI, Kaufman SL, Barth KH. Therapeutic embolization of the kidney with detachable silicone balloons. *J Urol* 1983;129:11–13.

Kalish M, Greenbaum L, Silber S, Goldstein H. Traumatic renal hemorrhage treatment by arterial embolization. *J Urol* 1974;112:138–141.

Katzen BT, Rossi P, Passariello R, Simonetti G. Transcatheter therapeutic arterial embolization. *Radiology* 1976;120:523–531.

Kaufman SL, Freeman C, Busky SM, White Jr. RI. Management of postoperative renal hemorrhage by transcatheter embolization. *J Urol* 1976;115:202–205.

Keller FS, Rosch J, Baur GM, Taylor LM, Dotter CT, Porter JM. Percutaneous angiographic embolization: a procedure of increasing usefulness: review of a decade of experience. *Am J Surg* 1981;142:5–11.

Kerber CW, Freeny PC, Cromwell L, Margolis MT, Correa Jr. RJ. Cyanoacrylate occlusion of a renal arteriovenous fistula. *Am J Roentgen* 1977;128:663–665.

Klamut M, Szczerbo-Trojanowska M, Kowalewski J, Nowakowski A. Transcatheter embolization in a haemophiliac with post-traumatic renal haemorrhage. Report of a case. *Acta Radiol* 1979;20:606–608.

Lea Thomas M, Lamb GHR. Selective arterial embolization in the management of post operative renal hemorrhage. *Acta Radiol* 1977;18:49–53.

Leiter E, Gribetz D, Cohen S. Arteriovenous fistula after percutaneous needle biopsy—surgical repair with preservation of renal function. *N Engl Med* 1972;287:971–972.

Marshall FF, White Jr. RI, Kaufman SL, Barth KH. Treatment of traumatic renal arteriovenous fistulas by detachable silicone balloon embolization. *J Urol* 1979;122:237–239.

Mathieu J, Schulman CC, Struyven J. Percutaneous embolic occlusion of an acquired bleeding intrarenal aneurysm. *Eur Urol* 1978;4:212–213.

Mazer MJ, Baltaxe HA, Wolf GL. Therapeutic embolization of the renal artery with Gianturco coils: limitations and technical pitfalls. *Radiology* 1981;138:37–46.

Meaney TF, Chicatelli PD. Obliteration of renal arteriovenous fistula by transcatheter clot embolization. Case report and experimental observations. *Cleveland Clin Q* 1974;41:33–38.

Pontes JR, Parekh N, McGuckin JT, Banks MD, Pierce JM. Percutaneous transfemoral embolization of arterio-infundibular-venous fistula. *J Urol* 1976;116:98–99.

Reuter SR, Pomeroy PR, Chuang VP, et al. Embolic control of hypertension caused by segmental renal artery stenosis. *AJR* 1976;127:389–392.

Richman SD, Green WM, Kroll R, Casarella WJ. Superselective transcatheter embolization of traumatic renal hemorrhage. *AJR* 1977;128:843–844.

Rizk GK, Atallah NK, Bridi GI. Renal arteriovenous fistula treated by catheter embolization. *Br J Radiol* 1973;46:222–224.

Rosen RJ, Feldman L, Wilson AR. Embolization for postbiopsy renal arteriovenous fistula: effective occlusion using homologous clot. *AJR* 1978;131:1072–1388.

Silber SJ, Clark RE. Treatment of massive hemorrhage after renal biopsy with angiographic injection of clot. *N Engl J Med* 1975;292:1387–1388.

Smith JN, Hinnan F. Intrarenal arterial aneurysms. *J Urol* 1967;97:990–996.

Tucci P, Doctor D, Diagonale A. Embolization of post-traumatic renal arteriovenous fistula. *Urology* 1979;13:192–194.

Tunner WS, Middleton RG, Watson RW, Marshall VF. Repair of an intrarenal arteriovenous fistula with preservation of the kidney. *J Urol* 1970;103:286–289.

Tynes WV, Devine Jr. CJ, Devine PC, Poutasse EF. Surgical treatment of renal arteriovenous fistulas: report of 5 cases. *J Urol* 1970;103:692–697.

Uflacker R. Radiologia intervencionista: uma especialidade emergente. *Rad Bras* 1983;16:71–85.

Uflacker R. Transcatheter embolization of arterial aneurysms. *Br J Radiol* 1986;59:317–324.

Uflacker R, Paolini RM, Lima S. Management of traumatic hematuria be selective renal artery embolization. *J Urol* 1984;132:662–667.

Uflacker R, Saadij. Transcatheter embolization of superior mesenteric arteriovenous fistula. *Am J Roentgen* 1982;139:1212–1214.

Wallace S, Gianturco C, Anderson JH, Goldstein HM, Davis LJ, Bree RL. Therapeutic vascular occlusion utilizing steel coil technique: clinical applications. *AJR* 1976;127:381–387.

Wallace S, Schwarten DE, Smith DC, Gerson LP, Davis LJ. Intrarenal arteriovenous fistulas: transcatheter steel coil occlusion. *J Urol* 1978;120:282–286.

Walter JF, Bookstein JJ, Kramer RA, Cannon WB, Trollope ML, Jamplis RW. Therapeutic angiography. Its value to the surgical patient. *Arch Surg* 1978;113:432–439.

White Jr. RI, Kaufman SL, Barth KH, DeCaprio V, Strandbert JD. Embolotherapy with detachable silicone balloons: technique and clinical results. *Radiology* 1979;131:619–627.

Zollikofer C, Castaneda-Zuniga W, Nath PH et al. Vascular pseudotumors of the kidney. *Radiologe* 1980;20:577–584.

Thoracic Embolization

RENAN UFLACKER

PULMONARY ARTERIOVENOUS FISTULAS

Pulmonary arteriovenous fistula (PAVF) is a vascular change characterized by abnormal communication between the arterial and venous systems, with absence of capillary circulation.

This abnormality may be either congenital or acquired. Congenital PAVF if more frequent, and almost 50 percent of patients with hereditary hemorrhagic telangiectasis (HHT) (Rendu-Osler-Weber disease) also have PAVF. HHT is an autosomal dominant disease characterized by vascular dysplasia, with the vascular wall reduced to endothelium, lacking any elastic support or contractility.

Acquired PAVF is related to trauma, pulmonary schistosomiasis, pulmonary metastases, or slowly developing hepatic cirrhosis. PAVF is more frequently located in the lower lobes of the lungs and in subpleural space. It is multiple in nature in 33 to 50 percent of patients, bilateral in 8 to 20 percent, and systemic in only 4 percent.

Pulmonary arteriovenous fistulas are conveniently classified as solitary, multiple with varying sizes, multiple with uniform size, and diffuse (telangiectatic). Morphologically, PAVF may be classified as simple or complex.

The simple type, which occurs in 79 percent of cases, is formed with only one pulmonary feeding artery, with direct communication through an aneurysm to a single pulmonary vein. (See Fig. 4.40.) The complex type, which occurs in 21 percent of cases, has multiple feeding arteries and drainage veins. The connection between artery and vein is aneurysmal; however, it is septated,

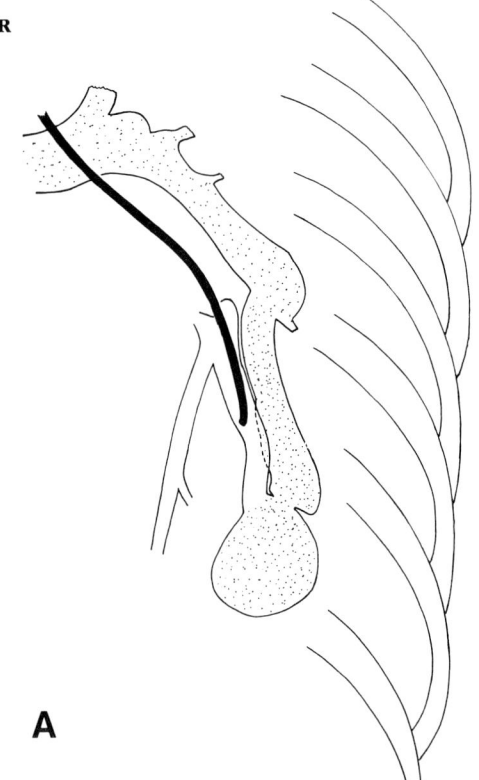

A

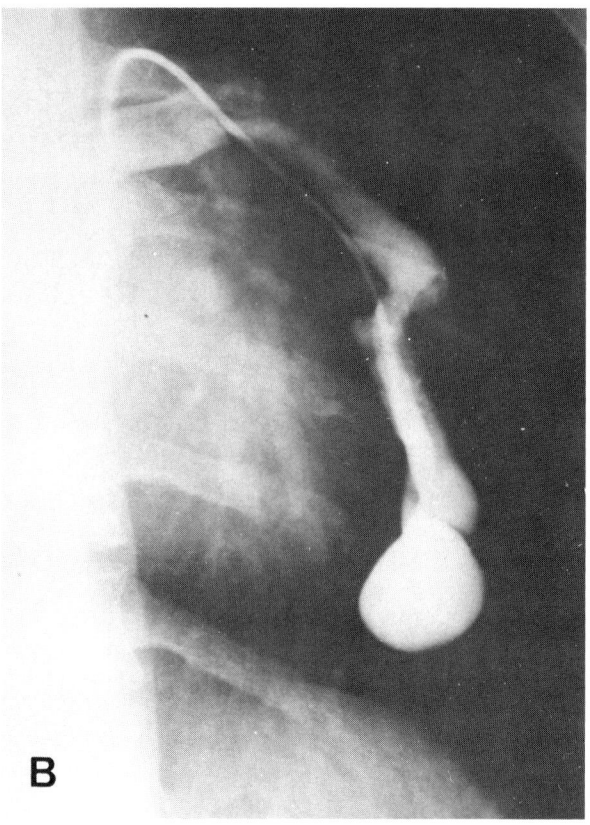

B

Figure 4.40 44-year-old patient with simple, bilateral, morphologic-type pulmonary arteriovenous fistula presenting with hemoptysis. At age 29 a right inferior lobectomy was performed.
(A) Schematic drawing of a simple PAVF. Note the single feeding artery, the single pulmonary drainage vein, and the large aneurysm. (B) A PAVF on the left lower lobe, with single artery and vein. (C) Postembolization angiogram showing occlusion of the fistula by a latex balloon (Debrun technique) (arrow) and, more proximally, by a Gianturco spring coil (arrows). (D) Angiogram showing a PAVF on the right upper lobe. (E) Same as (D), lateral view. (F) Postembolization angiogram showing occlusion of the right-upper-lobe fistula by a Gianturco spring coil (arrows).

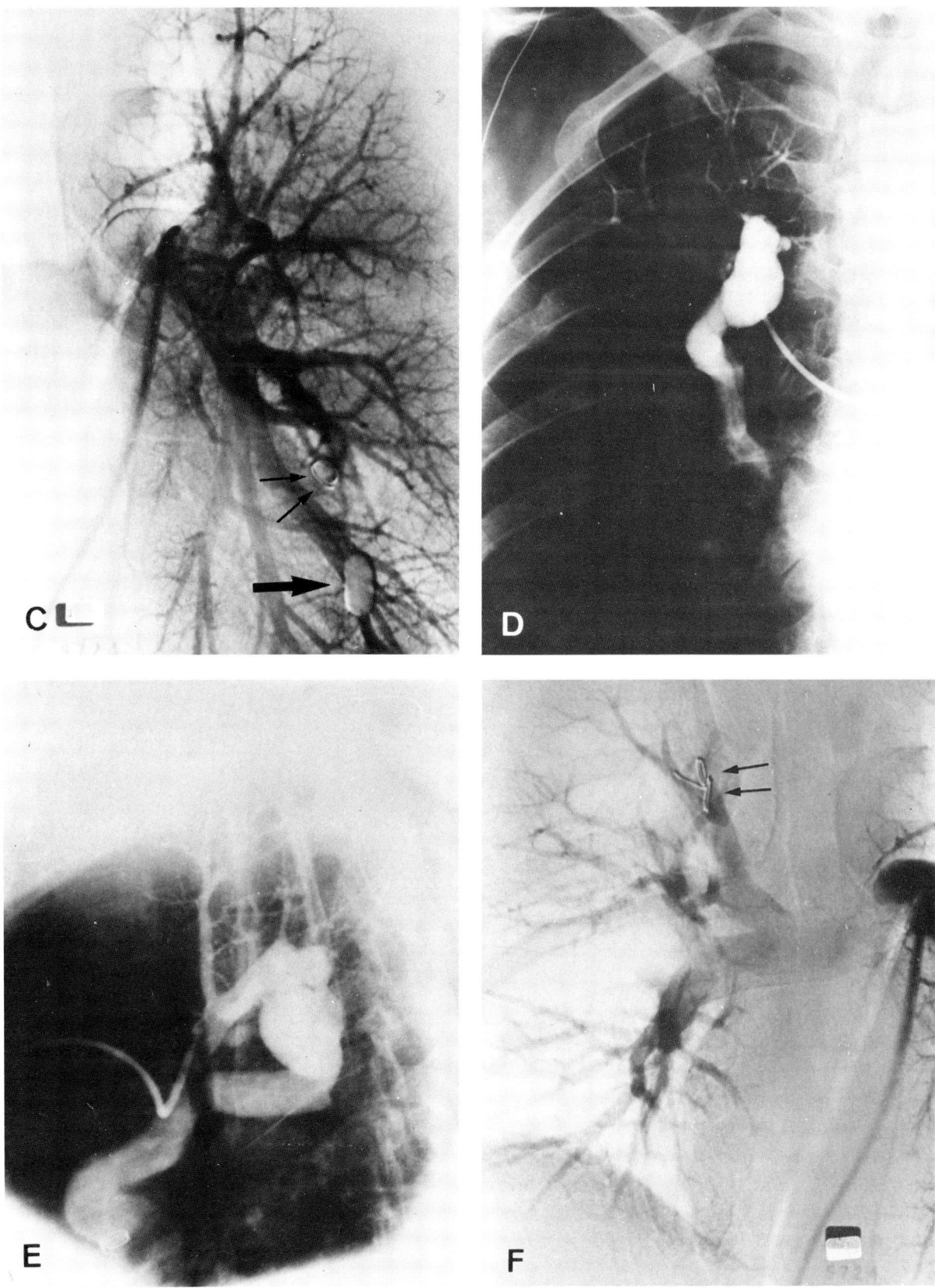

Figure 4.40 *Continued*

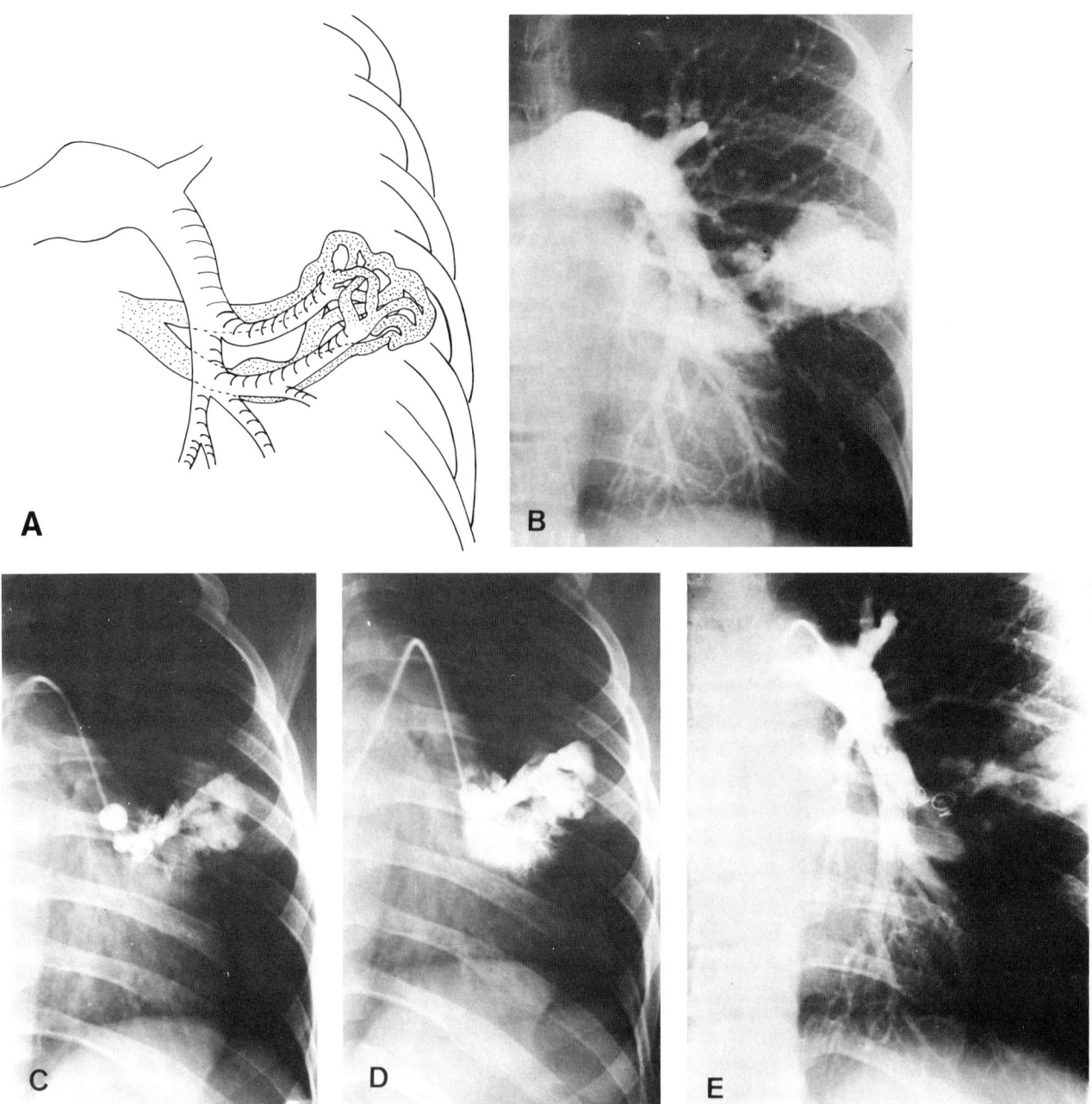

Figure 4.41 25-year-old patient with a single, complex PAVF on the left lung.
(A) Schematic drawing of a complex, cirsoid PAVF with two feeding arteries and several drainage drains. (B) Complex PAVF. (C,D) Selective catheterization of one of the arteries with an occluding balloon catheter for purposes of measurement. (E) Postembolization angiogram showing occlusion of the fistula by Gianturco spring coils.

with cirsoid appearance and divided into multiple vessels. (See Fig. 4.41.)

The most significant pathophysiologic change is related to the arteriovenous shunt. If the shunt is small, no change occurs. In fistulas with larger diameter and output, significant volumes of nonoxygenated blood get into the systemic circulation, causing cyanosis, digital clubbing, dyspnea, polycythemia, and an increase in red blood cell count. In contrast to cases of peripheral fistulas, pulmonary shunts do not cause hemodynamic changes; heart rate, arterial blood pressure, and cardiac output remain normal.

When PAVF is associated with Rendu-Osler-Weber disease, the presence of telangiectasia in other areas may lead to epistaxis, hematuria, and hematemesis.

Local and systemic complications of PAVF include hemoptysis, pulmonary hematoma, hemothorax, and hemorrhagic shock. Brain abscess and embolism, which are present in 33 to 41 percent of patients with HHT and in 18 percent of non-HHT patients, may be the first symptoms of PAVF.

Some authors offer surgery as a viable treatment for PAVF, even for asymptomatic lesions, but the presence of multiple and bilateral lesions makes surgical treatment a poor alternative, due to the fact that extensive pulmonary resection is impossible.

Recently, percutaneous transcatheter embolization has been used, with outstanding success, as the treatment of choice for these fistulas. Diagnostic angiography should be carefully performed, using selective catheterization and taking several anteroposterior and oblique views, in order to clearly distinguish the feeding vessel(s) from the venous drainage, which may be single or multiple (Figs. 4.40 and 4.41).

It is important to classify PAVF as simple or complex, since simple fistulas require only one large-diameter balloon for occlusion, while complex fistulas require several balloons or Gianturco coils.

In complex-type fistulas each vessel must be individually embolized. All symptomatic patients should undergo embolization, provided that the fistula has a diameter under 2 cm, which is the size limit of currently available detachable balloons. All PAVF over 3 mm in diameter should also be embolized, even if the patient is asymptomatic, to prevent stroke and brain abscess formation.

Embolization using a detachable balloon is very well suited for treating PAVF, because when the balloon is inflated, its diameter, location, and effectiveness of the occlusion may be adjusted before it is detached from the introducing catheter. Gianturco coils are a valid alternative and these may be used in conjunction with a balloon as a safety precaution against the unlikely occurrence of balloon deflation.

Complications are usually minimal, involving small infarctions due to occlusion of normal pulmonary arterial branches. If embolization is limited to those lesions of sizes compatible with the embolizing material, the embolizing material will not cross the fistula. There is no reference in the literature to systemic embolism due to PAVF embolization.

POSTSURGICAL THORACIC BLEEDING

Postsurgical thoracic bleeding is basically limited to three vascular territories: pulmonary artery and bronchial and thoracic wall circulation.

Postsurgical bleeding related to pulmonary circulation usually occurs in cases in which ablation surgery has been performed on one pulmonary lobe or segment and a dehiscence or fistula has occurred. In such cases bleeding may occur, particularly after physical effort (Fig. 4.42). Embolization with coils or detachable balloon is the best treatment option.

The bronchial arteries may bleed operatively or postoperatively, for example, in cases in which some areas in the lung have remained bloody after correction of an older inflammatory process, such as a bronchial fistula, (Fig. 4.43). In most cases embolization of the bronchial arteries with Gelfoam or coils effectively stops the bleeding.

The thoracic wall may present postoperative bleeding originating from the intercostal, internal mammary, and subclavian artery branches. Embolization of intercostal and internal mammary arteries with Gelfoam is effective in controlling this type of bleeding.

HEMOPTYSIS

Massive hemoptysis is a highly significant clinical and surgical problem. It is associated with a 50 to 100 percent mortality rate, death usually being due to asphyxia rather than to hypovolemia.

The primary cause of massive or repeated hemoptysis is active or residual pulmonary tuberculosis. Tuberculosis is generally cured by the use of tuberculostatic agents only. In 80 to 90 percent of patients, there are no significant complications. Of the 10 to 20 percent of patients who do develop chronic lung disease, a significant number experience massive hemoptysis. The main causes of massive hemoptysis other than tuberculosis are, in order of importance, bronchiectasis, pneumoconiosis, bronchial aspergilloma, carcinoma, and cystic fibrosis.

Surgery (thoracotomy) is the definitive treatment for massive hemoptysis; however, this is viable only for those few patients who present with a unilateral, highly localized disease. Surgery is contraindicated for patients with diffuse, advanced, and bilateral lung disease. In the past, treatment for such patients was limited to clinical maintenance: diagnosis of bleeding location through bronchoscopy, postural pulmonary drainage, rest, and volemic replacement. Today, embolization of bronchial arteries is the treatment of choice for control of hemoptoic bleeding. In fact, bronchial embolization is the primary method of treatment for massive or repeated hemoptysis, either isolated or associated with other treatment methods such as tuberculostatic agents or surgical resection.

Bronchial embolization has three well-defined objectives: (1) immediate control of bleeding in all cases; (2)

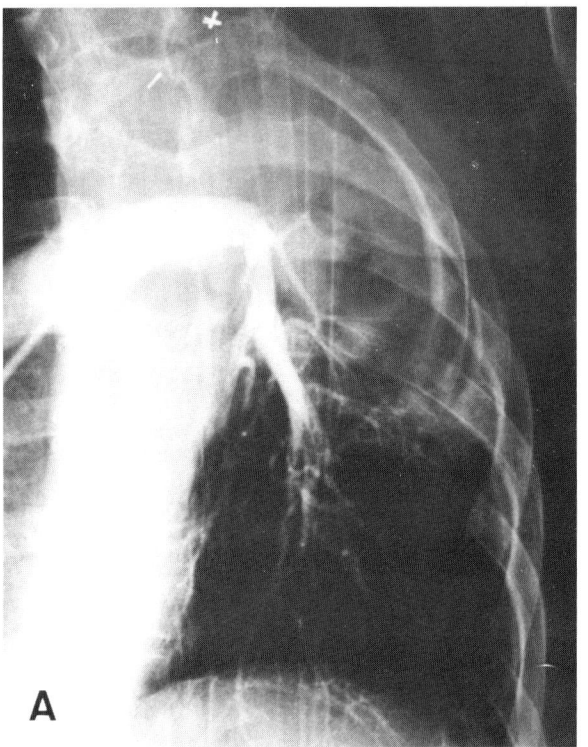 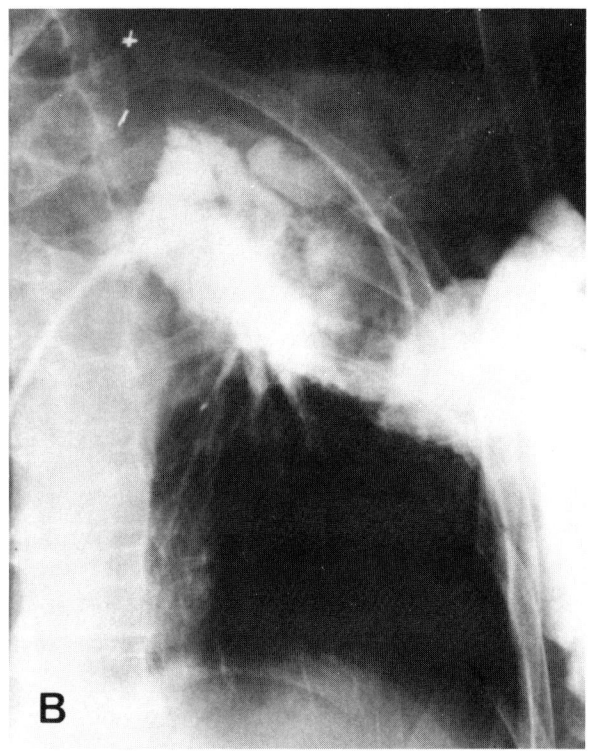

Figure 4.42 Patient immediately post left upper lobectomy, with bleeding through the surgical incision during coughing episodes.
(A) Amputation of left upper lobe branches of the pulmonary artery. Notice arterial wall irregularities. (B) There is a massive contrast medium extravasation inside and outside the thoracic wall during cough. Partial embolization of left pulmonary artery was performed with Gianturco coils (not shown). This improved but did not control bleeding, and corrective surgery became necessary (Courtesy of Dr. Flavio Aesse).

long-term control of bleeding in patients for whom surgery is contraindicated; and (3) improvement of the patient's clinical condition for prospective surgery.

It is well known that surgery during a massive hemoptysis episode results in high mortality and morbidity, with transoperative bleeding, asphyxia, bronchopleural fistula, and ventilation failure, and surgeons welcome any preoperative aid, or treatment which may make the surgical procedure unnecessary.

Highly detailed knowledge of the anatomy of the bronchial arteries is critical for performing bronchial angiography and embolization. According to Cauldwell's classic 1948 study, in 90 percent of cases bronchial artery anatomy is one of four types:

Type I: Two bronchial arteries on the left and one intercostal bronchial trunk (ICBT) on the right (40.6 percent)
Type II: One bronchial artery on the left and one ICBT on the right (21.3 percent)
Type III: Two bronchial arteries on the left and two on the right, one of which is an ICBT (20.6 percent)
Type IV: One bronchial artery on the left and two on the right, one of which is an ICBT (9.7 percent)

Cauldwell's classification was based on dissection. A different classification, on angiographic findings in 72 patients, is perhaps closer to reality (Fig. 4.44). Ten different arterial distribution patterns are described (Fig. 4.44):

Pattern I: One ICBT on the right and a bronchial artery on the left (30.5 percent)
Pattern II: One ICBT on the right, and a common trunk with a bronchial artery on the right, and one on the left (25.0 percent)
Pattern III: One ICBT on the right and two bronchial arteries on the left (12.5 percent)
Pattern IV: One ICBT on the right, one bronchial artery on the right, and one on the left (11.1 percent)
Pattern V: One ICBT on the right, one common bronchial trunk, and one left bronchial artery (8.3 percent)
Pattern VI: One ICBT on the right, one bronchial artery on the left, and one common bronchial trunk in caudal position (4.2 percent)
Pattern VII: Only one common bronchial trunk (2.8 percent)
Pattern VIII: One ICBT on the right, giving origin to a left bronchial artery, and one bronchial artery on the left (2.8 percent)

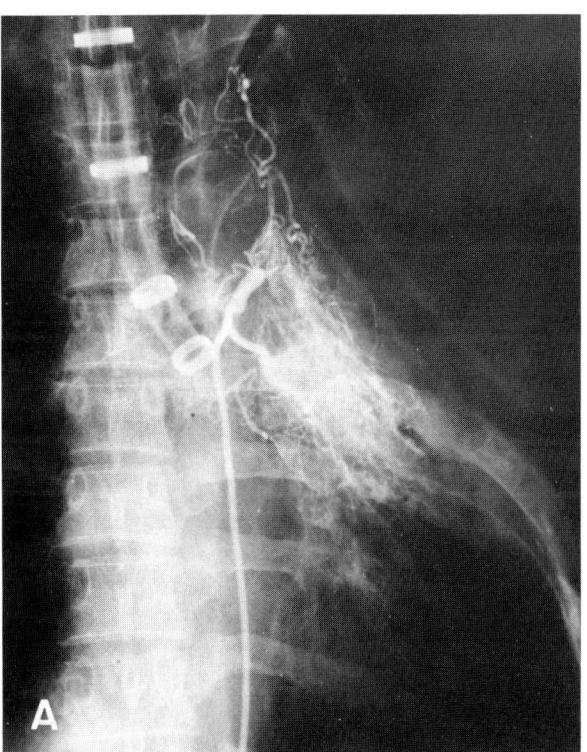 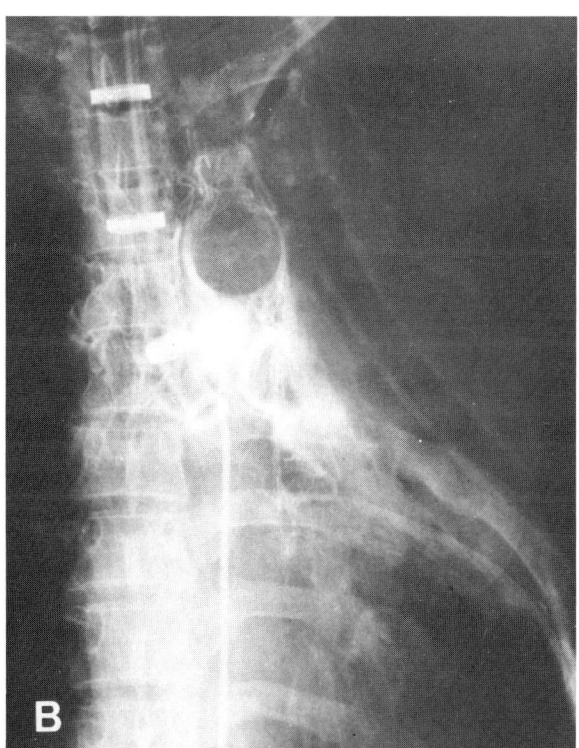

Figure 4.43 42-year-old patient showing a thoracoplasty (for tuberculosis) sequela on the left. Bronchial fistulas drained in the left pleural cavity. Massive hemoptysis occurred during surgical correction of bronchial fistulas. The patient was taken from the surgical room to the angiographic lab, and bronchial embolization was performed while the patient was still under general anesthesia.
(A) Injection into left bronchial artery. Notice the diffuse hypervascularity without demonstrable bleeding. (B) Angiogram immediately following bronchial embolization, which permanently controlled bleeding.

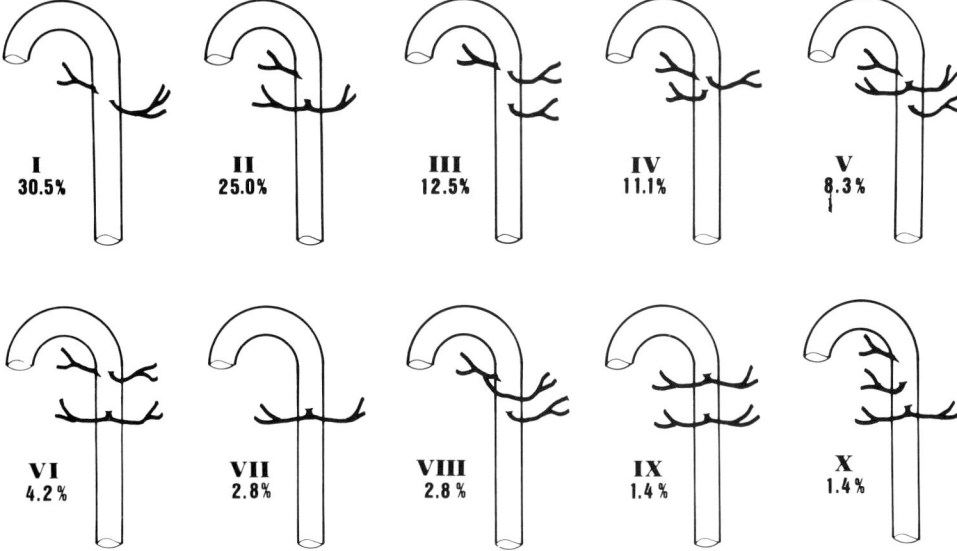

Figure 4.44 Diagram (ventral aspect) showing classification of the different types of bronchial arterial circulation, based on angiographic finding. The intercostal bronchial trunk has a lateral ventral origin. All other bronchial single arteries and common bronchial trunks have a ventral origin as related to the aorta.

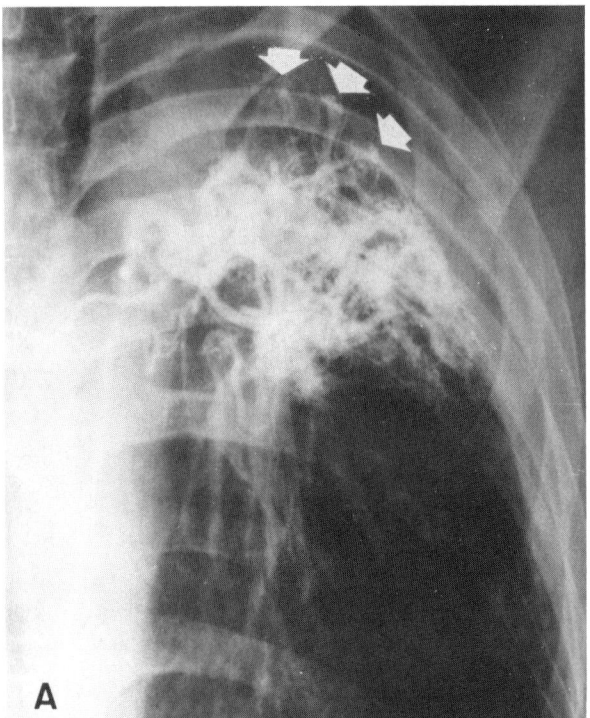
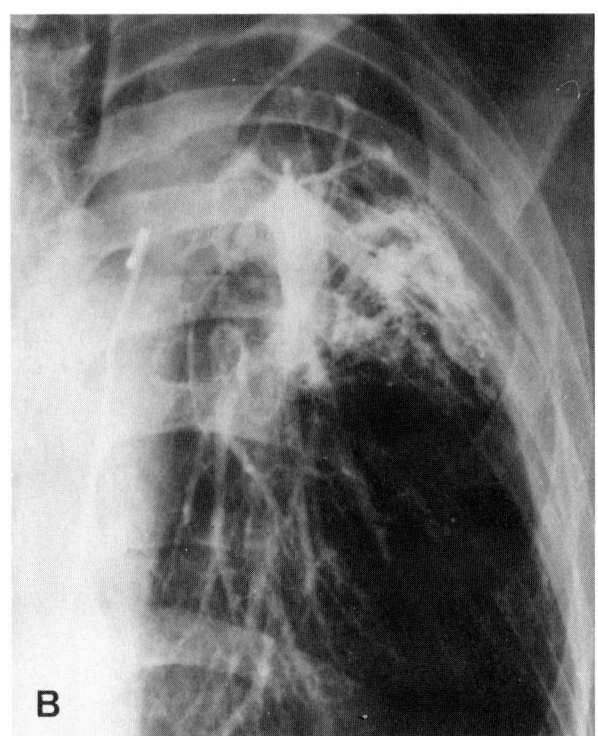

Figure 4.45 (A) Injection into the left bronchial artery showing a large hypervascular inflammatory lesion in the left lung. Notice the significant pleural thickening. The arrows show the vascular tufts in bronchiectases. (B) Massive pulmonary systemic arterial shunt with dense opacification of the left pulmonary artery. (C) Left lung tomogram showing bronchial changes and left upper lobe bronchiectases, corresponding to the vascular tufts shown in (A). (D) Postembolization angiogram showing total occlusion of the left bronchial artery. Massive hemoptysis was permanently controlled.

Pattern IX: Two common bronchial trunks giving origin to bronchial arteries on the right and on the left (1.4 percent)

Pattern X: One ICBT on the right, one bronchial artery on the right, and one common bronchial trunk origin to arteries on the right and on the left (1.4 percent)

Radicular arteries originating from the ICBT were seen in 58.3 percent of cases.

The effectiveness of bronchial embolization in controlling hemoptysis is shown in Table 4.1.

In general, Gelfoam particles are used, injected through a Mikaelsson-type catheter (Fig. 4.45) to occlude the bronchial artery or the ICBT (Fig. 4.46).

Table 4.1 – Results of bronchial arterial embolization in 64 patients

Treatment	Immediate Results		Long-Term		Lost to Follow-up	Total
	Good No. (%)	Poor No. (%)	Good No. (%)	Poor No. (%)		
Massive Hemoptysis (35 cases)						
Embolization only	17 (81.0)	4 (19.0)	13 (76.5)	4 (23.5)	4	
Embolization + chemotherapy + surgery	12 (85.7)	2 (14.3)	14	0	0	
Total	29 (82.8)	6	27 (87.0)	4	4	
Repetitive Hemoptysis (29 cases)						
Embolization only	16 (80.0)	4 (20.0)	11 (68.7)	5 (31.3)	4	41
Embolization + chemotherapy + surgery	4 (44.4)	5 (55.5)	8 (88.8)	1	0	23
Total	20 (68.9)	9	19 (76.0)	6	4	64

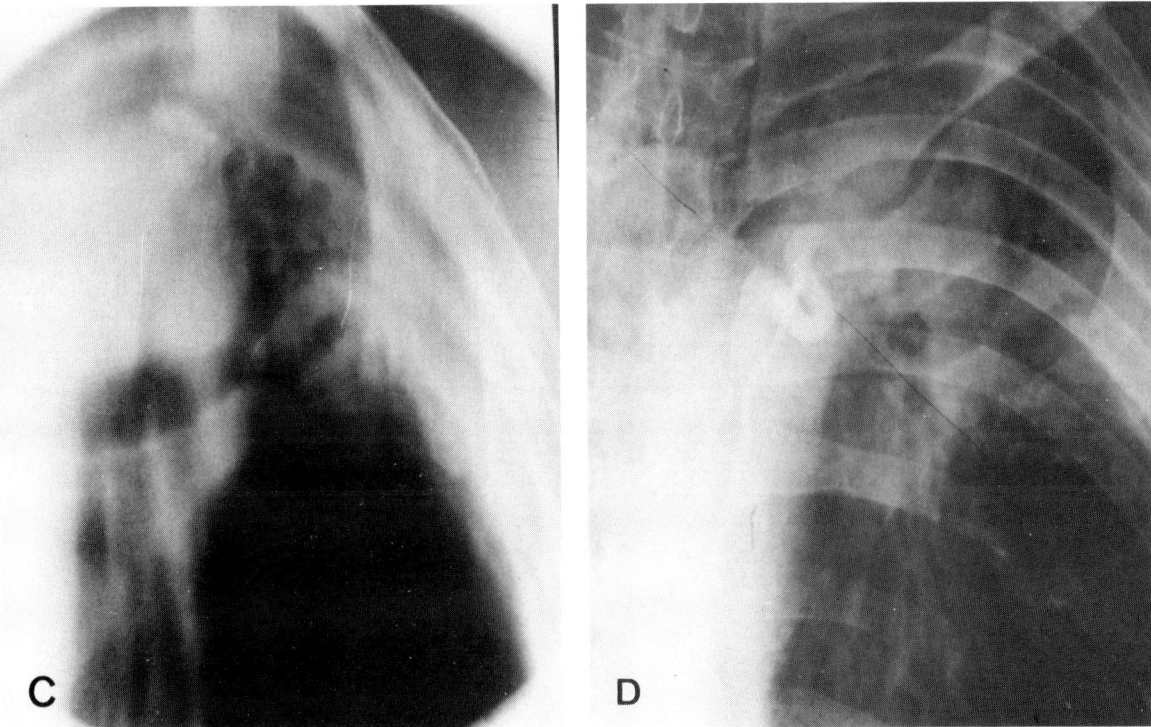

Figure 4.45 *Continued*

Figure 4.46 (A) Injection into intercostal bronchial trunk (ICBT) showing diffuse hypervascularity in sequela to right lung tuberculosis. Notice that the intercostal arteries have a normal diameter. A few radicular arteries are seen on the midline. (B) Control following embolization showing complete ICBT occlusion, resulting in cessation of hemoptysis. Bleeding has recurred. (C) Angiographic study performed 10 months following embolization. Angiogram shows persisting bronchial artery occlusion, and revascularization of the intercostals and of a peripheral bronchial branch (arrows). (D) After embolization was repeated, with intimal dissection resulting from catheter manipulation, arterial occlusion occurred. Recovery was free of hemoptysis.

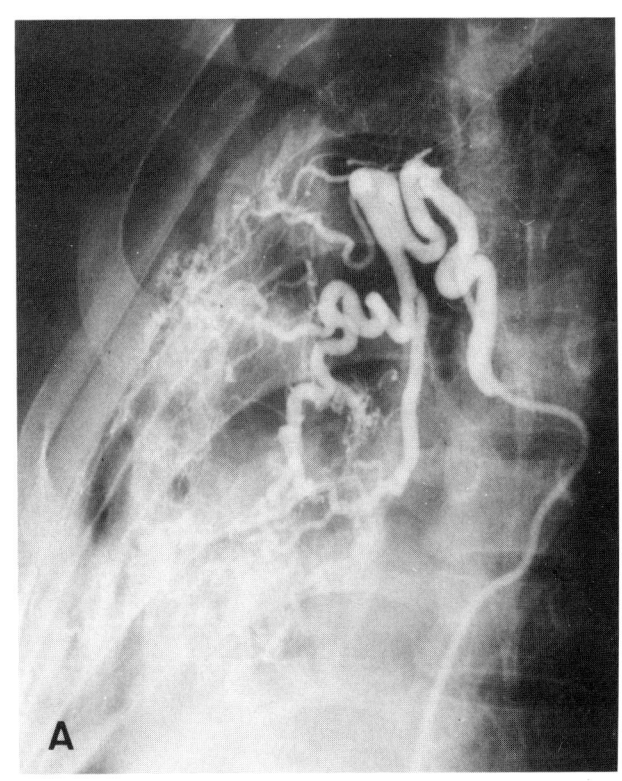

Figure 4.46 *Continued*

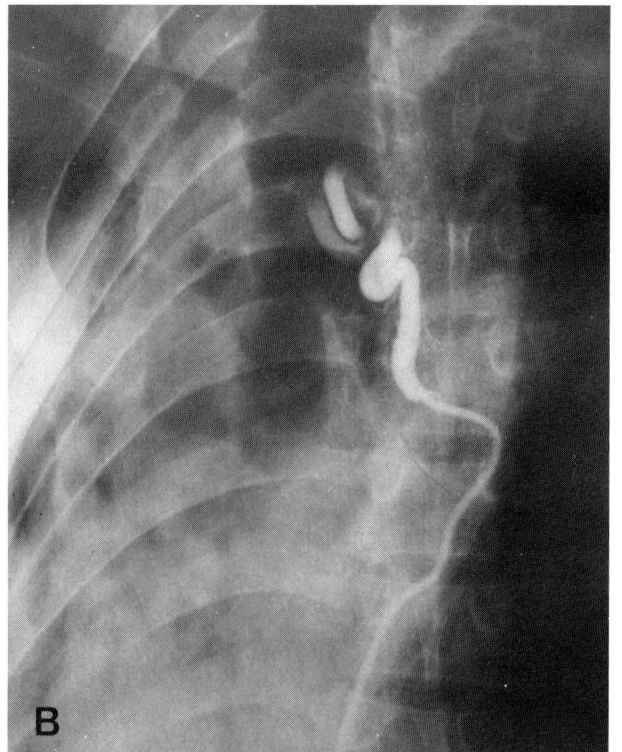

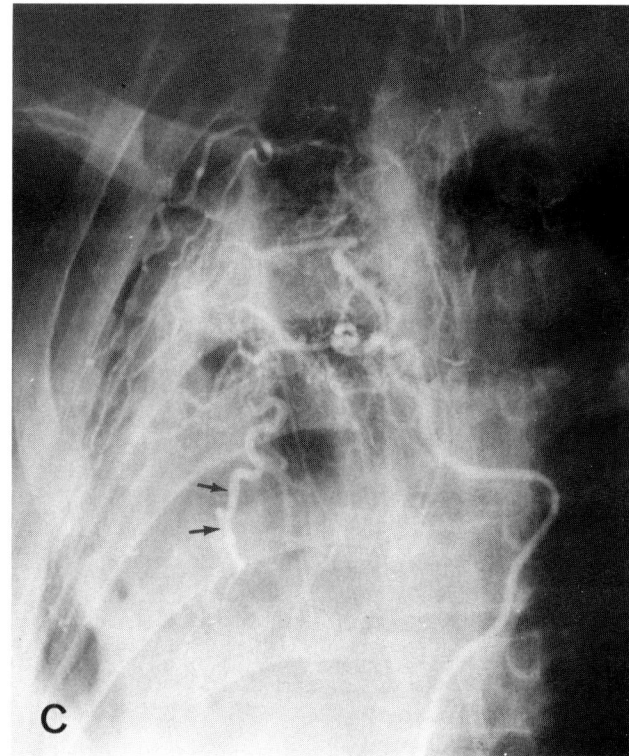

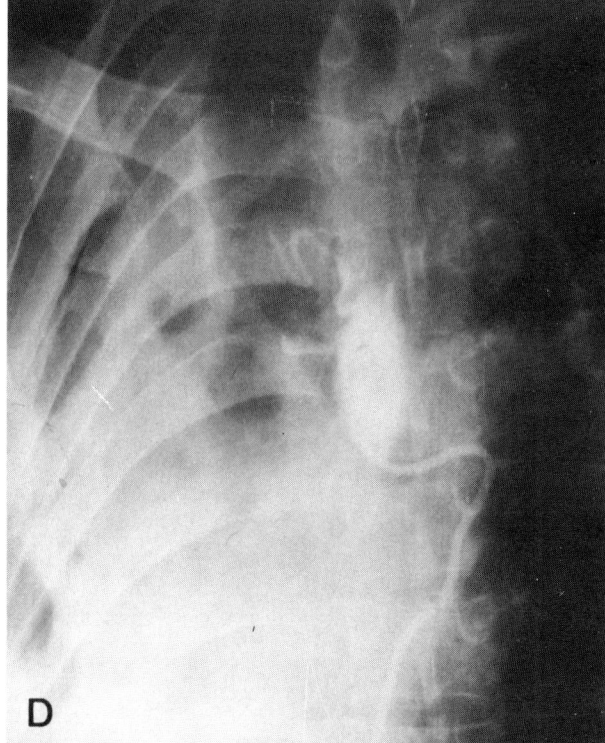

Embolization is initiated with 2- by 1-mm Gelfoam flow-directed particles; later, 3- by 5-mm particles are used to achieve a more proximal occlusion. Ivalon particles, 250 μm, may also be used for embolization.

Contrast medium extravasation may either be intracavitary (Fig. 4.47), or may occur inside the diseased parenchyma (Fig. 4.48). It is rarely seen at the bleeding site, either because it it intermittent or because the volume is small. Arterial systemic pulmonary shunts may also hide contrast extravasation, and scintigraphy can be useful in identifying the bleeding site.

Tubercular lung lesions may be associated with bronchiectases with apical tufts, which bleed readily during the course of an infectious process (Fig. 4.45). Embolization usually controls this condition effectively.

The use of digital angiographic equipment, with a low-viscosity (higher dilution), low osmolarity contrast medium, has made it possible to perform more rapid bronchial arteriographic studies. In addition, it allows better visualization of radicular and medullary arteries

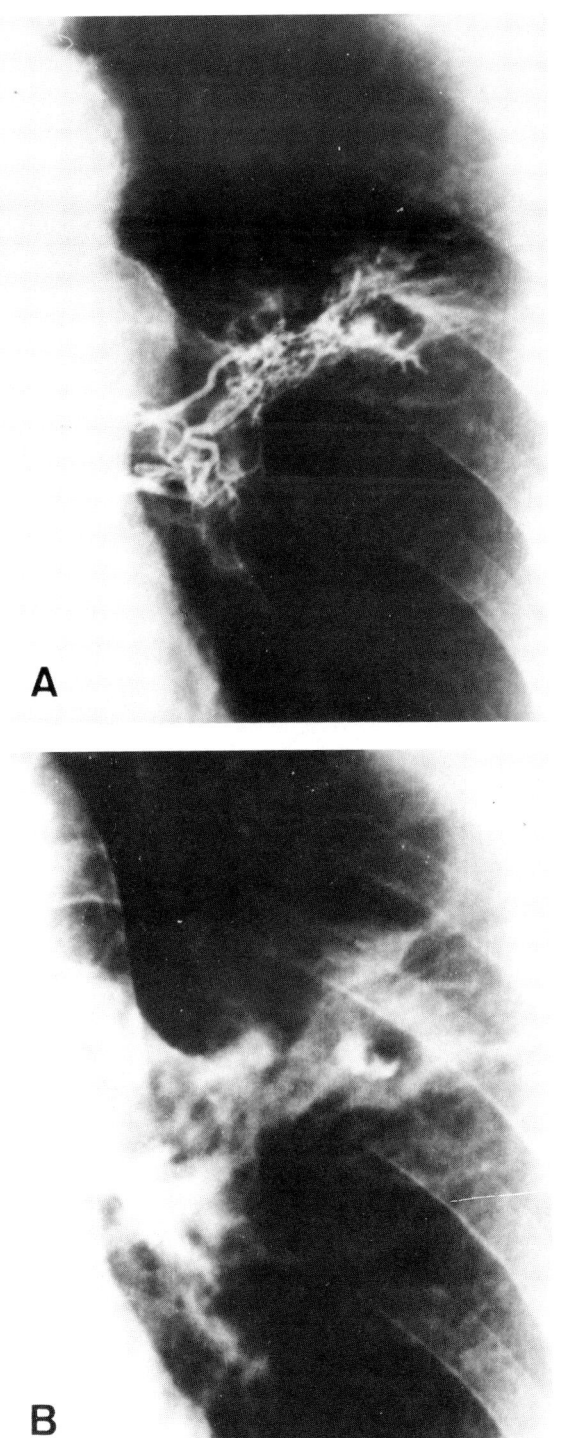

Figure 4.47 (A,B) Active bleeding inside a small pulmonary cavity on the left side. The later angiogram phase shows partial filling of the cavity with contrast medium.

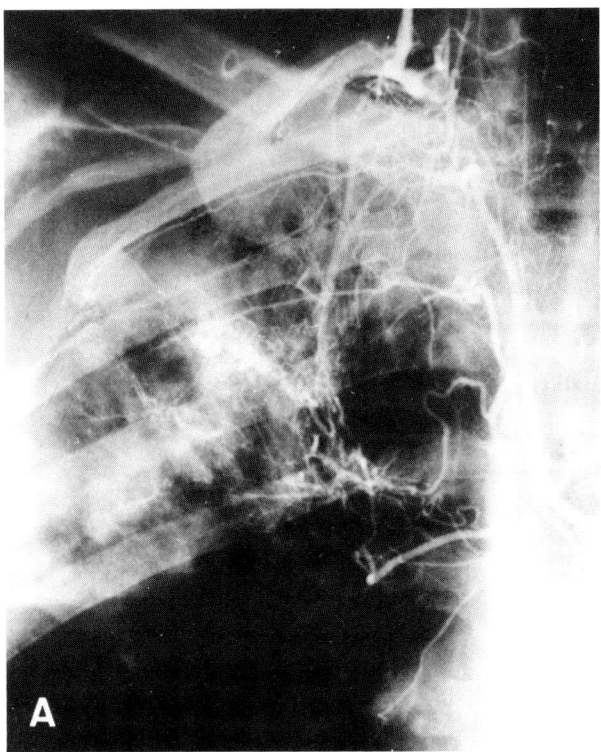
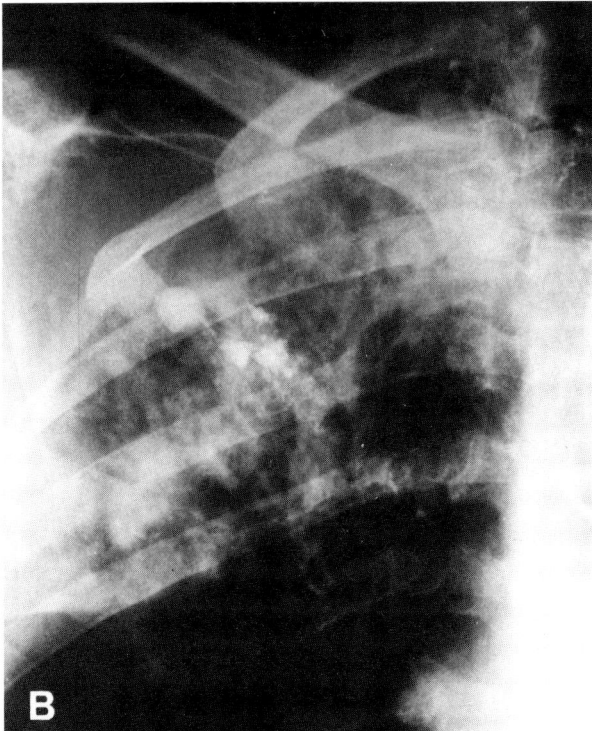

Figure 4.48 Intraparenchymal and intracavitary contrast medium extravasation during acute hemoptysis episode.
(A) Arterial phase showing the hypervascular right upper lobe inflammatory lesion and contrast medium extravasation. Notice the radicular circulation. (B) Later phase angiogram showing active parenchymal and cavitary bleeding. The intercostal bronchial trunk was embolized, and hemoptysis was controlled.

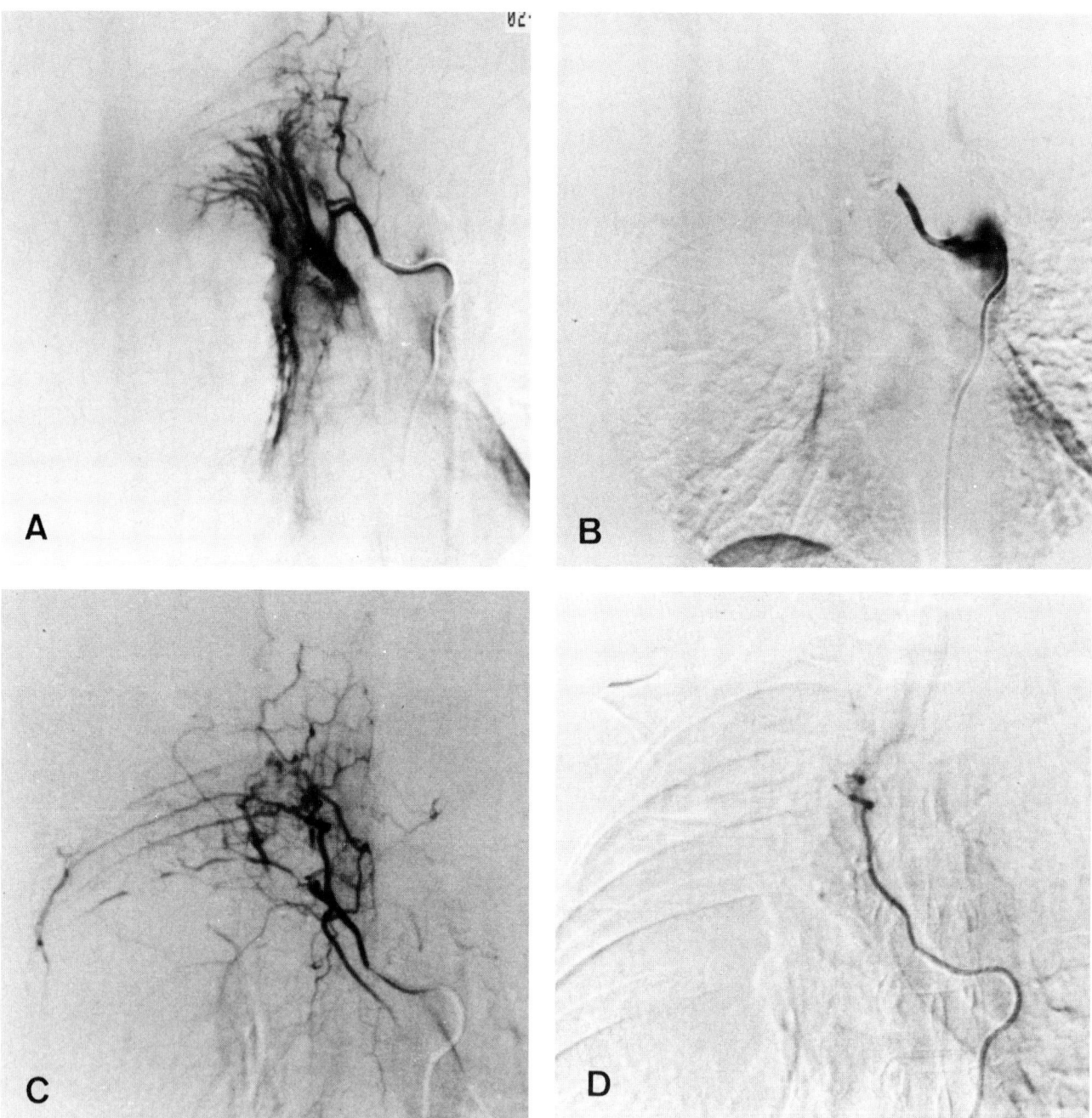

Figure 4.49 Digital angiogram of a patient with massive hemoptysis and history of right breast neoplasm, who has been operated on and irradiated.
(A) Inflammatory lesion secondary to radiation therapy in right upper lobe, with pulmonary systemic arterial fistula. The injection was into the intercostal bronchial trunk.
(B) Postembolization control showing intercostal bronchial trunk occlusion. (C) Injection into right intercostal artery with lesion involvement. (D) Control following embolization. Hemoptysis has stopped permanently. Observe the opacified radicular arteries in (A) and (C).

because of high-quality subtraction (Figs. 4.49 to 4.51). It should be stressed, however, that space resolution in digital angiography is lower than that obtained with the conventional process, particularly if geometric magnification and photographic subtraction are used. Nonionic or low-osmolarity contrast medium should be used whenever conventional angiography is performed.

Pulmonary lesions often involve the thoracic wall, particularly when the lesions are diffuse, causing transpleural collateral circulation that is frequently the cause

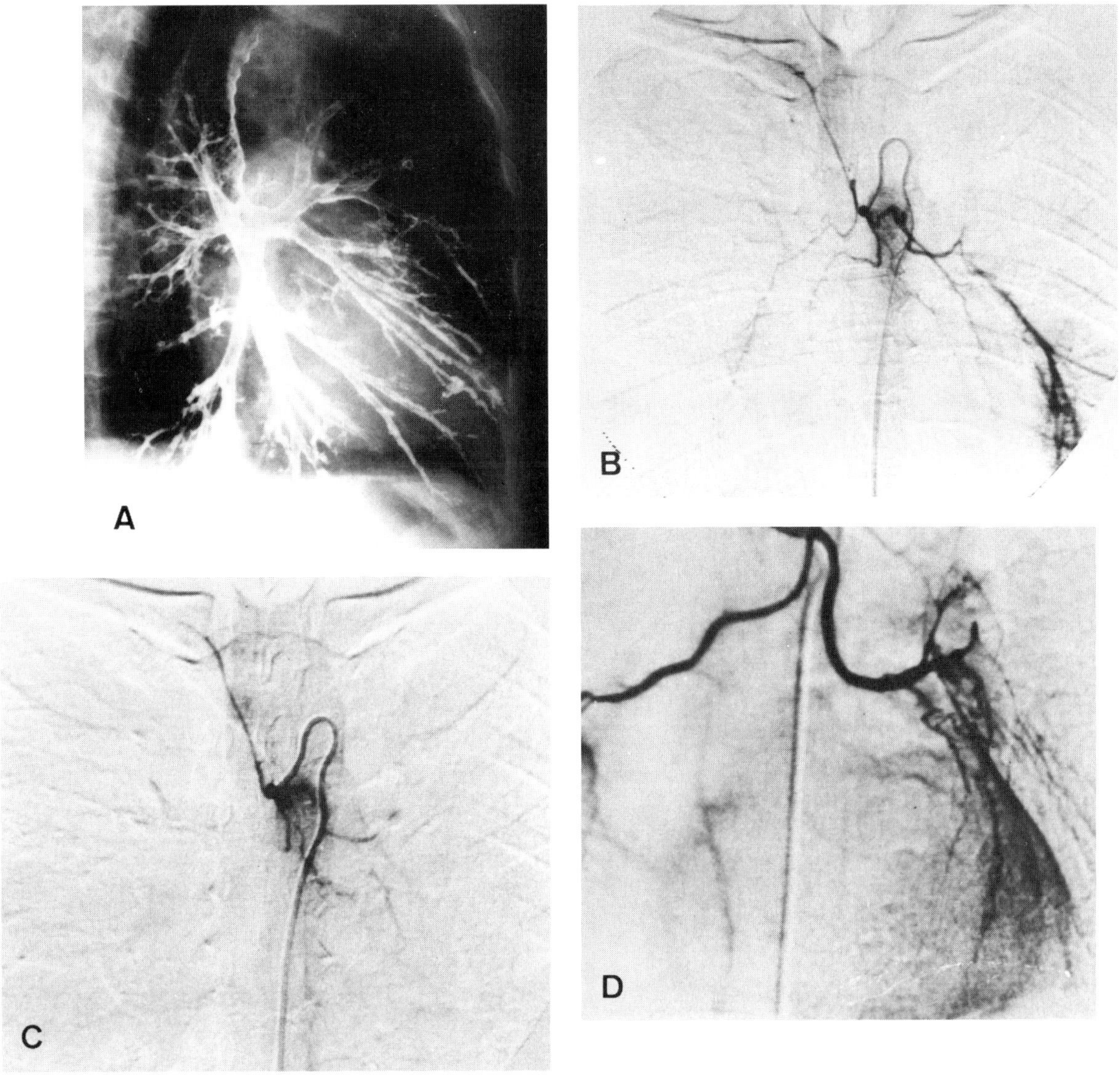

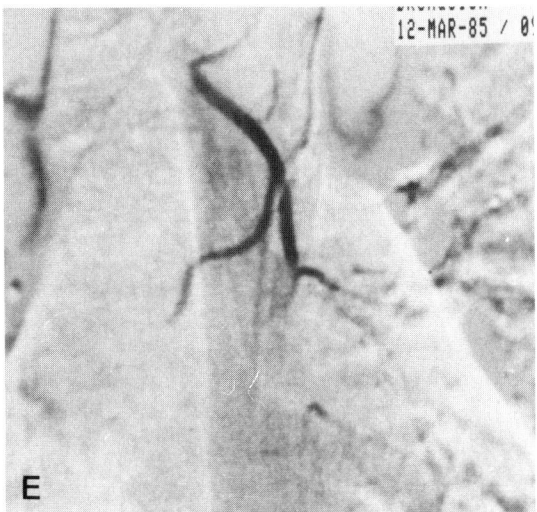

Figure 4.50 (A) Bronchogram in patient with hemoptysis and left lower lobe and lingular bronchiectases. (B) Digital angiogram showing a common bronchial trunk seen in B. (D) Digital angiogram showing a common bronchial trunk with abnormal vessels on the left lung. (E) Postembolization angiogram of the common trunk seen in (B).

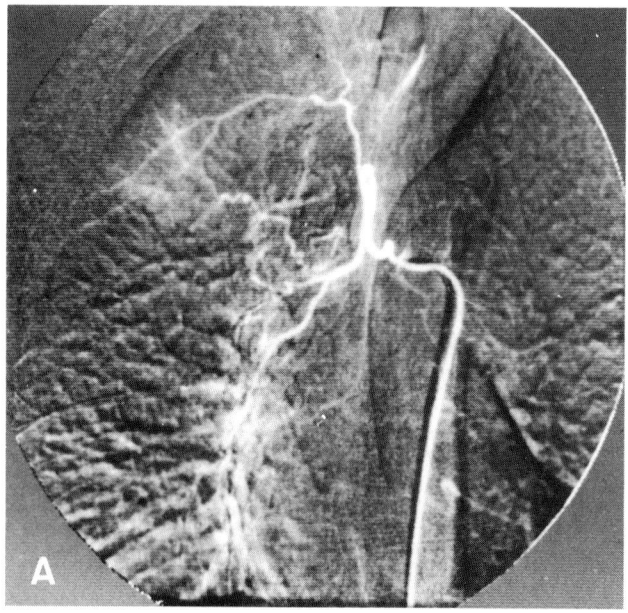
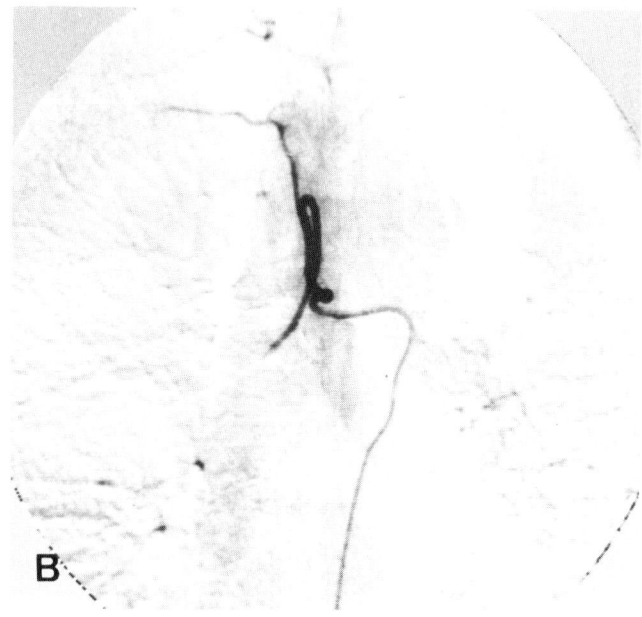

Figure 4.51 (A) Digital angiogram of patient with residual tuberculosis and hemoptysis involving the right lung. Notice the breathing artifacts in the background. The injection was into the intercostal bronchial trunk. (B) Control angiogram following embolization.

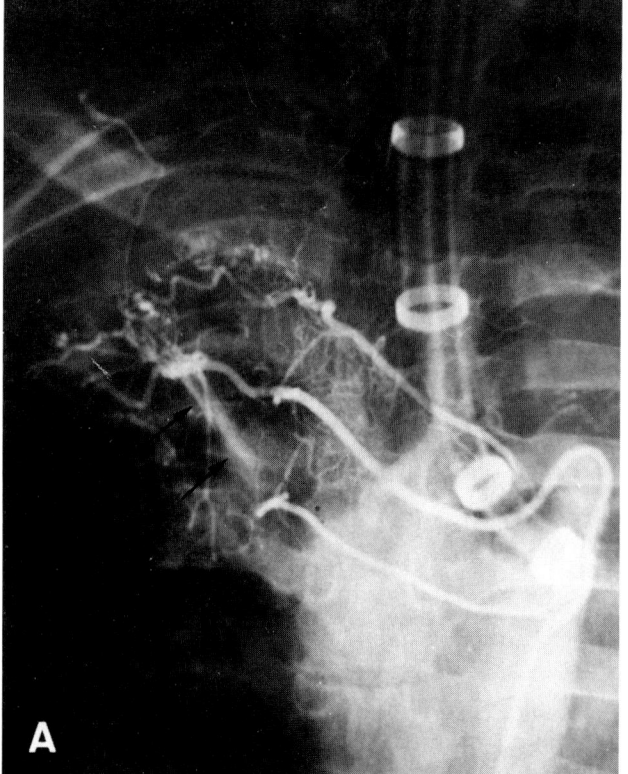
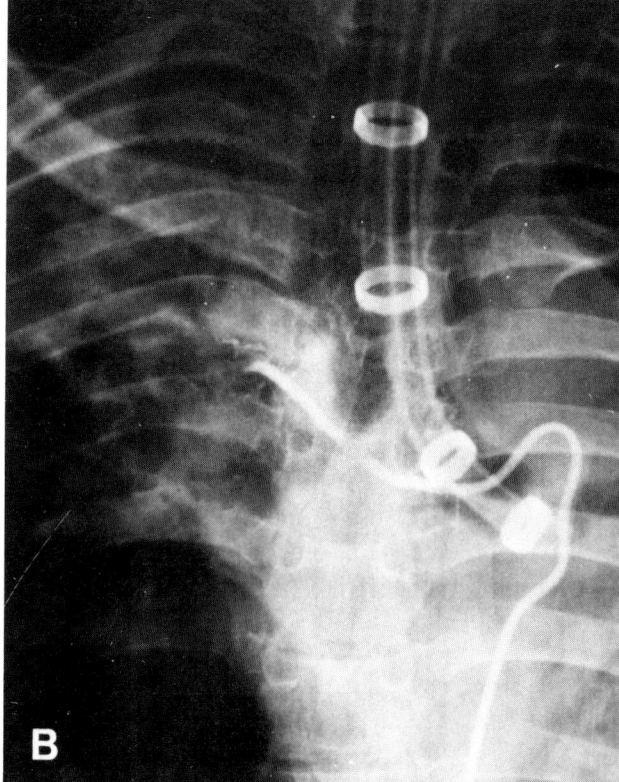

Figure 4.52 Involvement of intercostal arteries in a pulmonary inflammatory lesion.
(A) Selective injection into right intercostal artery showing communication with the pulmonary artery (arrows).
(B) Control following embolization with Gelfoam. In this case, the bronchial arteries were also embolized. Due to massive bleeding a Carlens tube was introduced to prevent contralateral overflowing.

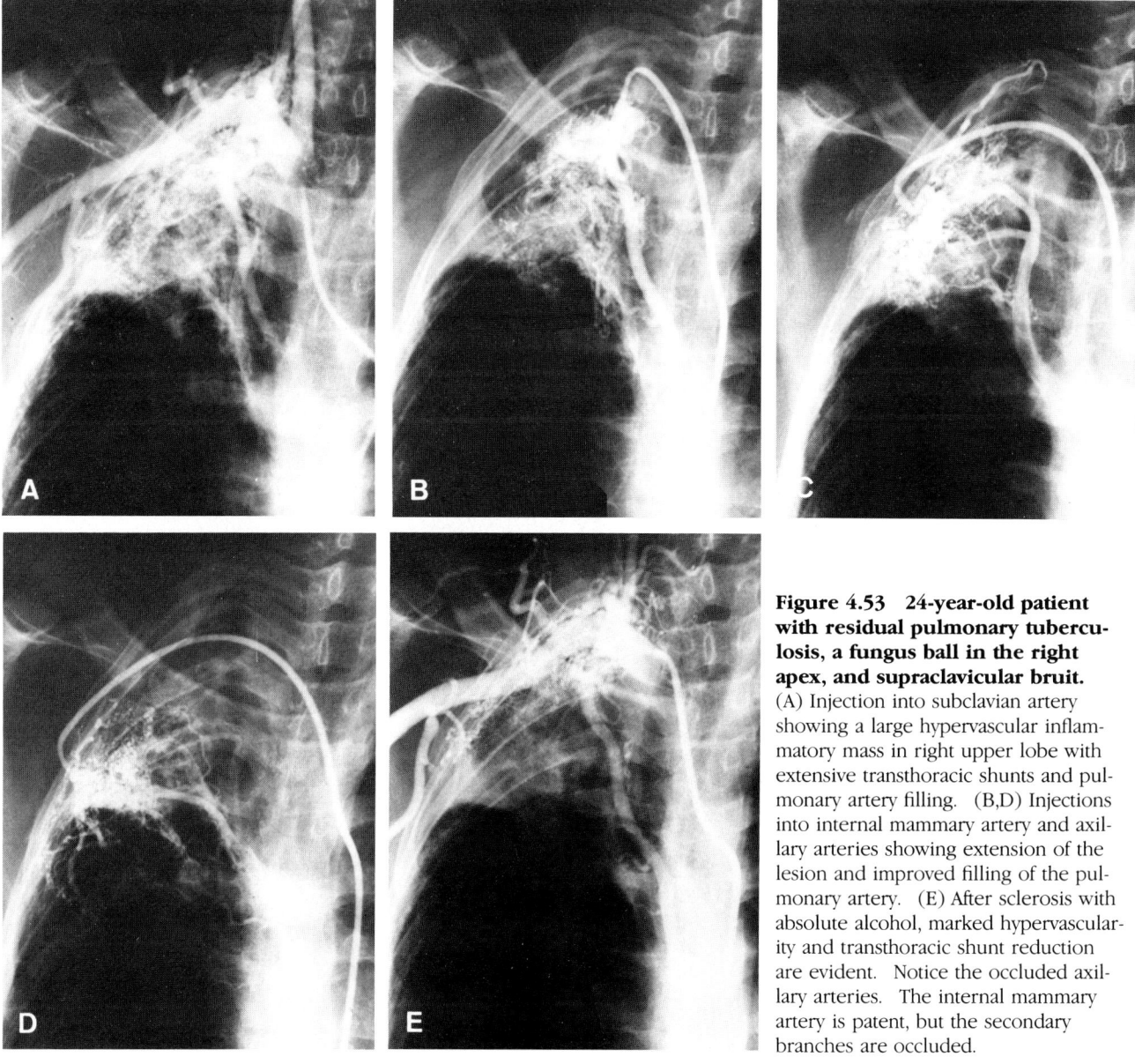

Figure 4.53 24-year-old patient with residual pulmonary tuberculosis, a fungus ball in the right apex, and supraclavicular bruit.
(A) Injection into subclavian artery showing a large hypervascular inflammatory mass in right upper lobe with extensive transthoracic shunts and pulmonary artery filling. (B,D) Injections into internal mammary artery and axillary arteries showing extension of the lesion and improved filling of the pulmonary artery. (E) After sclerosis with absolute alcohol, marked hypervascularity and transthoracic shunt reduction are evident. Notice the occluded axillary arteries. The internal mammary artery is patent, but the secondary branches are occluded.

of primary bleeding and recurring bleeding episodes.

Whenever bronchial angiography does not show the lesion, the study should be extended to the intercostal (Fig. 4.52), axillary, subclavian, and internal mammary arteries (Fig. 4.53).

Pulmonary arteriograms rarely show changes which are capable of causing bleeding, but they are useful in selected cases, for example, for localizing and embolizing a Rasmussen aneurysm (Fig. 4.54). Lesion recurrence in patients who have undergone surgery is frequent, with thoracic wall involvement and development of arterial systemic pulmonary shunts (Fig. 4.55).

The embolization of bronchial arteries involves risks, due both to the patient's poor general condition and to the vascular anatomy involved. Reflux of emboli into the aorta is the most immediate risk, and care should be taken to keep the catheter stable and to introduce it as deeply as possible into the bronchial artery. Flow in this artery is slower, but the force of the embolus injection should be adequate to the previously identified flow. Any artery located below the bronchial arteries may be inadvertently embolized. Esophageal symptoms, such as odynophagia and dysphasia, may well occur due to embolization of muscular arteries in this organ. Esophageal fistulization, though rare, may also occur. Intimal lesion in the vicinity of the bronchial artery ostium, due to manipulation and to the acute angle that may occur between the artery and the aorta, is also a possibility.

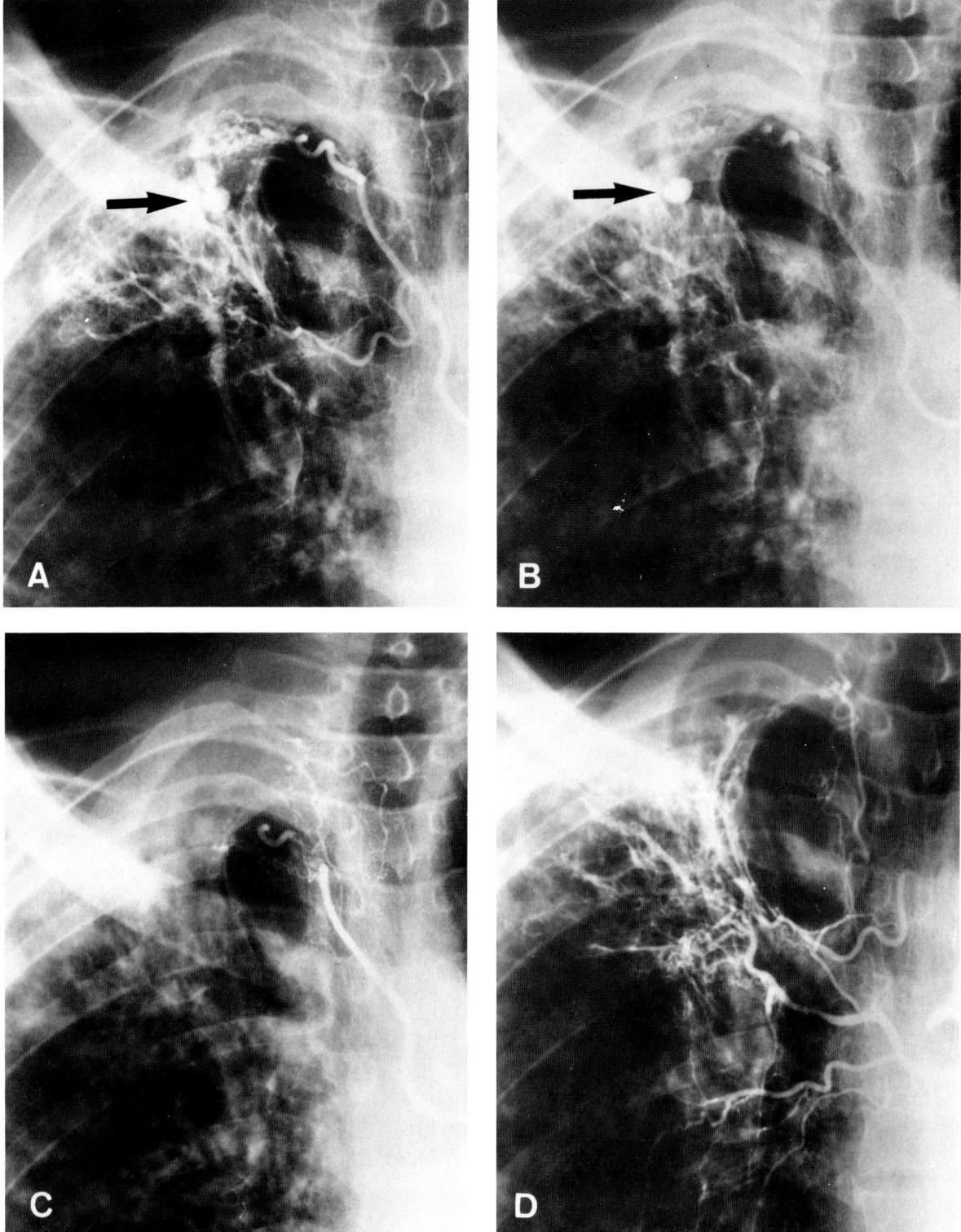

Figure 4.54 Demonstration of small Rasmussen aneurysm by arterial injection.
(A) Injection into the intercostal bronchial trunk showing a right apical inflammatory lesion, next to a cavity (medial), and an aneurysm in one of the pulmonary artery branches (arrow). (B) Lateral phase showing contrast stagnation inside the aneurysm following arterial emptying (arrow). (C) Control following embolization showing occlusion of the intercostal bronchial trunk. (D) Injection into a common bronchial axis with well-demarcated apical pulmonary cavity wall.

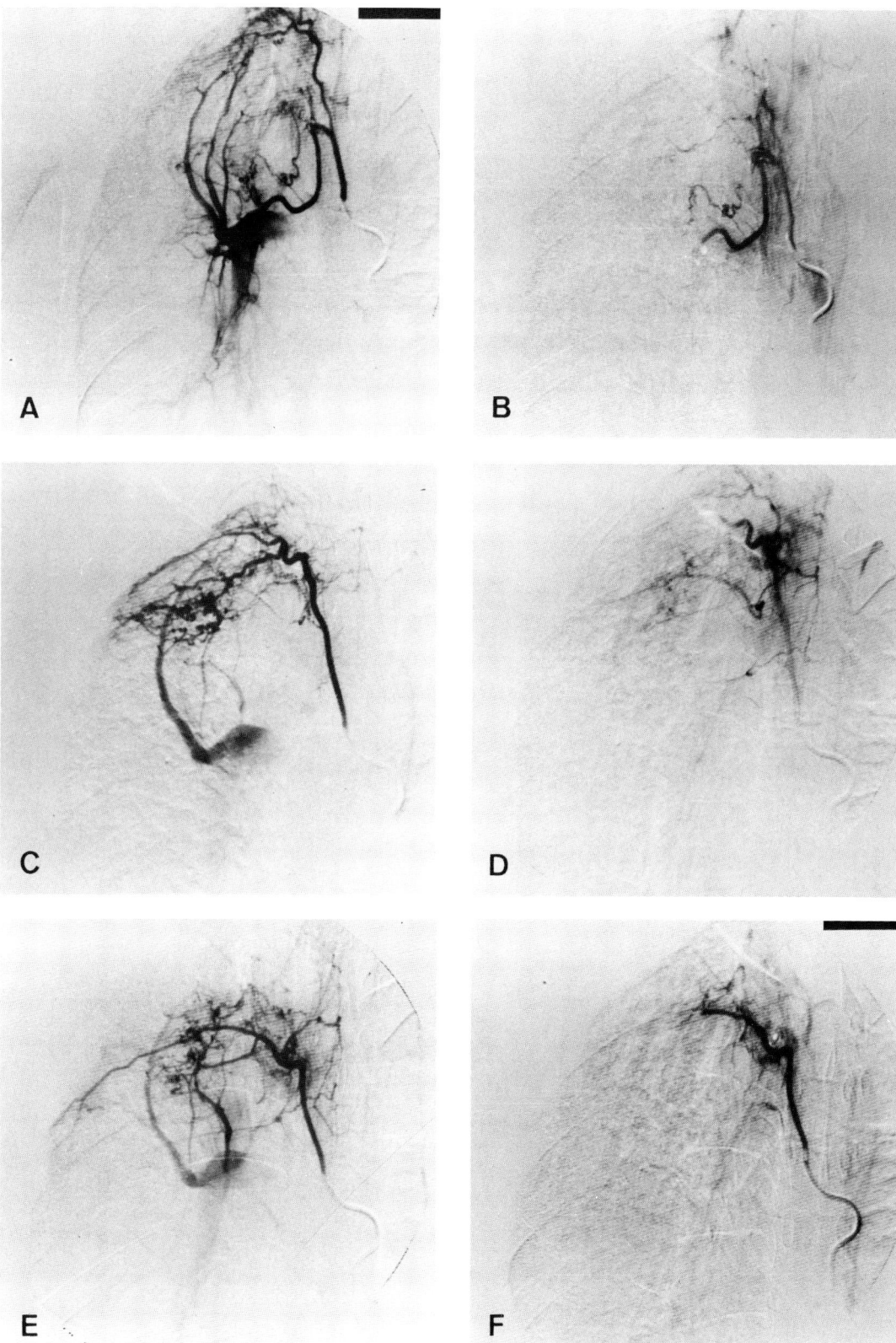

Figure 4.55 Bronchial digital angiogram showing a lesion in the upper portion of the right lung in a patient who has previously undergone lobectomy. The lesion has recurred, showing atypical mycobacterium, and has been insensitive to conventional treatment. The angiogram was performed after an acute hemoptysis episode.
(A,B) Pre- and postembolization of intercostal bronchial trunk showing extensive inflammatory lesion with involvement of the intercostal arteries. (C,D) Second and third intercostal arteries feeding the lesion (pre- and postembolization angiograms). (E,F) Pre- and postembolization angiograms showing fourth intercostal artery feeding the lesion. Bleeding was controlled, making it possible to continue the clinical treatment.

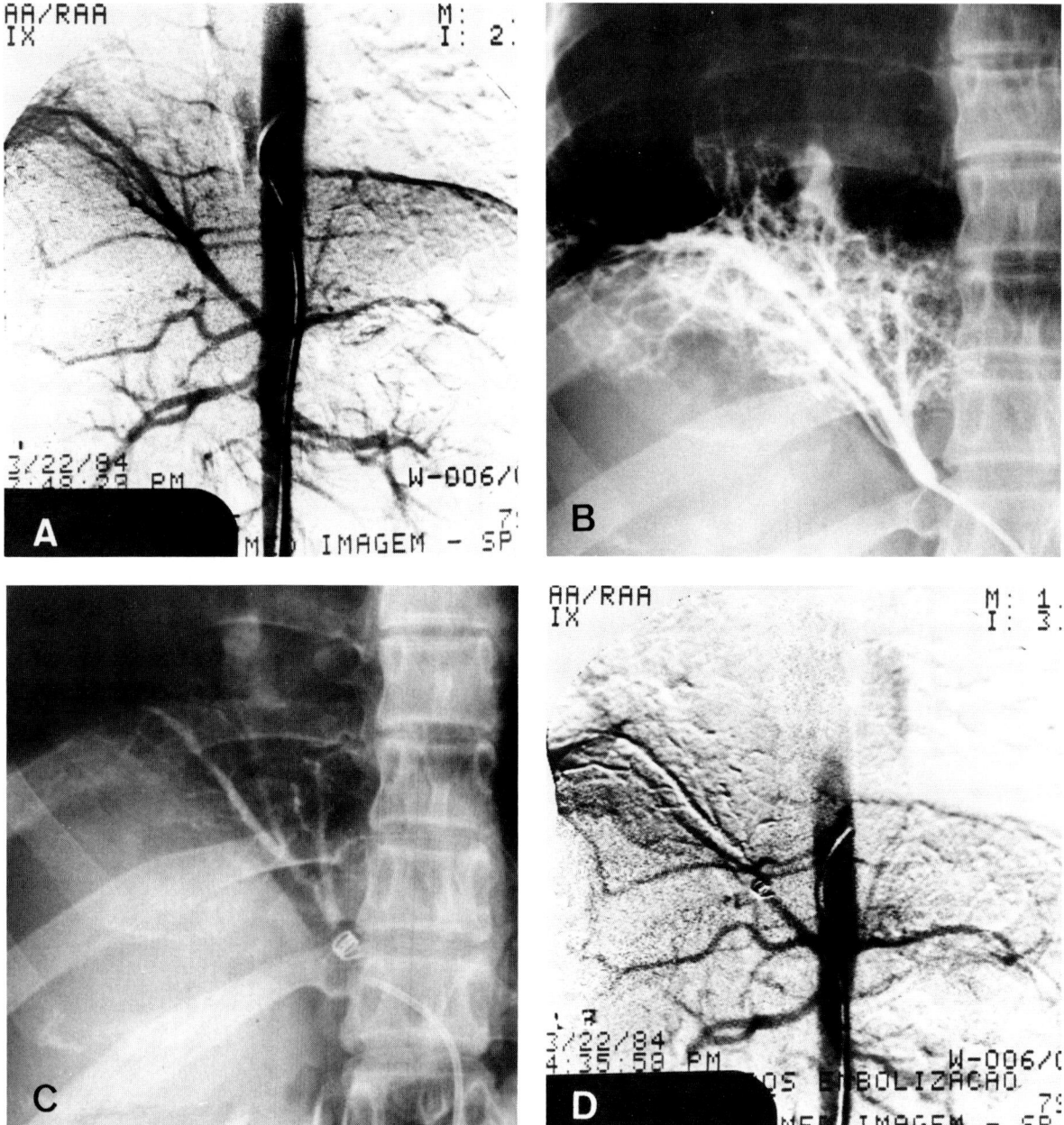

Figure 4.56 Pulmonary sequestration with massive and acute hemoptysis.
(A) Thoracic abdominal digital aortogram showing the abnormal artery on the right. (B) Selective injection into abnormal artery which vascularizes the right lung basal sequestration. (C) Injection of bucrylate as embolizing agent, using a Gianturco coil. (D) Control following embolization. Hemoptysis had stopped, permitting elective surgery.

Usually, pain is the only other problem noted in these cases.

There is no reference in the literature to medullary neurologic lesion following embolization of bronchial arteries. There are some reports of medullary lesions following the embolization of intercostal arteries. These are, however, probably more closely related to the use of hyperosmolar contrast medium than to the embolization itself, and the use of nonionic, low-osmolarity contrast medium should be encouraged in these cases because of its low neurotoxicity.

There are several possible causes of recurrence of hemoptysis following bronchial embolization. One of the most frequent is partial embolization.

Progress of the underlying disease is a serious problem, necessitating a multidisciplinary approach to hemoptysis. All the available therapeutic means, besides vascular embolization, should be utilized: antimicrobial therapy, antineoplastc therapy, radiotherapy, and surgery.

The presence of a fungus ball in a lung cavity is a significant cause of rebleeding, and one of the main causes of embolization failure. The use of corticosteroids and radiotherapy is a valid action in desperate cases. Bronchial embolization in patients with a fungus ball is necessarily palliative, as the ball must always be removed surgically.

PULMONARY SEQUESTRATION

Pulmonary sequestration is fed by a systemic artery originating from the aorta, above or below the diaphragm. In cases of intralobular sequestration, venous drainage is usually through the pulmonary veins; if sequestration is extralobular, drainage is through the systemic veins. Surgery is the treatment of choice.

Complications of this type of lesion usually involve repeated pulmonary infections in the thoracic mass, generally located at the base of the lung. A less frequent complication is intrabronchial bleeding (hemoptysis), usually during the course of an infectious process. Embolization of the systemic artery, which vascularizes the sequestration, can definitively stop the bleeding in such cases. A nonabsorbable embolic material such as bucrylate or Gianturco coils is used (Fig. 4.56).

It must be remembered that the area of sequestration is an infected territory, and the consequences of the infected territory being devitalized, in terms of contamination and sepsis, can be catastrophic. Emergency embolization should *only* be used as a preoperative procedure, to stop bleeding. However, elective systemic artery embolization may be useful as a measure for facilitating surgical resection, since the surgeon can proceed with the operation without having to first locate the abnormal artery.

REFERENCES

PULMONARY AV FISTULAS

Castaneda-Zuniga W, Epstein M, Zollikofer C, et al. Embolization in the management of congenital arteriovenous malformations. *Radiology* 1980;137:21–29.

Costa GPR, Cukier A, Lima SS, et al. Fistulas arterio-venosas pulmonares: Tratamento por embolizacao. *J Pneumol* 1986;12:180–183.

Hatfield DR, Fried AM. Therapeutic embolization of diffuse pulmonary arteriovenous malformations. *AJR* 1981;137:861–863.

Hewes RC, Auster M, White RI. Cerebral embolism: First manifestation of pulmonary arteriovenous malformation in patients with hereditary hemorrhagic telangiectasis. *Cardiovasc Intervent Radiol* 1985;8:151–155.

Prager RL, Lws KH, Bender HW. Arteriovenous fistula of the lung. *Ann Thorac Surg* 1983;36:231–239.

Terry PB, Barth KH, Kaufman SL, White RI. Balloon embolization for treatment of pulmonary arteriovenous fistulas. *N Engl J Med* 1980;302:1189–1190.

White RI, Mitchell SE, Barth KH, et al. Angioarchitecture of pulmonary arteriovenous malformations: An important consideration before embolotherapy. *AJR* 1983;140:681–686.

POSTOPERATIVE BLEEDING

Husted JN, Stock JR, Manella WJ. Traumatic anterior mediastinal hemorrhage: Control by internal mammary artery embolization. *Cardiovasc Intervent Radiol* 1982;5:268–270.

Keller F, Rosch J, Barker AF, Dotter CT. Percutaneous interventional catheter therapy for lesions of the chest and lungs. *Chest* 1982;81:407–412.

McClean GK, Mackie JA, Hartz WH, Friedman DB. Percutaneous alcohol for control of internal mammary bleeding. *AJR* 1983;141:181–182.

Sanchez FW, Freeland PN, Bailey GT, Vujic I. Embolotherapy of a mycotic pseudoaneurysm of the internal mammary artery in chronic granulomatous disease. *Cardiovasc Intervent Radiol* 1985;8:43–45.

Smity DC, Senae MD, Bailey LL. Embolotherapy of a ruptured internal mammary artery secondary to blunt chest trauma. *J Trauma* 1982;22:333–335.

TREATMENT OF HEMOPTYSIS

Arciniegas E, Lam CR. Management of massive hemoptysis. *Henry Ford Hosp Med J* 1969;16:283–288.

Aspelin P, Kalen N, Svanberg L. Treatment of severe haemoptysis by embolization of the bronchial artery. *Scand J Respir Dis* 1979;60:20–23.

Bookstein JJ, Moser KM, Kalafer ME, Higgins CB, Davis GB, James W. The role of bronchial arteriography and therapeutic embolization in hemoptysis. *Chest* 1977;72:658–661.

Botenga ASJ. *Selective Bronchial and Intercostal Angiography*. Stenfert Kroese NV, Leiden, 1970.

Bredin CP, Richardson RP, King TKC, Sniderman KW, Sos TA, Smith JP. Treatment of massive hemoptysis by combined occlusion of pulmonary and bronchial arteries. *Am Rev Respir Dis* 1979;117:969–973.

Cauldwell EW, Siekert RG, Lininger RE, Anson BJ. The bronchial arteries: An anatomic study of 150 human cadavers. *Surg Gynecol Obstet* 1948;86:395–412.

Crocco JA, Rooney JJ, Fankushen DS, DiBenedetto RJ, Lyons HA. Massive hemoptysis. *Arch Intern Med* 1968;121:495–498.

Di Chiro G. Unintentional spinal cord arteriography: A warning. *Radiology* 1974;112:231–233.

Feigelson HH, Ravin HA. Transverse myelitis following selective bronchial arteriography. *Radiology* 1965;85:663–665.

Fellows KE, Khaw KT, Schuster S, Shwachman HO. Bronchial artery embolization in cystic fibrosis: Technique and long term results. *J Pediatr* 1979;95:959–963.

Ferris EJ. Pulmonary hemorrhage: Vascular evaluation and interventional therapy. *Chest* 1981;80:710–714.

Garzon AA, Cerruti MM, Golding ME. Exsanguinating hemoptysis. *Thorac Cardiovasc Surg* 1982;84:829–833.

Garzon AA, Cerruti M, Gourin A, Karlson KE. Pulmonary resection for massive hemoptysis. *Surgery* 1970;67:633–638.

Gomfett RE, Liesemborgh L. New contrast media in cerebral angiography: Animal experiments and preliminary clinical studies. *Invest Radiol* 1980;15:270–274.

Greenfield AJ. Transcatheter vessel occlusion: Selection of methods and material. *Cardiovasc Intervent Radiol* 1980;4:26–32.

Grenier P, Cornud F, Lacombe P, Viau F, Nahum H. Bronchial artery occlusion of severe hemoptysis: Use of isobutyl-2 cyanoacrylate. *AJR* 1983;140:467–471.

Harley JD, Killien FC, Peck AG. Massive hemoptysis controlled by transcatheter embolization of the bronchial arteries. *AJR* 1977;128:302–304.

Heffernan JF, Nunn AJ, Peto J, et al. Tuberculosis in Scotland, a national sample survey (1968–1970): A two-year follow-up of newly diagnosed respiratory tuberculosis reported in 1968. *Tubercle* 1976;57:161–175.

Helenon CH, Chatel L, Bigot JM, Brocard H. Fistule oesophagobronchique gauche après embolization bronchique. *Nouv Presse Med* 1977;6:4209.

Ivanick MJ, Thorwarth W, Donohue J, Mandell V, Delany D, Jaques PF. Infarction of the left main stem bronchus: A complication of bronchial artery embolization. *AJR* 1983;141:535–537.

Kardjiev V, Symeonov A, Chankov I. Etiology, pathogenesis, and prevention of spinal cord lesions in selective angiography of bronchial and intercostal arteries. *Radiology* 1974;112:81–83.

Lamarque JL, Senac JP. Die therapeutische Angiographie bei Hamoptysen. *Radiologe* 1979;19:514–520.

MacErlean DP, Gray BJ, Fitzgerald MX. Bronchial artery embolization in the control of massive haemoptysis. *Br J Radiol* 1979;52:558–561.

Magillian Jr DJ, Ravipati S, Zayat P, Shetty PC, Bower G, Kvale P. Massive hemoptysis: Control by transcatheter bronchial artery embolization. *Ann Thorac Surg* 1981;32:380–392.

Naar CA, Soong J, Clore F, Hawkins Jr IF. Control of massive hemoptysis by bronchial artery embolization with absolute alcohol. *AJR* 1983;140:271–272.

Newton TH, Preger L. Selective bronchial arteriography. Radiology 1965;84:1043–1051.

Olson RR, Athanasoulis CA. Hemoptysis: Treatment with transcatheter embolization of the bronchial arteries. In *Interventional Radiology*, edited by Athanasoulis CA, Pfister RC, Greene RE, Roberson GH. Saunders, Philadelphia, 1982:196–202.

Remy J, Arnaud A, Fardou H, Giraud T, Voisin C. Treatment of hemoptysis by embolization of bronchial arteries. *Radiology* 1977;122:33–37.

Remy J, Voisin C, Dupius C, et al. Traitment des hemoptysies par embolization de la circulation systemique. *Ann Radiol* 1974;17:5–16.

Sebens AA. Pulmonary gas exchange. In *Taylor's Physiological Basis of Medical Practice*. 9th ed., edited by Brobec JR. Williams & Wilkins, Baltimore, 1973:20–21.

Shneerson JM, Emerson PA, Philips RH. Radiotherapy for massive hemoptysis from an aspergilloma. *Thorax* 1980;35:953–954.

Tadavarthy SM, Moller JH, Amplatz M. Polyvinyl alcohol (Ivalon): A new embolic material. *AJR* 1975;125:609–616.

Thoms NW, Wilson RE, Puro HE, Arbulu A. Life threatening hemoptysis in primary lung abscess. *Ann Thorac Surg* 1972;14:347–358.

Uflacker R, Kaemmerer A, Picon PD et al. Bronchial artery embolization in the management of hemoptysis: Technical aspects and long-term results. *Radiology* 1985;157:637–644.

Uflacker R, Kaemmerer A, Neves C, Picon PD. Management of massive hemoptysis by bronchial artery embolization. *Radiology* 1983;146:627–634.

Vujic I, Pyle R, Parker E, Mithoefer J. Control of massive hemoptysis by embolization of intercostal arteries. *Radiology* 1980;137:617–620.

Wholey MH, Chamorro HA, Rao G, Ford WB, Miller WH. Bronchial artery embolization for massive hemoptysis. *JAMA* 1976;236:2501–2504.

Winzelberg G, Wholey MH. Scintigraphic detection of pulmonary hemorrhage using Tc-99 sulfur colloid. *Clin Nucl Med* 1981;6:537–539.

Embolization in Cases of Varicocele

RENAN UFLACKER

BACKGROUND

One of the primary causes of infertility in male patients is oligospermia and spermatic motility dysfunction related to the presence of varicocele. Varicocele originates from a pathologic dilatation of the pampiniform venous complex which surrounds the testis caused by pressure elevation as a consequence of the absence or incompetence of the valves of the internal spermatic vein (primary), or of renal vein obstruction (secondary). Valvular insufficiency allows retrograde venous flow through the spermatic vein, causing venous ingurgitation and an increase in testicular temperature. Other symptoms associated with voluminous varicocele are pain and testicular edema.

Around 15 percent of males develop varicocele during puberty. It is most common on the left (about 90 percent); 8 percent of cases are bilateral, and only 2 percent occur on the right side. Thirty to forty percent of patients with varicocele present reduced spermatogenesis.

The surgical treatment of varicocele, involving suprainguinal or retroperitoneal ligation of the venous plexus, improves semen quality in many cases. Varicocele, however, recurs in 10 percent of cases, most frequently because of communication between the right and left plexus. In the past, venous catheterization was used primarily as a technique for the phlebographic demonstration of varicocele. Currently, spermatic vein occlusion is widely used as a practical, effective way to correct varicocele. It costs less than surgery and can be performed in the radiology department with topical anesthesia in all patients, either by the femoral or the jugular approach.

ANATOMIC CONSIDERATIONS

Figure 4.57 shows the basic anatomy of the spermatic venous system. Anatomic variations are common, and several venous collaterals may be found along the spermatic veins. The gonadal veins have anastomoses with the lumbar, retroperitoneal, ureteral, and capsular veins (Fig. 4.58). Very often there are anastomoses with the intrarenal venous system. Complete or segmental duplication of the spermatic veins is a common finding.

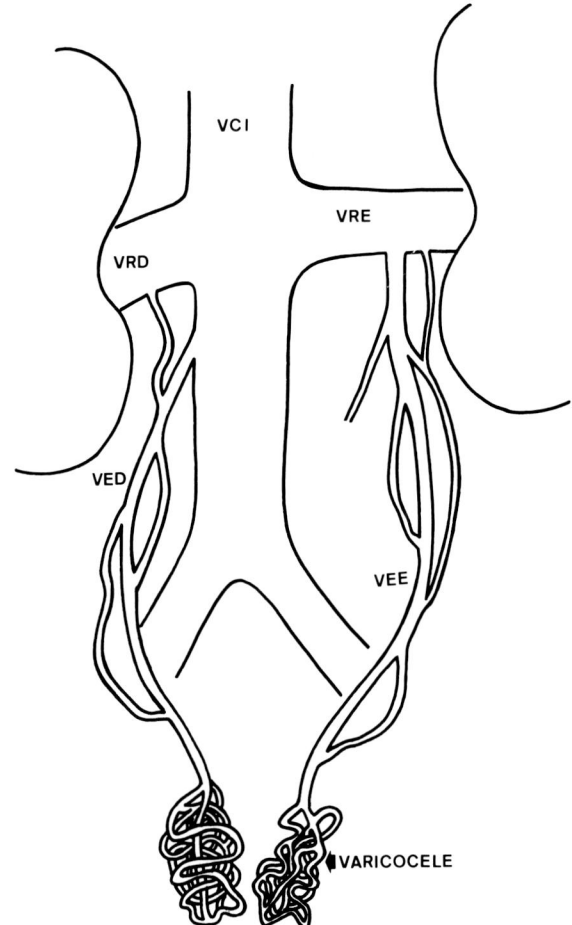

Figure 4.57 Schematic drawing of venous circulation in testes and varicocele drainage.
VCI—inferior vena cava (IVC); VRD—right renal vein (RRV); VRE—left renal vein (LRV); VED—right spermatic vein (RSV); VEE—left spermatic vein (LSV). The arrow points to the venous entanglement in the pampiniform plexus, which is the varicocele. Notice the confluence point of RSV directly on the lateral IVC wall, right below the RRV. The LSV opening into the LRV is a constant finding, although division of the LSV may occur, with several anastomoses. Notice the duplications and collaterals that exist along the left and right spermatic veins, as well as the anastomoses with the renal venous circulation.

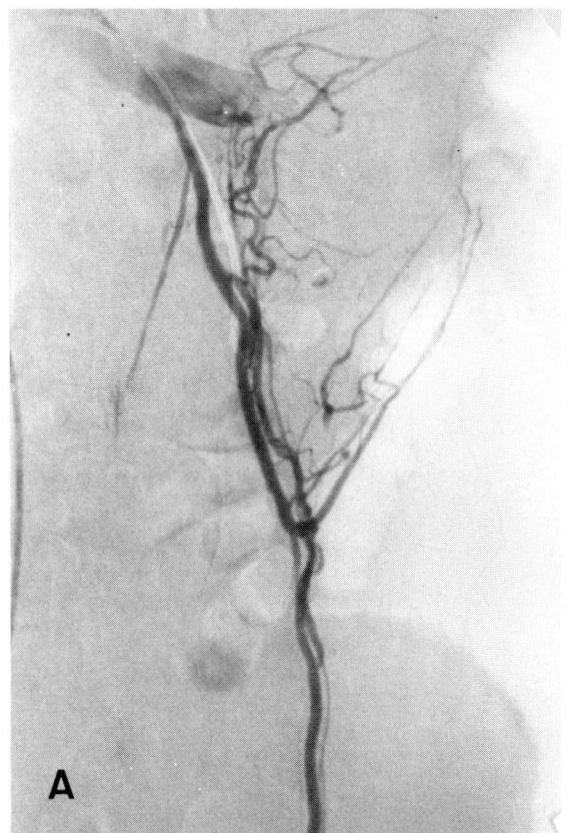
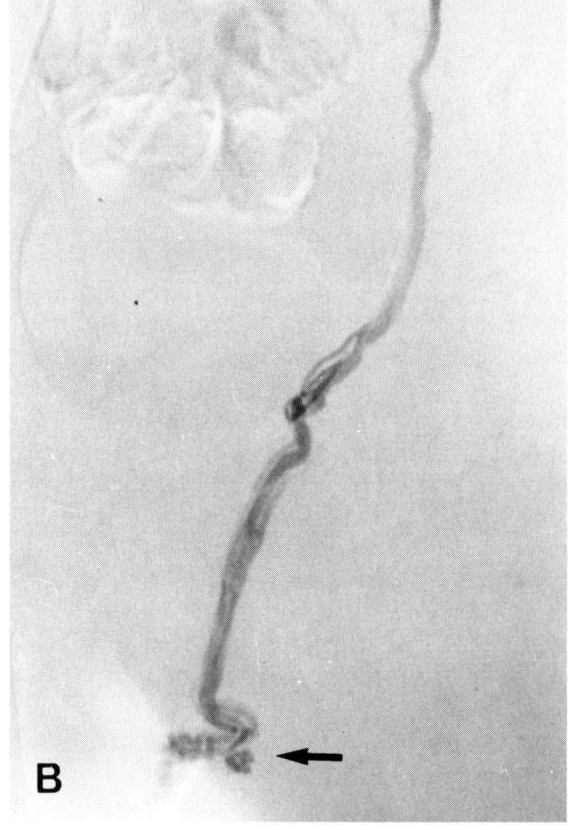
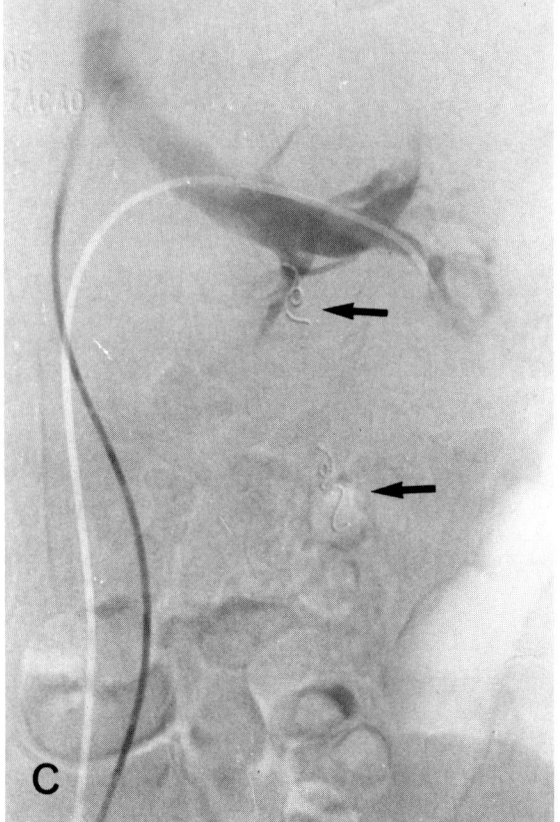

Figure 4.58 Spermatic phlebogram in young adult patient with infertility and varicocele.
(A) Injection into the left spermatic vein showing valvular incompetence or absence and abundant opacification of retroperitoneal collaterals, anastomosed with the left renal capsular circulation. (B) Proximal left spermatic vein segment showing the varicocele venous entanglement at scrotal level (arrow). (C) Postembolization control. Two Gianturco coils have been used at different levels (arrows), and a sclerosing agent employed for occlusion of collaterals.

Abnormal confluences with the renal vein on the left side, and with vena cava and renal vein on the right side, are occasionally found. It is common to find the right gonadal vein opening directly into the vena cava on the right, and the left gonadal vein opening into the left renal vein (Figs. 4.57 and 4.59).

TECHNIQUE

The most frequently used techniques are selective catheterization of the left spermatic vein with a Cobra-type catheter by the femoral route (Fig. 4.60), or with a specially curved catheter by the internal right jugular route.

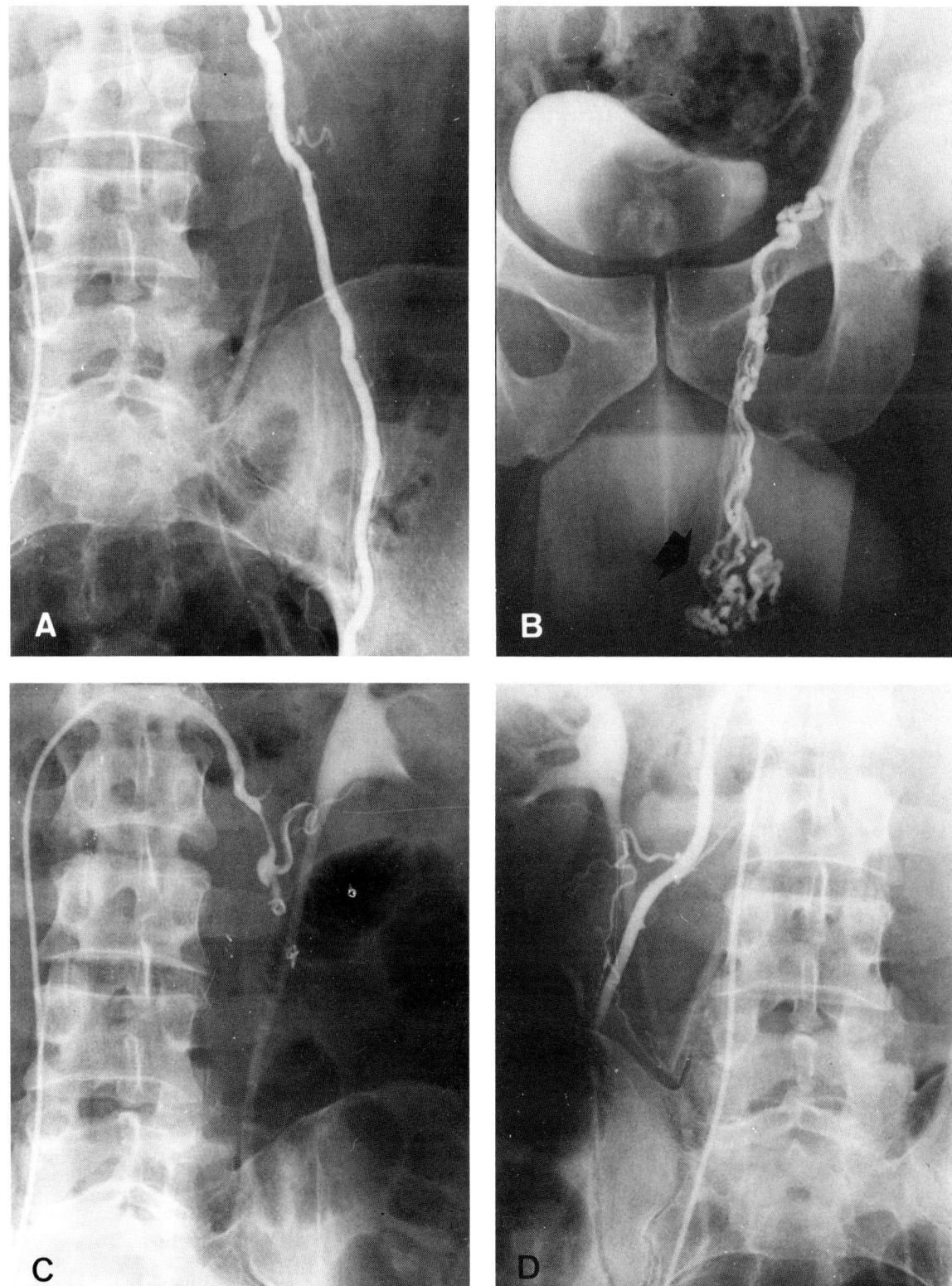

Figure 4.59 41-year-old patient who has presented with scrotal pouch pain and edema on the left related to varicocele on the same side.

(A) Injection into the left spermatic vein, showing valvular incompetence. (B) The vein's more proximal portion, showing the varicocele (arrow). (C) Control following embolization with two 3-mm coils at two levels. (D) Injection into the right spermatic vein showing valvular competence and opacification of the vein's distal third. Significant improvement in pain and edema was obtained after embolization, although testicular tenderness persisted.

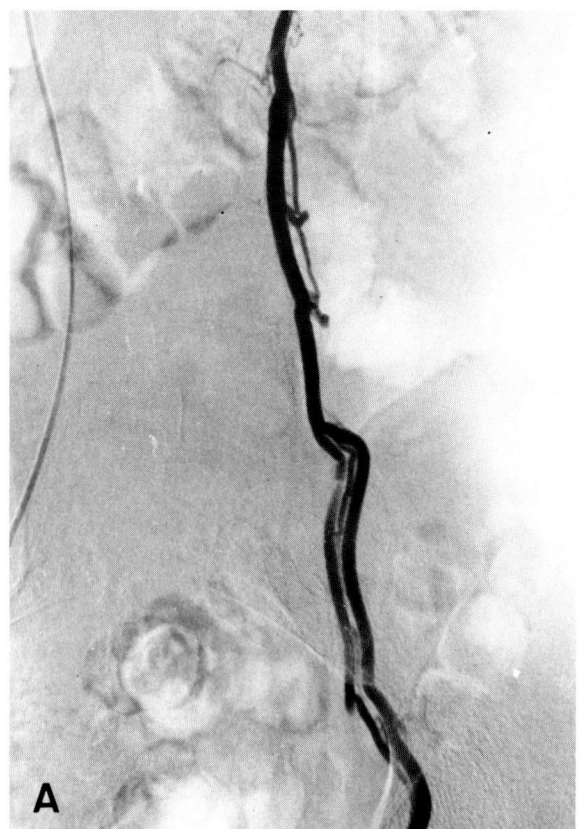
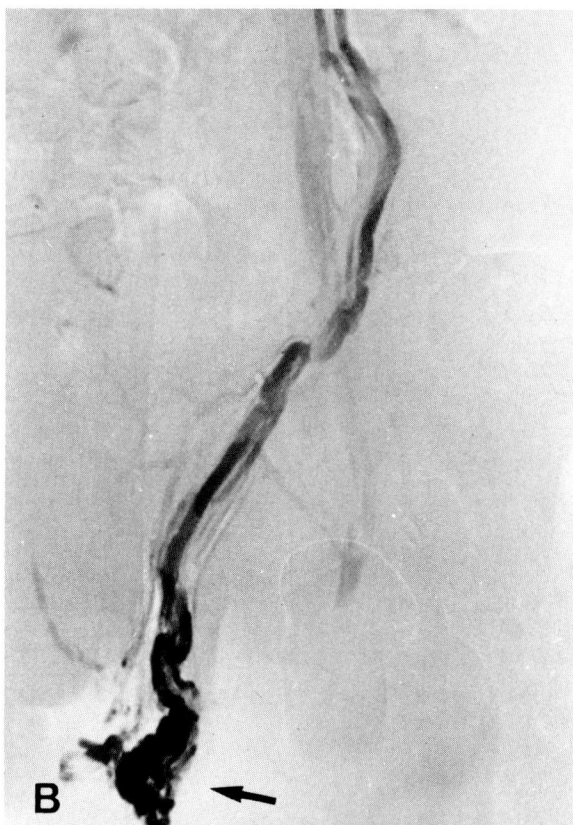
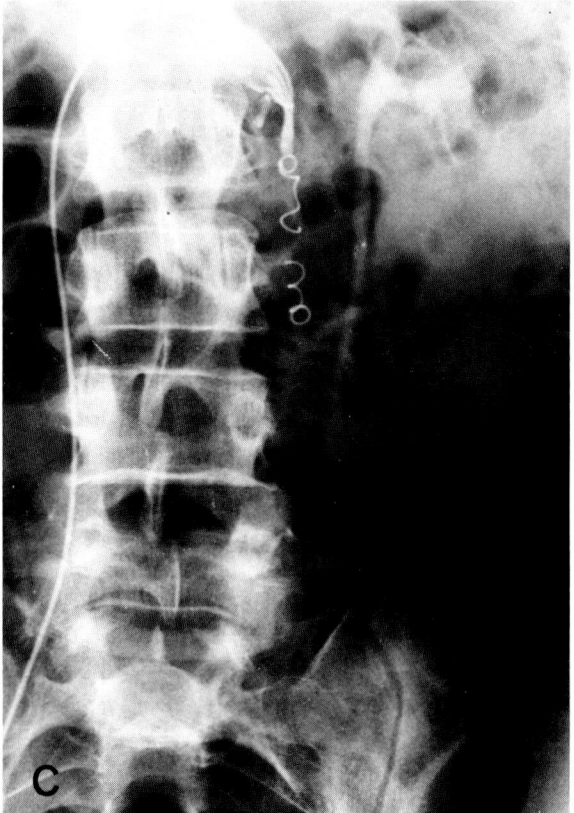

Figure 4.60 33-year-old patient with a 10-year history of infertility, exhibiting varicocele on the left.
(A) Injection into the left spermatic vein showing venous failure and retrograde opacification. Notice the segmental duplication. (B) Proximal portion of the vein, showing the varicocele (arrow). (C) Control following embolization with two Gianturco coils in the distal third. The spermogram improved, and pregnancy was achieved during a 14-month follow-up.

Once the left spermatic vein has been catheterized, a phlebogram of the whole system should be obtained to evaluate the anatomy and to check valvular competence (Fig. 4.58). After the phlebogram, a flexible-tip straight catheter is introduced deeply into the spermatic vein and advanced as far as possible; new radiographs may then be obtained for evaluation of the collaterals.

After the extent of collateralization and duplication has been identified, the catheter is positioned at a point where no duplication exists and embolization is performed (Fig. 4.56). If it is impossible to avoid collaterals and duplications, embolization must be performed at several different levels (Fig. 4.58).

Embolization should be bilaterally performed, since varicocele recurrence through left-right communications of venous collaterals not demonstrable angiographically may be as high as 10 percent.

If the jugular route is used, the same catheter may be used for both the right and the left spermatic vein catheterization. If the femoral route is used, a No. 2 or 3 long-tipped Simmons-type catheter is a better choice. However, it must be carefully manipulated during the catheterization maneuvers to avoid caval and right spermatic vein dissection and rupture (Fig. 4.56).

In general, any of the occlusive materials in common use are effective.

When sclerosing agents are used for spermatic vein occlusion, 5 to 10 mL of hypertonic (75 percent) glucose is injected one or more times into the gonadal vein, followed by 1 to 2 mL of ethanolamine oleate (Ethamolin), usually producing total venous occlusion. To prevent epididymitis, care should be taken to keep the sclerosing agent from reaching the pampiniform plexus.

One technique used is to inject the sclerosing agent preceded by an air bubble, which is followed under fluoroscopy to the proximal third of the gonadal vein (near the testis) and maintained in that position for 15 min, after which the sclerosing agent is immediately and totally aspirated. Another technique involves compressing the internal inguinal ring to occlude the spermatic vein while the sclerosing agent is being used, which prevents the agent from filling the pampiniform plexus. Sclerosis occludes the main vein, its collaterals, and the duplicated venous tracks.

Several different embolic materials have been used in spermatic vein occlusion, including Gianturco coils, detachable balloons, and bucrylate-type adhesives. After selective catheterization, the embolic agent should be introduced in accordance with the procedures described in Chap. 2.

Embolizing agents can be used in conjunction with sclerosing materials when difficulty is encountered in occluding the collaterals (Fig. 4.55).

RESULTS

Long-term results are encouraging; varicocele persists in only 10 to 15 percent of cases. Spermatic vein reconstitution through collaterals or duplication is the main cause of varicocele recurrence in patients treated by particulate emboli.

Side effects, which are minor, occur in about 12 percent of cases. The most common side effects of spermatic vein sclerosis are hypotension, contrast medium extravasation, pain during sclerotherapy, scrotal edema, and epididymitis.

In couples with male infertility problems, the pregnancy rate obtained after treatment is as high as 48 percent. The improvement in spermogram values (78 percent) is similar to the results obtained with surgery.

REFERENCES

Adams PE. Treatment of varicocels with detachable balloon embolization. *Radiol Technol* 1983;55:611–614.

Formaneck A, Rusnak B, Zollikofer C, et al. Embolization of the spermatic vein for treatment of infertility: A new approach. *Radiology* 1981;139:315–321.

Gonzales R, Narayan D, Castaneda-Zuniga WR, Amplatz K. Transvenous embolization of the internal spermatic vein for the treatment of varicocele scroti. *Urol Clin North Am* 1982;9:177–184.

Kaufman SL, Kadir S, Borth KH, et al. Mechanisms of recurrent varicocele after balloon occlusion or surgical ligation of the internal spermatic vein. *Radiology* 1983;147:435–440.

Lima S, Castro MP, Costa OF. A new method for the treatment of varicocele. *Andrologia* 1978;10:103–106.

Riedl P, Kumpan W, Maier U, et al. Long term results after sclerotherapy of the spermatic vein in patients with varicocele. *Cardiovasc Intervent Radiol* 1985;8:46–49.

Riedl P, Lunglmayr G, Stackl O. A new method of transfemoral testicular vein obliteration for varicocele using a balloon catheter. *Radiology* 1981;139:323–325.

Seyferth W, Jecht E, Zeitler E. Percutaneous sclerotherapy of varicocele. *Radiology* 1981;139:335–340.

Swerdloff RS, Boyers SP. Evaluation of the male partner of an infertile couple. *JAMA* 1982;247:2418–2422.

Walsh PC, White RI. Balloon occlusion of the internal spermatic vein for the treatment of varicocels. *JAMA* 1981;246:1701–1702.

White RI, Kaufman SL, Barth KH, et al. Occlusion of varicocels with detachable balloons. *Radiology* 1981;139:327–334.

Zeitler E, Jecht E, Richter EL, Seyferth W. Selective sclerotherapy of the internal spermatic vein in patients with varicocels. *Cardiovasc Intervent Radiol* 1980;3:166–169.

Embolization in Cases of Bleeding from Pelvic Organs

GUILLHERME DE SOUZA MAURÃO

BACKGROUND

Embolization of the hypogastric arteries for treatment of pelvic organ hemorrhage was introduced by Margolies, who in 1972 described the utilization of this procedure in the treatment of massive hemorrhage secondary to pelvic trauma. This method is now widely accepted, and is the method of choice for controlling pelvic hemorrhage of different etiologies, including pelvic trauma, bladder neoplasm, gynecologic neoplasms, pelvic organ post-irradiation sequelae, complications of urologic and orthopedic surgery, arteriovenous fistulas, and puerperal hemorrhages.

The transcatheter arterial embolization of pelvic vessels has proved particularly useful in cases of clinically uncontrolled vesical or vaginal hemorrhage, or when surgery is not a viable alternative.

ANATOMIC CONSIDERATIONS

The superiority of embolization over surgical ligation of hypogastric arteries for control of pelvic hemorrhage has long been recognized. Transcatheter embolization makes possible the occlusion of pathologic small-diameter vessels, thus eliminating the plexus of small precapillary collaterals, which are the primary cause of recurrences of bleeding. Burchell has shown that after bilateral surgical ligation, pulse pressure drops by 85 percent, but blood flow only by 48 percent, due to the abundant collateral circulation present in the pelvic region.

The peculiar anatomic layout of the vascular supply to the pelvis facilitates transcatheter arterial embolization. Arteries up to a more peripheral level may therefore be occluded. Embolization at this level should be performed with extreme care; of utmost importance is choosing the right moment to discontinue the procedure. Excessive embolization, even if unilateral, may lead to tissue damage, particularly in the bladder. In addition, the greater the number of emboli introduced, the higher the possibility of reflux into the systemic circulation.

TECHNIQUE

Catheterization should be as selective as possible, and, whenever possible, embolization should be unilateral (Fig. 4.61). This allows occlusion of small-diameter

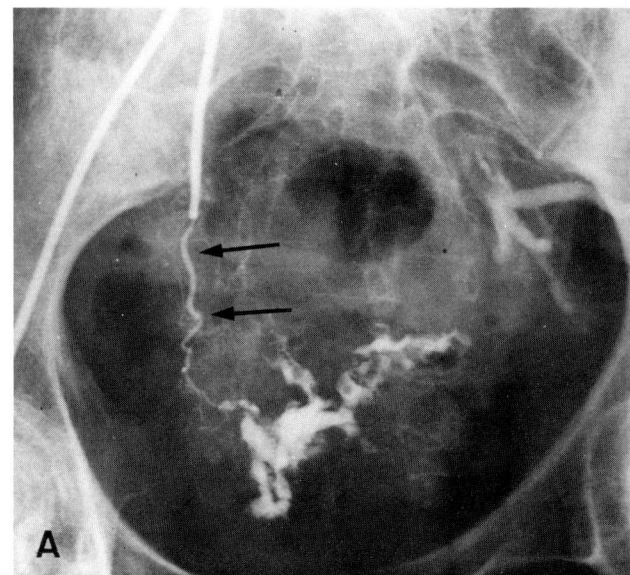

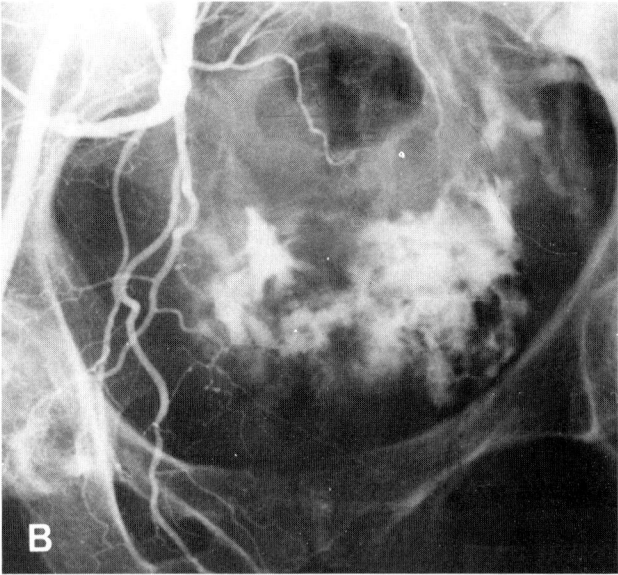

Figure 4.61 51-year-old patient with resected and irradiated uterine carcinoma and pelvic and vaginal hemorrhage.
(A) After left hypogastric embolization, a small artery, a right hypogastric anterior division branch (arrows), was embolized, and abundant contrast medium extravasation into the small pelvis is evident. (B) Embolization with Gelfoam particles resulted in occlusion of the responsible artery and control of bleeding. Notice the large quantity of residual contrast.

pathologic vessels, while maintaining sufficient tissue perfusion through collateral circulation. In cases of bladder tumor, embolization should always be bilateral, as the vessels on the contralateral side may cause a recurrence of bleeding.

COMPLICATIONS

Complications from embolization depend on the site in which the embolizing material is lodged. Possible complications are lower limb ischemia; necrosis of gluteal musculature, iliac bone, and sciatic and femoral nerves; and occlusion of radicular arteries (Fig. 4.62). Impotence is an undesirable complication, particularly in patients under 60 years of age, who may, for example, bleed after prostatectomy. Reports in the literature on neurologic complications following embolization of hypogastric arteries are scarce. Guiliani et al. have described the occurrence of Brown–Séquard's paralysis following hypogastric artery embolization for bladder carcinoma. Other reports exist of transient paresis without sequelae.

Neurologic accidents are probably closely related to blockage of blood supply to greater nerves, such as the sciatic or the femoral nerve, or to the distal spinal cord, as a result of occlusion of the radicular arteries (Fig. 4.62). Therefore, when the radicular arteries are identified, but at the same time it is not possible to selectively catheterize the anterior hypogastric artery axis, embolization should be avoided, except in extreme cases of hemorrhage (Fig. 4.63).

Anastomotic channels are known to exist between the iliolumbar and lateral sacral arteries, which are branches of the posterior division of the hypogastric artery, and the spinal arteries. Occlusion of the posterior branch of the hypogastric artery may compromise the vascular integrity not only of the cauda equina, but also of the sciatic nerve, and can lead to muscle necrosis in the gluteal region.

Hemorrhage is rarely demonstrable (Fig. 4.61), but this is not a problem because in most cases the bleeding site is not identified, and therefore all branches of the anterior division of the hypogastric artery must be embolized. Preferential blood flow to the pathologic vessels responsible for bleeding will ensure the desired effect, even when superselective embolization is not possible (Fig. 4.64).

A femoral entry can be used in most cases to obtain superselective catheterization; only in a few patients is it necessary to perform a bilateral femoral puncture or to use the axillary route.

Selection of an embolizing material will depend on the size of the vessels to be embolized, and on the desired occlusion time. Gelfoam is the most commonly used material. The particles must be of sufficient size to occlude the distal vessels without producing tissue necrosis; 2- by 2-mm particles are commonly utilized.

Proximal occlusion with Gianturco coils achieves permanent occlusion, the results being similar to those of surgical ligation. Gianturco coils are not adequate for effective bleeding control, as they do not prevent distal recanalization and rebleeding. Both embolization with coils and surgical ligation makes future distal embolization impossible.

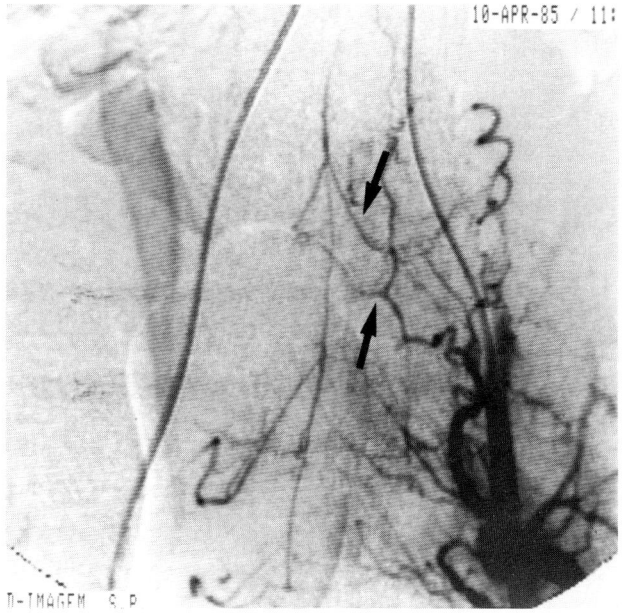

Figure 4.62 Digital angiogram of 70-year-old patient with hematuria from prostate adenocarcinoma.
Selective injection into the left hypogastric artery has caused radiculomedullary (arrows) and sacral lateral arterial filling. A later phase (not shown) showed filling of the anterior medullary artery. Because of the presence of these arteries, embolization was not performed.

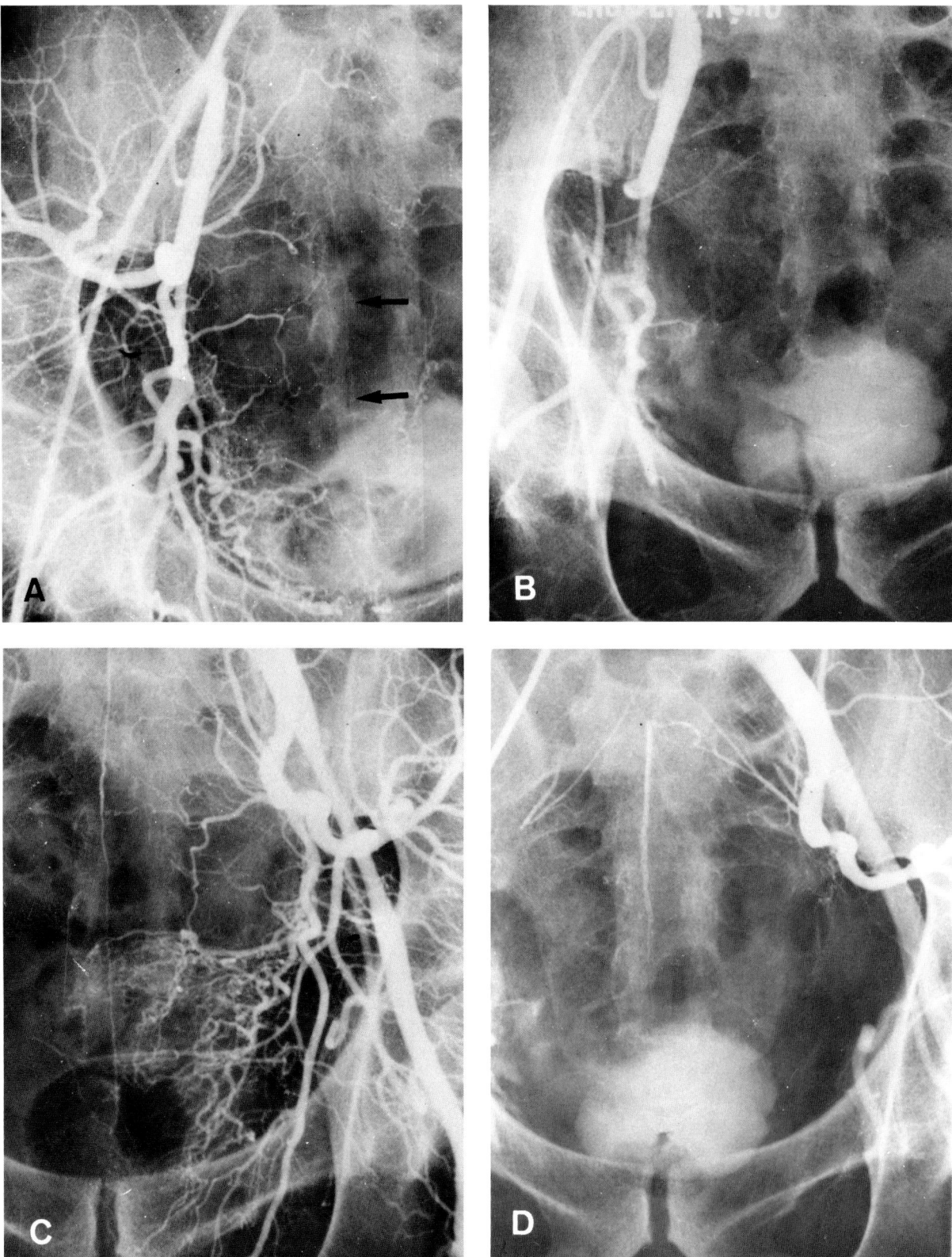

Figure 4.63 45-year-old patient with bladder carcinoma that has been resected and irradiated.
(A) Injection into the right hypogastric artery showing vesical wall hypervascularity and multiple radicular arteries feeding the sacral arteries (arrows). (B) Postembolization control on the right, showing extensive occlusion of right hypogastric branches without vesical wall vascularity. (C) Injection into the left hypogastric artery showing left vesical wall vascularity. Notice the presence of radicular arteries filling the middle sacral artery. (D) Control following embolization of left hypogastric artery showing total occlusion of its branches, including the radicular arteries. Note the opacification of the middle sacral artery. Permanent clinical control of bleeding was obtained, without sequelae.

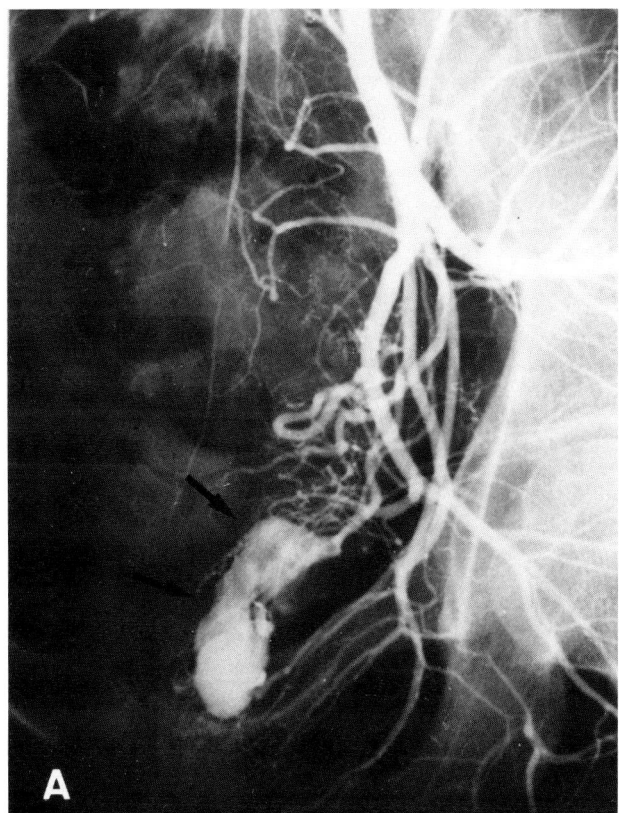
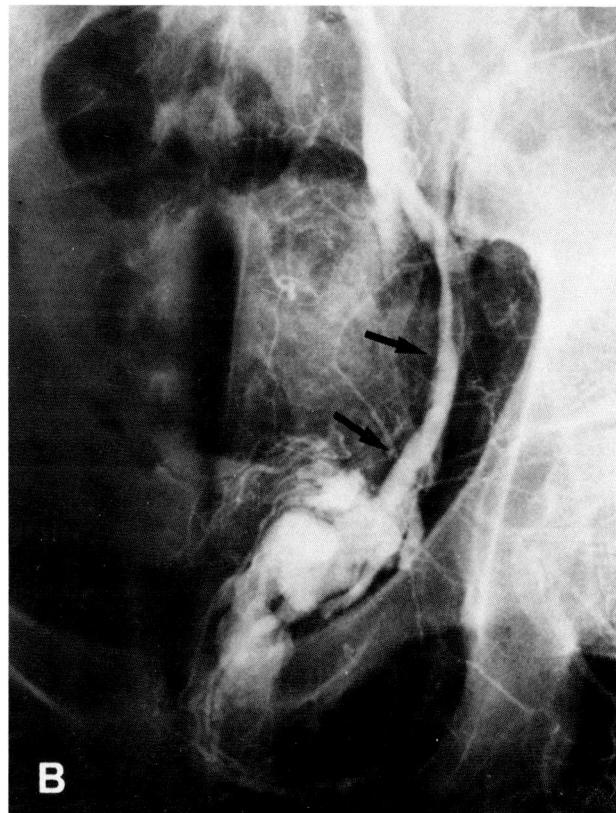
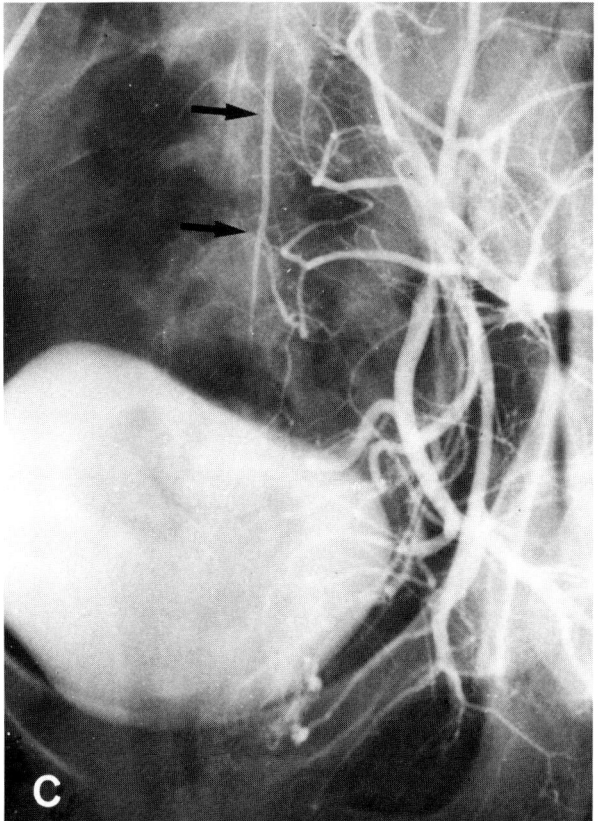

Figure 4.64 19-year-old patient operated on for hydatidiform mole presented massive vaginal bleeding.
(A) Arterial phase of left hypogastric injection showing active bleeding in pseudoaneurysm of the small pelvis (arrows). (B) Later phase of arterial injection showing arteriovenous fistula with early venous filling (arrows). (C) Postembolization control of hypogastric arterial branches. The pseudoaneurysm and the arteriovenous fistula have disappeared. Opacification has persisted following embolization of radicular and middle sacral arteries (arrows). Clinical control of bleeding was obtained.

REFERENCES

Amis ES Jr, Pfister RC, Yoder IC. Interventional radiology of the adult bladder and urethra. *Semin Roentgenol* 1983;18(4):322–330.

Burchell RC. Physiology of internal iliac artery ligation. *J Obstet Gynaecol Br Cwlth* 1968;75:642–651.

Diamond NG, Casarella WJ, Bachaman DM, Wolff M. Microfibrillar collagen hemostat: A new transcatheter embolization agent. *Radiology* 1979;133:775–779.

Dichiro G. Unintentional spinal cord arteriography: A warning. *Radiology* 1974;112:213–215.

Feldman L, Greendield AJ, Waltman CA, et al. Transcatheter vessel occlusion angiographic results versus clinical success. *Radiology* 1983;147:1–152.

Gianturco C, Anderson JH, Wallace S. Mechanical devices for arterial occlusion. *AJR* 1975;124:428–432.

Giuliani L, Carmignani G, Belgrano E, Pupo P. Gelatin form and isobutyl-2-cyanocrylate in the treatment of lifethreatening bladder haemorrhage by selective transcatheter embolization of the internal iliac arteries. *Br J Urol* 1979;51:125–128.

Hare WSC, Lond FRCR, Holland CJ. Paresis following internal iliac artery embolization. *Radiology* 1983;146:47–51.

Heaston DK, Mineau DE, Brown BJ, Miller Jr FJ. Transcatheter arterial embolization for control of persistent massive puerperal hemorrhage after bilateral surgical hypogastric artery ligation. *AJR* 1979;133:152–154.

Higgins CB, Bookstein JJ, et al. Therapeutic embolization for intractable chronic bleeding. *Radiology* 1977;122:152–154.

Jander PH, Russinovich NAE. Transcatheter Gelfoam embolization in abdominal, retroperitoneal and pelvic hemorrhage. *Radiology* 1980;136:337–340.

Kam J, Jackson H, Menachem YB. Vascular injuries in blunt pelvic trauma. *Radiol Clin North Am* 1981;19(1):171–180.

Kelemen J, Scultely S. Nemeth A, Szegvari M. Embolization of the arteria iliac interna as treatment of life endangering hemorrhages caused by intrapelvic malignant tumors. *Diagn Imag Clin Med* 1979;48:275–285.

Kobayashi T, Kusano S, Matsubayashi T, Uchida T. Selective embolization of the vesical artery in the management of massive bladder hemorrhage. *Radiology* 1980;136:345–348.

Lang EK. Transcatheter embolization of pelvic vessels for control of intractable hemorrhage. *Radiology* 1981;140:331–339.

Lang EK, Deutsch JS, Goodman JR, et al. Transcatheter embolization of intractable bladder hemorrhage. *J Urol* 1979;121:30–36.

Lang EK, Pisco M. Transcatheter embolization of hypogastric branch arteries in the management of intractable bladder hemorrhage. In Interventional Radiology, edited by Veiga-Pires JA. Excerpta Medica, Amsterdam, 1980;102–104.

Lazorthes G. Blood supply and vascular pathology of the spinal cord. In *Spinal Angiomas: Advances in Diagnosis* edited by Pia HW, Djindjian R. Springer-Verlag, Heidelberg, 1978;1–17.

Luzsa G. *X-ray Anatomy of the Vascular System*. Butterworth, London, 1974;294–296.

Margolies MN, Ring EJ, Waltman AC, et al. Arteriography in the management of hemorrhage from pelvic fractures. *N Engl J Med* 1972;287:317–320.

Mohri M, Hiramatsu K. Simplified bilateral selective catheterization of the uterine artery. *Radiology* 1981;129:239–241.

Mourao GS, Uflacker R, Piske RL, Lima SS. Embolizacao das arterias hipogastricas no tratamento de sangramento dos orgaos pelvicos. *Radiol Bras* 1985;18(3):175–181.

Nataf R, Jeanpierre R. Problemes et accidents de l'embolization arterielle hipogastric. *J Urol Nephrol* 1976;82:872–878.

Schwartz PE, Goldstein HM, Wallage S, Rutledge FN. Control of arterial hemorrhage using percutaneous arterial catheter techniques in patients with gynecologic malignancies. *Gynecol Oncol* 1975;3:276–286.

Smith Jr JC, Kerr WS, Athanasoulis CA, et al. Angiographic management of bleeding secondary to genitourinary tract surgery. *J Urol* 1975;113:89–92.

Steinhart L, Hlava A, Navratil P, Svab J. Indications for obliterations of pelvic arteries in bleeding lesions of pelvic organs. In *Intervention Radiology,* edited by Veiga-pires JA. Excerpta Medica, Amsterdam, 1980;111–117.

Thelen VM, Bruhl P. Arterielle kathetere embolization biem blutender blasen-karzinom. *Fortschr Rontgenstr* 1978;12:198–201.

Waneck VR, Lechner G, Powischer G. GefaBaembolisation bei urstillbarem tumor: Und strahlendedingten blutunger der harnblase. *Fortschr Rontgenstr* 1979;130:193–196.

Embolization in Traumatic and Aneurysmal Lesions

RENAN UFLACKER

BACKGROUND

Lesions of traumatic origin may involve neurologic problems, multiple organ failure, and bone fractures. In addition, they introduce hemorrhagic changes leading to hemodynamic instability and even to death. From the standpoint of angiography, two types of traumatic lesions are important: visceral lacerations and direct vascular lesions. Both are associated with bleeding.

Diagnostic and therapeutic angiographic procedures are becoming more and more significant in the management of patients with traumatic lesions, as they allow accurate location of hemorrhagic lesions, as well as hemostasis through catheterization.

In treating all cases of traumatic lesions, the following points should be remembered:

Death during hospitalization is often preventable.
Trauma patients often develop disseminated intravascular coagulation, exsanguinating more rapidly than expected.
Multiple, inessential radiographic studies are frequently the cause of death.
Peritoneal lavage and aspiration to detect intraperitoneal bleeding offer limited accuracy.
Understanding the underlying mechanism of trauma is essential for effective management of lesions.
Hemorrhage following trauma, whether surgical or nonsurgical, is basically a function of the mechanics of vascularization of lesions.
Angiographic studies should be performed early, and the decision regarding embolization of a bleeding lesion should be made immediately.
Embolization is a safer, frequently more effective, solution than surgical intervention.
To prevent exsanguination, bleeding should be controlled by surgery or embolization, even when the patient's general condition is unstable.

A few of the most common errors in the management of bleeding trauma patients include not proceeding with the investigation when initial findings are negative; not evaluating adequately the mechanisms of trauma; not realizing early enough the significance of postsurgical hemorrhage; inadequate assessment of the severity of the trauma; failing to move a patient who exhibits hemodynamic instability to the surgical center or angiography lab.

Lesions of traumatic origin involving the skull, face, cervical region, thorax, abdomen, pelvis, and limbs frequently cause severe bleeding episodes which are difficult to diagnose and to treat. Lacerated lesions in parenchymal organs may cause massive hemorrhage inside cavities (thorax and abdomen), in virtual spaces (e.g., retroperitoneum), or in natural pathways (such as hemoptysis in the bronchial tree or hematuria in the pelvis and ureters). Lesions on the face, neck, and limbs are more frequently related to direct vascular trauma with external bleeding or bleeding into the virtual spaces (muscle sheaths, etc.). Pseudoaneurysms, with or without arteriovenous fistula, may be formed at any of the above-mentioned locations.

The different aspects of embolization in cases of bleeding and arteriovenous fistulas in the head and neck are discussed in the section "Embolization in Head and Neck Lesions" in this chapter. The treatment of thoracic traumatic lesions was discussed under "Thoracic Embolization," also in this chapter. The embolization of traumatic lesions of the abdomen, pelvis, and limbs will be approached next, although illustrations and some specific aspects of the different organs have already been described in the sections "Embolization in the Liver," "Splenic Embolization," "Embolization in the Pancreas," "Renal Embolization," and "Embolization in Bleeding of Pelvic Organs."

ABDOMINAL ORGANS

Embolization of traumatized abdominal organs should be performed by femoral or axillary puncture through a valvulated, check-flow-type sheath, in order to facilitate the exchange of catheters of varying diameter during the procedure.

Even when the origin of bleeding is known, because abdominal trauma is frequently of multiple nature, it is desirable to perform an aortogram before embolization despite the fact that the source of hemorrhage is only shown through selective injection in most cases.

Embolization is indicated whenever trauma has caused a bleeding artery in the abdomen. Gelfoam particles and Gianturco coils are probably the most frequently used embolic materials. Powder Gelfoam, or any other small particle or fluid-state material, which may cause structural infarction, is not advisable in most cases.

Gelfoam particles (2- by 2-mm, or 3- by 3-mm) are utilized for occlusion of small-diameter arteries, as they preserve the microcirculation. Gianturco spiral coils are used for embolizing large and medium-sized arteries; they produce an overall reduction in arterial pressure in the embolized territory, making hemostasis possible.

Intraperitoneal hemorrhage due to contusive trauma is usually associated with hepatic and splenic laceration, but may also result from trauma to organs located in the retroperitoneum, such as the pancreas, kidneys, pelvis, and other retroperitoneal vessels. In cases of penetrating abdominal trauma, there is an additional danger of bleeding from mesenteric and larger abdominal vessels.

PELVIC LESIONS

Pelvic fractures, which are common in cases of massive trauma, are usually accompanied by lesions involving other organs. They are usually complex, may bleed copiously, and are associated with high morbidity and mortality rates.

Surgical treatment of bleeding pelvic lesions is usually ineffective, and may even exacerbate the hemorrhagic process. It may also cause infection. For these reasons, diagnostic and therapeutic angiographic studies through embolization are indicated in cases of traumatic pelvic lesions.

Angiography should be performed as early as possible in these patients, even simultaneously with resuscitation maneuvers. Bladder and urethral studies should not precede angiography, since the contrast medium used may prevent the visualization of arterial extravasation. After angiography, these studies may be performed without removing the patient from the table. Both abdomen and pelvis, including all soft tissue, should always be examined.

As in other situations involving trauma and hemorrhage, it is generally desirable to use a medium-duration embolizing material, which is absorbed after a few weeks, thus allowing tissue circulation to be restored after healing. If larger vessels are to be occluded, or if permanent occlusion is required, a nonabsorbable material should be used.

The arteries chosen for occlusion are preferably those which show active extravasation during examination. If however, anatomic considerations prevent superselective catheterization, the whole hypogastric artery may be closed on the bleeding side. This may also be done when several hypogastric branches are bleeding simultaneously and the patient will not stand a prolonged procedure.

It should be emphasized that embolization and angiography are only the beginning of a long and difficult treatment process, for both physician and patient, and special care is required to reduce mortality in patients with traumatic lesions of the pelvis.

LESIONS OF THE EXTREMITIES

Traumatic lesions to the extremities, with bleeding, pseudoaneurysms, or arteriovenous fistulas, are usually caused by penetrating knife or gunshot wounds. In rare instances, such lesions are due to contusion or bone fracture, or are surgical sequelae. From an angiographic standpoint, traumatic lesions of the limbs may be classified as acute or chronic.

Acute lesions are vascular lacerations with hemorrhage, thrombosis, or formation of acute arteriovenous fistula. These lesions occur more frequently in the thigh. Because locating a lesion of this type involves extensive surgical investigation, angiography, which may instantaneously show the lesion site, is indicated.

Figure 4.65 shows the result of an inadequate surgical exploration, with ligation ("treatment") of the wrong artery. Lesions in the subclavian artery are more dangerous than other lesions because of cervicocranial vascular involvement. Because the subclavian artery is a critical vessel for neurologic and upper limb viability, temporary occlusion with a balloon catheter may be a better alternative than definitive embolization. Surgical exploration is never easy under the best of circumstances, and it is particularly difficult to identify a vascular lesion inside a large, uncontrolled hematoma that has evolved with extensive tissue infiltration.

Another acute case involves limb bleeding due to surgical sequela, with formation of a compartment syndrome, and distal ischemia (Fig. 4.66). Hemorrhage usually originates from a muscular branch in which hemostasis has not been adequately achieved.

Chronic limb lesions are usually arteriovenous fistulas and/or pseudoaneurysms which were missed on the initial examination but which have developed progressively. The mechanism is either wall laceration of greater vessels or transection (artery and vein) with arterial pseudoaneurysm formation, which may or may not communicate with an adjacent vein.

Arteriovenous fistula flow tends to increase over time, causing distal ischemia due to flow stealing.

ANEURYSMAL LESIONS

Pseudoaneurysms cause a mass effect (Fig. 4.67). A pseudoaneurysm may also be a surgical sequela, the result of vascular suture dehiscence or of accidental injury to the greater vessel. Pseudoaneurysms may be secondary to arterial wall necrosis due to inflammatory process, proteolysis in the peripancreatic area, or radicular arteritis. Any artery may be involved, regardless of location or function. Surgical treatment is difficult, particularly when the affected area is hard to reach.

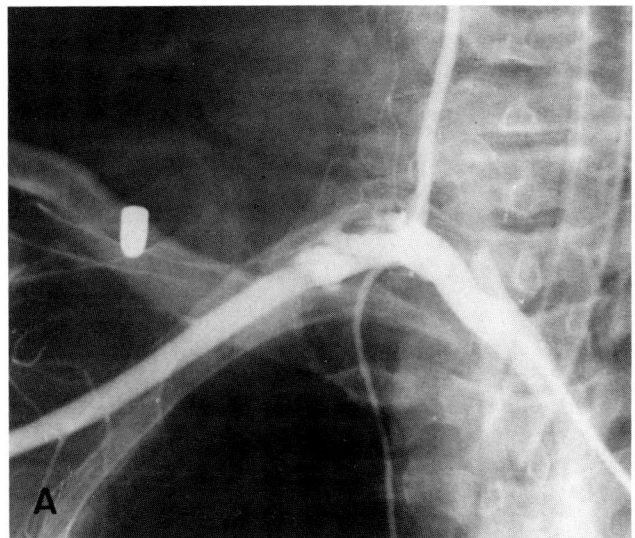
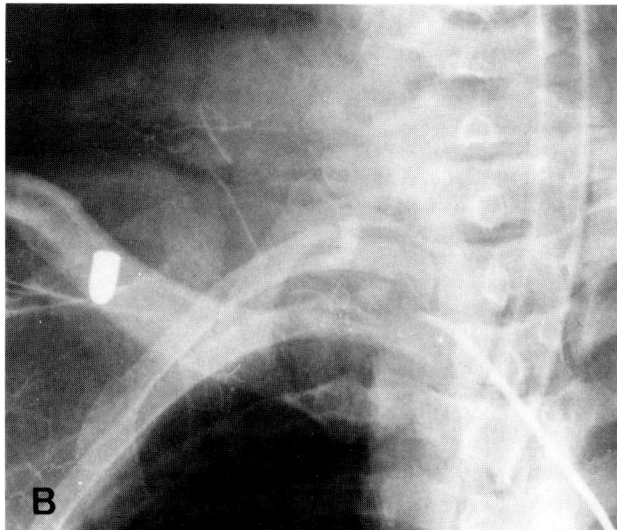
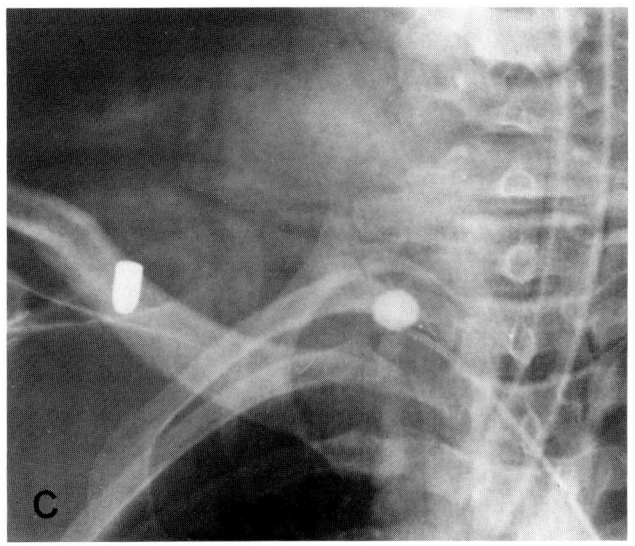

Figure 4.65 (A) Patient with right subclavian artery laceration produced by firearm bullet. Voluminous hematoma is present in the cervical and supraclavicular region. Notice the laceration of the arterial wall and the ligation of the right common carotid artery. (B) Later phase of injection showing small contrast medium collection outside the vessel.
(C) Temporary presurgical occlusion of right subclavian artery with occlusion balloon catheter. Arterial surgical repair was performed without significant blood loss.

Pseudoaneurysms may be embolized, but should be carefully approached due to wall fragility. A low-pressure embolization system should be used. When the artery is small (up to 3 mm), the embolizing material for pseudoaneurysms may be particulate (Gelfoam); spiral Gianturco coils should, however, be used for occlusion of main arteries. Traumatic arteriovenous fistulas are best treated with detachable balloons or Gianturco coils. Angiographers' personal experience will help them choose the most appropriate materials.

Embolization with coils may only reduce flow. However, if, because of high output, the vessel is not totally occluded, it is advisable to place other coils, with progressively smaller diameters, until obstruction is obtained. Addition of particulate Gelfoam to the system increases thrombogenicity. Occasionally, the pseudoaneurysm with or without arteriovenous fistula may be directly punctured percutaneously and embolized with Gianturco coils.

Radiation-induced pseudoaneurysm is rare. When it does occur it is most frequently seen in the carotid territory, and is associated in the high mortality rate due to bleeding. In this situation, embolization of the involved vessel may cure the bleeding permanently (Fig. 4.68).

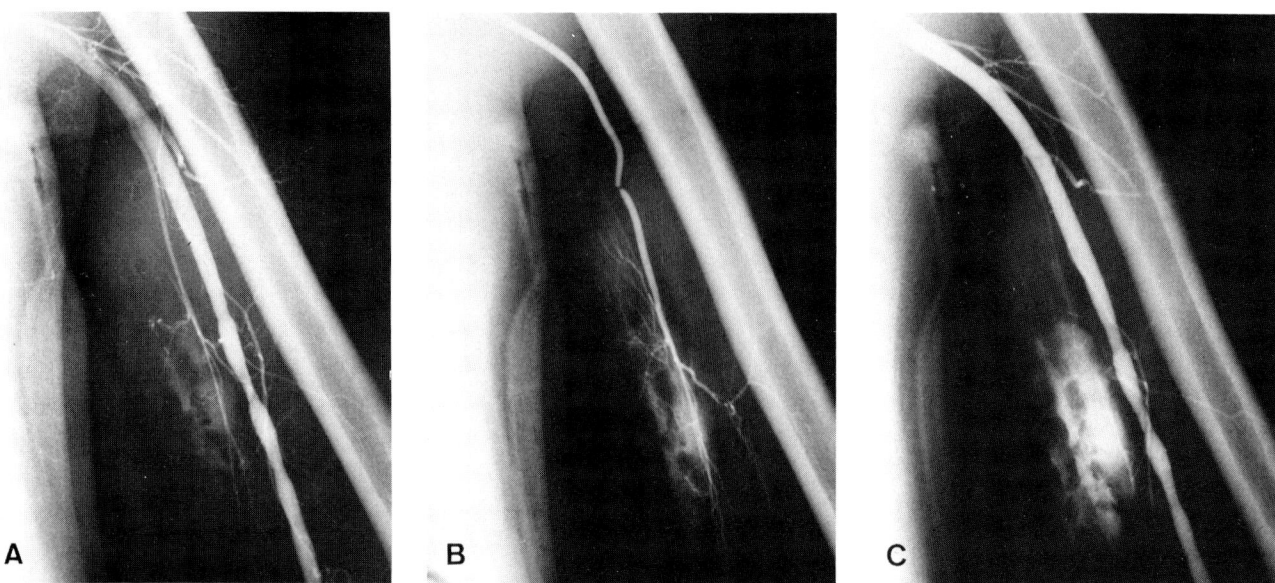

Figure 4.66 Left arm bleeding, after surgical embolectomy, with compartment syndrome and hand ischemia.
(A) Injection into the left subclavian artery showing contrast medium extravasation originating from a muscular artery (probably the subscapular artery). Notice the brachial artery spasm at the surgical site. (B) Superselective catheterization showing contrast collection at the surgical site. (C) Postembolization control showing occlusion of the bleeding artery. It was necessary to operate for decompression of the compartments of the left forearm.

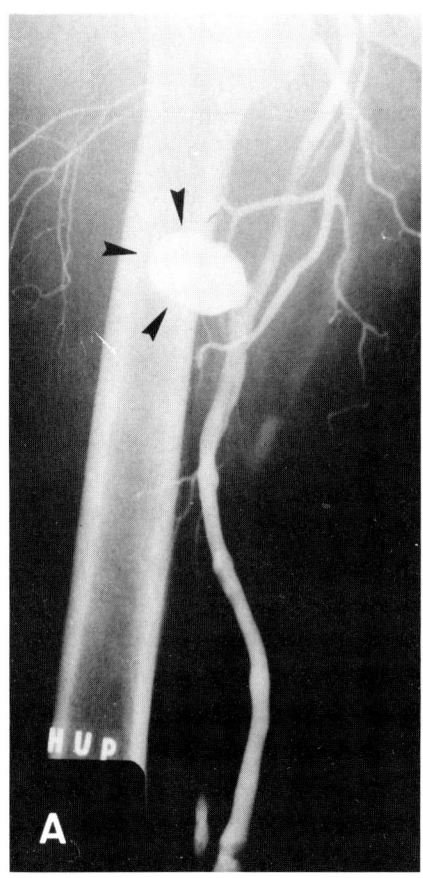
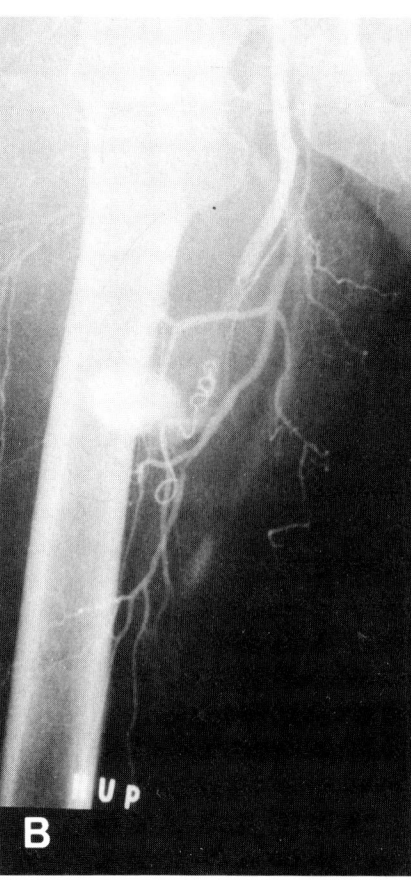

Figure 4.67 (A) Postsurgical pseudoaneurysm with femoropopliteal venous graft (arrowheads). (B) Control following embolization with Gianturco coils, occluding both graft and aneurysm (still filled with contrast). No distal ischemia occurred after occlusion. The graft was not effective in revascularizing the patient's foot. The contraindication for surgery in this case was uncontrolled diabetes and infected surgical incision.

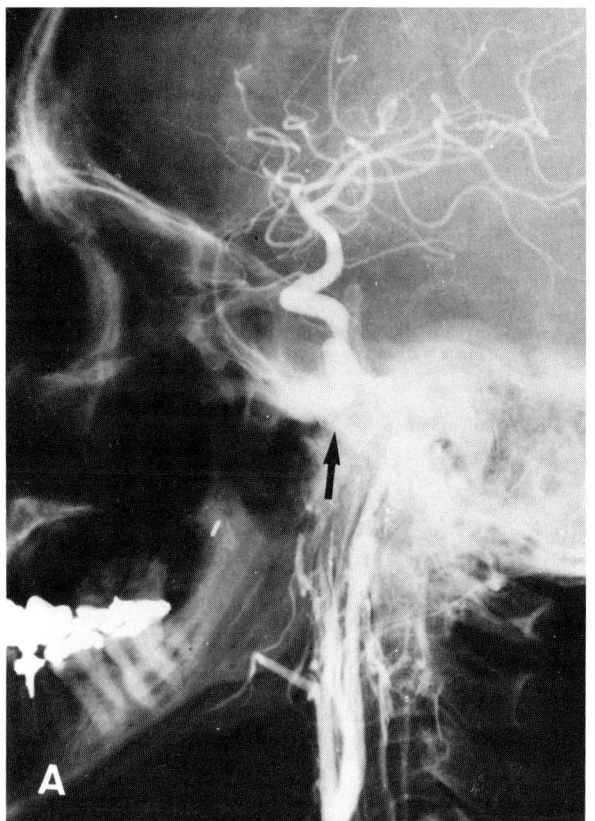

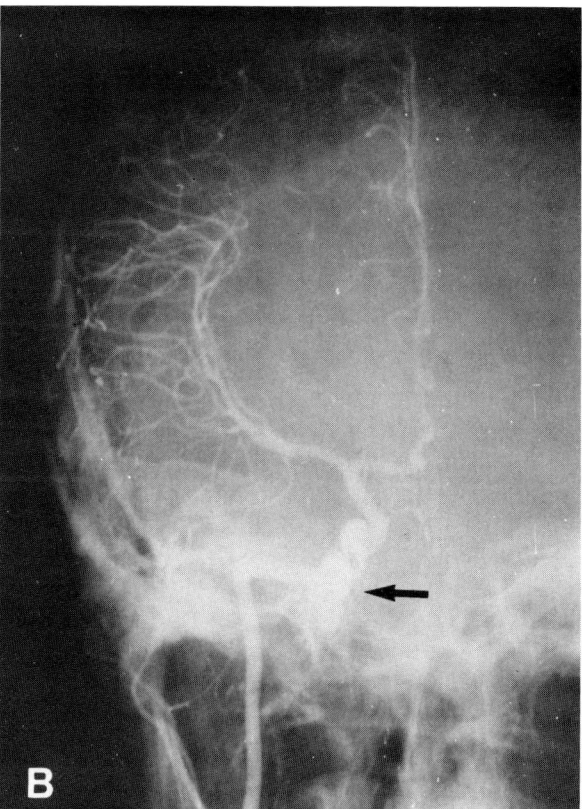

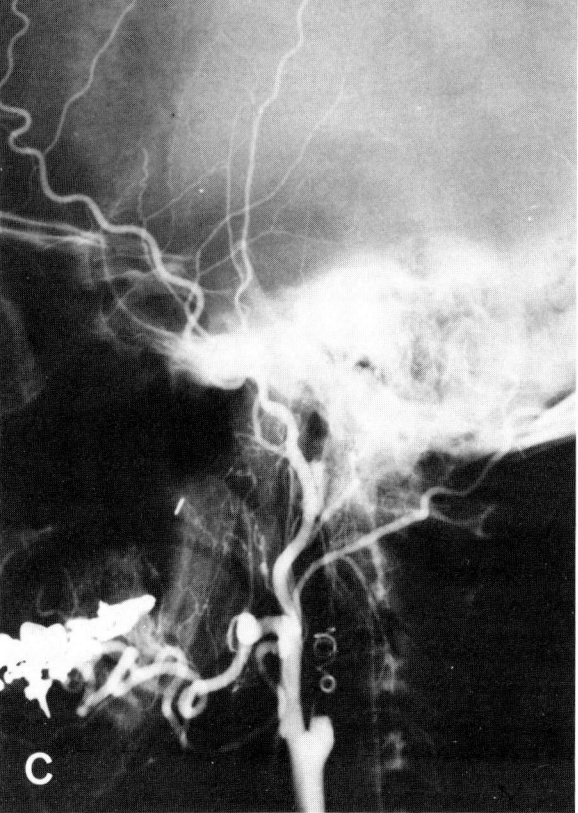

Figure 4.68 (A,B) Pseudoaneurysm (arrow) induced by radiation therapy in right internal carotid artery, with massive bleeding. (C) Control angiogram following embolization with one 5-mm and one 3-mm coil, showing occlusion of the right internal carotid artery. Permanent control of bleeding was obtained.

REFERENCES

Aakhus T, Enge I. Angiography in traumatic rupture of the spleen. *Br J Radiol* 1967;40:855–861.

Aakhus T, Enge I. Angiography in rupture of the liver. *Acta Radiol* 1971;11:353–362.

Ben-Menachen Y. *Angiography in Trauma: A Work Atlas.* Saunders, Philadelphia, 1981:62–94, 206–267, 416–419, 280–281, 446–451.

Ben-Menachen Y, Handel SF, Ray RD, Childs TL. Embolization procedures in trauma: The pelvis. *Semin Intervent Radiol* 1985;2:158–181.

Boijsen E, Judkins MP, Simay A. Angiographic diagnosis of hepatic rupture. *Radiology* 1966;86:66–72.

Clark RA, Gallant TE, Alexander ES. Angiography management of traumatic arteriovenous fistulas: Clinical results. *Radiology* 1983;147:9–13.

Elkin M, Meng C, DeParedes R. Roentgenologic evaluation of renal trauma with emphasis on renal angiography. *AJR* 1966;98:1–26.

Fajardo LF, Lee A. Rupture of major vessels after radiation. *Cancer* 1975;36:904–913.

Fischer RB, Ben-Menachen Y. Embolization procedures in trauma: The extremities—acute lesions. *Semin Intervent Radiol* 1985;2:118–124.

Fischer RG, Ben-Menachen Y. Embolization procedures in trauma: The abdomen—extraperitoneal. *Semin Intervent Radiol* 1985;2:148–157.

Grinnell VS, Flanagan KG, Mehringer CM et al. Occlusion of large fistulas with detachable valved balloons and the spider. *AJR* 1983;140:1259–1261.

Kim D, Guthaner DF, Walter JF, et al. Embolization of visceral arteriovenous fistulas with a modified steel wire technique. *AJR* 1984;142:1215–1218.

Sclafani SJA, Cooper R, Shaftan GW, et al. Arterial trauma: Diagnostic and therapeutic angiography. *Radiology* 1986;161:165–172.

Sclafani SJA, Shaptan GW. Transcatheter treatment of injuries to the profunda femoris artery. *AJR* 1982;138:463–466.

Sclafani SJA. Arteriographic treatment of chronic post-traumatic arteriovenous fistulas of the extremities. *Semin Intervent Radiol* 1985;2:125–129.

Sclafani SJA. Transcatheter control of arterial bleeding in the neck, mediastinum, and chest. *Semin Intervent Radiol* 1985;2:130–138.

Sclafani SJA. Angiography control of intraperitoneal hemorrhage caused by injuries to the liver and spleen. *Semin Intervent Radiol* 1985;1:139–147.

Silverberg GD, Britt RH, Goffinet DR. Radiation induced carotid artery disease. *Cancer* 1978;41:130–137.

Smith PL, Lim WN, Ferris EJ, et al. Emergency arteriography and extremity trauma: Assessment of indications. *AJR* 1981;137:803–807.

Uflacker R. Transcatheter embolization of arterial aneurysms. *Br J Radiol* 1986;59:317–324.

Uflacker R, Enge I. Avaliacao angiografica do trauma abdominal. *Rev Amrigs* 1978;22:38–46.

Uflacker R, Saadi J. Transcatheter embolization of superior mesenteric arteriovenous fistula. *AJR* 1982;139:1212–1214.

Tumoral Lesions in Soft Tissue and Bones

RENAN UFLACKER

BACKGROUND

Occlusive and infusion therapy offer an outstanding contribution to the management of primary and secondary lesions of the musculoskeletal system. Initially, these therapeutic techniques were palliative only, but they are now an integral part of the primary treatment in some institutions. They have been used in the treatment of malignant bone or soft tissue tumors, benign bone tumors, and metastatic lesions in bone or soft tissue.

TECHNIQUE

The catheterization of the arteries feeding the lesion is performed by a No. 5 French torque catheter. Depending on the location of the lesion, selective catheterization may be performed by the femoral or the axillary route. In bone or soft tissue lesions of the lower limbs, the femoral catheterization is performed in antegrade fashion.

A combination of occlusive materials is generally used: Gelfoam or Ivalon particles for peripheral intratumoral occlusion and Gianturco coils for central definitive occlusion. In lesions not directly related to cutaneous arteries, Gelfoam powder, absolute alcohol, or IBC may be used; these will all occlude at the microcirculation level. Flow-oriented embolization may be used with these materials.

Chemoinfusion has been successfully used to treat bone lesions. A drug such as cisplatin (CDDP) is given in doses ranging from 80 to 150 mg/m^2 over a 2-hour period. The patient is kept on a strict hydration regimen, including diuresis with mannitol, for the purpose of minimizing renal side effects. The procedure is repeated twice, 4 weeks and 8 weeks after the first course.

Adequate response is obtained in about 60 percent of osteosarcoma patients with disease remission. This technique may also be used for chondrosarcomas, malignant fibrous histiocytomas, and giant-cell malignant tumors. In sarcomatous soft tissue tumors, response has been obtained with infusion of cisplatin, adriamycin, and actinomycin D.

The action of embolization in the treatment of bone tumors has no clearly explained mechanism. However, it has been demonstrated that arterial occlusion of hypervascular lesions decreases lesion size and slows growth. A decrease in periosteal distension and nerve fiber stretching, which is responsible for pain accompanying these lesions, also occurs. Embolization has no precise indication for pain control (Fig. 4.69) in patients with bone tumor. Preoperative embolization reduces bleeding and facilitates resection (Fig. 4.70).

Bone metastases of renal carcinoma occur in 30 to 45 percent of patients, and are usually hypervascular. The vertebrae, pelvis, and skull are the sites most commonly involved by such neoplasms (Figs. 4.68 and 4.128). When radiotherapy fails or is contraindicated, embolization is an excellent alternative method for reducing mass volume and symptoms (Figs. 4.71 and 2.22).

Metastases of renal carcinoma may be embolized with particles when a sensitive territory is being treated, and with other materials, such as absolute alcohol and IBC, when less sensitive areas are involved (Fig. 2.22). Safe, superselective catheterization, as well as a careful evaluation of the territory to be occluded, is required for any of these procedures. Special care should be taken to avoid occlusion when the vessels are feeding nerve tissue, skin, or vital organs.

The embolization of soft tissue neoplasms has a predominantly preoperative or palliative application (Figs. 4.72 and 4.73). Embolization of organs with metastases may be used to control complications such as bleeding (Fig. 4.74).

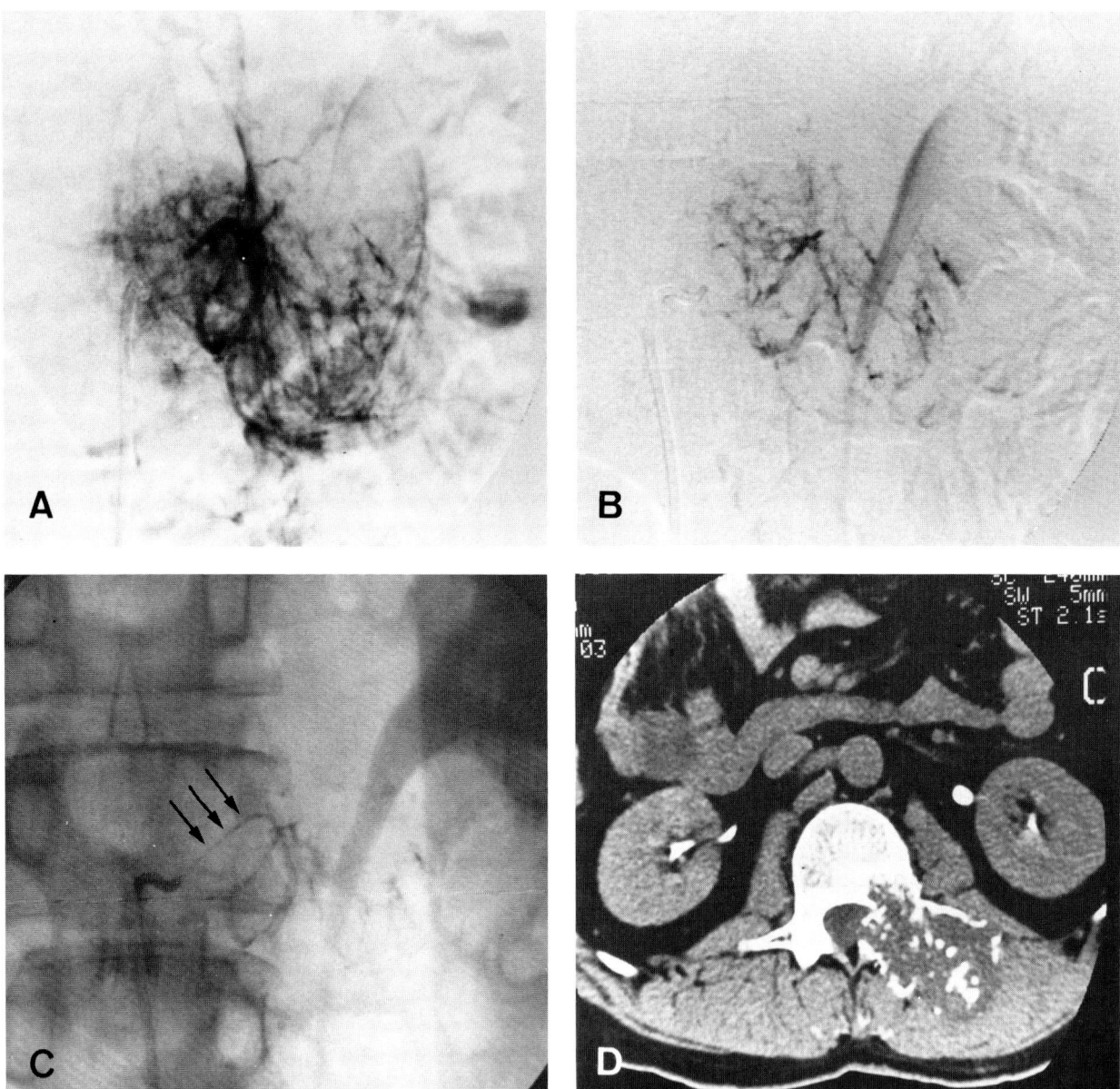

Figure 4.69 Patient with plasmocytoma lesion destroying the second lumbar vertebra on the left, with tumefacient mass of adjacent soft tissue.

(A) Digital angiogram showing injection into the second left lumbar artery, with the hypervascular lesion. (B) A view during IBC injection for embolization. Notice the excellent radiopacity obtained. (C) Digital radiograph showing Shepherd-Hook-type catheter (No. 6.3 French) and coaxial catheter (No. 3 French) (arrows) for IBC injection, and the material being injected into the lesion. (D) Control computer tomograph after embolization. Notice the radiopaque material (IBC) inside the lesion. The lesion was later operated on and treated with radiotherapy.

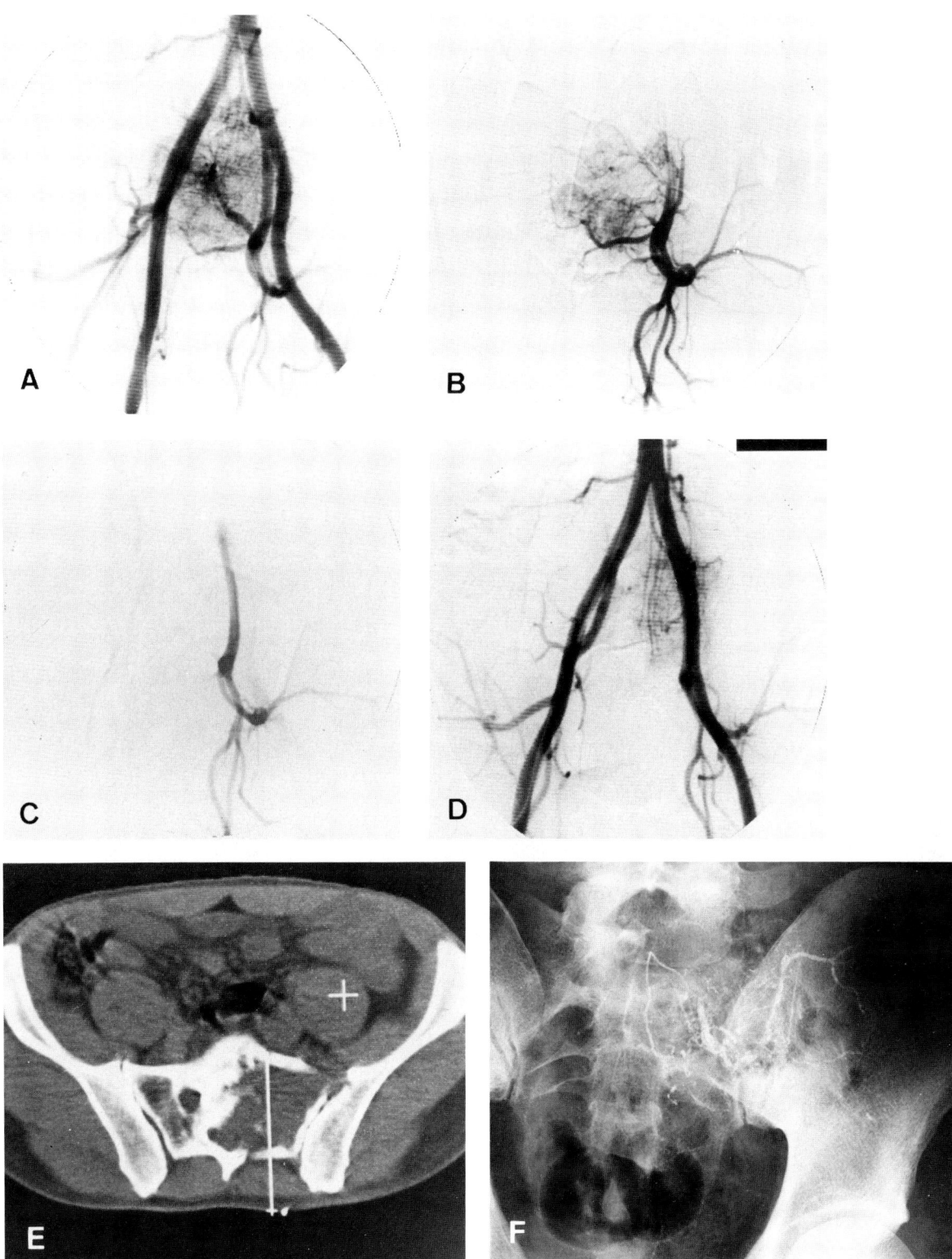

Figure 4.70 34-year-old patient with lumbar pain and osteolytic lesion in the sacrum on the left compatible with plasmocytoma.
(A) Aortogram showing that the lesion is hypervascular and fed by the posterior branches of the left hypogastric artery.
(B) Selective injection into the left hypogastric artery showing vascularization of the lesion. (C) Control following embolization of left hypogastric artery posterior branches with bucrylate (IBC). The anterior arteries remain opacified.
(D) Postembolization control aortogram showing partial vascularization of the lesion's upper border by the middle sacral artery. (E) Computed tomogram showing the lithic lesion in the sacrum, on the left. (F) Plain x-ray after embolization showing radiopaque IBC inside the lesion. Radiotherapy, curretage followed by bone graft, and lumbar and iliac osteosynthesis have been performed.

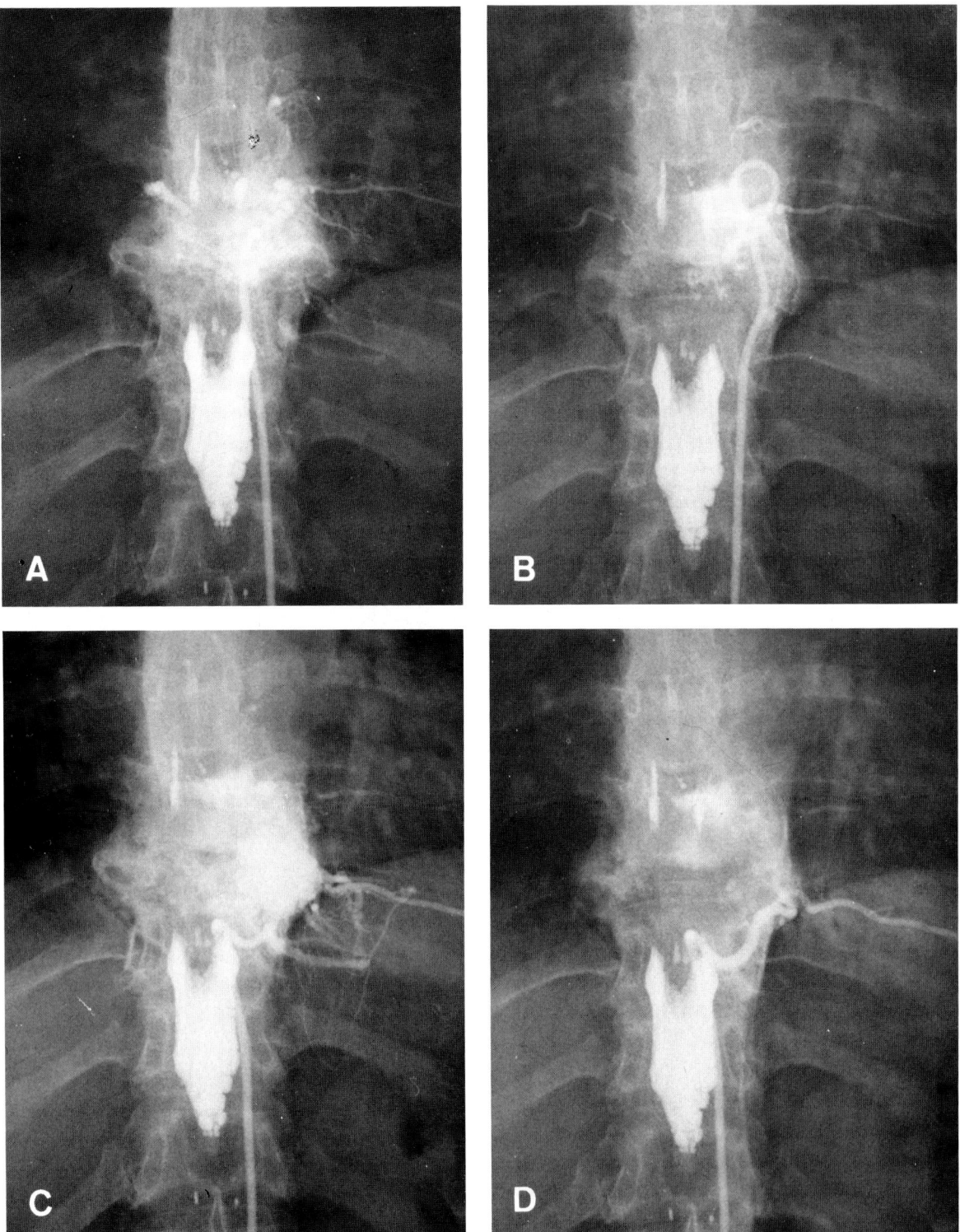

Figure 4.71 Renal carcinoma metastasis in T8, with vertebral collapse and medullary compression causing progressive paraplegia.

(A) Injection into the left intercostal artery. Notice the hypervascular lesion of the vertebral body. (B) Control following embolization with Gelfoam particles, showing devascularization of the lesion. (C) Injection into the ninth left intercostal artery, showing tumoral hypervascularity. (D) Control following embolization with Gelfoam. Notice that the intercostal artery is patent, and no tumor impregnation is seen. The eighth dorsal artery on the right has also been embolized. Notice the lipoiodinated contrast medium residue inside the spinal canal, which has incidentally shown the occlusion. The patient showed improvement at clinical follow-up, with return of leg movements after 24 hours and ambulation after 48.

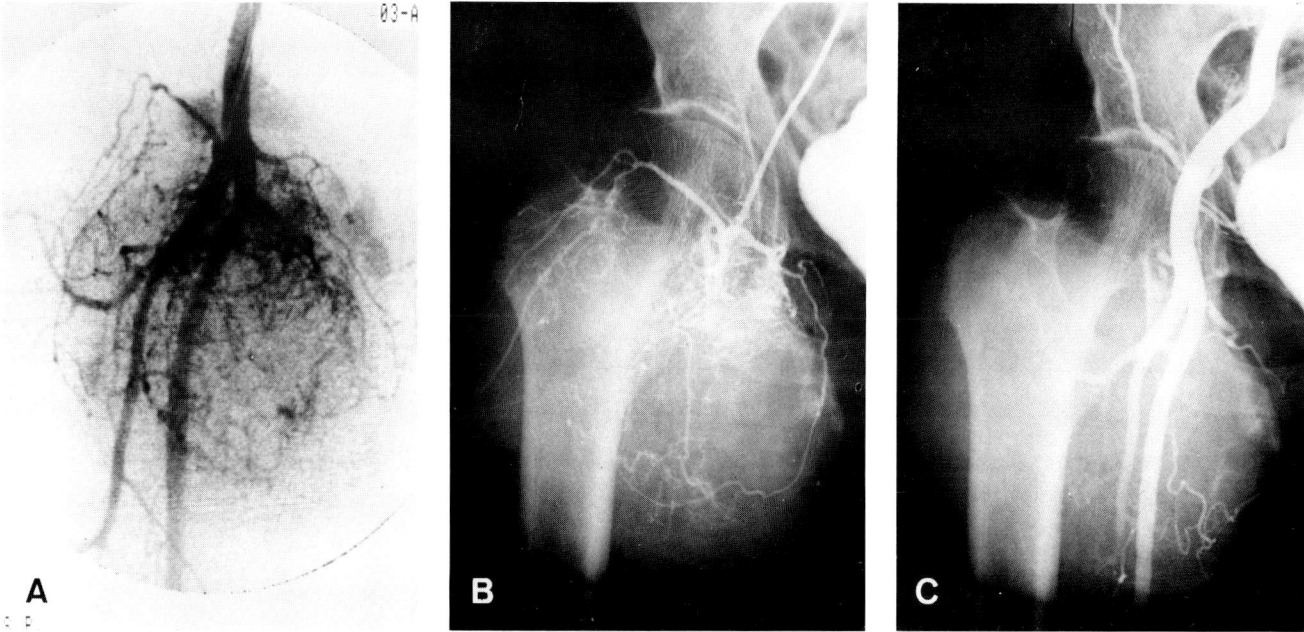

Figure 4.72 Patient with melanoma metastasis at right thigh root.
(A) Right common, deep, and superficial femoral artery digital angiogram showing hypervascular expansive lesion of the right thigh. (B) Superselective injection into right medial circumflex femoral artery showing its role in lesion vascularization. (C) Control angiogram following preoperative selective embolization of the lesion's several feeding branches with Gelfoam particles.

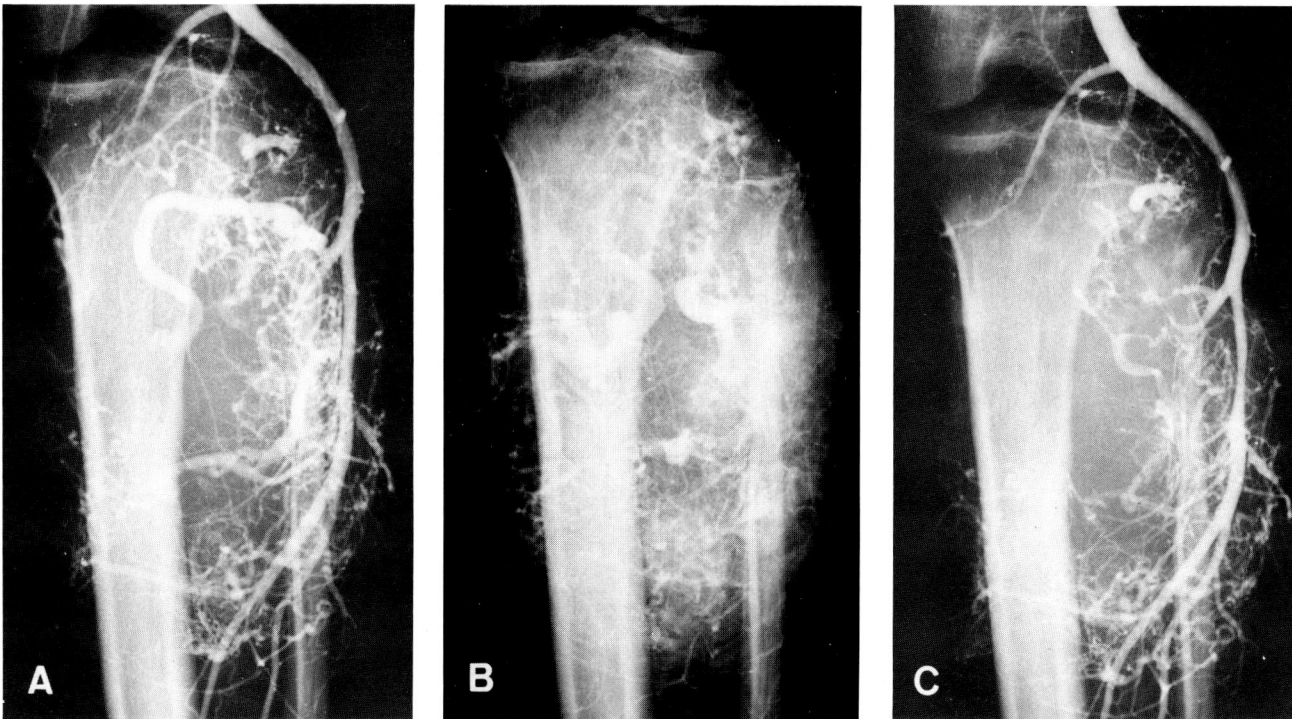

Figure 4.73 Patient with soft tissue fibrous sarcoma of the left leg.
(A) Injection into left popliteal artery showing the soft tissue hypervascular lesion. Notice the diastasis between the tibia and the peroneus. (B) Later phase of the same injection seen in (A), showing diffuse lesion impregnation. (C) Control injection following superselective occlusion, with absolute alcohol, of a few vessels involved by the lesion. Notice the partial devascularization of the tumoral mass.

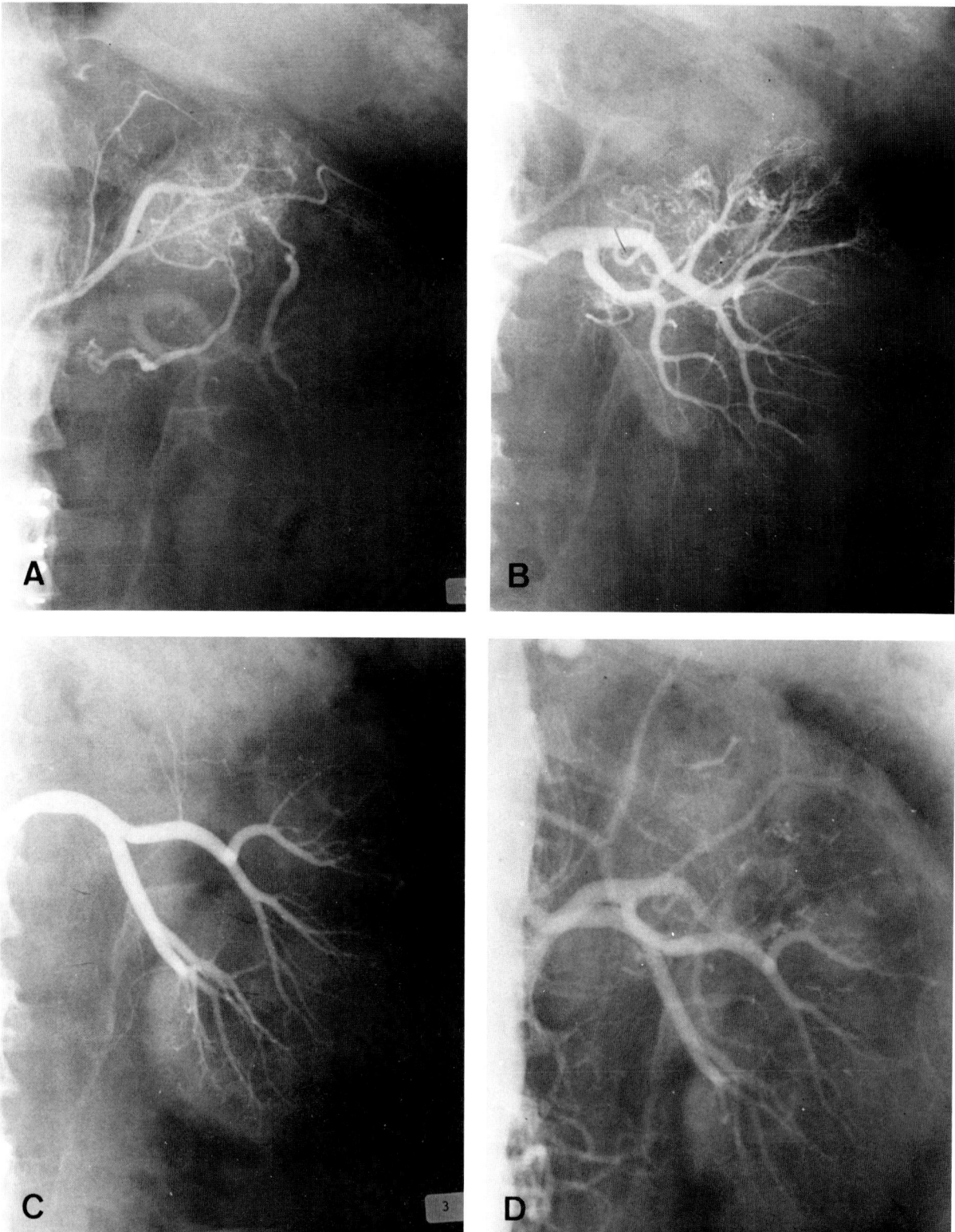

Figure 4.74 A patient who had undergone right nephrectomy 4 years previously presented with massive hematuria due to metastatic tumoral lesion in the left kidney.
(A,B,C) Selective injections into the three arteries of the left kidney. The two upper arteries (A,B) vascularize a hypervascular tumor lesion in the upper pole of the kidney. Superselective embolization of the two arteries identified in (A) and (B) was performed with lipiodol-impregnated Gelfoam particles. (D) Control angiogram following embolization. Notice the absence of tumor opacification, and the gelfoam particles with lipiodol inside the lesion. The renal function remained satisfactory, in spite of limited, although extensive, left renal parenchymal embolization.

Embolization in Hemangiomas, Arteriovenous Malformations, and Arteriovenous Fistulas

RENAN UFLACKER

CLASSIFICATION

Much confusion still exists concerning the proper classification of vascular skin lesions, with many different names being used to define the same entity. For example, the term "hemangioma" has been used to identify a whole range of vascular lesions with different etiologies and natural histories. This is obviously inadequate. The term "angiodysplasia" is similarly imprecise, and hybrid terms such as "lymphangiohemangioma" and "capillary cavernous hemangioma" only add to the confusion. The name "hamartoma," which refers to a congenital developmental defect, is too comprehensive.

Mulliken has recently used a cellular analysis to classify vascular lesions as either hemangiomas or vascular malformations. Hemangiomas show a high level of mitotic activity, characterized by alternating stages of proliferation and involution, while malformations are cellularly stable.

Infantile capillary hemangiomas, which are three times more common in females than in males, are the most common vascular tumors in childhood. These benign vascular tumors are characterized by hypercellularity at the expense of endothelial cell proliferation. When submitted to tissue culture medium, the cells of these tumors show the ability to form tubules. They form during fetal life or the early neonatal period, but are usually not visible at birth. Generally they become visible during the first 3 months of life. These lesions typically present a proliferative stage, in which rapid, sometimes frightening growth is observed, which lasts until the sixth or eighth month of life. Following this phase, most lesions evolve over a period lasting from the tenth, eleventh, or twelfth month of life to the fifth, sixth, or seventh year, at the end of which the tumor has regressed completely. The exact mechanism of regression is unknown; there is both a decrease in the number of endothelial cells and a gradual replacement of angiomatous tissue with fatty, fibrous stroma.

Childhood hemangiomas exhibit benign characteristics under angiography: mass effect; arterial feeding from branches of adjacent arteries, which are slightly enlarged in diameter; and intensive impregnation of tumoral tissue, which has a lobulated appearance. The dilated veins drain into normal systemic veins. Arteriovenous communications sometimes exist.

Vascular skin lesions that grow *pari passu* with the child, have normal endothelial mitotic activity, do not regress, and grow during or even after puberty should be classified as arteriovenous malformations (Table 4.2). Malformations are structural abnormalities resulting from inborn errors in vascular morphogenesis. Although they do not proliferate, they exhibit growth alterations, including changes in pressure and flow, and ectasia, and may form collaterals in fistulas. This type of malformation may expand secondary to hemodynamic changes induced by trauma or incomplete surgical excision, and may react to hormonal changes (e.g., puberty, the menstrual cycle, pregnancy, or oral contraceptives).

This general classification does not, however, include lesions that exhibit the characteristics both of neoplasms and malformations. For example, endothelial proliferation may establish a vascular network inside a hemangioma, which mimics a malformation, or a physiologic shunt. A hemodynamic classification based on angiographic studies separates such lesions into two groups: active, high-flow; and inactive, low-flow. This suggests the necessity of identifying arteriovenous fistulas as a

Table 4.2 – Angiographic classification of vascular lesions

Vascular tumors
   Hemangiomas (predominate in head and neck region)
     Capillary: infantile
     Cavernous: adult
     Associated syndromes
       Cardiac failure
       Kasabach-Merritt (thrombocytopenic purpura)
   Other tumors

Arteriovenous malformations
   Arterial: high-flow (with or without fistula)
   Capillary: average-flow
   Venous-capillary: low-flow
   Venous: low-flow

Arteriovenous fistulas
   Congenital
   Acquired
     Traumatic (nonsurgical)
     Surgical

Angiomatoses
   Rendu-Osler-Weber
   Klipper-Trenaunay-Weber
   Sturge-Weber

distinct entity. A truly comprehensive classification should include embryologic, clinical, angiographic, and cellular aspects of a lesion. Subcategories, such as "capillary," "cystic," and "cavernous," may also be necessary in some cases.

In this text, classification is based primarily on angiographic aspects. Childhood vascular tumoral lesions with strong mitotic activity, as well as adult cavernous hemangiomatous lesions presenting cell proliferation, will be classified as hemangiomas. Lesions that grow along with the patient, without mitotic activity, will be classified as arteriovenous malformations.

HEMANGIOMAS

Hemangiomas vary from small, innocuous skin blemishes to mutilating processes that are in some cases life-threatening. Embryologically, they start with a stop in differentiation on the thirtieth day of fetal development, the undifferentiated capillary network stage. An angiogenic factor is also involved in the process, which must be responsible for hemangiomatous proliferation.

Hemangiomas may be classified as capillary (infantile) (Figs. 4.75 and 4.76) and cavernous (adult), with high and low flow, respectively (Table 4.2).

Hemangiomas present a few functional syndromes associated with high flow (heart failure) (Fig. 4.75), and with stasis and sequestration of formed blood elements, causing thrombocytopenic purpura (Kasabach-Merritt syndrome) (Fig. 4.76). These require immediate treatment. Complications caused by evolution of hemangiomas that also require immediate therapeutic intervention are ulceration, hemorrhage, infection, and rapid growth of lesions in certain locations.

Ulceration is the most common complication of hemangiomas that are centrally located in larger ulcerations, occurring as a result of skin ischemia. The ulceration will not hasten involution, but results in permanent scars after lesion involution. Hemorrhage is usually not significant, although the rare cases of voluminous hemorrhage require emergency embolization or surgical treatment. Bleeding is more frequent in cases of trauma (in childhood) or deep ulceration that exposes a large-diameter vascular bed. Infection requires the conventional antiseptic care; elimination of infection accelerates the healing of ulceration. Trauma may lead to ulceration, with or without active bleeding. Lesions that are located on the eyelid, auditory canal, or the airway may suddenly grow, causing acute occlusion and requiring emergency treatment (Table 4.3).

When a hemangioma is located on the eyelid or in the orbit there is risk of development of amblyopia and strabismus. With deeper lesions, exopthalmos and optic nerve compression may occur. Involvement of slightly more than half the eyelid in a child leads to amblyopia in up to 60 percent of cases, occluding the sight for just a few days (5 to 8), and may lead to total sight loss. Amblyopia leads to blindness through stimulus deprivation. The treatment of sight-occluding eyelid lesions, therefore, constitutes a medical emergency (Table 4.3).

Table 4.3 – Indications for treating vascular lesions

Treatment Indicated	Treatment Not Indicated
Hemorrhage	Stable lesions
Traumatic	Aesthetically acceptable
Iatrogenic	No functional loss
Dentition	No associated syndromes
Ulceration	Immature hemangiomas
Mass effect	Nidus inaccessible by endovascular route (vascularization through ophthalmic artery branches, for instance)
Deformity (permanent sequelae)	
Functional problems (emergencies)	
Difficulty swallowing	
Difficulty breathing	
Amblyopia	
Professional dysfunction	
Rapid growth	
Ulceration	
Pain	
Infection	
Aesthetics (?)	
Associated syndromes	
Heart failure	
Kasabach-Merritt	
Preoperative	

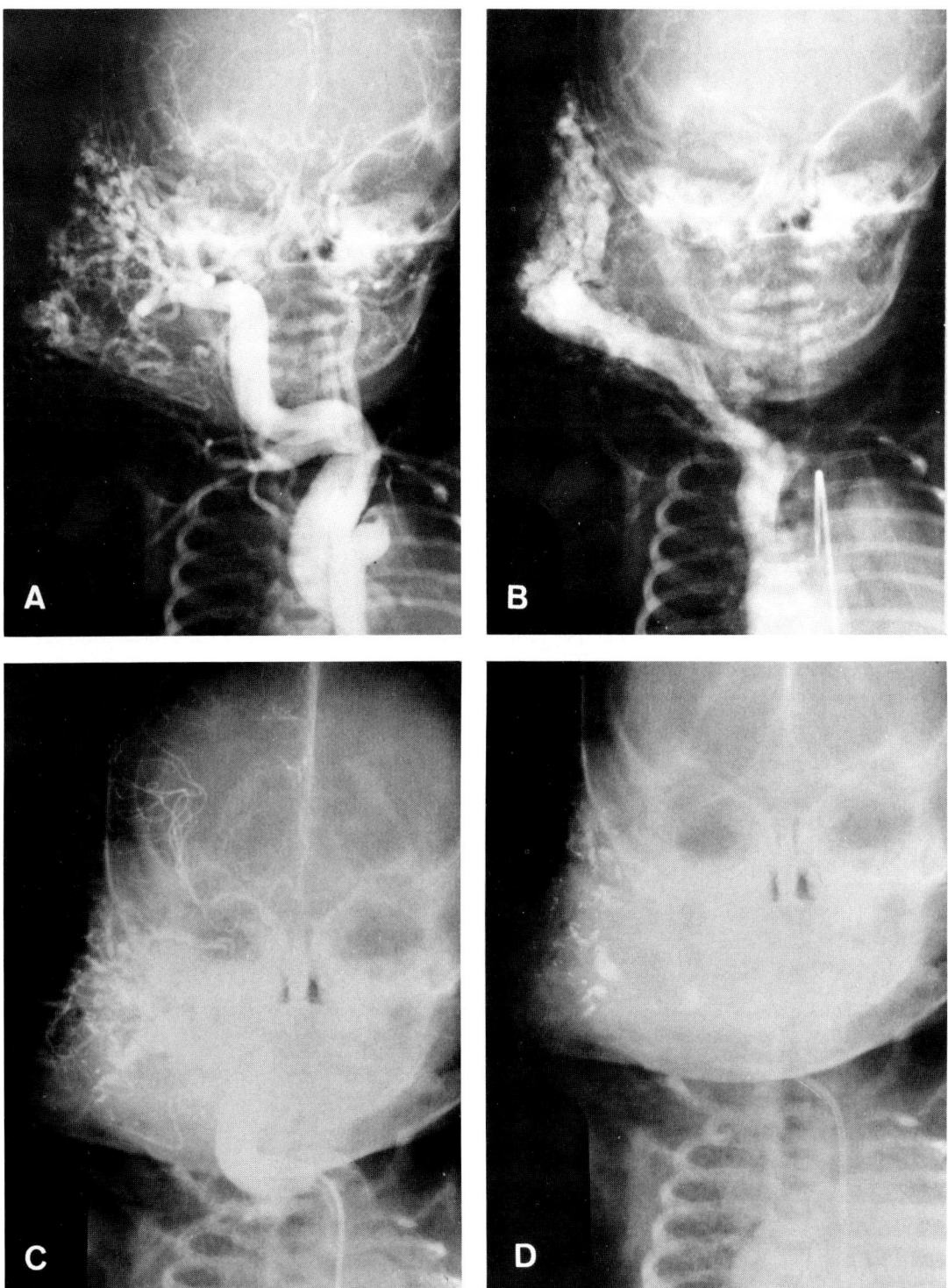

Figure 4.75 Five-day-old patient presenting with heart failure with high output due to right cervical capillary hemangioma with rich flow.

(A) Aortogram showing the extraordinary increase in diameter of the primitive carotid artery and the right external carotid, vascularizing a large hemangiomatous lesion in the right cervical region. (B) Later phase aortogram showing massive venous return by AV intratumoral shunts. (C) Selective control angiogram in right common carotid following embolization with Gelfoam soaked in Lipiodol, showing occlusion of circulation inside the lesion without noticeable AV shunt. (D) Later x-ray showing the radiopaque embolizing material inside the lesion. Heart failure was under control immediately following embolization, and the lesion regressed about 50 percent in 1 week. Later treatment with corticosteroids almost totally reduced the lesion.

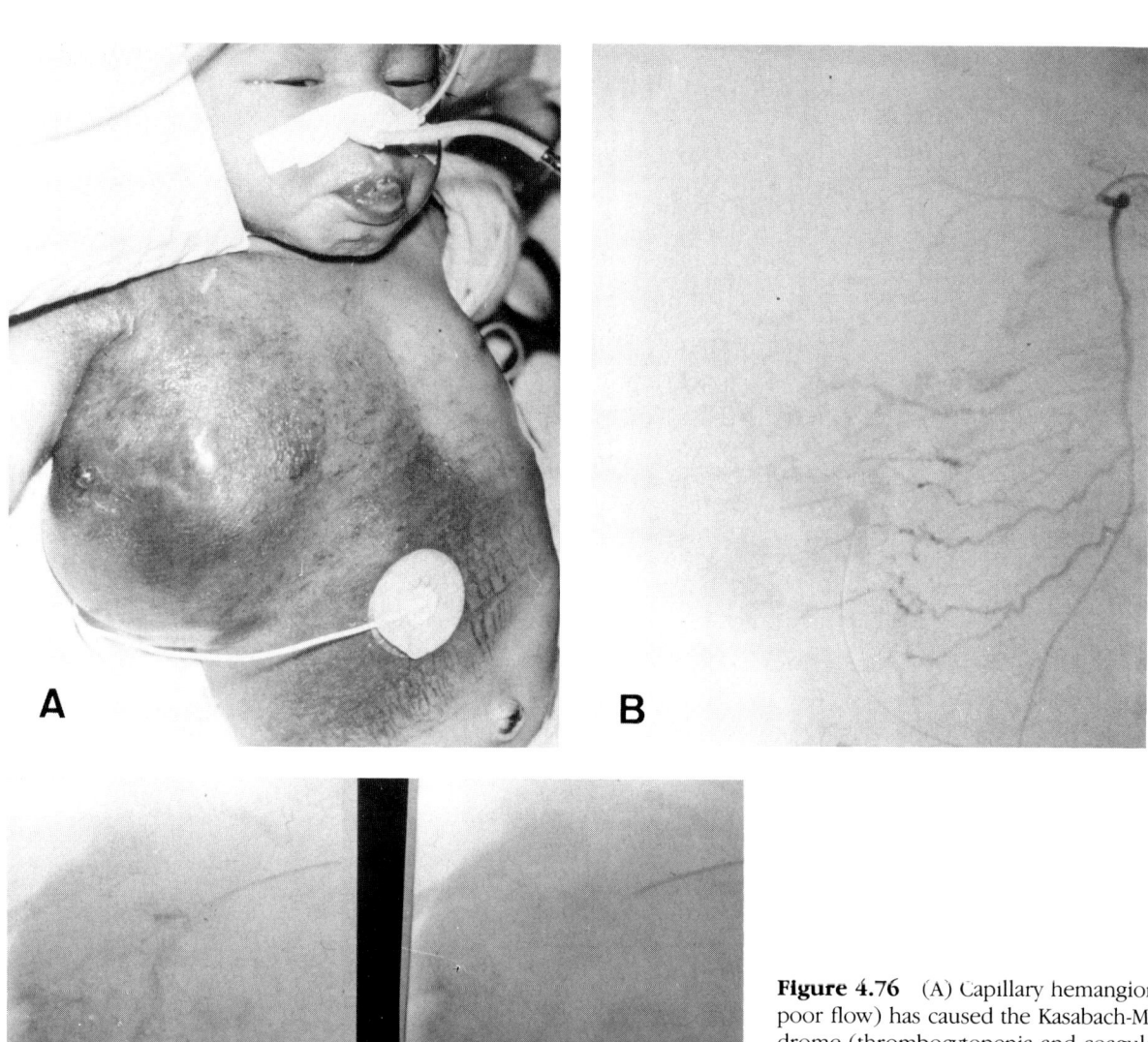

Figure 4.76 (A) Capillary hemangioma (with poor flow) has caused the Kasabach-Merrit syndrome (thrombocytopenia and coagulopathy) in a newborn baby. (B) Selective angiogram of internal mammary artery showing vascularization of the lesion on the right thoracic wall.
(C) Injection into axillary branches showing vascularization of the lesion. There is no significant AV shunt present. Embolization on two different occasions with polyvinyl alcohol particles permanently controlled thrombocytopenia.

ARTERIOVENOUS MALFORMATIONS

Arteriovenous (AV) malformations should not be mistaken for AV fistulas, which are direct arteriovenous shunts, although they may contain direct arteriovenous communications. AV malformations are vascular canals lined by mature endothelium without cell proliferation. They grow with the patient, and do not regress spontaneously. AV malformations may present any combination whatsoever of capillary, venous, arterial, and lymphatic components, with or without AV fistula.

Although these lesions are stable from a cellular standpoint, clinically they may be devastating, especially when harboring an arteriovenous shunt. There are four types of AV malformation (Table 4.2): high-flow (arterial) (Figs. 4.77 to 4.79), medium-flow (capillary) (Figs. 4.80

Figure 4.77 (A) Early arterial phase of arteriovenous malformation with high flow (arterial) on the plantar region of the left foot, which has caused pain and mass effect. Early arterial phase. (B) Later arterial phase showing massive AV shunt. (C) Control following highly selective embolization with Gelfoam particles soaked in Lipiodol injected into the pedis artery. Notice the significant reduction in shunt, which is still present. (D) Control following embolization of posterior tibial artery. Notice the reduction of shunt, with improvement of plantar circulation filling. Pain improved significantly, the volume of the lesion was reduced, and the digital circulation was not harmed.

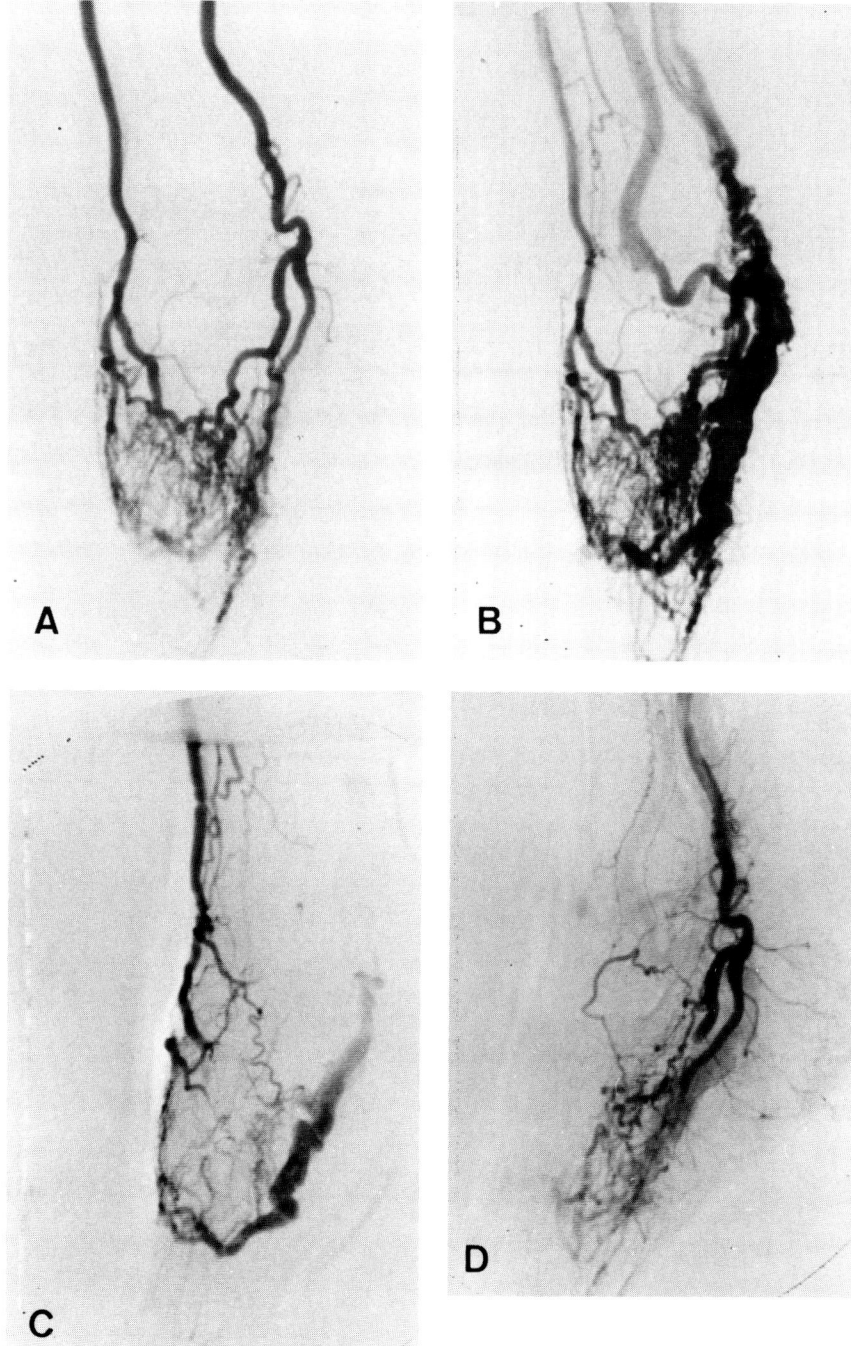

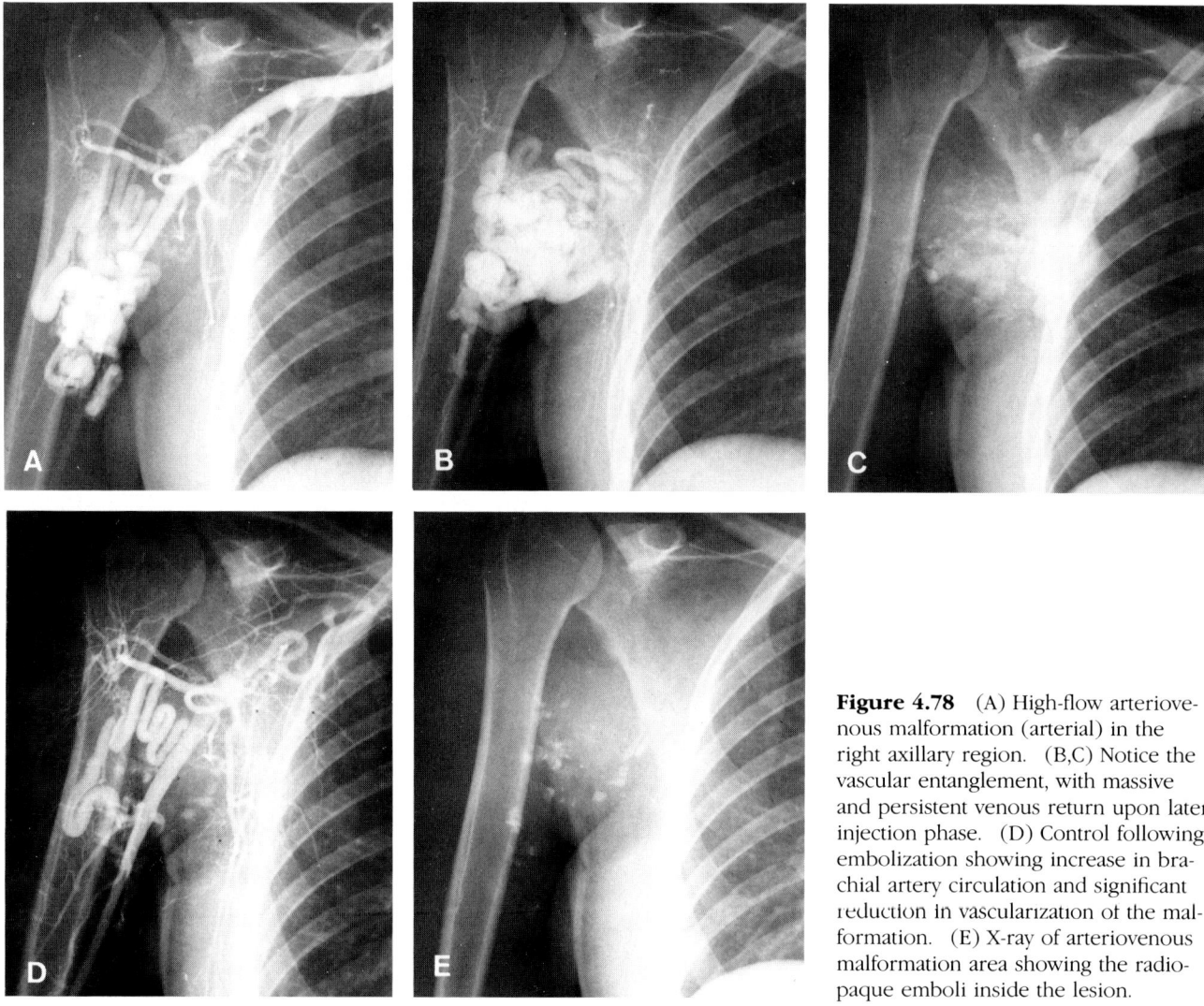

Figure 4.78 (A) High-flow arteriovenous malformation (arterial) in the right axillary region. (B,C) Notice the vascular entanglement, with massive and persistent venous return upon later injection phase. (D) Control following embolization showing increase in brachial artery circulation and significant reduction in vascularization of the malformation. (E) X-ray of arteriovenous malformation area showing the radiopaque emboli inside the lesion.

and 4.81), low-flow (capillary venous) (Fig. 4.82), and purely venous (Fig. 4.83).

ARTERIOVENOUS FISTULAS

AV fistulas are direct, abnormal communications between arteries and veins. Congenital AV fistulas are due to an arrest in embryonic development at a later fetal stage than the formation of hemangiomas. Embryonic vascular communications fail to regress.

Angiographically, AV fistulas are classified as macro or microfistulas. Microfistulas belong to an extensive vascular network with small communications. AV fistulas are further classified, according to their etiology, as congenital, traumatic, or surgical.

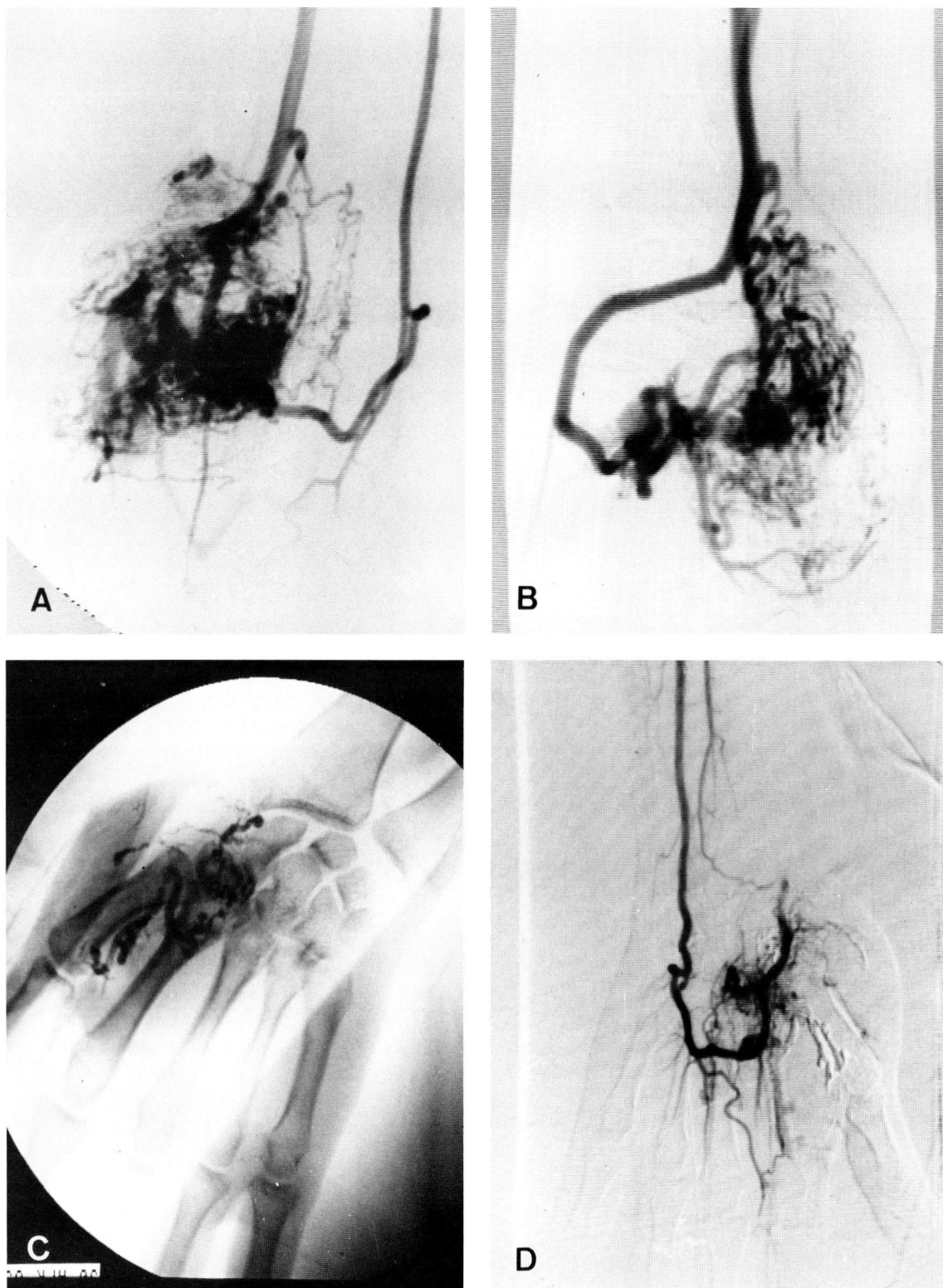

Figure 4.79 28-year-old patient with arteriovenous high-flow malformation (arterial) on the right hand.
(A) Frontal view, (B) profile. Embolization, which was indicated due to pain and lesion growth, was performed by puncture into the radial artery using a superselective coaxial catheterization system. C) Digital x-ray showing bucrylate (IBC) inside the lesion nidus. D) Control angiogram following embolization through injection into the ulnar artery. Notice the integral digital circulation at the origin of the malformed mass. The mass was permanently reduced.

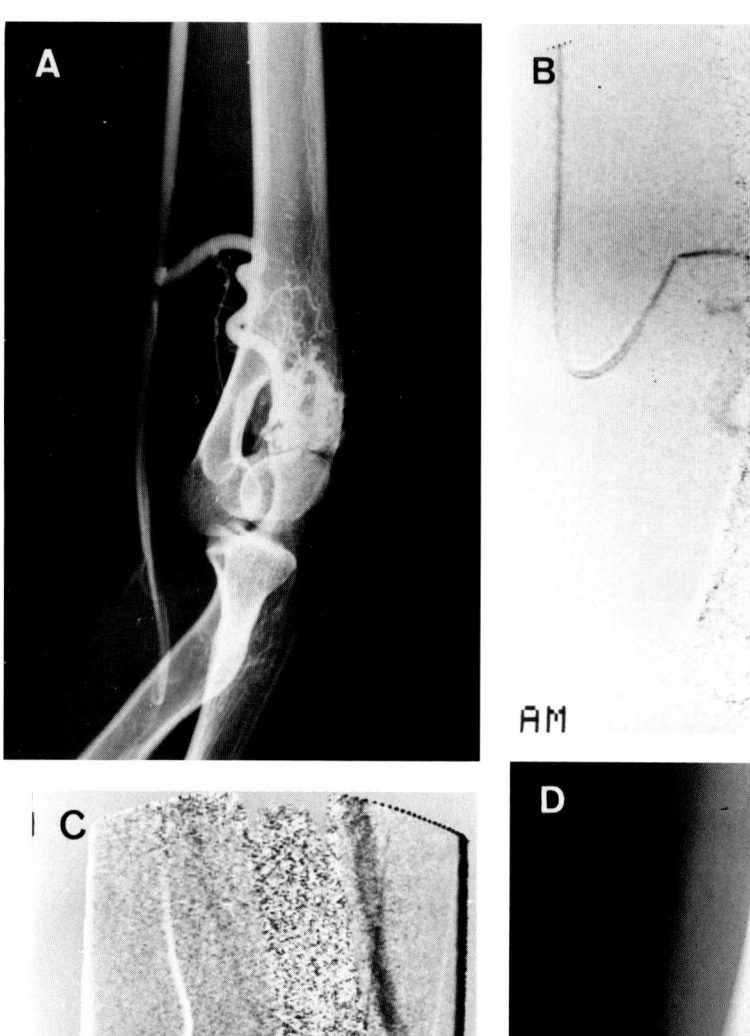
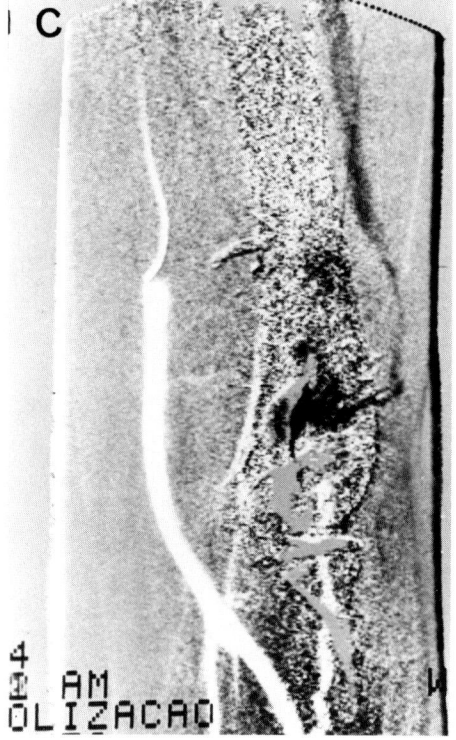
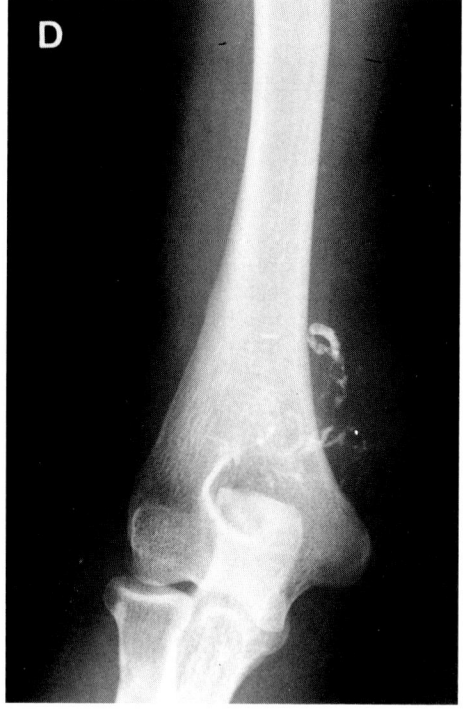

Figure 4.80 (A) Arteriovenous medium-flow malformation (capillary) involving the elbow. Embolization in this case was indicated for aesthetic correction due to professional needs. (B) Superselective coaxial catheterization with a No. 3 French catheter was used, and bucrylate (IBC) was injected into the nidus of the lesion. (C) Control angiogram following embolization showing that the lesion is no longer vascularized, due to nidus occlusion. (D) Plain x-ray following occlusion showing the radiopaque material (IBC) inside the lesion.

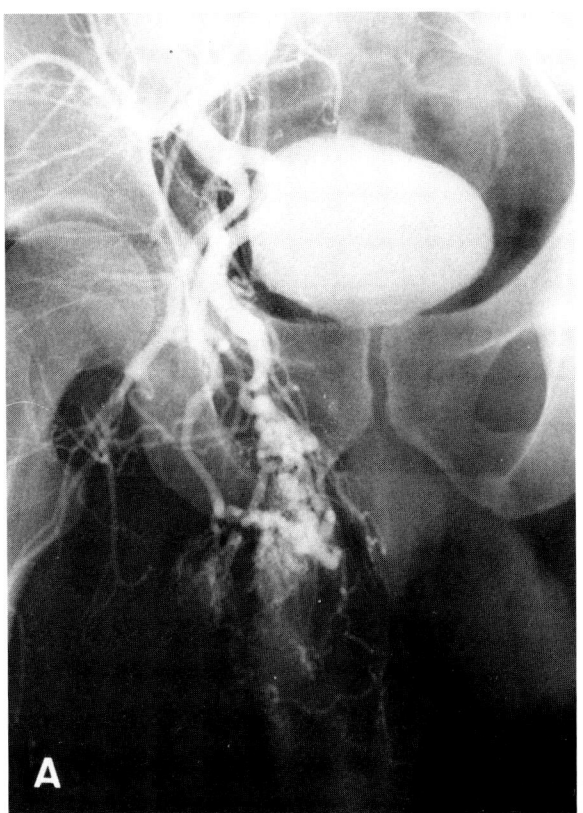
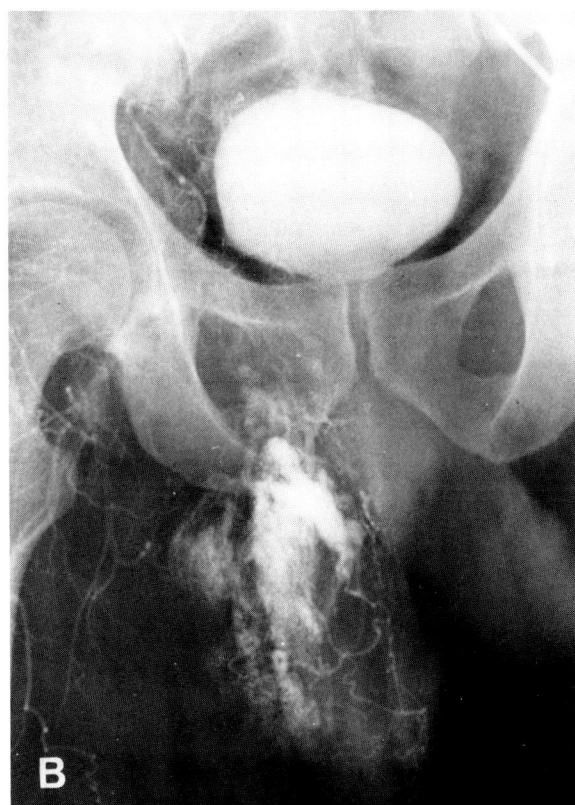
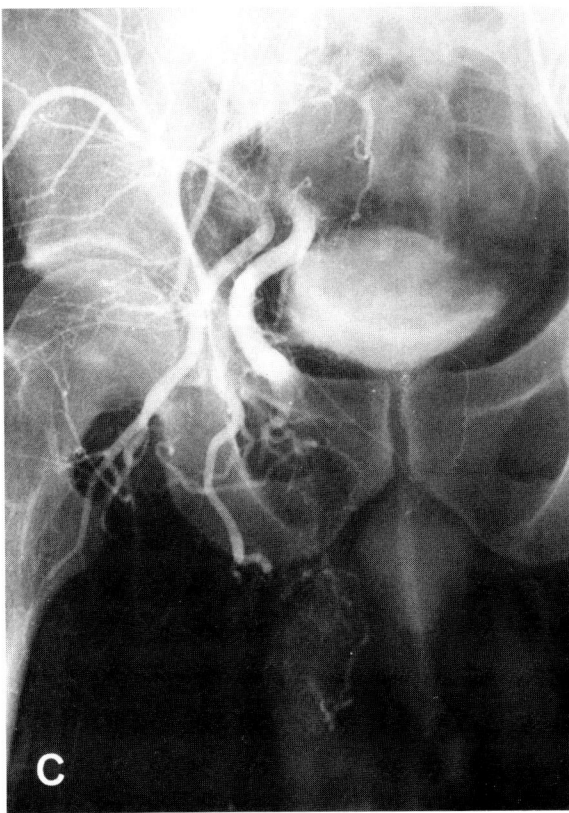

Figure 4.81 (A) Arteriovenous malformation with medium or low flow (venous-capillary) in the perineum, predominantly vascularized by branches of the superficial perineal artery. (B) Later phase showing intensive lesion blush and filling of vascular spaces, without venous return. (C) Embolization, which was indicated because of pain and lesion growth, was performed with Gelfoam. Notice the occlusion of the lesion's main arteries. The initial embolization reduced the mass, and further reduction was achieved by repeat embolization 1 year later.

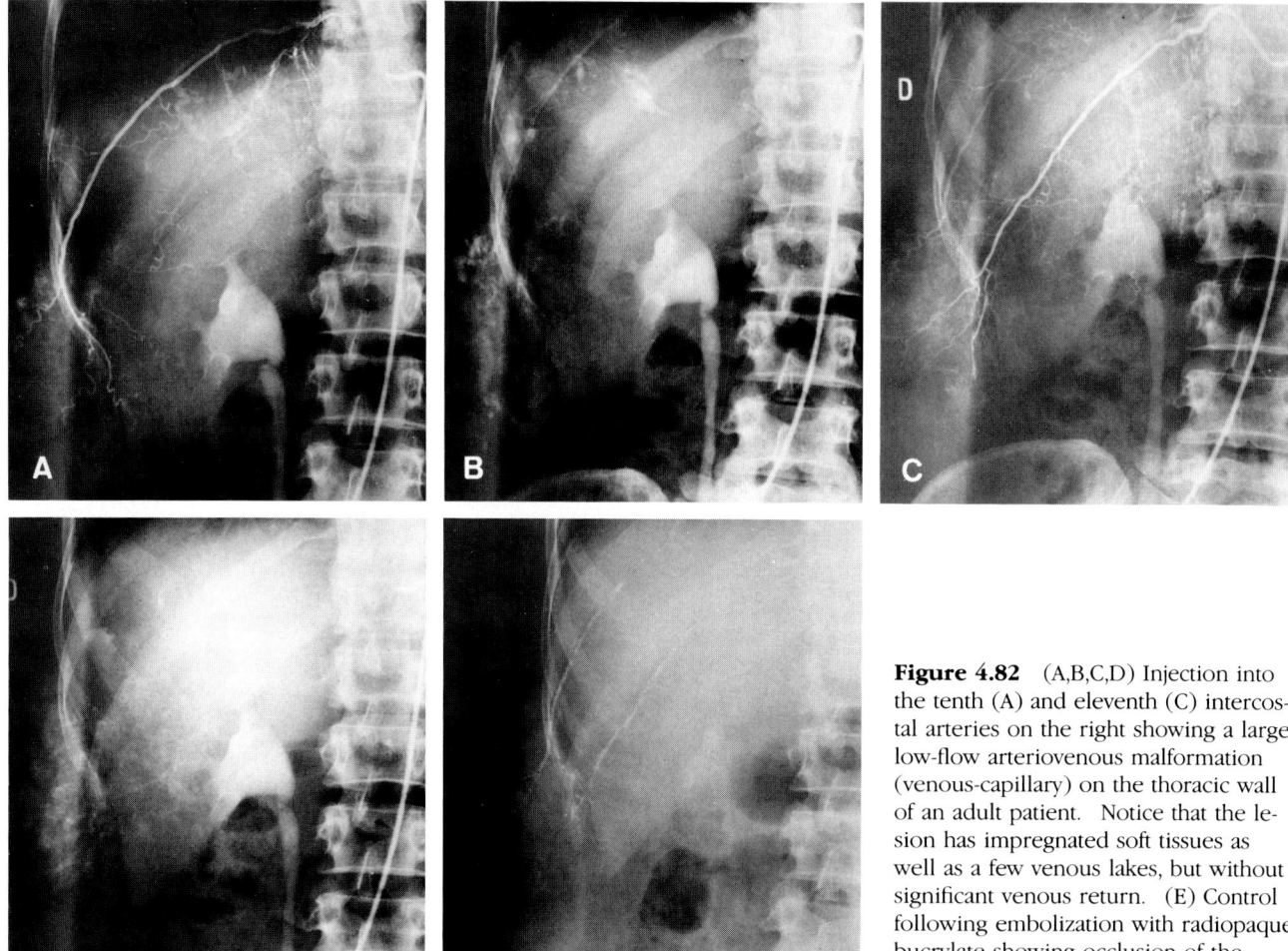

Figure 4.82 (A,B,C,D) Injection into the tenth (A) and eleventh (C) intercostal arteries on the right showing a large, low-flow arteriovenous malformation (venous-capillary) on the thoracic wall of an adult patient. Notice that the lesion has impregnated soft tissues as well as a few venous lakes, but without significant venous return. (E) Control following embolization with radiopaque bucrylate showing occlusion of the feeding vessels of the lesion and a small amount of material inside the nidus.

Congenital AV fistulas are most commonly located on the limbs (Fig. 4.84), most frequently in the legs. They may, however, occur anywhere, and are often found in the central nervous system.

The presence of heart failure due to high output is a relatively frequent occurrence in large congenital and traumatic fistulas, and treatment may become an urgent need (Fig. 4.85). Systemic hemodynamic effects are less pronounced with congenital lesions than with those produced by trauma or surgery. When splanchnic organs are affected by arteriovenous fistulas, symptoms caused by gastrointestinal malfunction, such as mesenteric angina and portal hypertension, may appear (Fig. 4.86).

Arteriovenous lesions are diagnosed by Doppler ultrasound examination and by angiographic studies which demonstrate the anatomy of the lesion and its afferent and efferent vessels.

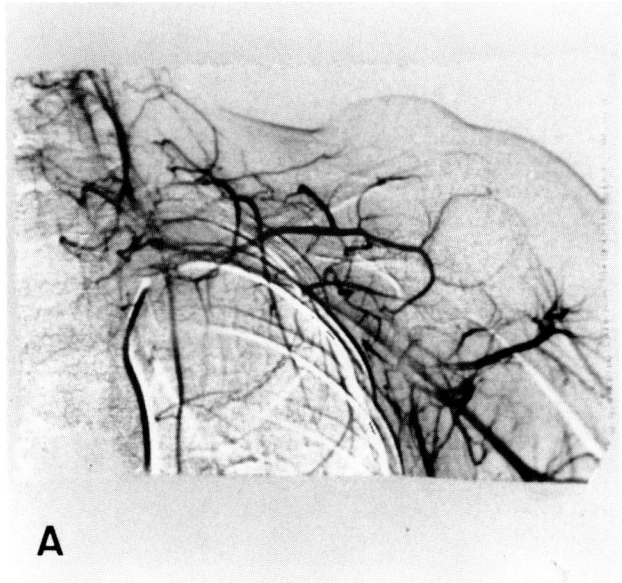
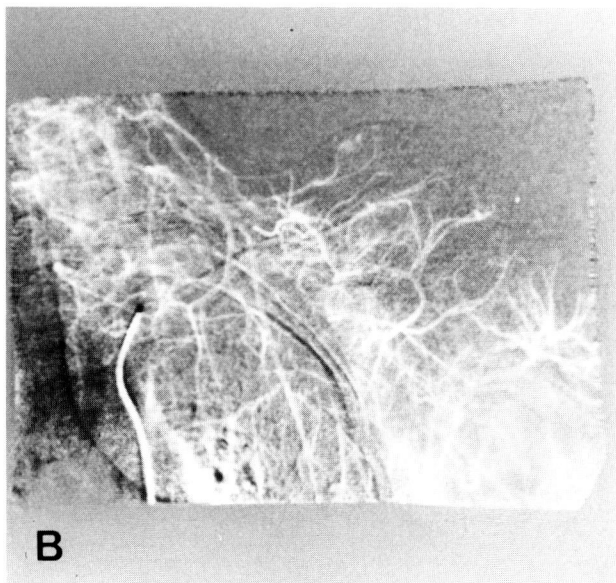
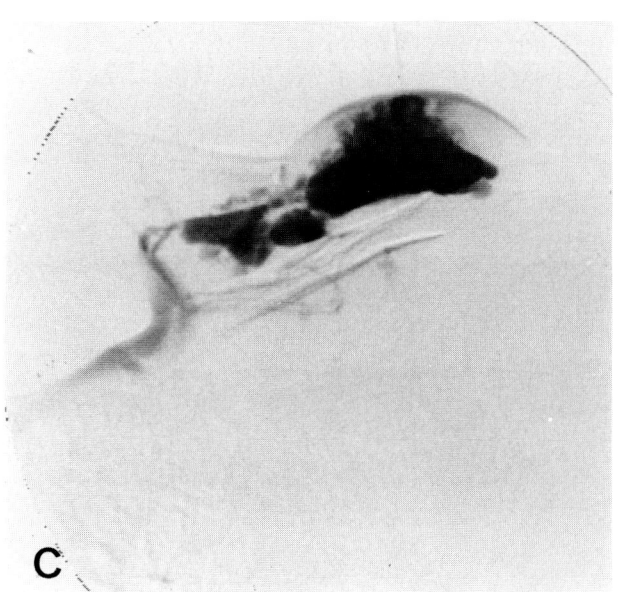
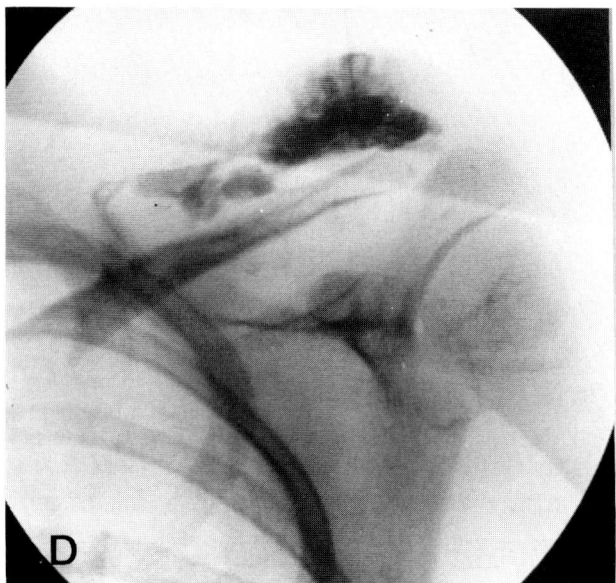

Figure 4.83 (A,B) Arteriogram of the left shoulder region. No soft tissue impregnation by the malformation in the supraclavicular region is evident. (C,D) Direct injection into the arteriovenous malformation (purely venous), showing lesion cavities and venous drainage, with and without digital subtraction. Sclerosis with absolute alcohol plus compression is the best treatment alternative in cases like this.

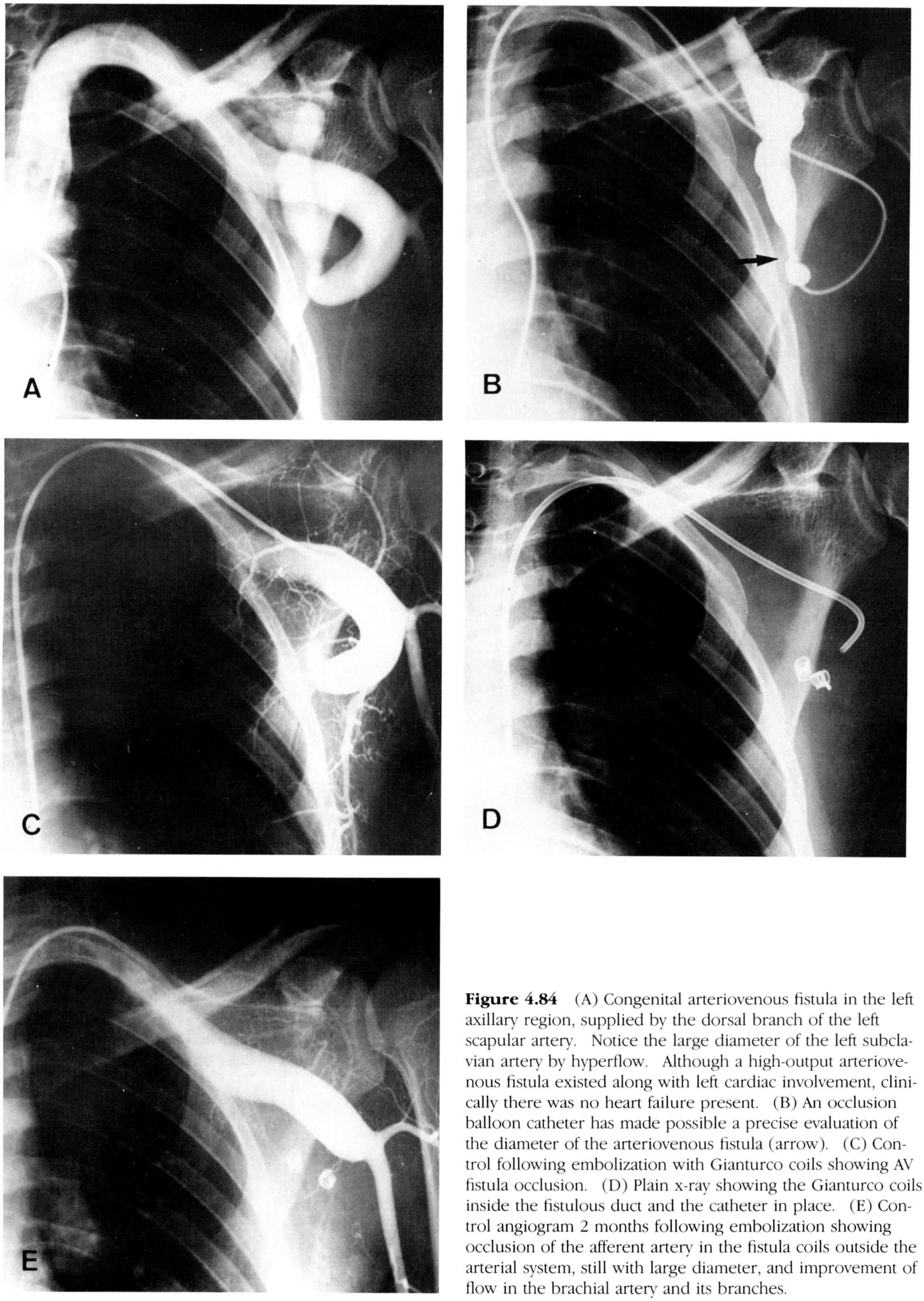

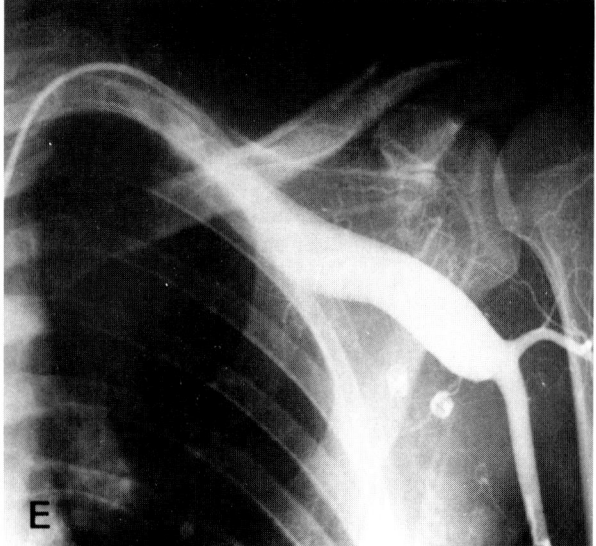

Figure 4.84 (A) Congenital arteriovenous fistula in the left axillary region, supplied by the dorsal branch of the left scapular artery. Notice the large diameter of the left subclavian artery by hyperflow. Although a high-output arteriovenous fistula existed along with left cardiac involvement, clinically there was no heart failure present. (B) An occlusion balloon catheter has made possible a precise evaluation of the diameter of the arteriovenous fistula (arrow). (C) Control following embolization with Gianturco coils showing AV fistula occlusion. (D) Plain x-ray showing the Gianturco coils inside the fistulous duct and the catheter in place. (E) Control angiogram 2 months following embolization showing occlusion of the afferent artery in the fistula coils outside the arterial system, still with large diameter, and improvement of flow in the brachial artery and its branches.

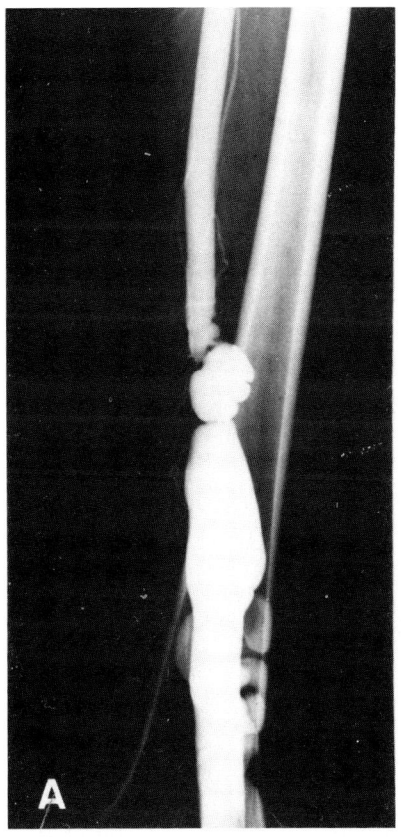
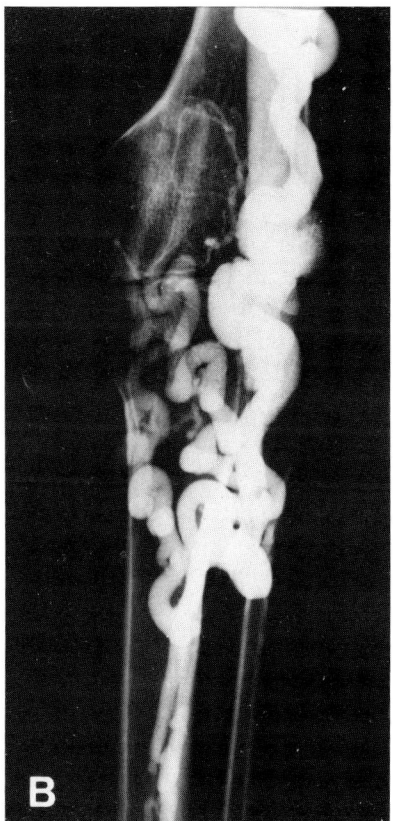
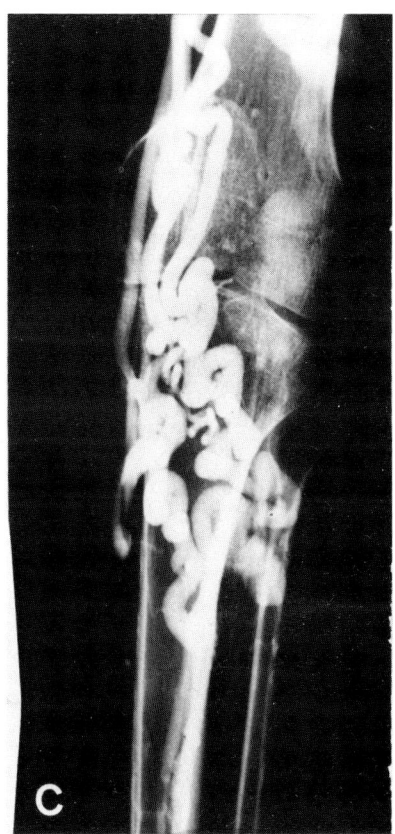
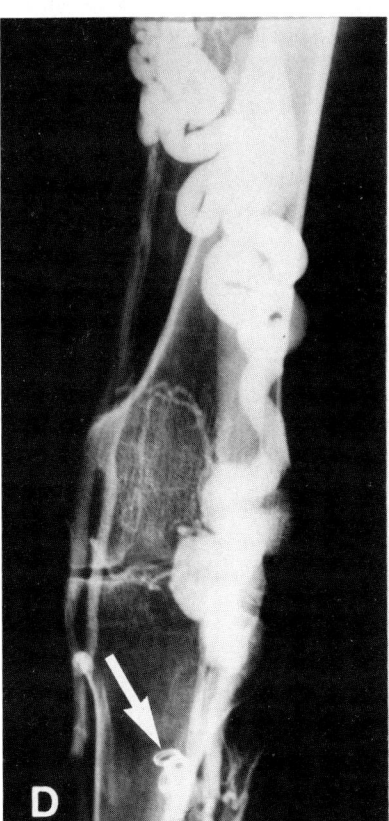
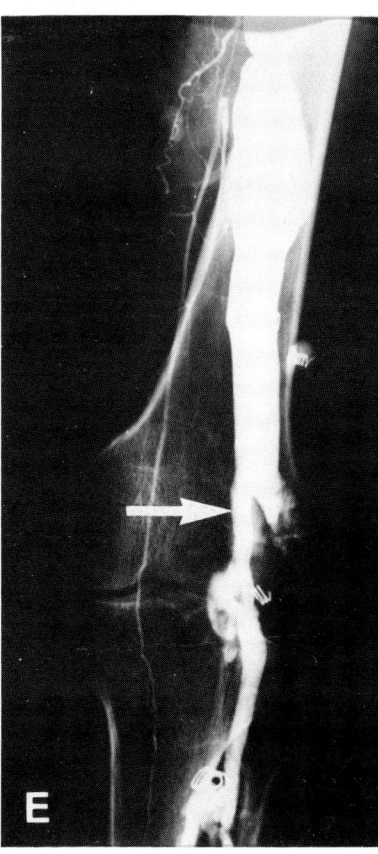

Figure 4.85 Arteriovenous fistula surgically created over 20 years ago in left popliteal artery to improve growth of a limb with poliomyelitis sequela.
(A) Femoral angiogram showing stenosis in large-diameter artery, with poststenotic dilatation. (B) Angiogram at popliteal level showing the fistula massive venous return, with significant reduction in distal flow, is evident. (C) Later phase angiogram showing the venous system more completely. Embolization was indicated in this case for limb ischemia caused by flow steal induced by arteriovenous fistula. (D) Control angiogram following partial embolization showing partial venous return and occlusion by Gianturco coils (arrows). (E) Control angiogram following complete embolization of fistula with Gianturco coils. Notice the occlusion of fistulous os (arrow). Significant improvement of distal ischemia was obtained after embolization, in spite of superficial leg and thigh phlebitis, which had been treated clinically.

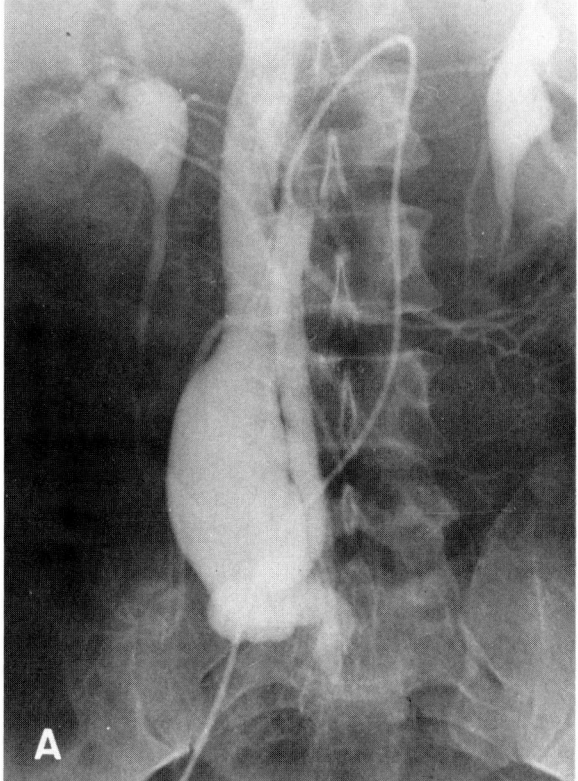 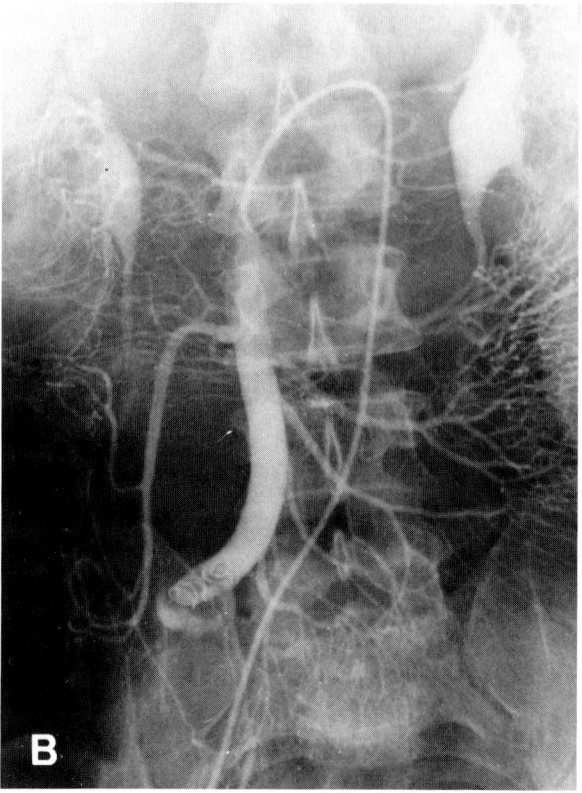

Figure 4.86 (A) Selective superior mesenteric artery angiogram showing high-output arteriovenous fistula with immediate and dense filling of the superior mesenteric and portal veins after multiple surgeries for small bowel resection. Notice the aneurysmal dilatation of the proximal mesenteric vein and the poor intestinal circulation filling, which has caused mesenteric angina. (B) Control following embolization showing arteriovenous fistula occlusion by Gianturco coils. Hyperkinetic portal hypertension and pain due to mesenteric angina have been corrected. The treatment was effective and definitive over a 4-year follow-up period.

ANGIOMATOSIS

Angiomatosis is a name given to certain clinical conditions closely associated with AV malformations and hemangiomas. The most important of these is Rendu-Osler-Weber disease (hereditary hemorrhagic telangiectasia) which is characterized by telangiectasia, which is present in different organs, and AV fistulas (particularly pulmonary) (Figs. 4.40, 4.41, 4.118, and 3.46). The Parkes-Weber syndrome associates AV fistulas with hypertrophy of one limb, varicosity, and superficial angioma. The Klippel-Trenaunay syndrome involves limb hypertrophy, AV fistulas, and venous varicosities, and Sturge-Weber (port wine) syndrome presents brain and facial angioma.

THERAPEUTIC APPROACH

Because of the extreme difficulties of managing patients with hemangiomas and AV malformations and fistulas, a multidisciplinary approach is indicated for examination and evaluation of the lesions and for establishing a treatment protocol for each case.

In deciding whether treatment is indicated, it should be kept in mind that 95 percent of all infantile hemangiomas evolve spontaneously as the patient grows, ultimately regressing. Asymptomatic, stable arteriovenous malformations, hemangiomas, and arteriovenous fistulas that are not a cosmetic problem (that is, are aesthetically acceptable) and do not pose an anatomic threat to adjacent areas or vital organs are not indicated for treatment (Table 4.3).

Some common indications for treatment are as follows.

Immediate intervention is required if an arteriovenous malformation or hemangioma sustains repetitive bleeding or massive hemorrhage, which cannot be controlled by usual means, putting the patient's life or any organ at risk. Treatment is also indicated for rapidly growing lesions, or those causing anatomic

or functional deformities which will leave permanent sequelae, for example, limb asymmetry, amblyopia, or facial deformity.
- Other indications for therapeutic intervention are pain, plethora, heart failure due to hyperflow, the syndromes described under "Angiomatosis," and Kasabach-Merritt syndrome (thrombocytopenic purpura).
- One major indication for treatment involves cases in which preoperative embolization can be used to reduce the volume of the lesion and reduce bleeding, thus facilitating dissection. Embolization is usually performed 3 or 4 days before surgery, with absorbable material. Partial embolization should probably not be attempted as the sole treatment, as it will result in an increase in vascularization through a different vascular territory. Embolization should be complete, even if multiple procedures are necessary.

It should be remembered that some lesions will remain unresectable even after embolization, and further treatment should be nonsurgical. Incomplete excision of a vascular lesion will create the potential for progressive malformation similar to that which might be caused by nonsurgical trauma (Table 4.3) and will prevent access for endovascular procedures (embolization).

TREATMENT

Observation

As stated previously, most lesions do not require treatment, and an attitude of expectant observation is therefore highly effective. However, the evolution of all such lesions should be closely followed so that intervention, if it becomes necessary, will be timely.

Corticosteroids

Corticosteroids should be used to treat infantile hemangioma when one or more of the following conditions exists:

Obstruction of airways
Hemorrhage and ulceration, with or without thrombocytopenia
Cardiovascular failure due to hyperflow
Rapid and uncontrolled lesion growth
Deformity

Corticosteroids can be used anytime during childhood for treating hemangiomas; however, they are more effective during the first year of life and in cases not previously treated.

Corticosteroids act through arteriolar constriction and narrowing of precapillary sphincters, causing a decrease in blood flow.

Within 2 to 3 weeks following the initiation of therapy, a partial regression of the lesion is observed. Reduction is progressive over a period of 30 to 90 days. Ulcerations usually heal within about 2 weeks.

A 1- to 2-mg/kg dose of predinisone (Meticorten) can be used every other day for 30 days. Prednisolone (Meticortelone) can also be used, at an average daily dose of 20 mg/day over 3- to 8-week periods, the dose being gradually reduced to 2.5 mg/day before medication is discontinued.

Results obtained from using corticosteroids are encouraging (satisfactory responses have been obtained in up to 90 percent of cases), and the treatment of hemangiomas in children probably should always start this way.

Radiotherapy

Presently, there is no place for radiotherapy in the treatment of vascular malformations or hemangiomas. The complications of radiotherapy include bone growth retardation, radiodermatitis, the risk of neoplasm, and possible sterility.

Compression Treatment

Recent experimental findings have shown that mast cells are present in large numbers in proliferating hemangiomas but are scarce in regressed hemangiomas and vascular malformations. A high-molecular-weight heparin released by the mast cells probably creates a local anticoagulation state, which in conjunction with coagulopathy states associated with hemangiomas (thrombocytopenia) may serve to protect the lesions from intravascular thrombosis.

Because of this, there is no spontaneous thrombosis in angiomatous vascular lesions, in spite of the low-flow or stasis conditions that exist in some of these cases.

A few years ago, the literature described some success using a technique involving intermittent compression with bandages to "release the platelets" from the hemangioma, thus promoting thrombosis. Success of this treatment method was confirmed by several subsequent papers. The most significant mechanism is probably vessel collapse, which, in combination with stasis, causes thrombus formation.

In order for the compressive therapy to be effective and safe, it is necessary that the pressure transmitted by the compressive bandage be lower than that of the local artery, to avoid ischemia of normal tissue and of the skin surrounding the angiomatous lesion.

Superficial hemangiomatous lesions seem to respond relatively uniformly to prolonged intermittent compression, which produces accelerated regression and volume decrease. Corticosteroids have no effect upon nonregressed hemangiomas, but compression improves those cases through volume reduction.

Compression does not cause lesions to disappear completely, but it significantly reduces their volume, at least temporarily. Ease of application depends upon the anatomic location of the lesion. In the trunk and limbs, compression is achieved with elastic bands or tight clothes made from some elastic material. Effective compression is more difficult when the lesions involve the face, neck, or scalp. Bands are useless, but in the case of facial lesions, a mask constructed from elastic fabric produces effective and uniform pressure.

Probably the best methods involve compression used in conjunction with other forms of treatment, such as corticosteroids, embolization, sclerosis, or resection. In considering compression therapy, two things should be kept in mind. First, even when the lesions are benign, the cosmetic improvement afforded by this simple therapeutic technique can mean a great deal to the parents. Second, because the parents, rather than the physician, apply the compression treatments, they become actively involved and are likely to accept the results obtained more readily.

There are two major indications for compression therapy: (1) newborn babies with hemangioma and thrombocytopenic purpura, and (2) older children with rapidly growing hemangioma or children above 6 years of age in whom the hemangioma has not receded.

Sclerosing Agents

Sclerosing injections may be used in patients with lesions located in areas difficult to access surgically, such as the base of the tongue, floor of the mouth, and pharyngeal wall. Some skin lesions are also helped by sclerosis, particularly cavernous-type lesions or those predominantly venous in nature. Percutaneous puncture of a lesion may be used simultaneously for diagnostic and therapeutic purposes (Fig. 4.83).

Percutaneous approach to the lesion should be obtained through the healthy skin surrounding the mass, the needle being introduced into the malformation or hemangiomatous cavity. Contrast medium may be injected in order to obtain x-ray films; this is followed by injection of the sclerosing agent and temporary compression of the area. The most commonly used sclerosing agents are absolute alcohol and ethanolamine oleate (Ethamolin). Percutaneous sclerosis of a hemangioma may be followed by surgical resection if necessary.

Embolization

Embolization can be used to treat hemangiomas, AV malformations, and fistulas directly, or as adjuvant therapy designed to change the evolution of the lesion. Although embolization is an effective way to manage certain complications of vascular malformations, it does not, as a rule, cure them. When hemangioma is present, with malformed canals inside a tumor acting as a high-output AV shunt, hyperflow and heart failure may be present. In such situations, usually occurring in newborns or low-birth-weight infants, immediate intervention is necessary to stop the shunt and to improve the patient's general condition. Corticosteroids do not act quickly enough, and surgical excision of the lesion is appropriate only when the patient would tolerate the surgical act. Embolization of this type of lesion leads to prompt recovery of the hemodynamic status without massive AV fistula (Fig. 4.75).

Superselective catheterization of the involved arteries should be performed by the femoral route, and embolization carried out with nonabsorbable particulate or long-duration material (PVA plus Gelfoam). In cases of limb malformation, it is sometimes necessary to puncture the regional arteries in order to carry out embolization.

It is possible to treat large hemangiomas presenting with Kasabach-Merritt's syndrome (thrombocytopenia) and severe coagulopathy by surgical excision, compression, or corticosteroid therapy. Embolization, however, immediately reduces the blood supply to the lesion, decreasing platelet sequestration and reversing the clinical condition within a few days (Fig. 4.76). After a few weeks it may be necessary to repeat the procedure with relative frequency.

Embolization should be flow-oriented, with polyvinyl alcohol (Ivalon) microparticles and Gelfoam powder being used. Permanent occlusion of the vessels and part of the lesion's nidus is thus achieved. The expected result is that the beginning of mass regression will be accelerated by embolization and enhanced by the simultaneous use of corticosteroids and compression. Cyanoacrylate glues are also extremely valuable for embolization of such lesions when the purpose is to occlude the nidus and not the artery.

AV malformations start to develop symptoms and complications later than hemangiomas, but embolization can also play a significant role in either curative or palliative treatment of these symptoms.

AV malformations are usually first noticed when they have grown to the point at which they cause discomfort due to mass effect or to the presence of AV communications which have become symptomatic (Figs. 4.77 to 4.79). These lesions frequently involve extremities, causing pain, bleeding, and deformity, and embolization must be carefully performed, as the occlusion of distal arteries may cause new necrotic areas to be formed in healthy tissue (especially digital). Selective catheterization is always required, using either particulate or fluid embolizing material. Gelfoam and PVA (Ivalon) are the two most frequently used particulate materials for such cases (Fig. 4.77), although bucrylate glue also has a significant role to play (Fig. 4.79).

It is absolutely essential that the nidus of the lesion be occluded, and occasionally for that purpose a highly

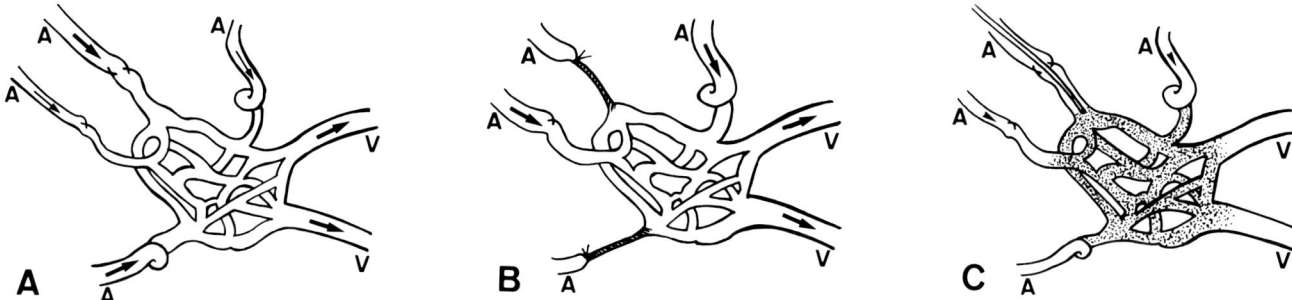

Figure 4.87 Schematic illustration of the use of embolizing material occluding the nidus of a vascular lesion (IBC).
(A) Arteriovenous malformations with four feeding arteries, two of which have significant flow (large arrows), and two of which have smaller flow (small arrows). Venous drainage is performed by two high-output veins (V) (large arrows).
(B) If surgical ligation of the main arteries shown in (A) were performed, immediate flow redistribution would occur through the secondary arteries (A) (large arrows), the venous drainage being maintained (V). (C) If superselective catheterization of the main artery were performed (A), and a polymerizing fluid injected into the lesion, the nidus would be occluded, resulting in a drastic reduction in accessory arterial flow, as well as occlusion or reduction of venous flow to normal (V). (Modified from Athanasoulis et al., *Interventional Radiology,* Saunders, Philadelphia, 1982.)

selective coaxial system will be required for catheterization (Fig. 4.87). Proximal embolization is ineffective in treating these vascular malformations; indeed, it will be equivalent to surgical ligation, as illustrated in Fig. 4.87.

When the limbs are involved, puncture and catheterization of regional arteries may be necessary to reach the nidus (Fig. 4.79). In malformations of average flow, it is also possible to reach the nidus with a coaxial system, using either bucrylate (Fig. 4.80) or particulate material (Fig. 4.81). In malformations with low flow, percutaneous direct sclerosis may be required to reach the lesion nidus (Fig. 4.82).

Some malformations may be embolized with particles or fluid material through direct percutaneous puncture when the vascular anatomy will not allow a catheter approach. The vascular malformations best suited for treatment by embolization are AV fistulas. In contrast to cases of hemangioma and AV malformation, where treatment is mainly to manage complications, AV fistulas are always candidates for catheterization. In choosing a material that will result in adequate occlusion, the size and type of the AV fistula must be taken into account.

Congenital AV fistulas may include one or more communications. It is always advisable to test the diameter and number of communications with an occlusion balloon catheter before selecting the size of the embolic material to be used (Fig. 4.84). The most frequently used materials in AV fistula occlusion are detachable balloons and Gianturco coils (Fig. 4.88). In surgical (Fig.

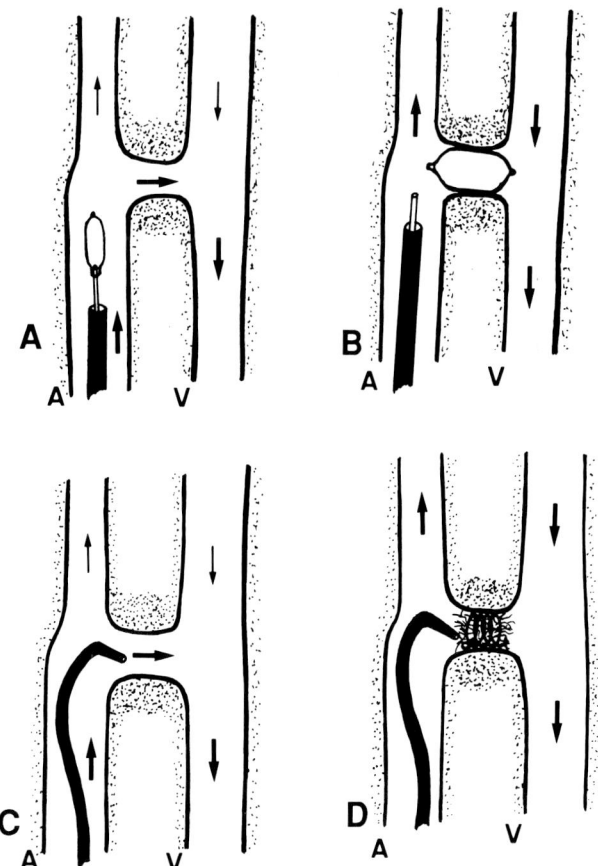

Figure 4.88 Schematic drawings showing the use of detachable balloon and Gianturco coil for occlusion of large-diameter AV fistula and flow changes before and after occlusion (A = artery; V = vein).
(A) Large AV fistula. Notice the large arrows in the afferent vessel of the AV fistula and in the efferent vessel. Flow is decreased in the artery and vein distally to the AV fistula. A detachable balloon is in position for release. (B) Following balloon release, occlusion of the AV fistula, and flow changes (observe the arrows), occur. (C) The fistula is as described in (A). However, the occlusion technique being used involves Gianturco coils and a Cobra-type catheter selectively positioned. (D) Gianturco coil occluding the fistula.

4.85) or traumatic (Fig. 4.86) fistulas, the AV communication is usually larger, requiring larger embolic materials.

AV fistulas are a primary cause of distally located flow steal, particularly in the extremities and in the mesenteric system, which causes digital and mesenteric ischemia, respectively. Occlusion of the AV fistula by catheterization allows the fistula to be conservatively closed, increases distal circulation, and prevents hemodynamic complications (Fig. 4.86).

REFERENCES

Andrews GC, Domonkos AN, Torres-Rodriguez VM, Bem-Benista J. Hemangiomas: Treated and untreated. *JAMA* 1957;165:1114–1117.

Argenta LC, Bishop E, Cho KJ, Andrews AF, Coran AC. Complete resolution of life-threatening hemangioma by embolization and corticosteroids. *Plast Reconstr Surg* 1982;70:739–744.

Athanasoulis CA. Transcatheter arterial occlusion for arteriovenous fistulas and malformations of the trunk, pelvis, and extremity. In *Interventional Radiology,* edited by Athanasoulis CA, Pfister RC, Greene RE, Roberson GH. Saunders, Philadelphia, 1982:203–222.

Bennett JE, Zook EG. Treatment of arteriovenous fistulas in cavernous hemangiomas of face by muscle embolization. *Plast Reconstr Surg* 1972;50:84–87.

Cohen SR, Wang CI. Steroid treatment of hemangioma of the head and neck in children. *Ann Otol* 1972;81:584–590.

Edgerton ME. The treatment of hemangiomas: With special reference to the role of steroid therapy. *Ann Surg* 1976;183:517–532.

Flye MW, Jordan BP, Schwartz MS. Management of congenital arteriovenous malformations. *Surgery* 1983;94:740–747.

Forbes G, Earnest F, Jackson IT, Marsh WR, Jack CR, Cross SA. Therapeutic embolization angiography for extra-axial lesions in the head. *Mayo Clin Proc* 1986;61:427–441.

Gomes AS, Busuttil RW, Baker DJ, Oppenheim W et al. Congenital arteriovenous malformations: The role of transcatheter embolization. *Arch Surg* 1983;118:817–825.

Leikensohn JR, Epstein LI, Varconeg LO. Superselective embolization and surgery of noninvoluting hemangiomas and AV malformations. *Plast Reconstr Surg* 1981;68:143–152.

Mangus DJ. Continuous compression treatment of hemangiomata. *Plast Reconstr Surg* 1972;49:490–493.

Merland JJ, Riche MC, Melki JP. Selective arteriography and embolization in vascular malformations of the limbs. In *Interventional Radiology,* edited by Wilkins RA, Viamonte M. Blackwell, Oxford, 1982:51–61.

Miller SH, Smith RL, Shochat SJ. Compression treatment of hemangiomas. *Plast Reconstr Surg* 1976;58:573–579.

Moore AW. Pressure in the treatment of giant hemangioma with purpura. *Plast Reconstr Surg* 1964;31:606–611.

Mulliken JB, Glowacki J. Hemangiomas and vascular malformations in infants and children: A classification based on endothelial characteristics. *Plast Reconstr Surg* 1982;69:412–420.

Natali J, Merland JJ. Superselective arteriography and therapeutic embolization for vascular malformations (angiodysplasias). *J Cardiovasc Surg* 1976;17:465–472.

Olcott C, Newton TH, Stoney RJ, Ehrenfeld WK. Intraarterial embolization in the management of arteriovenous malformations. *Surgery* 1976;79:3–12.

Pritchard DA, Maloney JD, Bernatz PE, Symmonds RE, Stanson AW. Surgical treatment of congenital pelvic arteriovenous malformation. *Mayo Clin Proc* 1978;53:607–611.

Smith CJ, Clark SK. Cervical congenital arteriovenous malformation. *Laryngoscope* 1978;88:1522–1528.

Stanley RJ, Cubillo E. Nonsurgical treatment of arteriovenous malformations of the trunk and limb by transcatheter arterial embolization. *Radiology* 1975;115:609–612.

Thomson HG, Ward CM, Crawford JS, Stigmar G. Hemangiomas of the eyelid: Visual complications and prophylactic concepts. *Plast Reconstr Surg* 1979;63:641–647.

Vinters HV, Lundie MJ, Kaufmann JCE. Long-term pathological follow-up of cerebral arteriovenous malformations by embolization with bucrylate. *N Engl J Med* 1986;314:477–483.

Weber TR, West KW, Cohen M, Grosfield JL. Massive hemangioma in infants: Therapeutic considerations. *J Vasc Surg* 1984;1:423–428.

Wisnick JL. Hemangiomas and vascular malformations. *Ann Plast Surg* 1984;14:41–59.

Zarem HA, Edgerton MT. Induced resolution of cavernous hemangiomas following prednisolone therapy. *Plast Reconstr Surg* 1967;39:76–83.

Embolization of Lesions in the Head and Neck

MARCIO SAMPAIO
RONIE LEO PISKE

TRAUMATIC ARTERIOVENOUS FISTULAS

Traumatic AV fistulas are abnormal, direct communications between arteries and veins formed as a consequence either of trauma, with or without fracture to the base of the skull, or of a direct vascular lesion as a consequence of contusive or penetrating trauma.

Angiographically, AV traumatic fistulas are identified by the presence of one or more arterial pedicles, frequently dilated and tortuous, causing early drainage and vein opacification.

Carotid Cavernous Fistulas

The cavernous sinuses are venous (Fig. 4.89), extradural compartments, with bilateral parasellar location. They communicate through the coronary sinuses, transversely interposed on the anterior, inferior, and posterior sella turcica walls and receive drainage from the orbit, cranial base, meninges, diploe, and temporal cortex.

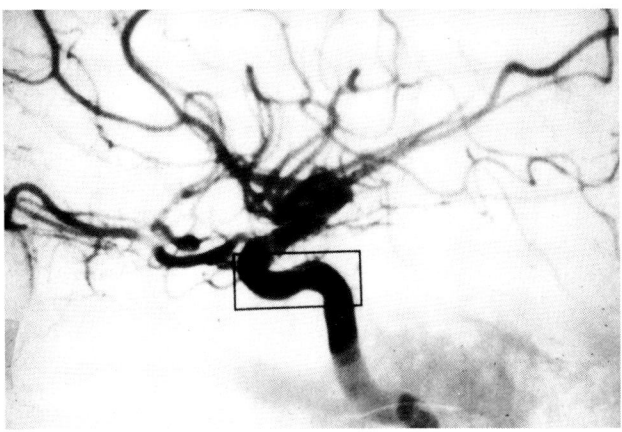

Figure 4.90 Internal carotid artery arteriogram, lateral view. The rectangle represents the intracavernous segment of the carotid siphon.

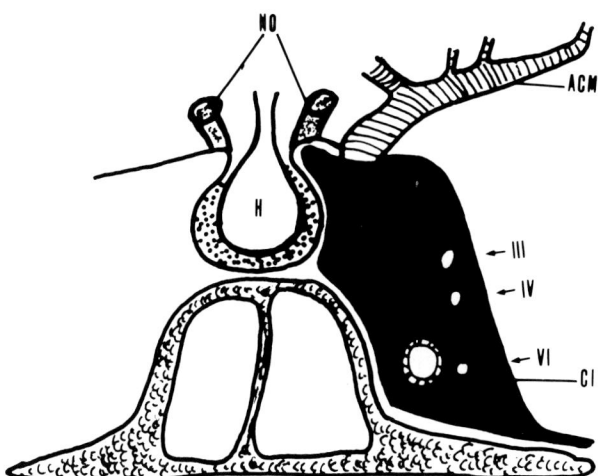

Figure 4.89 Schematic drawing showing the cavernous sinus (in black), and its relation with the cranial nerves (III, IV, and VI) and with the internal carotid artery (IC). H, hypophysis; ON, optic nerves; MCA, middle cerebral artery.

When the internal carotid artery enters the midcranial fossa, it traverses the cavernous sinus in a short horizontal segment (Fig. 4.90), its external walls (adventitia) being bathed with venous blood. During this course, it is in close connection with the common motor oculi nerve (III), as well as the trochlear (IV), abducent (VI), and ophthalmic nerves, which before entering the orbit will pass through the cavernous sinus as well.

Carotid rupture inside the cavernous sinus results in injection of high-pressure blood into a low-pressure compartment, reversing the physiologically centripetal venous blood flow and causing it to become centrifugal (Fig. 4.91). Thus the veins which normally drain into the cavernous sinus start receiving arterial blood directly. The clinical manifestations of this phenomenon, which are a consequence of ophthalmic venous hypertension, are generally externalized in the orbit. They are characterized by exophthalmos, which is almost invariably pulsatile; progressive vision deficit; conjunctival congestion; chemosis; orbital systolic murmur; and associated or isolated paralysis of the cranial nerves that cross the cavernous sinus. The clinical manifestations may, rarely, be contralateral to the lesion. When this is the case, the ophthalmic vein abnormality will always be ipsilateral to the fistula (Fig. 4.91).

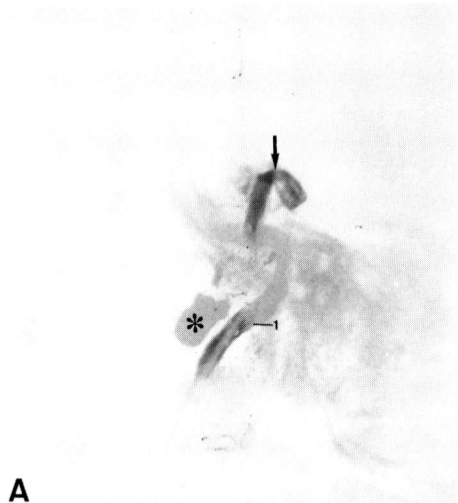
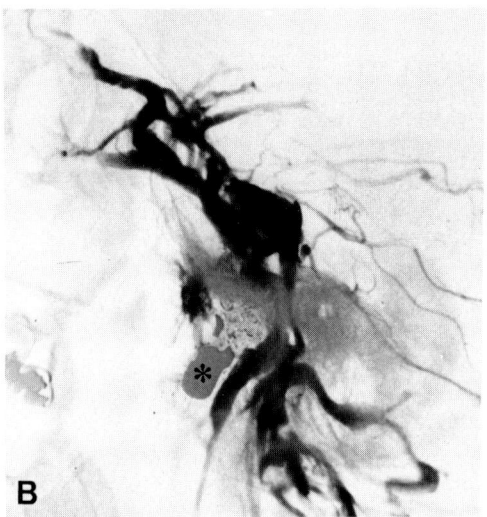
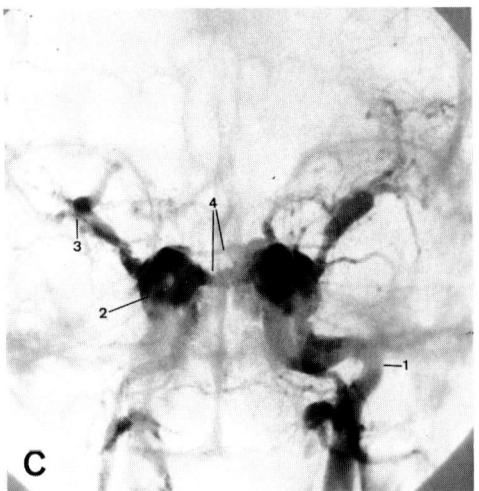

Figure 4.91 Showing left carotid cavernous high-output fistula following trauma caused by gunshot wound.
(A,B) Left internal carotid arteriograms, lateral view, early and later phase, respectively. The fistulous track (arrow) is only visible on the early phase. 1, internal carotid; (*), firearm bullet. (C) Internal carotid arteriogram (1), anteroposterior view, on the same side as the fistula (left). Cavernous sinus opacification (2); opacification of the ophthalmic vein (3) on the opposite side of the lesion, through the coronary sinus (4). (D) internal carotid arteriogram on side opposite to the fistula (right). Anteroposterior view with simultaneous compression of the primitive carotid on the fistula side. The anterior communicating artery (arrow) is patent. Retrograde opacification of the fistula (arrowhead) is evident (E) Skull x-ray. The arrow shows positioning of the balloon; an asterisk (*) indicates the bullet. (F) Left internal carotid arteriogram, lateral view. Immediate postembolization control showing completely closed fistula and patent carotid flow.

Angiographic Protocol

Angiographic evaluation should include both the internal carotids and the vertebral and external carotid arteries on the same side as the fistula. The internal carotid contralateral to the fistula is studied in order to evaluate the patency of the anterior communicating artery. Thus if it becomes necessary during treatment to sacrifice the carotid artery, information on whether the two hemispheres are fed by only one carotid axis will be available.

Injection into the vertebral artery shows, via the posterior communicating artery, retrograde filling of the fistula, in most cases, pinpointing the position of the fistulous track.

In addition to direct communication between the carotid and the cavernous sinus some fistulas involve the participation of external carotid branches. The protocol for selective study of these branches is as follows:

1. Internal carotid artery on the opposite side of the fistula: AP view, with simultaneous compression of the common carotid, on the same side as the fistula
2. Vertebral: lateral view, with simultaneous compression

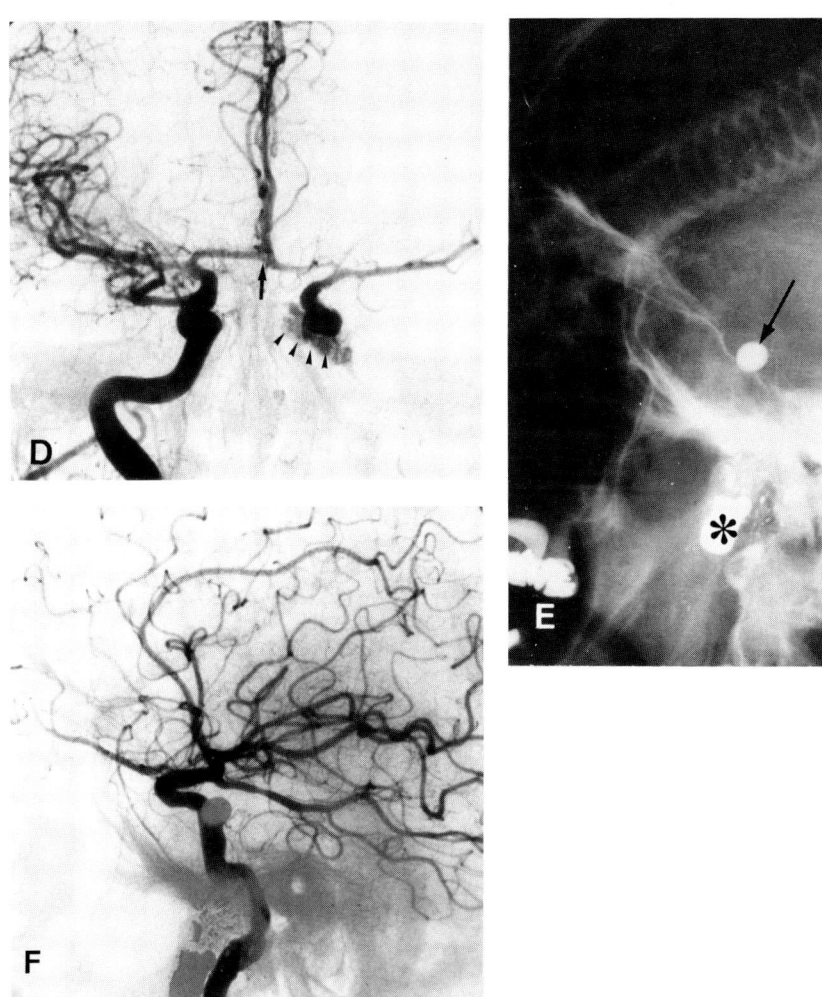

Figure 4.91 *Continued*

of the common carotid on the same side as the fistula
3. External carotid ipsilateral to the fistula: lateral view
4. Internal carotid ipsilateral to the fistula: AP and lateral views

Treatment

The therapeutic objective is to obliterate the fistulous track, while maintaining the carotid flow intact (Fig. 4.92).

Surgical approach to traumatic AV fistulas of the head or neck is a difficult procedure. However, surgical ligations of intra and supracavernous internal carotid segments (trapping procedure) have obtained satisfactory results in a large number of cases. This method, which requires two different surgical accesses, does not directly obliterate the fistula. Therefore, there may be recurrence through collateral circulation developed by the external carotid system and by the posterior communicating artery.

Currently, treatment of these fistulas through endovascular embolization seems to be the first choice. The main advantage of embolization is that in most cases the internal carotid artery remains patent (Fig. 4.93).

For fistulas related to the internal carotid, detachable balloons are used (Fig. 4.93). With mixed fistulas, particles can be used; for those pedicles depending upon the external carotid, fluid embolus (bucrylate) is appropriate.

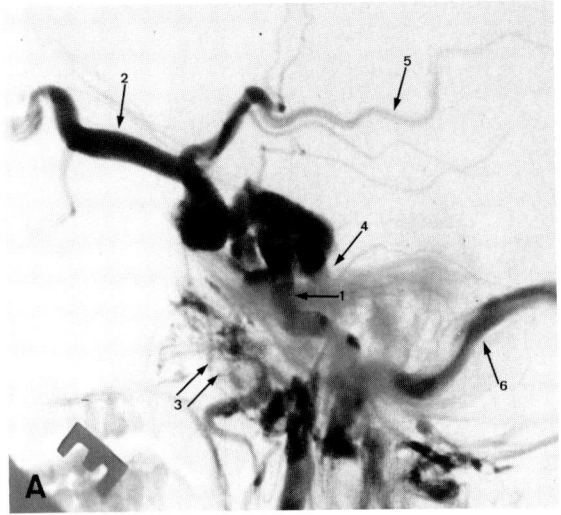
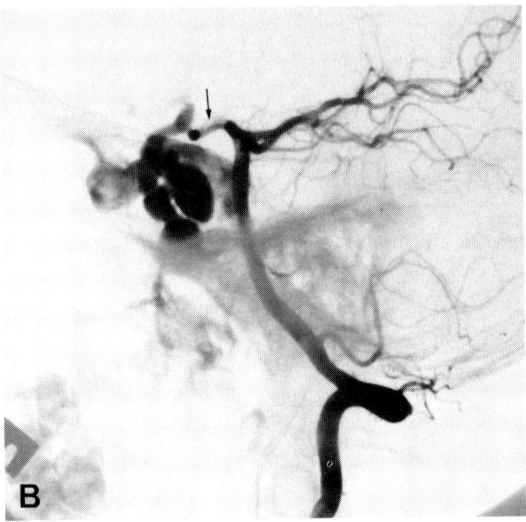
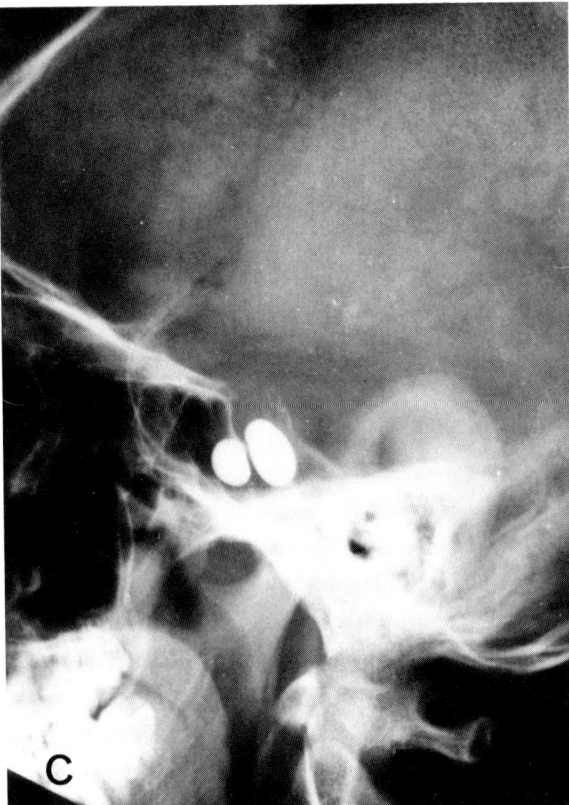
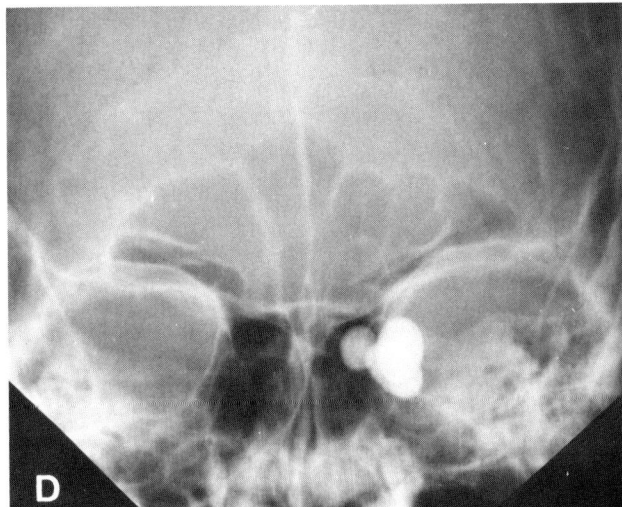

Figure 4.92 Cavernous high-output carotid fistula, arterial approach.

(A) Left internal carotid arteriogram, profile view. Internal carotid artery (1), superior opthalmic vein (2), pterygoid plexus (3), upper petrous sinus (4), temporal veins (5), and lateral sinus (6). Venous steal is so significant that there is no opacification of the cerebral arteries. (B) Vertebral arteriogram, lateral view, with simultaneous compression of the primitive carotid, showing retrograde opacification of fistula via the posterior communicating artery (arrow) is evident. (C,D) Skull x-rays showing the three balloons in position inside the cavernous sinus. (E) Left internal carotid arteriogram, lateral view. Immediate postembolization control showing significant reduction in fistulous output, with partial ophthalmic vein thrombosis (arrowheads). (F) Lateral skull x-ray. As a safety measure, a fourth balloon (arrowheads) was introduced into the intracavernous carotid siphon. (G) Arteriogram of the primitive carotid, profile view. The arrow shows internal carotid thrombosis (arrow). (H) Vertebral arteriogram, profile view, showing obliterated fistula. 1, posterior communicating artery; 2, supracavernous carotid siphon. Compare with (B).

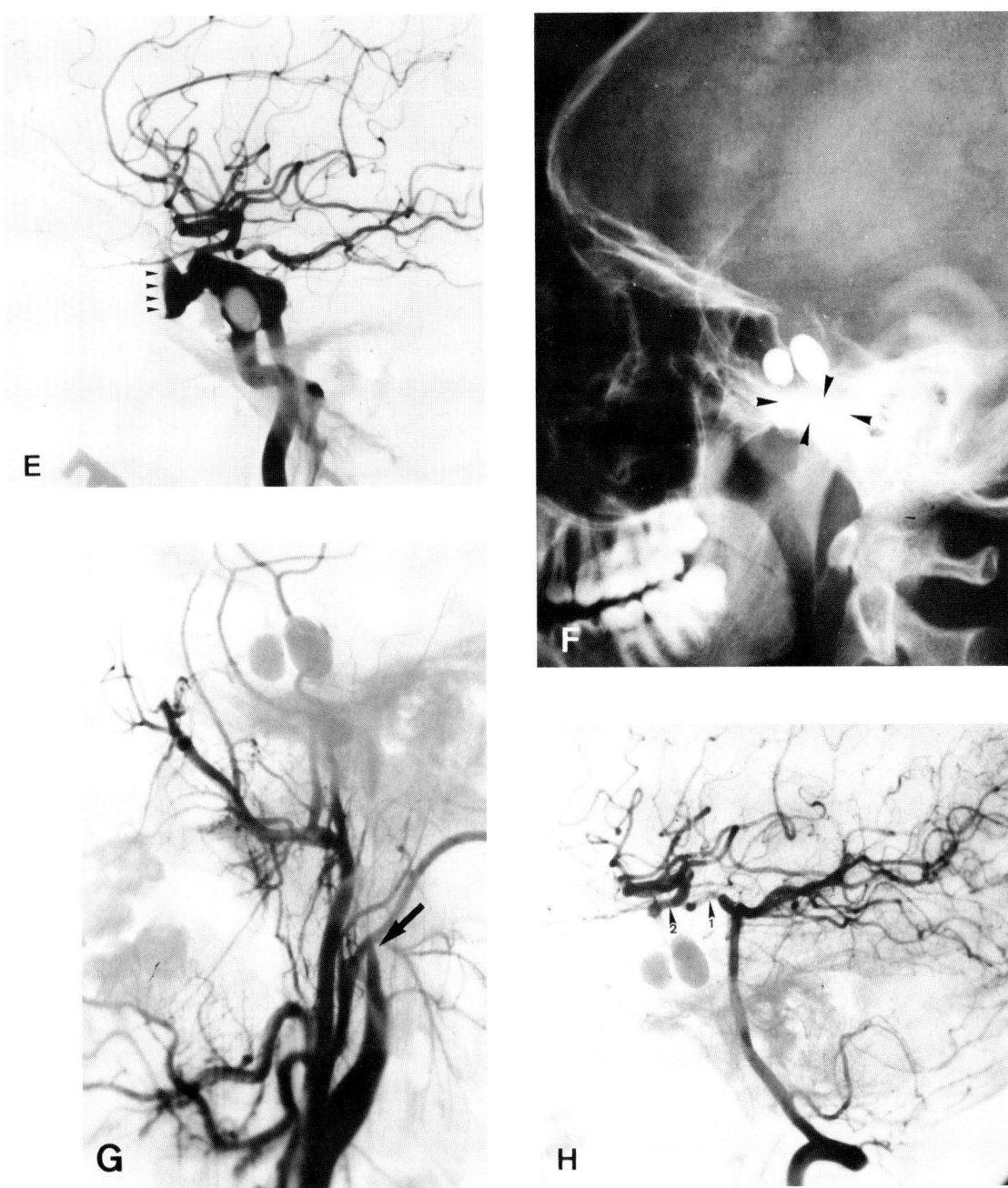

Figure 4.92 *Continued*

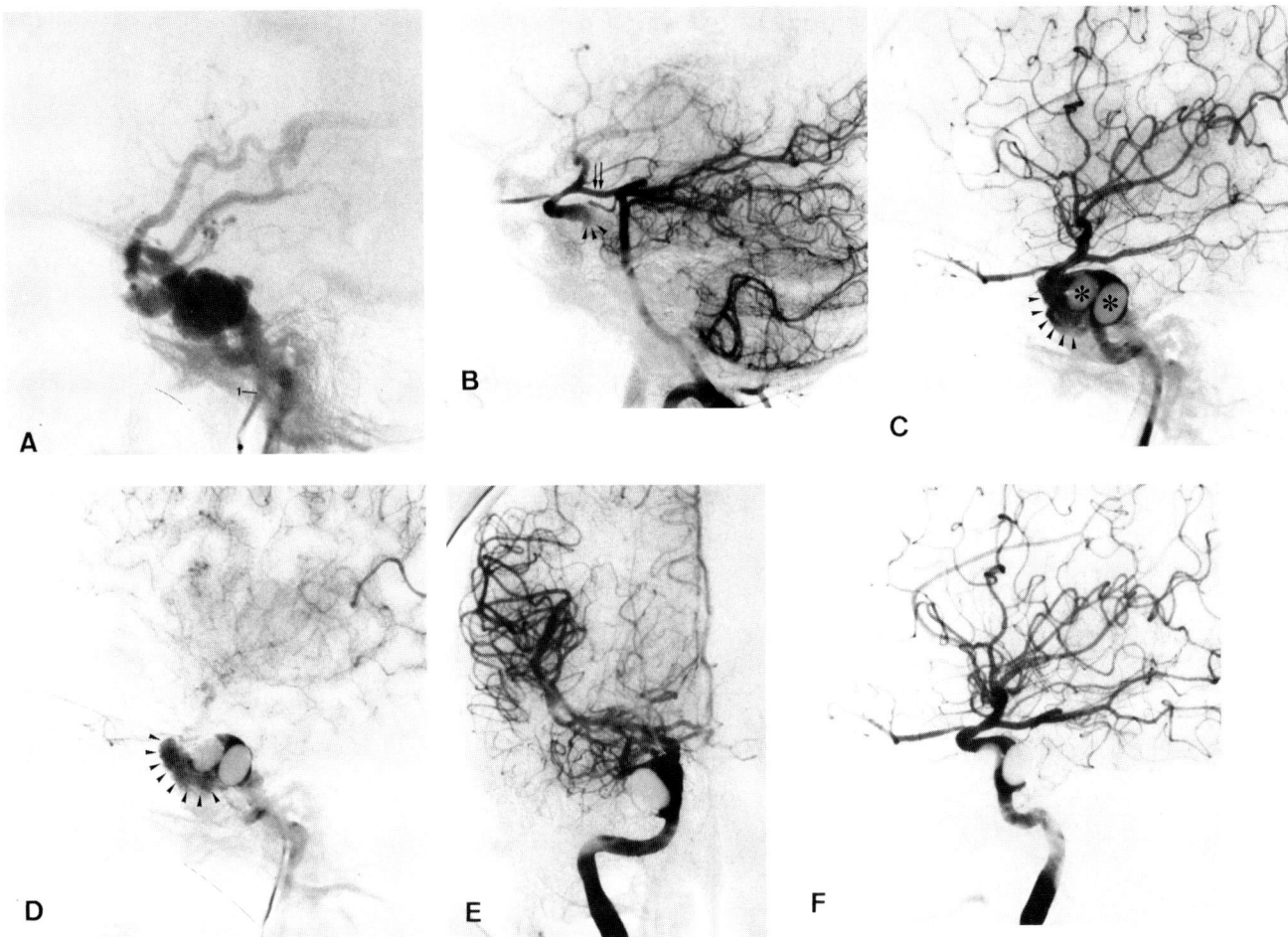

Figure 4.93 (A) Early-phase internal carotid arteriogram lateral view. It is not possible to identify the fistulous tract level. 1, internal carotid artery; (*), catheter. (B) Vertebral arteriogram, lateral view, without simultaneous compression of the primitive carotid artery on the same side of the fistula. The double arrow indicates retrograde filling through the posterior communicating artery, and the arrowheads pinpoint the location of a fistula inside the C5 siphon segment. (C,D) Early and later-phase internal carotid arteriograms, lateral view. Immediate control was obtained following embolization with two detachable balloons (*). Partial closure of the fistula is shown with venous drainage system in partially thrombosed drainage veins (arrowheads). (E,F) Internal carotid arteriograms, frontal and lateral views, respectively. Control angiogram 3 days following manual and intermittent compression of the primitive carotid showed that the fistula was completely closed and carotid flow was maintained.

Latex detachable balloons (Fig. 4.94) are available in different sizes. They contain a silver microsphere which serves as a radioscopic guide during catheterization of the fistula. The balloons are assembled and tied with elastic thread on a No. 2 French catheter, which is introduced through a coaxial system into a No. 3 French catheter (Fig. 4.95). Recently, balloons with valves have been developed which allow the procedure to be performed more easily and more rapidly.

When the approach is made by direct carotid puncture, the system is introduced through a 14- or 16-gauge Jelco-type needle catheter.

Arterial Access

When access is arterial, the system is introduced by the femoral route, through a previously positioned No. 6 French or No. 7 French fine-wall guiding catheter, into the internal carotid artery. Once the carotid siphon has been reached, the balloon should be carefully directed toward the fistulous track. Distending the balloon with small infusions of contrast medium will facilitate its

Figure 4.94 Four different types of detachable balloons utilized according to Debrun's technique.

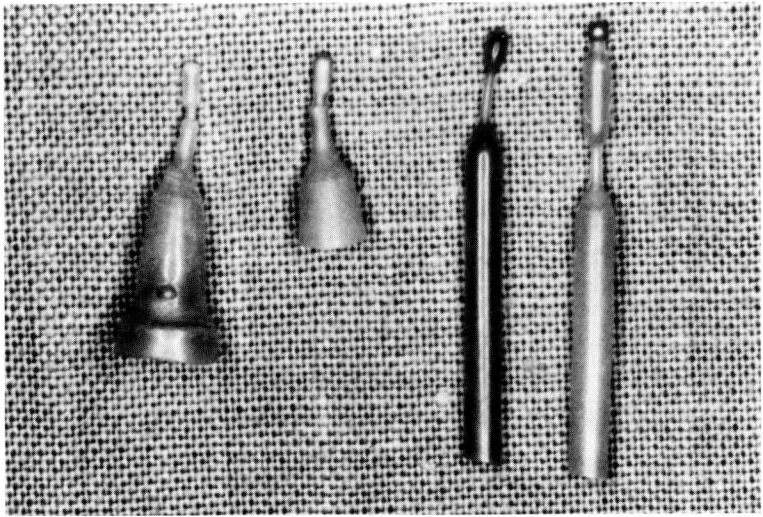

advancement. When the balloon has penetrated the fistula, it is filled with isosmolar contrast medium or with silicone. Before releasing the balloon, one should make certain that it is well positioned inside the fistula, a control angiogram being performed through one of the system's perfusion routes. Release of the balloon is accomplished through a simple maneuver. The No. 3 French catheter is firmly held, while the No. 2 French catheter is gently pulled. As ligation is performed with elastic thread, the moment the No. 2 French catheter is removed, the normal elastic retraction over the balloon neck acts as a valve, preventing deflation. For occluding voluminous fistulas, it is frequently necessary to leave more than one balloon in, and it is not always possible to preserve carotid flow. As a safety measure in such cases, another balloon should be introduced to occlude the segment of the internal carotid below the fistula, thus preventing the eventual migration of one of the balloons positioned in the siphon to cerebral arteries.

Spectacular clinical results are obtained if treatment is adequately performed. Within a few hours, progressive regression of symptoms is perceived, and ocular manifestations usually have disappeared after a few days.

Recurrent cases, which have previously been treated by carotid ligation (trapping), may be approached by the venous route or by the external carotid route. The choice depends on which route offers the easiest, least risky access.

Figure 4.95 Microcatheter with detachable balloon for embolization (Debrun system).
1, No. 2 French catheter; 2, No. 3 French catheter; 3, No. 6 French catheter; 4, inflated latex balloon; 5, antireflux valve; 6, coaxial system perfusion (arrow); 7, contrast injection port (arrow); 8, balloon inflation port (arrow).

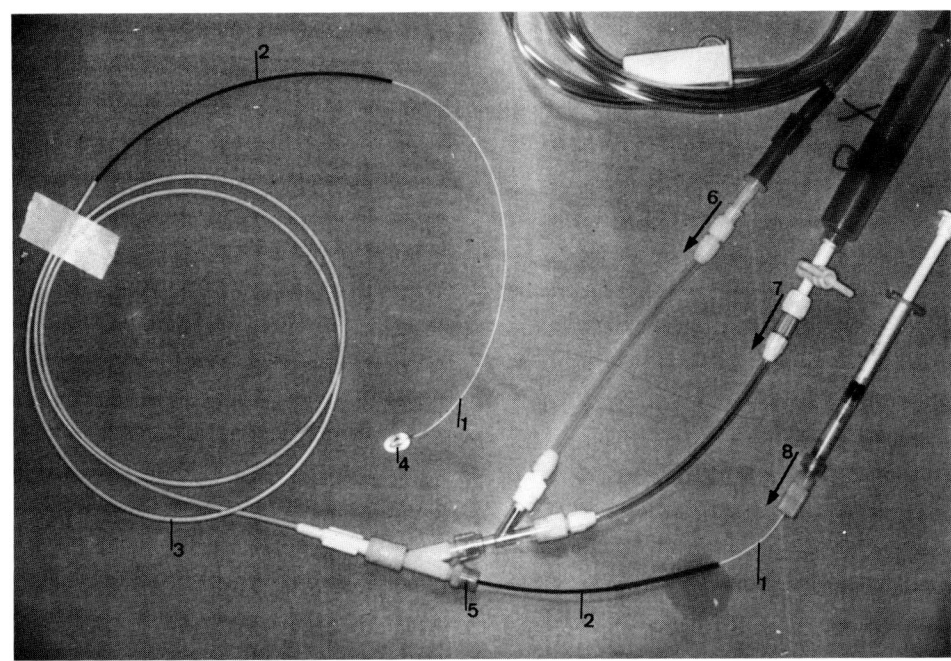

Venous Access

Two different types of venous access may be utilized:

1. If preferred drainage is toward the posterior compartment, i.e., toward the petrous sinuses, the balloon system may be retrogradely introduced via femoral vein or direct jugular puncture. There has been little clinical experience with this method.
2. If preferred drainage is toward the anterior compartment, the ophthalmic vein is utilized. Under general anesthesia, the vein is surgically exposed on the superior internal orbital border, and a small (2-cm) incision, following the eyebrow fold, is made.

After direct venous puncture the balloon system may be introduced directly by phlebotomy or through the catheter needle (Fig. 4.96).

Before proceeding with embolization of pedicles originating from the external carotid, certain criteria should be followed. One should always check for the presence of any dangerous anastomoses existing between distal branches of the internal maxillary and ophthalmic

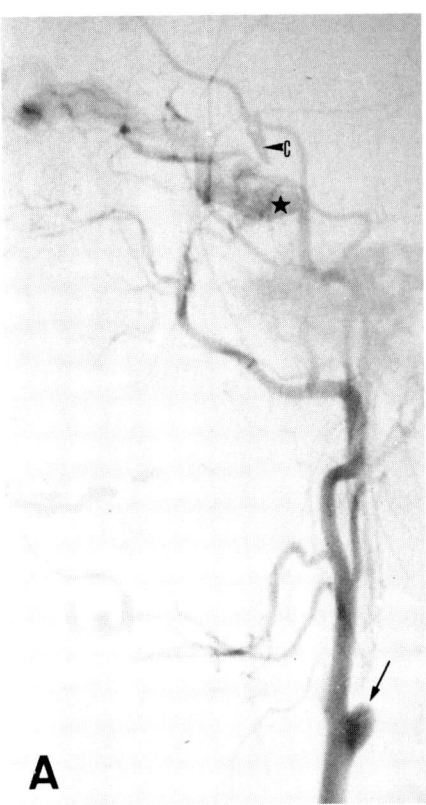

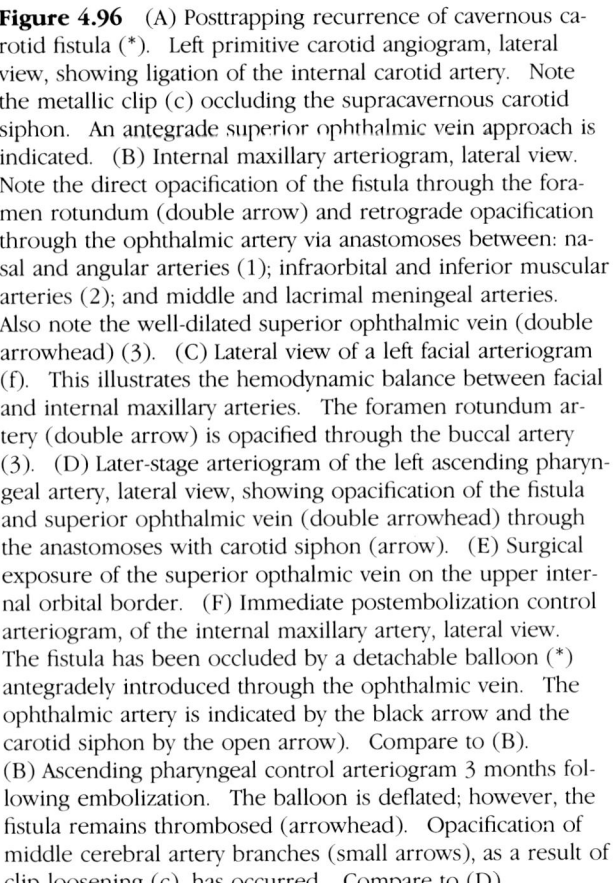

Figure 4.96 (A) Posttrapping recurrence of cavernous carotid fistula (*). Left primitive carotid angiogram, lateral view, showing ligation of the internal carotid artery. Note the metallic clip (c) occluding the supracavernous carotid siphon. An antegrade superior ophthalmic vein approach is indicated. (B) Internal maxillary arteriogram, lateral view. Note the direct opacification of the fistula through the foramen rotundum (double arrow) and retrograde opacification through the ophthalmic artery via anastomoses between: nasal and angular arteries (1); infraorbital and inferior muscular arteries (2); and middle and lacrimal meningeal arteries. Also note the well-dilated superior ophthalmic vein (double arrowhead) (3). (C) Lateral view of a left facial arteriogram (f). This illustrates the hemodynamic balance between facial and internal maxillary arteries. The foramen rotundum artery (double arrow) is opacified through the buccal artery (3). (D) Later-stage arteriogram of the left ascending pharyngeal artery, lateral view, showing opacification of the fistula and superior ophthalmic vein (double arrowhead) through the anastomoses with carotid siphon (arrow). (E) Surgical exposure of the superior opthalmic vein on the upper internal orbital border. (F) Immediate postembolization control arteriogram, of the internal maxillary artery, lateral view. The fistula has been occluded by a detachable balloon (*) antegradely introduced through the ophthalmic vein. The ophthalmic artery is indicated by the black arrow and the carotid siphon by the open arrow). Compare to (B).
(B) Ascending pharyngeal control arteriogram 3 months following embolization. The balloon is deflated; however, the fistula remains thrombosed (arrowhead). Opacification of middle cerebral artery branches (small arrows), as a result of clip loosening (c), has occurred. Compare to (D).

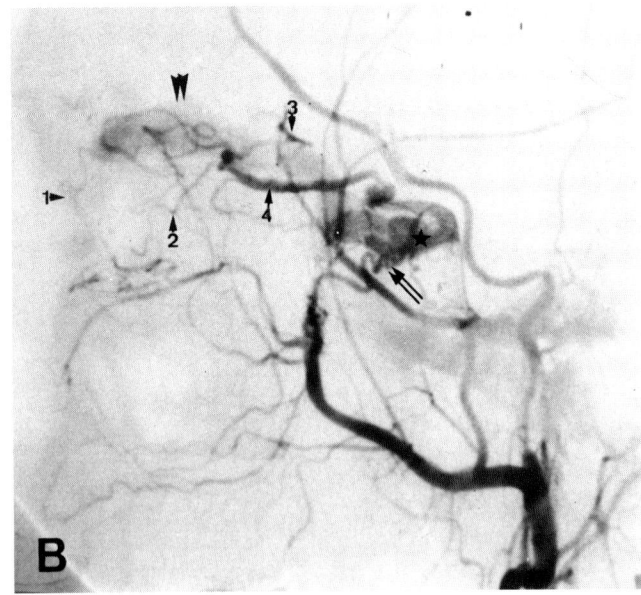

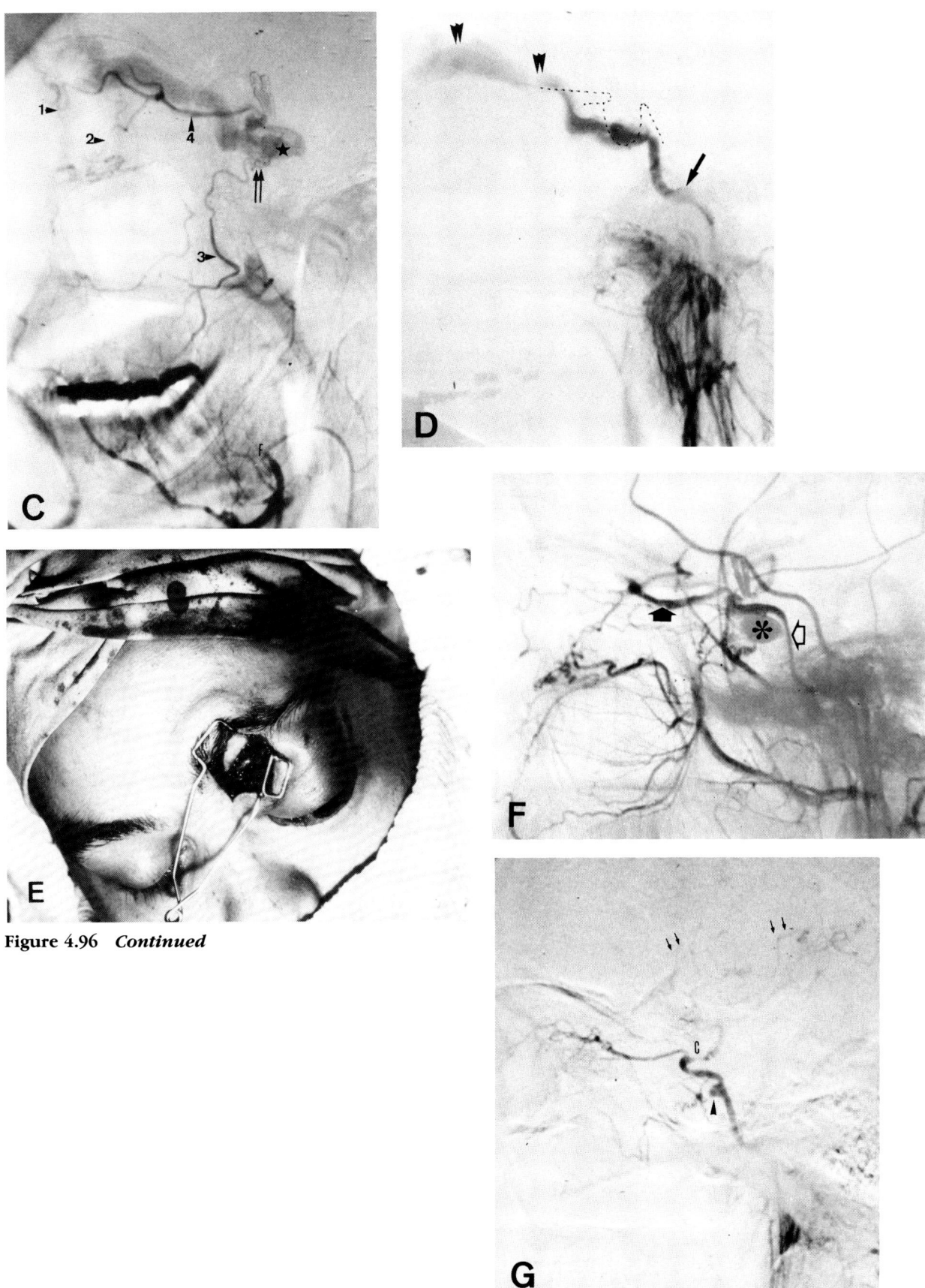

Figure 4.96 *Continued*

arteries, or between the ascending pharyngeal and vertebral arteries. Embolization with bucrylate can only be performed if the pedicle is selectively catheterized. Because bucrylate is a material with great emboligenic power, it cannot be injected remotely into healthy arterial axes. If due to technical or anatomic difficulties, the pedicle is not selectively catheterized, particles of nonabsorbable material should be used (Ivalon or Lyodura).

Arteriovenous Fistulas of the Face, Neck, and Scalp

Arteriovenous fistulas of the face, neck, and scalp are those lesions which depend upon external carotid branches and ascending subclavian artery branches, including vertebrovertebral and vertebrojugular fistulas.

Uni- or multipedicled fistulas related to the external carotid artery are most effectively embolized with bucrylate (Figs. 4.97 and 4.98). Vertebrovertebral and vertebrojugular fistulas are generally direct, with high output. For these fistulas, methods employing detachable balloons are indicated, the same system being utilized as that used for carotid cavernous fistulas (Debrun's technique).

Some superficial segmental fistulas may be directly punctured using a fine needle and afterward embolized with bucrylate. In these cases the bucrylate should not be mixed with Lipiodol, so that its polymerization will be instantaneous. Otherwise there is the risk of accidental migration into the drainage venous system and subsequent lodging in the lung (Fig. 4.99).

ANGIOMATOUS LESIONS

Intracerebral Arteriovenous Angiomas

Intracerebral arteriovenous angiomas are vascular malformations morphologically characterized by three basic components: a uni- or multipedicled afferent arterial system, an angiomatous nidus, and a venous drainage system.

Brain angiomas are benign lesions of uncertain evolution and natural history. They may remain asymptomatic for a long period of time, or may manifest themselves through cerebromeningeal hemorrhages of varying intensity. Frequently, these angiomas are discovered during investigations for cephalalgia, convulsive episodes, transient or progressive motor deficit, or intellectual or mental deterioration.

From the therapeutic standpoint, several different techniques may be utilized: localized radiotherapy, surgery, preoperative embolization, embolization by superselective catheterization, or a combination of these methods. The choice depends not only on lesion size and location, but also on the experience and theoretical background of the clinical team.

Embolization

Although worldwide experience with the use of embolization by superselective catheterization to treat brain angiomas is still limited, the recent literature describes highly satisfactory results. The potential utility of the procedure is enormous: It may be curative; may reduce the volume of the lesion significantly, thus facilitating surgery or making previously inoperable lesions operable; or may control symptoms associated with voluminous lesions that would otherwise be considered intractable. Here we provide a brief introduction to this sophisticated technique, which permits access to small-diameter intracerebral arteries.

Embolization of brain angiomas requires perfect control over the coaxial catheterization system by the angiographer. A latex balloon (calibrated leak balloon), with a perforated distal tip, is mounted on an extremely flexible microcatheter. The whole set is then introduced into a No. 6 French catheter that has previously been positioned inside the internal carotid or vertebral artery. The system is activated by a hydraulic pressure mechanism obtained through a hermetically sealed reservoir with its inlet and outlet controlled by antireflux valves (propulsion chamber) (Fig. 4.100). Once the balloon is distended, it is passively taken away by the preferential blood flow. The distal orifice of the balloon allows the injection of contrast medium or fluid emboli. Once it has been positioned in the feeding pedicle, an arteriogram is performed through the balloon, allowing an evaluation to be made of the volume of embolization material that will occlude the arterial pedicle (Fig. 4.101).

Immediately after embolization, the balloon–microcatheter–catheter system should be removed. For subsequent embolization of another pedicle, the whole operation should be repeated from the beginning, special care being taken not to use again any material which may have already been in contact with bucrylate.

Embolization of intracerebral angiomas requires all the usual precautions and support used for elective surgery (Fig. 4.102), including constant parenteral heparinization.

The patient is given deep analgesia, but should be kept conscious in order to inform the surgical team of any neurologic problem that may occur during the procedure.

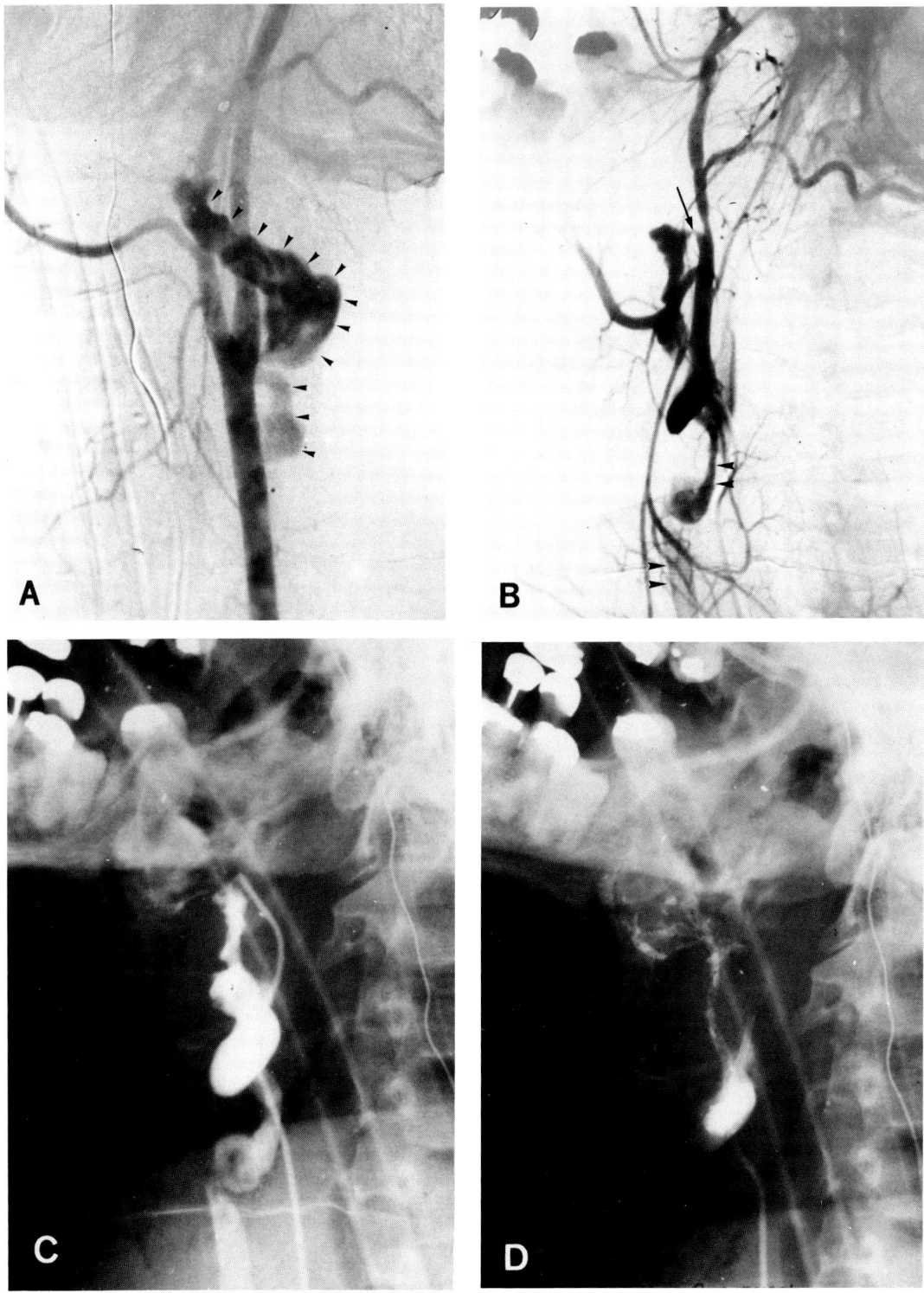

Figure 4.97 Arteriovenous fistula following trauma caused by gunshot wound.
(A) Primitive carotid arteriogram, oblique view, showing contrast extravasation into the soft parts of the neck (arrowheads). (B) External carotid arteriogram, oblique view, demonstrating origin of the fistula at the facial artery (arrow), with drainage to the jugular vein (arrowheads). (C) Selective facial artery catheterization. (D) Plain x-ray. Control was performed following embolization with isobutyl and Lipiodol. The embolizing material is seen inside the fistulous track and on the proximal venous outlet.

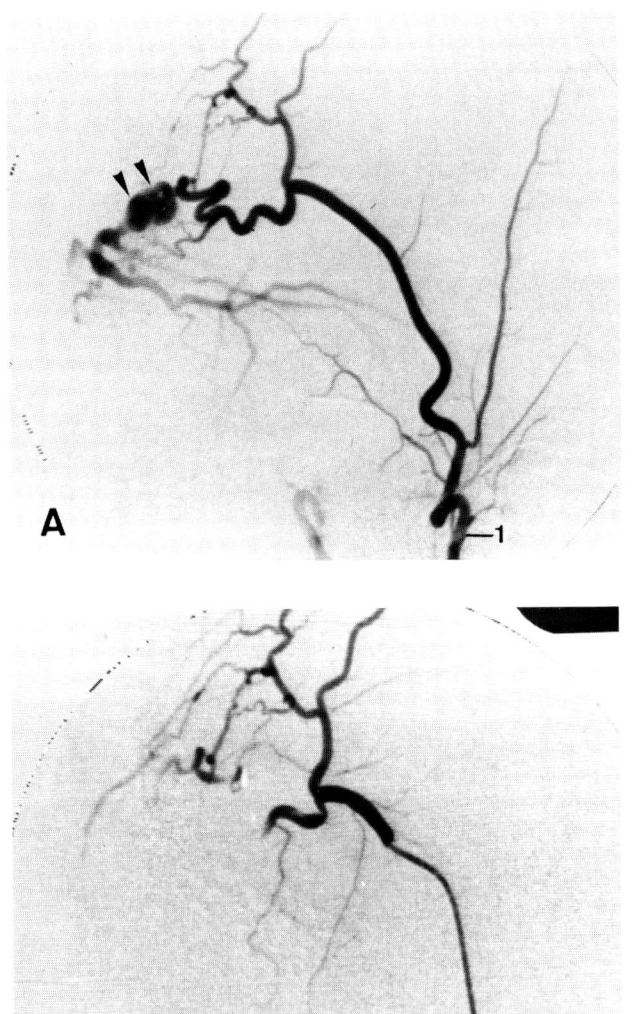
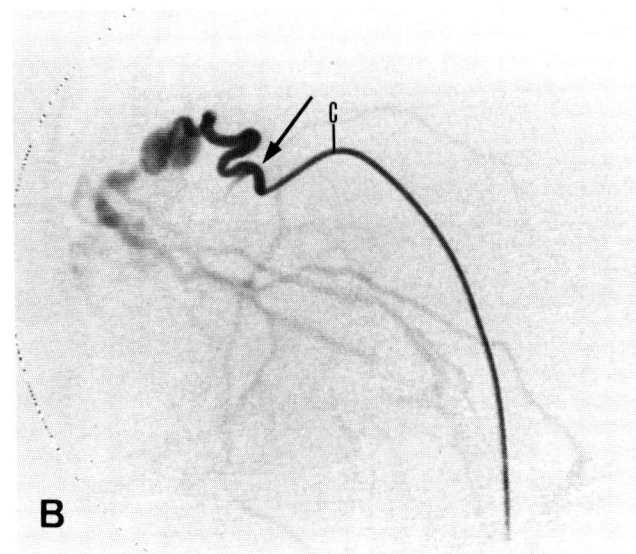

Figure 4.98 Posttraumatic frontal tegumental arteriovenous fistula (arrowheads).
(A) Selective temporal superficial arteriogram (1). (B) Superselective catheterization of the afferent pedicle (arrow); the catheter is labeled (c). (C) Immediate postembolization control with 0.3 mL of isobutyl.

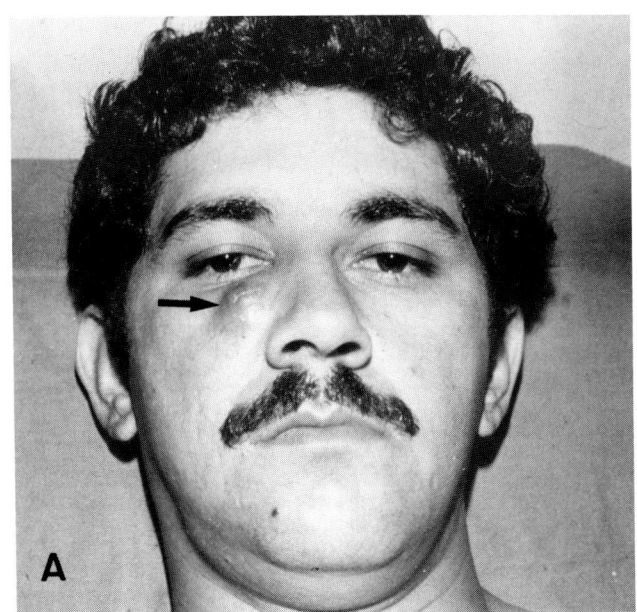

Figure 4.99 Posttrauma (beesting) cutaneous arteriovenous fistula.
(A) Picture of the lesion (arrow). (B,C) Right distal external carotid and facial arteriograms, respectively, profile view, showing lesion opacification (arrowheads) through cutaneous branches. (D) Direct puncture of the fistula with fine needle (arrow). (E) Postembolization control with bucrylate plus Lipiodol. Digital plain x-ray of face, lateral view. Observe the embolizing material occupying the lesion (arrowheads). (F,G) Right distal external carotid and facial arteriograms, respectively, lateral view. Postembolization control showed occlusion of the fistula (*), with preservation of the external carotid artery circulation.

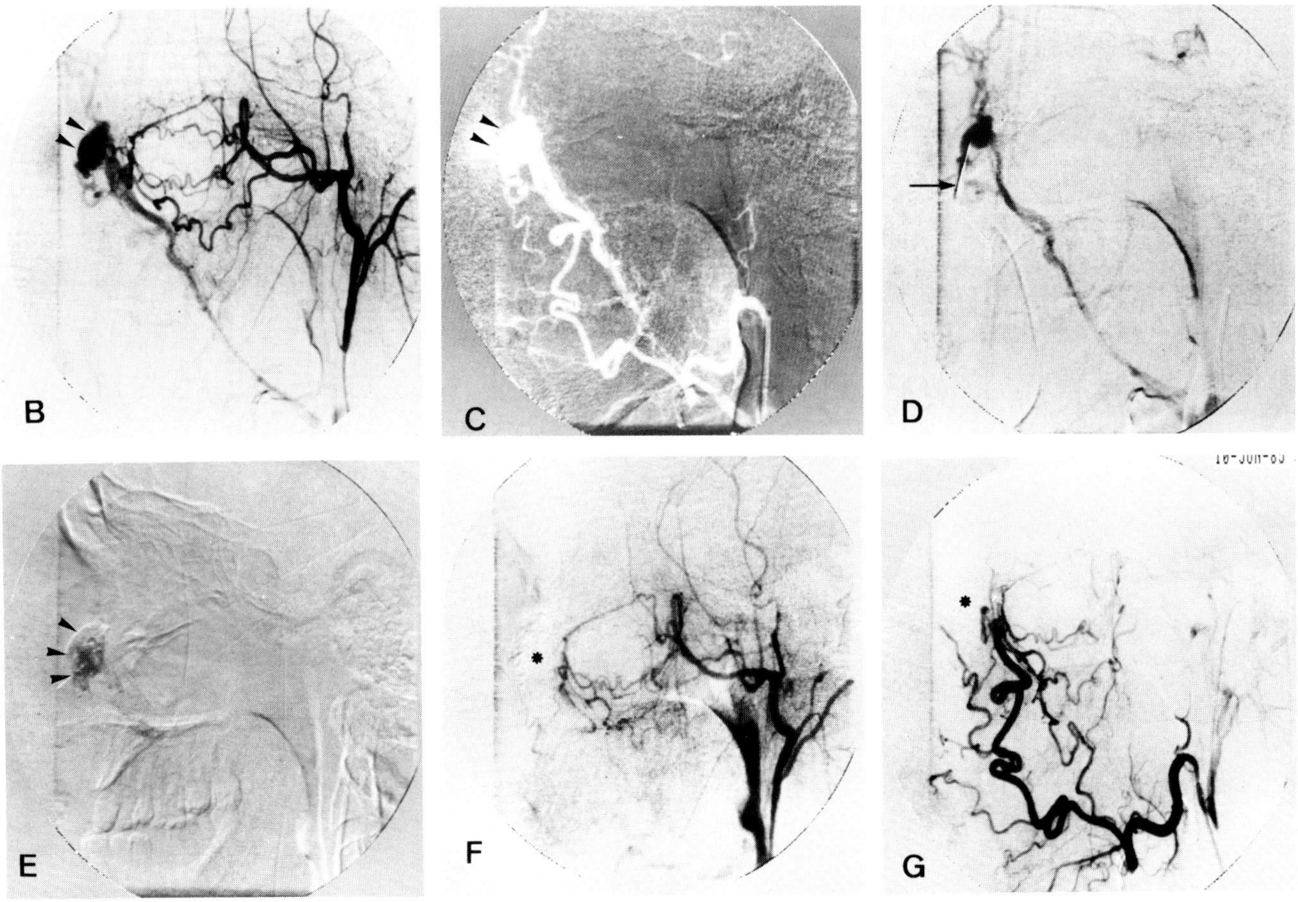

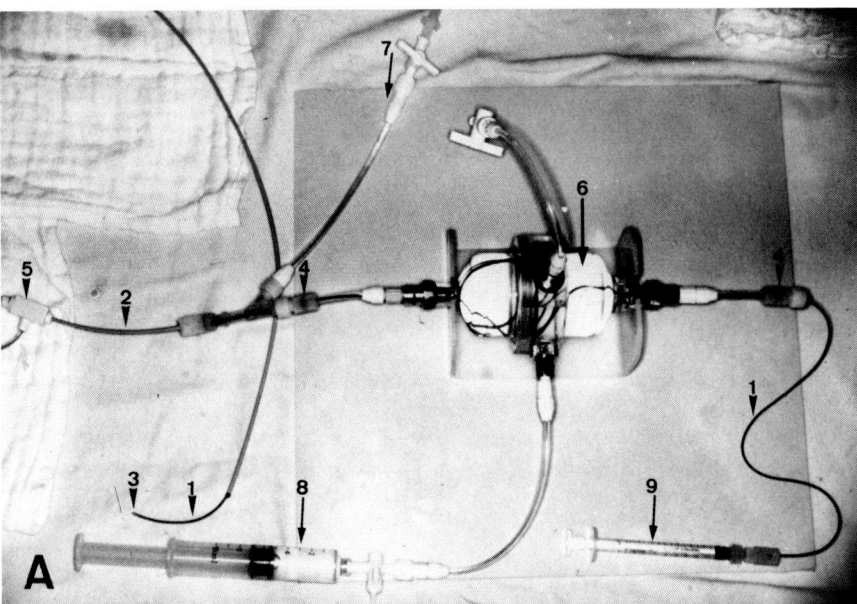
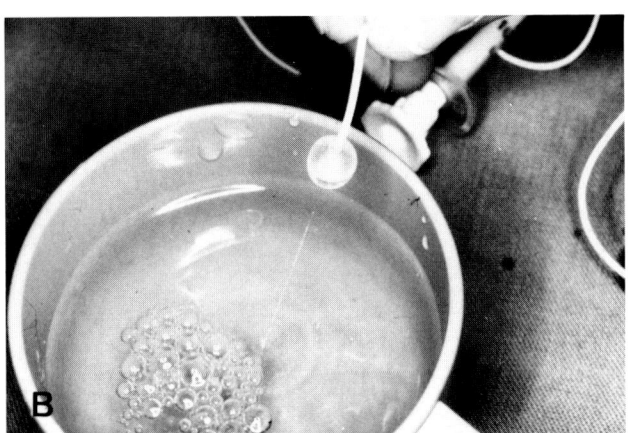

Figure 4.100 (A) Propulsion chamber. 1, microcatheter; 2, No. 6 French catheter; 3, perforated latex balloon; 4, antireflux valves; 5, arterial introducer, 6, hydraulic reservoir; 7, coaxial system perfusion; 8, hydraulic pressure route; 9, contrast medium or fluid embolus part. (B) Injection through partially distended calibrated leaking balloon, showing material leaving through the distal hole.

Vascular Lesions of the Face and Neck

The number of indications for endovascular therapy has grown in the last few years because of several factors: the increasing sophistication of hyperselective catheterization techniques, the utilization of digital or photographic subtraction, a better understanding of vascular anatomy, and the formation of specialized teams. Hyperselective angiography, in addition to providing a better topographic image of the lesion and defining its uni- or pluricompartmental character, also allows the visualization of any dangerous anastomoses present between the internal and external carotid branches or between the ophthalmic and internal maxillary arteries. This avoids many complications previously associated with the procedure. Embolization performed on the basis of hyperselective catheterization is also more effective in taking the embolus inside the lesion, thus avoiding embolization of adjacent territories.

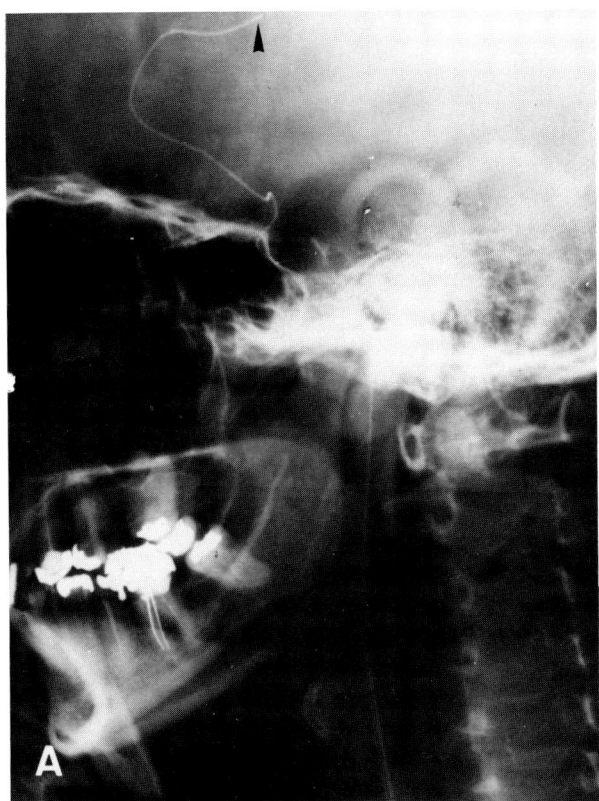
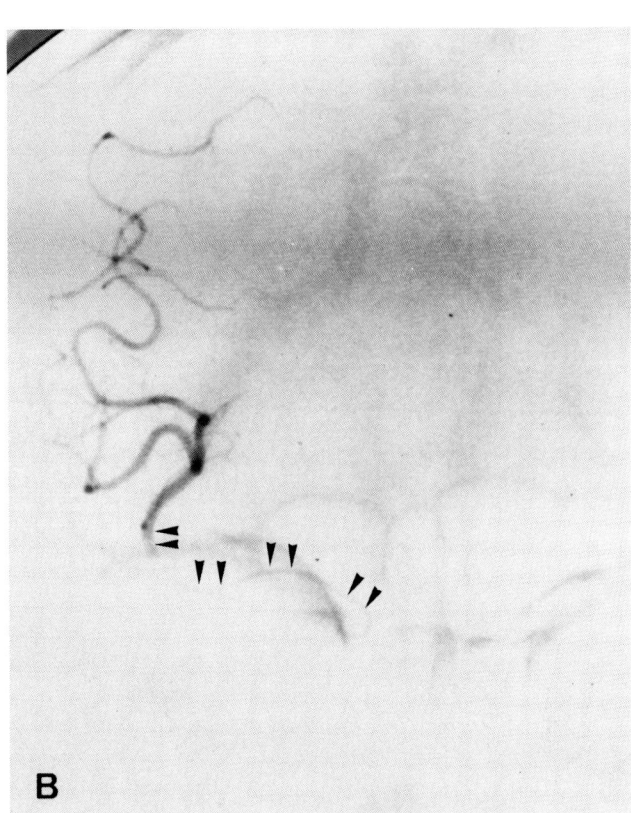

Figure 4.101 (A) Balloon microcatheter positioned in the pericallosal artery (arrowhead). (B) Superselective injection into the middle cerebral artery branch, anteroposterior view (arrowheads).

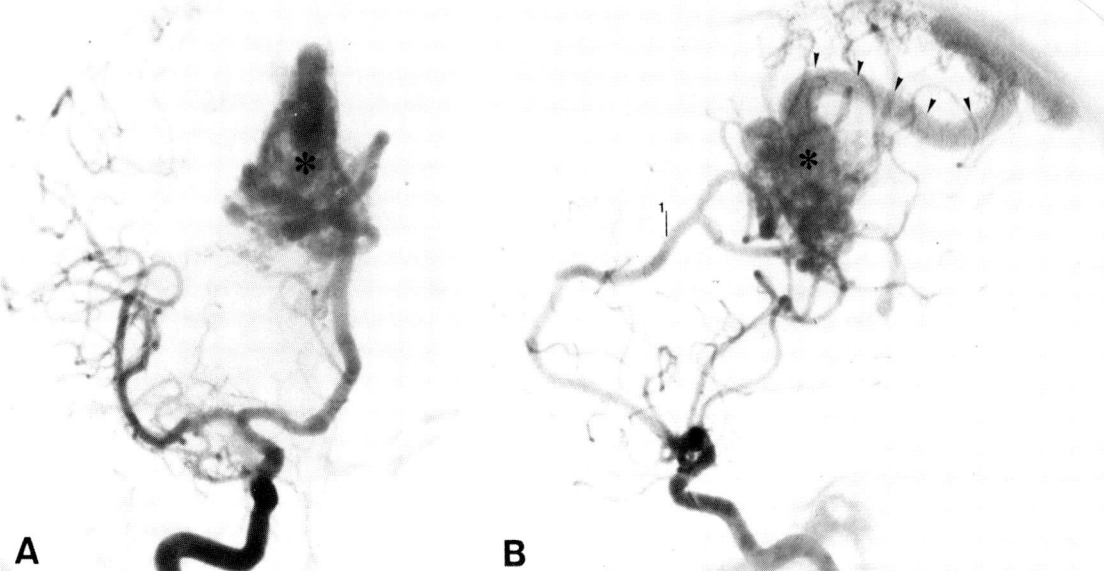

Figure 4.102 Deep right parasaggital parietal intracerebral arteriovenous angioma. Embolization resulted in total symptom recovery.

(A,B) Internal carotid arteriograms, anteroposterior and lateral views, respectively. The lesion is fed by two branches of the pericallosal artery (1). The angiomatous nidus is indicated by an asterisk (*). Drainage veins (arrowheads) appeared very early. (C,D,E) Superselective catheterization with balloon microcatheter (arrow) of upper and lower pedicles. (F) Plain skull x-ray following embolization with isobutyl plus Lipiodol plus powder tantalum. Embolizing material is present inside the feeding arteries and the angiomatous nidus. (G,H) Early and later-phase internal carotid arteriograms, lateral view. Occlusion of the angiomatous mass has been practically total. The drainage vein is less intensively opacified than it was before embolization [Compare to (B)].

Figure 4.102 *Continued*

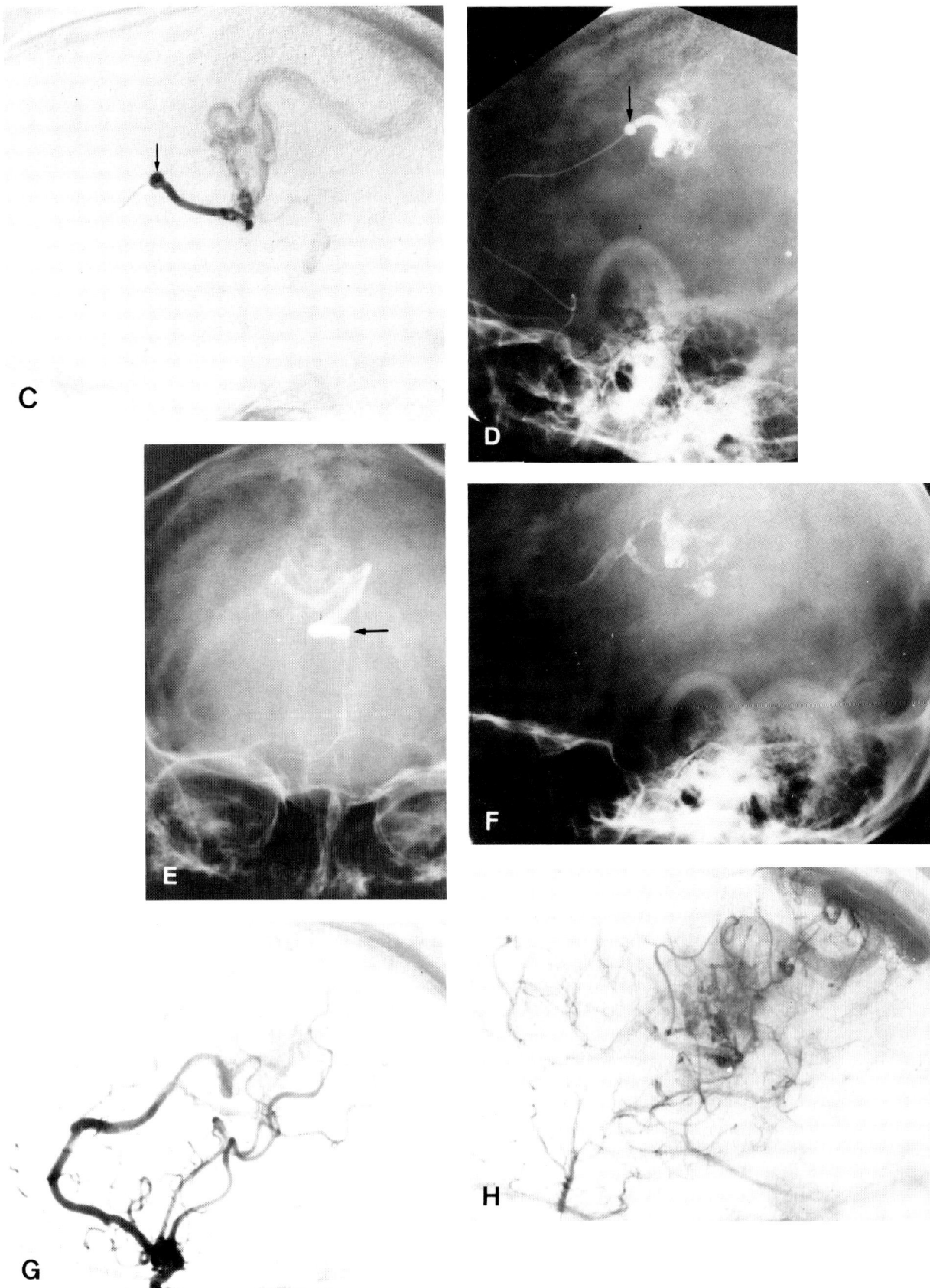

Table 4.4 – Classification of craniofacial vascular lesions

Malformations
   Arterial with or without fistula
   Capillary
   Venous-capillary
   Venous

Vascular tumors
   Hemangiomas
      Capillary (in children)
      Cavernous (in adults)
   Hemangiopericytoma
   Hemangioendothelioma
   Kaposi's syndrome

Lymphangiomas

Hemolymphangiomas

Table 4.5 – Complex vascular lesions of the head and neck

Multifocal arteriovenous malformations

Multiple ectasias

Arteriovenous malformation and ectasia associations

Angiodysplastic syndromes:
   Sturge-Weber (metameric)
   Rendu-Osler-Weber (systemic)
   Wiburn-Mason (functional)
   Recklinghausen
   Ehlers-Danlos
   Fibromuscular dysplasia

The classification of vascular lesions has been extensively discussed in a previous section. Tables 4.4 and 4.5 present a practical classification of vascular lesions of the face and neck based on the clinical behavior of these lesions.

Vascular Tumors

The most effective nonsurgical methods for treating vascular tumors are corticotherapy and embolization. At the beginning of therapy, corticosteroids are generally used, although these are not always effective and may not be well tolerated. In the case of childhood hemangiomas, most of which regress without leaving sequelae, treatment is conservative unless complications are present. This is often difficult for the patient's family to accept, especially in cases involving disfigurement.

With certain forms of lesion, active therapy is necessary, sometimes on an emergency basis (Table 4.6).

Tumors occluding the eyelid, for example, may lead to blindness within 7 to 10 days if left untreated (Fig. 4.103). Other situations which require immediate treatment are hemorrhage (Figs. 4.104 and 4.105), heart failure (Fig. 4.75), and coagulopathy (Kasabach-Merrit syndrome) (Fig. 4.76). Because these are benign, spontaneously regressing lesions, in most cases embolization should be the first aggressive treatment of choice. Surgery is indicated for lesions that are either inaccessible or only partially accessible to embolization techniques. Embolization should, however, be performed whenever possible as a preoperative measure (Fig. 4.103).

Cavernous adult hemangiomas do not usually regress, their histologic behavior and etiology being different from the infantile form of hemangioma. On the angiogram, avascular masses may be encountered, and the angiogram may be negative or show only a slight blush or filling of venous vascular spaces.

Vascular Malformations

The evolution of vascular malformations depends on the nature of the vessels involved and on the hemodynamic secondary effects. These lesions may produce minimal aesthetic problems, or may cause significant deformities, with or without functional change (swallowing, breathing, eyesight, mastication) or maxillofacial growth dysfunction. Bleeding, pain, ulceration, bruits, glaucoma, heart failure, and thrombophlebitis may be present. The following factors may reveal, or may complicate, a venous arterial malformation by promoting hemorrhage: direct trauma (oral hygiene, eating, shaving, biopsy-caused iatrogenesis, surgery, tooth extraction, oral prosthesis),

Table 4.6 – Indications for treatment of vascular lesions in children

Cases Requiring Emergency Treatment
   Hemorrhage
   Respiratory obstruction (subglottic tumors)
   Occular occlusion
   Heart failure (overload)
   Cerebral complications
   Coagulopathy (thrombocytopenic purpura; Kasabach-Merrit Syndrome)
   Traumatic lesions

Urgent Cases
   Facial skeletal function or development loss
   Interference with nutrition (oral tumors)
   Potential cerebral complications
   Chronic bleeding

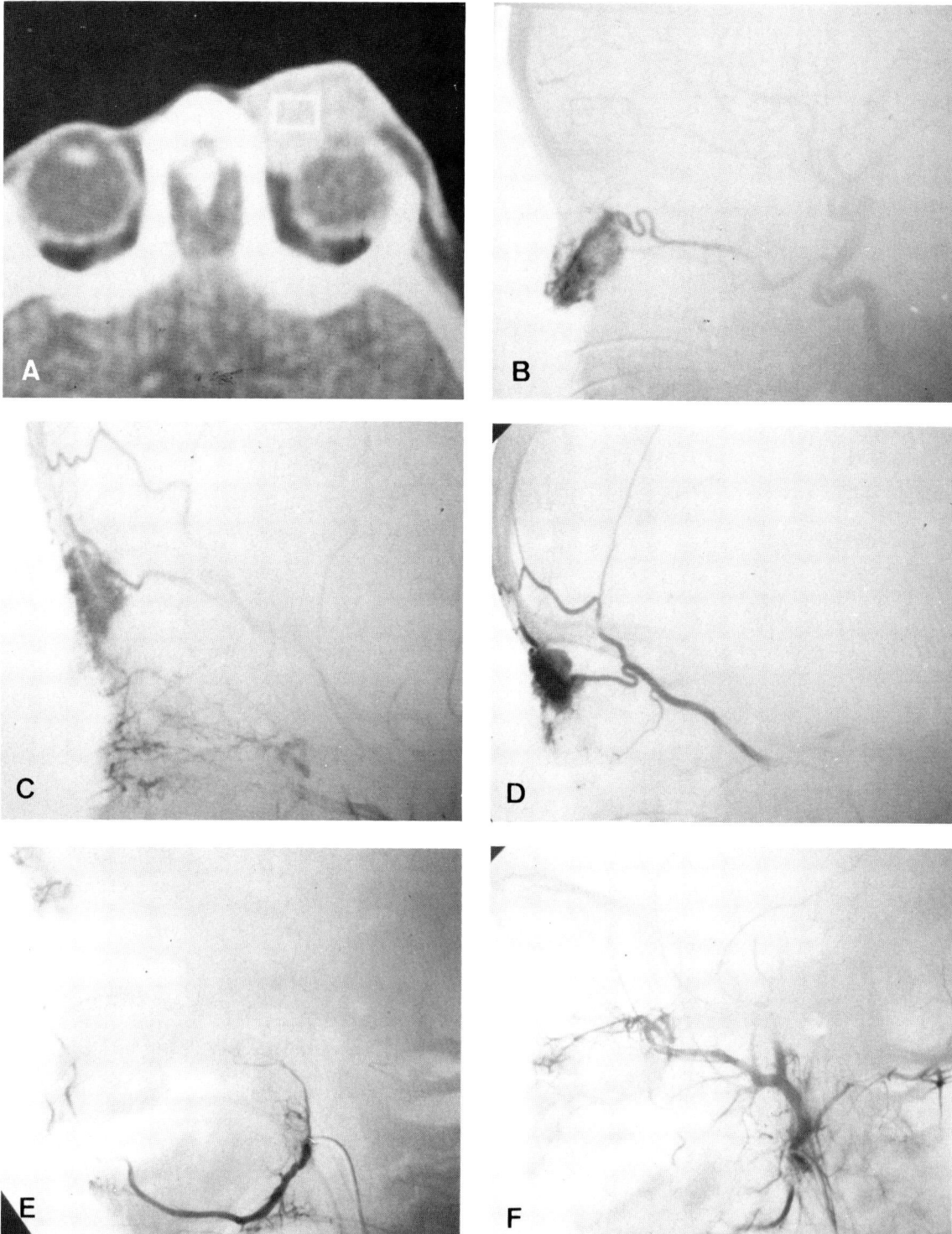

Figure 4.103 2½-year-old girl with vascular lesion on the eyelid. The lesion was first seen a few days after birth and was progressively increasing in volume until treatment with corticoids. Corticosteroids produced moderate volume regression after 3 days. At that point, treatment did not promote further regression. The left eye was partially occluded.

(A) Computed tomography shows the location of the lesion; there is no retrooccular involvement. (B) Injection into the left internal carotid artery showing enlarged ophthalmic artery and lesion vascularization by the superior palpebral artery, a branch of the ophthalmic artery. The lesion is of the arteriolar type, with significant homogeneous impregnation, and is still evolving. (C) View of the superficial temporal artery with lesion vascularization from the superior palpebral branches. The artery was embolized with 160-μm Ivalon.

(D) Control angiogram 2 years after (C). The superficial temporal artery still irrigates the lesion. New embolization was performed with 160-μm Ivalon. (E) Control of the facial artery showing its moderate participation in the malformation. This artery was also embolized with Ivalon. (F) Control of the external carotid, showing that the lesion is no longer opacified. The patient has been operated on due to vascularization by ophthalmic artery branches inaccessible to embolization.

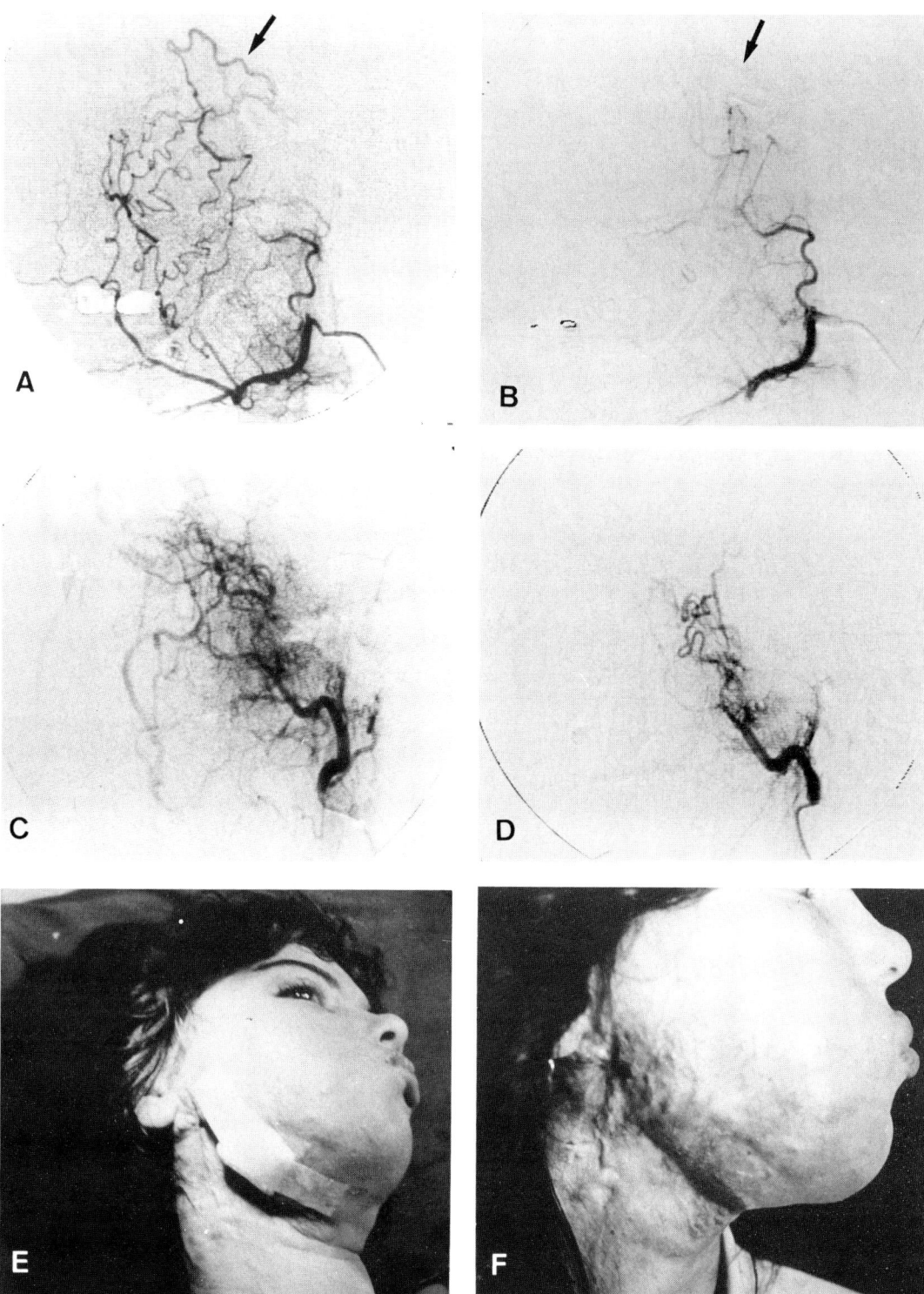

Figure 4.104 Partially regressed right hemangioma in 18-year-old patient bleeding from ulceration of the lesion. The lesion caused amblyopia during childhood due to right eye occlusion, and the patient does not have vision in the right eye. The external carotid artery was surgically ligated 1 year earlier.

(A) Injection into the left facial artery showing anastomoses with contralateral lesion, and possible anastomosis with the ophthalmic artery (arrow). (B) Control following embolization with Gelfoam and Lipiodol showing occlusion of the vascularization of the lesion. Partial ophthalmic opacification still persists (arrow). (C) Injection into the proximal internal maxillary artery showing the hemangioma only partially. (D) Postembolization control showing complete devascularization of the lesion from that artery. (E) The patient before embolization; the hemorrhagic ulceration is partially covered by dressing. (F) Aspect 1 month following embolization showing ulcer healing with bleeding under control. The lesion volume was moderately reduced. A visual field deficit occurred on the left, probably related to ophthalmic artery embolization, but this receded after 4 weeks.

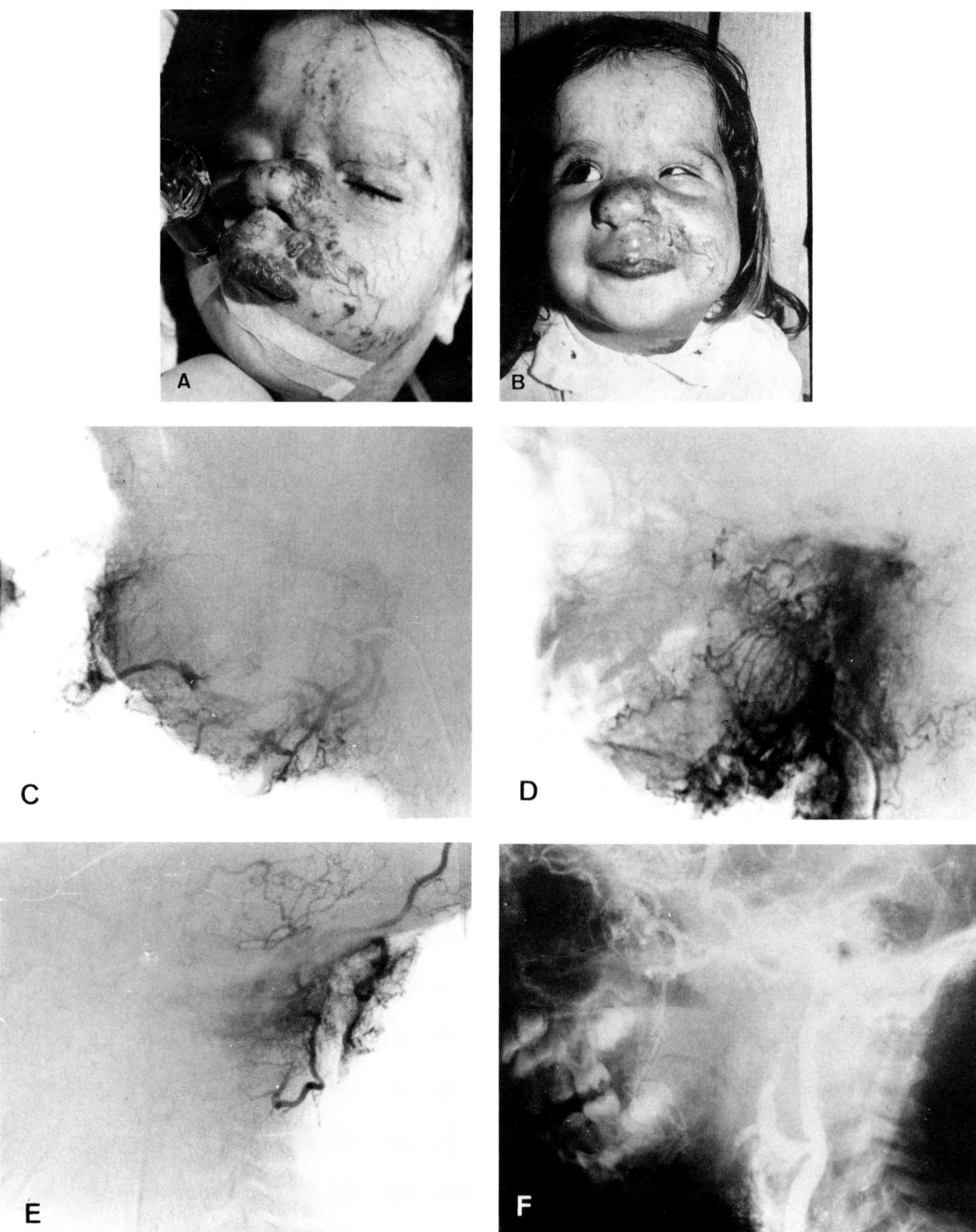

Figure 4.105 (A) 3-year-old girl with hemangioma involving the face, cervical region, body, and left upper limb. The lesion exhibited rapid growth despite treatment with corticosteroids. Embolization was performed to correct uncontrollable left orbital bleeding that occurred upon mild effort. (B) Control 2 months after embolization showing moderate reduction of mass effect, and reepithelialization of several facial and labial lesions. Orbital bleeding was permanently controlled. (C) Injection into left facial artery showing abnormal circulation on the left cheek, lips, nose, and orbital floor. (D) Injection into proximal internal maxillary artery showing lesions of the oropharyngeal and mental lesions. (E) Injection into the occipital artery showing lesion of the left retroauricular and occipital region. (F) Control following embolization with Gelfoam showing occlusion of the left external carotid arterial branches. The left ophthalmic artery is also enlarged.

local infection, tooth exchange during infancy, hormones (e.g., oral contraceptives), stress, arterial and/or venous hypertension, and exposure to sunshine.

Pretherapeutic angiography study will determine the exact location of the lesion, the type and output of the vessels involved, the presence or absence of fistulas, and the aspect of the nidus. All these must be taken into account in deciding upon the therapeutic regimen to be followed, including the type of embolic material to be utilized.

Treatment

In the absence of complications, treatment in childhood should be conservative. Better results are obtained by reconstruction after complete development of the maxillofacial complex.

One should not try to excise maxillofacial vascular malformations unless total excision is feasible. Embolization in these cases is a preoperative procedure, reducing bleeding and mass effect and making it easier to extirpate these lesions. The best results are obtained when surgery is performed 2 to 3 days following embolization (Figs. 4.106 and 4.107).

In some cases, partial (Fig. 4.108) or total (Fig. 4.106) embolization, either as the sole therapeutic option or in conjunction with others, can be used successfully to treat symptoms (Figs. 4.109, 4.110, and 4.112). In such cases, embolization should be performed before surgery is resorted to. Surgical procedures alone cannot identify anatomic variations, and blind vessel ligation may cause a proximal occlusion, leading to immediate development of collateral circulation, which will prevent satisfactory endovascular procedures from being performed subsequently (Fig. 4.113). In addition to producing good immediate results, embolization does not aggravate the lesion, and so does not preclude other therapeutic procedures including reembolization.

Other significant benefits from embolization include a reduction of pain, either of vascular origin or due to mass effect (Figs. 4.111 and 4.114). Embolization may also be beneficial in terms of mass-effect phenomena such as difficulties in respiration or swallowing, cosmetic problems or deformities (Fig. 4.111), bone growth dysfunctions, ocular occlusion, and bruits (Fig. 4.114), which in some cases may be so severe that the patient is not able to lead a normal life.

The material to be used in embolization depends on the type of vessels involved. When high-output lesions are present, with direct arteriovenous fistulas, isobutyl-2-cyanoacrylate (IBC) is generally used. In medium- to low-flow lesions, Ivalon is presently being utilized, and this should be slowly and progressively injected. Superselective catheterization makes it possible to more

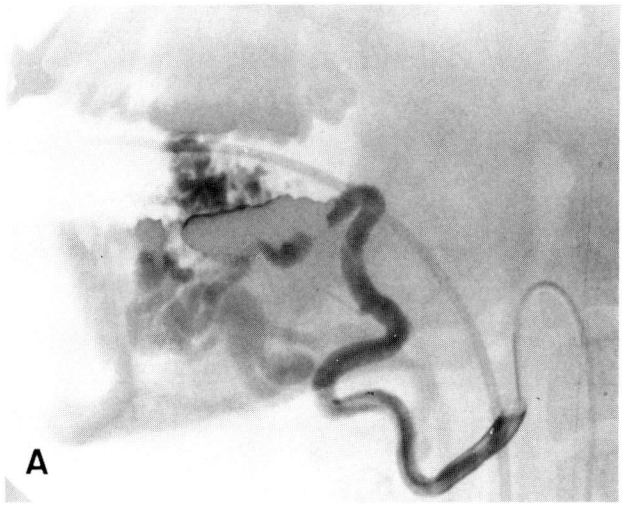

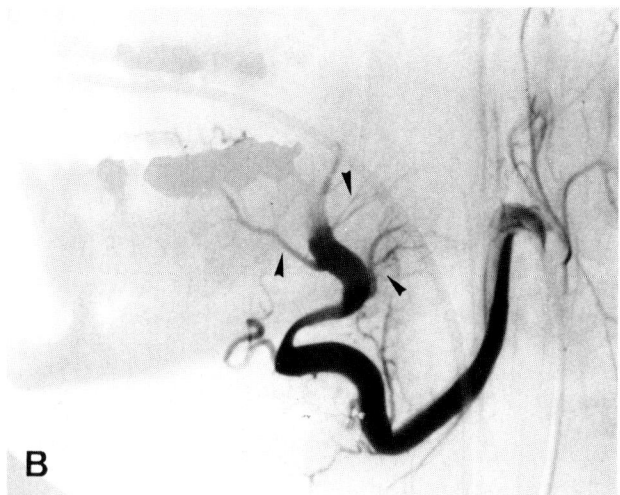

Figure 4.106 30-year-old man with arteriovenous malformation on the base of the tongue. Several hemorrhage episodes were recorded due to trauma while eating. Embolization is preoperative.
(A) Injection into the lingual artery, showing the high-output arteriovenous malformation. (B) Immediate postembolization control showing preservation of normal muscular branches (arrowheads), and occlusion of lesion nidus only. The embolization was performed with Ivalon powder and Gelfoam. The patient was operated on 2 days following the procedure; the lesion was completely excised, without bleeding.

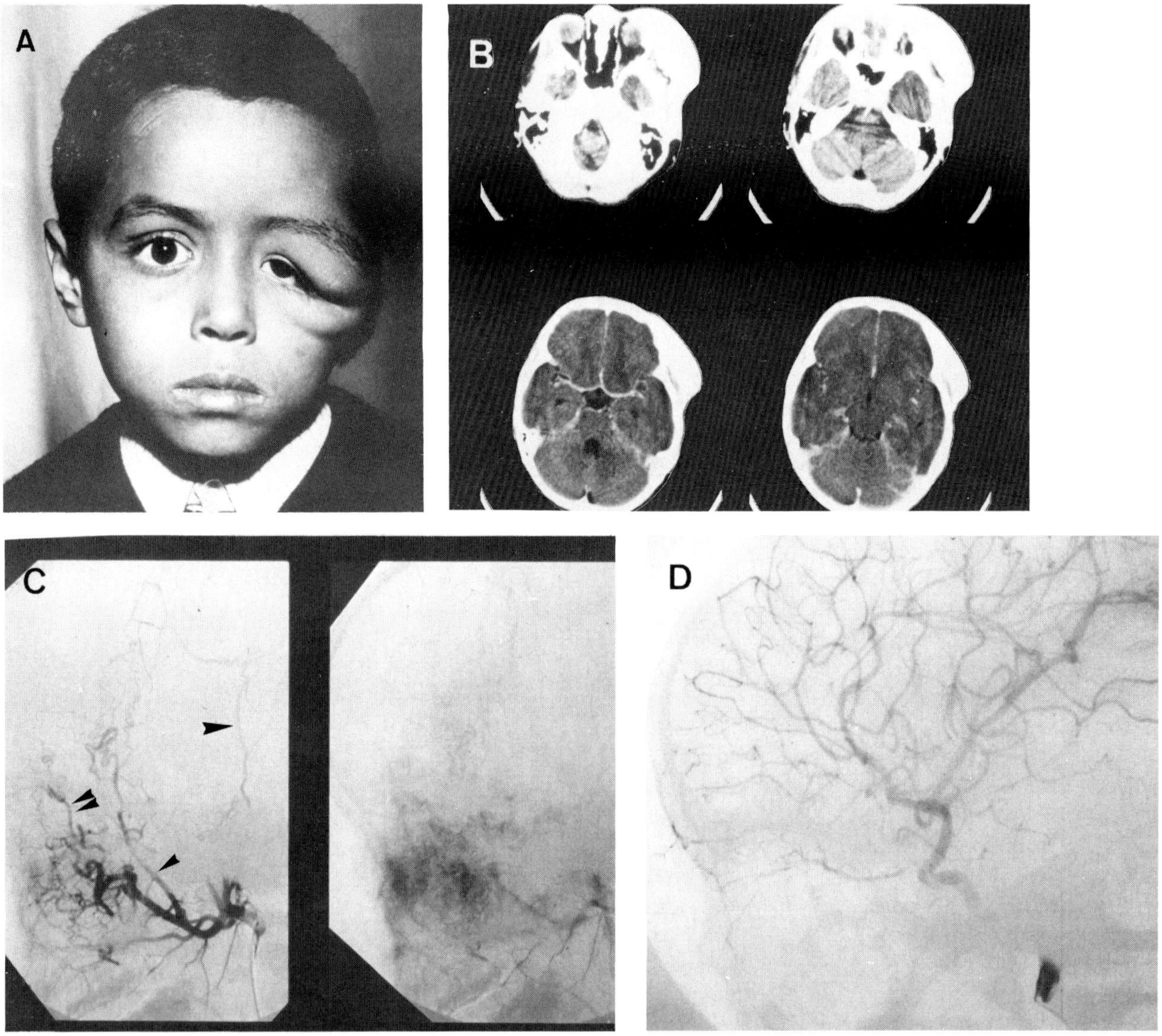

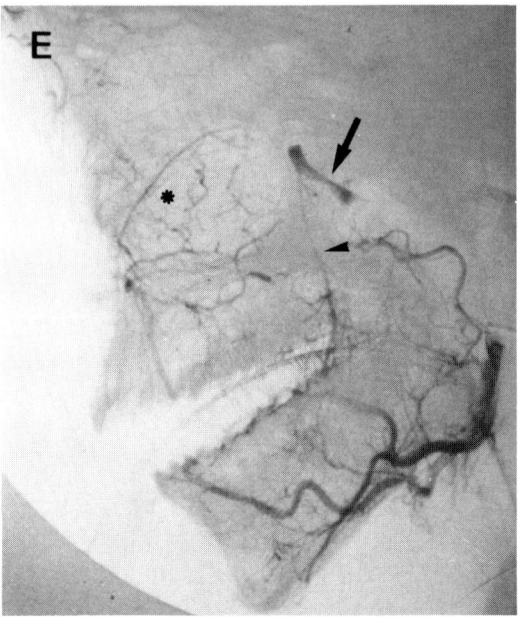

Figure 4.107 (A) 11-year-old boy with a facial deformity on the left temporal region and on the eyelids. The lesion was evident at birth, and volume increased after 2 years of age. He was operated on at that time, but the lesion recurred. The embolization procedure described here is preoperative. (B) Computed tomography showing extension of the lesion internally to the bone plate. (C) Arterial and later-phase injections into the proximal internal maxillary artery, showing the hypoplastic superficial temporal artery (large arrowhead), with vascularization coming from the middle deep temporal (small arrowhead) and anterior (double arrowhead) arteries. The malformation is of capillary type, without arteriovenous shunt. Peripheral embolization was performed with 160-μm Ivalon, and truncal embolization with Gelfoam particles. (D) Postembolization control with injection into the internal carotid artery showing no vascularization from ophthalmic anastomoses [anterior deep temporalis branches], confirming that embolization has been distal to the lesion nidus. (E) Injection into the facial artery showing opacification of the internal maxillary (*) artery branches, and of the middle third (arrow) of the facial artery through the buccal artery (arrowhead). (Courtesy Dr. P. Lasjaunias.)

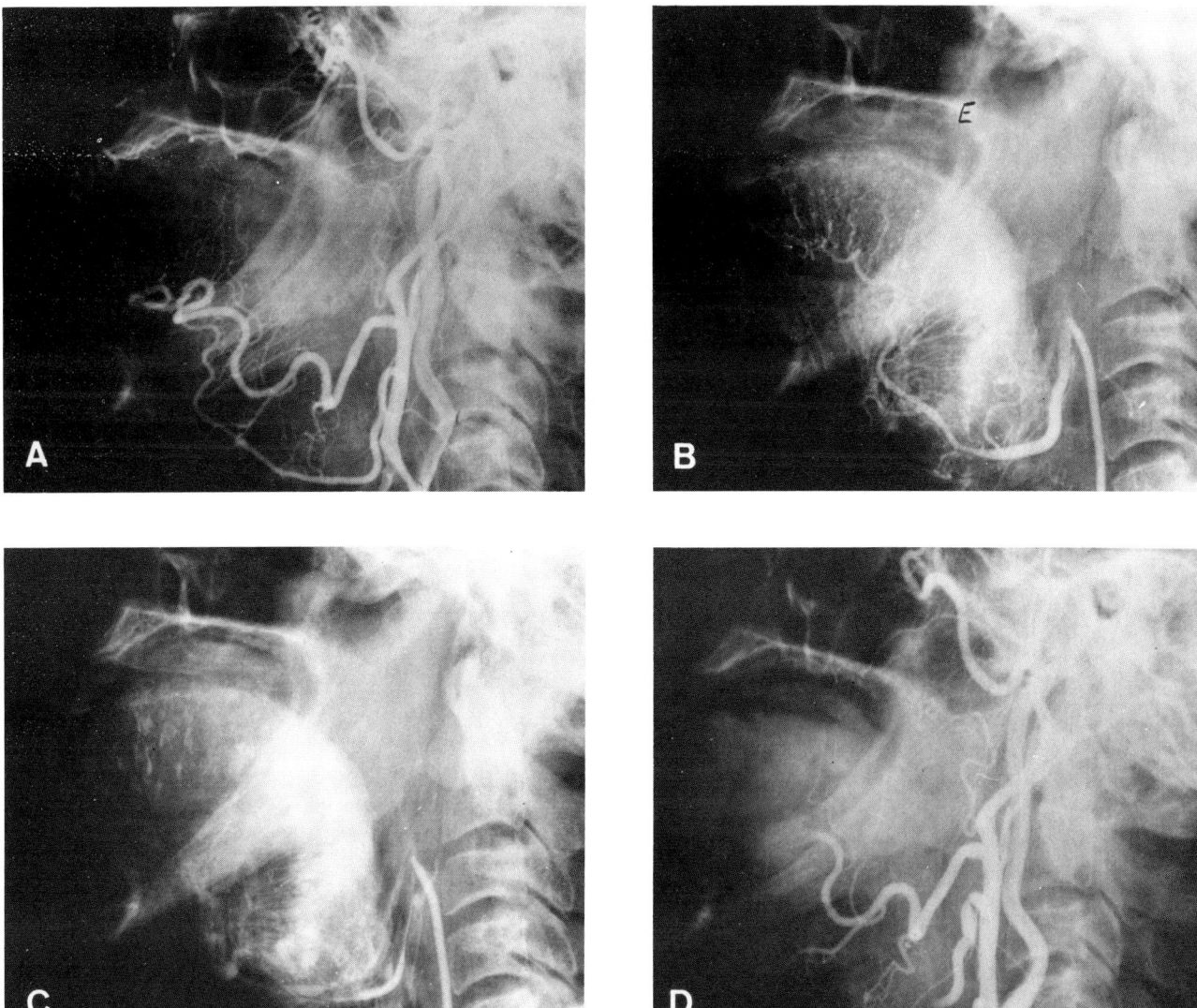

Figure 4.108 58-year-old man with large arteriovenous malformation involving the whole tongue and part of the left cheek. There have been repeated bleeding episodes due to trauma while eating or during oral hygiene. The embolization was performed using Gelfoam.

(A) Injection into the left external carotid; abundant lesion vascularization is not evident. (B) Selective injection into the lingual artery showing diffuse, large-volume malformation. (C) Later phase showing impregnation of arteriovenous malformation in the tongue. (D) Control following embolization showing lingual and left facial artery occlusion. (E) Selective injection into the right lingual artery showing significant tongue hypervascularity. (F) Later phase showing dense impregnation of the whole tongue, with areas of contrast collection. (G) Control following right lingual artery embolization showing devascularization of the whole tongue. Follow-up has shown volume reduction in some areas of the tongue; bleeding has been under permanent control for 4 years.

Figure 4.108 *Continued*

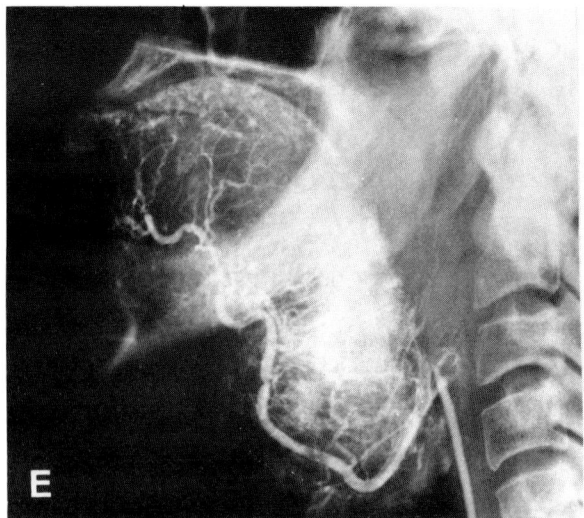
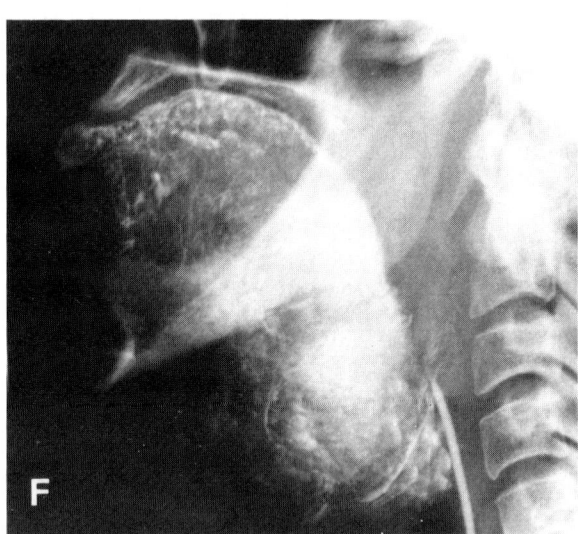
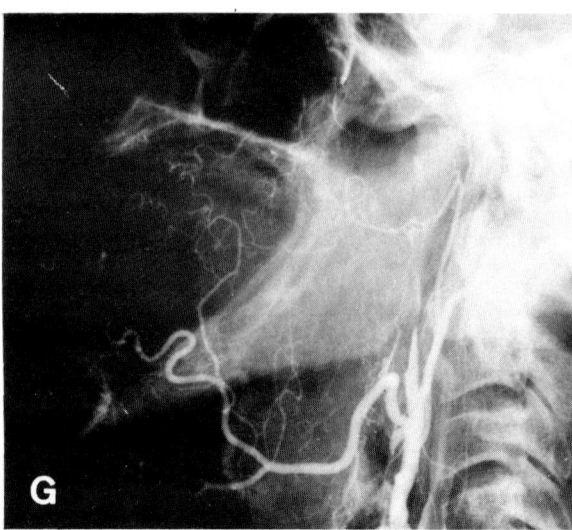
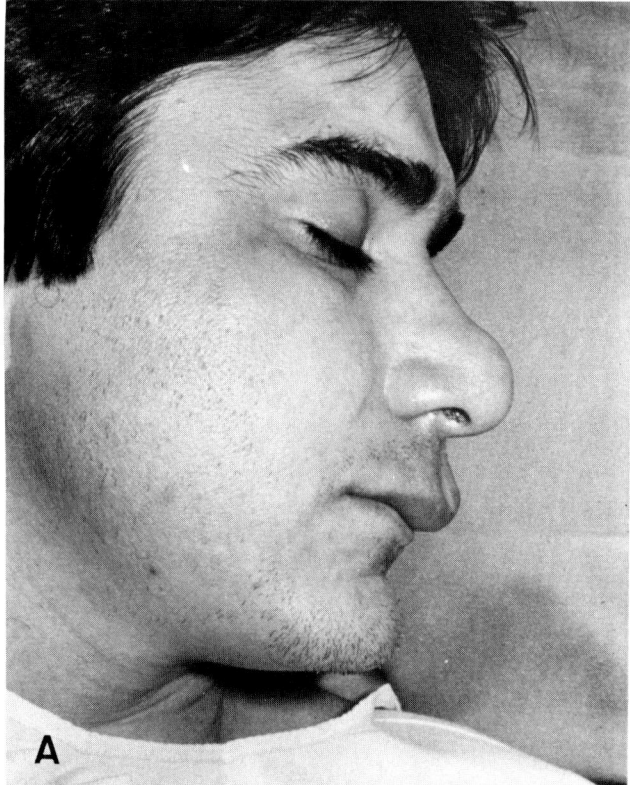

Figure 4.109 (A) 35-year-old patient with arteriovenous malformation of the upper lip (childhood) and nose (post-childhood) who presented with accelerated growth (during the previous 6 months) and bruit. The treatment objectives were to minimize the bruit and the mass effect. It was considered that surgery would result in unacceptable deformity. (B) Injection into the left distal external carotid artery showing anastomoses with the upper labial territory from the distal internal maxillary artery. (C) Control following embolization with Gelfoam particles soaked in Lipiodol. (D) Injection into the left facial artery showing two pedicles to the upper lip originating from this artery (arrows). (E) Control following embolization of the left facial artery. (F) Injection into the right internal maxillary artery vascularizing the upper lip. (G) Control following embolization of the distal branches of the right internal maxillary artery. (H) Injection into the right facial artery producing upper lip and nasal tip vascularization. (I) Control following embolization of the facial artery showing distal branch occlusion in the lesion.

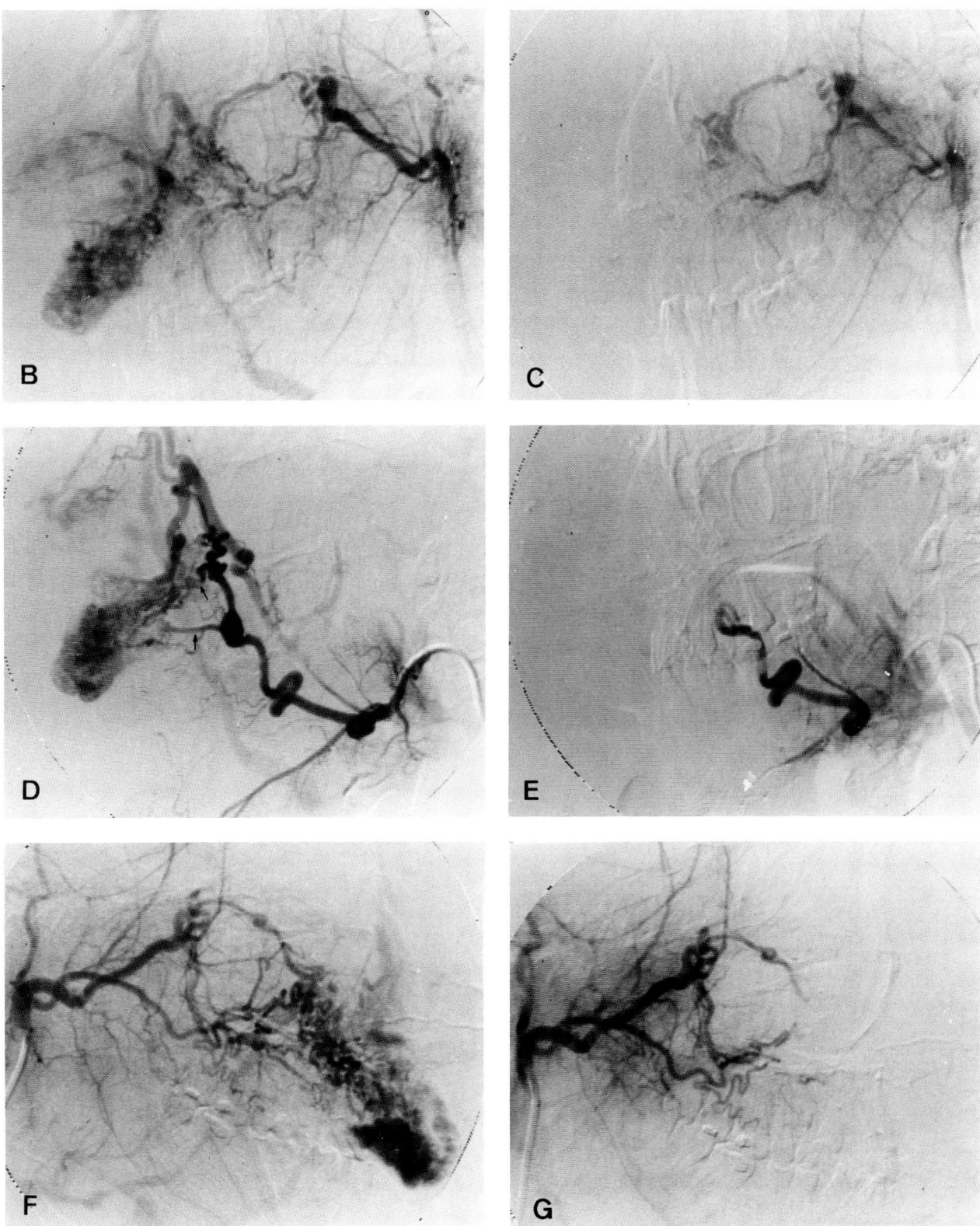

Figure 4.109 *Continued*

Figure 4.109 *Continued*

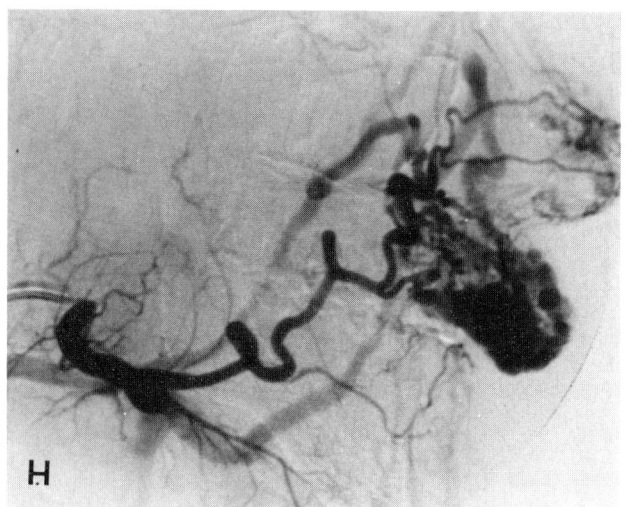
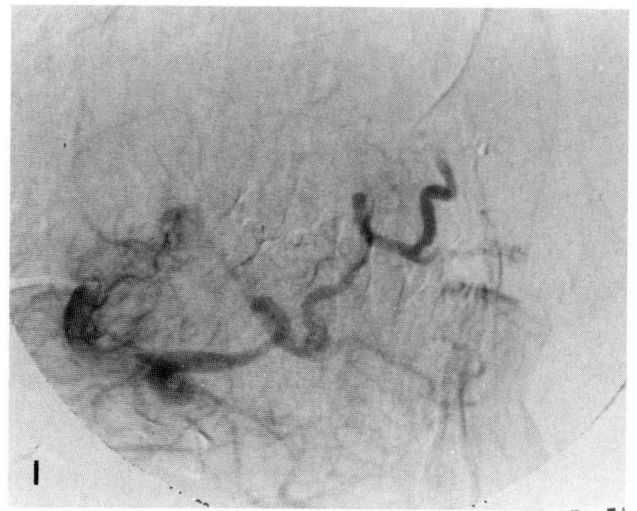

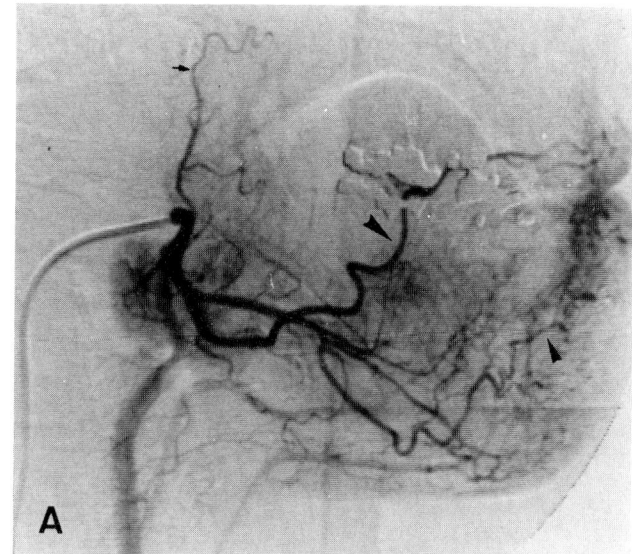

Figure 4.110 40-year-old patient with lower lip malformation, present since childhood, who presented with bruit. There had been slight growth during the previous year. Embolization was performed with Gelfoam soaked in Lipiodol.

(A) Posterior jugal variant of the facial artery (large arrowhead). The supply to the lower lip and to the arteriovenous malformation comes from mental branches (small arrowhead). Notice the origin of the facial artery in the soft palate (arrowheads). (B) The axis of the main facial artery was preserved after embolization (arrowhead). (C) Faciolingual common axis, with hypoplastic facial artery ending at the lower lip artery (small arrowhead). Lingual artery (large arrowhead), with lower flow than the facial artery due to the presence of the malformation. (D) Control after embolization showing distal occlusion of the facial artery (small arrowhead), with total preservation of the lingual artery (large arrowhead). (E) Radiopaque emboli inside the malformation (arrow).

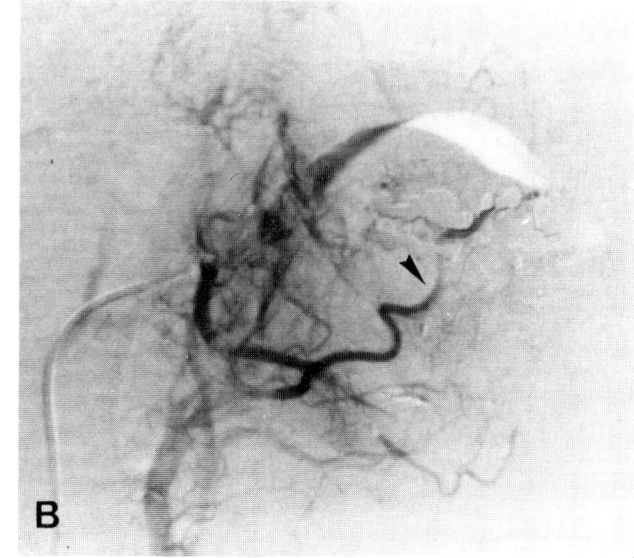

Figure 4.110 *Continued*

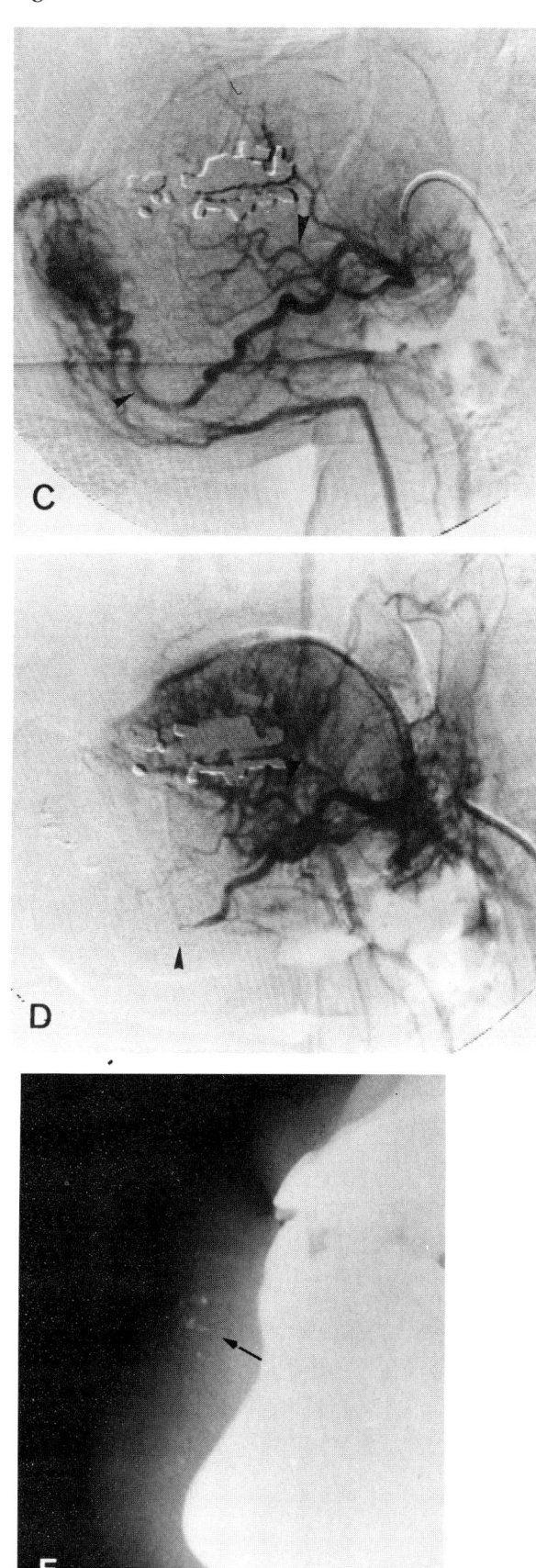

Figure 4.111 31-year-old patient with facial malformation that has been growing since adolescence, with alternating periods of volume increase and reduction. Embolization is to be performed for cosmetic purposes.

(A) Preembolization aspect. (B) Patient about 1 month after embolization. (C) Hypoplastic right facial artery; the soft palate artery is indicated by an asterisk (*). Malformation of the floor of the mouth, with extension to the lower lip, is evident. (D) Irregular impregnation of the lesion with cavities. (E) Control following embolization showing facial artery occlusion. The soft palate (ascending palatine) artery is indicated with an asterisk (*). (F) Right lingual artery showing extension of the lesion to the tongue. (G) Same irregular aspect, but seen on later-phase image. (H) Control following embolization showing preservation of the mental branch (asterisk). (I) Injection into the left facial artery showing the farthest posterior part of the lesion (submandibular gland). (J) Later-phase facial injection. (K) Control following left facial artery embolization. Injection at the left lingual artery shows tongue lesion on the left side. (M) Later phase showing irregular impregnation of the tongue. (N) Control following embolization showing complete occlusion of the lingual artery. Some improvement in lesion size occurred at medium term. The picture in (B), 1 month later, shows a certain volume decrease. An angiogram performed about 1 year after embolization showed little recanalization of embolized vessels.

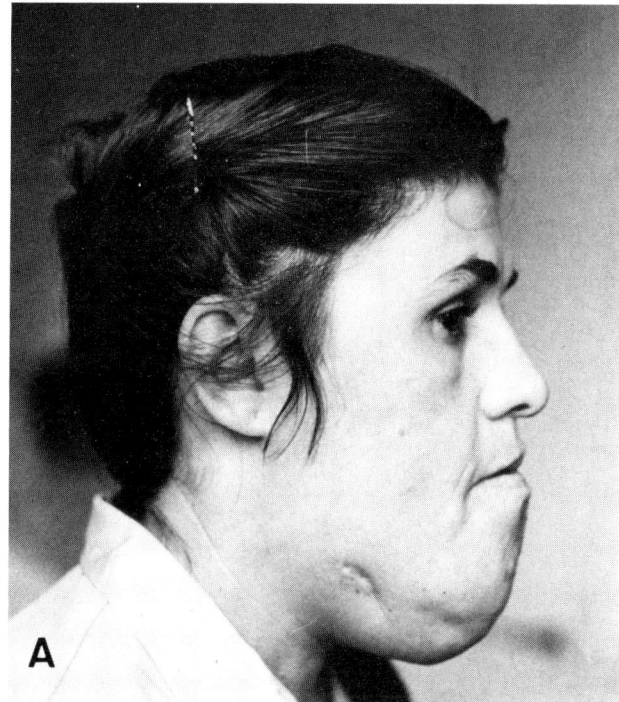

Figure 4.111 *Continued*

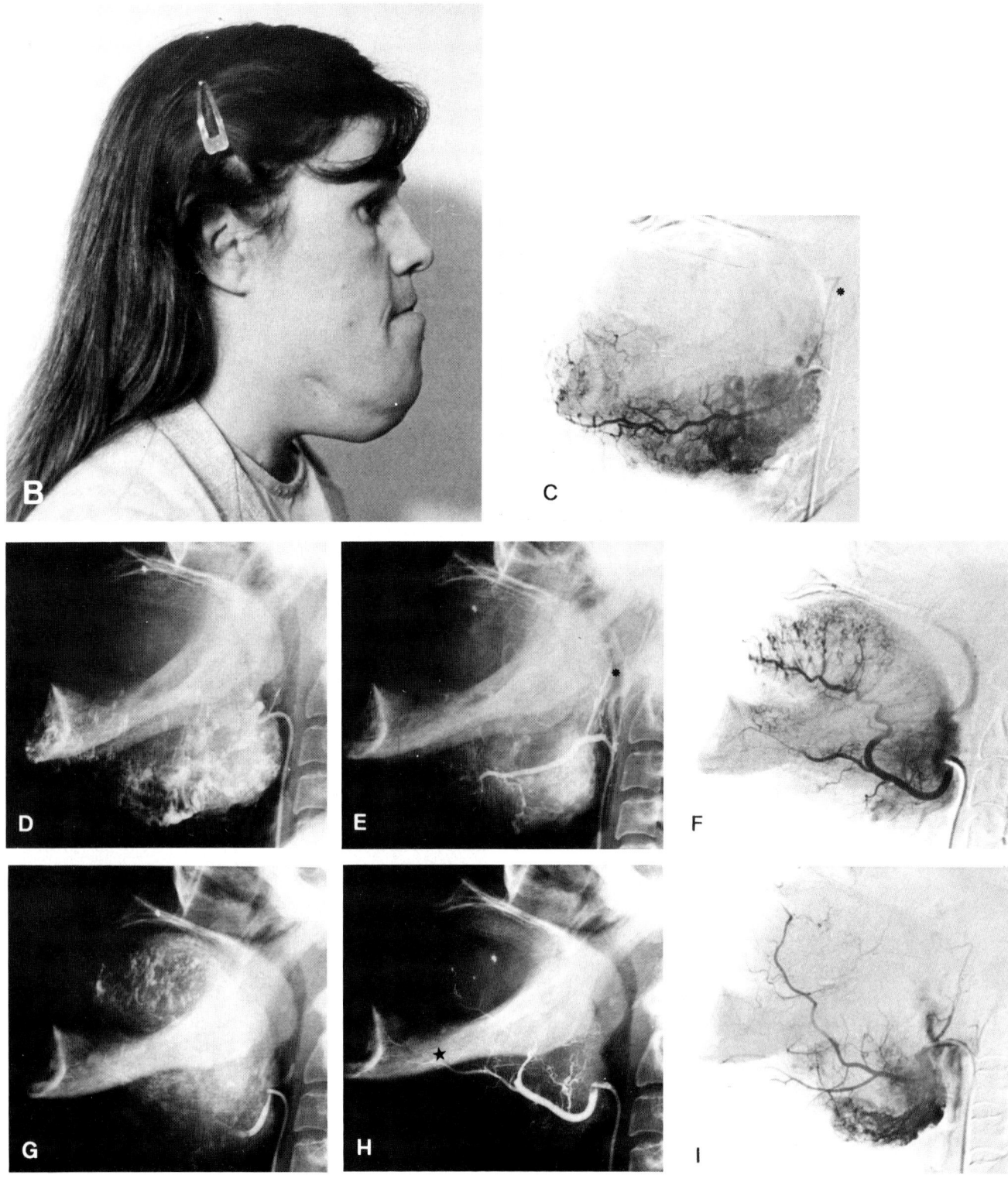

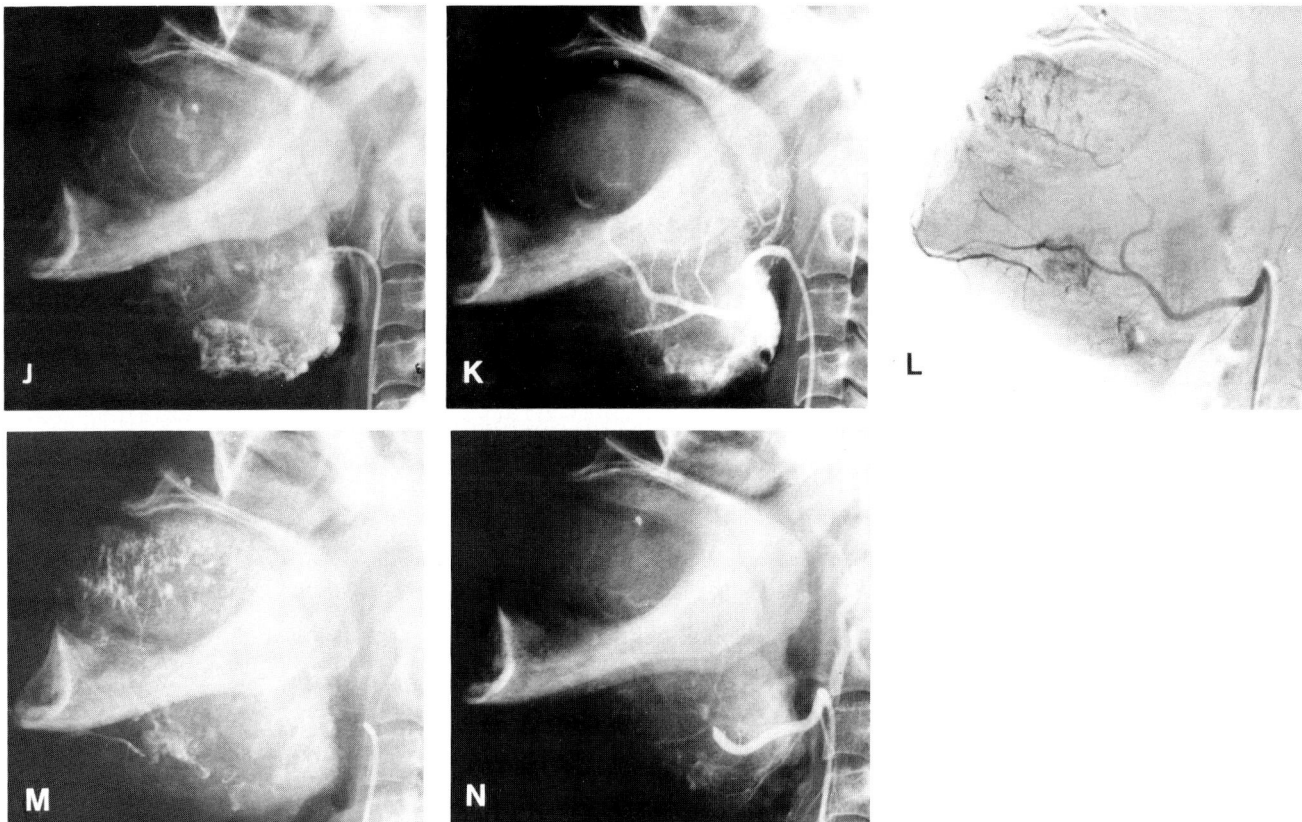

Figure 4.111 *Continued*

Figure 4.112 **Sublingual hemangioma in 3-month-old boy who presented with massive bleeding, shock, and respiratory obstruction.**
(A,B) Injection into left lingual artery showing angiomatous lesion of the tongue and base of the tongue. (C) Control following lingual artery embolization showing occlusion of the same artery and reflux into the internal carotid.
(D) Injection into the external carotid artery showing patency of the other arteries, with contrast stagnated in the lingual artery (arrow head). (E) Notice the lesion on the base of the tongue, and the bruises on the face caused by bleeding.

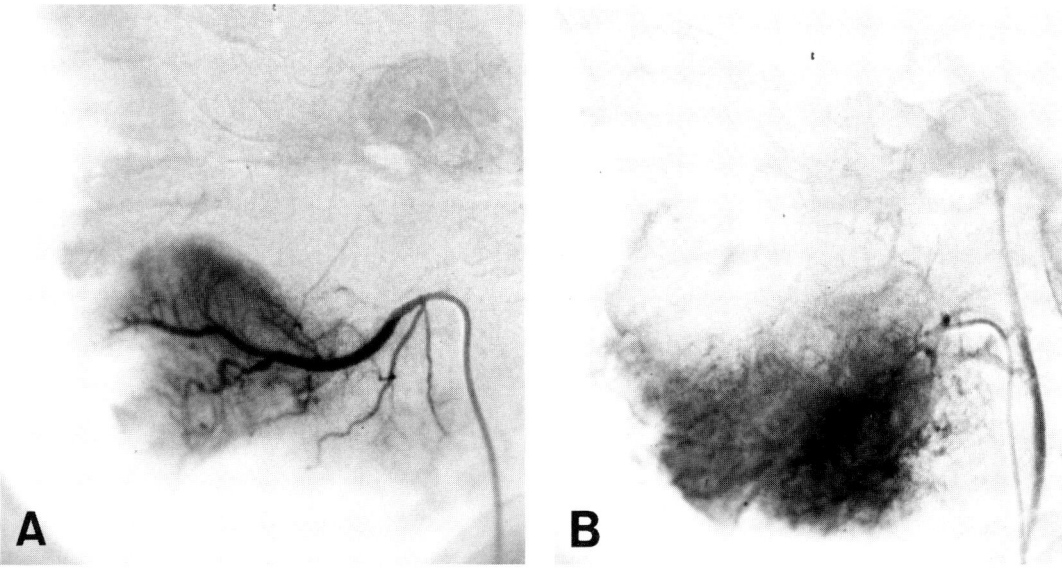

Figure 4.112 *Continued*

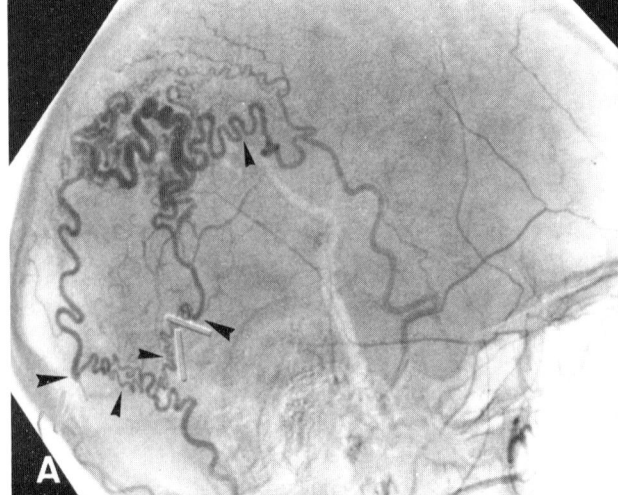
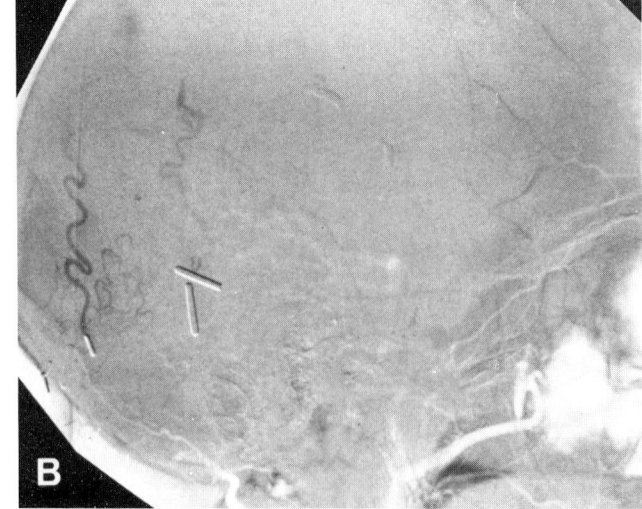

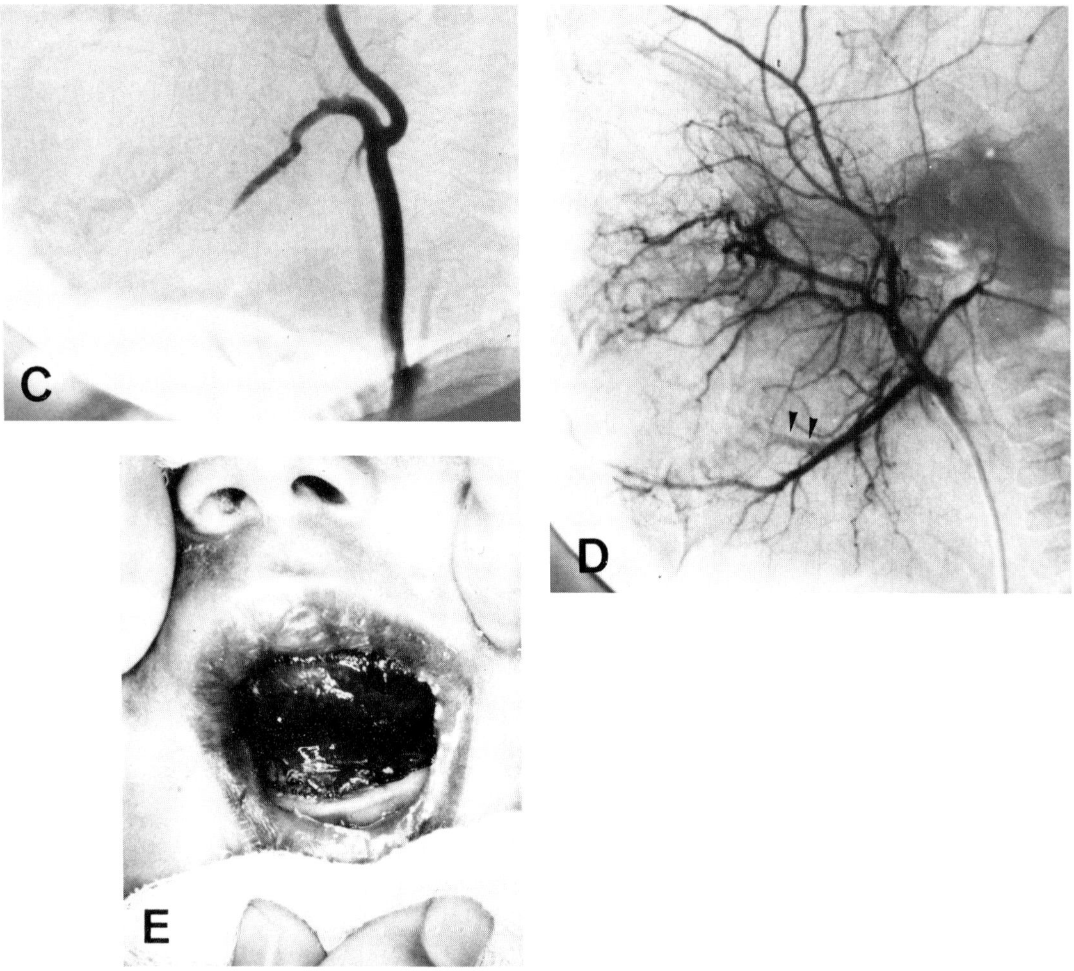

Figure 4.113 21-year-old man with arteriovenous malformation of the scalp that was partially resected 2 years previously but has since grown.
(A) Abundant collateral circulation (large arrowheads) producing malformation filling. (B) Control angiogram following presurgical embolization with Gelfoam. Surgical resection was performed without significant bleeding.

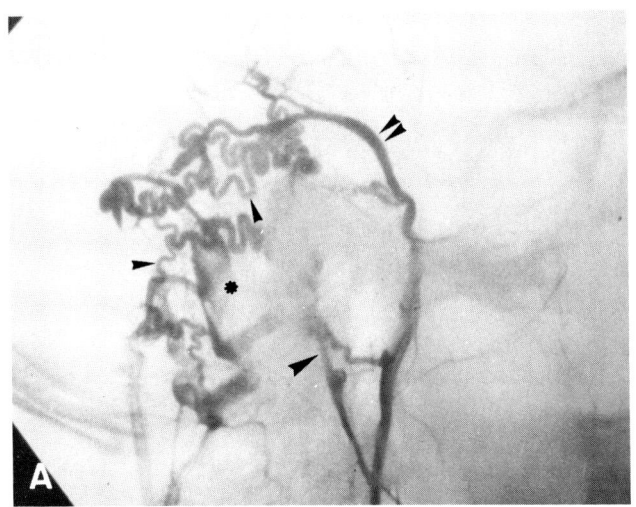

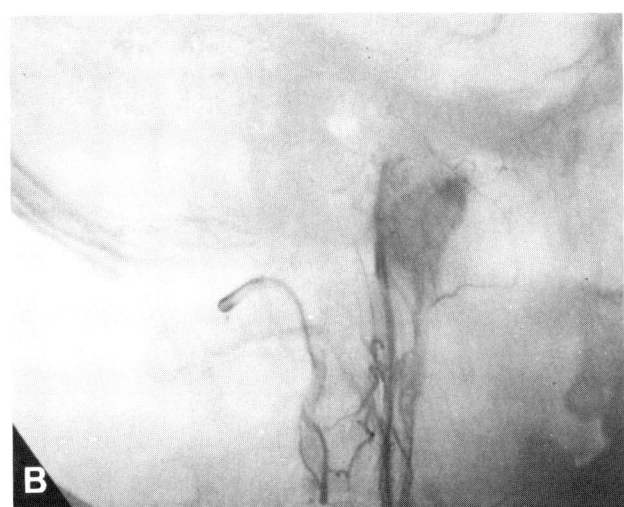

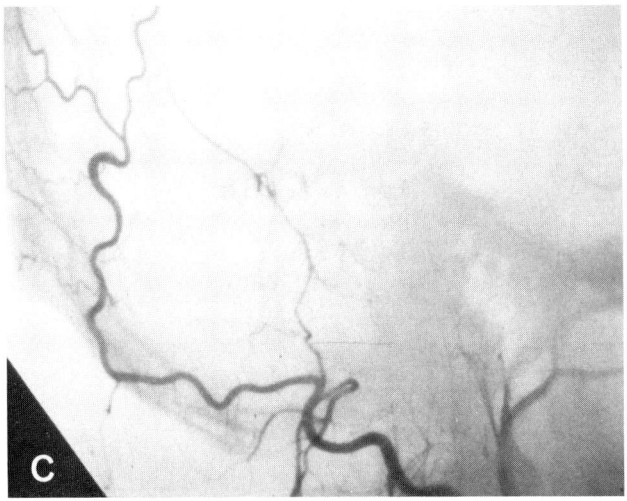

Figure 4.114 23-year-old man, with a painful pulsatile mass noted after direct trauma, presenting with pain and sleep-disruptive bruit.
(A) Angiogram of the posterior auricular artery (large arrowhead) showing the arteriovenous malformation with high-flow arteriovenous fistulas at the mastoid bone. Note the superficial venous drainage (small arrowheads), the anterior auricular vein (double arrowheads), and filling of the sigmoid sinus (*). Embolization was performed with 150-μm Ivalon particles and Gelfoam powder. (B) Normal ascending pharyngeal artery. (C) Normal occipital artery. After embolization, pain and bruit subsided.

easily reach the nidus, thus avoiding embolization of adjacent healthy tissue (Figs. 4.115 and 4.116).

Purely venous malformations (Fig. 4.117) do not communicate with the arteriocapillary system and may not be visible on the arterial angiogram. Hemorrhage is rare, its manifestations being mainly related to mass effect. Venous malformations are enlarged by Valsalva's maneuver, excessive crying, and physical strain. They may be studied by direct puncture (Fig. 4.117), or by multiple punctures in cases of multiple venous lakes without communication between them. Puncture of the lesion produces arterial-type blood, which makes it possible to determine the volume of the lesion and its drainage into the normal venous system. These lesions are easily emptied under manual compression. They may be treated by means of sclerosis with absolute alcohol, special care being taken to minimize the risk of necrosis due to extravasation into healthy tissue.

Hemolymphangiomas and Lymphangiomas

Hemolymphangiomas and lymphangiomas are manifested soon after birth, and may be either partially or totally regressible. Lymphangiomas are more common in the neck. When they do occur in the tongue, they have a pinkish appearance. Embolization is not an effective treatment for lymphangiomas of the tongue. The most common location of hemolymphangiomas is the tongue, where they present with a black mucosal mass, which may be of such volume that mouth closure is prevented. Treatment is, of course, mandatory in cases of hemorrhage, but embolization is also often indicated when feeding difficulties exist and when the deformity will damage the osteodental system due to mass effect. If embolization does not reduce the tumoral mass, surgery should be performed.

In cases of lymphangioma, embolization is ineffective.

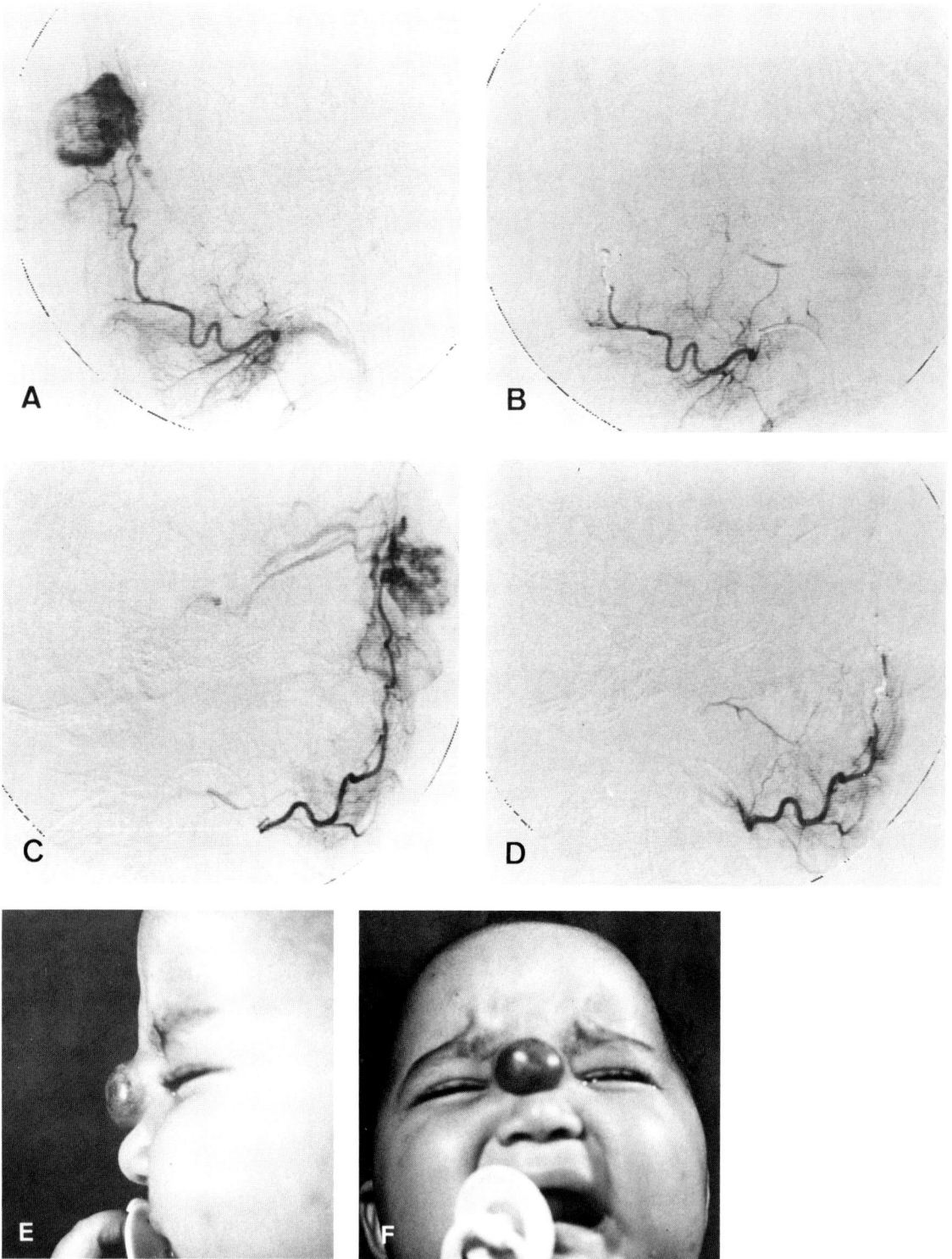

Figure 4.115 20-month-old boy with a glabelar hemangioma that had been growing rapidly since birth. Corticosteroids had not been used.
(A) Angiogram of the left facial artery showing opacification of the lesion. (B) Postembolization angiogram showing occlusion of the left facial artery. (C) Angiogram of the right facial artery showing opacification of the lesion. (D) Postembolization angiogram showing occlusion of the right facial artery. (E,F) Lateral and frontal views of the lesion. After embolization, the hemangioma was reduced in size by 30 to 40 percent, and the red color darkened.

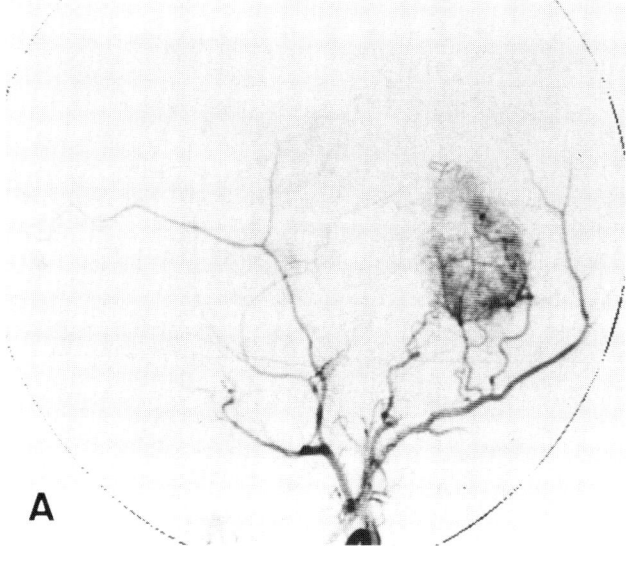

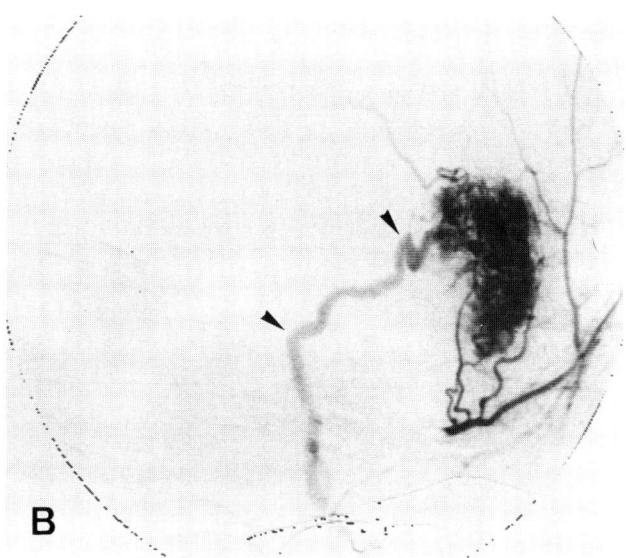

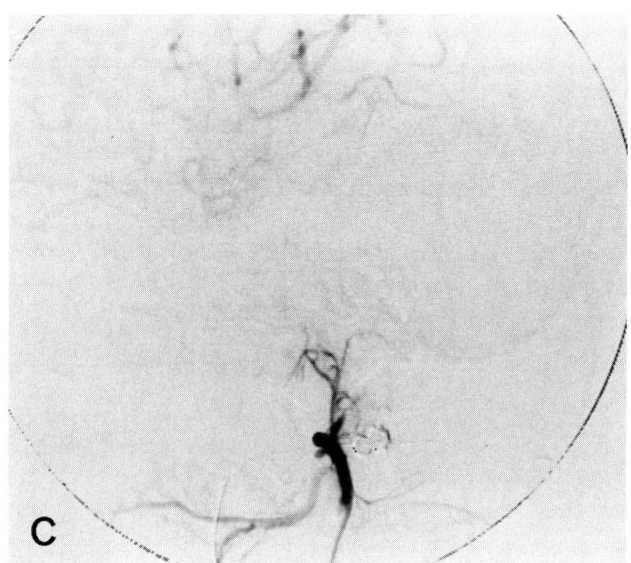

Figure 4.116 17-month-old boy with retroauricular and left frontal hemangioma.
(A) Injection into the left external carotid artery showing a retroauricular hypervascular lesion. (B) Injection into the left occipital artery, which vascularizes the lesion directly. Observe the venous return (arrowheads). (C) Control following embolization with collagen suspension (0.3 mL) showing total occlusion of the embolized arteries. Right hemiparesis sequela has occurred with good posterior clinical evolution.

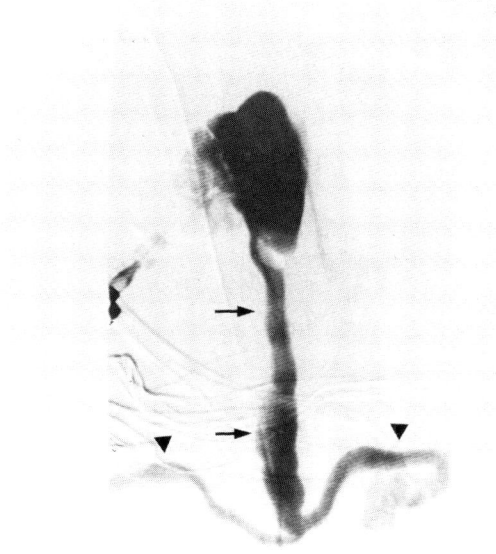

Figure 4.117 11-year-old child with a cervical mass which appeared 3 years earlier on the higher portion of the neck (anterior midline) and which increased in volume with crying, defecation effort, and physical exercise. The mass was easily emptied through manual compression. Angiogram with selective anterior injections into the region was normal. Direct puncture of the lesion demonstrated a vascular malformation of the purely venous and unicompartmental type, draining through a sole median vein (arrows) into the subclavian veins (arrowheads).

Angiomatoses

Of the angiomatoses, Rendu-Osler-Weber disease is the one of greatest importance in the maxillofacial territory. It is a well-known entity, epistaxis being its most frequent clinical manifestation. A family history of nasal hemorrhage and the presence of skin telangiectasia suggest the diagnosis. The angiographic study does not always reveal telangiectasia, and in cases of copious bleeding which has persisted even after anterior and posterior tamponading of the nasal fossae, embolization should be performed even when no angiographic lesions have been identified.

Arterial ligation is contraindicated. It is ineffective and may lead to the development of collateral circulation which will often be inaccessible to catheterization (for example, the ophthalmic artery may revascularize the internal maxillary artery and its branches). Medium-duration embolization will produce excellent results, and may be repeated whenever epistaxis reappears during the natural course of the disease (Fig. 4.118).

The angiographic evaluation of epistaxis should include the study of both of the internal carotid arteries, the internal maxillary artery, and both of the facial arteries. This protocol permits evaluation of all the possible causes of epistaxis: tumoral (e.g., nasopharyngeal fibroma), Rendu-Osler-Weber disease, isolated arteriovenous malformation, internal carotid aneurysm, coagulation dysfunction (congenital, hepatic, or toxic type), and arterial hypertension.

Except in cases of internal carotid aneurysm, embolization should always be bilateral, in both the internal maxillary and facial arteries. It should start from the bleeding site or, in case of bilateral bleeding, from the side in which bleeding is more severe. The nasal tampons should be removed immediately following embolization, still at the angiography lab, before the catheter is removed. Immediate results are excellent in a high percentage of cases, particularly in patients who have not been submitted to different therapeutic procedures previously.

Dural Arteriovenous Malformations

Dural arteriovenous malformations (DAVMs) are acquired lesions which represent the irreversible opening of arteriovenous physiologic shunts existing in the dura mater, particularly in the lining of the dural sinuses. The pathogenesis of these lesions requires the existence of a factor for poor development of the arterial and dural venous systems. Thrombosis and/or dural sinus thrombophlebitis then act to trigger the opening of a physiologic shunt. (Note that thrombosis and thrombophlebitis may

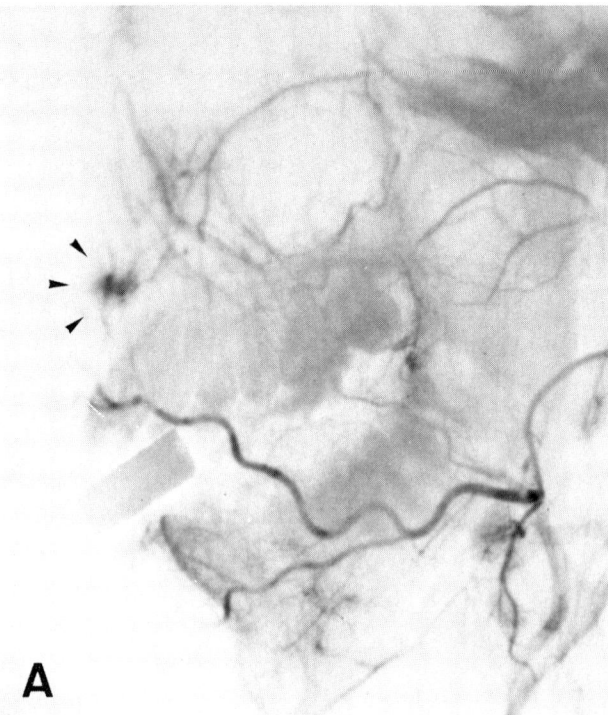
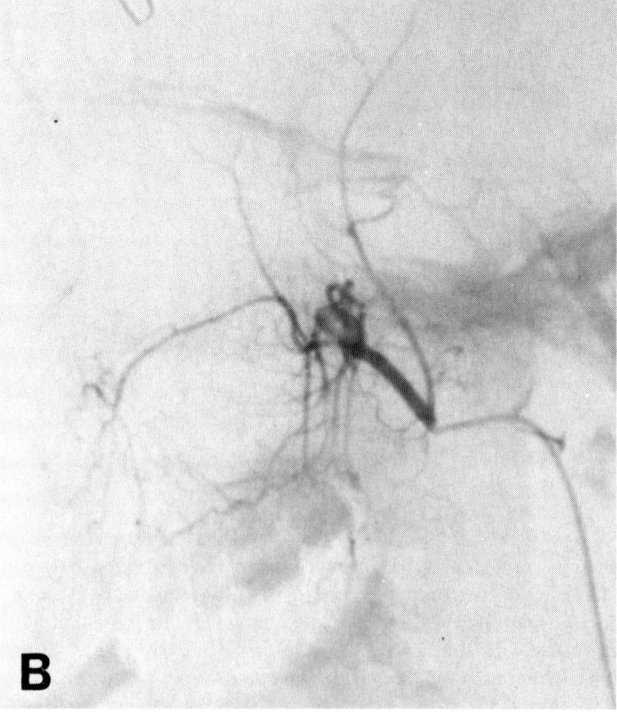

Figure 4.118 Untreatable epistaxis, caused by hereditary hemorrhagic telangiectasia, controlled by embolization. (A) Right facial arteriogram, profile view, showing small hypervascular lesion in the right nasal fossa (arrowheads) (telangiectasia). (B) Internal maxillary control arteriogram, profile view, following embolization of the facial artery with microgranular Ivalon.

be transient conditions, not always demonstrable angiographically.) Because several conditions can lead to dural sinus thrombosis, and these conditions rarely lead to DAVM, thrombosis alone is not sufficient to make a diagnosis, and it may be necessary to invoke the poor development factor.

DAVMs are usually found on the sigmoid, lateral, cavernous, or longitudinal sinuses; on the torcula; on the free and insertion tentorial borders; or on the anterior cranial fossa floor. The most practical classification of DAVMs is on the basis of type of venous drainage—to a dural sinus, to cerebral veins, or to both. Identification of the drainage type may clarify the symptoms and potential complications and suggest the best therapeutic strategy, including how aggressive the treatment should be. DAVMs with venous drainage to the dural sinus (Fig. 4.119) are manifested by proptosis, cranial nerve palsy, visual symptoms (exophthalmos), changes in intracranial

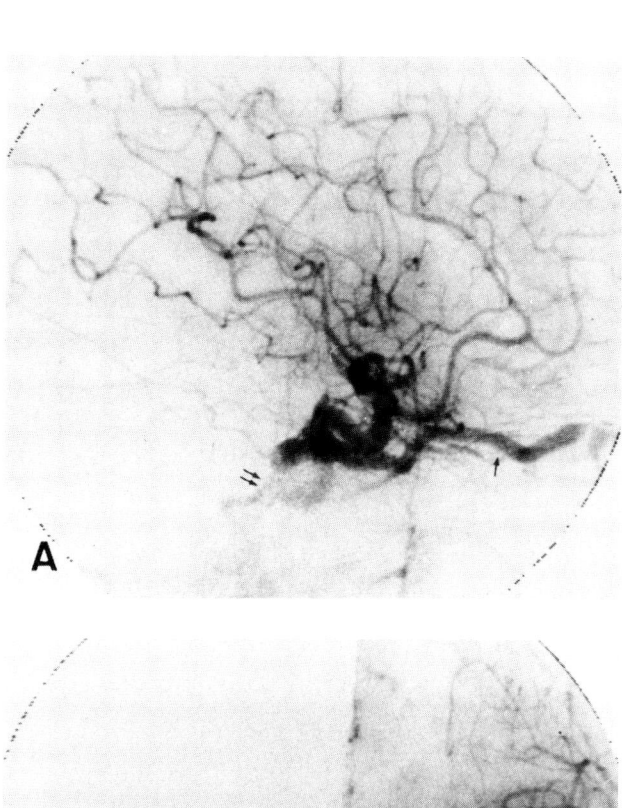

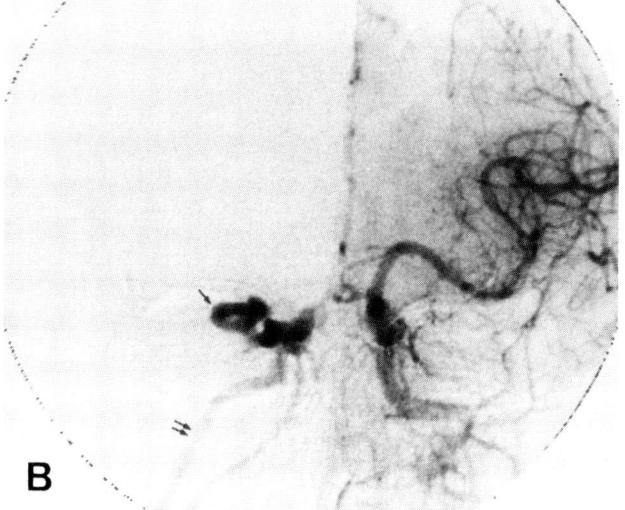

Figure 4.119 A 58-year-old female patient was seen 10 months ago for sudden headache and loss of vision in the right eye (exophthalmos with conjunctival hyperemia). Cephalalgia persisted for 3 months, then became episodic, and partial recovery of sight in the right eye occurred. Bruit in the right ear was becoming progressively more pronounced.
(A,B) Angiographic study revealed the presence of a DAVM on the left posterior portion of the cavernous sinus, draining into the right ophthalmic vein (arrow) and the right inferior petrous sinus (double arrow) in A. After the angiographic study was performed, the clinical picture (bruit, headache, and exophthalmos) improved. Left carotid compression maneuvers with the right hand were performed by the patient, who 3 weeks later was asymptomatic, with almost total recovery of visual acuity. On the fifth week after angiography, bruit and headache suddenly reappeared. (C) An angiographic study was performed for therapeutic purposes. Capsular branches of the left internal carotid artery vascularize the lesion, which drains only into the inferior petrosal sinus [double arrow, compare with (A)], superior ophthalmic vein thrombosis having occurred, as expected. (D) Injection into the distal left external carotid artery showing the malformation vascularized by cavernous regional branches and anastomosed to the lower lateral axis: foramen rotundum artery (large arrowhead), intracranial accessory meningeal artery branches (small arrowhead), and cavernous branches of the middle meningeal artery originating from its anterior and petrous branch (double black arrows). Embolization was performed in this position with Ivalon particles, until these arteries were no longer visible. This was followed by truncal embolization with large cylindrical fragments of Gelfoam soaked in ε-amino-caproic acid. (E) Angiogram of the left ascending pharyngeal artery, after embolization in the same manner as in (D), but with Ivalon and Gelfoam, showing the malformation being vascularized through the lower tympanic branch (black arrow) and lateral clival artery. (F) Angiogram of anterior right ascending pharyngeal branch, after embolization with the same material, showing vascularization through the carotid branch (black arrow). The inferior petrosal sinus is indicated by the double arrow. (G) Angiogram of the distal right external carotid artery, other pedicles not being seen. Truncal embolization was performed with Gelfoam. Postembolization control in right internal carotid. (H) Injection into the left primitive carotid artery showing almost no lesion visualization on the left side, significant flow reduction, as with the right internal carotid, and slight opacification of the lower petrosal sinus (double arrow). Following this procedure, the patient remained asymptomatic, without any bruit or headache, during a 3-month follow-up.

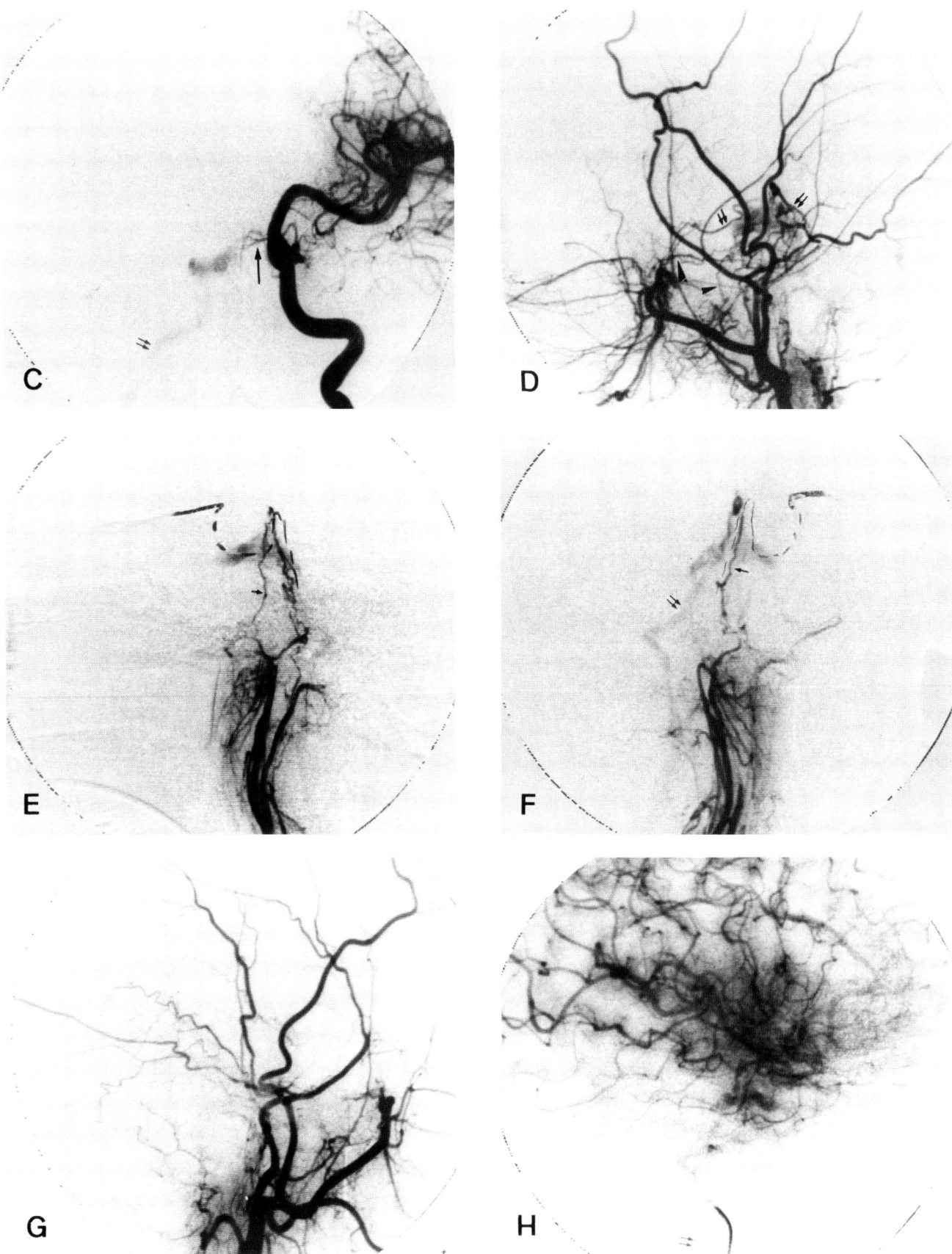

Figure 4.119 Continued

pressure, or bruit, depending on nidus location and flow intensity. Those malformations with venous drainage to adjacent cortical veins (Fig. 4.120) present intradural bleeding (hematoma, meningeal hemorrhage), focal CNS deficit, convulsion, and other transient symptoms. Such symptoms may also occur if the lesion is drained to the dural sinus.

DAVMs that are located on the anterior cranial fossa floor and on the tentorium almost invariably drain to the cortical veins; these malformations thus present the highest rate of intradural hemorrhage. Several different mechanisms are involved in the pathophysiology of the symptoms accompanying DAVMs. Most of them involve chronic retrograde venous hypertension in drainage veins due to hyperflow present in the arteriovenous shunt. In malformations not related to the cavernous sinus, cranial nerve palsy will be the only symptom related to the lesion's arterial aspect, due to the steal phenomenon. Bruits, which are due to turbulence inside the nidus, are more frequent in those lesions near the petrous pyramid, and these are more intense in higher-output lesions.

The therapeutic strategy for DAVMs depends on a consideration of both the clinical picture and the type of drainage present (Table 4.7). Spontaneous or postangiography DAVM thrombosis is amply described in the literature. In cases in which an aggressive therapy is not indicated, carotid compression maneuvers on the neck may lead to thrombosis. This maneuver is first used by the physician to make sure that there is adequate collateral circulation to supply the brain. Later the patient can apply the technique, compressing the common carotid with one hand (on the lesion side), for 1 minute every hour, for 1 month. In a recent case, partial thrombosis occurred after 3 weeks.

The decision as to the type of therapeutic strategy to be adopted must be multidisciplinary, and at an early stage the patient and the patient's family must be made aware of treatment objectives and potential risks. A detailed angiographic study of the lesion is preferably performed before decisions regarding procedures, scheduling, etc., are made.

Superselective catheterization of the arteries vascularizing the lesion and a thorough demonstration of vascular anatomy make it possible to locate the nidus precisely, establish the importance of each artery in the vascularization system, and visualize any dangerous branches or anastomoses. If only one or two pedicles are embolized, thrombosis of the whole nidus may result, preventing the embolization of arteries vascularizing the cranial nerves, or those which have dangerous anastomoses, which can lead to disastrous complications. These studies are made under general anesthesia, in order to obtain images of the best quality possible and amass the most information. This will facilitate effective embolization, as well as ensure that the procedure involves the least amount of discomfort possible for the patient. Superselective injection into the small arteries can be quite painful, and spontaneous head movement by the patient can make the radiologist's job more difficult.

The material to be used in the embolization of each artery is chosen on the basis of the angiographic study. Whenever IBC is utilized, superselective catheterization with a coaxial system should be used, in order to prevent complications in noninvolved arteries.

When establishing the treatment regimen, endovascular therapy should be the first aggressive method tried, and surgery at this stage should have the objective of restoring the patency of the major arteries feeding the lesion, making them accessible for endovascular therapy. When anatomic cure of the lesion cannot be obtained by embolization, surgery is an option.

After embolization, the patient is followed through visits to the radiologist. In cases in which intradural hemorrhage has occurred, a control angiographic study should be performed 6 months after the initial embolization in order to check its stability. If necessary, embolization can be repeated.

Table 4.7 – Therapeutic strategy for dural arteriovenous malformations

Clinical Picture and Drainage	Treatment Strategy
DAVM with sinusal venous drainage Subjective, moderate, well-tolerated bruit	Not treated; patient followed clinically
Objective bruit, with other symptoms	Embolization with particles or IBCA, depending on anatomic type and on significance of symptoms
DAVM with cortical venous drainage Headache, convulsions	Embolization with IBCA, aimed at cure or reduction of symptoms
Hemorrhagic accidents or CNS deficits	Embolization with IBCA, aimed at anatomic cure

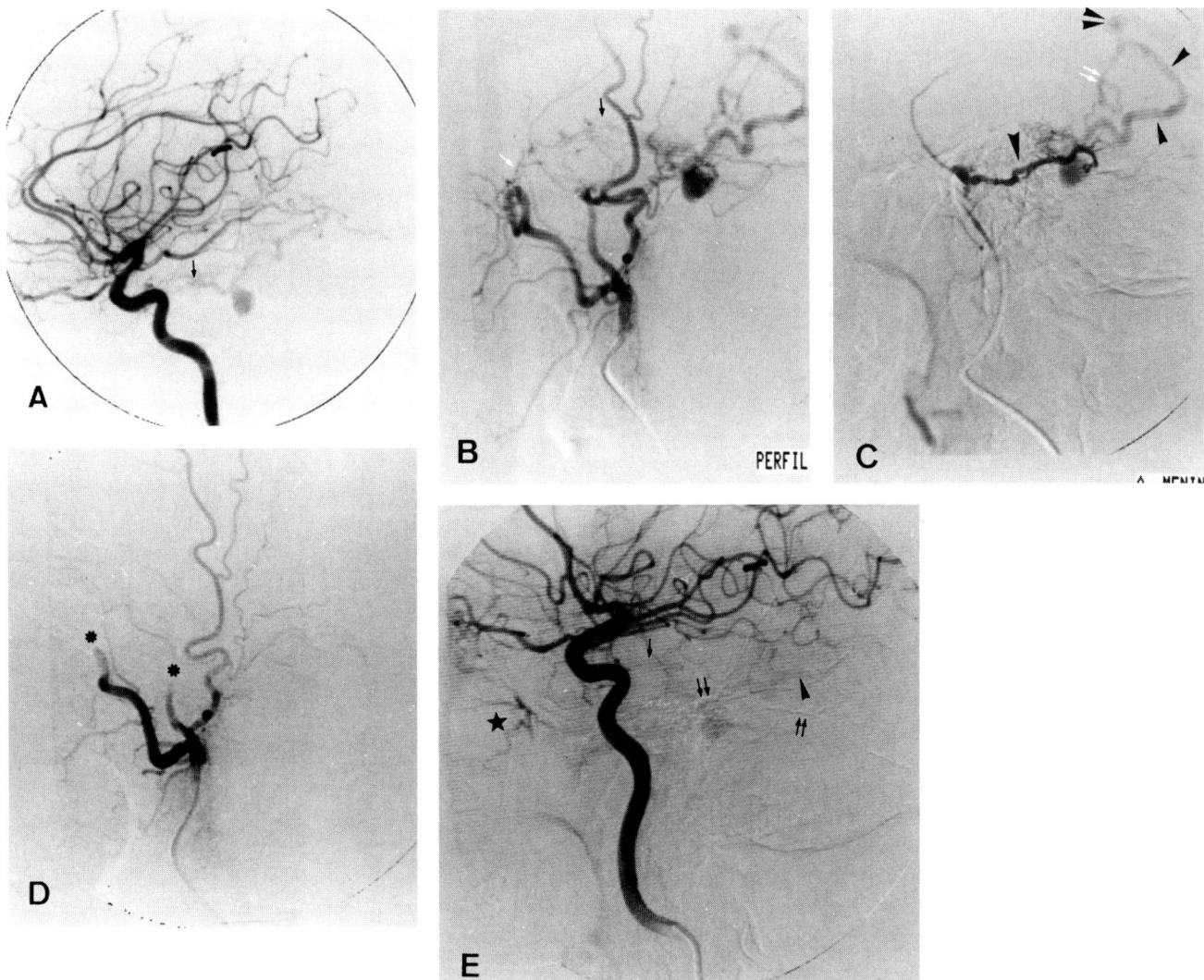

Figure 4.120 42-year-old male patient who presented with typical clinical picture of meningeal hemorrhage. Computed tomography showed evidence of blood in the subarachnoid space but no other changes.

(A,B) Angiograms (internal and distal external carotid, respectively) showing a DAVM vascularized by meningeal branches of the cavernous internal carotid artery (black arrow), which are feeding the territory of the lesion. These branches are also visualized from the anastomosis between them and the foramen rotundum artery (white arrow in B), originating from the distal internal maxillary artery through the inferior lateral axis. Here the foramen rotundum artery is the main feeding vessel of the inferior lateral axis, without direct communication with the internal carotid artery cavernous portion, and it was possible to reach the internal carotid meningeal branches and the nidus with a fluid embolus (bucrylate), without risk of reflux into the internal carotid. The postembolization control performed in the internal carotid (E) shows opacification of the internal maxillary distal branches (asterisk) from anastomoses with the ophthalmic artery, as well as a significant decrease in number and flow of internal carotid meningeal branches (arrow). This is an illustration of the effectiveness of very distal embolization, with emboli in the nidus and in feeding arteries, preserving those arteries not involved with the malformation. (C) Superselective catheterization of the middle meningeal artery with a coaxial system (Berenstein No. 7 to No. 5 French catheter plus No. 3 French coaxial catheter), showing that the main feeding source of the lesion is the petrosal branch of this artery (large arrowhead). The malformation is thus located on the insertion border of the territory, on the transition between the squamous and petrosal portions of the temporal bone. Venous drainage, as is common in this territory, is done by the cerebral veins. The superior cerebellar vein, together with the superior vermian vein (small arrowheads), joined by an anastomotic vein (double white arrow), will drain into the vein of Galen (double arrowheads) and eventually into the straight sinus. Embolization was performed in this position with bucrylate. (D) Injection into the distal external carotid showing middle meningeal and distal maxillary occlusion (*). (E) Bucrylate is seen inside the nidus of the lesion and in the distal branches of the middle meningeal artery (double black arrows). Slight opacification of a drainage vein is also still seen (small arrowhead). With bucrylate present inside the nidus, subsequent thrombosis is expected due to the slow flow within the remaining nidus and drainage veins.

TUMORS

Embolization is appropriate for treatment of some hypervascular tumors, either benign or malignant, primary or metastatic, developing in the skull, meninges, or the facial complex, when their vascularization depends to a large extent on the external carotid system. The objective of embolization is generally to produce tumor ischemia and reduce volume. In most cases, the procedure is performed as a preoperative measure, as it offers a better cleavage plane and reduces hemorrhage during surgery. However, it may be a palliative measure in patients in whom surgery is contraindicated, or for highly vascularized tumors involving vital structures.

Angiographic Protocol

The treatment of nasopharyngeal angiofibromas and tympanojugular paragangliomas, which have a definite topography, follows a preestablished protocol. The treatment of other hypervascular tumors depends on the region in which they are located.

Meningiomas

Meningiomas are benign tumors originating from the meninges; they account for 15 percent of all intracranial tumors. There are many different histologic types of meningiomas. Two of them, because of their hypervascularity, are viable candidates for embolization: endotheliomatous and angiodysplastic meningiomas.

Meningiomas are fed by two different arterial systems (Fig. 4.121). The first is made up of the meningeal arteries or arterial branches. These vascularize the center of the tumor; they are the insertion pedicle, and are extraaxial. The second is comprised of the pial branches of the cerebral or cerebellar arteries; they feed the tumor peripherally and are intraaxial (Fig. 4.122).

Meningiomas may be divided into three groups according to location:

- At the convexity: These represent 50 percent of all intracranial meningiomas, including parasaggital meningiomas and those on the falx cerebri (Fig. 4.121). They have extraaxial feeding pedicles from the distal branches of the middle meningeal artery, falx cerebri artery, and transosseous branches of the superficial temporal and occipital arteries.
- At the base: These represent 40 percent of the total and include those originating from the olfactory trough, the sellar tubercle, the tentorial incisure, and petrous bone surfaces. They have extraaxial feeding pedicles from the ethmoidal branches of the opthalmic artery, anterior deep temporal artery, cavernous branches of the carotid siphon, accessory meningeal artery, the foramen rotundum artery, cavernous branches, petrosal and petrosquamous branches, and meningeal branches of the vertebral pharyngeal arteries.
- Intraventricular: These comprise the remaining 10 percent; they are basically fed by the choroidal arteries. Those of the foramen rotundum and those of the jugular foramen have the meningeal branches of the vertebral and ascending pharyngeal arteries as dominant pedicles.

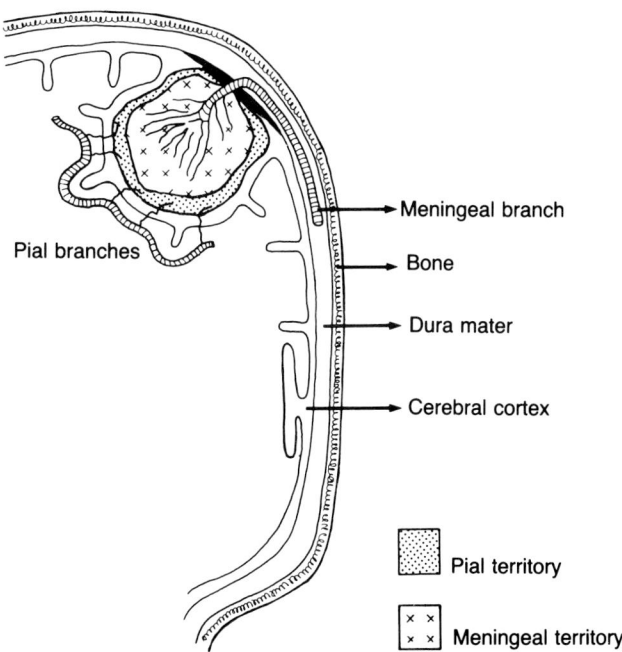

Figure 4.121 Schematic representation of convexity meningioma vascularization showing the meningeal and pial vascularization territories.

Embolization

The decision to embolize a meningioma as a presurgical procedure will depend very much on the neurosurgeon's point of view. For the cases shown in Figs. 4.122, 4.123, and 4.124, embolization was definitely beneficial.

All the feeding pedicles accessible to the catheter should be embolized. Because the procedure is preoperative, the material to be used should be reabsorbable. For superselective embolization, Gelfoam powder or 150-μm Ivalon is utilized, which produces effective distal embolization. If for technical reasons a superselective procedure cannot be performed, smaller particles of the same material should be used. Embolization will be less effective, but the procedure will involve less risk of ischemia in healthy tissue.

The embolizing material should be injected in solution with the conventional contrast medium material, or, when using Gelfoam, soaked in Lipiodol.

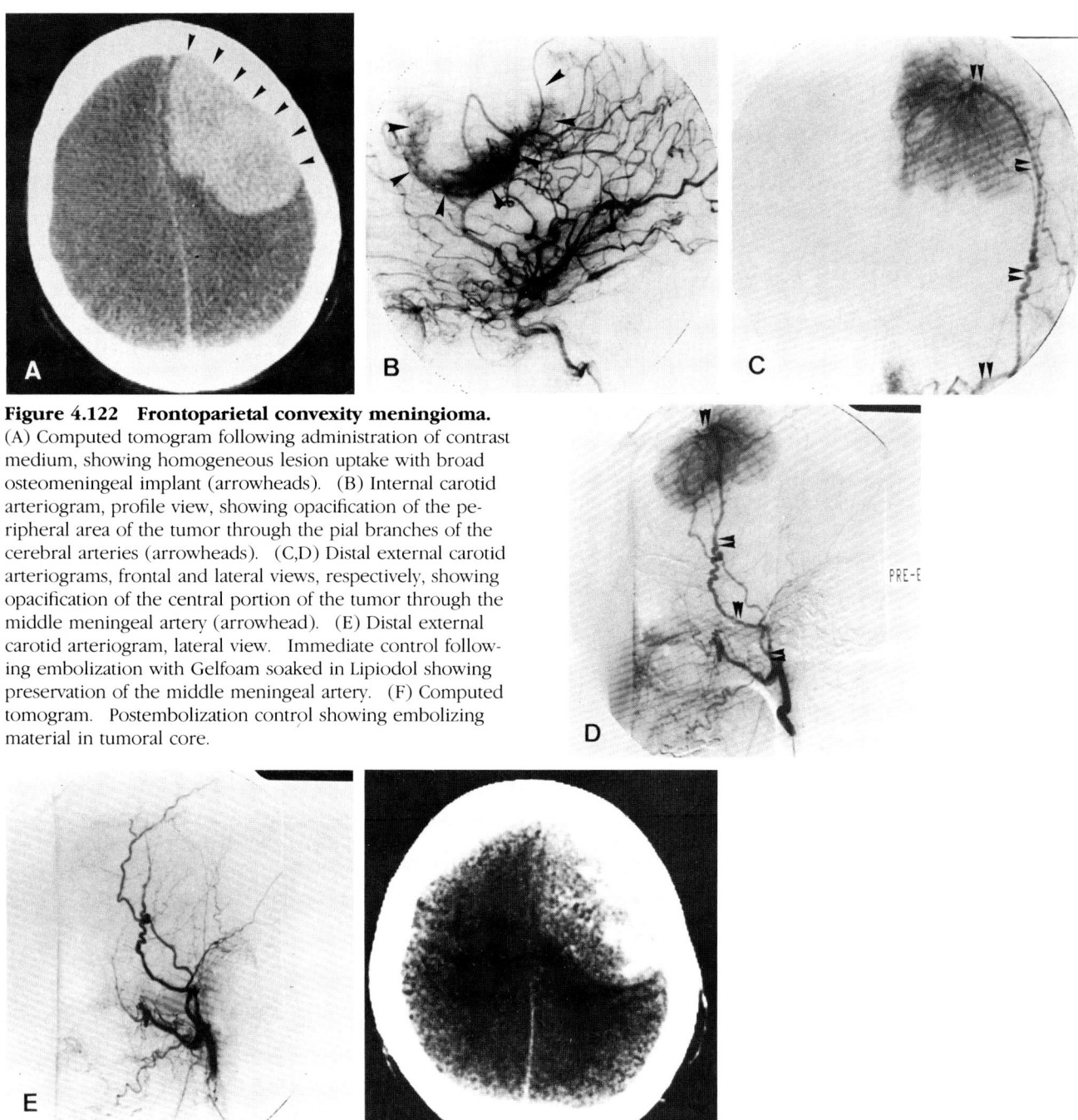

Figure 4.122 Frontoparietal convexity meningioma.
(A) Computed tomogram following administration of contrast medium, showing homogeneous lesion uptake with broad osteomeningeal implant (arrowheads). (B) Internal carotid arteriogram, profile view, showing opacification of the peripheral area of the tumor through the pial branches of the cerebral arteries (arrowheads). (C,D) Distal external carotid arteriograms, frontal and lateral views, respectively, showing opacification of the central portion of the tumor through the middle meningeal artery (arrowhead). (E) Distal external carotid arteriogram, lateral view. Immediate control following embolization with Gelfoam soaked in Lipiodol showing preservation of the middle meningeal artery. (F) Computed tomogram. Postembolization control showing embolizing material in tumoral core.

Nasopharyngeal Angiofibromas

Nasopharyngeal angiofibromas are benign, highly vascularized, slow-growing tumors originating from the posterior compartment of the nasal fossa. They may extend to the maxillary sinus, pterygopalatine fossa, cavum, base of the skull, orbit, and midcranial fossa. They frequently extend beyond the midline, occupying the nasopharynx bilaterally.

Nasopharyngeal angiofibromas usually appear in young male patients presenting with epistaxis and symptoms of nasal obstruction. Other associated clinical manifestations are purulent rhinorrhea, facial deformity, anosmia, and, less frequently, exophthalmos and hypoacousia. They are rarely found in female patients.

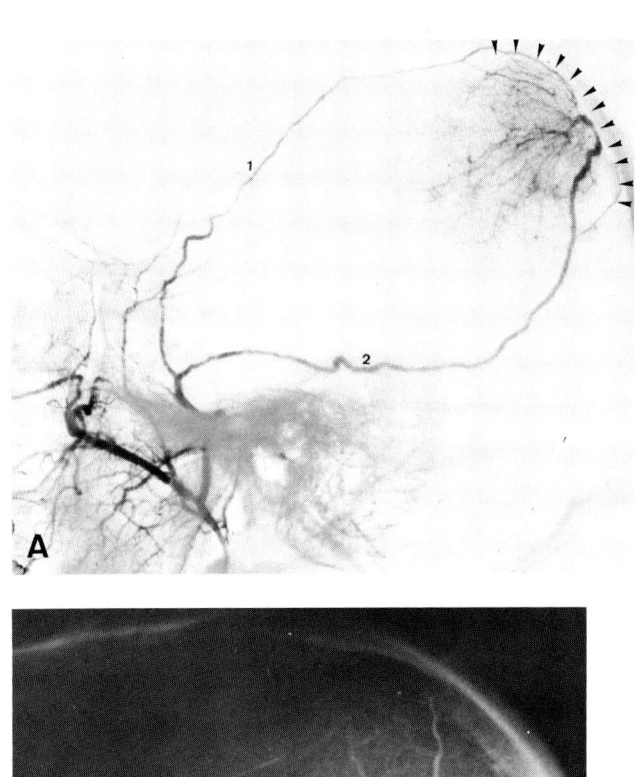

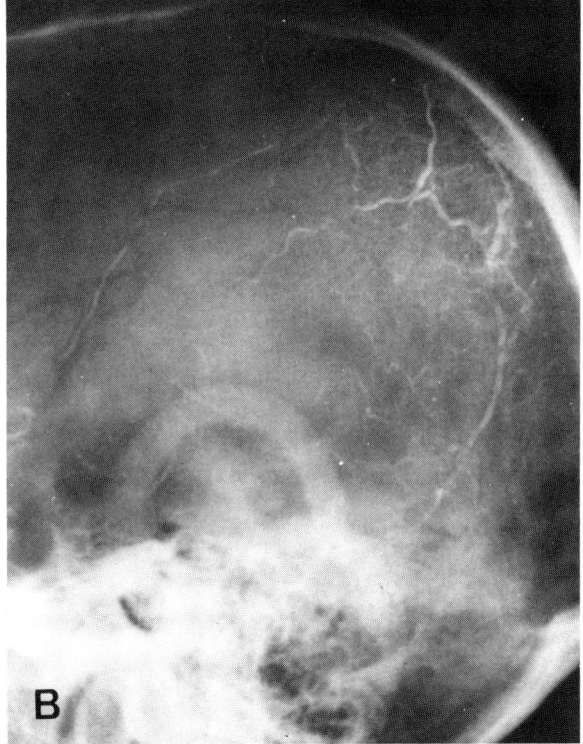

Figure 4.123 Parietal convexity meningioma.
(A) Middle meningeal selective arteriogram, profile view, showing opacification of the central portion and tumor insertion (arrowheads) through two dilated branches (1 and 2). (B) Plain lateral skull x-ray. Control following embolization with Lipiodol-soaked emboli.

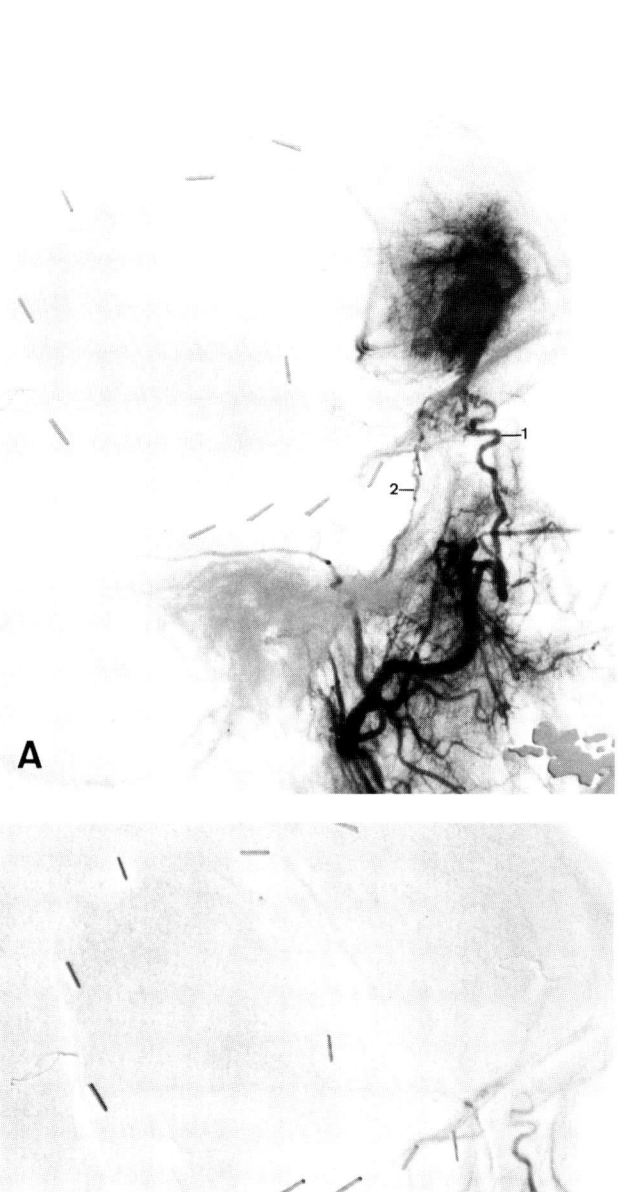

Figure 4.124 Recurrent frontal meningioma.
(A) Internal maxillary arteriogram, lateral view, showing the tumor being fed by the anterior deep temporal artery (1) and branches of the middle meningeal artery (2). (B) Control following embolization with Gelfoam fragments.

Angiographic Protocol

The angiographic study has the objective of confirming the diagnosis, showing the relationship between the tumor and the internal carotid and the ophthalmic arteries in cases of intracranial and orbital expansion, and demonstrating the feeding pedicles and any dangerous anastomoses. The protocol should basically be determined by information previously obtained through conventional and/or computed tomography. Because this type of lesion frequently advances beyond the midline, the study should include lateral views for pedicles on the dominant side of the lesion and anteroposterior views for pedicles on the opposite side. The following arteries should be explored: the internal carotid, internal maxillary, ascending pharyngeal, and facial (including the ascending palatine).

Embolization

Embolization should be performed up to 5 days prior to surgery. In most cases, reabsorbable emboli are utilized and finely particulate or powder Gelfoam is the best choice. For inoperable cases nonreabsorbable emboli (Lyodura or Ivalon) are preferred.

The internal maxillary artery should be the first pedicle to be occluded. Then an angiographic control should be immediately performed in the facial and ascending pharyngeal arteries in order to evaluate non-embolized tumor compartments. Subsequent embolizations in these arteries are frequently necessary. The effectiveness of embolization should be demonstrated by contralateral arterial injection without opacification of the lesion (Fig. 4.125).

The potential benefits of preoperative embolization of nasopharyngeal angiofibromas are now universally recognized. Embolization reduces tumoral volume and vascularization, making the surgical procedure safer and decreasing the number of blood transfusions required. Because this procedure is, in most cases, performed in young patients with a healthy arterial system, it is not generally technically difficult.

Paragangliomas

Paragangliomas are infrequent, well-vascularized tumors which originate from glomic structures. They are also called chemodectomas and glomic tumors.

Since these tumors originate from cells which are part of the neural crest and of the APUD system, they are able to secrete vasoactive substances. They may be located anywhere in the body, although they are most often found in the tympanic region, jugular gulf, vagal glomus, carotid body, and retropharynx.

Clinical manifestations include symptoms of compression on the base of the skull, particularly involving the cranial nerves, or the presence of a palpable cervical

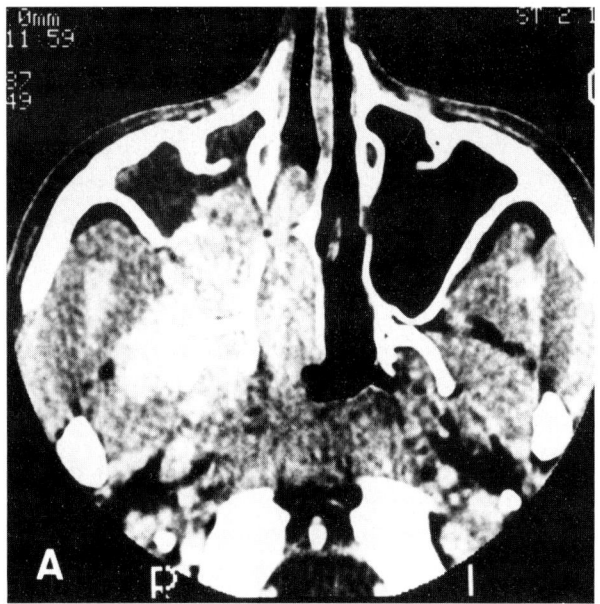

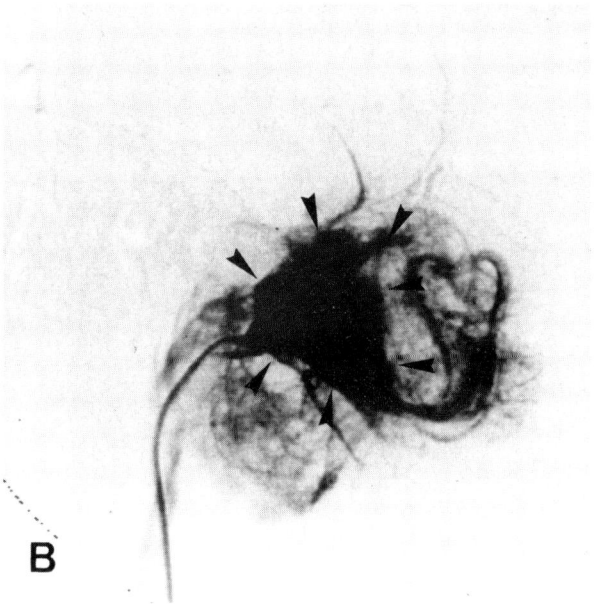

Figure 4.125 Juvenile angiofibroma.
(A) Computed axial tomogram following contrast-medium administration showing tumoral mass in the nasopharynx, pterygoid fossa, and part of the maxillary sinus. (B) Selective distal internal maxillary arteriogram. (C) Ascending pharyngeal artery. (D) Ascending palatine artery, lateral view, showing opacification of tumoral compartments (arrowhead). (E) External carotid global arteriogram, lateral view. Control immediately following embolization. (F) Internal maxillary arteriogram on the side opposite to the lesion, frontal view. (G) Ascending pharyngeal arteriogram on the side opposite to the lesion, lateral view. Control following embolization of pedicles on the same side of the lesion shows opacification of small residual tumoral nodule (arrowheads) and a normal pharyngeal parenchymogram (*).

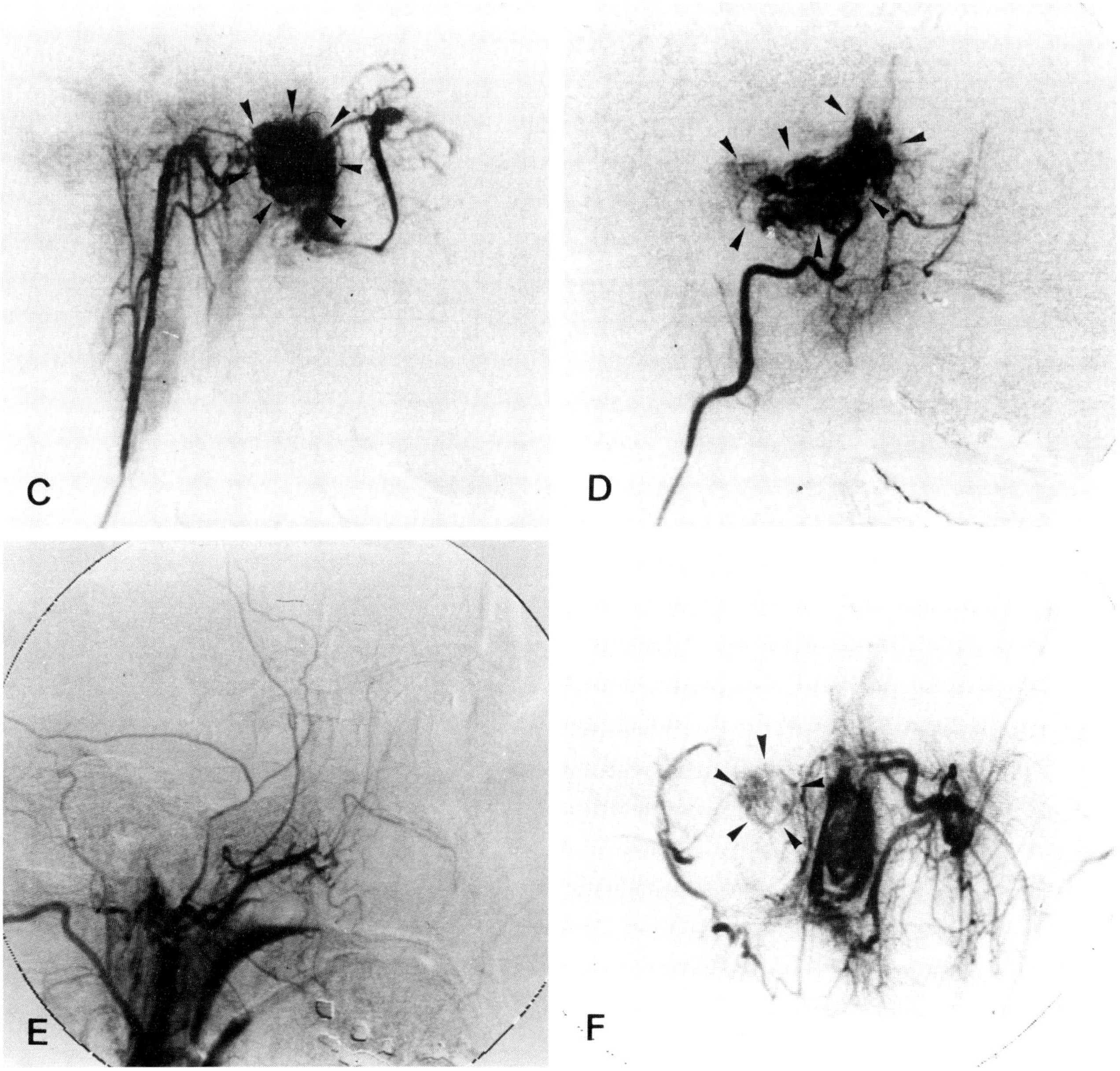

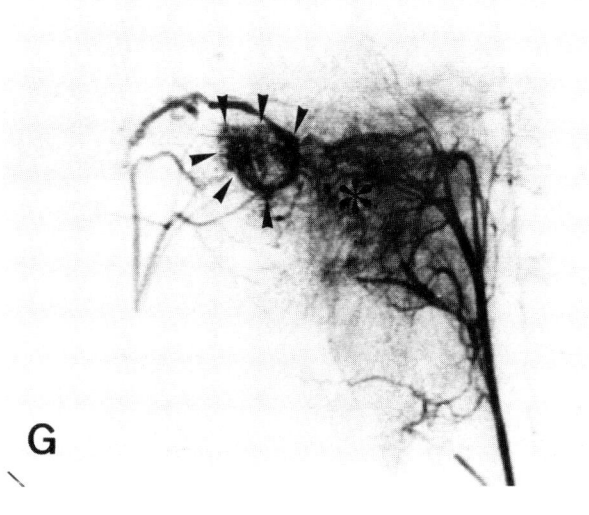

Figure 4.125 *Continued*

mass. Due to their excretory ability, these tumors may also produce symptoms similar to those of pheochromocytomas or carcinoid tumors.

Angiographic Protocol

The objectives of angiography are to confirm the diagnosis; define topography and the relationship between the tumor and vital vascular structures, showing any association with another glomic tumor undetected by routine studies; and evaluate the technical possibilities for embolization.

A complete angiographic protocol should be per-

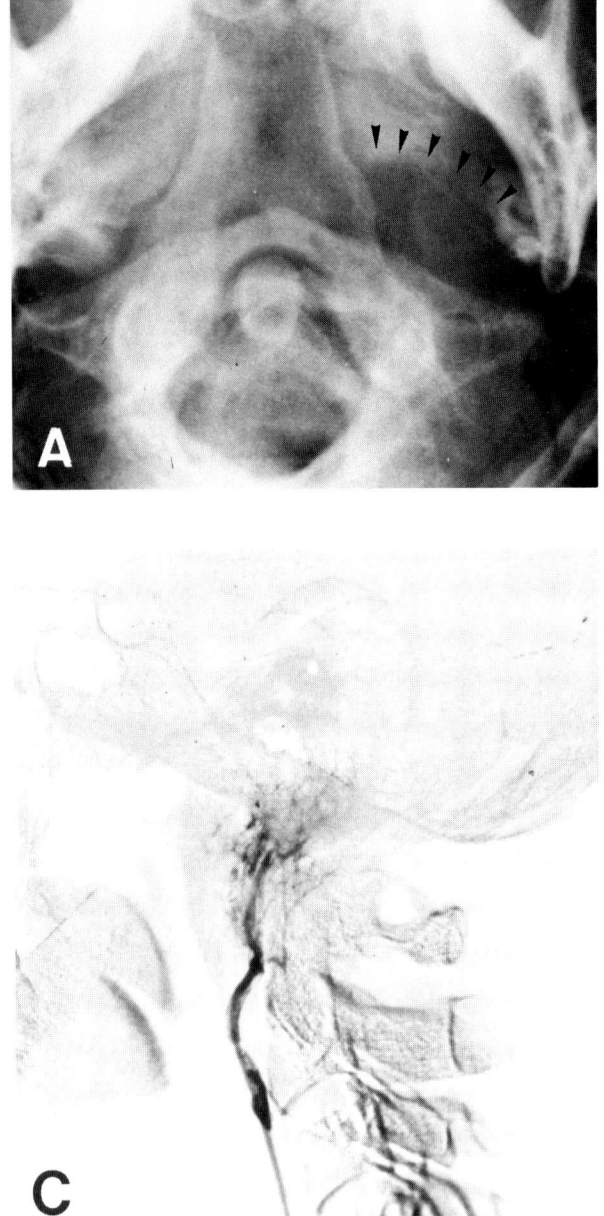
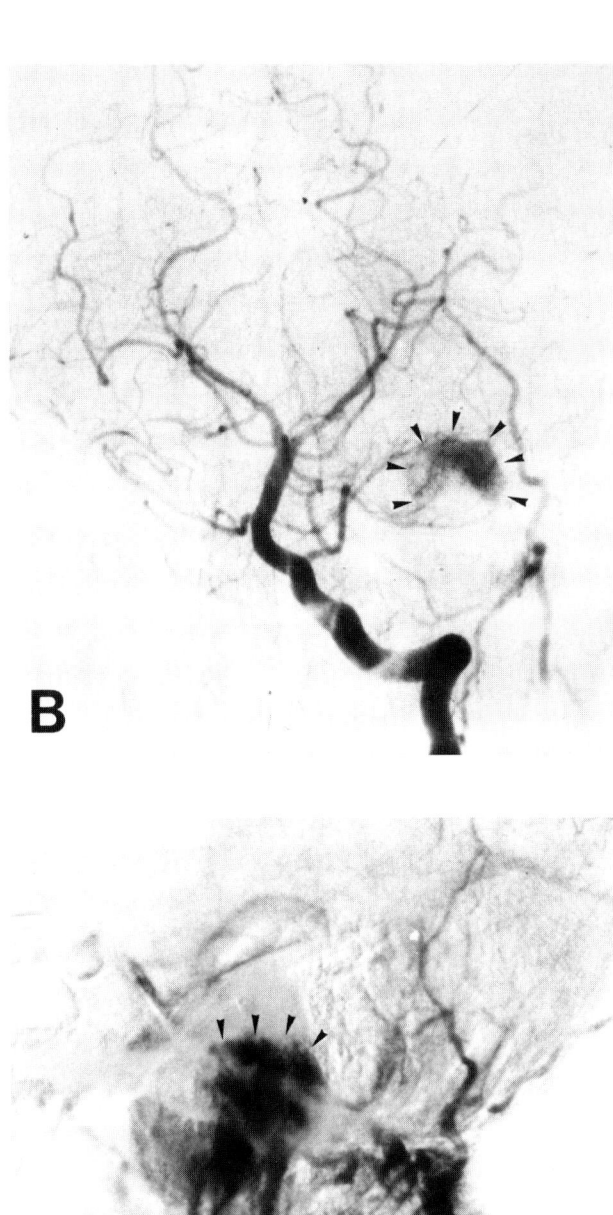

Figure 4.126 Tympanojugular paraganglioma with extension to the posterior fossa.
(A) Plain x-ray of skull base showing partial destruction of petrous bone base, with enlargement of the foramen jugulare and deformity (arrowheads). (B) Vertebral arteriogram, anteroposterior view, showing tumor extension into the posterior fossa (arrowhead). (C,D) Ascending pharyngeal arteriogram, lateral views. (E) Injection at the level of the posterior auricular artery origin (double arrow), showing participation of this artery in tumor feeding (arrowheads). (F) Occipital arteriogram (1), lateral view showing participation of the stylomastoid artery (2); presence of muscular branches between the occipital and vertebral arteries (the arrows indicate flow direction) and the basilar artery (3). (G) Primitive carotid arteriogram, lateral view. Control immediately following successive embolization of the tumor feeding arteries. (H) Postembolization vertebral control arteriogram, lateral view.

formed, including the following arteries: bilateral ascending pharyngeal, anteroposterior view of the side opposite to the lesion; lateral view of the same side as the lesion; AP and lateral view of the vertebral artery; lateral or Stenvers view of the internal carotid artery; lateral view of the occipital artery; lateral view of the internal maxillary artery; lateral view of the posterior auricular artery.

Figure 4.126 *Continued*

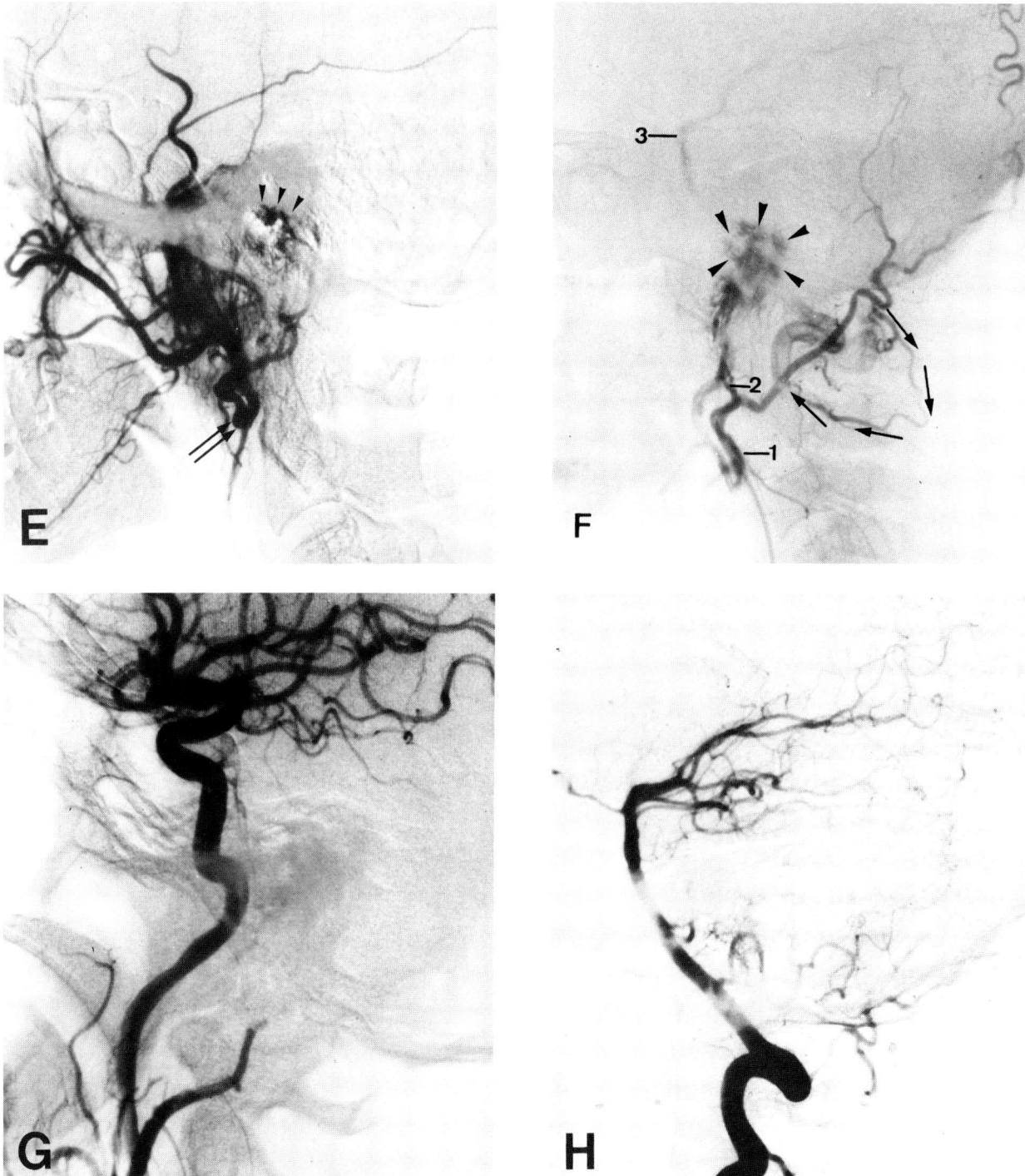

Embolization

Paragangliomas are a major indication for embolization (Fig. 4.126). In cases considered inoperable, embolization may be carried out with the purpose of controlling the symptoms, decreasing the mass effect, and stabilizing tumoral growth. Each pedicle feeding the lesion, and depending upon the external carotid artery, should be selectively embolized.

For operable lesions, powder or fine particulate Gelfoam is the preferred material. For nonsurgical cases in which palliation is the goal, nonreabsorbable materials are utilized.

The angiographic control, which is used to evaluate the effect of embolization, should be performed in vertebral arteries and in the internal and proximal external carotid arteries on the same side as the lesion.

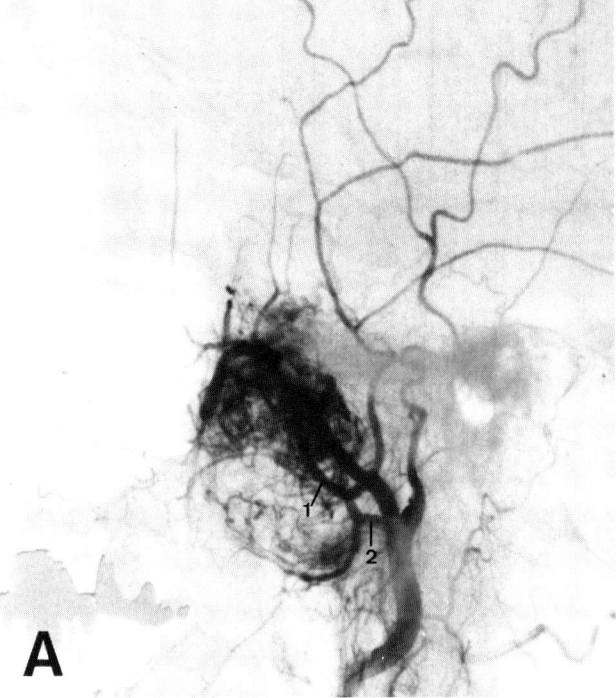

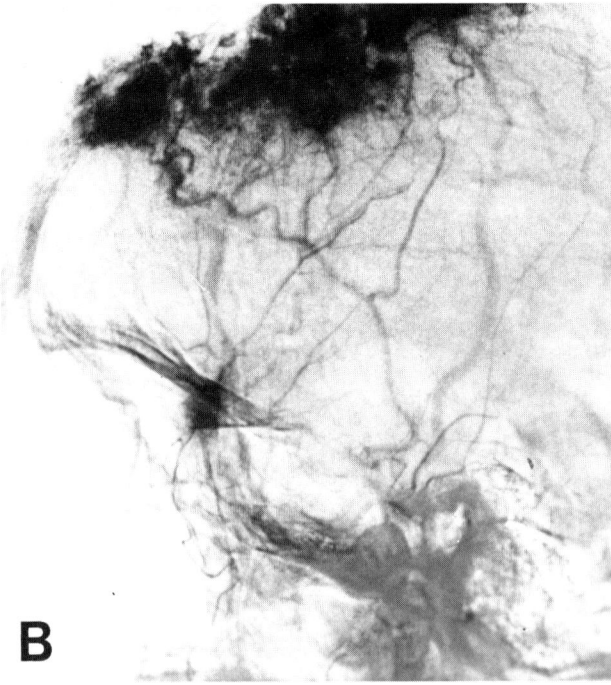

Figure 4.127 Facial hypernephroma metastasis.
(A) Internal maxillary arteriogram, lateral view, showing that the hypervascular lesion is basically fed by the middle deep temporal and facial transverse arteries (2). (B) Control following embolization with Ivalon microparticles.

If the ascending pharyngeal artery contralateral to the lesion side has not been embolized, it should be included in the control.

Other Tumors

Hypervascular metastases of renal carcinomas (Figs. 4.127 and 4.128), thyroid tumors and neuroblastomas (Fig. 4.129), and certain rare tumors, such as hemangiopericytomas (Fig. 4.130), may benefit from embolization as a palliative or preoperative measure.

If the tumor is sensitive to chemotherapy, conventional embolization is contraindicated because it will deprive the lesion of its vascularization, thereby preventing the chemotherapeutic agent from acting. A combination of embolization and radiotherapy can be an effective palliative therapeutic option, in those lesions considered inoperable.

Embolization in these cases follows the same basic principles used for lesions. However, with malignant lesions, it is preferable that nonreabsorbable emboli be utilized, even when the procedure is preoperative.

Some centers are presently developing chemoembolization techniques in which selective embolization utilizes both embolic particles and a chemotherapeutic drug. The results have been quite satisfactory, even better than those obtained with conventional embolization.

Epistaxis

Angiography is the least used of the therapeutic procedures for control of epistaxis in the craniofacial territory.

Anterior nasal hemorrhage is easily controlled by the specialist through conventional methods. Posterior epistaxes, which do not always respond to posterior tamponading, are a more complex problem.

With the exception of epistaxes of tumoral origin or those caused by rupture of a vascular malformation (e.g., Rendu-Osler-Weber), the vessel responsible for bleeding is very seldom angiographically identified. Angiographic study of epistaxis, be it of spontaneous, traumatic, or postoperative origin, will rarely reveal any pathologic vessels or abnormal contrast-medium extravasation. When angiography is used, it is of fundamental importance that the ear, nose, and throat specialist identify for the angiographer the probable site of bleeding, as well as its etiology.

Angiographic Protocol and Embolization

A complete series of the vascular territories from which epistaxis may originate from should be performed, including the internal carotid artery, the internal maxillary, and the facial artery on both sides. In doubtful cases, or when a pathologic image is identified, a complementary anteroposterior or mentonasal view may be required for further clarification.

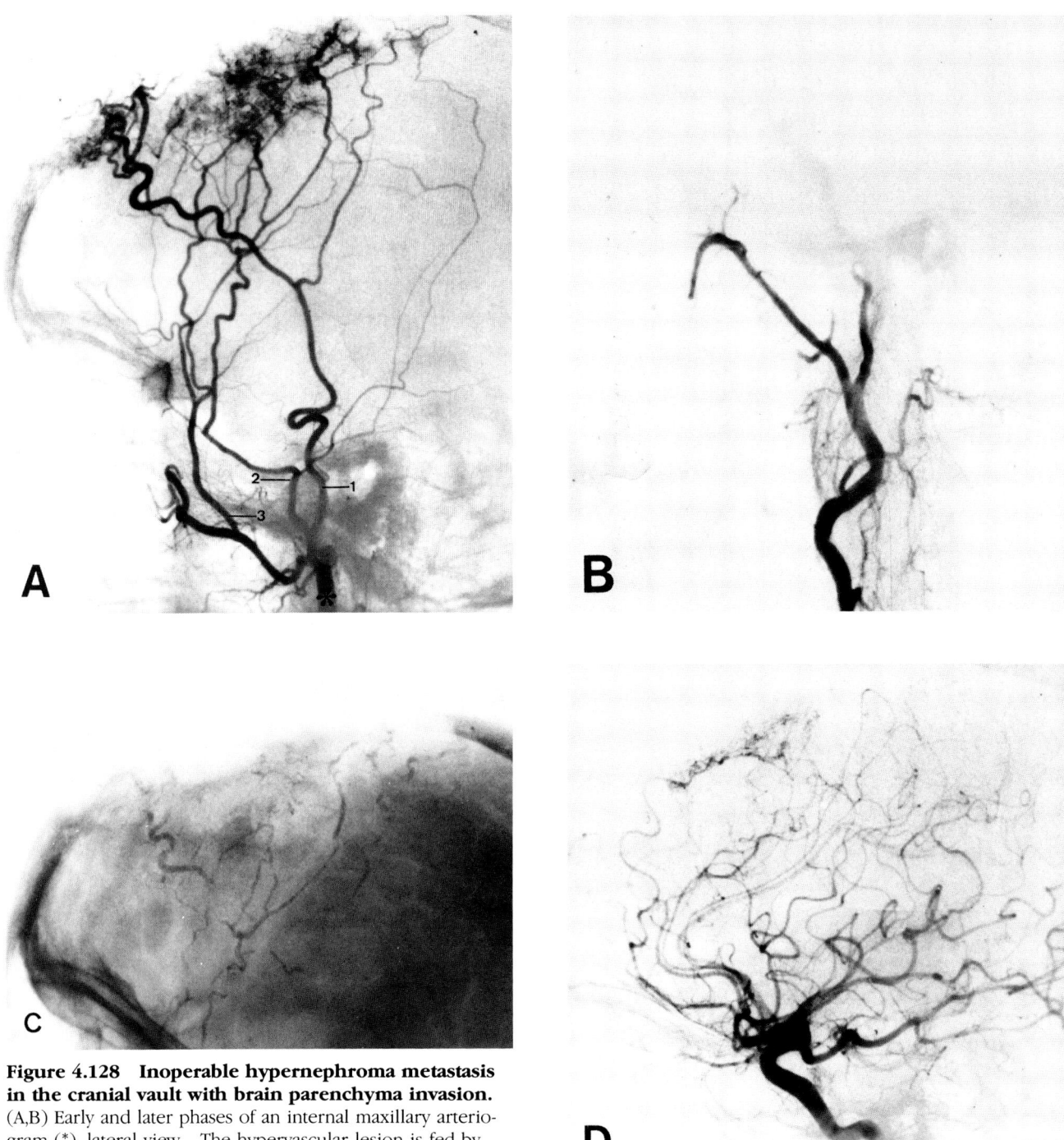

Figure 4.128 Inoperable hypernephroma metastasis in the cranial vault with brain parenchyma invasion.
(A,B) Early and later phases of an internal maxillary arteriogram (*), lateral view. The hypervascular lesion is fed by superficial temporal (1), middle meningeal (2), and middle deep temporal (3) arteries. C) Plain skull x-ray, lateral view. Control following embolization with isobutyl and Lipiodol. (D) Internal carotid arteriogram, lateral view. Control following embolization of external carotid pedicles. Small hypervascular tumoral area, supplied by the anterior frontal artery, persists.

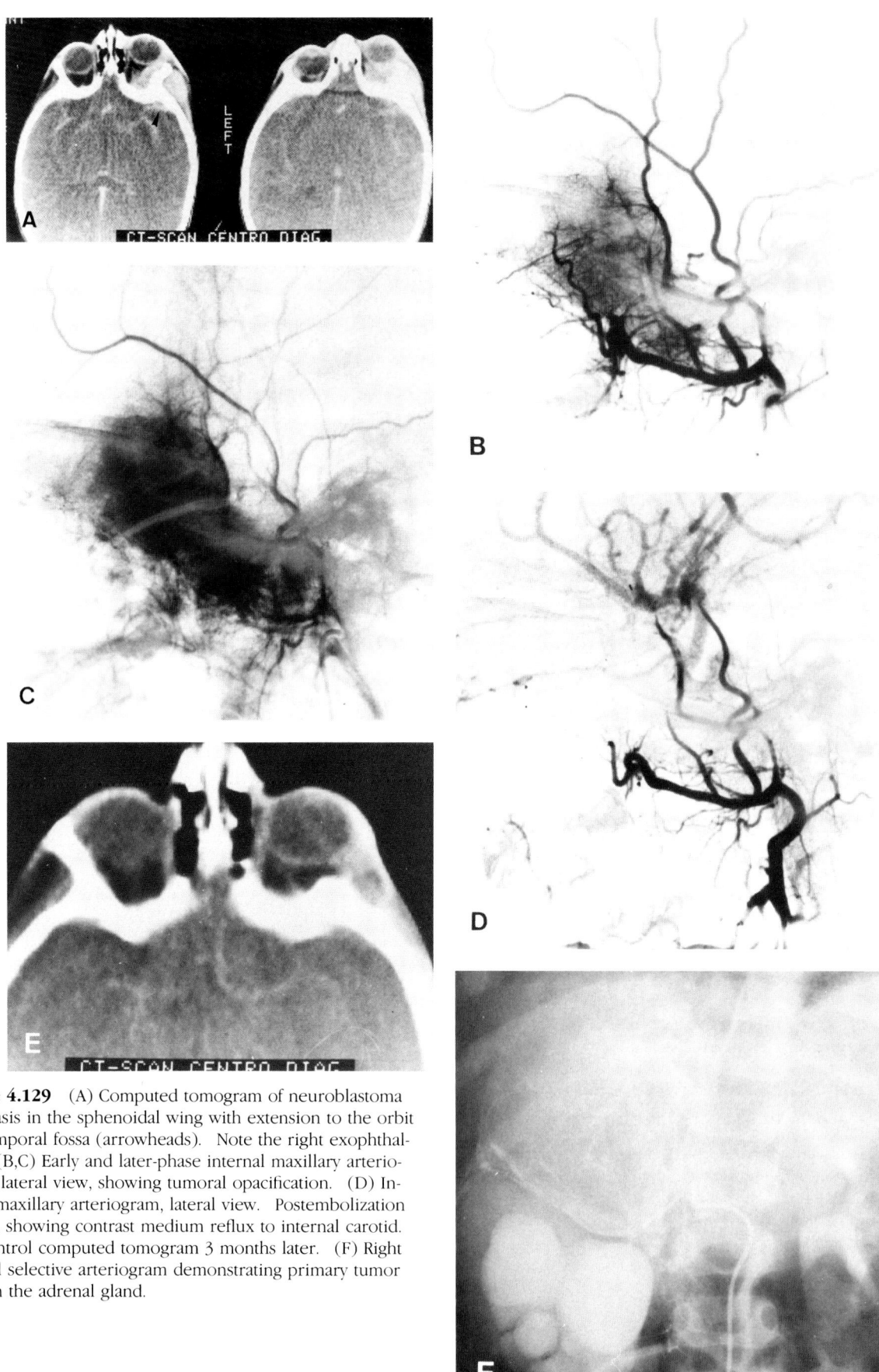

Figure 4.129 (A) Computed tomogram of neuroblastoma metastasis in the sphenoidal wing with extension to the orbit and temporal fossa (arrowheads). Note the right exophthalmos. (B,C) Early and later-phase internal maxillary arteriograms, lateral view, showing tumoral opacification. (D) Internal maxillary arteriogram, lateral view. Postembolization control showing contrast medium reflux to internal carotid. (E) Control computed tomogram 3 months later. (F) Right adrenal selective arteriogram demonstrating primary tumor mass in the adrenal gland.

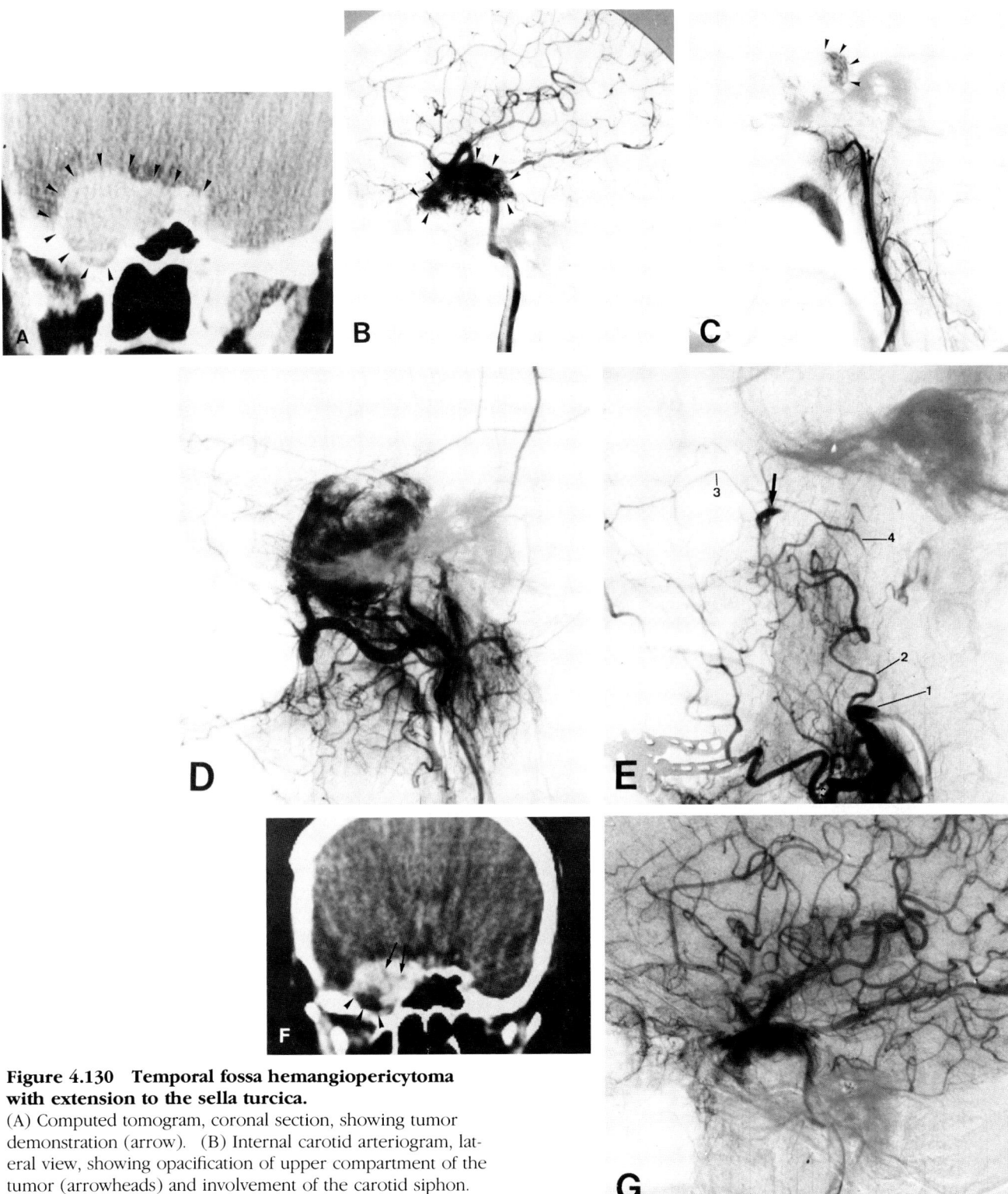

Figure 4.130 Temporal fossa hemangiopericytoma with extension to the sella turcica.
(A) Computed tomogram, coronal section, showing tumor demonstration (arrow). (B) Internal carotid arteriogram, lateral view, showing opacification of upper compartment of the tumor (arrowheads) and involvement of the carotid siphon. (C) Ascending pharyngeal arteriogram, lateral view, showing preferential opacification of the upper compartment (arrowheads). D) Internal maxillary arteriogram, lateral view, showing opacification of lower compartment of the tumor. (E) Facial arteriogram, lateral view. 1, facial artery; 2, ascending palatine artery; 3, infraorbital artery; 4, facial transverse artery. Control was performed immediately following embolization of internal maxillary and ascending pharyngeal arteries with Ivalon particles. Note the filling of the distal internal maxillary artery (arrow) without tumoral opacification. (F) Computed tomogram, coronal section. Control was performed 3 days after embolization. Note the intratumoral necrotic areas (arrows). Devascularization of the lower compartment and (arrowheads), as compared with (A). (G) Postembolization internal carotid control arteriogram showing significant tumoral volume reduction as compared with (B).

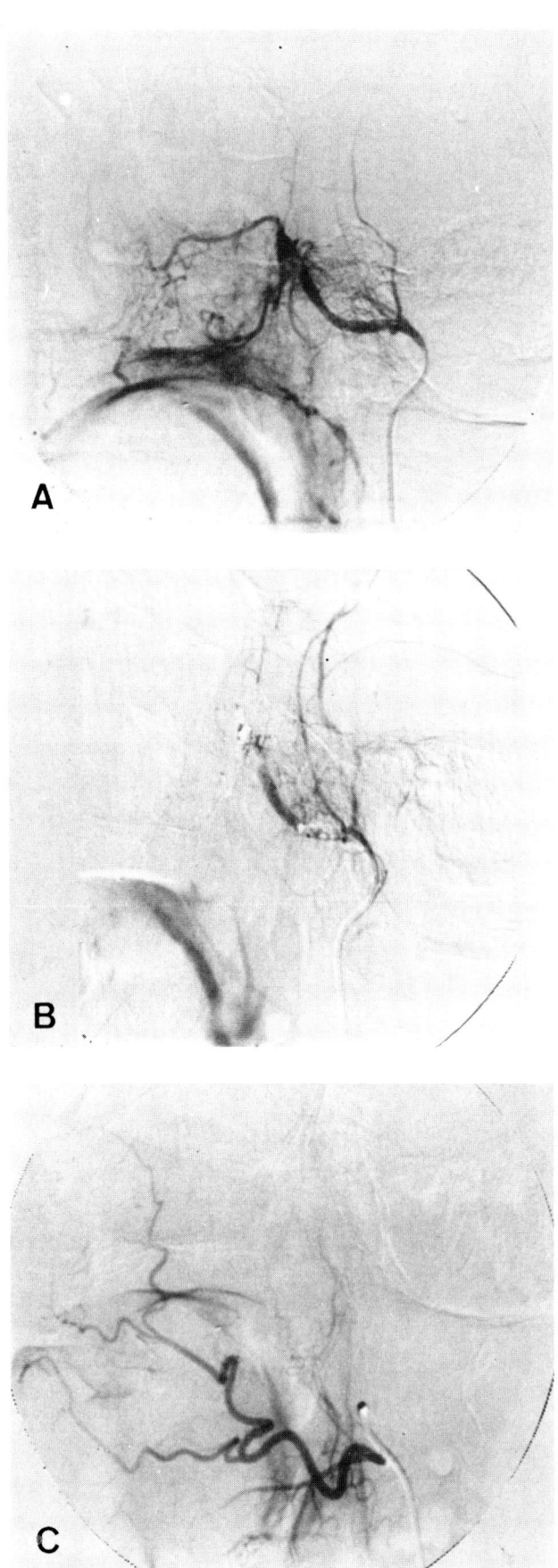

Angiography in a patient with epistaxis should be performed only after all conventional methods of hemostasis have proved ineffective. The complete protocol described here may be abbreviated or adapted in accordance with clinical information or as a result of pathologic conditions found during early series.

The decision to embolize, and the material to be used, will depend on bleeding site, origin, and volume.

In cases of epistaxis in which normal images are obtained, embolization should be performed with reabsorbable material in the internal maxillary artery. In cases of hereditary hemorrhagic telangiectasia, a permanent embolic material should be used. The angiographic control will be performed in the facial artery, on the same side. If control over hemorrhage is not achieved, complementary embolizations in the facial artery and in the internal maxillary artery on the opposite side may be required (Fig. 4.131).

In cases of epistaxis of traumatic origin, particularly in large craniofacial disjoining type lesions (LeFort III fractures), where bleeding may be catastrophic and lethal, embolization may be performed at first with Gelfoam, and the more proximal artery then occluded with bucrylate or a Gianturco coil (Fig. 4.132), in order to ensure definitive hemostasis.

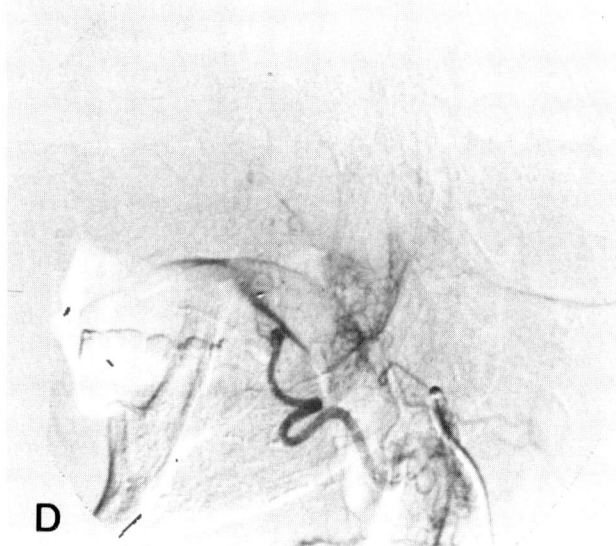

Figure 4.131 Spontaneous massive epistaxis in a patient with hypertensive crisis.
(A) Internal maxillary arteriogram, lateral view, showing absence of pathologic or contrast extravasation images.
(B) Internal maxillary arteriogram, lateral view. Control was performed immediately following embolization with Gelfoam particles soaked with Lipiodol. (C) Facial arteriogram, lateral view. Control was performed after embolization of the internal maxillary artery. (D) Facial arteriogram, lateral view. Final control performed after embolization with the same material. Permanent control of epistaxis was obtained with this procedure.

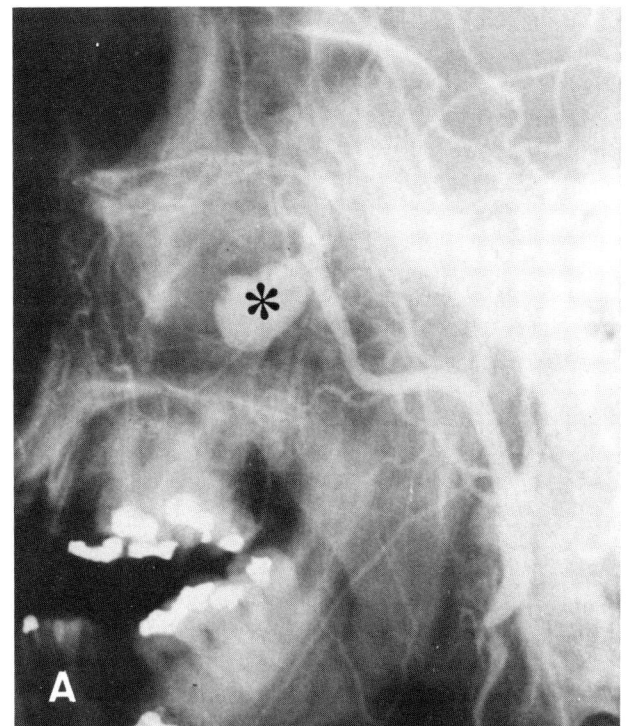 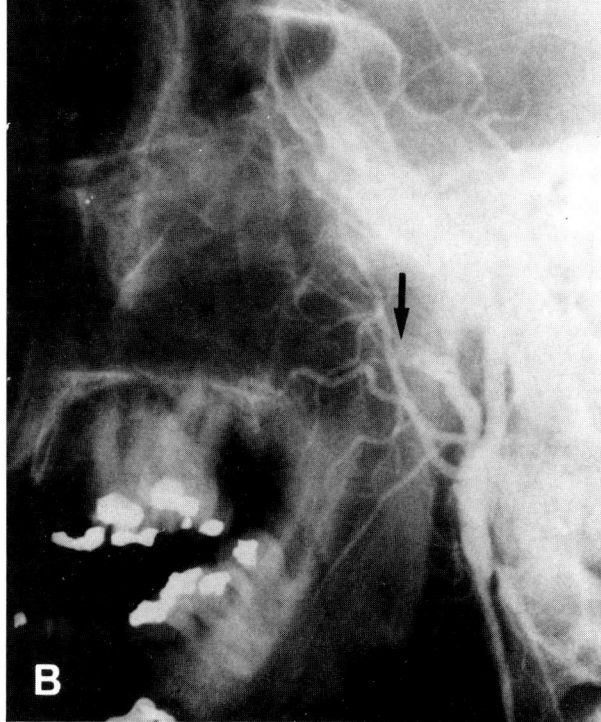

Figure 4.132 Massive epistaxis following craniofacial trauma (Leford III).
(A) Internal maxillary arteriogram, lateral view, showing a pseudoaneurysm (*) in the distal segment of the internal maxillary artery. (B) Permanent control of bleeding was obtained following distal embolization with Gelfoam particles and a more proximal 3-mm Gianturco coil (arrow).

REFERENCES

Head and Neck

Aminoff MJ. Vascular anomalies in the intracranial dura mater. *Brain* 1973;96:601–612.

Andre JM, Picard L, Fays J, et al. Angiomatose de Rendu-Osler: Etude clinique et pathogenique. Aspects angiographiques des localizations viscerales. *J Neuroradiol* 1974;1:233–255.

Athanasoulis CA, Pfister RC, Greene RE, Roberson GH. The central nervous system. In *Interventional Radiology,* edited by Athanasoulis CA. Saunders, Philadelphia, 1982.

Bank WO, Kerber C, Cromwell LD. Treatment of intracerebral arteriovenous malformations with isobutyl-2-cyanoacrylate: Initial clinical experience. *Radiology* 1981;139:606–616.

Bank WO, Kerber CW, et al. Carotid cavernous fistula: Endarterial cyanoacrylate occlusion with preservation of carotid flow. *J Neuroradiol* 1978;5:279–285.

Berenstein A, Kricheff II. Catheter and material selection for transarterial embolization. Technical considerations II: Materials. *Radiology* 1979;132:619–631.

Berenstein A, Kricheff II. Catheter and material selection for transarterial embolization. Technical considerations II: Materials. *Radiology* 1979;132:631–641.

Brian M, Tress MB, et al. Management of carotid cavernous fistulas by surgery combined with interventional radiology. *J Neurosurg* 1983;59:1076–1081.

Brainin M, Samee P. Venous hemodynamics of arteriovenous meningeal fistulas in the posterior fossa. *Neuroradiology* 1983;15:161–169.

Braun IF, Levy S, Hoffman JC. The use of transarterial microembolization in the management of hemangiomas of the perioral region. *J Oral Maxillofac Surg* 1985;43:239–248.

Burrows PE, Mulliken JB, Fello KE et al. Childhood hemangiomas and vascular malformations: Angiographic differentiation. *AJR* 1983;141:483–488.

Castaigne P, Bories J, Brunet P, et al. Les fistules arterioveineuses maningees pures a drainage veineaux cortical. *Rev Neurol* 1976;132:169–181.

Chaudhary MY, Sachdev VP, Cho SH, et al. Dural arteriovenous malformations of the major venous sinuses: An acquired lesion. *AJNR* 1982;3:13–19.

Chiras J, Bories J, Leger JM et al. CT scan of dural arteriovenous fistulas. *Neuroradiology* 1982;23:185–194.

Davis KR. Embolization of epistaxis and juvenile nasopharyngeal angiofibromas. *AJNR* 1986;7:953–962.

Debrun G, Davis KR, Hochberg FH. Superselective injection of BCNU through a latex calibrated leak balloon. *AJNR* 1983;4:399–400.

Debrun G, Lacour P, et al. Treatment of 54 traumatic carotic cavernous fistulas. *J Neurosurg* 1981;55:678–692.

Debrun G, Vinuela F, Fox A, Drake CG, et al. Embolization of cerebral arteriovenous malformations with Bucrylate: Experience in 46 cases. *J Neurosurg* 1982;56:615–627.

Djindjian R, Cophingnon J, et al. Plymorphieme neuroradiologique des fistulas carotido-cavernueses. *Neurochirurgie* 1968;14:881–890.

Djindjian R, Merland JJ. *Superselective Arteriography of the External Carotid Artery.* Springer-Verlag, New York, 1978.

Doyon D, Lasjaunias P, Manelfe C, Merland JJ, Moret J, Picard L, Theron J. Analysis of the complications of therapeutical angiography: Review of 850 cases. XI Symposium, Wiesbaden, June 1978.

Gigaud M. L'embolization par catheterisme percutane en pathologie neurochirurgicale. Theses pour la doctorat d'etat en Medecine. Universita Paul-Sabatier, Toulouse, 1976.

Grisoli F, Vincentelli F, Fuchs S et al. Surgical treatment of tentorial arteriovenous malformations draining into the subarachnoid space: Report of four cases. *J Neurosurg* 1984;60:1059–1066.

Hayes GJ. External carotid cavernous sinus fistulas. *J Neurosurg* 1963;20:692–700.

Houser OW, Baker Jr HL, Rhoton Al Jr, et al. Intracranial dural arteriovenous malformations. *Radiology* 1972;105:55–64.

Humeau F, Fourre D, LeRoquais P, Lesaint JN. Embolization arterielle dans le traitement des tumeurs neoplasiques. *Presse Medicale* 1975;4:1709–1715.

Ito J, Imamura H, Kobayashi K, et al. Dural arteriovenous malformations of the base of the anterior cranial fossa. *Neuroradiology* 1983;24:149–154.

Kataoka K, Taneda M. Angiographic disappearance of multiple dural arteriovenous malformations: Case report. *J Neurosurg* 1984;60:1275–1278.

Kerber CW. Intracranial cyanoacrylate, a new catheter therapy for arteriovenous malformation. *Invest Radiol* 1975;10:536–538.

Kosnik EJ, Hunt WE, Miller CA. Dural arteriovenous malformations. *J Neurosurg* 1974;40:322–229.

Krayenbuhl H, Yasargil I. *Cerebral Angiography.* Georg Thieme Verlag, Stuttgart, 1982.

Kuhner A, Krastel A, Stoll W. Arteriovenous malformations of the transverse dural sinus. *J Neurosurg* 1976;45:12–19.

Lamas E, Lobato RD, Esparza J, et al. Dural posterior fossa AVM producing raised sagittal sinus pressure: Case report. *J Neurosurg* 1977;46:804–810.

Lapresle J, Lasjaunias P. Cranial nerve ischemic arterial syndromes: A review. *Brain* 1986;109:207–215.

Lasjaunias P. *Craniofacial and Upper Cervical Arteries: Collateral Circulation and Angiograph Protocols.* Williams & Wilkins, Baltimore, 1983.

Lasjaunias P, Appel B, Carriere T. Maladie de Rendu-Osler-Weber: Evaluation diagnostique et therapeutique par l'angiographie. *Ann Otolaryngol Chir Cervicofac (Paris)* 1983;100:203–215.

Lasjaunias P, Berenstein A. *Surgical Neuroangiography,* Vol I. *Functional Anatomy of Craniofacial Arteries.* Springer-Verlag, New York, 1986.

Lasjaunias P, Berenstein A. *Surgical Neuroangiography,* Vol II. *Craniofacial Embolization.* Springer-Verlag, New York, 1986.

Lasjaunias P, Deffez JP, Fellus P, et al. Les malformations vasculaires linguales: Leurs consequences sur la croissance de letage inferieur. *Rev Stomatol Chir Maxillofac* 1985–86;2:99–102.

Lasjaunias P, Doyon D. L'artere pharyngienne ascendante dans la vascularization des dernieres paires craniennes. *J Neuroradiol* 1978;5:287–301.

Lasjaunias P, Doyon D. Embolization in tumours and vascular malformations of the head and neck. *Ann Acad Med* 1980;9:332–341.

Lasjaunias P, Doyon D. L'angiographie das les malformations de la cavite buccale. *Rev Stomatol Chir Maxillofac* 1982–83;2/3:111–115.

Lasjaunias P, Halim P, Lopez-Ibor, et al. Traitment endovasculaire des malformations vasculaires durales (MVD) pures "spontanees": Revue de 23 cas explores et traites entre Mai 1980 et Octobre 1983. *Neurochirurgie* 1984;30:207–223.

Lasjaunias P, Lopez-Ibor L, Abanou A, et al. Radiological anatomy of the vascularization of cranial dural arteriovenous malformations. *Anat Clin* 1984;6:87–99.

Lasjaunias P, Marsot-Dupuch K, Doyon D. Bases radioanatomiques de l'embolisation arterielle au cours des epistaxis. *J Neuroradiol* 1979;6:45–53.

Lasjaunias P, Menu Y, Bonnel D, Doyon D. Nonchromaffin paragangliomas of the head and neck. *J Neuroradiol* 1981;8:281–199.

Lasjaunias P, Ming C, Brugge KT, et al. Neurological manifestations of intracranial dural arteriovenous malformations. *J Neurosurg* 1986;64:724–730.

Lasjaunias P, Picard L, Manelfe D, Moret J, Doyon D. Angiofibrome naso-pharyngien: Review de 53 cas avec embolization. *J Neuroradiol* 1980;7:73–95.

Lee YY, Walace S, Dimery I, Goepfert H. Intraarterial chemotherapy of head and neck tumors. *AJNR* 1986;7:343–348.

Leikensohn JR, Epstein LI, Vasconez LO. Superselective embolization and surgery of noninvoluting hemangiomas and AV malformations. *Plast Reconstr Surg* 1981;68:143–152.

Manelfe C, Berenstein A. Traitement des fistules carote-caverneuses par voie veineuse: A propos d'un cas. *J Neuroradiol* 1980;7:13–20.

Manelfe C, Guiraud B et al. Embolization par catheterisme des meninguiomes intra-craniens. *Rev Neurol (Paris)* 1973;128:339–351.

Merland JJ, Djindjian R. Manifestations cerebrales de la maladie de Rendu-Osler. *J Neuroradiol* 1974;1:257–285.

Miyasaka K, Takei H, Nomura M et al. Computerized tomography findings in dural arteriovenous malformations: Report of three cases. *J Neurosurg* 1980;53:698–702.

Moret J. La vascularization de l'appareil auditif: Normal variantes, tumerus glomiques. *J Neuroradiol* 1982;9:209–260.

Mulliken JB, Glowacki J. Hemangiomas and vascular malformations in infants and children: A classification based on endothelial characteristics. *Plast Reconstr Surg* 1982;69:412–420.

Mulliken JB, Zetter BR, Folkman J. In vitro characteristics of endothelium from hemangiomas and vascular malformations. *Surgery* 1982;92:348–352.

Obrador S, Soto M, Silvela J. Clinical syndromes of arteriovenous malformations of the transverse sigmoid sinus. *J Neurol Neurosurg Psychiatry* 1975;38:436–541.

Parkinson D. Carotid cavernous fistula: Direct repair with preservation of the carotid artery. Technical note. *J Neurosurg* 1976;38:99–106.

Pasyk KA, Dingman RO, Argenta LC, et al. The management of hemangiomas of the eyelid and orbit. *Head Neck Surg* 1984;6:851–857.

Picard L, Manelfe C, et al. Embolizations et occlusions par bollonnets dans les lesions vasculaires cranio-faciales. *J Neuroradiol* 1978;16:393–394.

Picard L, Moret J, LePoire J. Traitement endovasculaire des angiomes arterio-veineus intracerebraux. *J Neuroradiol* 1984;11:9–28.

Piske RL, Lasjaunias P. Extrasinusal dural arteriovenous malformations: Report of three cases. In press.

Popescu V. Intratumoral ligation in the management of orofacial cavernous hemangiomas. *J Oral Maxillofac Surg* 1985;13:99–107.

Rey A, Cophignon J, Djindjian R, Houdart R. Traitement des fistules carotido-caverneuses. *Neurochirurgie* 1973;19:111–122.

Riche CW. Intracranial cyanoacrylate, a new catheter therapy for arteriovenous malformation. *Invest Radiol* 1975;10:536–538.

Sampaio MM, Couto BA, et al. Fistula carotido-cavernosa: Tratamento por oclusao endovascular. *Rev Bras Neurol* 1983;19:5–8.

Serbinenko FA. Balloon catheterization and occlusion of major cerebral vessels. *J Neurosurg* 1974;41:125–145.

Spiegel SM, Vinuela F, Goldwasser MJ, Fox AJ, Pelz DM. Adjusting the polimerization time of isobutyl-2-cyanoacrylate. *AJNR* 1986;7:109–112.

Tazi Z, Lasjaunias P, Doyon D. Malformations vasculaires invasives de la face et du scalp: Evaluation diagnostique et therapeutique par l'angiographie. Revue de 32 cas entre 1977–1980. *Rev Stomatol Chir Maxillofac* 1982;83:24–35.

Terada T, Kikuchi H, Karasawai et al. Intracerebral arteriovenous malformation fed by the anterior ethmoidal artery: Case report. *Neurosurgery* 1984;14:578–582.

Theron J. Les affluents du plexus caverneaux. *Neurochirurgie* 1972;18:623–638.

Theron J, Chevalier D et al. Diagnosis of small and micro pituitary adenomas by intercavernous sinus venography: A preliminary report. *Neuroradiology* 1979;18:23–30.

Theron J, Lasjaunias P, Moret J, Merland JJ. Vascularization des meninges de la fossa posterieure. *J Neuroradiol* 1977;4:203–224.

Theron J, Olivier A, Melancon D, Ethier R. Left carotid cavernous fistula with right exophthalmos: Treatment by detachable balloon. Case report and literature review. *Neuroradiology* 1985;27:349–353.

Thomason HG, Ward CM, Crawford JS, et al. Hemangiomas of the eyelid: Visual complications and prophylactic concepts. *Plast Reconstr Surg* 1979;1:641–647.

Toppozada H, Michaels L, Toppozada M, et al. The human respiratory nasal mucosa in pregnancy: An electron microscopic and histochemical study. *J Laryngol Otol* 1982;976:613–626.

Uflacker R. Transcatheter embolization of arterial aneurysms. *Br J Radiol* 1986;59:317–324.

Uflacker R, Lima S, Ribas GC, Piske RL. Carotid cavernous fistulas: Embolization through the superior ophthalmic vein approach. *Radiology* 1986;159:175–179.

Wisnicki FL. Hemangiomas and vascular malformations. *Ann Plast Surg* 1984;12:41–58.

Chapter Five
Interventional Radiology in the Biliary Tract
RENAN UFLACKER

INTRODUCTION

The introduction of percutaneous transhepatic cholangiography has allowed greater efficiency in the exploration of the biliary tree in patients with obstructive jaundice. The use of a fine needle (Chiba needle) has significantly lowered the morbidity associated with this procedure. When a fine needle is used, the biliary tree can be visualized adequately in practically 100 percent of patients when it is dilated and in 70 to 80 percent of patients when it is not dilated.

In icteric patients with a biliary tree of normal diameter, a percutaneous cholangiogram can safely exclude the presence of biliary obstruction. In patients with obstructive jaundice, the site of obstruction can be identified, along with the cause of obstruction, in many cases. However, the cause of obstructive jaundice is best identified by means of associated diagnostic procedures, such as computed tomography (CT), ultrasound, and selective arteriography of the celiac axis and superior mesenteric artery.

The next step in the development of biliary tree manipulation was external biliary drainage, which alleviates jaundice, reducing the morbidity rate compared with percutaneous large-needle cholangiography. This method of external drainage was utilized as a preoperative technique in patients with malignant and benign biliary obstruction. The technique of internal biliary drainage, which was developed later, allows the passage of bile into the duodenal lumen. However, this technique required special skills in catheterization and the manipulation of guidewires and catheters inside the biliary tree. Significant improvements in the material used for percutaneous manipulation of the biliary tree followed, with the introduction of more rigid guidewires especially suited for catheter exchange and guidewires with torque control and tip rotation that allow the physician to catheterize orifices and tracks inside the biliary tree and pass beyond the obstruction. Catheters for internal and external drainage as well as endoprostheses for internal drainage were also improved, supplying the interventional radiologist with a new therapeutic armamentarium.

The great value of biliary drainage by the percutaneous route is that it provides an alternative for patients with malignant nonresectable lesions, avoiding the morbidity and mortality rates associated with the merely palliative surgical procedure of biliary tree shunt.

INDICATIONS AND CONTRAINDICATIONS

Palliation of obstructive unresectable lesions is a major indication for percutaneous biliary drainage in patients with malignant lesions. Biliary drainage performed through a catheter or with an endoprosthesis implant is used to counteract the complications caused by the biliary obstructive process and cholestasis, including pain in the right hypochondrium, the hyposthenic syndrome, pruritus, anorexia, and weight loss. General and specific indications for this procedure are listed in Table 5.1.

Table 5.1 – Indications for Internal-External Percutaneous Biliary Drainage or the Placement of an Endoprosthesis

General
   Extrahepatic obstruction
     Pruritus
     Cholangitis, hepatic microabscesses, sepsis
     Hepatic dysfunction
       hemorrhagic syndromes
       hepatic coma
Specific
   Palliative (unresectable malignant neoplasm)
   Presurgical preparation
   Acute suppurative cholangitis (usually associated with lithiasis)
   Dilatation of biliary tree stenoses
   Stenoses of a biliary-digestive anastomosis
   Removal of residual biliary tree calculi

The most simple use of percutaneous drainage of the biliary tree is to improve the general condition of patients with biliary obstruction and improve the quality of survival in patients with malignant lesions. The timing, duration, and type of biliary drainage performed depend on the patient's general condition, the etiology of the obstruction, and any complications that have occurred as a consequence of the obstructive process.

In a common bile duct obstruction in a patient with lithiasis, there is no indication for biliary tree drainage except when acute suppurative cholangitis is associated with the obstruction. In this case, external drainage with a minimum of manipulation is the least aggressive and most effective procedure. In a second stage, after the septic period is over, internal-external drainage may be instituted prior to surgery. A percutaneous removal or lysis of stones is sometimes performed.

In patients with other types of benign obstructions, postsurgical stenosis, or common bile duct diaphragm without signs of infection, internal-external drainage should be instituted immediately. In patients with benign postoperative stenoses, dilatation with a balloon catheter is effective in the recovery process of this difficult surgical procedure. The most common use of biliary tree drainage is to provide palliative treatment of biliary obstructions caused by malignant neoplasms, either primary or metastatic to the portahepatis; 80 percent of these patients present with an unresectable lesion when the diagnosis is made, and the chances of a surgical cure are practically nil.

There are only a few contraindications for percutaneous drainage of the biliary tree, because this technique is most frequently used in patients who are too ill for surgery. Relative contraindications include hemorrhagic diathesis and diffuse or massive hepatic metastases. The presence of ascites is not a serious contraindication. However, ascites may hinder the procedure significantly in a number of patients as a result of hepatic mobility, which creates a distance between the abdominal wall and the hepatic surface, preventing the catheter and guidewire from advancing in a linear fashion. This difficulty can be overcome by the use of rigid metallic wires and Teflon dilators and Desilet-Hoffman–type sheaths.

A prothrombin time below 50 percent should be improved by the use of vitamin K for at least 2 days before drainage is performed. The platelet count should be above 50,000 mm^3; it can be corrected by infusion of platelets or fresh blood.

The presence of sepsis and coma, although indicating a bad prognosis, is not an absolute contraindication for drainage. Breaking the continence of infected bile in the biliary tree may improve the patient's general condition. However, it is true that the complications of biliary drainage are much greater in septic patients.

PATIENT PREPARATION

Once the coagulation parameters have been corrected, prophylactic coverage with antibiotics should be initiated 72 h before the procedure. Intramuscular (IM) gentamicin (80 mg every 8 h) and intravenous (IV) Cefoxetin (1 g every 6 h) can be used in these patients.

Adequate hydration can be achieved with a 5% or 10% glucose solution. Preinterventional medication is also required. Usually, a diazepam tablet (10 mg) is given 1 h before the procedure and an opiate analgesis is administered IV during the procedure in fractionated doses, varying according to the individual patient. A fast-acting short-duration fentanyl-type drug is given at a dose of 2 mL IV every hour or at shorter intervals. Sedation should not be too liberal, as these are usually debilitated, septic patients who may suffer respiratory arrest. Therefore, the use of shorter-duration drugs or drugs whose effects are easily reversed is generally advisable.

MATERIALS

For a biliary drainage of any type to be performed effectively, the radiology department should have an x-ray apparatus with a high-quality TV monitor and image intensifier, along with a whole range of materials, including catheters of different types and models and metallic guidewires of many different types.

The following list gives the minimum materials necessary for performing percutaneous drainage of the biliary tree.

1. Contrast medium diluted to 50%.
2. A No. 22 or 23 Chiba needle, 15 cm long, with an external diameter of 0.8 or 0.9 mm.
3. Connector tubes with plastic hubs.
4. A 25-cm-long needle with a No. 5 French radiopaque Teflon sheath.
5. A 0.038-in. straight guidewire with torque control and a shapeable tip with memory (Lunderquist guidewire).
6. A 0.038-in. straight guidewire with a flexible tip and rigid shaft (Lunderquist) for catheter exchange.
7. A 0.038-in. guidewire with a 3-mm J-tip and heavy-duty resistance.
8. A pigtail No. 10 French catheter for external drainage.
9. A pigtail No. 8.3 French Ring-type catheter or a Cope-type catheter (No. 8, 10, or 12 French) for internal-external drainage.
10. Endoprosthesis equipment in all its different presentations for internal drainage (the Pereiras, Coons, Hoevels, and Burcharth types), varying from No. 7 to

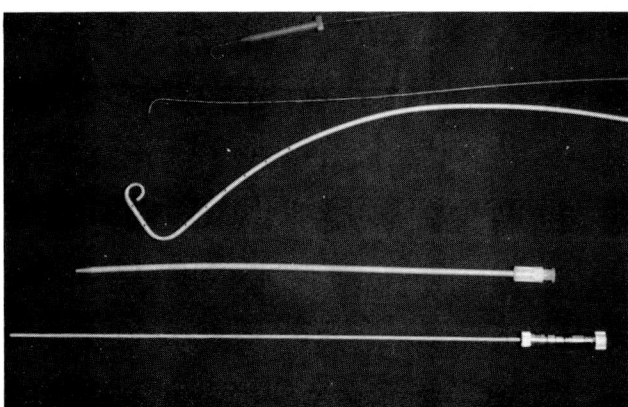

Figure 5.1 Minimum required materials for biliary drainage. From top to bottom: 3-mm J-guidewire; Lunderquist guidewire with torque and a shapable tip; internal-external drainage type catheter of the ring type with lateral orifices and a pigtail tip; No. 8 and No. 10 French Teflon dilators; needle with a metallic trocar and a No. 5 French Teflon sheath.

No. 14 French in diameter. The Gianturco Z stent is also useful. These plastic endoprostheses can be purchased ready for use or can be made from the large-diameter fine-walled tubes that are readily available in any angiography laboratory.

There are many other variations in the types and sizes of these materials, and changes in existing products are frequently introduced. However, these basic materials can be used to solve the great majority of problems that arise during biliary drainage (Fig. 5.1).

TECHNIQUE

Technically, biliary tree drainage always starts with a percutaneous cholangiogram with a Chiba needle, which opacifies the biliary tree, defines the site of obstruction, and selects the most convenient biliary duct for puncturing to initiate catheterization. The puncture site should be caudal to the costophrenic sinus in its maximal inspiration. However, the pleural recess sometimes extends up to the 9th and 10th costal arches at the level of the right midaxillary line. In this situation, the pleural space is always violated in the course of the procedure (Fig. 5.2).

The puncture site should be located on the midaxillary line, just above the upper border of the 9th or 10th rib, with the needle introduced toward the T11 vertebral body. The bevel angulation of the Chiba needle can be utilized to direct the puncture.

Once the liver has been punctured and the trocar has been removed, the needle is slowly pulled back, with simultaneous injection of contrast medium, until one of the intrahepatic biliary ducts is opacified. The Chiba needle is flexible and bends very easily, and so its track inside the liver can be controlled better if a quick and firm puncture is performed all at once instead of a slow and hesitating progression toward T11. Fast, high-volume contrast injection should not be done, as extravasation and parenchymal cavitation due to contrast medium can cause serious problems in regard to the visualization of structures under fluoroscopy.

When the Chiba need is pulled back during contrast injection, several structures may be visualized. Portal radicles appear as large, branched structures which are quickly emptied of injected contrast, although they are very similar to biliary ducts. Apart from that, the flow follows a peripheral direction, almost always impregnating the parenchyma on the segment which has been injected. Hepatic arteries have a small diameter with a smaller number of branches and are very rapidly emptied after injection, causing less parenchymal impregnation.

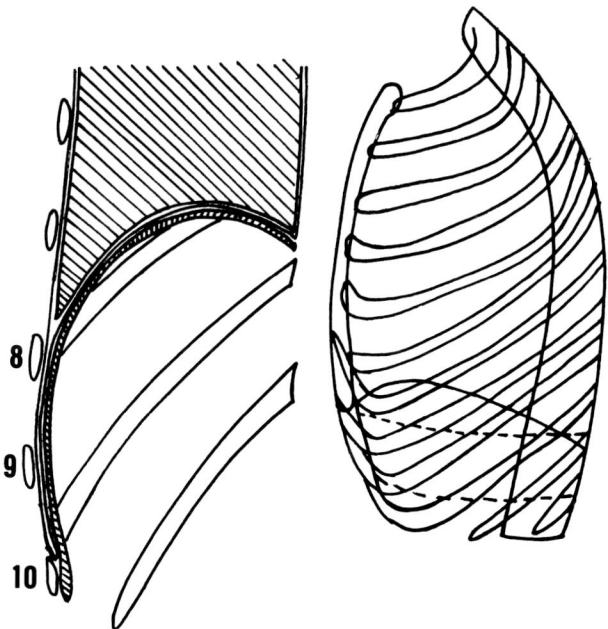

Figure 5.2 Schematic drawing of the frontal and lateral views of position relative to the costophrenic sinus and the actual pleural recess with the lower costal arches. The puncture site is necessarily located at the level of the intercostal spaces, between the 8th and 9th ribs and between the 9th and 10th ribs (arrowheads). Note that puncture at the levels indicated by the arrowheads always violates the pleural space, even several centimeters below the radiologic costophrenic sinus.

Visualization of lymphatics results from intraparenchymal injection of contrast medium, with these vessels appearing as fine, serpentlike irregular structures which do not produce any branches and drain in a hilar direction, remaining opacified for some time.

Hepatic veins are tubular, usually with a large diameter and without visible ramifications, following an oblique path as compared with the remaining vascular structures. They are rapidly emptied cranial, oriented toward the right atrium.

In some cases, periportal extravasation with tubular dissection occurs, delineating the portal radicles in negative. This is a common finding in patients with diseases that cause periportal thickening as a result of fibrosis.

The biliary ducts are immediately identifiable when opacified. When dilated, they have larger diameters and spread out in branches; in this case contrast opacifies them in a slow fashion, preferably in a peripheral direction, without mixing immediately with the bile. If the injection is interrupted, contrast remains stable inside the biliary tree. If the tree is not dilated, the ducts have a smaller diameter, and contrast-medium flow, although slow, follows a hilar direction, with immediate opacification of the hepatic duct and filling of the duodenal lumen. Once one is sure that the needle is inside the lumen of the biliary duct, a sufficient volume of contrast medium is injected to partially opacify the biliary tree and locate the site of obstruction.

If the etiology and level of obstruction are already known, only partial filling of the biliary tree by means of cholangiography is necessary. If the diagnosis is unknown, the biliary tree should be filled to the point of obstruction, and the type of obstruction should be evaluated using Owen's criteria (Fig. 5.3). The point of obstruction can be located in almost 90 percent of all patients through the cholangiogram alone, and a correct diagnosis can be achieved with cholangiography alone in 71 percent of patients. The use of other associated imaging methods will significantly increase dignostic accuracy regarding the etiology of the obstruction.

The biliary tree should not be excessively dilated, causing an increase of intraductal pressure, during a diagnostic cholangiographic procedure, since this will increase the risk of bacterial dissemination into the bloodstream. Elevating the table or changing the patient's position may improve visualization of the hilar region and the hepatic duct.

It is difficult to aspirate bile through a Chiba needle; however, whenever possible, partial emptying of the biliary tree should be attempted. If biliary obstruction

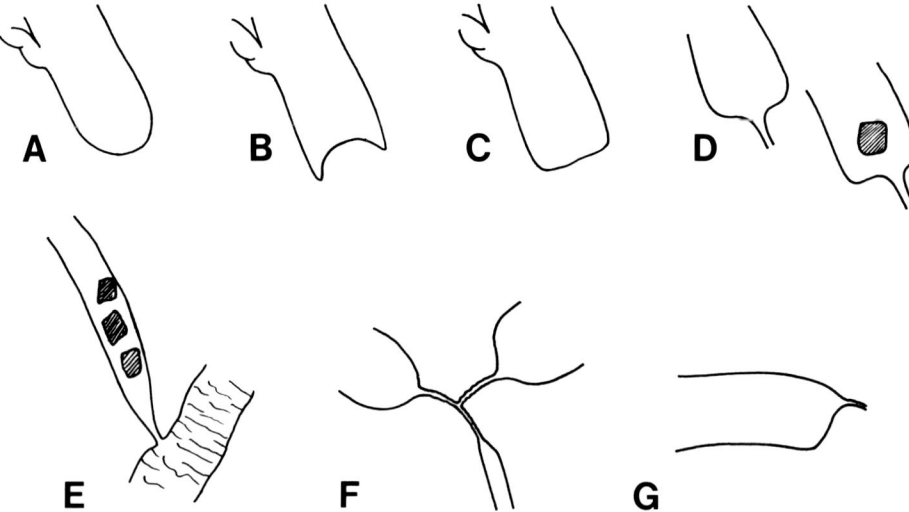

Figure 5.3 Schematic drawing of the different patterns of extrahepatic obstruction of the biliary tree in different groups of diseases.

(A) Convexity in the caudal direction, seen frequently in carcinoma of the pancreatic head. (B) Convexity in the cranial direction (image of inverted meniscus), common in impacted stones. (C) Abrupt interruption ("cut-off") with irregular borders. This is found frequently in carcinoma of the pancreatic head and hilar metastases. (D) Biconcave obstruction in the caudal direction, with or without calculi. This is seen in lithiasis with an associated inflammatory process and chronic pancreatitis (usually of the more elongated, pencil-tip type), is found frequently in ductal primary neoplasms, and is found occasionally in carcinoma of the pancreatic head. (E) Nonimpacted calculi with a normal or moderately dilated common bile duct. (F) Biconcave obstruction of the right and left ducts, with a common hepatic duct of normal diameter. This is characteristic of cholangiocarcinoma (Klatzkin's tumor). (G) Sudden biconcave eccentric obstruction and a horizontal common bile duct, seen frequently in carcinoma of the head of the pancreas and hilar metastases with extension into the retroduodenal space.

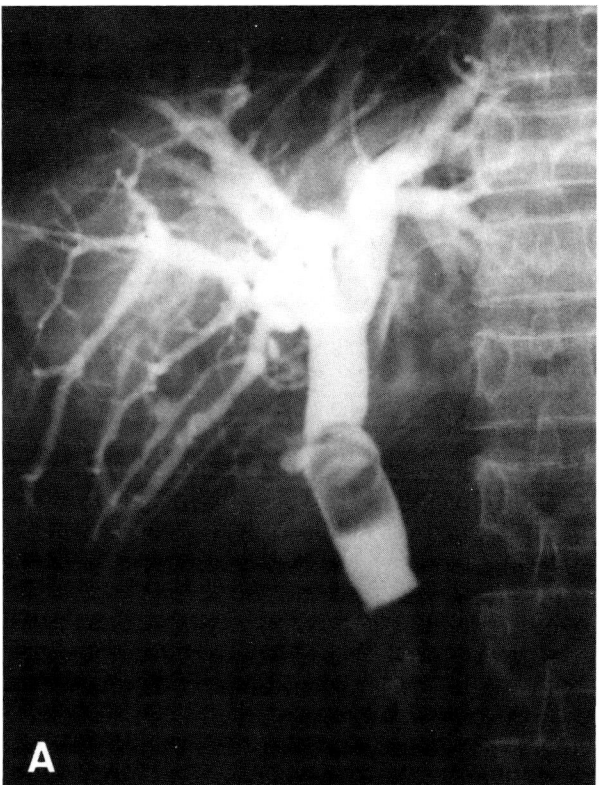
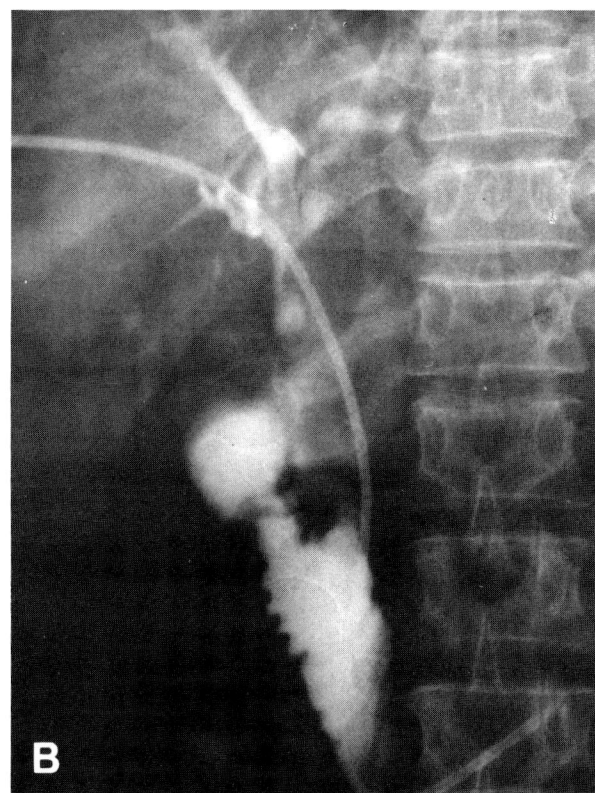

Figure 5.4 A 48-year-old patient with lithiasis of the common bile duct producing biliary obstruction and cholangitis.
(A) A percutaneous cholangiogram shows a dilated biliary tree, intracholedochal stones, and abrupt obstruction.
(B) Internal-external drainage with a No. 8.5 French catheter decompressing the biliary tree and improvement of cholangitis as a preoperative measure. In this patient, since the drainage system was easily passed into the duodenum, simple external drainage was not performed, as is advisable in most cases.

is due to the presence of stones and there are no signs of sepsis, the procedure can be terminated at this diagnostic stage. However, if the procedure is indicated for obstruction and lithisiac cholangitis, external drainage should be performed (Fig. 5.4), and if the obstruction is caused by a malignant lesion, percutaneous biliary drainage should be carried out.

To perform biliary drainage, a puncture should be made with a polyethylene or Teflon-sheathed needle which can accommodate inside its lumen a 0.038-in. J-guidewire. Puncture with a sheathed needle 20 to 25 cm long and around 1.6 mm in diameter (No. 5 French) is made toward a peripheral intrahepatic biliary duct with a large diameter and is directed as horizontally as possible with regard to the puncture needle. The less the parenchyma is penetrated between the hepatic capsule and the punctured duct, the lower the chance of complications such as hemorrhage and bile leakage into the peritoneum developing.

If puncture of the biliary duct is not successful on the first attempt, it should be repeated by redirecting the needle caudally and dorsally or ventrally. Normally, when the duct is adequately punctured, a wall deformity is seen under fluoroscopy, and upon removal of the trocar, bile flows freely through the catheter. At this point, a J-guidewire or a Lundérquist guidewire with torque control and a shapable tip is introduced and carefully advanced inside the biliary tree, toward the hepatic hilum (Fig. 5.5).

The confluence of the right and left ducts should be avoided during puncture; it is usually extrahepatic, and perforation may cause extensive bile effusion into the peritoneum. If a right lobe duct is not adequate for drainage, the puncture should be made into the left lobe, using an anterior subcostal approach.

When the lumen of the biliary tree is catheterized, the needle sheath is advanced inside the biliary track, and an attempt is made to pass beyond the obstruction.

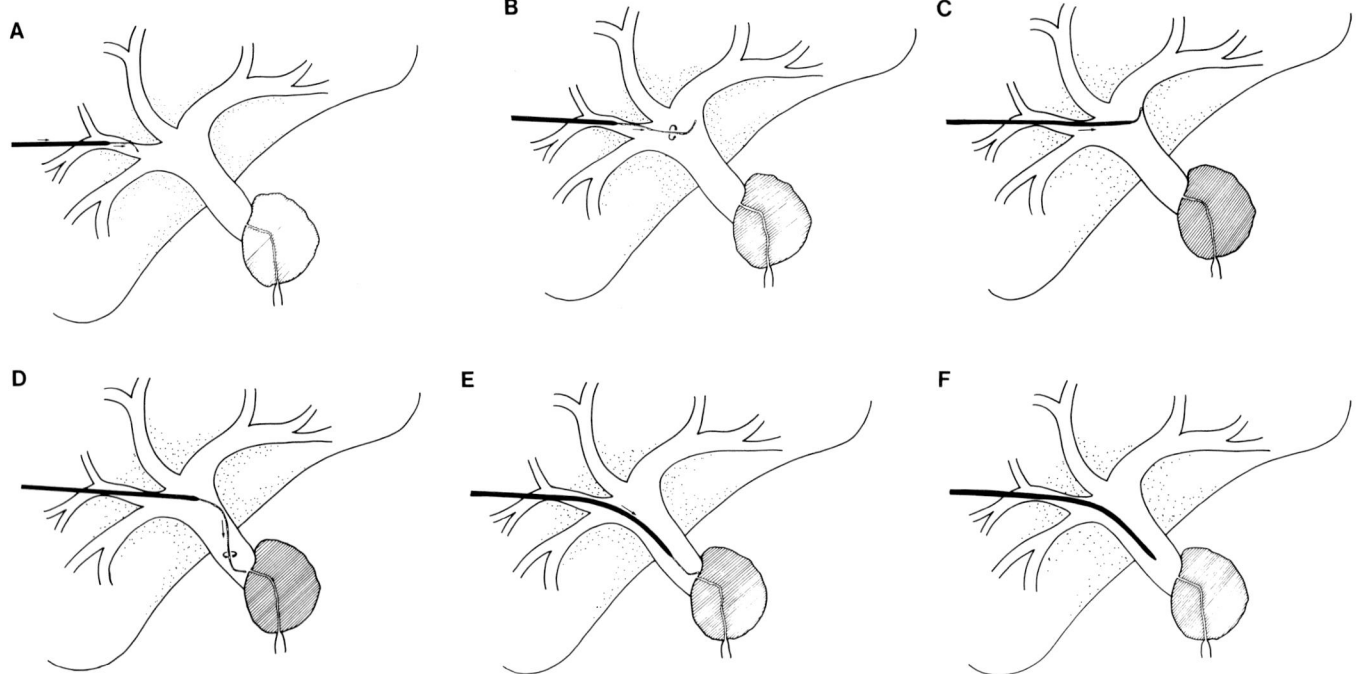

Figure 5.5 Procedure for guidewire and catheter manipulation to catheterize the biliary tree by the percutaneous route.

(A) Selecting a peripheral duct parallel to the axis of the puncture needle to achieve penetration into the biliary tree. The guidewire is introduced through the needle sheath, using the J-guidewire. (B) Rotating and advancing the guidewire into the biliary duct to the confluence. (C) Advancing the needle sheath up to the confluence. (D) Manipulating the guidewire again in an attempt to advance it to the point of obstruction. (E) Advancing the sheath as far as the common bile duct at the level of the obstruction. (F) Removing the guidewire, partially draining the bile, and making a new injection of diluted contrast for documentation and better visualization of the point of obstruction.

There are three basic types of percutaneous biliary drainage: external (Fig. 5.6), internal-external (combined) (Fig. 5.7), and internal (endoprosthesis) (Fig. 5.8).

External Biliary Drainage

Once the biliary tree has been opacified and punctured, a J-guidewire is advanced as deeply as possible inside the tree. The needle sheath is then removed, and progressive track dilatation is done over the guidewire with rigid Teflon Nos. 6, 7, 8, and 10 French dilators. Then a pigtail-type catheter for external drainage is advanced over the guidewire. This catheter, which has lateral holes, is fixed onto the skin and maintained with or without continuous aspiration (Fig. 5.6).

This type of drainage is effective in lowering bilirubin levels in a relatively short time but may cause severe hydroelectrolytic depletion if it is maintained permanently. Some measures can be used to restore the biliary salts, such as adding bile to fruit juices to be swallowed later, or introducing bile into the duodenum via a nasogastric tube. Some people freeze bile for later addition to beverages. This procedure may be done as a temporary presurgicial measure for biliary obstruction and should constitute the initial treatment for suppurative cholangitis, since it does not require prolonged hepatic manipulation and is easily performed.

Figure 5.9 shows a patient in whom only external drainage was performed because the obstruction could not be catheterized. Figure 5.10 shows a patient who received multiple external drainage for a diffuse biliary tree obstruction that made it impossible to go beyond the lesion and prevented drainage through a single tube.

Internal-External Biliary Drainage

After a percutaneous cholangiogram with opacification of the biliary tree, a puncture is made into a right lobe duct with a sheathed needle while the most rectilinear orientation possible is maintained in relation to the site of obstruction (Figs. 5.5 and 5.7). The guidewire is advanced to a point near the obstruction, usually at the

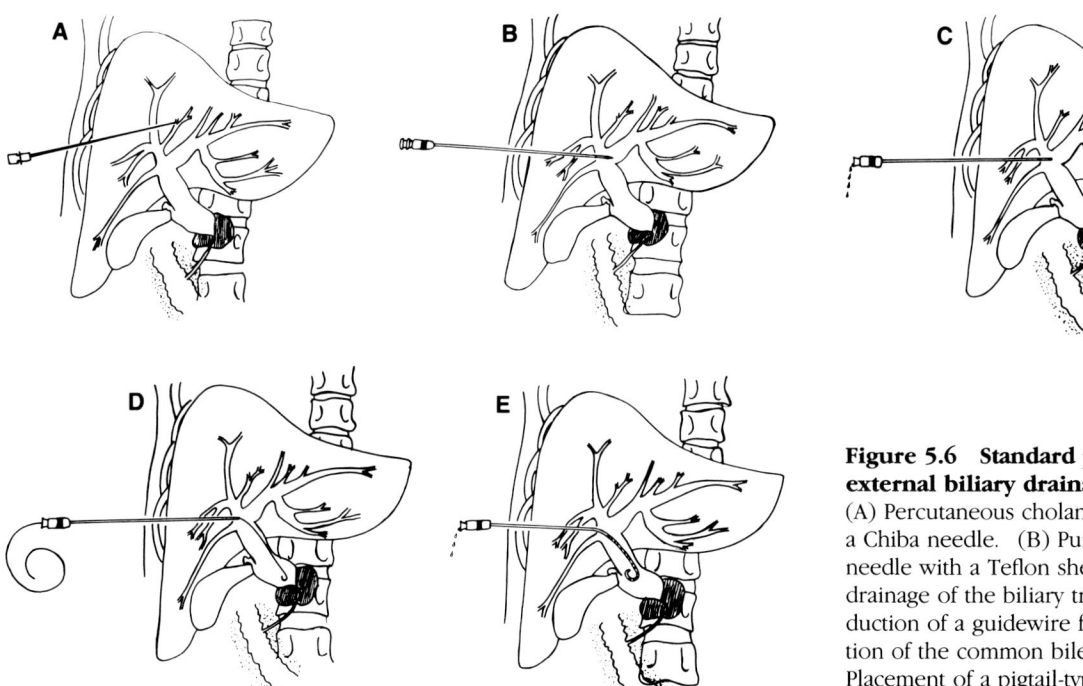

Figure 5.6 Standard procedure for external biliary drainage.
(A) Percutaneous cholangiography with a Chiba needle. (B) Puncture with a needle with a Teflon sheath. (C) Partial drainage of the biliary tree. (D) Introduction of a guidewire for catheterization of the common bile duct. (E) Placement of a pigtail-type catheter for external drainage.

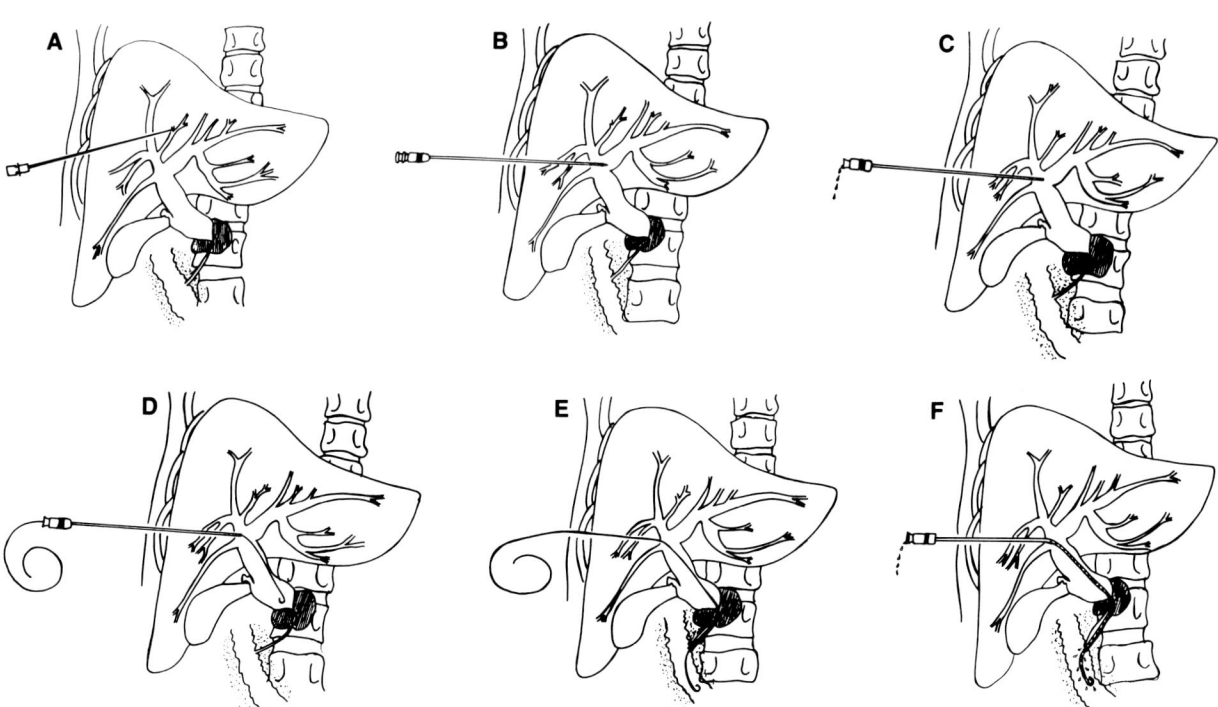

Figure 5.7 Standard procedure for internal-external biliary drainage.
(A) Percutaneous cholangiography with a Chiba needle. (B) Puncture with a needle with a Teflon sheath. (C) Partial drainage of the biliary tree. (D) Introduction of a guidewire for catheterization of the common bile duct. (E) Going beyond the obstruction with the guidewire, reaching the duodenum. (F) An internal-external Ring-type drainage catheter in the draining position, connecting the biliary tree to the duodenum.

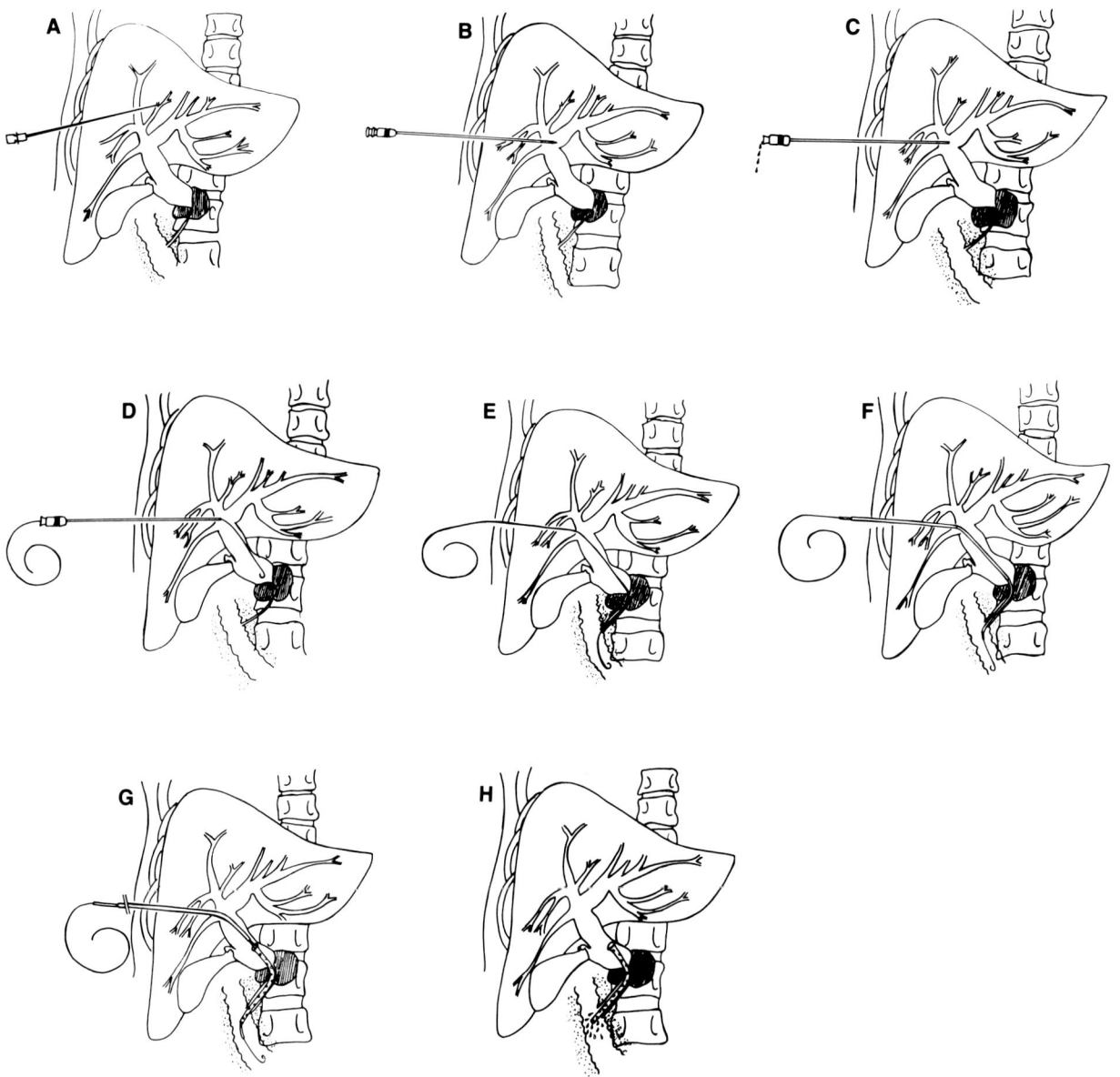

Figure 5.8 Standard procedure for internal biliary drainage (endoprosthesis).
(A) A percutaneous cholangiogram with a Chiba needle.
(B) Puncture with a needle with a Teflon sheath. (C) Partial drainage of the biliary tree. (D) Guidewire introduced for catheterization of the common bile duct. (E) Going beyond the obstruction with a guidewire, reaching the duodenum. (F) After passing beyond the obstructive lesion, the track is dilated by the coaxial introduction system of the endoprosthesis to the duodenum. (G) Placing a No. 12 French endoprosthesis over the No. 8 French guidewire and pushing it with the introducing catheter until it reaches its position through the obstruction. (H) An endoprosthesis in position for internal drainage, buried inside the biliary tree.

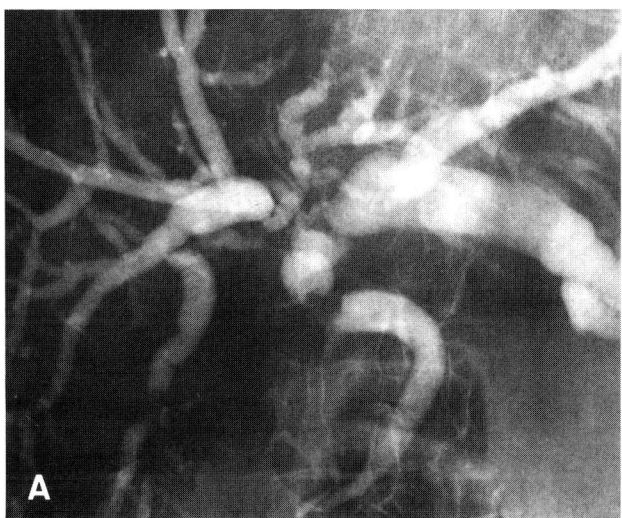
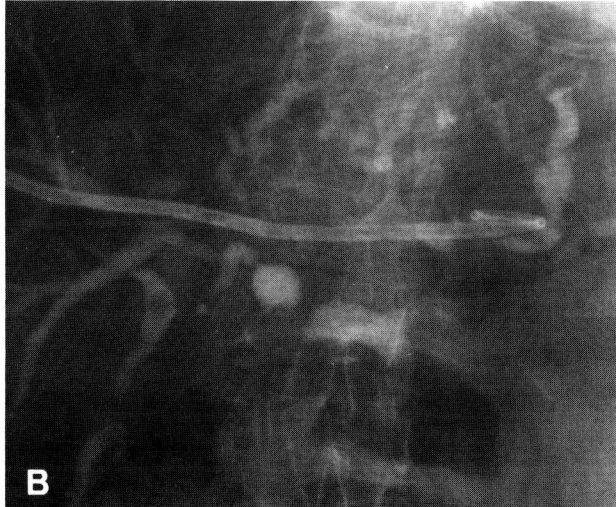

Figure 5.9 A 79-year-old patient with obstruction of the biliary tree caused by cholangiocarcinoma on the hepatic ducts and the common bile duct confluence.
(A) A percutaneous cholangiogram shows the tortuous, irregular, complex biliary obstruction. At this time it was not possible to pass beyond the obstruction and an external drainage catheter had been left in place. (B) Control cholangiography after 5 days, with reduction of biliary tree diameter; it still was not possible to go beyond the obstruction. The external drainage catheter was maintained, decompressing both liver lobes.

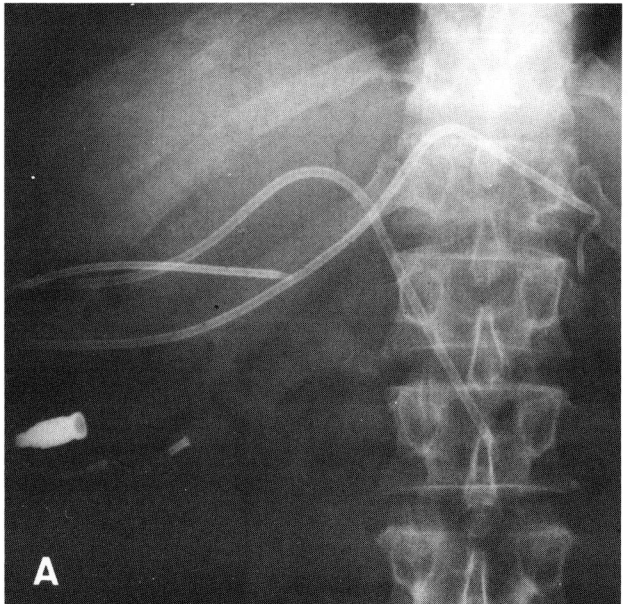
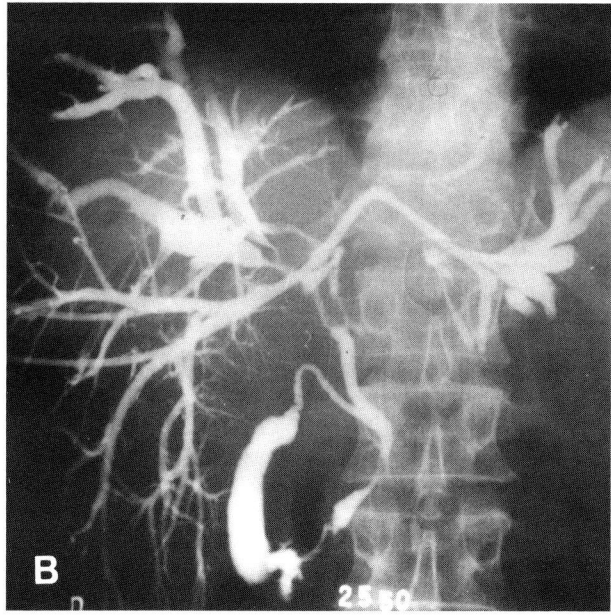

Figure 5.10 A 48-year-old patient with cholangiocarcinoma diffusely obstructing the biliary tree.
(A) Multiple catheters (three) were required to drain the different biliary tree segments. (B) A control cholangiogram after drainage shows the positioning of several catheters in relation to the different compartments formed inside the biliary tree. Even with three drainage catheters, a few compartments remain occluded. This kind of procedure is no longer recommended.

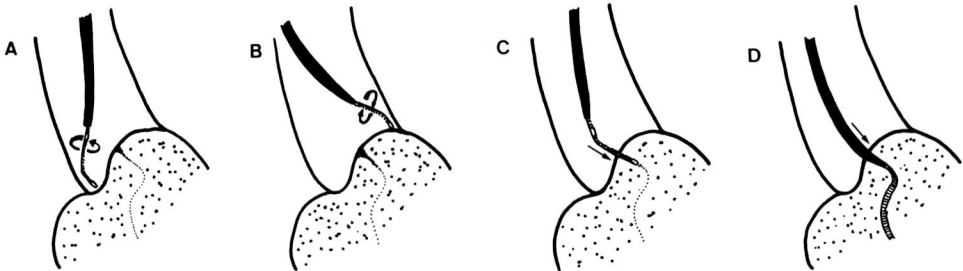

Figure 5.11 Maneuvers used to catheterize the virtual lumen which exists inside the tumor mass. There is always a track available, but the position of the orifice varies. Cul-de-sac locations in the acute angle are usually not related to the orifice of the intratumoral track. (A) A catheter with a Lunderquist torque guidewire probing the blunt portion of the obstruction. (B) A catheter and torque guidewire probing the sharp portion of the obstruction. Notice the rotational and longitudinal movement of the guidewire. (C) Multiple movements of the angulated tip of the guidewire end up "palpating" and penetrating into the orifice of the intratumoral track. (D) The catheter is advanced over the guidewire, which is then removed. Contrast injection is done, outlining the track inside the tumor.

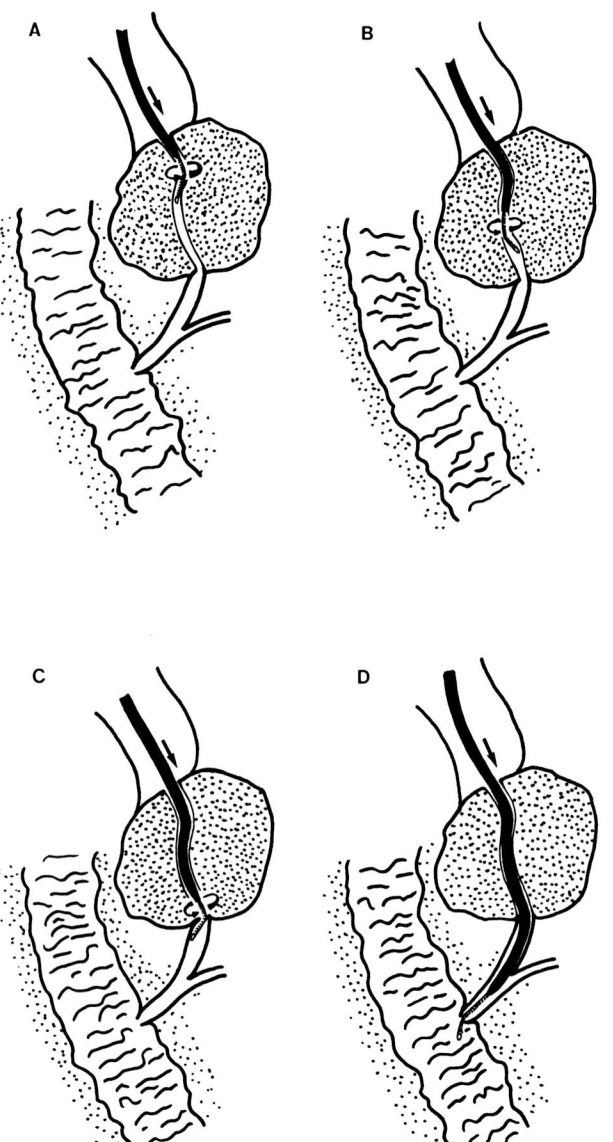

level of the common bile duct, and an attempt is made to pass it through the obstruction (Fig. 5.11). There is always a virtual lumen present inside the tumoral obstruction or the infiltrated common bile duct. The difficulty lies in finding it and passing beyond the tumoral mass. If it is not possible to pass beyond the obstruction during the first attempts, some maneuvers may be performed to catheterize it (Figs. 5.11 and 5.12), using a Lunderquist guidewire with a shapable tip and torque control. As this guidewire can have its distal tip rotated while the tip is advanced and pulled back, as shown in Fig. 5.11, the orifice is "palpated" with the tip of the guidewire. Usually, when the tip of the guidewire "finds" the orifice in the obstruction, one immediately feels that it is possible to advance the guidewire inside the virtual track which is present there.

Note, however, that the orifice of the virtual track inside the obstructive lesion is not usually found in the most obvious site or found on the tapered and eccentric tip which is formed in one of the extremities of the obstruction at the level of the hepatic duct or dilated common bile duct, as shown in Fig. 5.11. Rather, it is usually located on the midthird of the obstruction, in a position which is difficult to approach with a catheter. Therefore care must be taken to avoid following a false track, in a necrotic lesion, or perforating the tumoral mass. Even if this occurs, pulling the catheter, then immediately injecting contrast, may reidentify the true track. This true track may be found after another manipulation of the guidewire, although in most cases it

Figure 5.12 After the intratumoral track is visualized, the Lunderquist torque guidewire is advanced with careful and progressive rotational and longitudinal movements until the duodenal lumen is reached through the papilla (A through D).

is advisable to perform external drainage and manipulate only after 48 h of drainage.

Going beyond the obstructive lesion is the critical issue in internal-external biliary drainage. The ability or inability to pass beyond the obstruction will determine the success or failure of the procedure (Figs. 5.11 and 5.12).

The papilla usually causes some difficulty when the guidewire and catheter are introduced, especially if the use of analgesia with opiate narcotics results in spasm and sphincteric closure. As a rule, however, it is easy to pass beyond the papilla of Vater and Oddi's sphincter by using the advancement and rotation technique, with a Lunderquist guidewire, described above. Once the duodenal lumen has been reached, the same care in manipulation should be taken, producing rotation at the guidewire tip while simultaneously advancing both the guidewire and the catheter toward the third and fourth portions of the duodenum.

It is worth mentioning here a few maneuvers necessary in catheterizion and manipulation of the catheter and guidewire through tortuous biliary ducts or in puncturing a peripheral biliary duct perpendicular to the axis of the common bile duct.

If a puncture of the left duct is accidentally performed with a right approach, it is generally advisable to perform a new puncture in a more favorable position, as it is difficult, although not impossible, to catheterize the site of obstruction through a closed bend of both the guidewire and the puncture catheter (Fig. 5.13). In such cases, it is extremely difficult to go beyond the lesion, dilate the track, and position a catheter for internal-external drainage. As it has already been mentioned, it is quicker and easier to select another point for puncture. However, while looking for a new position, one should leave the needle inside the liver parenchyma, thus avoiding the presence of bile in the peritoneum and intraperitoneal bleeding.

If it is difficult to introduce the guidewire and catheter tip all the way down to the common bile duct, the following maneuver can be utilized. The tip of the guidewire is advanced into a left hepatic lobe duct with a continuous progression while the catheter is kept stationary so that its curve is formed inside the dilated hepatic duct. When enough curvature has been obtained, the catheter is advanced to a point at which it reaches a better position for catheterization of the obstruction (Fig. 5.14).

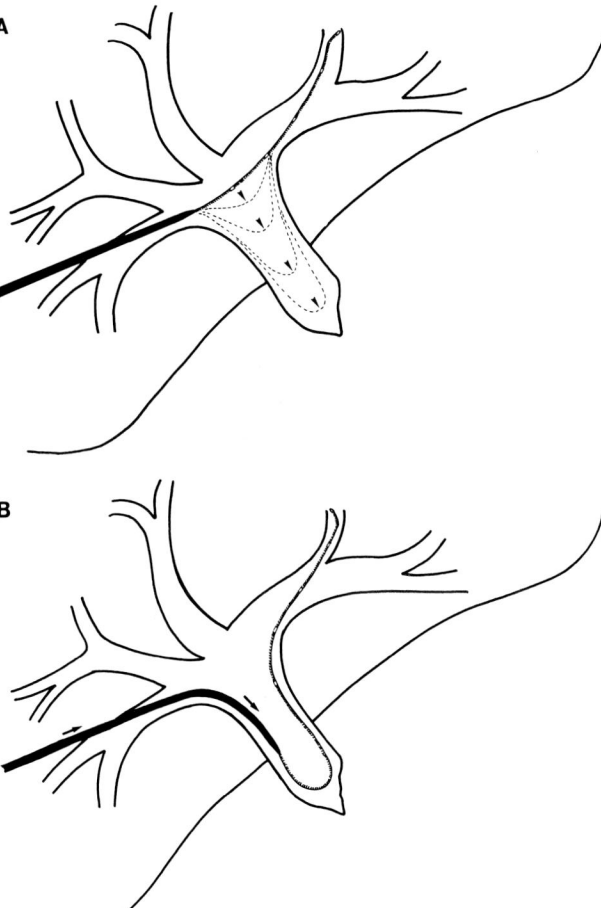

Figure 5.14 How to proceed if the guidewire does not go down to the common bile duct by the conventional maneuvers of rotation and tip progression.
(A) Introducing the guidewire to a left lobe duct and pushing the system while progressively bending the wire until the dilated common bile duct is penetrated with this bend. (B) Advancing the catheter over the guidewire until the obstruction site is reached. When the guidewire is removed, the catheter remains near the obstruction.

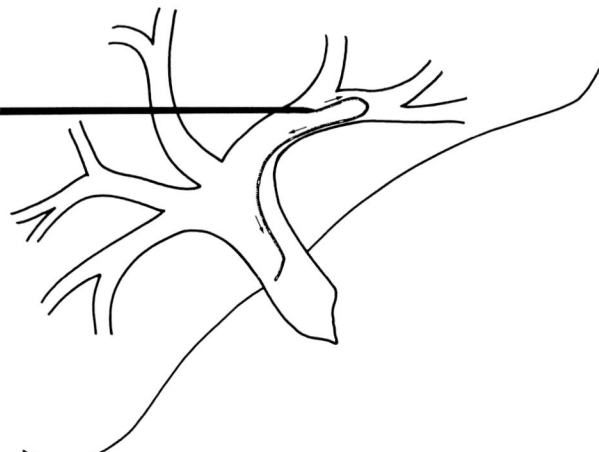

Figure 5.13 Puncture of a left biliary duct by the right approach may allow catheterization of the common bile duct and common hepatic duct. However, the angulation of the guide and catheter will prevent adequate control of manipulation and may even prevent catheterizing and passing beyond the obstruction. The track should be as rectilinear as possible and should be parallel to the common bile duct.

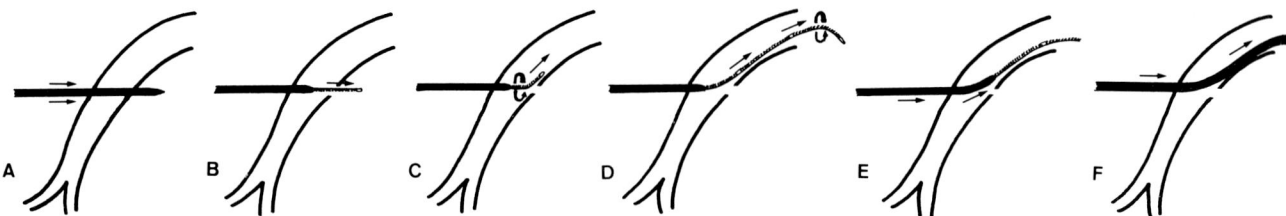

Figure 5.15 The procedure for puncturing a peripheral biliary duct.
(A) Introduce a needle with a Teflon sheath toward an opacified peripheral duct in a continuous manner without interrupting the introduction in the middle of the track. When duct wall is touched, a certain degree of wall deformity will be seen by means of fluoroscopy under the pressure of the needle tip, which will finally yield when perforated.
(B) After perforation, the trocar is removed, with a small volume of bile being aspirated. A straight guidewire will not get inside the biliary lumen, always tending to go beyond the duct and leaving through the hole in the contralateral wall.
(C) The use of a J or torque guidewire with a bent tip will permit easy penetration in the desired direction. (D) The guide is advanced into the biliary lumen as far as possible and is followed by the catheter. (E,F) New manipulation of the guidewire and catheter makes it possible to advance the catheter inside the biliary tree.

Puncture of a biliary duct which is peripherally located and not parallel to the common bile duct (Fig. 5.15) requires additional manipulation with the guidewire and puncture needle sheath, as will be seen later in this chapter.

When a verticalized biliary duct is punctured, the needle tip usually goes beyond the two walls. The use of a straight guidewire will prevent the lumen of the biliary tree from being catheterized. It is then necessary to use a J-guidewire or a Lunderquist guidewire with torque control and a shapable tip so that the tip can be reoriented toward the interior of the biliary tree. If one uses the technique of rotation and progressive advances, the needle sheath system of the guidewire can be pushed into the lumen of the biliary tree, away from the puncture site.

When the biliary tree is dilated and tortuous (Fig. 5.16), a Lunderquist guidewire with torque should be used to manipulate and advance beyond the curves in the biliary ducts. The rotation and progressive advancement technique should always be used to introduce the guidewire in accordance with the difficulties and obstacles encountered. In this situation, it is often convenient to leave in a temporary catheter for external drainage for 24 to 48 h and only then to attempt to go past the obstruction. After external drainage there will be a reduction in the tortuosity and diameter of the biliary ducts as well as a reduction of the edema in the area of obstruction (Fig. 5.17). Contrast injection into the virtual lumen inside the tumor will show the track in most cases while opacifying the distal common bile duct. This provides an excellent guide for catheterization (Fig. 5.18).

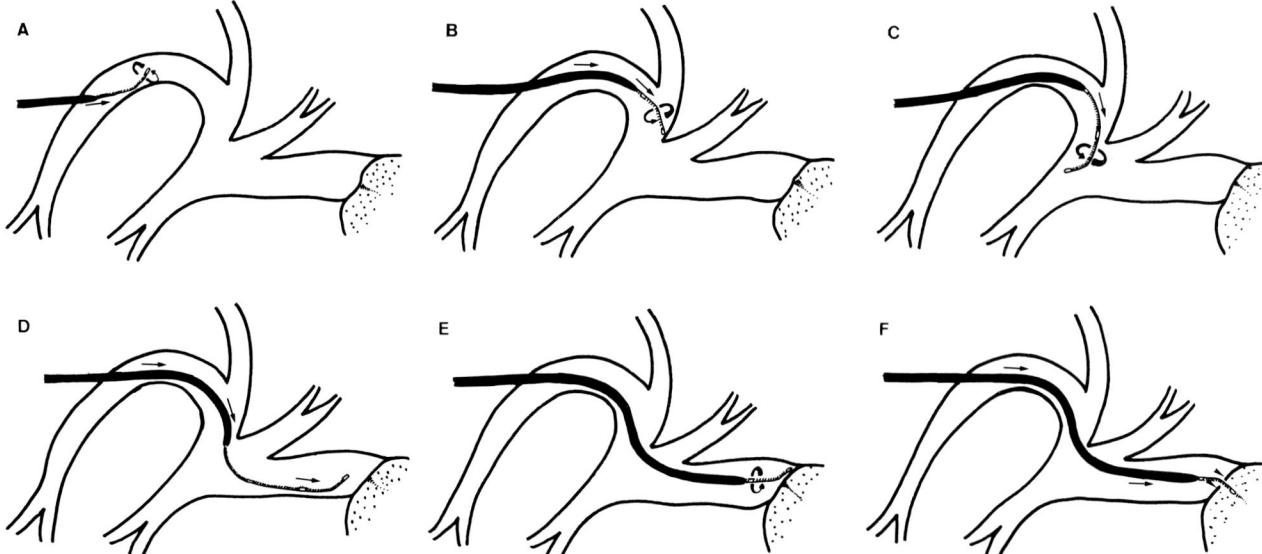

Figure 5.16 (A through D) Catheterization of a tortuous and dilated biliary tree using the technique of catheter rotation and progressive advancement with a Lunderquist torque guidewire. (E,F) Once the common bile duct has been reached, the procedure is similar to the one shown in Fig. 5.11. The orifice is sought until the intratumoral track is penetrated with the guidewire tip.

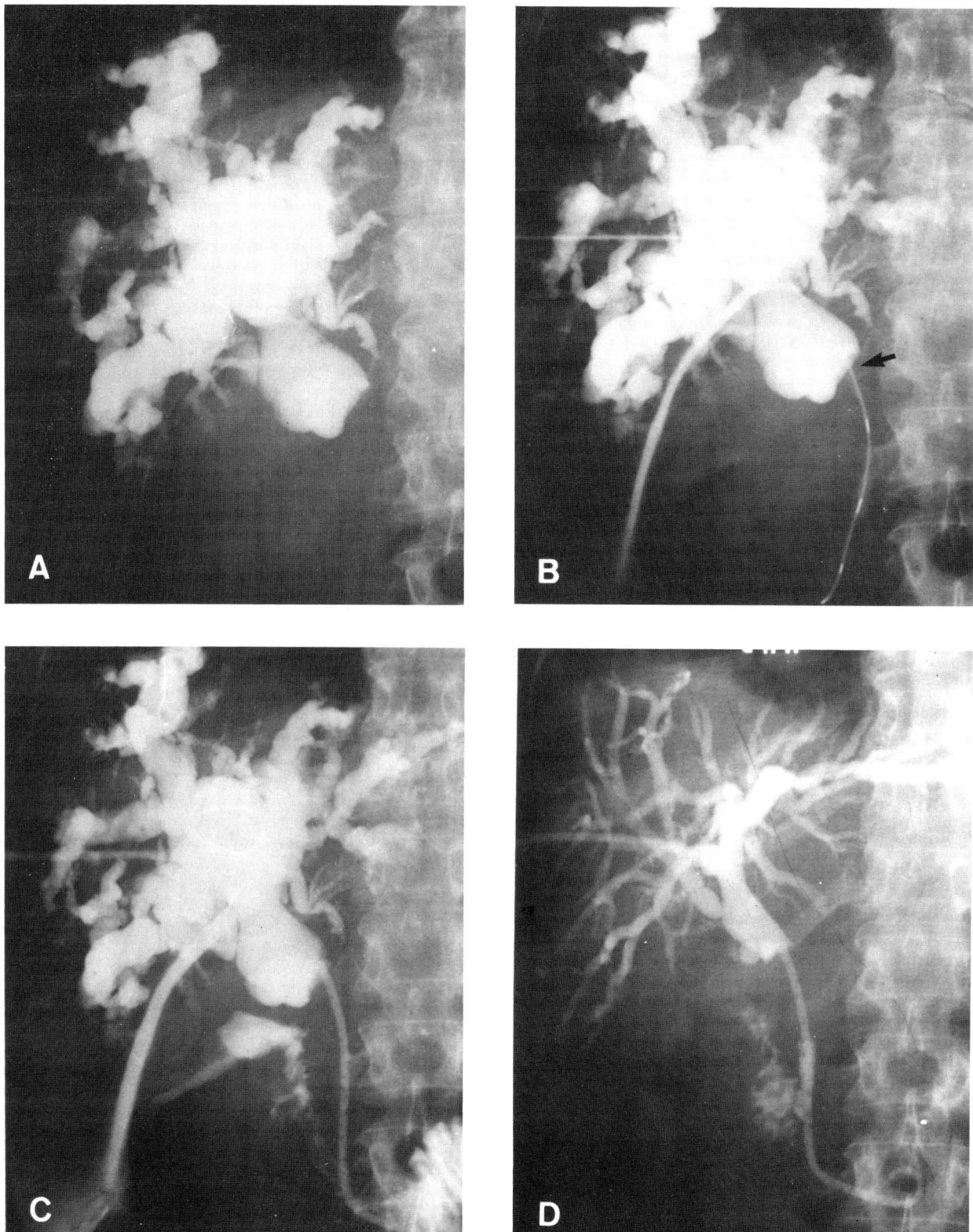

Figure 5.17 A 49-year-old female patient with gallbladder carcinoma with obstruction of the biliary tree and cholangitis. Note the effect of 72-h drainage on reduction of biliary tree diameter and tortuosity.
(A) Note the significant biliary dilatation with deformity of the intrahepatic ducts by tumoral obstruction. (B) After a long search, the orifice was found on the midthird of the obstruction (arrow), with a Lunderquist guidewire having been introduced into the duodenum. (C) A Ring catheter for internal-external drainage already in position, connecting the intrahepatic biliary tree to the duodenum. (D) A control cholangiogram shows thinning of the hepatic biliary tree with significant reduction in the tortuosity of the intrahepatic ducts.

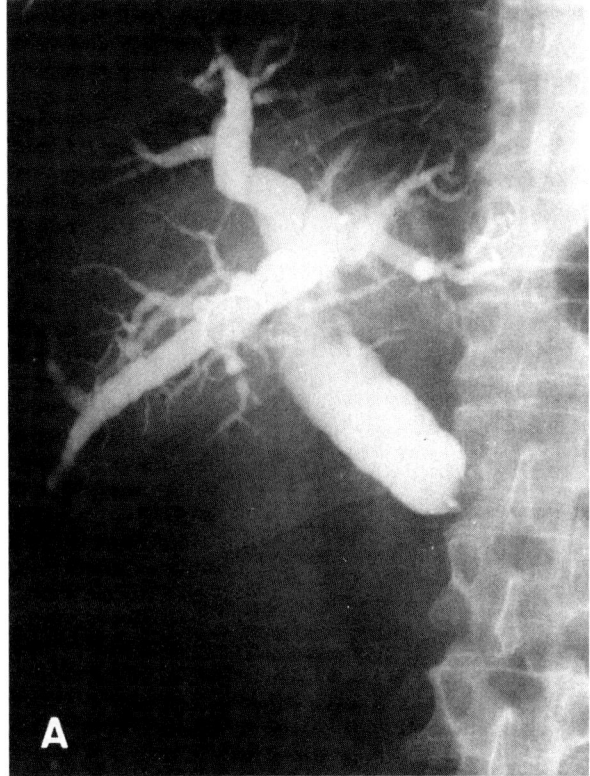

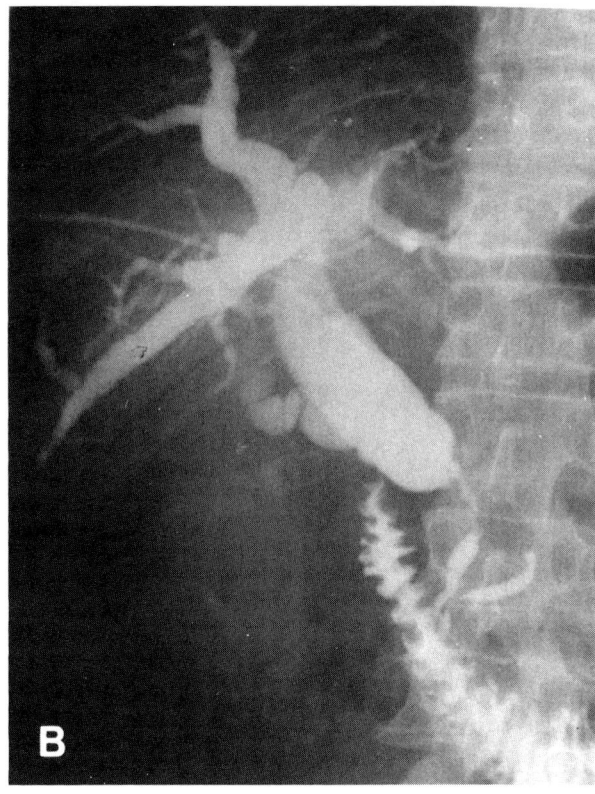

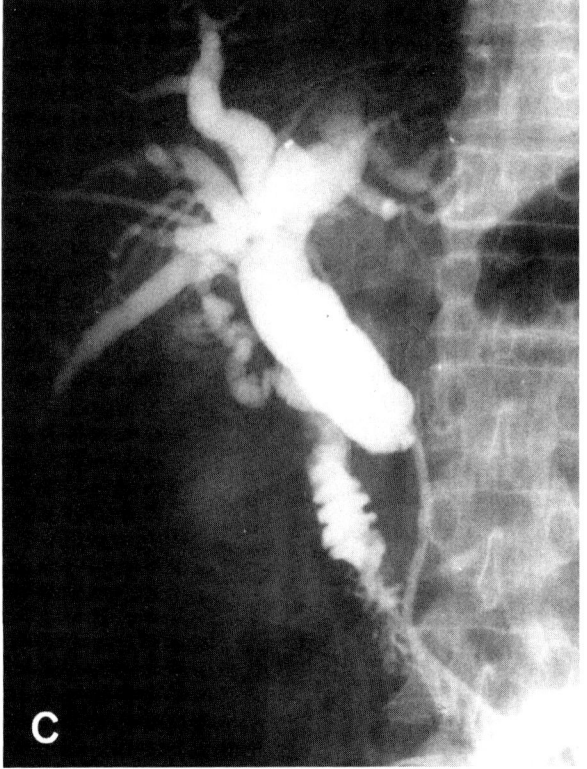

Figure 5.18 A 65-year-old male patient with carcinoma of the pancreatic head.
(A) A percutaneous cholangiogram shows significant dilatation of the biliary tree caused by obstruction at the level of the distal common bile duct with an image of umbilication at the obstruction site. (B) Catheterization of the obstructed track shows its patency to contrast injection, with opacification of the common bile duct. (C) Control cholangiography immediately after internal-external drainage with a Ring catheter.

After the duodenal lumen has been reached with a guidewire and needle sheath, the most difficult part of the procedure is over. The next step is to perform internal-external drainage.

Advancing the guidewire and the polyethylene or Teflon needle sheath provides a safe element that allows one to exchange the guidewire for a more rigid one which also was developed by Lunderquist (Fig. 5.19). This is a steel wire with a flexible tip that has the same gauge as the guidewire used previously. This type of guidewire allows progressive dilatation of the track with Teflon dilators up to one French number larger than the catheter used for drainage. It also facilitates the introduction of less rigid drainage catheters through tortuosities.

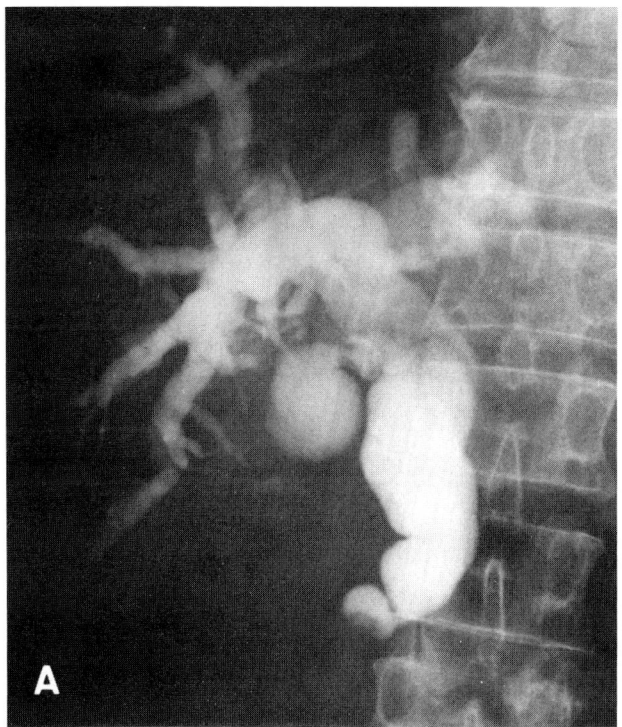
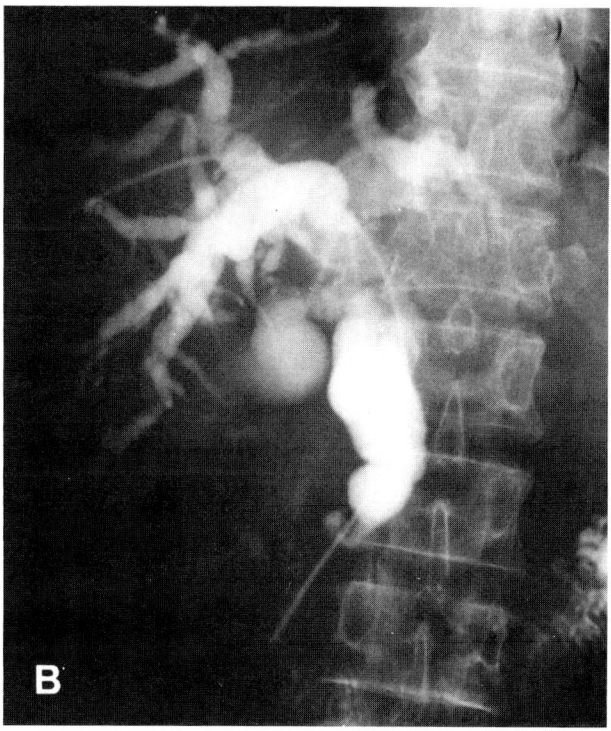

Figure 5.19 A 68-year-old male patient with papillary carcinoma.
(A) A percutaneous cholangiogram shows biliary tree dilatation by obstruction of the distal common bile duct. (B) Catheterization through the obstruction with a sheathed needle. This type of catheterization allows the Lunderquist exchange guidewire to be passed, making catheter introduction easier. (C) Control cholangiogram immediately after internal-external drainage was performed as a presurgical measure.

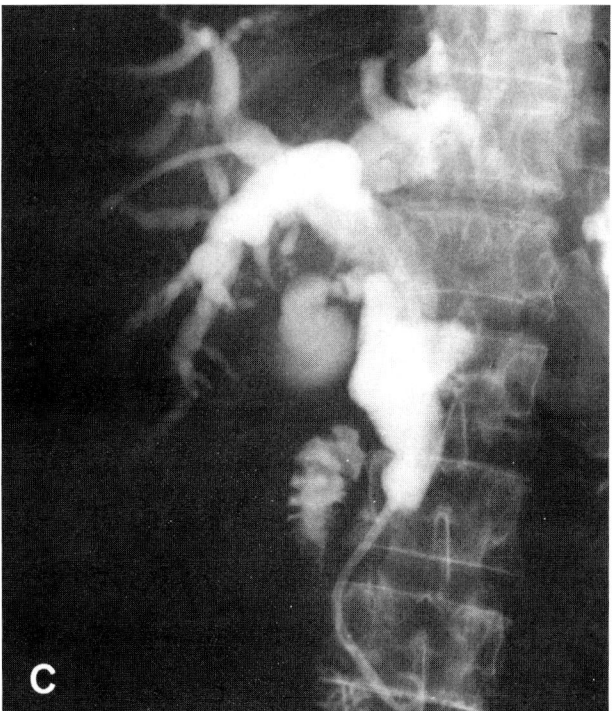

It is important to select the right drainage catheter. The most practical material is a Ring catheter with adequate curvature, a pigtail-shaped tip, and side holes which can drain most proximal or distal obstructions (Fig.5.20). Additional holes, however, may be opened to match the catheter size to the level of the obstruction. It is not difficult to localize the main orifices. With the needle sheath inside the duodenum, an old guidewire is pulled until its tip is at the same level as the papilla. The guidewire is then bent against the catheter connector at this point. Immediately afterward, the guidewire is pulled even farther, till its tip is at the level of the entry point to the peripheral hepatic duct; at this point a second bend is made in the guidewire. The distance between the guidewire bends will correspond exactly to the space

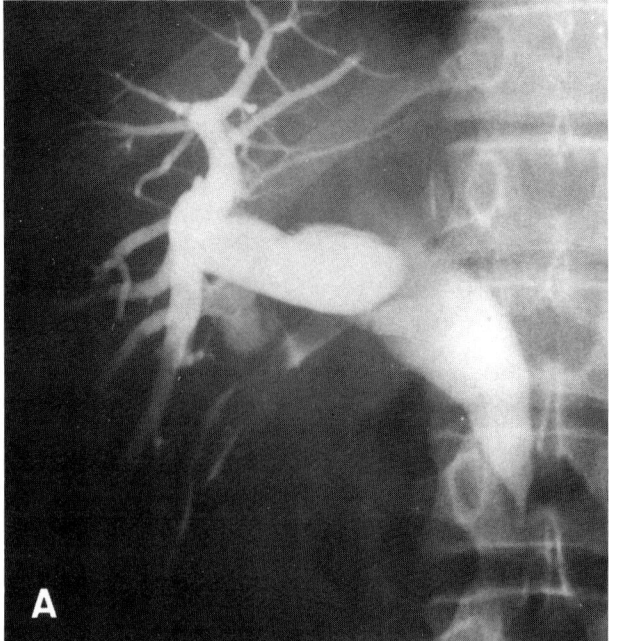
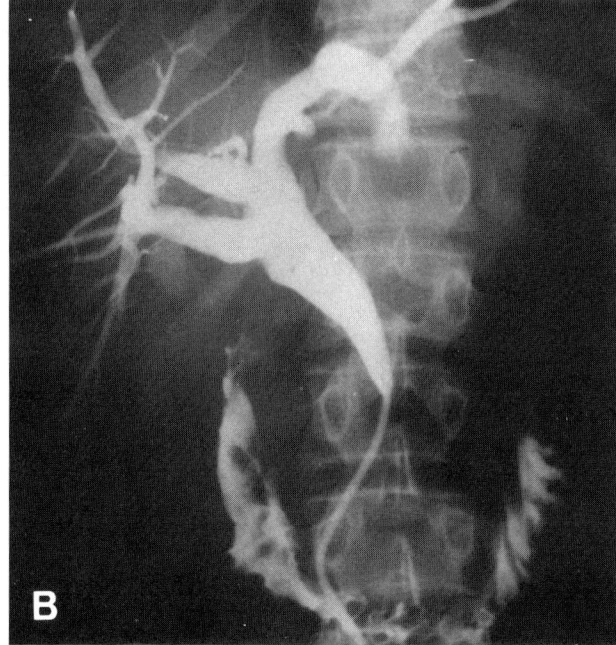
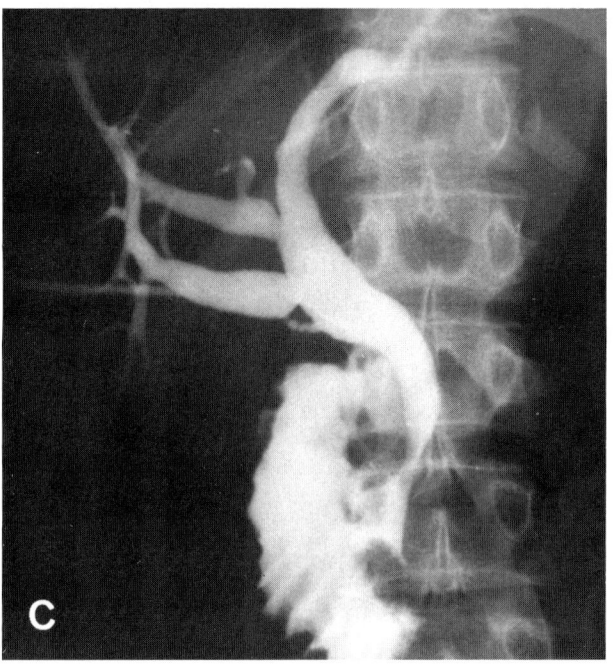

Figure 5.20 A 17-year-old male patient with duodenal lymphoma.
(A) Obstruction of the biliary tree by a duodenal lesion involving the head of the pancreas and the distal common bile duct. (B) Cholangiogram 48 h after internal-external drainage of the biliary tree. (C) Dramatic regression of biliary obstruction after systemic chemotherapy with recanalization of the common bile duct, which allowed drainage removal within 1 month. Chemotherapy can be given only after bilirubin levels have returned to normal and after improvement of liver function.

from the first lateral hole to the last lateral hole in the drainage catheter inside the biliary tree. Another option is to use a Cope-type catheter, which will remain firmly static in the ideal position; a loop can be produced in its tip by pulling the suture sling which is incorporated in its structure. No sutures are needed to fix this type of catheter onto the skin; the Ring catheter requires some kind of additional fixation system and is usually sutured to the skin.

Several techniques can be used to fix the catheter to the patient. The safest one is a suture thread between the catheter and the skin. A Molnar disk can be used, or sutures can be attached to the catheter and to an adhesive tape, instead of suturing the catheter directly to the skin.

Displacement of a catheter positioning the side holes inside the liver parenchyma may lead to bleeding and obstruction. This is discussed in "Complications."

Internal-external drainage always begins with external drainage, simultaneously with internal drainage, in an open or closed system. The use of a closed system will prevent external contamination of the biliary tree for the first 48 h.

Temporary internal-external drainage is particularly useful when a treatment alternative such as chemotherapy cannot be used because the patient has jaundice. Once this contraindication has ceased, chemotherapy can be started; upon regression of the lesion, the biliary drainage can be removed (Fig. 5.20). Low output or cessation of external drainage may be related to bad positioning of the catheter, catheter occlusion, dehydration of the patient, or reduced liver function due to diffuse disease.

The volume of bile during 24 h usually ranges from 400 to 600 mL; occasionally, several liters of bile may be drained during the first 2 or 3 days causing what is called "biluresis" from a poorly determined cause. Drainage of 3 to 4 liters of bile per day is not uncommon in these patients. This may cause severe hydroelectrolytic depletion and hypotension, requiring aggressive replacement as long as the condition lasts.

After 2 or 3 days of external drainage, the external catheter is closed, establishing internal or antegrade drainage. In most cases occlusion of the external catheter will cause bile to flow into the duodenum. In about 15 percent of cases internal drainage is not immediately established. There are four potential causes of internal drainage failure:

1. Few lateral holes above or below the obstruction.
2. The use of a catheter with a lumen diameter that is insufficient for the viscosity of the bile that will be drained. Bile does not behave like a Newtonian fluid, such as water. Because of its micellar composition and high viscosity (especially during and immediately after biliary tree obstruction), bile behaves like a Binghan plastic fluid, which does not flow until a minimum pressure gradient is reached. As bile viscosity decreases, the plastic fluid behavior also changes, approaching that of a Newtonian fluid. Bile viscosity is higher at the time of drainage, and the lower limit of the pressure gradient for flowing will decrease progressively until it reaches a plateau at around the fifth day after decompression.
3. A pressure gradient between the biliary tree and the duodenal lumen that is very small. In this case, the gradient may be insufficient to establish bile flow to the duodenum. Biliary secretion pressure ranges from 30 to 35 cmH$_2$O, and duodenal pressure at rest ranges from 10 to 15 cmH$_2$O. This relatively small gradient may disappear when duodenal pressure is increased because of distal obstruction. Patients with gastric resection and Bilroth type II anastomoses are prone to difficulties of this type, and in these cases there may be a need for permanent external drainage. One option is transhepatic catheterization of the afferent loop with intragastric positioning or catheterization of the efferent loop of the distal extremity of the drainage catheter.
4. No. 10 to No. 12 French catheters of the nasogastric tube type or vesical vinyl tubes are good alternatives for long-term drainage used by some authors. Because they are less susceptible to occlusion by thick bile and are softer than Ring-type polyethylene catheters, these catheters are usually more comfortable for the patient.

Note that the tubes cited in No. 4 above should not be introduced until 10 to 15 days after the original procedure, when a well-organized fistulous track has been formed around the initial catheter. It is always necessary in these cases to use a coaxial system with a No. 6 French polyethylene catheter to guide the soft vinyl catheter.

Percutaneous Biopsy

If a histologic diagnosis of obstructive lesion has not been made, an aspiration biopsy puncture should be performed, using a fine 19- to 22-gauge needle and utilizing the cholangiogram as a map (Fig. 5.21). The

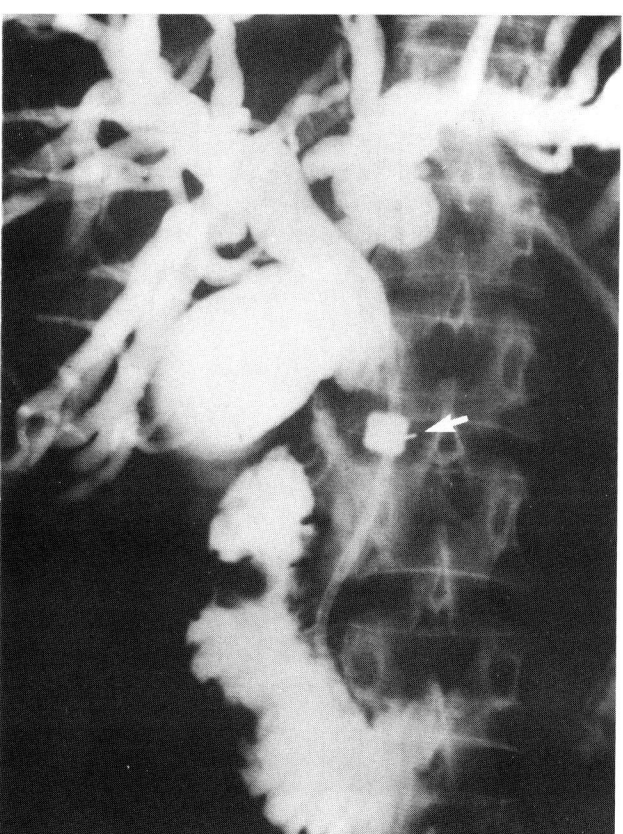

Figure 5.21 A 52-year-old female patient with carcinoma of the pancreatic head confirmed by percutaneous aspiration biopsy puncture.
Definitive placement of a Ring catheter was performed to achieve internal-external drainage. Note that the needle tip is very close to the drainage tube, which passes inside the tumoral lesion (arrow). A cell sample obtained with a Chiba needle, as in this case, is generally scarce, although other needles for removing larger fragments are available.

biopsy puncture can be made either at the time of the first procedure or during one of the control cholangiographic studies. Anteroposterior, lateral-view, or two-plane fluoroscopy can be used as an aid when available. Computed tomography may be extremely valuable as a guide to reference points in some cases, but fluoroscopy is often indispensable for needle positioning.

The needle is directed from the anterior abdominal wall, perpendicular to the area adjacent to the point of obstruction, as visualized in a transhepatic or catheter cholangiogram (Fig. 5.21). Lateral-view fluoroscopy is used to determine the depth of the needle tip. If necessary, the patient can be turned safely to a lateral position to achieve better orientation. When the needle penetrates the tumor, the sensation is that of penetrating a rigid material. Once the lesion has been localized and punctured, aspiration with disposable 20-mL syringe is done while the needle is advanced and rotated a few millimeters. This technique may vary considerably depending on the biopsy needle available. The needle is removed immediately afterward without any suction. Three to five punctures usually must be performed to obtain adequate material.

Preparation of materials for cystopathologic analysis varies from institution to institution and from cytologist to cytologist. This preparation should be integrated with the biopsy procedure to achieve better results.

Cytopathologic study of the bile aspirated during drainage is frequently useful in defining the type of lesion. Brushing the lesion through drainage catheters with bronchial biopsy brushes has become a useful method for defining the lesion from a diagnostic standpoint.

Internal Biliary Drainage (Endoprosthesis)

External and combined biliary drainage may cause a few inconveniences, such as pain at the site of catheter penetration (accentuated by breathing movements), bacterial colonization in the catheter and its track, and consequent development of cholangitis. The patient may be incapacitated for normal physical activity, and this in turn can generate psychological problems. The most serious inconvenience, however, involves patients who are unable to cooperate or who cooperate minimally, for example, those living far away from hospitals, and those from lower social and economic levels, who frequently do not take care of their biliary drainage or fail to return for quarterly catheter exchange and drainage revision.

To prevent these inconveniences, a new type of biliary endoprosthesis was first used around 1978–1979 (Fig. 5.8). These prostheses promote internal biliary drainage by connecting the intrahepatic biliary tree to the duodenal

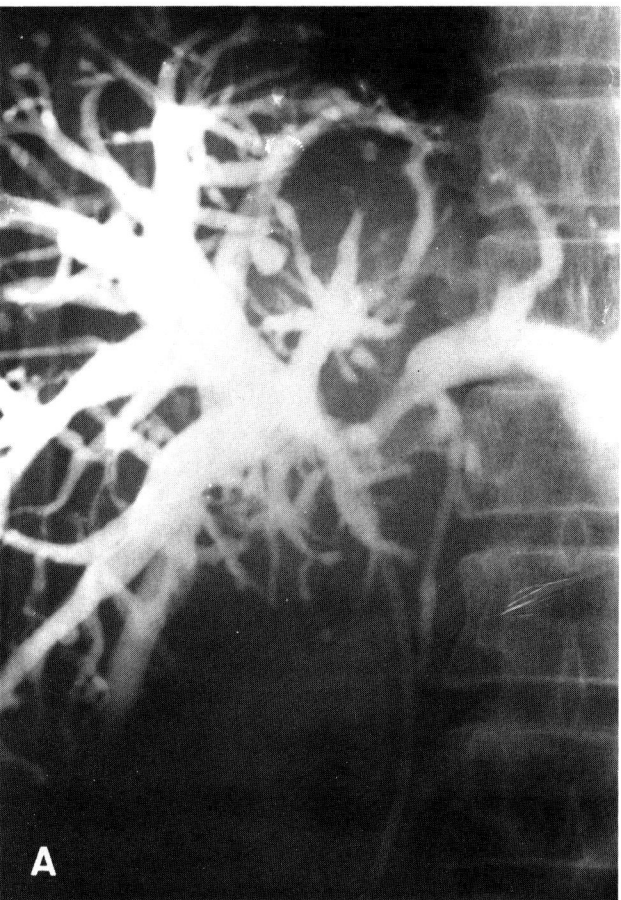

Figure 5.22 (A) A patient with high obstruction of the biliary tree dilatation, and multiple peripheral abscesses. The fine catheter goes beyond the obstruction, reaching the duodenum. (B) A control cholangiogram after placement of a Lunderquist-Hoevels–type endoprosthesis shows adequate drainage and a diminished diameter of the biliary tree. (C) A Lunderquist endoprosthesis in position after biliary tree drainage.

lumen. The first type of endoprosthesis used was the one described by Lunderquist and Hoevels in 1978. This was a short, thick endoprosthesis with a proximal flange that prevents migration (Fig. 5.22).

A few basic types of endoprostheses are in current use. One type is a large-gauge (No. 12 to No. 14 French) long prosthesis with or without lateral holes, depending on the manufacturer, which promotes full drainage of the biliary tree into the duodenum (Fig. 5.23). Another type is a fine (No. 7 to No. 8 French) long (12 to 15 cm) endoprosthesis which is very easily positioned and can be introduced in varying numbers (two, three, or four) (Fig. 5.24).

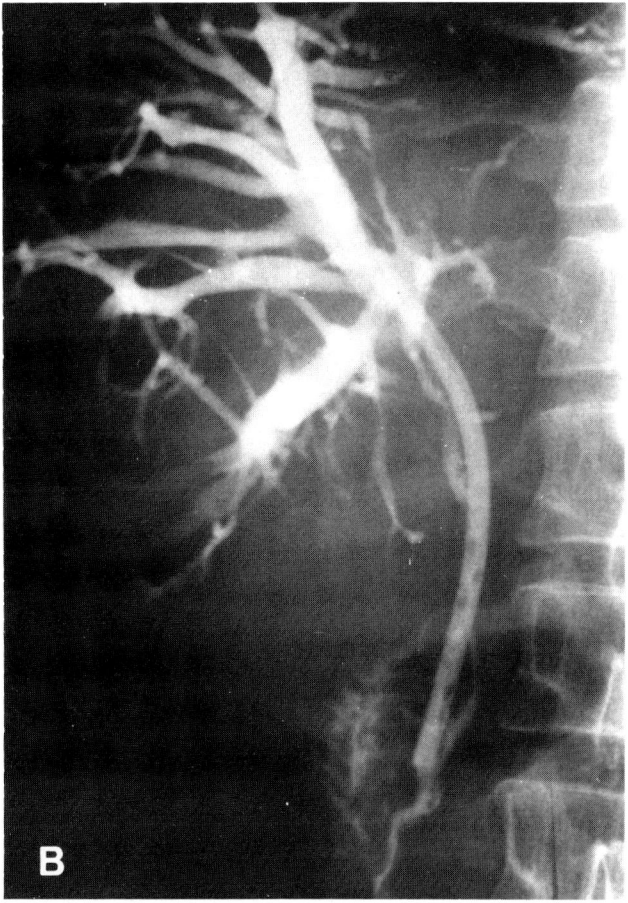
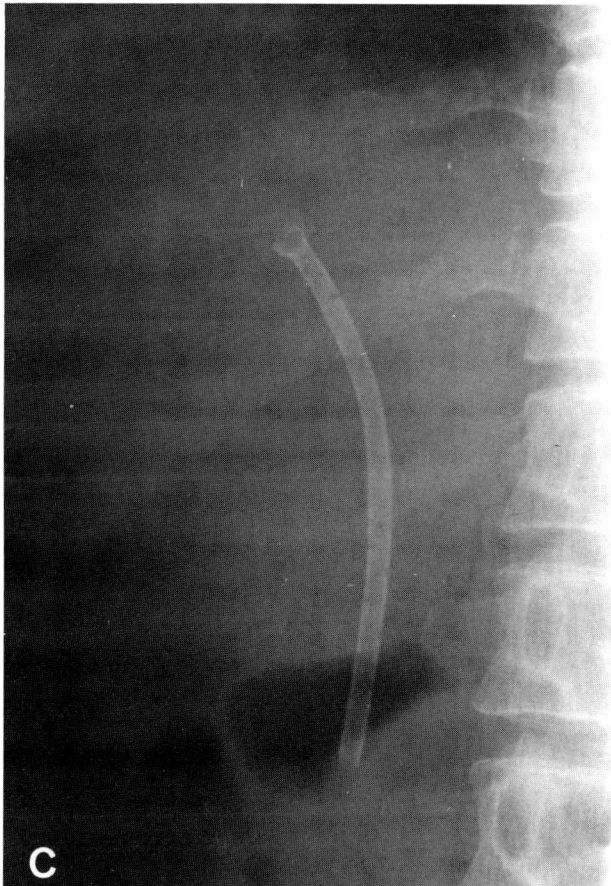

Figure 5.22 *Continued*

The Carry-Coons endoprosthesis is another alternative for biliary drainage. Made of the soft material Percuflex, it has a J shape and is very stable when held by a sling thread attached to a button placed in the subcutaneous tissue. More recently, the Muller double-mushroom biliary endoprosthesis became available; it is made of polyethylene and is available in several different lengths and diameters. It is easily introduced through a long Teflon sheath.

Internal biliary drainage is the end objective of all nonsurgical decompression procedures involving the biliary tree because it is more physiologic, allowing the patient to avoid using external drainage systems while preventing contamination of the biliary tree by exogenous germs.

A biliary tree endoprosthesis is indicated for patients with inoperable malignant biliary obstruction and a lesion in whom the prognosis for survival is short (6 months to 1 year). The rationale for the use of an endoprosthesis is the extraordinary improvement in the quality of life of the patient that results from effective drainage during the patient's expected survival, depending on the type of lesion causing biliary obstruction. Thus, endoprostheses are indicated for patients with carcinoma of the head of the pancreas, gallbladder carcinoma, some malignant lesions of the biliary ducts (cholangiocarcinomas), and some types of metastases which do not respond to chemotherapy or radiotherapy and which involve the porta hepatis.

In most cases, the endoprosthesis will "outlive" the patient without occluding. However, if it is used in patients with less aggressive lesions and a longer survival prognosis, the chances of prosthesis occlusion are greatly increased. In these cases it is better to leave the internal-external catheter in place and exchange it every 3 months, allowing permanent access to the biliary tree. Although most larger-diameter prostheses can be recanalized when occluded, this procedure demands a certain degree of expertise. It requires a great deal of effort to clean the tube, then a new biliary puncture must be performed and the whole catheterization procedure repeated.

The technique by which the biliary tree is catheterized

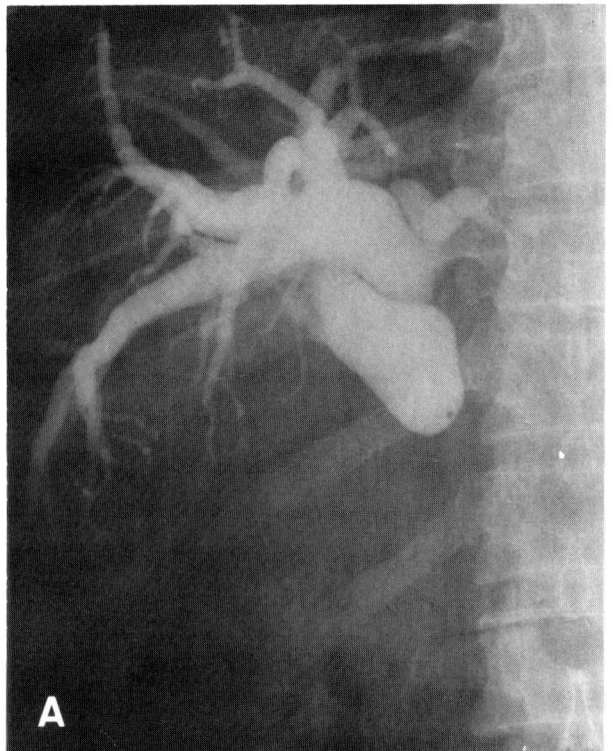
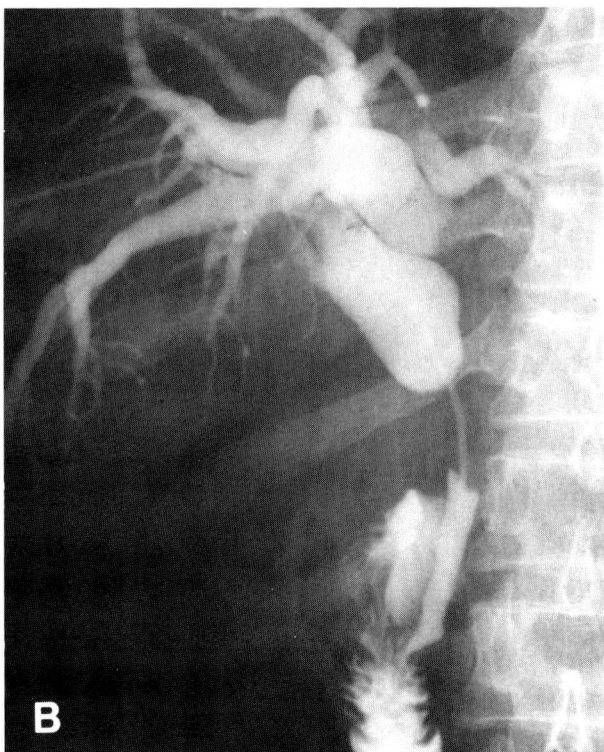
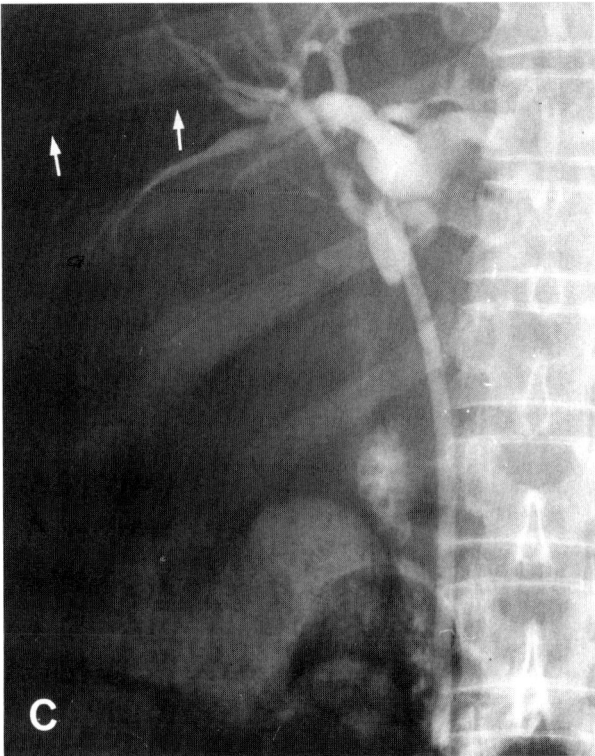

Figure 5.23 A 56-year-old female patient with carcinoma of the gallbladder drained with a modified long Coons endoprosthesis.
(A) Significant dilatation of intra- and extrahepatic bile ducts by hepatic duct occlusion. Note the central umbilication on the point of obstruction. (B) A catheter cholangiogram soon after catheterization of the obstruction track shows the precise extension of the lesion after opacification of the distal stump of the common bile duct down to the papilla of Vater. (C) A large-diameter (No. 12 French) long (15 cm) endoprosthesis was used in this patient for definitive and palliative internal drainage of the obstruction. Note the significant reduction in the size of the intrahepatic biliary tree after drainage for 24 h. The percutaneous catheterization track is still visible (arrows). This type of modified Coons endoprosthesis rests against the antipapillary duodenal wall, preventing displacement.

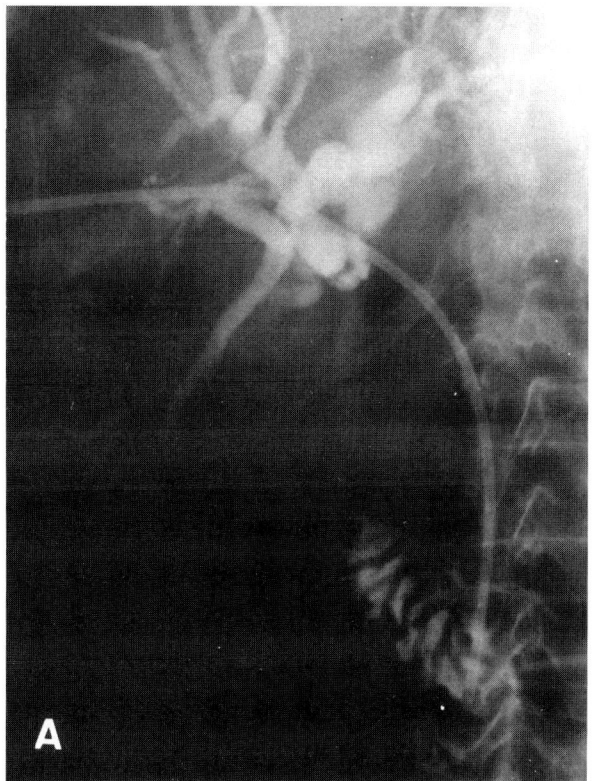
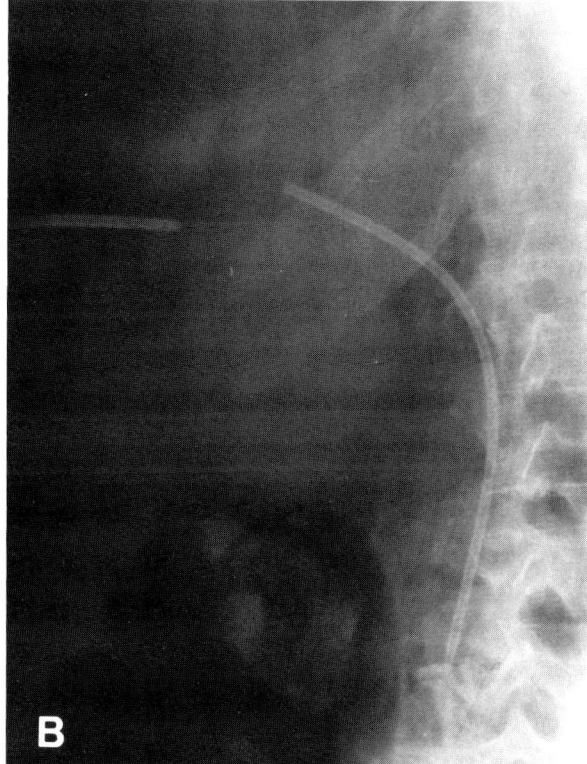
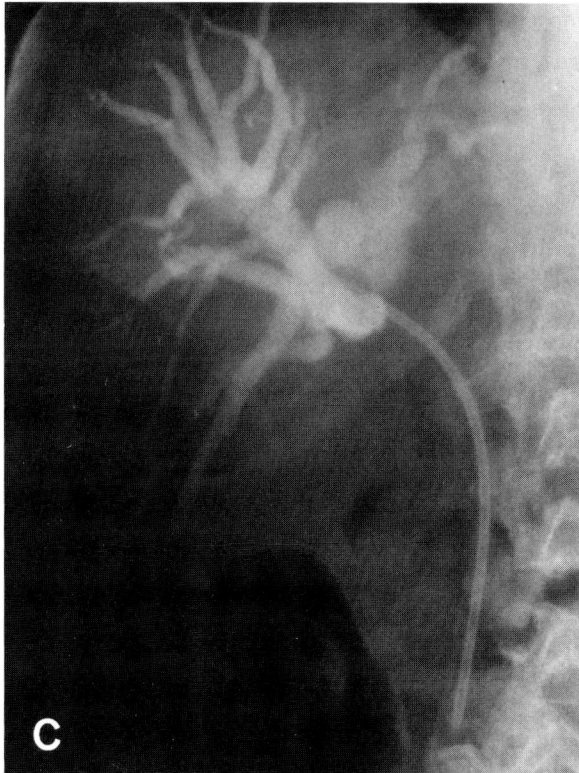

Figure 5.24 A 60-year-old patient with carinoma of the gallbladder drained with a Burcharth endoprosthesis.
(A) A cholangiogram through the catheter soon after a fine (No. 8 French) long (15 cm) endoprosthesis was placed. Note passage of contrast through the duodenum. (B) A plain x-ray before removal of the percutaneous catheter shows a well-positioned endoprosthesis. (C) Control immediately after removal of the percutaneous catheter shows the relationship between the endoprosthesis and the biliary tree.

and the guidewire and catheter are advanced through the obstruction to reach the duodenal lumen was described in "Internal-External Drainage."

The technique for endoprosthesis placement is as follows: After the needle sheath has reached the duodenum, it is exchanged for a semirigid Lunderquist guidewire with a flexible tip that is advanced to the duodenal fourth portion; the sheath is then removed. The track is dilated with a No. 8 French Teflon catheter, which reaches the duodenum; immediately afterward, a No. 12 French Teflon catheter is passed in a coaxial manner over the No. 8 French tube (Fig. 5.8).

The large-gauge prosthesis is made from a No. 12 or No. 14 French Teflon tube. A 12- to 15-cm tube segment is cut, the distal tip is tapered to fit over the No. 8 French tubing, and a flange is made on the proximal extremity. Multiple side holes are then opened in a helicoid distribution along the prosthesis. The proximal flange is not always needed, and it is difficult to construct in Teflon tubes. The longer the prosthesis is, the more stable it will be and the less likely to migrate. It is convenient to use a suture thread of the 0 or 00 mononylon type to anchor the prosthesis in order to allow repositioning of the endoprosthesis when it is inside the patient's biliary tree.

The No. 12 French endoprosthesis is introduced inside the biliary tree while the anchorage suture sling is kept outside, held by a forceps over the No. 8 French guide catheter. Then it is pushed through the No. 12 French introducing catheter to its final position, which can be adjusted by using the introducing catheter for pushing and the anchorage suture sling for pulling.

The No. 8 French guide catheter is removed along with the anchorage suture sling, and the guidewire is pulled to a position above the prosthesis while being kept inside the biliary tree and redirected to the common bile duct or left duct. An external drainage catheter, usually of the pigtail type, is then introduced into the biliary tree and is kept open to a flask for 2 or 3 days. Before this catheter is removed, a cholangiogram is performed to evaluate the position of the endoprosthesis. If the position has changed, some manipulation may be performed to reposition the endoprosthesis. Alternatively, it can be pushed into the duodenum, from which it can be removed through the gastrointestinal (GI) tract without causing further problems.

Special Techniques for Biliary Drainage

Anterior Approach

The anterior approach through the left hepatic lobe is very useful when there is an obstruction which involves the confluence of the right and left hepatic ducts. This is easier than an approach through the right lobe, but the radiation doses are significantly higher for the physician performing the procedure.

The puncture site is laterally located to the left of the midline, below the costal border and the xiphoid appendix. Through this approach, the cholangiogram is performed with a fine needle, and the biliary tree is punctured. This is followed by the same procedure performed on the right side (Figs. 5.25 and 5.26).

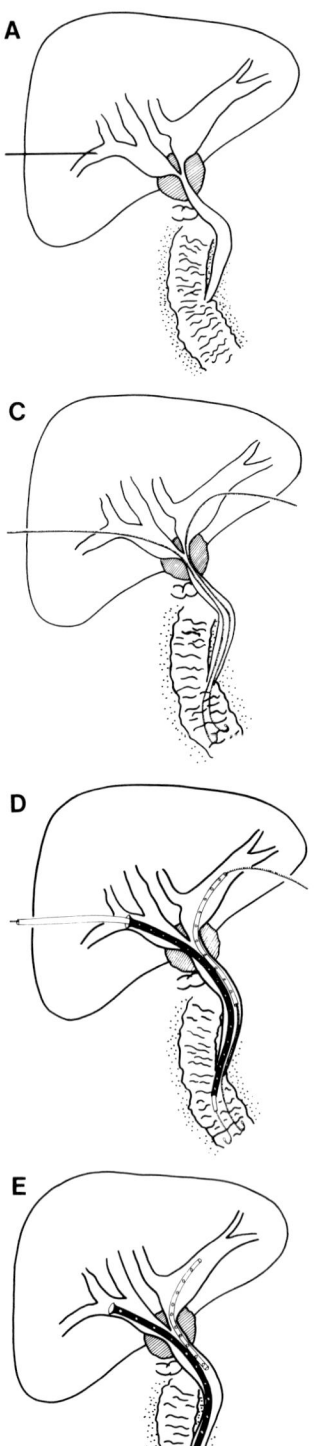

Figure 5.25 Schematic drawing of the anterior left biliary approach done simultaneously with a right lateral approach in a patient with high biliary tree obstruction.
(A) A percutaneous cholangiogram with a Chiba needle, using the right lateral approach with puncturing of the midaxillary line. (B) After biliary tree opacification and filling up of the duodenum is performed, puncture of the left biliary tree is done with a needle with a Teflon sheath. (C) The obstruction is catheterized using both approaches. (D) Once the main endoprosthesis or Ring catheter has been placed from the right side, a biliary endoprosthesis is introduced from the left duct to the common bile duct. (E) Final aspect of biliary drainage by the right lateral and left anterior route. Left duct drainage is done into the common bile duct, and the whole biliary tree is drained by the main endoprosthesis or catheter on the right.

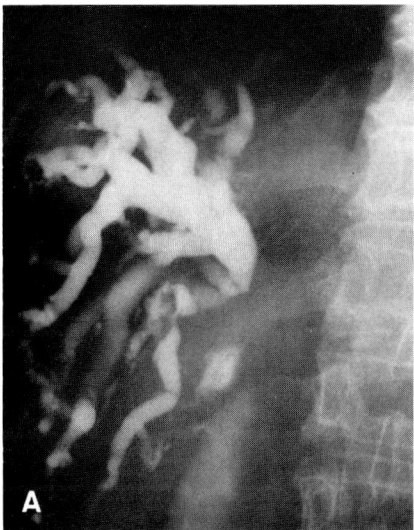 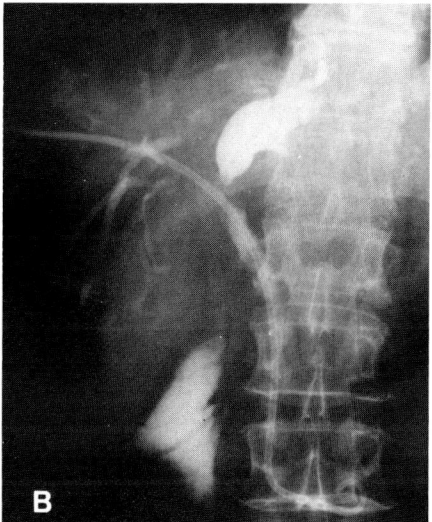 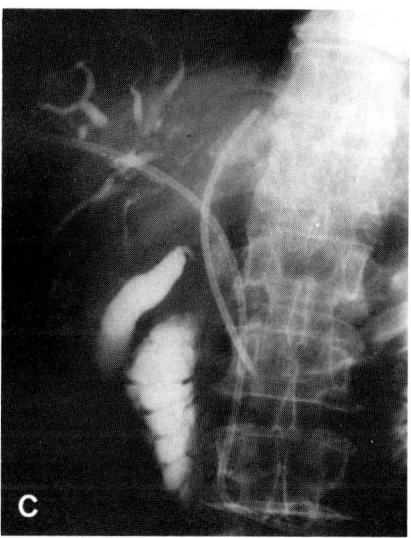

Figure 5.26 A 52-year-old patient with cholangiocarcinoma and high biliary obstruction.
(A) A cholangiogram shows obstruction on the confluence of the right and left ducts by a Klatzkin's tumor. (B) After drainage of the right lobe, cholangitis occurred as a result of bacterial colonization of the left biliary tree. Note the severe stenosis and dilatation of the left duct after abundant drainage on the right. (C) From an anterior approach, No. 8 French endoprosthesis was placed, connecting the left duct to the common bile duct, as shown schematically in Fig. 5.25.

Puncturing under apnea in inspiration is a useful technique for reaching the liver and the biliary tree from below the rib cage and sternum (Fig. 5.27). Held inspiration for a few seconds is usually enough for puncture and opacification of the left biliary duct. It will make the puncture more vertical than when the puncture is made while the patient holds breathing under expiration.

Placing Endoprostheses or Multiple Catheters

Several endoprostheses or biliary tree drainage catheters can be used to drain multiple independent segments of the biliary tree. This can be done using the simultaneous lateral and anterior approach technique or the lateral double approach technique with placement of a Y-shaped endoprosthesis.

In using the simultaneous anterior and lateral approach, one should proceed as in the lateral approach, draining the right biliary tree into the duodenum (Fig. 5.25). With additional puncture of the left biliary tree, using the technique that has been described above, an endoprosthesis is introduced that can connect the left hepatic duct to the common bile duct without going beyond the papilla. Figure 5.28 illustrates the use of two endoprostheses in these conditions.

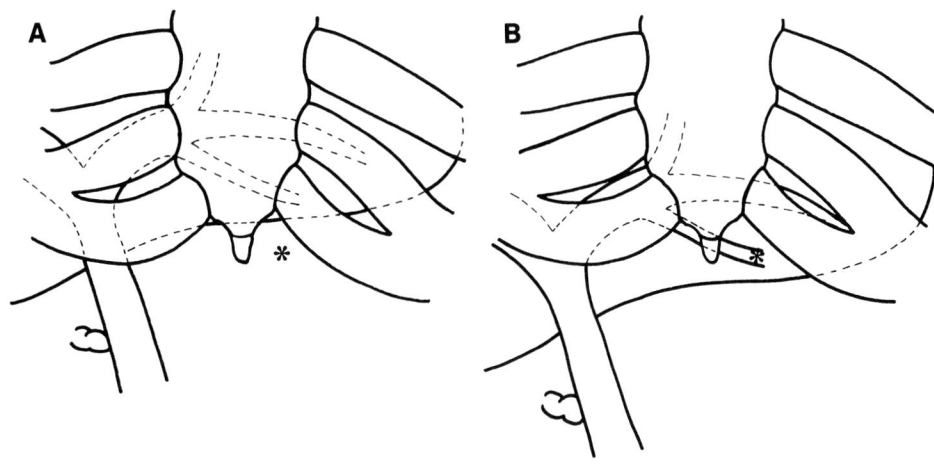

Figure 5.27 Importance of the respiratory phase in biliary duct puncture of the left liver lobe.
(A) During expiration, the left liver lobe hides behind the costal cage and sternum. Asterisk shows the ideal puncture site, lateral to the xiphoid appendix and below the substernal angle of the left costal border formed by the seventh costal cartilage. (B) During inspiration, the whole left liver lobe is caudally displaced and the left biliary tree remains at the level of the ideal puncture site.

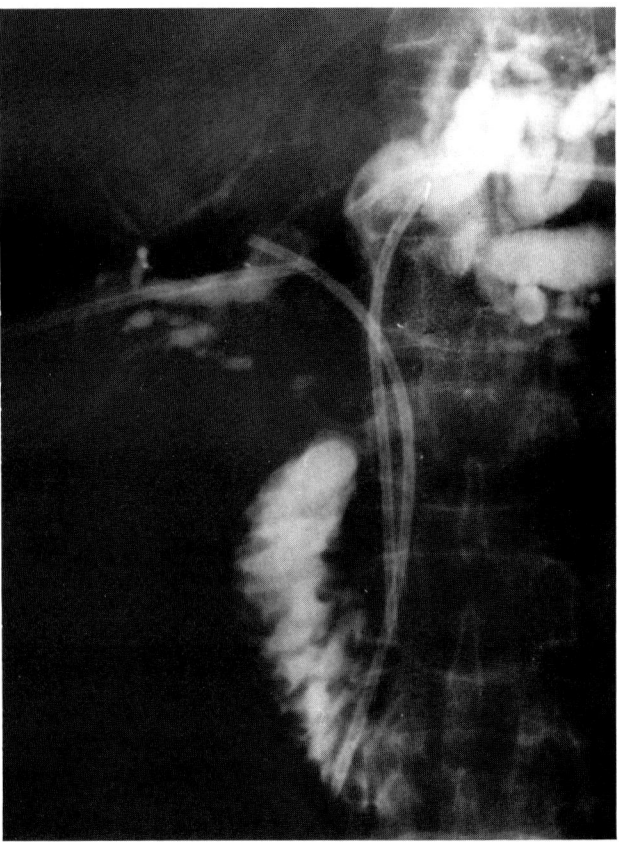

Figure 5.28 A patient with cholangiocarcinoma on the confluence of the hepatic ducts.
Two Burcharth-type endoprostheses were placed using the right lateral and left anterior approach. Note that the left prosthesis connects the left duct to the common bile duct and that the right prosthesis connects the right biliary tree to the common bile duct, going beyond the papilla to the duodenum.

An alternative to the Y-shaped endoprosthesis is the conventional right lateral approach followed by transhepatic right-left interductal puncture, with placement of an internal-external endoprosthesis from the left duct to the right duct. This prosthesis is drained into the duodenum by the conventional endoprosthesis. Alternatively, an internal-external drainage catheter can be used to decompress the right lobe (Figs. 5.29 and 5.30).

Another method for draining both biliary tree segments in a patient with confluential occlusion is retrograde catheterization of the left duct with a Simmons-type catheter. After a conventional right lateral approach, a Simmons type 1 catheter is introduced and bent inside the duodenum. The papillary orifice, as well as the left duct orifice, is retrogradely catheterized, with a guidewire passed to the left duct. Once the guidewire is anchored inside the left biliary tree, the Simmons catheter is pulled; it penetrates the biliary tree while dilating the track inside the tumor in the porta hepatis. The Simmons catheter is then exchanged for an internal-internal endoprosthesis, which connect's the left duct to the common duct and the right duct (Figs. 5.31 and 5.32). An endoprosthesis or internal-external drainage catheter can be used in the conventional fashion to drain the right duct.

Draining both sides of the biliary tree is not always necessary in patient's with Klatzkin's tumor, since decompression of the right lobe alone will keep most of these patients both anicteric and free of complications. However, violating the biliary tree while connecting it to the duodenum may lead to bacterial colonization of the biliary bed, with stasis and formation of severe suppurative cholangitis in the left occluded segment. In these cases, additional manipulation should be performed, as

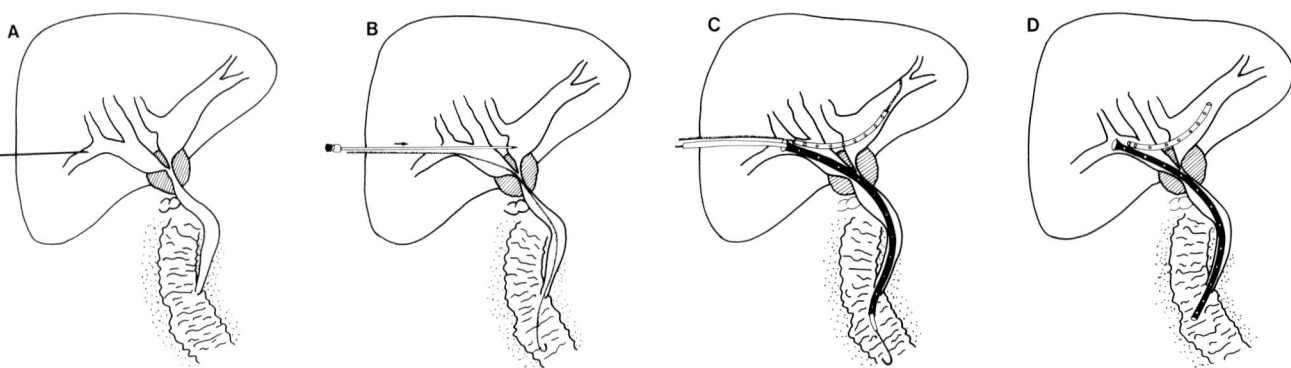

Figure 5.29 Schematic drawing of the right lateral approach with interductal puncture by placement of a Y endoprosthesis.
(A) Puncture of the right biliary tree for a cholangiogram with a Chiba needle. (B) Interductal puncture by the right approach with a needle with a Teflon sheath after passing beyond the obstruction, reaching the duodenum, and placing a safety guidewire. (C) After catheterization of the left duct, an internal-internal endoprosthesis is placed, connecting the left and right ducts and the main internal endoprosthesis that connects the right lobe ducts to the common bile duct and duodenum. (D) Final aspect shows the two endoprostheses in place after removal of the introducing system.

Figure 5.30 A 55-year-old patient with gallbladder carcinoma in whom the interductal technique was used.
(A) A cholangiogram after drainage of the right biliary tree and the occurrence of cholangitis in the left duct.
(B) After puncture and interductal catheterization, the main endoprosthesis is placed.
(C) After both endoprostheses are in place, a contrast injection shows abundant drainage of the whole biliary system into the duodenum. (D) Final aspect after Y endoprostheses have been placed and the introducing system has been removed.

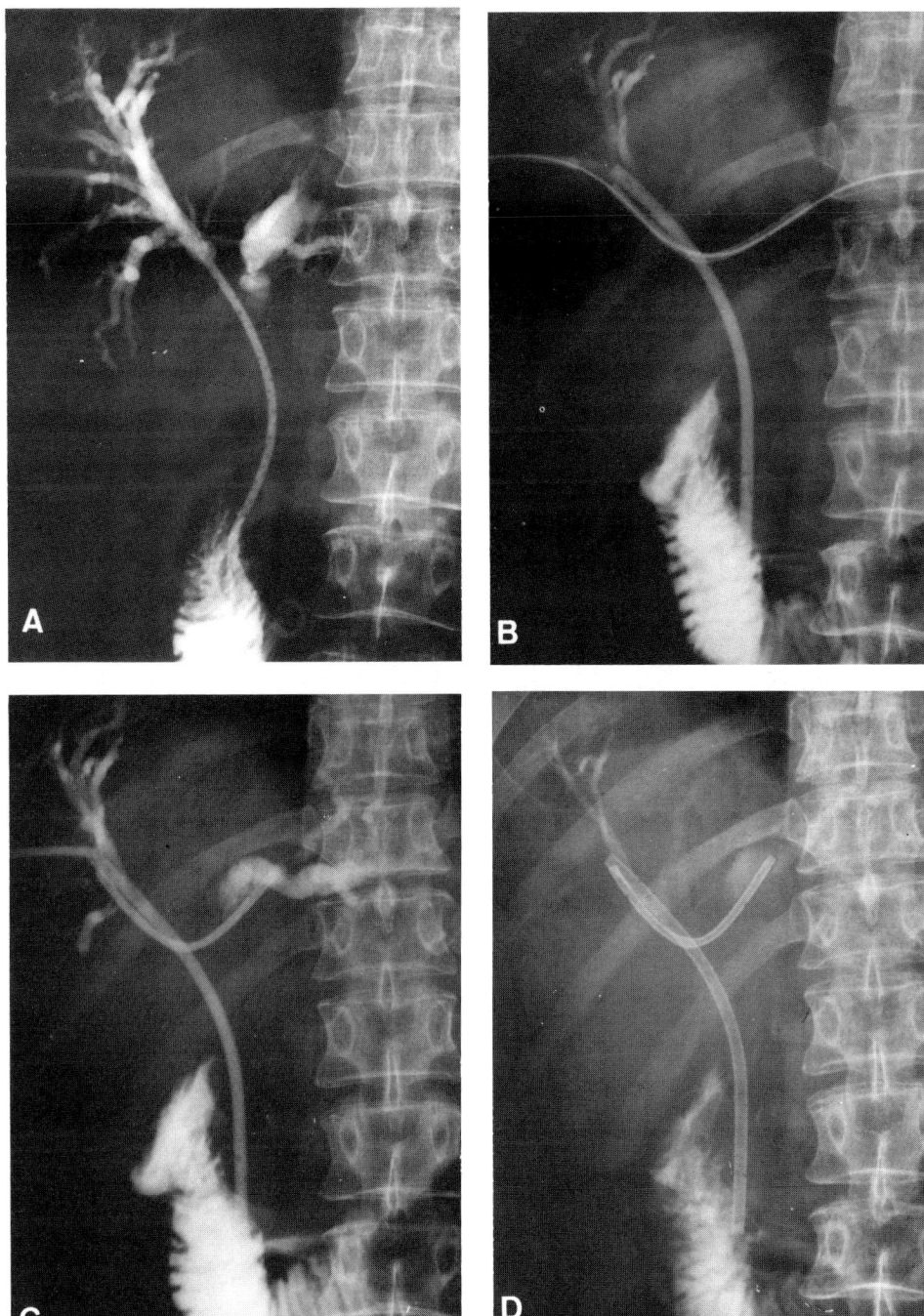

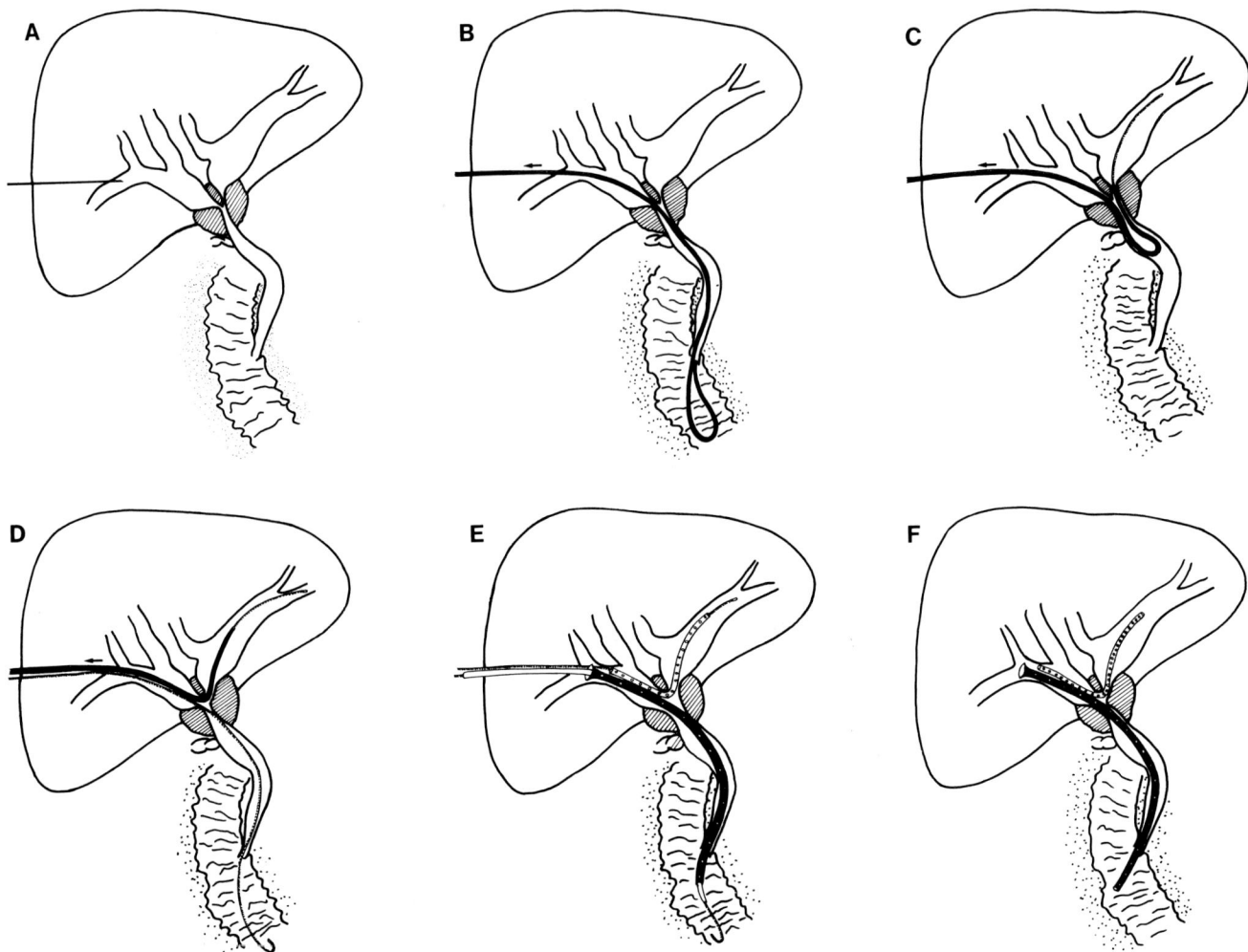

Figure 5.31 Schematic drawing of retrograde catheterization of the left biliary duct.
(A) A percutaneous cholangiogram with a Chiba needle introduced through the right approach in a patient with high obstruction. (B) After the lesion has been passed, the duodenum is catheterized with a Simmons-type catheter, which is reshaped to its original form inside the duodenal lumen. After this, the papilla is catheterized retrogradely and the catheter is pulled inside the common bile duct. (C) Once inside the common bile duct, the Simmons catheter is used to penetrate the left duct orifice; a guidewire is then introduced deeply into the left lobe ducts. (D) Soon afterward, the Simmons catheter is pulled back, and its distal tip penetrates the left duct. (E) The internal-internal endoprosthesis is then introduced from right to left, with the main endoprosthesis or Ring catheter introduced into the right duct. (F) Final aspect of the Y endoprosthesis.

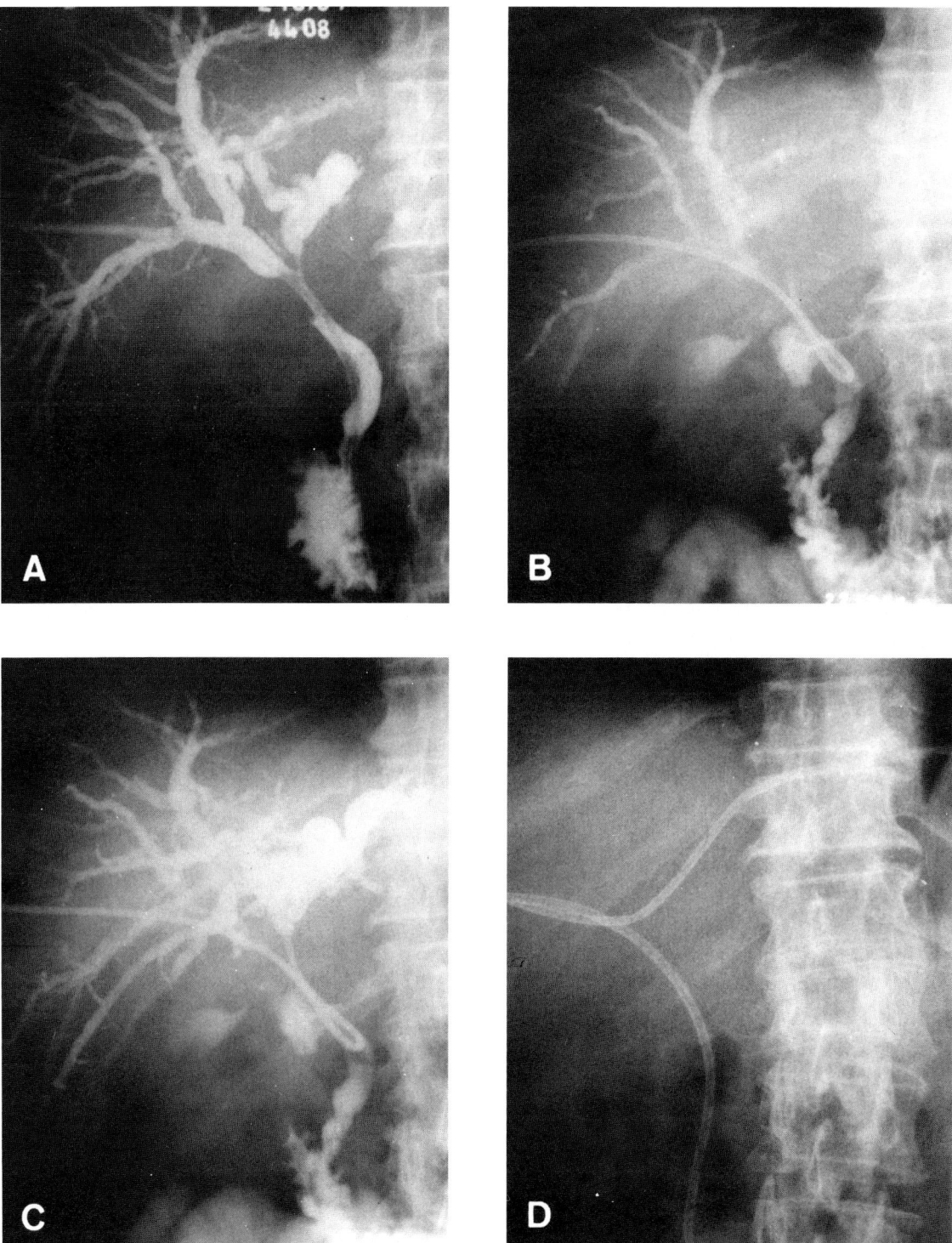

Figure 5.32 Patient with cholangiocarcinoma in the porta hepatis.
(A) A cholangiogram through a Ring catheter which adequately drains only the right lobe. (B) A Simmons catheter already inside the orifice of the left duct. (C) Selective contrast injection into the left duct. (D) Final aspect shows the internal-internal endoprosthesis connecting the left and right ducts and a Ring catheter placed through the right lateral approach for internal-external drainage.

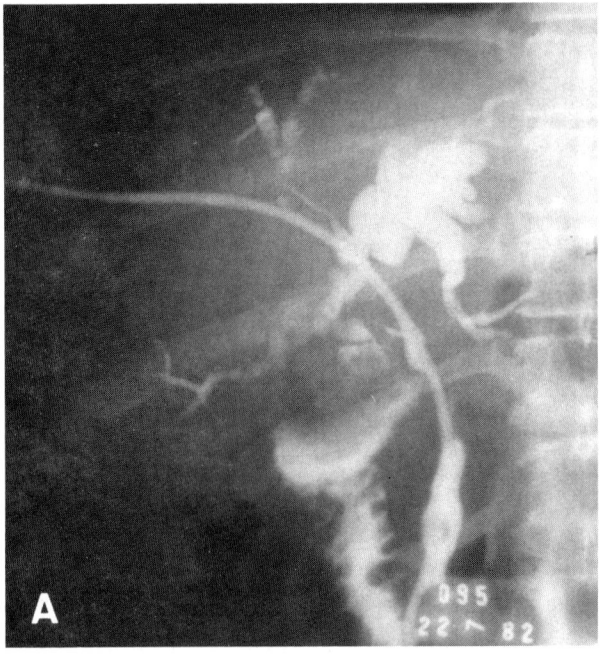
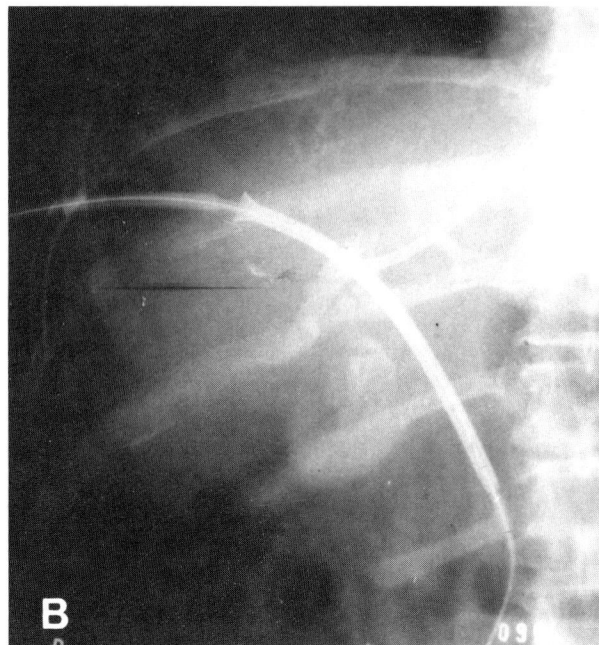
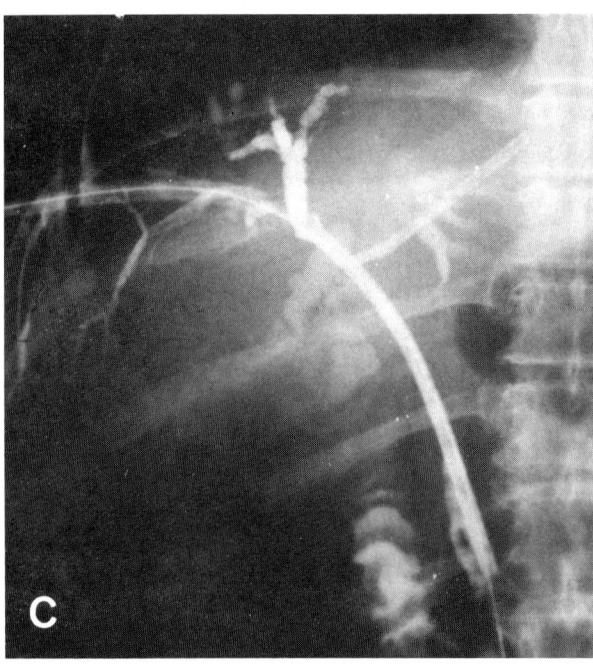

Figure 5.33 A 40-year-old patient with cholangiocarcinoma of the porta hepatis.
(A) Internal-external drainage with a Ring catheter of the right liver lobe only. (B) A Lunderquist-Hoevels–type endoprosthesis is placed with the flange's proximal tip associated with a small internal-internal No. 8 French endoprosthesis. (C) Note that the main endoprosthesis is placed with its distal tip above the papilla, preserving the sphincteric mechanism.

already described. The easiest alternative in these patients is the anterior approach through the left lobe (Figs. 5.25 and 5.26). However, the option of approaching only from the right should always be considered when a Y-shaped endoprosthesis is placed (Fig. 5.33) or when a catheter is used with an endoprosthesis (Fig. 5.34).

Should the distal tip of the endoprosthesis be above or below the papilla? Placing the distal tip above the papilla offers the obvious advantage of preserving the functional sphincteric mechanism very close to its physiologic condition, i.e., preventing backflow of duodenal contents into the biliary tree, which can cause cholangitis (Fig. 5.33). This position, however, may lead to perforation of the common bile duct inside the pancreatic head as a result of the continuous pressure imposed by the tip of the endoprosthesis on the wall of the common bile duct. This perforation usually does not create inconveniences, but it may cause pancreatitis and/or bleeding. For this reason, it is convenient to place the distal tip of the endoprosthesis inside the duodenal lumen, where in most cases the risk of structural lesion is lower.

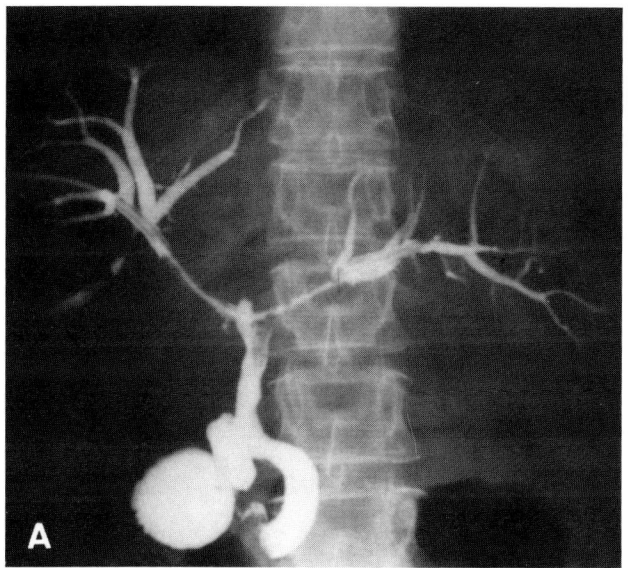
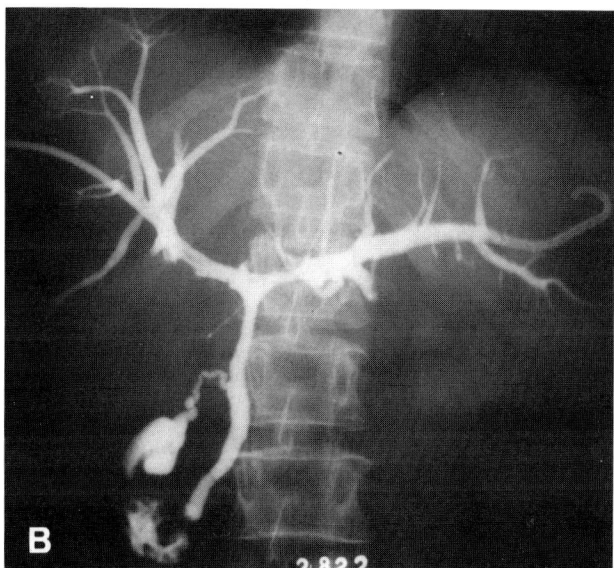
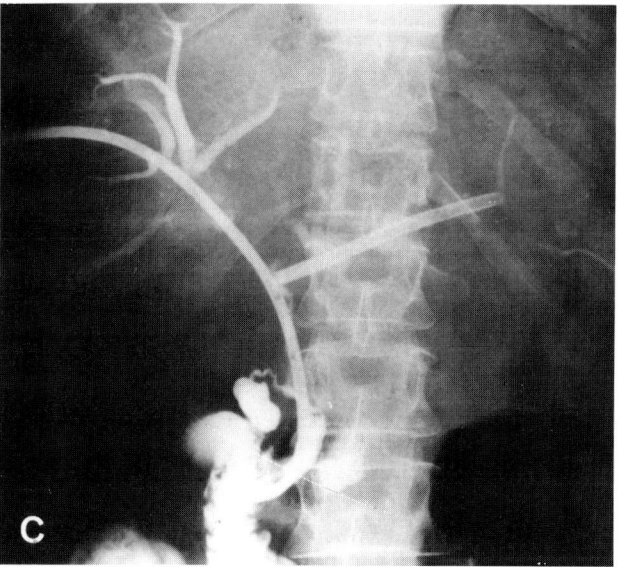

Figure 5.34 A 72-year-old female patient with hilar metastases of colon carcinoma.
(A) High obstruction of the biliary tree, which was previously drained externally. (B) A Ring catheter connecting the left and right hepatic ducts. (C) An internal-external drainage catheter was later placed on the right side, and a large-gauge internal-internal endoprosthesis formed the Y.

Metastatic Disease of the Porta Hepatis

Metastatic involvement of lymph nodes in the porta hepatis is one of the most common causes of malignant biliary obstruction. These tumors usually originate in the digestive tract, but other primary lesions, such as those of the breast and lung, may also involve the porta hepatis and cause biliary obstruction (Fig. 5.34).

Some of these metastases respond well to chemotherapy and radiotherapy, with excellent results in terms of regression. However, the application of these different therapies is hindered by the patient's debilitated condition and by liver dysfunction caused by biliary obstruction. These metastatic lesions are not generally suitable for surgical biliary decompression, because the obstruction occurs at a site that provides poor access for bile-enteric shunting and because these patients are placed at high risk by surgery.

Percutaneous biliary drainage has one of its major indications in these patients since it interrupts the progressive process of anorexia, pruritus, coagulopathy, and other symptoms. Effective percutaneous biliary drainage in patients with metastases in the porta hepatis often creates the possibility for additional treatment with chemotherapy and/or radiotherapy because of the clinical improvement obtained. The major benefit, however, is improvement in symptoms and quality of life. Survival in these patients is, however, limited. The average survival is approximately 5 months, although some patients have survived for more than a year.

A biliary endoprosthesis is a good alternative in patients with metastatic disease of the porta hepatis with the primary lesion in the digestive tract because these patients clearly do not respond to either chemotherapy or radiotherapy and thus have a very limited prognosis for survival. In all other patients with primary tumors in the breast or lungs, an internal-external drainage catheter should be used, since in these patients survival will probably be longer and obstruction may regress. After adequate treatment, the drainage tube can be removed.

Pancreatic Carcinoma

In spite of recent progress in imaging methods, along with extraordinary improvement in the diagnosis of pancreatic lesions, in most cases pancreatic tumors remain unresectable by the time the diagnosis is made. Surgical resection can be performed in just 10 to 15 percent of patients, with a 5-year survival rate below 15 percent for operated patients.

The average survival of patients with carcinoma of the pancreas is 5.4 months after diagnosis. Half the deaths caused by pancreatic carcinoma occur within 3 months of the onset of symptoms, with the remaining patients surviving up to 6 or 8 months. Palliative surgical decompression of the biliary tree represents a high risk for this group of patients, with 16 to 59 percent mortality rates in some series.

Percutaneous biliary decompression is therefore a significant nonsurgical alternative for treating patients with an unresectable tumor. Palliation of symptoms can be obtained quickly with a procedure that has a low mortality rate, such as percutaneous drainage (Fig. 5.18). Because of their short survival these patients are the primary candidates for placement of a permanent internal drainage endoprosthesis.

A short stay in the hospital (3 days to 1 week) is an additional benefit for patients with a prognosis of a short survival. Another indication for percutaneous drainage in these patients is an unsuccessful previous surgical procedure for decompression.

Aspiration biopsy is always indicated for patients with masses on the head of the pancreas because of the need to establish a definitive diagnosis of the lesion while excluding other pathologies, such as pancreatitis and lymphomas, which may mimic a pancreatic carcinoma (Fig. 5.21).

Cholangiocarcinoma

Primary tumors of the biliary ducts are the least aggressive malignant lesions involving obstruction in the biliary tree. Distal tumors are frequently resectable, with a cure obtained in up to 30 percent of patients. When the tumoral lesion involves the common hepatic duct and the confluence of the right and left hepatic ducts—the so-called Klatzkin's tumor—resection is less frequently feasible. In only 10 percent of cases are these lesions resectable because they are usually far advanced by the time of diagnosis.

The natural history of these lesions, however, is one of slow growth, with progressive local infiltration and without distant metastatic lesions. Prolonged survival is not uncommon among these patients, since the biliary obstruction and consequent complications can be alleviated. Average survival is up to 13 months after diagnosis, although survival times of 2, 3, or 4 years have been recorded. The surgical treatment of these patients usually includes some type of permanent tube drainage, and in most cases percutaneous internal-external biliary tree drainage appears to be an adequate alternative (Figs. 5.18, 5.26, and 5.32).

In these patients, with only rare exceptions, internal-external drainage with one or two percutaneous catheters is the best choice, leading to longer survival. This makes it possible to exchange the catheters every 3 months, keeping the system adequate and permeable for several years. The transductal Y-shaped endoprosthesis should be considered an option in cases where it is necessary to drain both hepatic lobes (Fig. 5.35).

Brachytherapy has more recently been associated with antegrade drainage. Radioactive seeds are used to irradiate the Klatzkin's tumor, with promising results (see "Brachytherapy").

Carcinoma of the Gallbladder

Gallbladder carcinomas are extremely aggressive malignant lesions, but they are characterized by predominantly local dissemination. The diagnosis is usually late, and extensive areas of the liver may be invaded before biliary obstruction occurs.

The vast majority of patients die within 6 months after diagnosis. Tumor resection during cholecystectomy only occasionally leads to longer survival or cure of the carcinoma. Enlarged resections associated with partial hepatectomy increase the morbidity and mortality of the surgical procedure without significantly prolonging patient survival. These are of course the patients who will benefit from the use of percutaneous biliary drainage to decompress the cholestasis and improve the general condition. In these cases there is a firm indication for the use of an endoprosthesis for internal drainage alone, improving the quality of patients' life (Figs. 5.17 and 5.23).

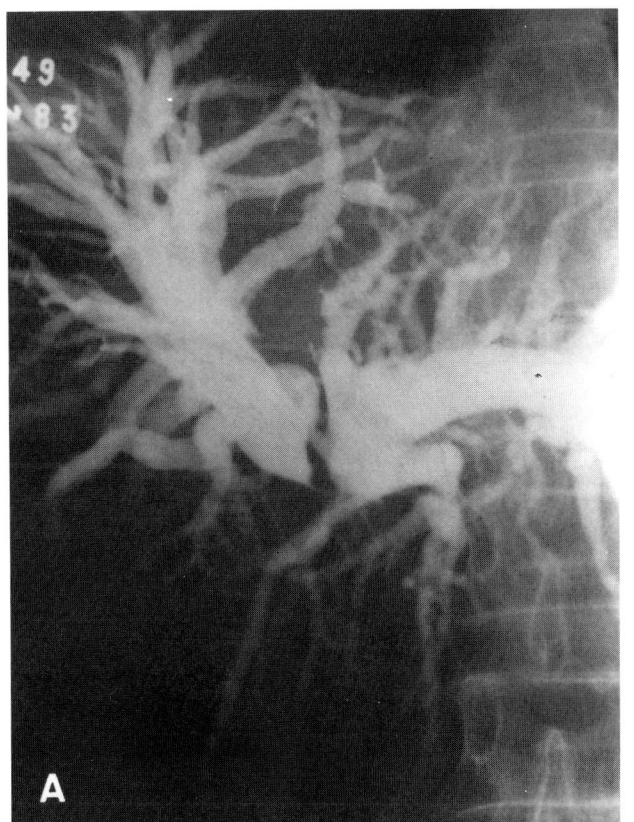
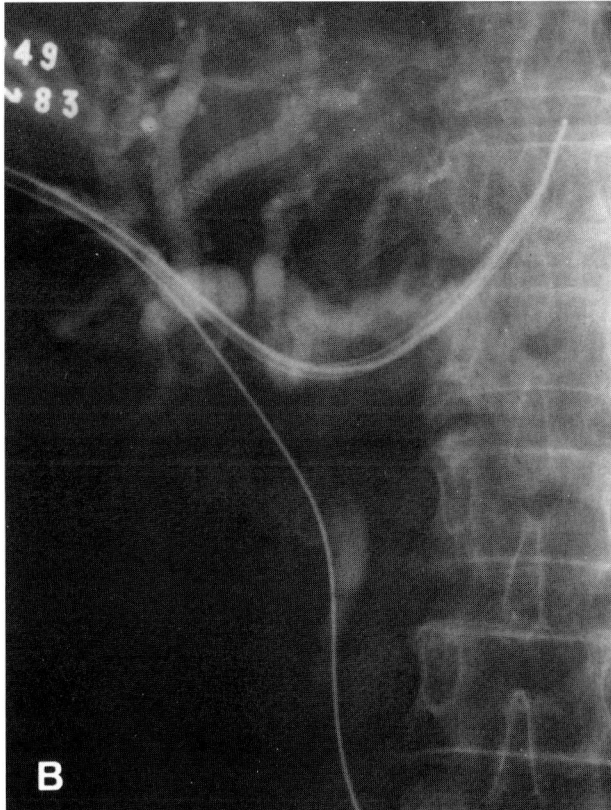
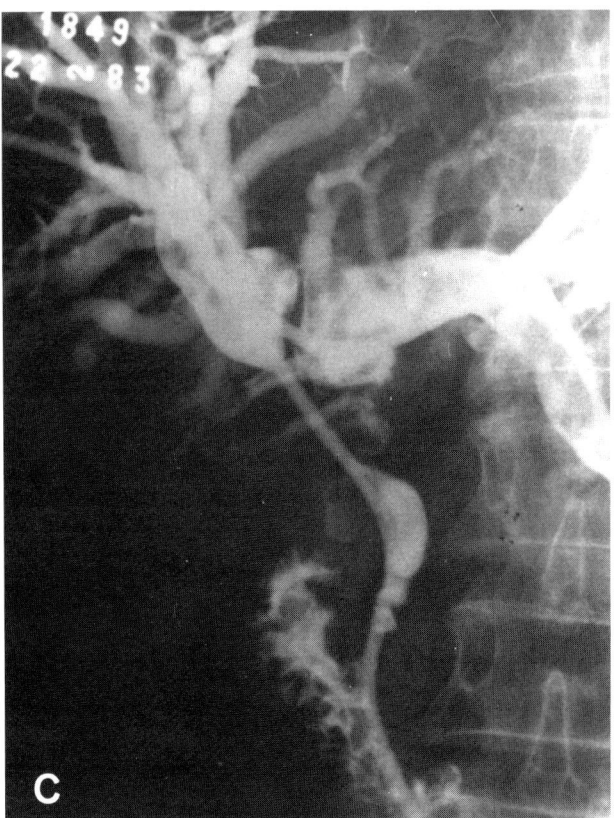

Figure 5.35 A patient with cholangiocarcinoma on the confluence of the right and left ducts.
(A) A percutaneous cholangiogram shows a dilated biliary tree and the obstruction on the confluence. (B) An internal prosthesis between the right and left ducts being placed. Note the guidewire passing through the lesion and reaching the duodenum. (C) Final aspect of internal-external drainage with a Ring catheter associated with a transductal endoprosthesis forming a Y.

Complications

Table 5.2 shows the incidence of several complications in a series of 105 patients. Mortality related to percutaneous biliary drainage is rare, generally associated with the patient's poor general condition, i.e., sepsis and blood dyscrasias followed by bleeding. The mortality rate for the percutaneous biliary drainage procedure is less than 2 percent. These complications as a whole affected around 23.1 percent of these 105 patients, or 16.7 percent of 152 procedures. Acute complications such as hemorrhage and sepsis occur in about 3 to 5 percent of patients according to the literature. Mortality caused by biliary drainage in patients with sepsis stays at approximately 10 to 17 percent, while the surgical mortality rate in the same population is approximately 50 to 75 percent.

Among the most common immediate problems related to percutaneous drainage of the biliary tree, pain during the procedure is the most serious, routinely requiring heavy sedation and analgesia. General anesthesia can be used, but it adds to the morbidity rate, particularly among septic patients. Some authors recommend the use of nitrous oxide gas with self-application by the patient if pain becomes severe or unbearable.

Complications associated with biliary tree drainage are as follows.

Table 5.2 – Complications in 105 Patients

Complication	Patients No.	%
Occlusion	6	5.7
Respiratory arrest	1	0.9
Fracture of endoprosthesis	1	0.9
Displacement		
Proximal	1	0.9
Distal	4	3.8
Sepsis	2*	1.8
Skin fistula	1	0.9
Portal-biliary fistula	1	0.9
Duodenal perforation	1	0.9
Common bile duct perforation	3	2.8
Hemorrhage	2	1.8
Pleural effusion	2	1.8
Total	25	23.7

*Associated with death in one patient.

Complications Caused by the Catheter

Occlusion

The presence of a biliary thrombus, clots, or debris originating from the duodenum or resulting from accelerated tumor growth may occlude the biliary drainage catheter. Such an alteration can be detected through contrast injection into the catheter, with a cholangiogram performed through the drain itself. When an endoprosthesis is obstructed, a percutaneous transparietal cholangiogram will be necessary (Fig. 5.36). In patients with mucus-producing pancreatic carcinoma, obstruction of the biliary tree endoprosthesis may occur as a result of mucous impaction (Fig. 5.40).

When obstruction occurs, the clinical picture deteriorates, with recurrence of pruritus, jaundice, and pain in the right hypochondrium or even fever and shivering caused by cholangitis. This picture is accompanied by elevations in bilirubin, alkaline phosphatase, and γ-glutamyltransferase values.

Failure of antegrade drainage of the biliary tree after adequate catheterization is associated with several different causes and factors related to the position and number of lateral catheter holes, a catheter diameter that is inadequate for the viscosity and volume of bile to be drained, and the gradient between bile secretion pressures and duodenal intraluminal pressure (see "Internal-External Biliary Drainage").

Replacing a catheter with another with the same diameter or a larger diameter, repositioning the catheter, or, in the case of an endoprosthesis, disobstructing or repositioning the stent or exchanging it will overcome most problems caused by obstruction. Occasionally, endoprosthesis obstruction may be due to perforation of the common bile duct and duodenum (Figs. 5.37 and 5.38) or fracture of a polyethylene tube (Fig. 5.39).

Relieving endoprosthesis obstruction can be rather cumbersome, necessitating the use of a "roto-rooter" system to remove the debris from inside the endoprosthesis (Fig. 5.36). Endoscopic biopsy brushes as well as torque-controlled guidewires can be used to achieve this objective (Fig. 5.36).

Displacement of a large-gauge endoprosthesis can be corrected by recatheterizing the biliary tree, passing a guidewire through the endoprosthesis, and using an angioplasty 4-mm balloon catheter that is inflated inside the endoprosthesis. This technique is so effective that it is now possible to remove the endoprosthesis by the percutaneous route through the newly created track.

In mucus-producing pancreatic carcinomas, the large volume of mucus may occlude the biliary-digestive an-

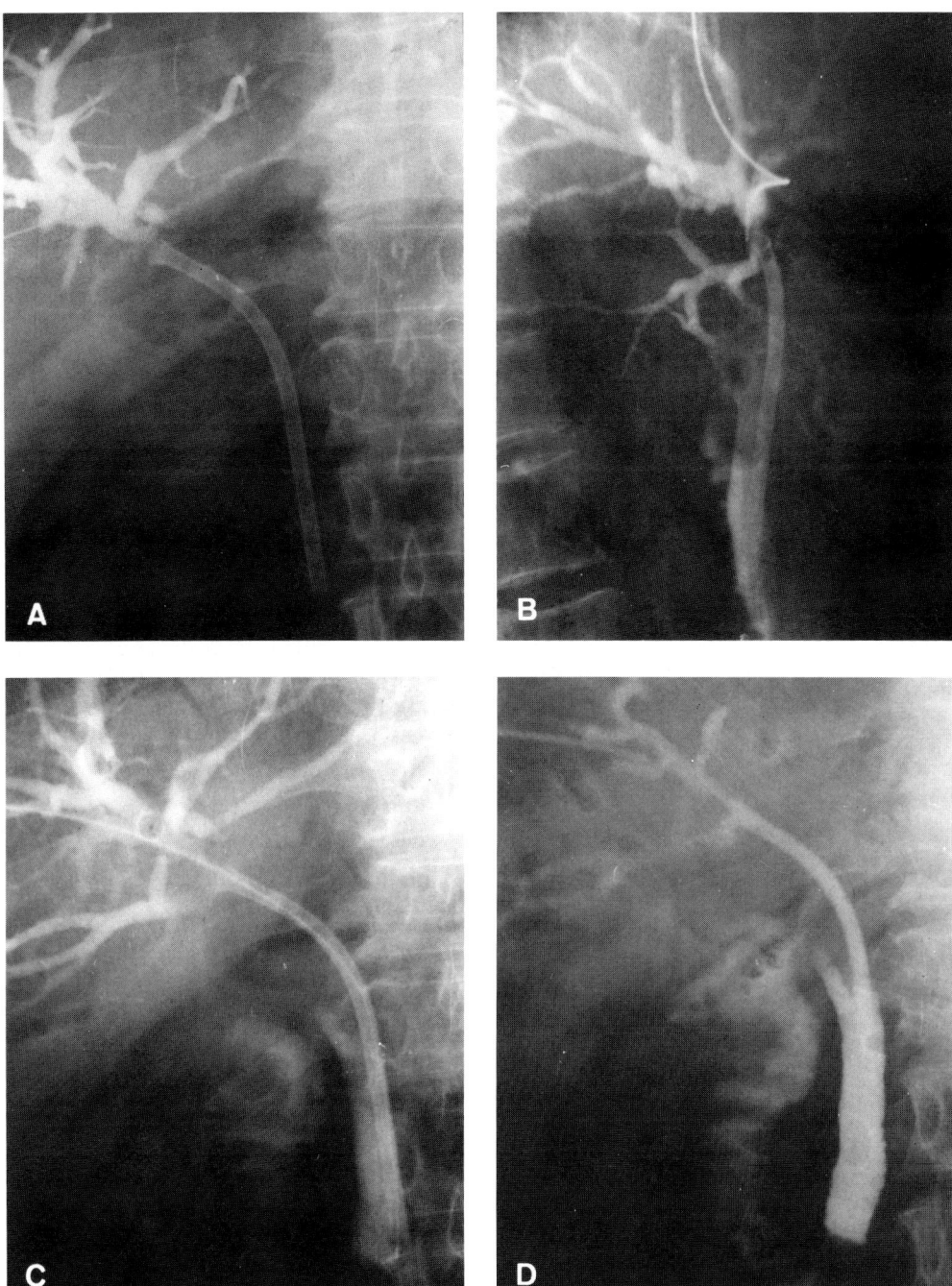

Figure 5.36 A Lunderquist-Hoevels–type endoprosthesis that occluded after being in place for a few months. (A) A percutaneous cholangiogram shows occlusion of the endoprosthesis. (B) Lateral view shows the guidewire at the beginning of disobstruction. Note the filling defects inside the endoprosthesis. (C) A guidewire inside the endoprosthesis while it is being cleaned. (D) Control of endoprosthesis patency after disobstruction.

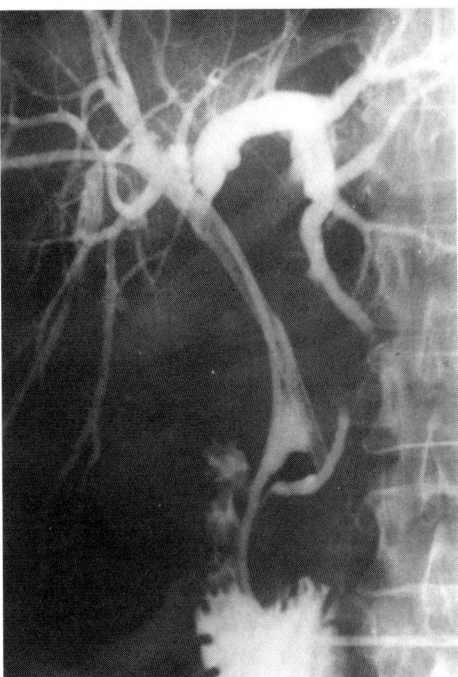

Figure 5.37 Perforation of the common bile duct by a large-gauge endoprosthesis.
The likely mechanism of perforation is mucosal compression and ischemia with rupture. Note the Ring internal-external drainage catheter in addition to the prosthesis.

Figure 5.38 Duodenal perforation by migration of an endoprosthesis in a patient with cholangiocarcinoma.
(A) Control after two endoprostheses have been installed for drainage of both hepatic ducts, using the lateral and anterior approach. (B) A control cholangiogram 48 h later shows migration of the right endoprosthesis with duodenal perforation (arrow). (C) An internal-external drainage catheter was introduced for drainage of the right biliary tree. Further migration of the endoprosthesis occurred with manipulation.

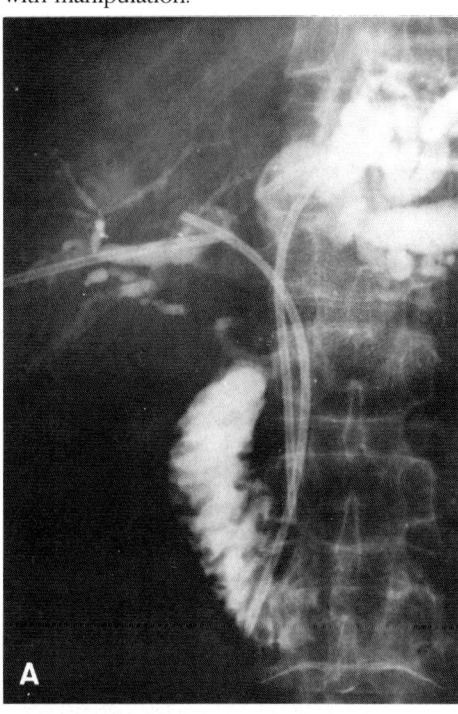

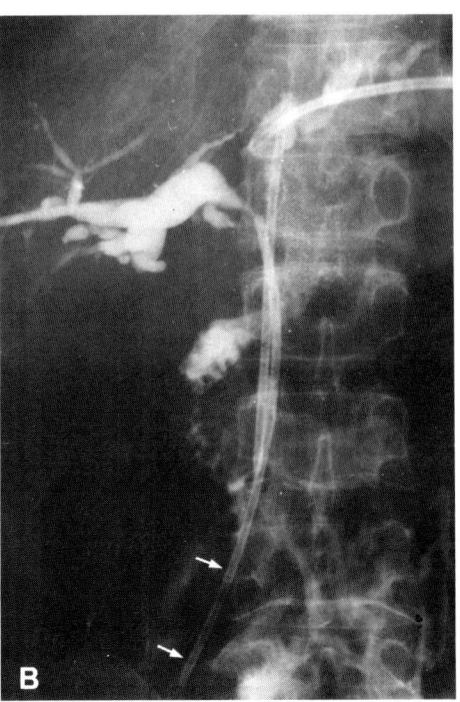

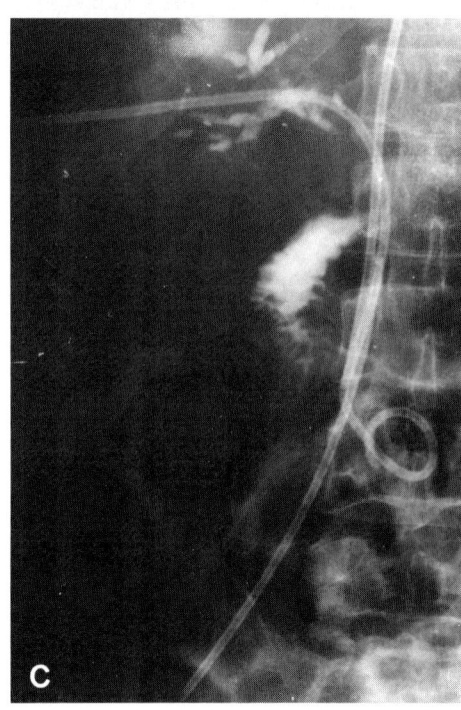

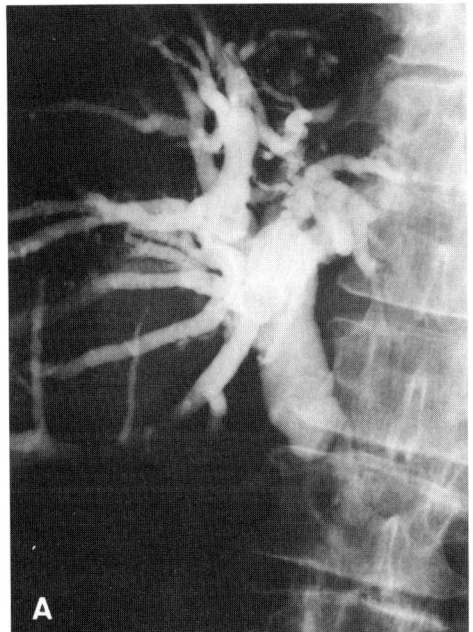
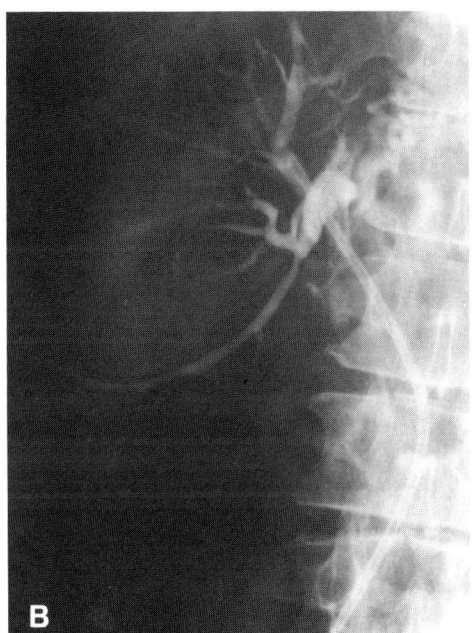
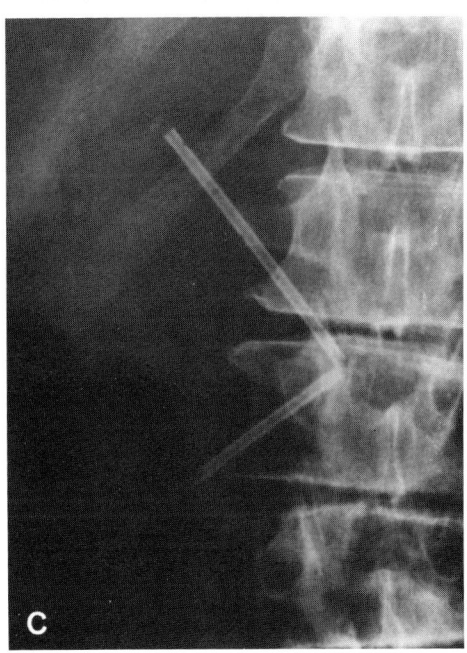

Figure 5.39 A patient with pancreatic carcinoma.
(A) Obstruction of the proximal common bile duct by a neoplasm. (B) Drainage was effective after a No. 8 French endoprosthesis was installed. (C) Jaundice recurred 2 months later. There was in situ fracture of the endoprosthesis, after which definitive external biliary drainage was performed.

astomosis and the catheter regardless of the available diameter (Fig. 5.40).

Hemmorrhage

Hemobilia is the most frequent hemorrhagic event among bleeding complications related to catheterization. The presence of blood in the drainage catheter most frequently reflects bad positioning, with side holes located in the liver parenchyma near the hepatic veins, the portal vein, or, less frequently, an extensive tumoral necrosis (Fig. 5.41). The formation of an arterial pseudoaneurysm by vascular trauma during the procedure is rare, although vascular lesions were found after biliary drainage in 20 to 30 percent of patients in recent series in which celiac axis arteriography was performed (Fig. 5.42). Embolization should control most cases of catheter-related hemobilia due to a pseudoaneurysm.

When bleeding is of venous origin, merely repositioning the catheter will control most accidents of this type. When bleeding originates from tumoral necrosis, frequent washing of the catheter and clinical observation,

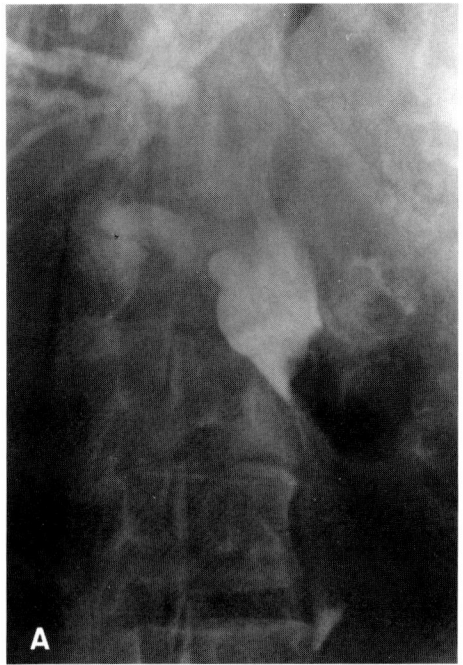
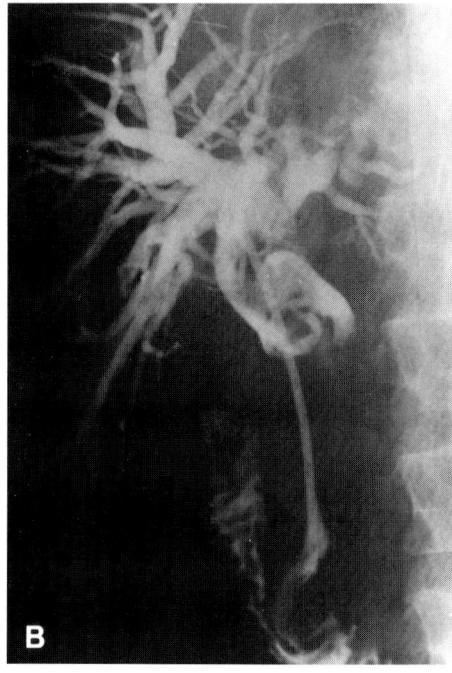
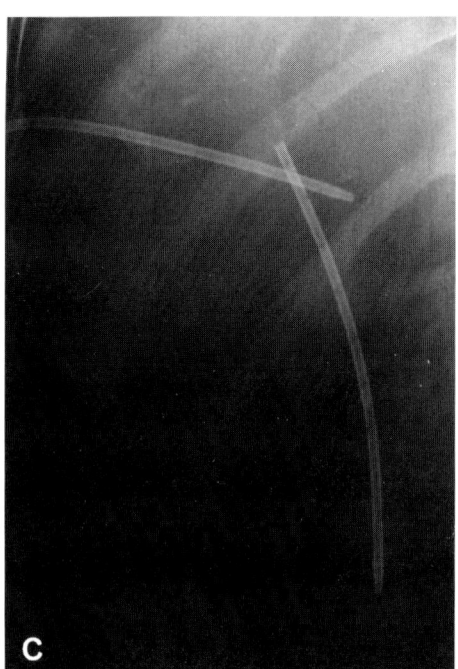
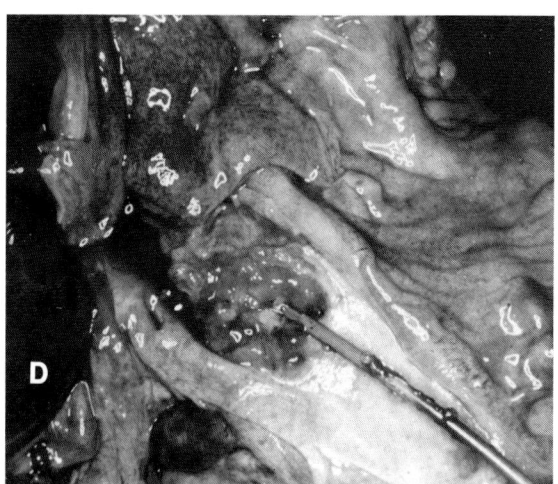

Figure 5.40 A 54-year-old patient with a mucus-producing pancreatic carcinoma.
(A) Occlusion of the common bile duct by an irregular expansive mass. (B) After an endoprosthesis was placed, good drainage was obtained for 15 days. Note the multiple filling defects inside the common bile duct caused by the presence of mucus. A biliary-digestive anastomosis with the gallbladder had previously been occluded. (C) View of a properly placed endoprosthesis. (D) View of an occluded endoprosthesis at necropsy. Note the large quantity of mucus inside the biliary tree.

with or without blood replacement, should control the majority of cases (Fig. 5.41). In rare situations, tumoral embolization may be the only way to control the hemorrhage. During severe bleeding due to an arterial pseudoaneurysm or arteriovenous (AV) fistula, immediate action should be taken. One option is immediate buffering of the drainage track with occlusion balloon catheters above and below the point of bleeding or even on the site of the pseudoaneurysm. This measure should always be followed by selective arterial embolization after the bleeding point has been carefully localized by means of angiography (Fig. 5.42). Embolization has become the standard technique for controlling this type of intrahepatic bleeding. Peripheral puncture of the biliary duct has been advocated as a way to prevent this complication.

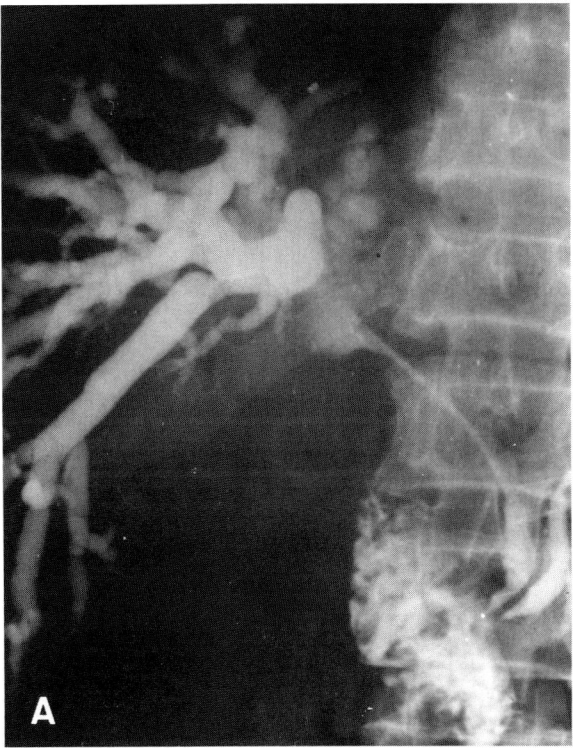
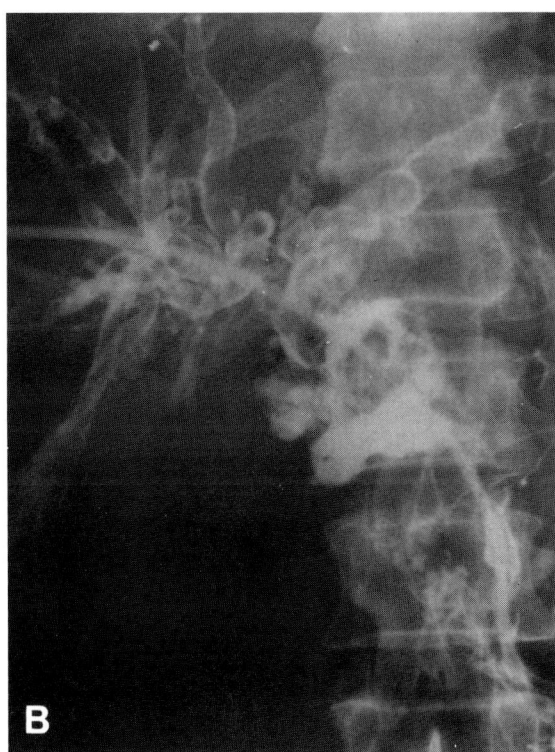

Figure 5.41 Obstruction of the biliary tree by metastasis of a gastric neoplasm to the porta hepatis.
(A) A long tumoral stenosis in the common bile duct.
(B) Two months after drainage acute bleeding occurred as a result of tumoral necrosis. Note tumor cavitation and double contrast inside the biliary tree as a result of clots. Bleeding resolved spontaneously with only blood replacement being required.

Perforation of Hollow Viscera

Perforation of the common bile duct or duodenum is a rare situation which results from inexperience in handling the rigid drainage guidewires and catheters or from unexpected displacement of a tapered endoprosthesis (Figs. 5.37 and 5.38).

Two different situations must be considered. The first is perforation of the biliary tree or duodenum during manipulation for biliary drainage. In these cases, once the viscera has been perforated, it is important that complete drainage of the area be performed with catheters for 7 to 10 days. In a patient with duodenal perforation, which is usually retroperitoneal, oral feeding should be discontinued, with a nasoduodenal tube used for decompression, along with antibiotic coverage (Fig. 5.38). In the second situation, visceral perforation occurs later, caused by displacement or continuous compression over the wall of the common bile duct or duodenum as a result of ischemic necrosis with perforation (Fig. 5.37).

If it is positioned above the papilla, a large-diameter rigid endoprosthesis of the biliary tree may lead to perforation of the common bile duct and penetration into the pancreas, causing pancreatitis. No action is usually required unless there is a loss of antegrade biliary drainage (Fig. 5.37). In some cases visceral perforation is complicated by significant bleeding, depending on the structures involved, or by abscess formation in the retroperitoneum or between the bowel loops.

Catheter Displacement

Displacement of a catheter or biliary tree endoprosthesis is a frequent complication. The most common effect of displacement is obstruction or a decrease in drainage efficiency due to bad positioning of the side holes in the internal-external drainage catheter or endoprosthesis in relation to the level of obstruction. In the case of internal-external drainage, catheter repositioning or exchange is a quick procedure; however, this is not the case with an endoprosthesis buried inside the biliary tree. If the endoprosthesis has a large diameter (No. 12 or No. 14 French), it may be easily catheterized in its lumen by the percutaneous route and repositioned utilizing a catheter with an inflated balloon inside it. If a fine endoprosthesis has been used (No. 7, 8, or 9 French), manipulation for repositioning is more difficult;

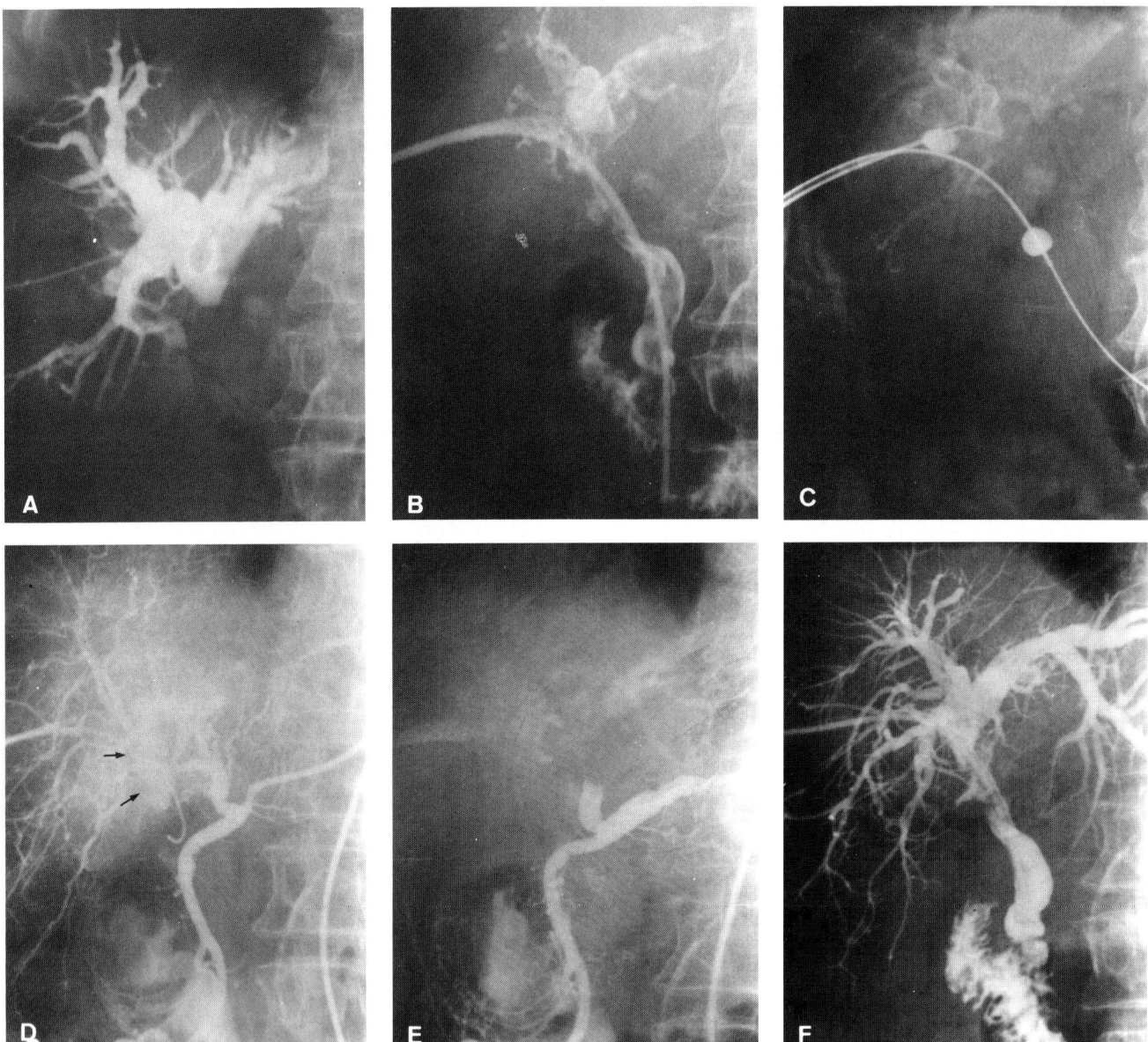

Figure 5.42 Cholangiocarcinoma of the porta hepatis.
(A) High obstruction of the common bile duct. (B) Intrabiliary bleeding (hemobilia) occurred 4 weeks after internal-external biliary drainage. Double contrast image inside the biliary tree. (C) Massive bleeding. Two balloon catheters were placed above and below the bleeding site, achieving a buffering effect. (D) A common hepatic selective angiogram shows a pseudoaneurysm in the right hepatic artery near the track of the drainage catheter (arrows). (E) Control after embolization of the right hepatic artery, with bleeding having stopped completely. (F) Control cholangiogram 5 days after bleeding stopped.

frequently the endoprosthesis is pushed into the duodenal lumen, and another prosthesis with a larger diameter is placed. The endoprosthesis in the duodenum may then migrate freely, or can be removed by means of endoscopy (Fig. 5.43).

Thoracic Complications of Biliary Drainage

Biliary drainage tubes may cross the pleural space more frequently than is usually thought in spite of the use of careful technique. This is caused by the extremely caudal position of the pleural recess, particularly in its lateral and posterior aspect (Fig. 5.2). Even if the lung and the

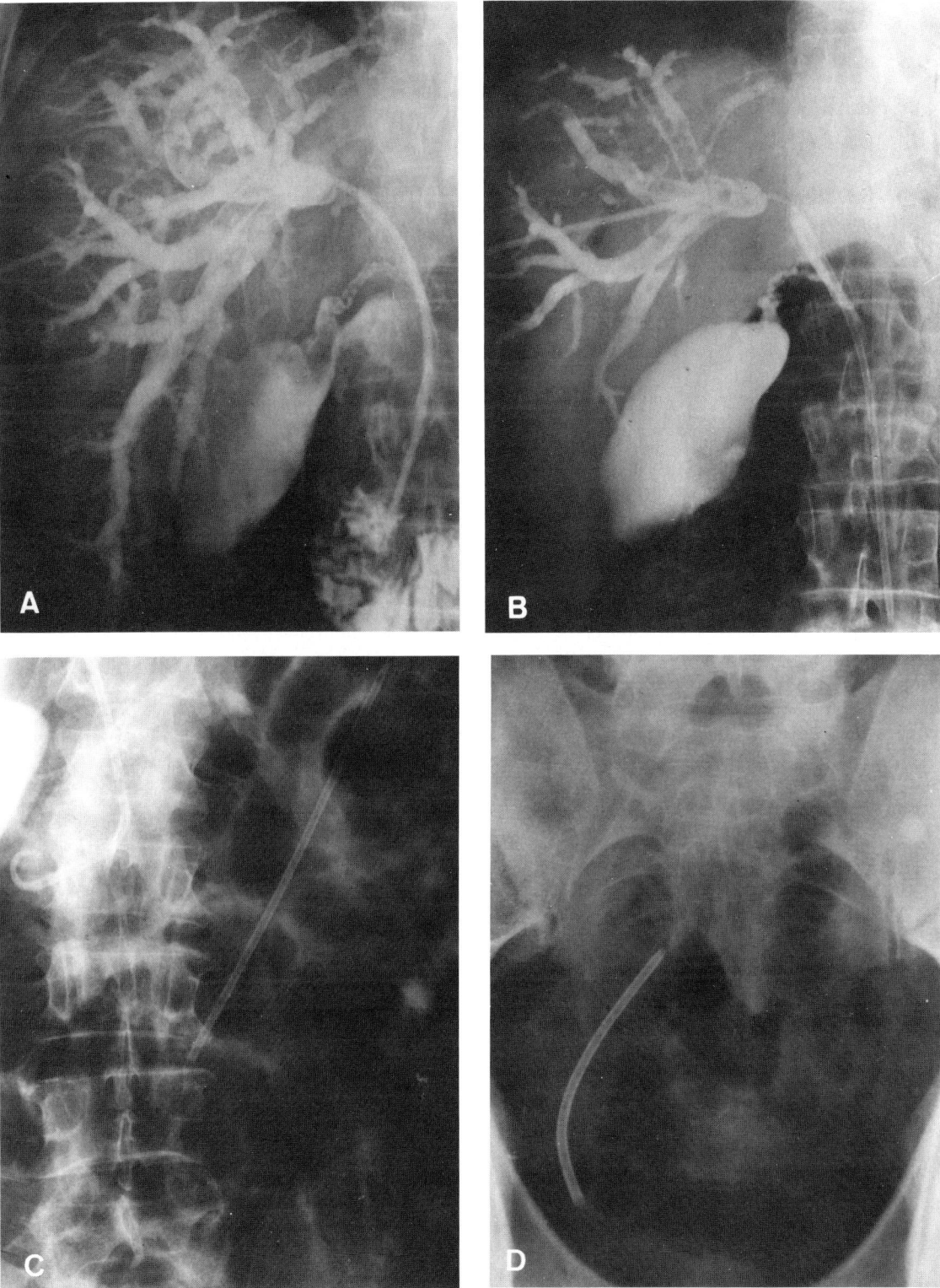

Figure 5.43 A 65-year-old patient with cholangiocarcinoma of the porta hepatis obstructing the common duct.
(A) Control immediately after internal drainage with a No. 8 French long prosthesis. Note the intrabiliary bleeding due to manipulation. (B) Control 48 h after drainage shows distal migration of the endoprosthesis. (C) The prosthesis migrating inside the third and fourth portions of the duodenal loop after it was displaced together with the internal-external drainage catheter. The endoscopist was not able to remove the endoprosthesis from the duodenum. (D) Endoprosthesis inside the terminal ileus. The tube was spontaneously evacuated later.

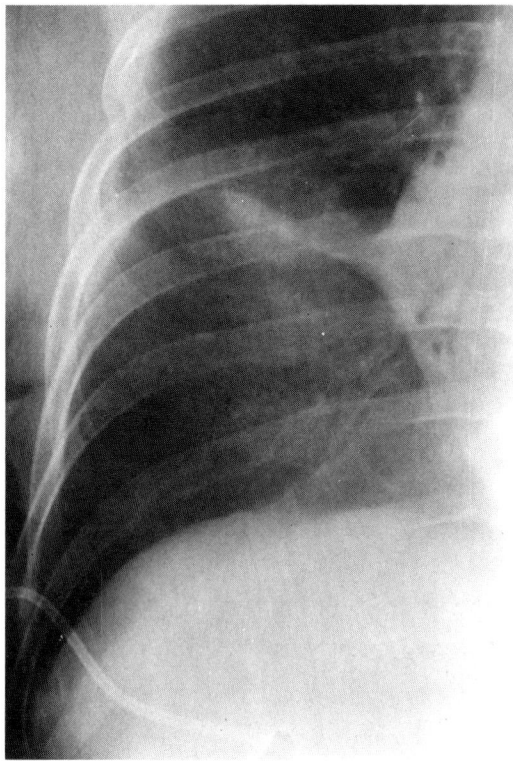

Figure 5.44 A 56-year-old patient with metastatic biliary tree obstruction of unknown origin at the level of the porta hepatis.
The patient presented with significant ascites and sepsis upon examination with an endoscopic retrograde cholangiographic procedure. Percutaneous puncture was performed, transfixing the right costophrenic sinus. Abundant pleural effusion developed. The patient had a poor evolution with pulmonary infection by *Pneumocystis carinii* and peritonitis and finally died of septicemia.

Tumoral dissemination along the puncture and drainage track, with tumoral implant on the skin, has seldom been observed. There was no track dissemination in any of our patients. Hemothorax with a serious or fatal evolution has rarely been reported in the literature.

Sepsis

Bile infection may have existed previously or may develop after biliary drainage. It is common to find infected bile in patients with biliary lithiasis and obstruction (Fig. 5.4). In these cases, manipulation of the biliary tree may result in severe systemic infection. In patients with tumoral obstruction, infection previous to drainage is seen less frequently; however, in patients who have been studied by retrograde endoscopic cholangiography, development of infection in the biliary bed has been found frequently, sometimes requiring emergency biliary drainage. The formation of a biliary cutaneous fistula caused by obstruction of biliary drainage can lead to serious septic complications in some patients (Fig. 5.45).

Acute cholangitis may establish itself after partial or total obstruction, sometimes followed by suppurative cholangitis. The most commonly found bacteria are *Escherichia coli, Streptococcus faecalis,* and *Klebsiella aerogenes*. When suppuration is present, the prognosis becomes significantly worse. In this situation, percutaneous decompression is mandatory.

Cholangitis that occurs while internal drainage is being performed with an internal-external drainage catheter should be treated with an aggressive antibiotic therapy protocol and the opening of external drainage into a flask.

costophrenic sinus are shown to be higher than the puncture site by fluoroscopy, it is always possible to reach the pleura during puncture. Although they are not frequent complications, hemothorax and pleural effusion of the biliary type may occur, along with pneumothorax (Fig. 5.44). Inadequate positioning of a catheter with lateral holes outside the liver parenchyma is the most frequent cause of these complications.

Complications Caused by the Technique

In patients with biliary drainage, organic complications caused by the technique may occur, including choleperitoneum, hemoperitoneum, sepsis, hemobilia, and the development of intrahepatic fistulas. Most of these complications can be prevented by improvement in the design and materials used to build the drainage system, by the use of antibiotics, and by greater experience on the part of the radiologist.

RESULTS

It was possible to go beyond the obstruction in 87 percent of the 105 patients in our first series of patients with biliary tree percutaneous drainage due to obstructive jaundice. Recently, success improved to about 96 percent.

The following causes of biliary obstruction were found: cholangiocarcinoma, 23 cases; metastases in the porta hepatis, 28; carcinoma of the pancreas, 21; gallbladder carcinoma, 19; papillary carcinoma, 3; periampullary lymphoma, 2; biliary-digestive fistula, 2; postoperative restenosis, 1; lithiasis of the common bile duct, 4; biliary tree laceration by a firearm, 1; parasitic cholangitis with stenosis, 1; surgical ligation of the common bile duct, 1; liver abscess, 1; and Caroli's disease, 1. There were 105 patients and 152 procedures in this series.

The obstructions found were high in 50 patients

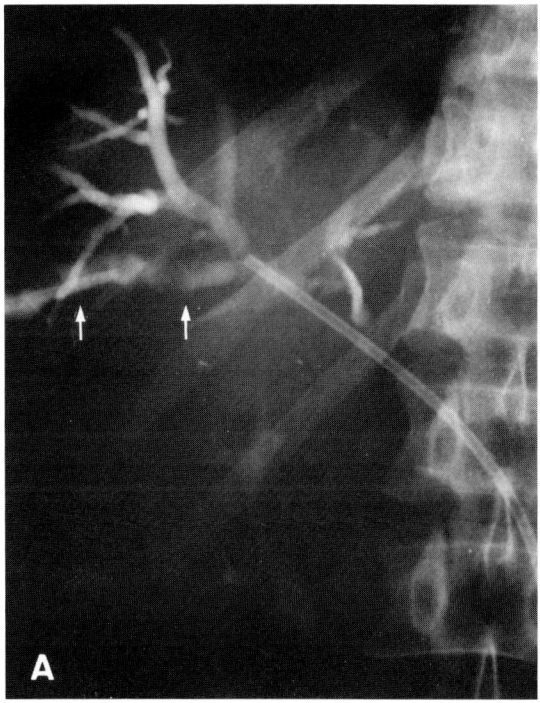 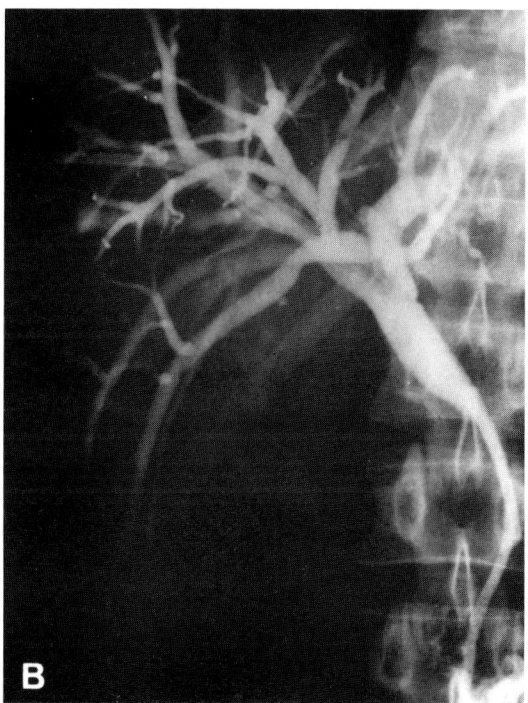

Figure 5.45 A biliary cutaneous fistula after migration and obstruction of an endoprosthesis.
(A) After removal of the external catheter, the external fistula remained open. This infected the patient, who later developed sepsis (arrows). (B) Internal-external drainage at another site (above the fistula) to drain the biliary tree and close the fistula. Sepsis was controlled by effective drainage and aggressive therapy with antibiotics. A culture of secretion showed *Klebsiella* sp. growth.

(47.62 percent), median in 37 (35.24 percent), and low in 18 (17.14 percent). Fifty biliary endoprostheses were used in the first 105 patients. Fifteen were Lunderquist-type endoprostheses, 19 were of the long modified Coons type, 13 were of the Burcharth type, and 3 were of the Y type. There were 25 complications (23.8 percent) (Table 5.2).

Death occurred as a consequence of these complications in two patients. Fatal complications were related to septic problems in a patient with immune deficiency due to neoplasm and postretrograde cholangioendoscopy suppurative cholangitis, and another patient with lithiasis and postretrograde endoscopic cholangiography developed suppurative cholangitis. Endoscopic papillotomy and impaction of the stone removal basket inside the common bile duct had caused the problem in the second patient.

In most patients in whom drainage was successful, there was significant improvement of the clinical condition, with reduction of jaundice, a decrease in bilirubin levels, and control of pruritus. The survival of patients with biliary neoplasm and percutaneous biliary drainage does not seem to be prolonged by this procedure, although there is obviously a reduction in hospital stay compared with biliary decompression surgery.

Some recent statistical studies have indicated that there would have been an extension in survival time in patients contraindicated for surgery, because of their poor general condition if they had been treated with biliary decompression by the percutaneous route.

REFERENCES

Adson MA, Farnell MB. Hepatobiliary cancer—surgical considerations. *Mayo Clin Proc* 1981;56:686–699.

Berquist TH, Mau GR, Johnson CM, et al. Percutaneous biliary decompression: Internal and external drainage in 50 patients. *AJR* 1981;136:901–906.

Bonnel D, Ferrucci JT, Mueller PR, Locaine F, Peterson HF. Surgical and radiological decompression in malignant biliary obstruction: A retrospective study using multivariate risk factor analysis. *Radiology* 1984;154:347–351.

Burcharth F. A new endoprosthesis for non-operative intubation of the biliary tract in malignant obstructive jaundice. *Surg Gynecol Obstet* 1978;146:76–78.

Burcharth F, Jensen LI, Olesen K. Endoprosthesis for internal drainage of the biliary tract: Technique and results in 48 cases. *Gastroenterology* 1979;77:133–137.

Burcharth F, Efsen F, Christiansen LA, et al. Nonsurgical internal biliary drainage by endoprosthesis. *Surg Gynecol Obstet* 1981;153: 857–860.

Burcharth F, Nielbo N. Percutaneous transhepatic cholangiography with selective catheterization of the common bile duct. *AJR* 1976;127:409–412.

Carrasco CH, Zornoza J, Bechtel WJ. Malignant biliary obstruction: Complications of percutaneous biliary drainage. *Radiology* 1984;152:343–346.

Castaneda-Zuniga WR, Tadavarthy SM. Anterior approach for biliary duct drainage. *Radiology* 1981;139:746–747.

Coons HG, Carey PH. Large-bore, long biliary endoprostheses (biliary stents) for improved drainage. *Radiology* 1983;148:89–94.

Dawson SL, Neff CC, Mueller PR, et al. Fatal hemothorax after inadvertant transpleural biliary drainage. *AJR* 1983;141:33–34.

Dawson S, Papanicolau N, Mueller PR, Ferrucci JT. Preserving access during percutaneous catheterizations using a double guidewire technique. *AJR* 1983;141:407.

Dooley JS, Dick R, Irving D, Sherlock S. Relief of bile duct obstruction by the percutaneous transhepatic insertion of an endoprosthesis. *Clin Radiol* 1981;32:163–172.

Druy EM. Hepatic artery biliary fistula following percutaneous transhepatic biliary drainage. *Radiology* 1981;141:369–370.

Edis A. Kiernan PD, Taylor WF. Attempted curative resection of ductal carcinoma of the pancreas. *Mayo Clin Proc* 1980;55:531–536.

Ferrucci JT, Adson MA, Mueller PR, Stanley RJ, Stewart ET. Advances in the radiology of jaundice: A symposium and review. *AJR* 1983;141: 1–20.

Ferrucci JT, Mueller PR. Interventional radiology of the biliary tract. *Gastroenterology* 1982;82:974–985.

Gobien RP, Stanley JH, Soucek CD, Anderson MC, Vujic I, Gobien BS. Routine preoperative biliary drainage: Effect on management of obstructive jaundice. *Radiology* 1984;152:353–356.

Gouma DJ, Wesdorp RIC, Oostenbroek RJ, Soeters PB, Greep JM. Percutaneous transhepatic drainage and insertion of an endoprosthesis for obstructive jaundice. *Am J Surg* 1983;145:763–768.

Gundry SR, Strodel WE, Knol JA, et al. Efficacy of preoperative biliary tract decompression in patients with obstructive jaundice. *Arch Surg* 1984;119:703–708.

Hamlin JA, Friedman M, Stein MG, Bray JF. Percutaneous biliary drainage: Complications of 118 consecutive catheterizations. *Radiology* 1986;158:199–202.

Hansson JA, Hoevels J, Simert G, Tylen U, Vang J. Clinical aspects of nonsurgical percutaneous transhepatic bile drainage on obstructive lesions of the extrahepatic bile ducts. *Ann Surg* 1979;198:58–61.

Hatfield AR, Terblanche J, Fataar S, et al. Preoperative external biliary drainage in obstructive jaundice. *Lancet* 1982;ii:896–899.

Hoevels J, Ihse I. Percutaneous transhepatic insertion of a permanent endoprosthesis in obstructive lesions of the extrahepatic bile ducts. *Gastrointest Radiol* 1979;4:367–377.

Hoevels J, Lunderquist A, Owman T, et al. Large-bore Teflon endoprosthesis with side holes for nonoperative decompression of the biliary tract in malignant obstructive jaundice. *Gastrointest Radiol* 1980;5:361–166.

Hoevels J, Nilsson U. Intrahepatic vascular lesions following nonsurgical percutaneous transhepatic bile duct intubation. *Gastrointest Radiol* 1980;5:127–135.

Honickman SP, Mueller PR, Ferrucci JT, Van Sonnenberg E, Kopaus DB. Malpositioned biliary endoprosthesis: Retrieval using a vascular balloon catheter. *Radiology* 1982;144:423–425.

Huibrectse K, Tytgat GN. Palliative treatment of obstructive jaundice by transpapillary introduction of large bore bile duct endoprosthesis. *Gut* 1982;23:371–375.

Jaques PF, Mandell VS, Delaney DJ, Nath PH. Percutaneous transhepatic biliary drainage: Advantages of the left lobe subxiphoid approach. *Radiology* 1982;145:534–536.

Jonsson K, Hellekant CAG. Percutaneous insertion of an endoprosthesis in obstructive jaundice. *Radiology* 1981; 139:749–750.

Kadir S, Ba'Assiria A, Barth KH, et al. Percutaneous biliary drainage in the management of biliary sepsis. *AJR* 1982;138:25–29.

Kaufman SL, Cameron JL, Adams PE, et al. Management of surgically placed silastic transhepatic biliary items. *AJR* 1984;142:347–350.

Kerlan RK, Pogany AC, Goldberg H, Ring EJ. Percutaneous biliary drainage in the management of cholangiocarcinoma. *AJR* 1983;141:1295–1298.

Kerlan RK, Stimac G, Pogany AC, et al. Bile flow through drainage catheters: An in vitro study. *AJR 1984*;143:1085–1087.

Kerlan RK, Ring EJ, Pogany AC, Jeffrey RB. Radiology biliary endoprostheses insertion on using a combined peroral-transhepatic method. *Radiology* 1984;150:828–830.

Leung JWC, Emergy R, Cotton PB, et al. Management of malignant obstructive jaundice at the Middlesex Hospital. *Br J Surg* 1983;70:584–586.

McPherson GAD, Benjamin IS, Hodgson HJF, et al. Preoperative percutaneous transhepatic biliary drainage: The results of a controlled trial. *Br J Surg* 1984;71:371–375.

Mendez G Jr, Russel E, LePage JP, et al. Abandonment of endoprosthetic drainage technique in malignant biliary obstruction. *AJR* 1984;143:617–622.

Miller GA, Hearton DK, Moore AV, et al. Peritoneal seeding of cholangiocarcinoma in patients with percutaneous biliary drainage. *AJR* 1983;141:561–562.

Mitchell SE, Schuman L, Kaufman SL, Chang R, Kadir S, Kinnison M. Biliary catheter drainage complicated by embolia: Treatment by balloon embolotherapy. *Radiology* 1985;157:645–652.

Mori K, Misumi A, Sugiyama M, et al. Percutaneous transhepatic bile drainage. *Ann Surg* 1977;185:111–115.

Mueller PR, VanSonnenberg E, Simeone JF. Fine-needle transhepatic cholangiography. *Ann Intern Med* 1982;97:567–572.

Mueller, PR, Van Sonnenberg E, Ferrucci JT. Percutaneous biliary drainage: Technical and catheter related problems in 200 procedures. *AJR* 1982;138:17–23.

Mueller PR, Ferrucci JT, Van Sonnenberg E, Warshaw AL, Simeone JF, Cronan JJ, Neff CC, Butch RJ. Obstruction of the left hepatic duct: Diagnosis and treatment by selective fine-needle cholangiography and percutaneous biliary drainage. *Radiology* 1982;145:297–303.

Mueller PR, Ferrucci JT, Teplick SK, Van Sonnenberg E, Haskin PH, Butch RJ, Papanicolau N. Biliary stent endoprosthesis analysis of complications in 113 patients. *Radiology* 1985;156:637–639.

Nichols DM, Cooperberg PL, Golding RH, et al. Safe intercostal approach? Pleural complications in abdominal interventional radiology. *AJR* 1984;142:1013–1018.

Nilsson U, Evander A, Ihse I, et al. Percutaneous cholangiography and drainage: Risks and complications. *Acta Radiol [Diagn] (Stockh)* 1983;24:433–439.

Norlander A, Kalin B, Sundblad R. Effect of percutaneous transhepatic drainage upon liver function and postoperative mortality. *Surg Gynecol Obstet* 1982;155:161–166.

Oleaga JA, Ring EJ. Interventional biliary radiology. *Semin Roentgenol* 1981;16:116–134.

Okuda K, Tanikawa K, Takeshi E, et al. Nonsurgical percutaneous transhepatic cholangiography—diagnostic significance in medical problems of the liver. *Am J Dig Dis* 1974;19:21–36.

Owen P. Analysis of the signs of common bile duct obstruction at percutaneous transhepatic cholangiography. *Clin Radiol* 1980;31:271–276.

Owman T, Lunderquist A. Sling retraction for proximal placement of percutaneous transhepatic biliary endoprosthesis. *Radiology* 1983;146:228–229.

Passariello R, Pavone P, Rossi P, Simonetti G, Modini C, Lasagni RP, Manella P, Gazzaniga GM, Paolini RM, Iacarino V, Feltrin GP, Roversi R, Mallarino G. Percutaneous biliary drainage in neoplastic jaundice: Statistical data from a computerized multicenter investigation: *Acta Radiol* 1985;26:681–688.

Pereiras R, Rheingold OJ, Hutron D, et al. Relief of malignant obstructive jaundice by percutaneous insertion of a permanent prosthesis in the biliary tree. *Ann Intern Med* 1978;89:589–593.

Ring EJ, Oleaga JA, Freiman DB, Husted JW, Lunderquist A. Therapeutic applications of catheter cholangiography. *Radiology* 1978;128:333–338.

Ring EJ, Kerlan, RK. Interventional biliary radiology. *AJR* 1984;142:31–34.

Scharschmidt BF, Goldberg HI, Schmid R. Approach to the patient with cholestatic jaundice. *N Eng J Med* 1983;308:1515–1519.

Shorvon PJ, Leung JWC, Corcoran M, Mason RR, Coton PB. Cutaneous seeding of malignant tumors after insertion of percutaneous prosthesis for obstructive jaundice. *Br J Surg* 1984;71:694–695.

Sibbtt RR, Palmay JC, Caplan RE, Page CP, Garcia F. Percutaneous biliary drainage with an enteric feeding tube. *Radiology* 1985;157:819.

Sniderman KW, Morse SS, Rapoport S, Ross GR. Hemobilia following transhepatic biliary drainage: Occlusion of an hepato-portal fistula by balloon tamponade. *Radiology* 1985;154:827.

Stambuck EC, Pitt HA, Paris O, Mann LL, Lois JF, Gomes AS. Percutaneous transhepatic drainage: Risk and benefits. *Arch Surg* 1983;118:1388–1394.

Stanley J, Gobien RP, Cunninghan J, Andriole J. Biliary decompression: An institutional comparison of percutaneous and endoscopic methods. *Radiology* 1986;148:195–197.

Teplick SK, Haskin PH, Goldstein RC, et al. New biliary endoprosthesis. *AJR* 1983;141:799–801.

Tylen U, Hoevels J, Nilsson U. Computed tomography of iattrogenic hepatic lesions following percutaneous transhepatic cholangiography and portography. *J Comput Assist Tomogr* 1980;5:15–18.

Uflacker R, Wholey MH, Amaral NM, Lima S. Parasitic and mycotic causes of biliary obstruction. *Gastrointest Radiol* 1982;7:173–179.

Uflacker R. Valor diagnostico da colangiografia trans-hepatica percutanea e da angiografia seletiva visceral na ictericia obstructiva. Dissertacao para obstenção de grau de Mestre em Medicina area de concentração em Gastroenterologia. Universidade Federal do Rio Grande do Sul. Faculdade de Medicina. Porto Alegre, 1981;1–123.

Uflacker R. Radiologia intervencionista: Uma especialidade emergente. *Radiol Bras* 1983;16:71–86.

Uflacker R, Lima SS, Pereira EC, Oliveira E, Silva A. Tratamento não cirúrgico das ictéricias obstrutivas. In *Hepatologia Clínica e Cirúrgica*. Ed Oliveria Silva A, D'Albuquerque LC. Sarvier, Sao Pãulo 1986:273–287.

Van Sonnenberg E, Ferrucci JT, Neff CC, Mueller PR, Simeone JF. Biliary pressure: Manometric and perfusion studies at percutaneous transhepatic cholangiography and percutaneous biliary drainage. *Radiology* 1983;148:41–50.

Extraction of Residual Stones from the Common Bile Duct

RENAN UFLACKER

Approximately 4 to 8 percent of patients who receive surgery for biliary lithiasis develop residual stones in the common bile duct. Until relatively recently, in most cases the only option in such cases was to repeat the surgical procedure. A major turning point was the development of the steerable catheter technique, which is used in patients in whom a T-tube exists. This percutaneous procedure, which has been successful in 95 percent of the more than 660 cases reported in the literature, can be performed in an outpatient clinic without anesthesia and with minimum morbidity.

In patients without a T-tube drain who have residual biliary tree stones, the most adequate options may be endoscopic papillotomy with stone extraction, stone dissolution with methyl *tert*-butyl ether (MTBE), and stone fragmentation with the extracorporeal shock wave lithotripsy (ESWL) technique. Only if these methods fail is surgical intervention in the biliary tree justified. Nevertheless, there have been reports in the literature of successful percutaneous transhepatic removal of stones from the common bile duct.

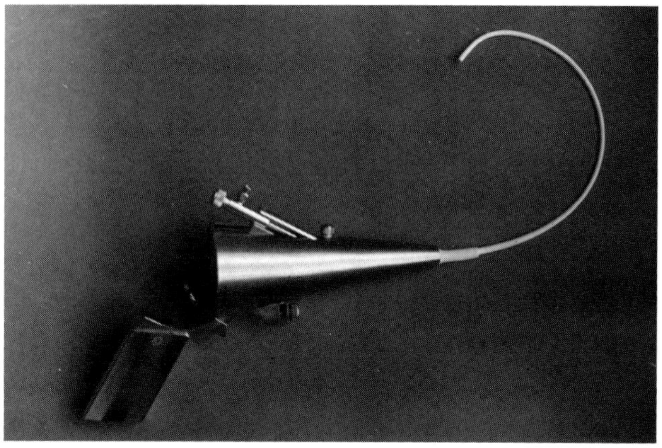

Figure 5.46 Instruments for percutaneous removal of residual stones in the common bile duct.
The photograph shows the manipulation handle of a Medi-Tech catheter. Note the upper entry point of the guidewire with a side-washing nozzle. The catheter is manipulated by a lever which is behind the gun. The white catheter is coupled to the gun, which is shown with its tip turned upward; the control lever is turned downward. This is a Medi-Tech catheter which was developed by Burhenne.

METHODOLOGY

After residual stones in the common bile duct have been identified, a waiting period is required. It takes about 5 weeks for a firm, thick, and well-delineated fistulous track to form around the drain. For smaller T-tubes, the waiting period should be extended to 7 weeks, both because it takes longer to form fistula walls with finer-diameter tubes and because the procedure itself is usually more difficult, requiring a more adequate fistula.

Some observations from the extensive experience gained by the authors who developed this technique are given here:

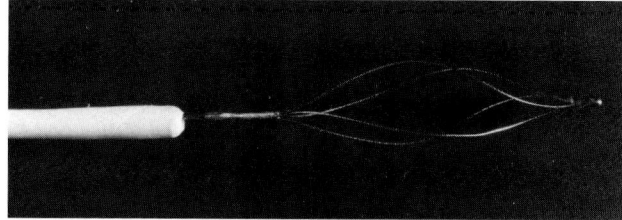

Figure 5.47 Instrument used for the extraction of residual stones in the common bile duct.
A Dormia-type basket is exteriorized on the directional tip of the catheter. This basket is manufactured by Cook.

1. Generally, a steerable-tip catheter of gauge No. 8, 10, or 12 French is used, coupled to a manipulation handle manufactured by Medi-Tech (Fig. 5.46). The Dormia-type stone basket, which is available in several diameters and sizes (Fig. 5.47), is used in conjunction with the steerable catheter.
2. The track used is the biliary cutaneous fistula formed by the T-tube drain.
3. The T-tube drain should be removed, but a guidewire should be kept inside the track. A cholangiogram performed before the drain is removed may show the stones in a position different from the actual position after T-tube removal, since wide lateral movement of the common bile duct occurs when the tube is pulled out.
4. After the steerable-tip catheter is introduced through the fistula until it reaches the site of the stone, a low-pressure cholangiogram should be performed. The

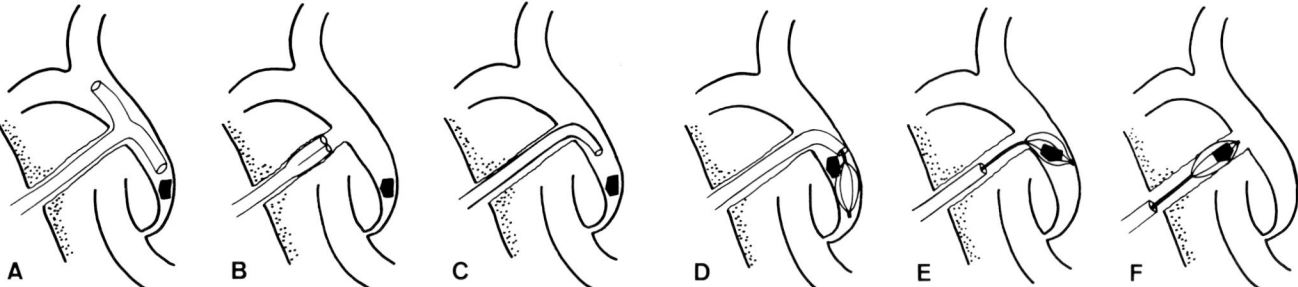

Figure 5.48 Schematic drawing and sequential detailed illustration of residual stones extracted from the common bile duct.
(A) A cholangiogram through the T-tube drain shows a residual stone inside the common bile duct. (B) Drain retrieval by pulling the T-tube. (C) Introduction of the catheter with a directional tip shown in Fig. 5.46. (D) Introduction of the Dormia basket beyond the stone. (E) Basket being pulled with rotational movement, with a stone trapped inside. (F) The Dormia basket is pulled through the biliary cutaneous fistula with the stone inside.

closed Dormia basket is advanced through the large-gauge catheter, going beyond its tip and the stone inside the biliary duct. The Dormia basket should be advanced only if the angle between the catheter and the duct wall is obtuse or, preferably, if the catheter is parallel to the duct axis (Fig. 5.48).

5. After it passes beyond the stone, the Dormia basket is expanded by pulling its catheter, and then the open basket is pulled gently with a rotational movement until the stone is trapped inside the basket (Fig. 5.49). Closing the Dormia basket will cause stone fragmentation in most cases, making the procedure more difficult. When the stone is trapped, the basket should be pulled out with the whole system through the hepatic duct and fistula. Slow traction, however, will result in the loss of small calculi in the track. If the stone is large or the fistula has a small diameter, it will be difficult to cross the fistula with the whole system, requiring greater pulling force. This may result in pain and/or rupture of the fistulous track.

The typical patient with a residual stone in the common bile duct has only one stone; this is the case in over 70 percent of patients (Fig. 5.50). It is not uncommon to remove multiple stones during several sessions; this occurs in about 40 percent of cases. Originally, a lack of experience with the method led to attempts to remove all the stones at the same time. This, however, is a more cumbersome and time-consuming procedure and is also related to high radiation doses; frequently it is impossible to complete the procedure because of the presence of air, clots, and spasm in the biliary ductal system. It is preferable to perform a good control cholangiogram a few days later to evaluate the results of a prolonged procedure, with care always taken to maintain a large-diameter tube inside the fistulous tract so that access is maintained.

INDICATIONS

Indications for selecting patients who may require multiple sessions include the following.

1. Large stones require fragmentation. The larger ones are removed during the first session, and the smaller ones are left in the biliary tree. Practically all fragments smaller than 3 mm spontaneously cross the papilla into the duodenum.
2. Patients with multiple intra- and extrahepatic calculi are better treated with several procedures because of the risk of fistula laceration caused by multiple extraction of stones in a single procedure.
3. Stones which remain lodged inside the cystic duct stump are difficult to extract, and multiple sessions are usually required to mobilize such stones and finally extract them. In certain circumstances, the stone remains ouside the cystic stump only when the patient is in the orthostatic posture.
4. Small-diameter fistulas with a T-tube drain smaller than No. 14 French usually require track dilatation, with stone extraction performed during a second or third procedure.
5. Impacted stones are often spontaneously dislodged

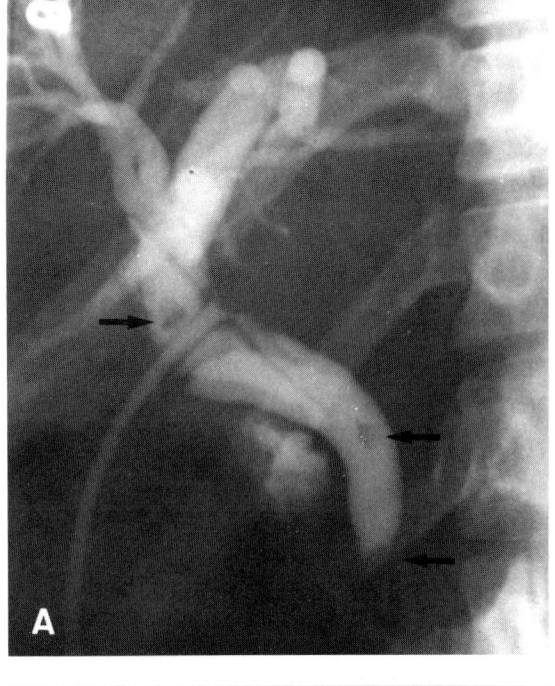
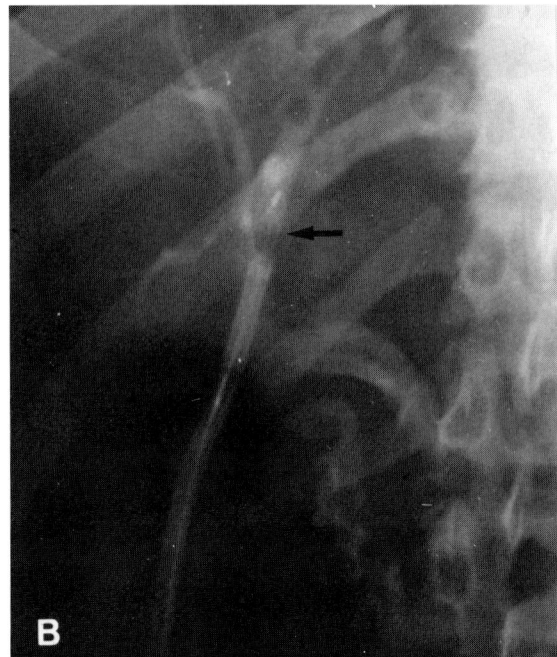
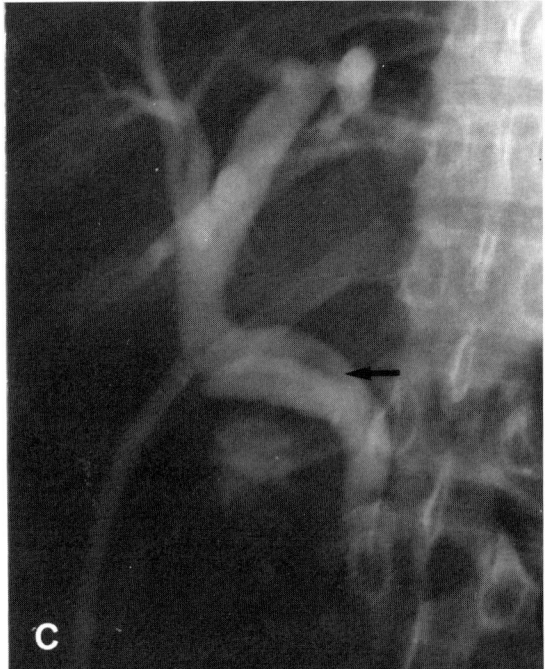
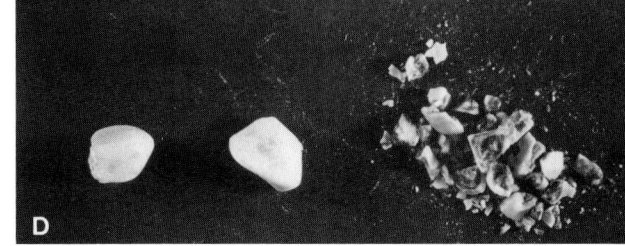

Figure 5.49 Removal of multiple stones in different positions.
(A) A cholangiogram through the T-tube drain shows three stones inside the biliary tree, one of which is impacted in the distal common bile duct (arrows). (B) After drain removal, the directional-tip catheter is seen inside the left hepatic duct, with the basket closed around the stone (arrow); the basket is about to be removed through the fistula. (C) A control cholangiogram after stone extraction shows that the biliary tree is free of stones. A round image which indicates the presence of air inside the biliary tree is seen (arrow). (D) A photograph of the biliary tree stones after their extraction from the biliary tree. One stone was fragmented. Note the regular aspect of the stones, with corners and angulations, as opposed to the round aspect of the air bubble shown in (C).

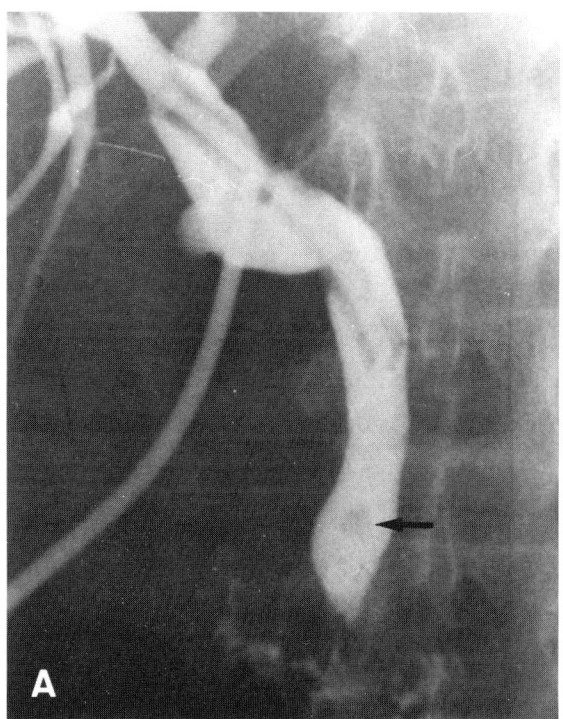
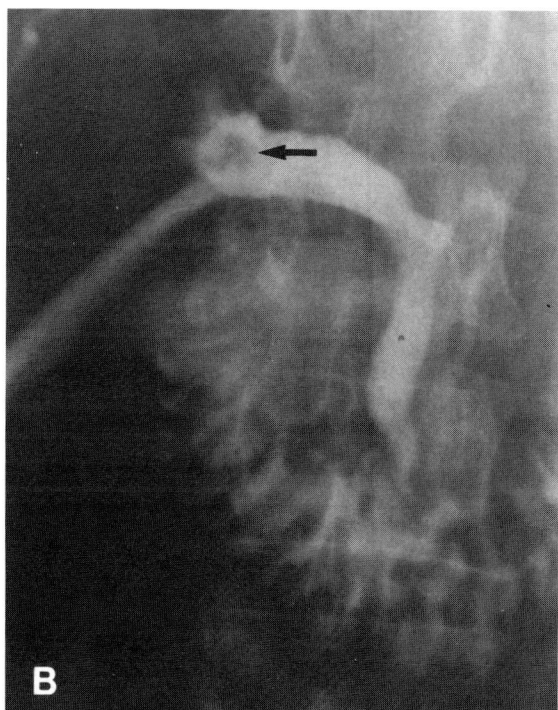

between one procedure and another, facilitating extraction with a basket (Fig. 5.51).
6. Peripheral stenoses of the biliary tree are usually treated during several dilatation sessions before final stone extraction.

STONE SIZE

Small stones usually pass into the duodenum without problem. Stones larger than 3 mm, however, should be extracted. In the case of a single stone, one session is generally sufficient; in the case of multiple stones, at least two procedures are required. Forced passage of small fragments through the papilla is a useful method in treating some patients.

The size of the Dormia basket used depends more on the size of the duct inside which it will be manipulated than on stone size. The basket should touch the duct walls independently of stone size.

Large stones up to 6 mm in size cross easily through a No. 14 French tube fistula. Calculi up to 8 mm require a No. 16 French tube fistula. If the stones are larger, fragmentation should be performed with a Dormia basket, removing as many of the larger fragments as possible without manipulation. Stone dissolution with MTBE may also be used for stone debulking before extraction.

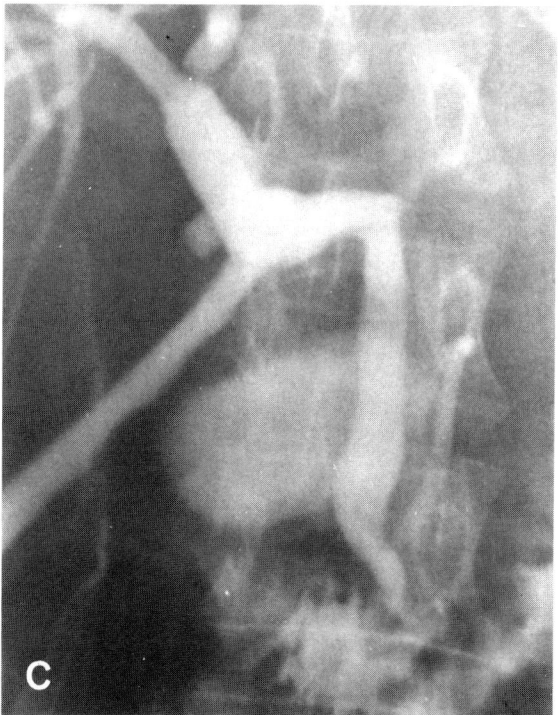

Figure 5.50 Usually a single residual stone is found in the common bile duct.
(A) A single nonimpacted stone in the distal common bile duct (arrow). (B) After mobilization, the stone is near the fistula (arrow). (C) A control cholangiogram shows a stone-free biliary tree.

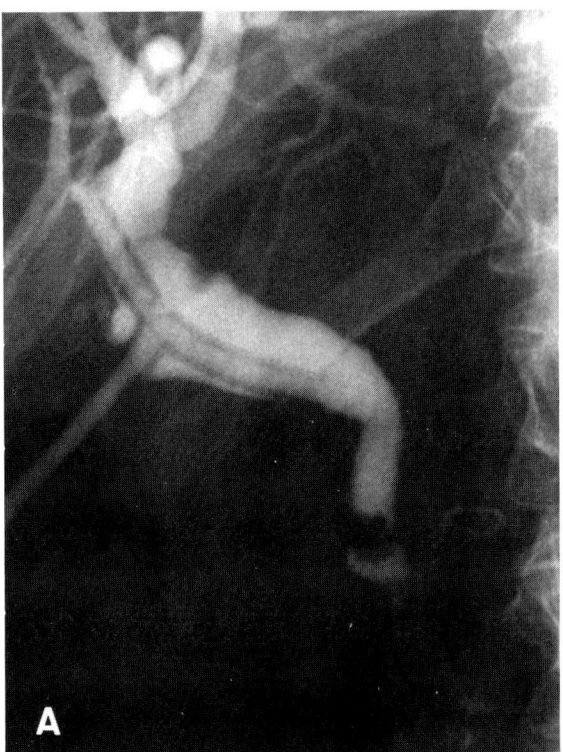
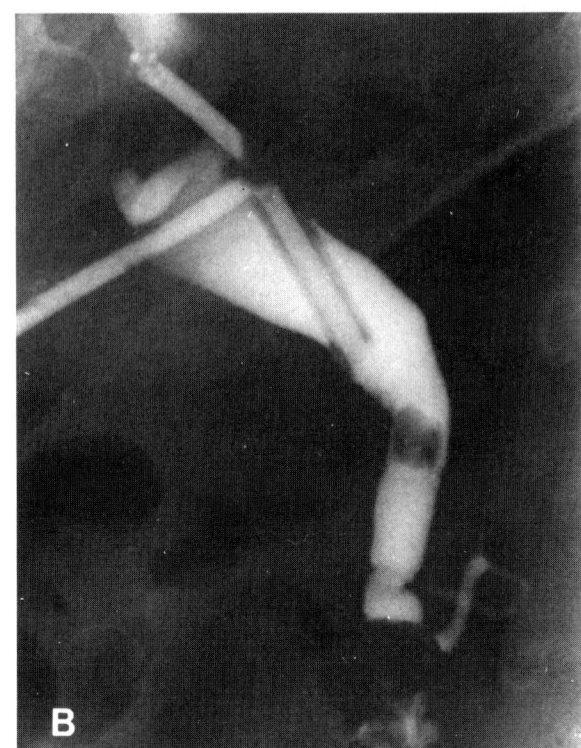
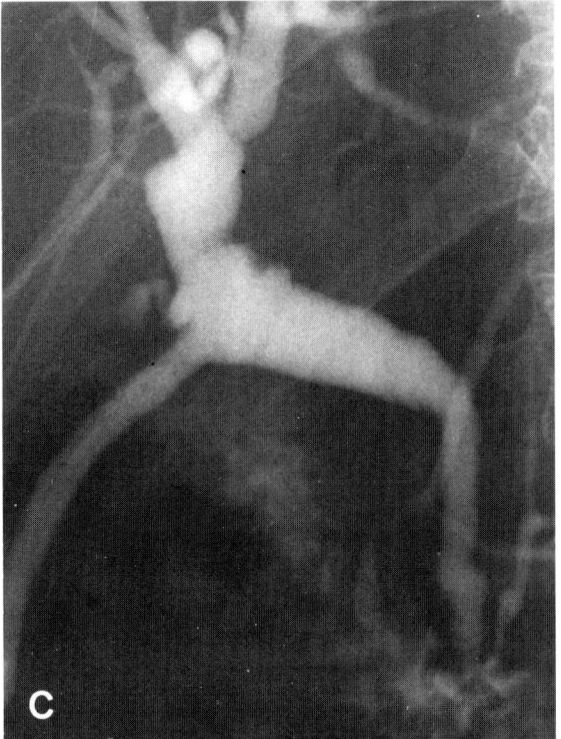

Figure 5.51 During the waiting period, the impacted calculus in the distal common bile duct usually is mobilized.
(A) A cholangiogram through T-tube drain shows an impacted stone in the common bile duct. Note that contrast passes around the stone. (B) After a few days, the stone is free inside the common bile duct. (C) Control after the extraction of a single stone shows the normal diameter of the biliary tree without filling defects.

Waiting a few days will show that most fragments have passed into the duodenum. A few percutaneous extraction sessions may be necessary to remove multiple fragments.

STONE IMPACTION

Impacted stones in the common and intrahepatic ducts represent a difficult technical problem. The Dormia basket cannot usually open itself and capture the stone even if it is passed beyond the stone. These stones should be mobilized first. Usually, calculi move spontaneously during the waiting period. Some maneuvers, however, may be tried, including distal contrast injection under pressure, aspiration of a stone with a large-diameter catheter, and the use of a balloon catheter to pull the stone.

Stones impacted in the intrahepatic biliary ducts are a little more difficult to manipulate, and this procedure has a higher failure rate (Fig. 5.52). Intrahepatic stones in general, however, are retained by the T-tube tip, and removal of the tube will mobilize the stones into the common bile duct (Fig. 5.53). If multiple intrahepatic stones are present, several sessions will be necessary. Intrahepatic stones in a very peripheral location require

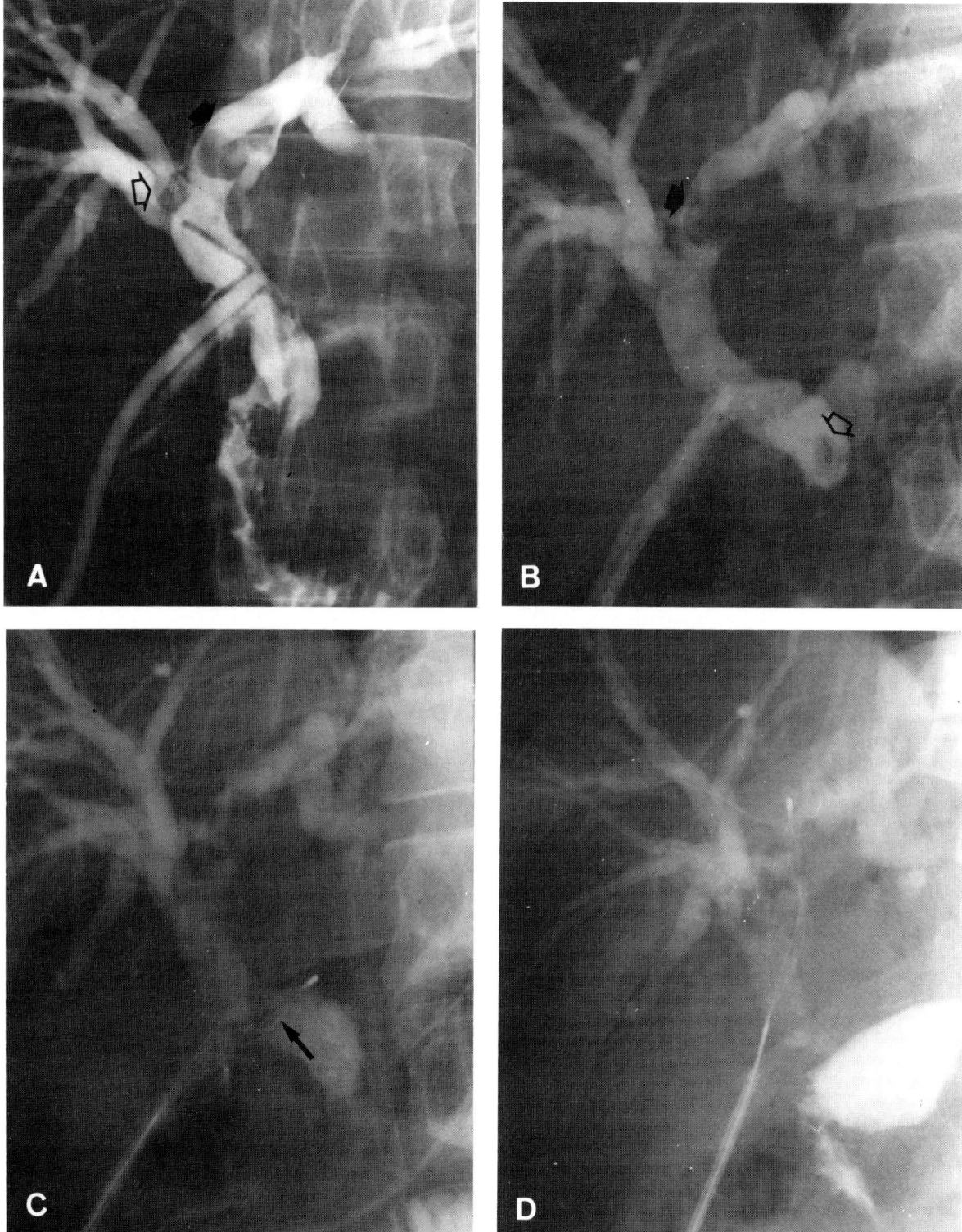

Figure 5.52 Not all stones can be removed by the percutaneous route.
(A) A cholangiogram through the T-tube drain shows a large impacted stone in the left biliary duct (black arrow) and a smaller stone in the right biliary duct, which is maintained there by the tip of the T-tube drain (white arrow). (B) After the drain was removed, the small stone migrated into the distal common bile duct (white arrow) while the large stone remained impacted (black arrow). (C) A Dormia basket extracting the smaller stone (arrow). (D) The Dormia basket is not able to involve the large impacted left duct stone completely. It was not possible at that time to mobilize the stone.

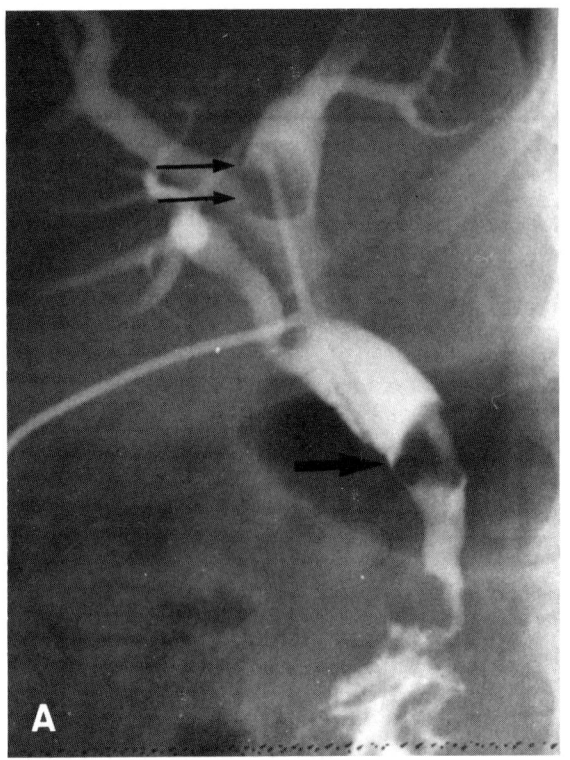
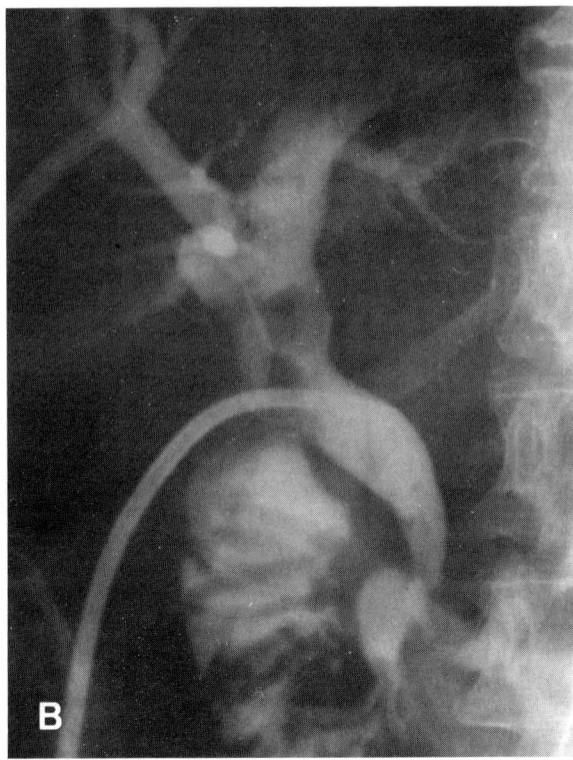
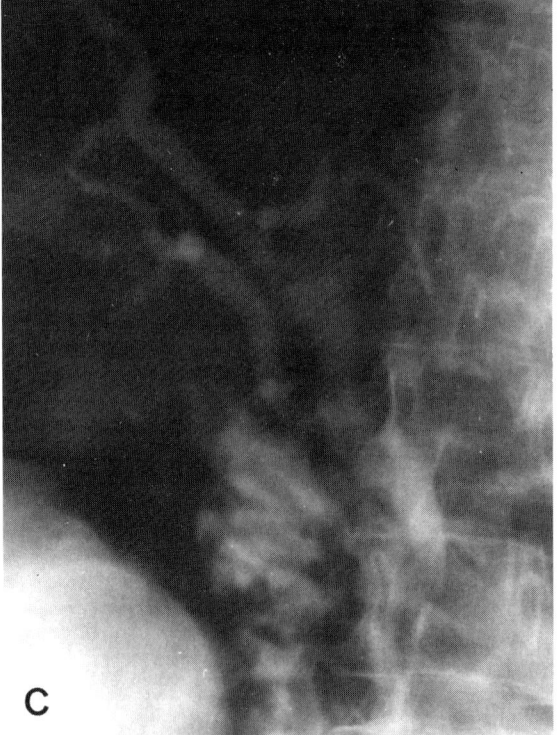

Figure 5.53 (A) A 60-year-old female patient with two large residual stones. One stone is seen in the left duct (arrows), kept in place by the T-tube drain; the other is in the common bile duct (arrow). (B) Control after extraction of a stone from the common bile duct. (C) Image after extraction of the second stone, which has escaped from the basket, remaining inside the fistulous track.

more time for manipulation and smaller-diameter baskets, but they can be removed in spite of adjacent strictures (Fig. 5.54).

RESULTS

As stated above, these procedures are successful in about 95 percent of cases. We had only one failure, which occurred when a large impacted stone could not be removed from an intrahepatic duct. Our experience is, however, less extensive than that which has been reported by major authors.

One of the main causes of failure is a narrow and tortuous fistulous track, which may prevent adequate biliary tree catheterization and stone extraction. Another difficulty is caused by the presence of an inflammatory process in the fistula that leads to wall brittleness.

COMPLICATIONS

These procedures cause few complications, but the incidence of complications is approximately 4 percent in the largest series available. Pancreatitis due to ma-

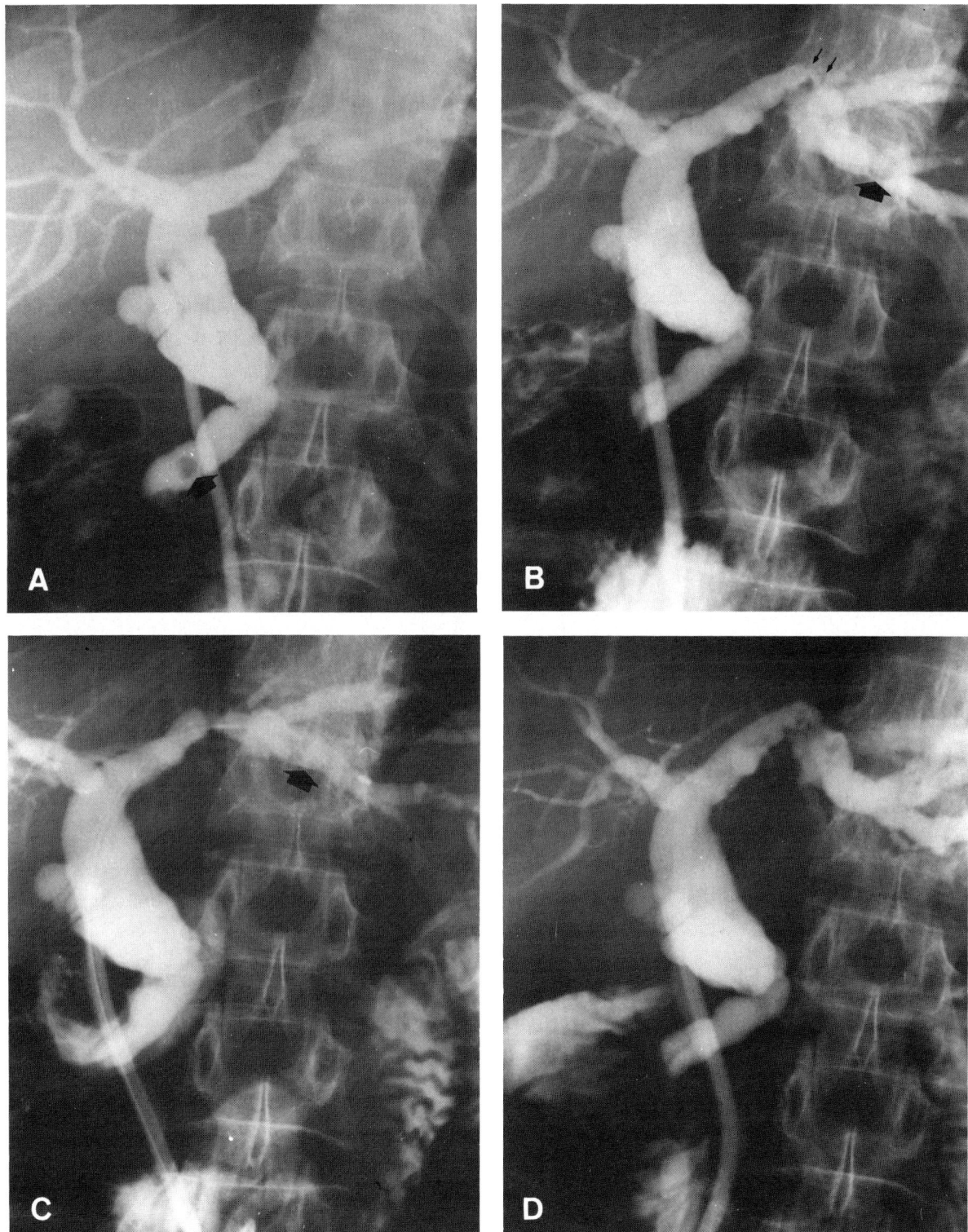

Figure 5.54 A 50-year-old male patient with a residual stone in the common bile duct.
(A) Only one stone is visible inside the distal common bile duct (arrow); it was later extracted. (B) Upon control cholangiography, after extraction of the stone from the common bile duct, an area of stricture was identified in the left biliary duct (arrows), along with a peripheral stone in the left duct (arrow). (C) A Dormia basket in the peripheral portion of the left duct seizing the residual stone (arrow). (D) Control after extraction of two residual stones from the biliary tree; a few air bubbles are seen in the left duct.

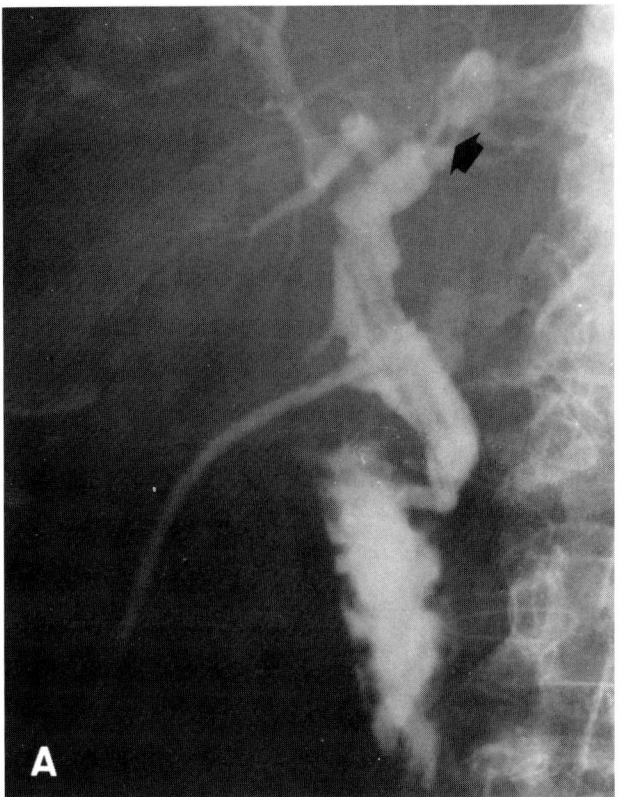 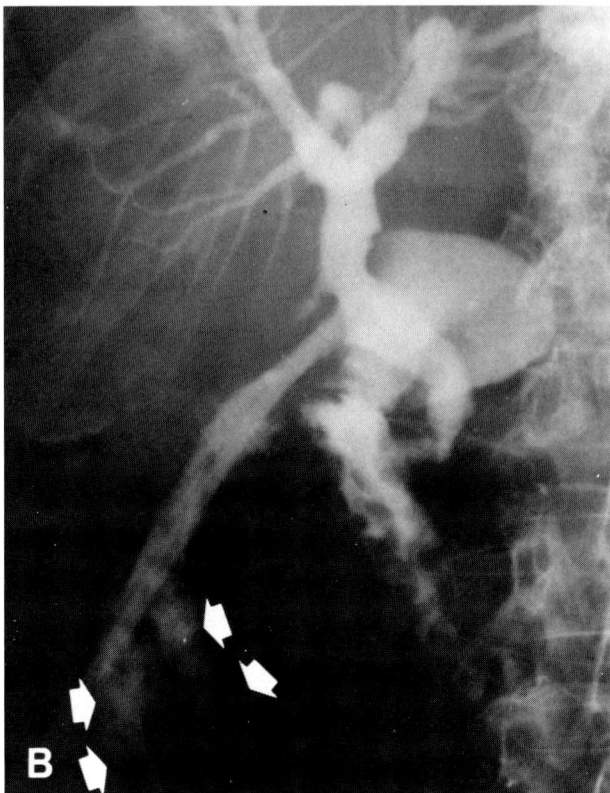

Figure 5.55 (A) A cholangiogram through a T-tube drain shows a small residual stone in the left hepatic duct (arrow) in a 75-year-old patient with severe ischemic heart disease, uncompensated diabetes, and pulmonary emphysema. The stone was easily removed through the fistula after a 6-week maturation period. (B) A control cholangiogram after extraction of the residual stone shows extravasation due to rupture of the walls of the fistulous track (arrows). The patient developed purulent collections in the abdomen, which later required surgical treatment.

nipulation occurs infrequently but is probably the most serious complication. Other complications include fistulous track rupture, bile in the peritoneum, formation of bilomas, and fever or sepsis following manipulation.

The mortality rate should be zero for this type of procedure. Large volumes of potentially contaminated bile leaking into the peritoneal cavity should be treated surgically, particularly in diabetic patients (Fig. 5.55).

REFERENCES

Burhenne HJ. Nonoperative roentgenologic instrumentation technics of the postoperative biliary tract. *Am J Surg* 1974;128:111–117.

Burhenne HJ. Percutaneous extraction of retained biliary tract stones: 661 patients. *AJR* 1980;134:888–898.

Burhenne HJ. Interventional radiology through the T-tube tract and retained biliary stone removal. In *Interventional Radiology*, edited by Wilkins RA, Viamonte M. Blackwell, Oxford, 1982:295–307.

Clouse ME, Falchuh KR. Percutaneous transhepatic removal of common duct stones: Report of ten patients. *Gastroenterology* 1983;85:815–819.

Kadir S, Kaufman SL, Barth KH, White RI. Therapeutic procedures in the biliary tract. In *Selected Techniques in Interventional Radiology*, edited by Kadir S, Kaufman SI, Barth KH, White RI. Saunders, Philadelphia, 1982:104–141.

Dilatation of Benign Biliary Stenoses

ROSA MARIA PAOLINI
RENAN UFLACKER

Dilatation of benign stenoses through a transhepatic approach has been used in the last few years to treat stenoses in biliary anastomoses or as palliative treatment in patients with sclerosing cholangitis.

Benign biliary stenoses are usually caused by surgical trauma. Although they are classified as benign, these stenoses result in chronic disease with an evolution that may be considered malignant. The outcome depends on the severity of the primary stenosis, and, secondarily, on the evolution of the stenosis into sclerosing cholangitis, hepatic failure, and sepsis. Dilatation of these stenoses with a Grutzig balloon introduced by means of a percutaneous transhepatic puncture has been quite successful (Fig. 5.56).

TECHNIQUE

The dilatation of benign stenoses is performed in two main steps. Initially, the biliary tree is drained with an internal-external drainage catheter (Fig. 5.7). After decompression of the biliary tree for approximately 48 h, dilatation is performed (Fig. 5.57).

After skin asepsis is established, a J-guidewire is introduced through an internal-external drainage catheter which is placed deeply into a bowel loop. The drainage catheter is removed, and a sheath (No. 10 or 12 French) with a dilator is introduced. The sheath protects the pleura, which often is transfixed during puncture, from injury when the balloon is introduced or removed. Bile is drained through the sheath while the balloon remains inflated.

The dilator is removed, and a balloon catheter is introduced; under fluoroscopy, the catheter is positioned through the stenosis, where it is then inflated for at least 30 min up to 6 h. An adhesive collecting bag is placed on the skin to prevent contamination, and the patient is taken to the recovery room, where he or she remains during the period stipulated for dilatation. High-pressure Blue Max (Medi-Tech) and PE Plus (USCI) balloon catheters are used (Fig. 5.57). The balloon size must be compatible with the stenosis; usually the balloon has a diameter of 6, 8, 9, or 10 mm and is 3 to 4 cm long (Fig. 5.56).

The balloon catheter is removed after the dilatation period, together with the sheath. A drainage catheter is then introduced over the guidewire, which is soon removed. Large-diameter catheters, No. 9 or 10 French, of the nasogastric tube type are used for postdilation drainage. This catheter is removed after 45 days to 6 months, depending on case evolution.

This technique has been successful in 85 percent of cases according to a recently published study. The results are better in patients with primary lesions of the common bile duct and worse in patients with hepatojejunostomy.

RESULTS

Immediate or later recurrence of stenosis may occur. The success of dilatation depends on the pathogenesis of the stenosis. Stenosis of a biliary anastomosis and some primary stenoses of the common bile duct result from ischemia, presenting with a circumferential scar on the site of stricture. Stenoses frequently occur after clamping of the common bile duct or as a result of inadvertent suture of its lateral wall, which is mistaken for the base of the cystic duct. In these cases the lesion is eccentric. When the balloon is inflated on the site of an eccentric stenosis, normal soft tissue displacement will occur if adequate pressure is not applied directly over the scar. Dilatation in these cases is insufficient, involving the possibility of restenosis.

When the stenosis is circumferential, pressure from the inflated balloon is applied directly over the entire scar area, leading to more successful dilatation. A new dilatation is frequently required because of insufficient efficacy of the first procedure or recurrence of the fibrotic process.

Dilatation of a benign anastomotic stenosis using this method is the procedure of choice when the stenosis cannot be surgically reconstructed or when the stenosed segment is surgically inaccessible. Based on our experience and on data from the literature, we believe that percutaneous transhepatic dilatation of the biliary tree should be considered a primary therapeutic method for patients with postoperative stenoses.

The use of transjejunal percutaneous biliary dilatation has been proposed recently for the management of primary biliary stenosis, either through a surgically created access with a jejunal loop or by direct percutaneous

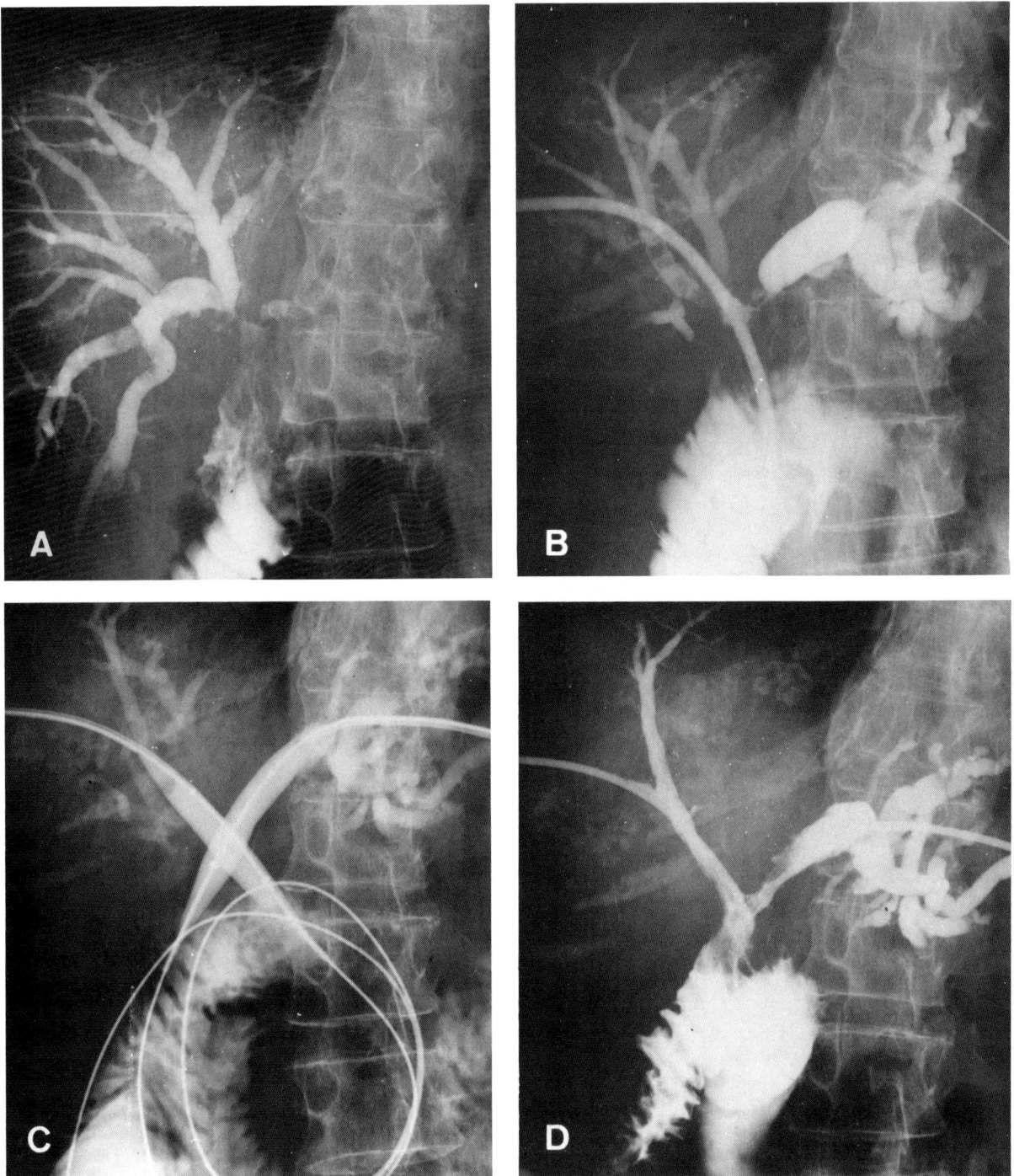

Figure 5.56 A biliary anastomosis of the right and left hepatic ducts with a small bowel loop after resection of a cholangiocarcinoma in the duct confluence.

(A) A percutaneous cholangiogram with a Chiba needle shows moderate biliary dilatation and severe stenosis of the anastomosis. (B) After the right duct was drained, a percutaneous left duct cholangiogram was performed; this also showed stenosis of the anastomosis on the left. (C) Dilatation with 8-mm kissing balloons for 6 h. (D) Control after dilatation shows biliary tree patency in the anastomosis on both sides.

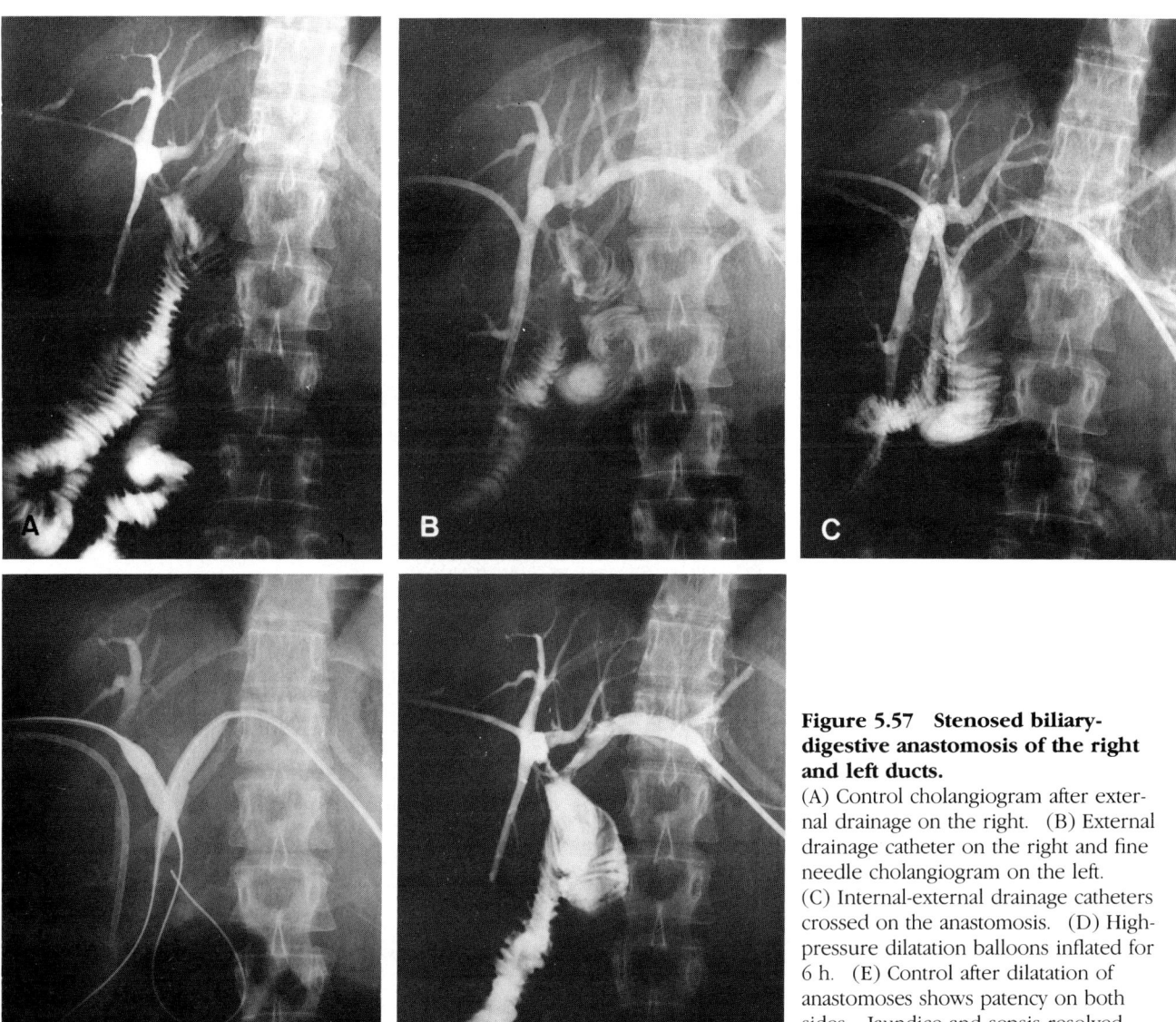

Figure 5.57 Stenosed biliary-digestive anastomosis of the right and left ducts.
(A) Control cholangiogram after external drainage on the right. (B) External drainage catheter on the right and fine needle cholangiogram on the left. (C) Internal-external drainage catheters crossed on the anastomosis. (D) High-pressure dilatation balloons inflated for 6 h. (E) Control after dilatation of anastomoses shows patency on both sides. Jaundice and sepsis resolved during a 6-month follow-up without drainage catheters.

puncture of the jejunal loop under fluoroscopic guidance. Ths technique provides easy access for repeated dilatations, which may be necessary in patients with certain types of evolutionary although benign lesions, such as sclerosing cholangitis and traumatic lesions of the biliary tree. More recently, however, the self-expandable Gianturco Z-stent has been used successfully to keep dilated anastomoses or strictures open for long periods of time in patients with sclerosing cholangitis and benign strictures.

REFERENCES

Clouse ME, Falchuk KR. Percutaneous transhepatic removal of common duct stones: Report of ten patients. *Gastroenterology* 1983;85:815–819.

Gallacker DT, Kadir S, Kaufman SL, Mitchell SE, Kinnison ML, Chang R, Adams P, White RI, Cameron NO. Nonoperative management of benign postoperative biliary strictures. *Radiology* 1985;156:625–629.

Kaufman SL, Kadir S, Mitchell SE, et al. Percutaneous transhepatic biliary drainage for bile leaks and fistulas. *AJR* 1985;144:1055–1058.

Russel E, Yrizarry JM, Huber JS, Nunes D, et al. Percutaneous transjejunal biliary dilatation: Alternate management for benign strictures. *Radiology* 1986;159:209–214.

Salomonowitz E, Castaneda-Zuniga WR, Lund G, et al. Balloon dilatation of benign biliary strictures. *Radiology* 1984;151:613–616.

Schwarz, W, Rosen RJ, Fitts WT, et al. Percutaneous transhepatic drainage preoperatively from benign biliary strictures. *Surg Gynecol Obstet* 1981;152:466–468.

Brachytherapy with Iridium-192 Wire in the Management of Cholangiocarcinoma

ROSA MARIA PAOLINI

Cholangiocarcinomas are slow-growing tumors which tend to remain localized. These tumors usually grow at the junction of the right and left hepatic ducts, in the intrahepatic biliary ducts, and in the common bile duct.

The tumor often is unresectable because of its location. When radical surgery is not possible, palliative treatment for the obstruction may be achieved through a biliary-digestive anastomosis or by external-internal transhepatic percutaneous biliary drainage or endoprosthesis. Another option is brachytherapy. To ensure a high dose of local radiation inside the tumor, iridium-192 wire is used for radiotherapy of cholangiocarcinomas.

TECHNIQUE

After biliary decompression with external-internal transhepatic percutaneous drainage, using a No. 9 French polyethylene catheter with side holes below and above the stenosis, the iridium-192 wire is introduced into the drainage catheter and positioned inside the tumor under fluoroscopic view. This wire (Amersham International Ltd.) is made of platinum-iridium alloy. It has a diameter of 3 mm and is surrounded by a platinum 0.1-mm sheath placed inside a 0.5-mm-diameter nylon tube. Wire length is adjusted according to the extension of the tumor. The total intratumoral radiation dose is 60 Gy (6000 rad), and the duration of brachytherapy depends on isotopic activity. The isodose is calculated by the physics department, indicating the ideal dose with direct local action on the tumor site and progressive decay of radiation in adjacent tissues (Fig. 5.58). During brachytherapy, the drainage catheter is not infused and the patient wears a plumbic apron when in contact with other people. As the total dose is achieved, the iridium-192 wire is retrieved and the drainage catheter is changed.

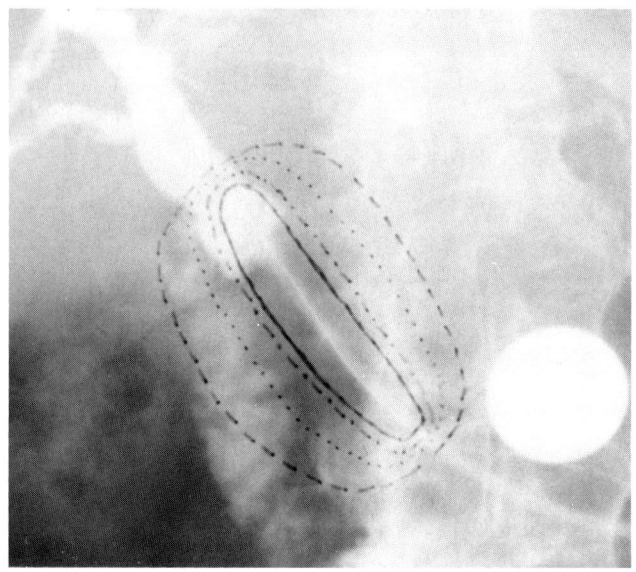

Figure 5.58 Isodose curves and dose distribution in the locale of tumor brachytherapy with iridium-192 wire.
After percutaneous biliary drainage, the iridium-192 wire was introduced inside the tumor through the drainage catheter.
————, 60 Gy; —.—.—, 40 Gy; ....., 20 Gy; -----, 10 Gy.

Patients with cholangiocarcinoma are submitted to treatment with iridium wire in an attempt to prolong and improve the quality of survival. Patients who receive brachytherapy are usually in poor general condition. Those who have smaller tumors and are in better condition usually receive radical tumoral resection.

In a series of 12 patients observed for 3 years the following results were recorded. Survival quality was improved in 10 of the 12 patients; in one case, the drainage catheter was removed and the patient died 6

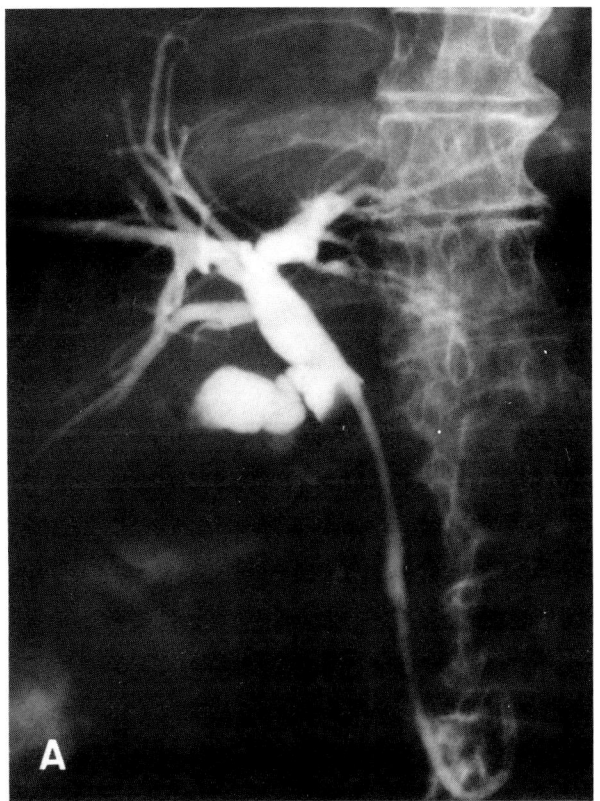 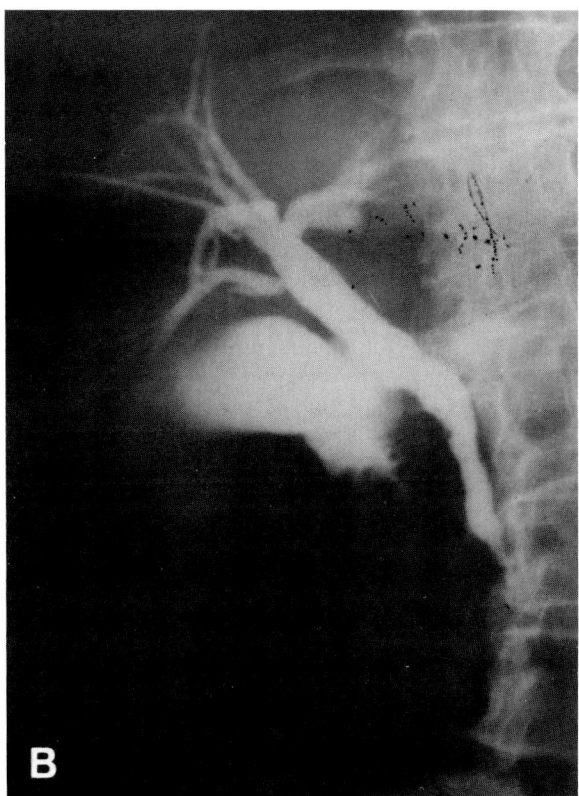

Figure 5.59 Result of brachytherapy in a cholangiocarcinoma of the common bile duct.
(A) Internal-external drainage catheter in position. (B) Excellent results from brachytherapy with total recanalization of the common bile duct.

months after brachytherapy without having developed jaundice. In seven patients, the drainage catheter was maintained without any problems, and an endoprosthesis was placed in four of these patients. In the same series, three patients died from metastasis without jaundice and two died from metastasis plus jaundice. Survival among these patients varied from 3 to 19 months.

Radical surgery is the best treatment for cholangiocarcinoma, but if it cannot be performed, palliative percutaneous biliary drainage should be done in association with brachytherapy (Fig. 5.59). The average rate of survival has been encouraging, and it is now recommended that patients with cholangiocarcinoma receive brachytherapy as well as conventional treatment.

Irradiation does not cause identifiable systemic effects, and side effects of radiotherapy have not been seen in patients submitted to brachytherapy. Quality of life is certainly improved in these patients.

Biliary Duct Reconstruction

Renan Uflacker

Benign biliary strictures are iatrogenic in 97 percent of patients. Surgical reconstruction of the bile ducts has morbidity and mortality rates of approximately 13 percent and 4 percent, respectively. Percutaneous nonsurgical alternatives represent a great improvement for patients with these difficult problems.

Percutaneous biliary drainage has undergone significant evolution in its relatively short existence. Percutaneous transhepatic biliary drainage has been extended and refined to the point where it is now a simple and safe procedure. Initially devised to treat malignant obstruction of the bile ducts, it is now applicable to a broad range of diseases. It was recognized early that percutaneous biliary drainage can also be used to treat benign lesions of the bile ducts such as postsurgical obstructions, sclerosing cholangitis, biliary fistulas, and biliary lacerations. Not only drainage but also balloon dilatation of a bile duct stenosis and the introduction of a variety of endoprostheses for bile duct remodeling can be done through the percutaneous tract.

Remodeling of the bile ducts may be done simply by means of balloon dilatation and the placement of an indwelling catheter for the required period of time. The stainless steel expandable stent provides a new alternative for the management of recurrent benign strictures. Because they support the bile wall, these stents offer the potential for long-term patency in recurrent strictures. Multiple stents can be placed through a single access, allowing treatment of multiple duct obstruction.

There are three basic problems associated with the bile ducts that require reconstruction and remodeling. The first, which is not the most common cause of biliary obstruction, is sclerosing cholangitis. The natural history of this disease involves alternating periods of relapsing and improvement. There is no specific treatment. Patients with marked inflammatory components may have an impressive response to oral corticosteroids, but the treatment focuses more on direct attempts at relieving the strictures by means of percutaneous techniques. Dilatation of one or more dominant stricture leads to striking improvement in some patients. The recurrence rate of strictures, however, is quite high, and some internal support is desirable in most cases to keep the reconstructed bile duct open. The best current way to provide internal support for a reconstructed stricture of the bile duct in a patient with sclerosing cholangitis is to use a stainless steel stent, either the so-called Gianturco Z-stent (Fig. 5.60) or the Palmaz stent. Multiple catheterizations of the bile ducts may be necessary to allow the introduction of the stent sheath into the periphery of the duct.

TECHNIQUE

The lesion is initially crossed with a guidewire and is dilated with an angioplasty balloon of appropriate size. A No. 10 French sheath is advanced beyond the distal end of the lesion, and the dilator is removed, leaving the guidewire and sheath in place. The Z-stent is compressed and fitted inside the sheath over the guidewire. A blunt-tip No. 8 French catheter is used to push the stent all the way through the sheath under fluoroscopic guidance. With the guidewire in place and with the pusher and stent kept still, the sheath is gently withdrawn until the stent is released.

When multiple stents are used, stent positioning should always follow the periphery to the center. The most distal stent should be placed first, followed by the more proximal stents. The movement of the sheath of a new stent that is advanced through a previously placed stent will often displace the first stent. When multiple ducts are occluded and join together at the same point, it is necessary to place a guidewire across each obstruction; otherwise, as the first stent expands, it may close the opening of the neighboring ducts, making them impossible to reach. After stent placement, a single catheter is left in the main duct that communicates with the common duct. If tight bends prove difficult to negotiate, a coaxial system with a large sheath may be necessary. A Gianturco Z-stent can also be used to reconstruct or recanalize tumoral occlusion of the bile duct. However, tumoral ingrowth within the stent between the struts may limit the life span of the stent.

The same general principles that guide the use of a Gianturco Z-stent are applicable to the Palmaz stent. The Palmaz stent, however, is not self-expandable, and balloon expansion is required to expand this stent to the desired size.

The second problem related to the bile ducts that may require percutaneous reconstruction involves postsurgical obstructions related to fistulas. Postoperative biliary lesions are usually associated with extensive surgical dissection of the bile ducts which causes ischemic necrosis of the wall of the bile duct; this is followed by the development of fibrotic scarring and stenosis, frequently leading to the formation of fistulas. Additional surgeries are usually not feasible, and a percutaneous

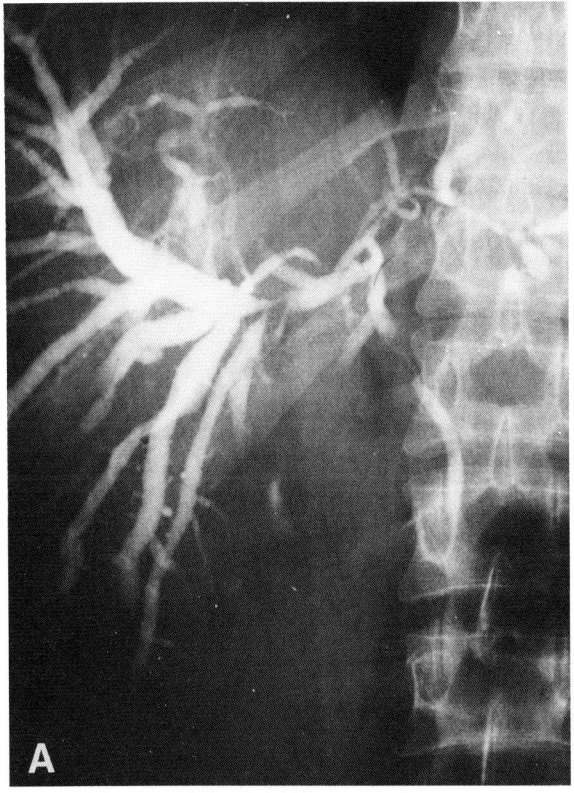
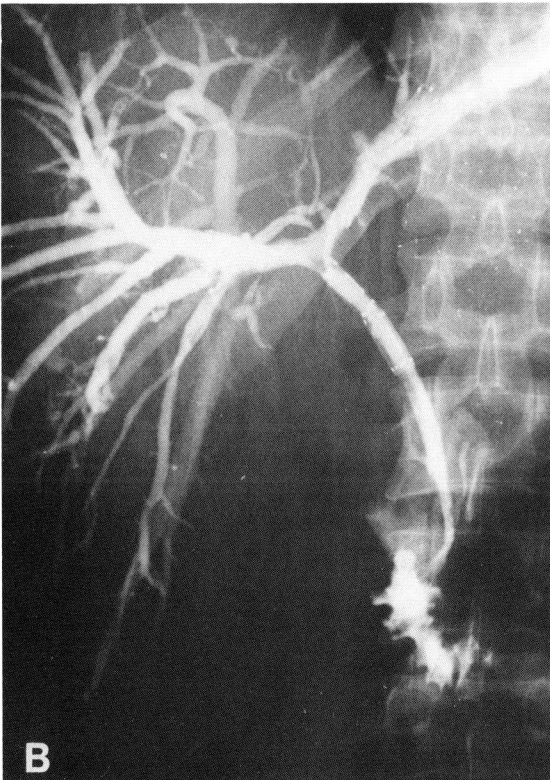
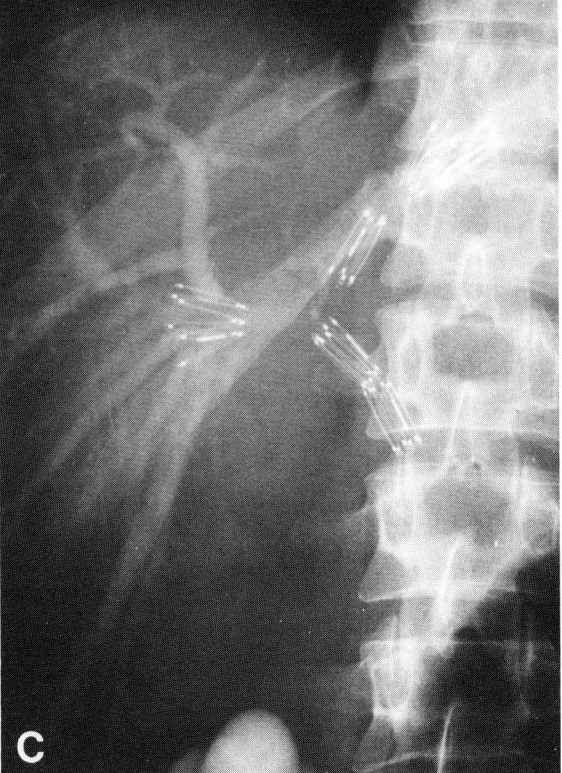

Figure 5.60 (A) Percutaneous cholangiography in a 28-year-old patient with sclerosing cholangitis. Note the characteristic aspect of diffuse strictures on the right lobe and left lobe of the bile ducts and on the common bile duct. (B) After percutaneous catheterization of the right and left bile ducts and dilatation of the common bile duct with a 6-mm balloon catheter was performed, six Z-stents were placed: three in the left duct, two in the common duct, and one in the right duct. Note the adequate patency of the stented ducts. (C) Radiography obtained a few hours after the cholangiographic procedure. Note the Z-stents positioned within the bile ducts. A stent in the left duct was distally displaced during manipulation and overlapped the distal, adequately positioned stent. The stent in the right duct was overexpanded because the suture was cut. Biliary drainage was adequate, and the patient remained asymptomatic.

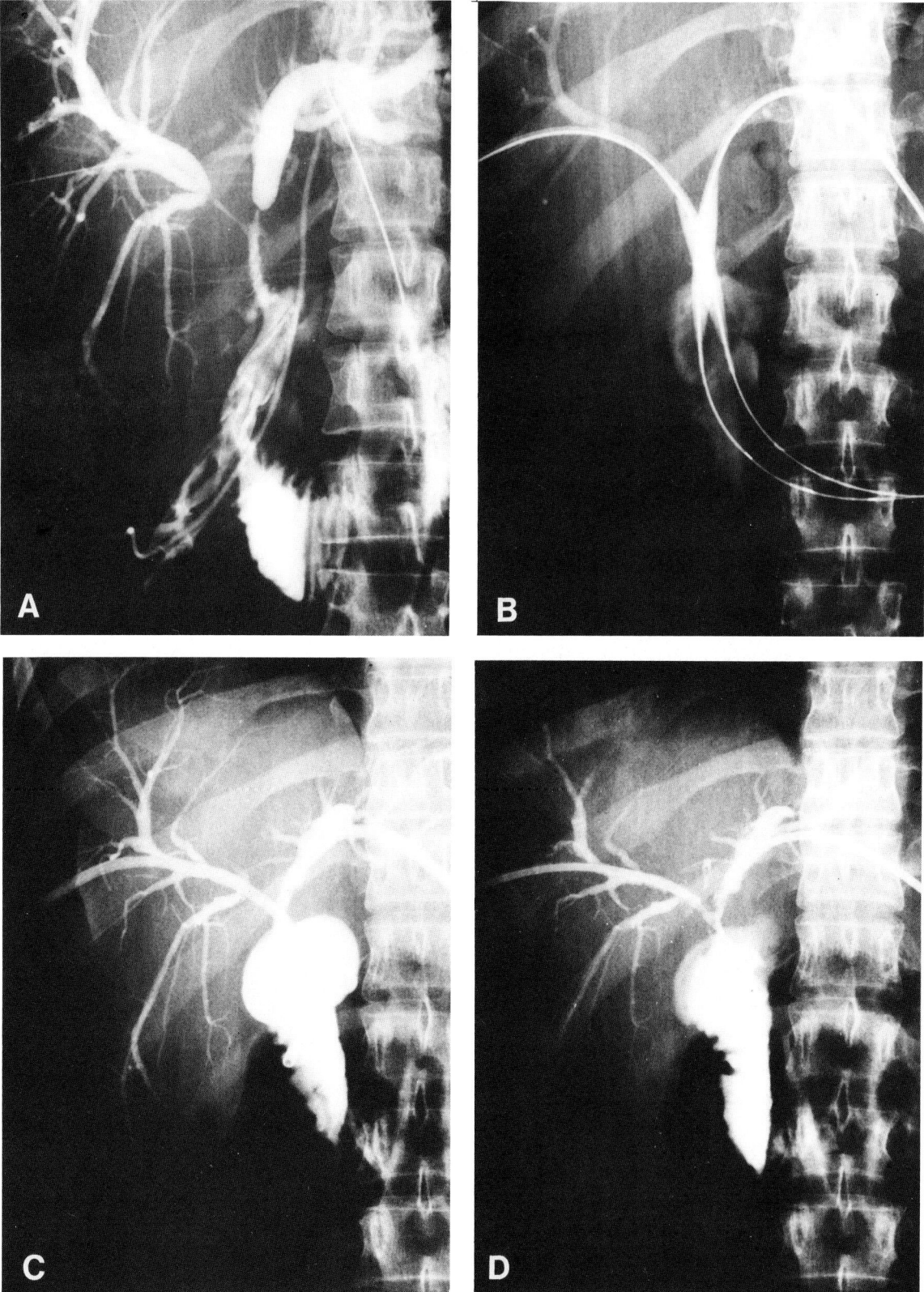

Figure 5.61 (A) Postoperative stenosis of the bile ducts associated with a fistula at the point of anastomosis. Bilateral puncture was performed, followed by catheterization through the obstructions. (B) Two 6-mm balloon catheters were used to dilate the stenosis. (C) Two indwelling drainage catheters were maintained through the dilated stenosis for 6 months. (D) Control cholangiogram after withdrawal of the drainage catheter shows the patent bile ducts.

approach is generally appropriate. The approach for percutaneous drainage may be either unilateral or bilateral. Internal-external drainage should be attempted. If this is not possible, only external drainage should be performed to overcome infection and allow the fistula to close. If it is possible to cross the stenosis, a catheter can be used for internal-external drainage. Effective drainage will close the fistulas in 1 or 2 weeks.

Percutaneous balloon dilatation of the stenosis should be attempted when the fistula is closed and infection has been controlled (Fig. 5.61). Balloon dilation should be performed for at least 10 to 20 min, and a large catheter (No. 10 to 20 French) should be maintained across the dilated stenosis for reconstruction and remodeling of the bile duct walls, acting as an inner cast. The length of time the catheter should be kept inside the dilated duct is controversial. Currently it seems that 4 to 6 months is a reasonable time. In some cases the treatment may be markedly improved if a Z-stent is used for internal support of the dilated bile duct wall.

Traumatic lesions of the bile ducts with lacerations and fistulas—the third problem—differ from surgical lesions when extensive dissections are followed by ischemia and necrosis. On the contrary, the traumatized biliary duct usually has a viable wall with a localized laceration or perforation.

Infection, fistulas, and obstruction are common findings in patients with bile duct trauma (Fig. 5.62). Per-

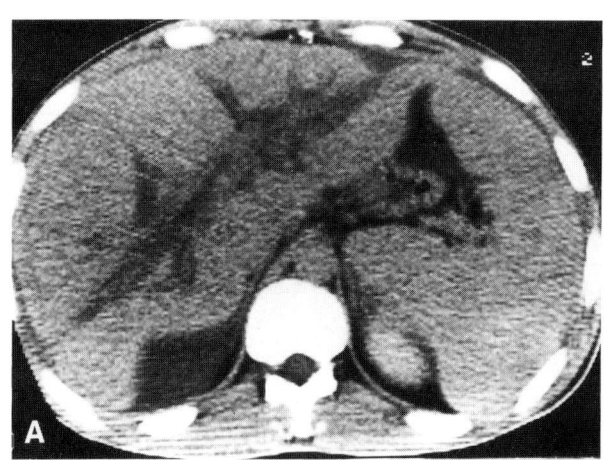
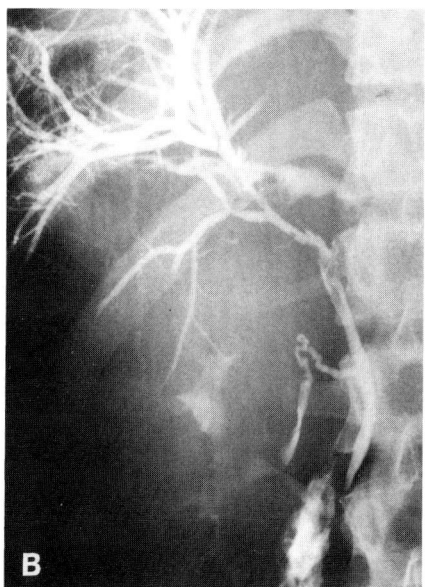

Figure 5.62 (A) A 22-year-old man with hepatic trauma due to a gunshot wound. Note the liver laceration on CT. The patient presented with cholangitis, fever, and moderate jaundice. (B) Percutaneous cholangiography showed mild dilatation of the intrahepatic bile ducts and small peripheral abscesses (not shown here) plus laceration of the common bile duct and a central cavity within the liver. The left hepatic duct is not opacified because of traumatic disconnection. Percutaneous internal-external drainage of the right side was performed. (C) Simultaneous injection in the drainage catheter and fistulous track shows the connection between the left duct, the fistula, and the central cavity. (D) Injection through the fistulous track to opacify the left duct for puncture. (E) After left duct puncture, the steerable guidewire follows the fistulous track. Note a small notch on the cavity wall which corresponds to the laceration path (arrow). (F) The steerable guidewire finally reaches the main common bile duct. (G) Internal-external drainage was also performed on the left side. The fistulous track was still patent but was embolized with glue. (H) Control cholangiogram through the drainage catheters several months after drainage shows regression of the central cavity and the fistulous track. (I) Control after catheter withdrawal from the right side. (J) Control just before catheter withdrawal from the left side. (K) Percutaneous cholangiography 3 months after catheter withdrawal shows patency of the bile ducts. Left side not opacified. (L) Percutaneous digital splenoportography shows occlusion of the portal vein and the development of collaterals. Total treatment time of 18 months for bile duct reconstruction. The patient was asymptomatic during a 3-year follow up.

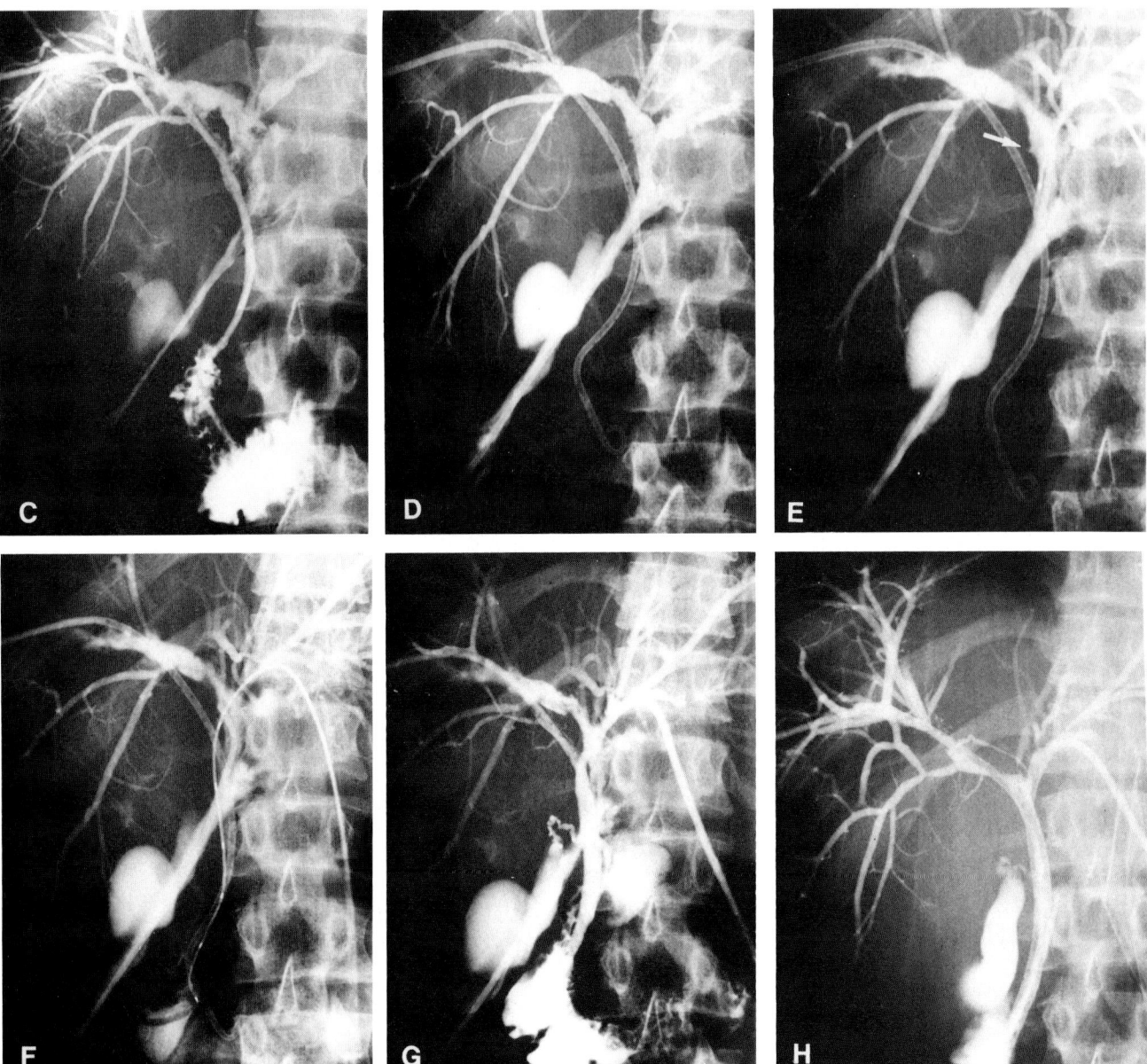

Figure 5.62 *Continued*

cutaneous drainage for the treatment of infection and obstruction is usually successful. The outcome of treatment of lacerations and bile duct disconnections may depend on the success of catheterization of the duct system in reestablishing the continuity of the traumatized ducts. Long-term drainage must be established. Embolization with glue of some of the fistulous tracks may be necessary when the output is very high. The association of a vascular trauma such as portal vein thrombosis precludes any form of surgical treatment and may increase the morbidity of the trauma and treatment.

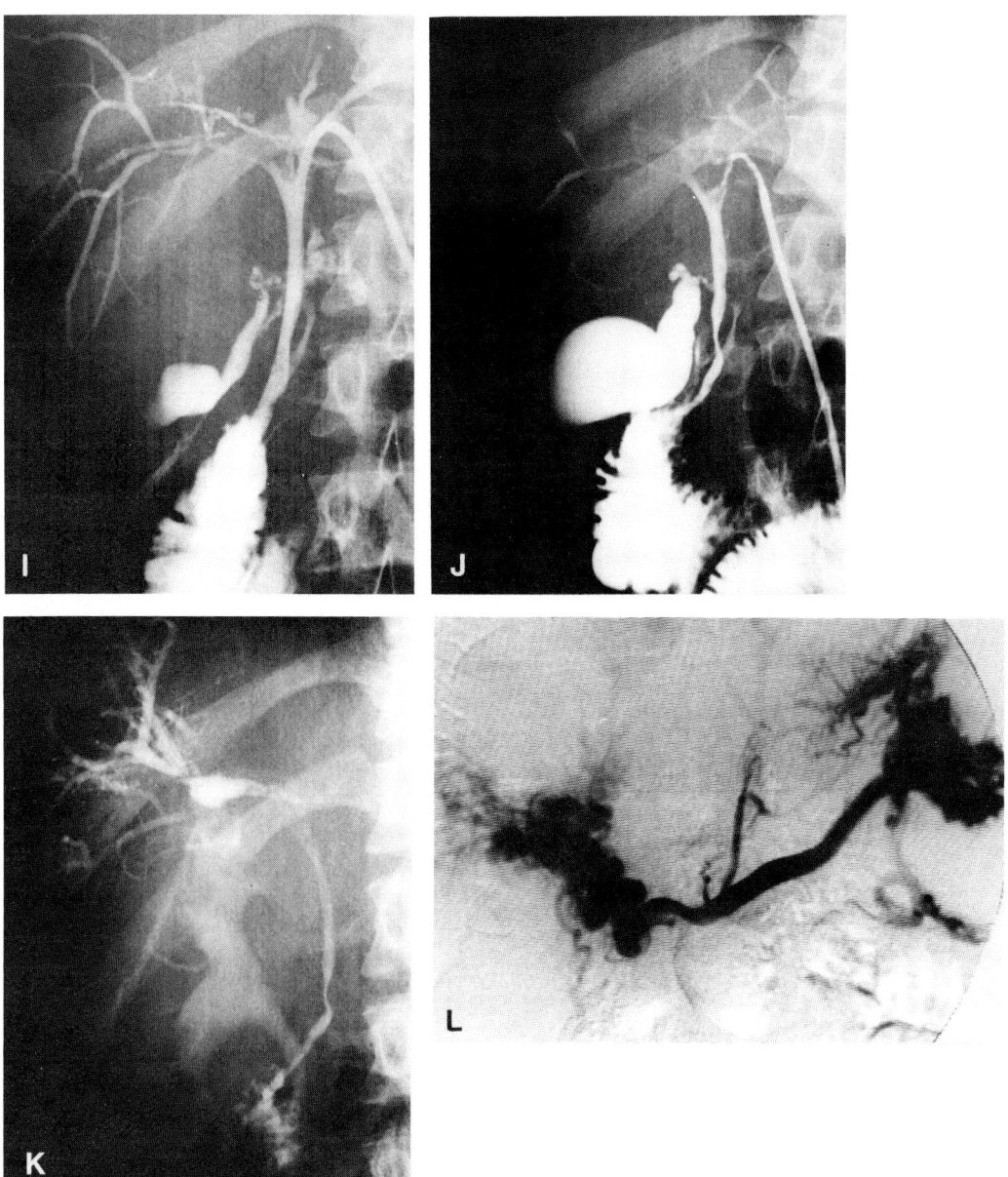

Figure 5.62 *Continued*

REFERENCES

Alvarado R, Palmaz JC, Garcia OJ, Tio FO, Rees CR. Evaluation of polymer coated balloon expandable stents in bile ducts. *Radiology* 1989;170:975–978.

Browder IW, Dowling JB, Koontz KK, Litwin MS. Early management of operative injuries of the extrahepatic biliary tract. *Ann Surg* 1987;205:649–658.

Coons HG. Self expanding stainless steel biliary stents. *Radiology* 1989;170:979–983.

Genest JF, Nanos E, Grundfest-Broniatowski S, Vogt D, Hemann RE. Benign biliary strictures: An analytic review. *Surgery* 1986;99:409–413.

Lindor KD, Wiesner RH, LaRusso NF. Recent advances in the management of primary sclerosing cholangitis. *Semin Liver Dis* 1987;7:322–327.

Mendez G, Russel E, LePage JP, et al. Abandonment of endoprosthetic drainage technique in biliary obstruction. *AJR* 1984;143:617–622.

McLean GK, Burke DR. Role of endoprosthesis in the management of malignant biliary obstruction. *Radiology* 1989;170:961–967.

Uflacker R, Mourao GS, Piske RL, Lima S. Percutaneous transhepatic biliary drainage: Alternatives in left hepatic duct obstruction. *Gastrointest Radiol* 1989;14:137–142.

Vogel SB, Howard RJ, Caridi J, Hawkins IF. Evaluation of percutaneous transhepatic balloon dilatation of benign biliary stricture in high-risk patients. *Am J Surg* 1985;149:73–79.

Treatment of Biliary Stones

RENAN UFLACKER

Elective cholecystectomy is an effective treatment for cholelithiasis but has a morbidity rate of 22 percent and a mortality rate of 2 percent in elderly patients. In high-risk groups, emergency cholecystectomy has a morbidity rate of 44 percent and a mortality rate of 10 percent. For elective cholecystectomy in chronic cholecystitis the mortality rate is only 1 percent. The development of a viable nonsurgical form of treatment was obviously necessary for the high-risk population. However, this is a formidable task because of the efficacy of surgical techniques, and procedures involving the gallbladder remain within the domain of surgery in most centers. However, a few early reports documented the feasibility of performing percutaneous gallbladder procedures, and more recently, a variety of therapeutic alternatives to cholecystectomy have become available, including percutaneous cholecystostomy; oral bile salts; contact dissolution of biliary stones; pulverization of stones with rotational devices, ultrasound, or a laser; and extracorporeal shock wave lithotripsy (ESWL). It has been established that not all patients with cholelithiasis should receive cholecystectomy, because many of these patients have no specific symptoms, refuse surgical treatment, or have a major contraindication to surgery. Patients with acute pyogenic cholecystitis are probably best treated by percutaneous cholecystostomy before surgical ablation of the gallbladder.

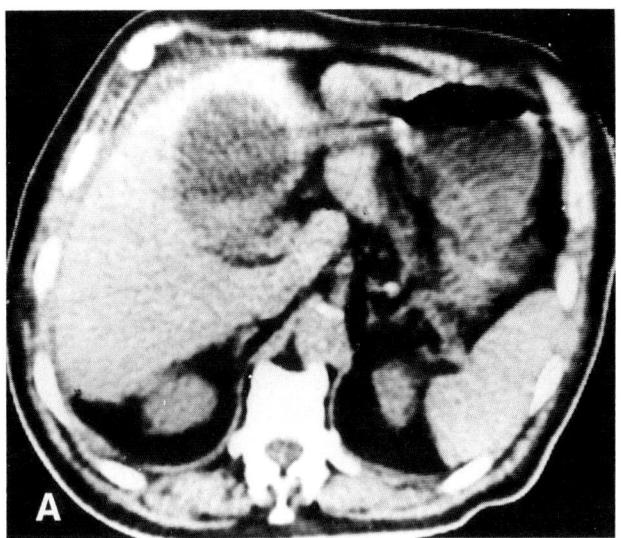

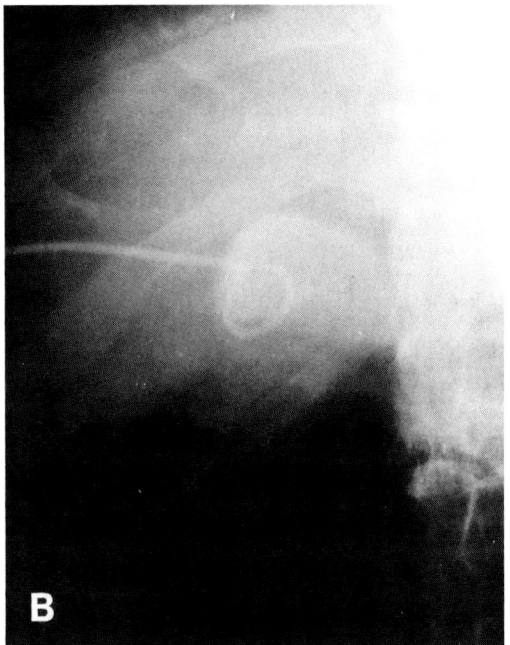

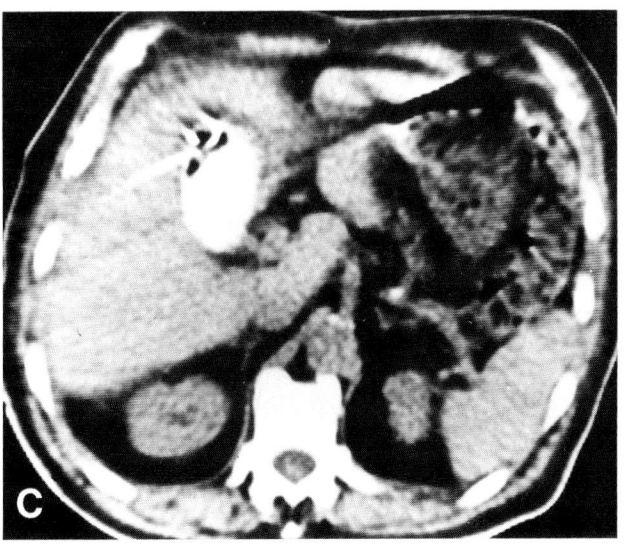

Figure 5.63 (A) Computed tomography (CT) in an 80-year-old patient with acalculous acute cholecystitis. Note the enlargement of the gallbladder. (B) Percutaneous puncture was oriented by CT, and external drainage was started. Cholangiography 48 h after drainage shows that the gallbladder is free of stones. (C) CT after transcatheter cholangiography shows a reduction in the size of the gallbladder and some peripheral edema. The patient was cured by percutaneous drainage, eliminating the need for surgery.

PERCUTANEOUS CHOLECYSTOSTOMY

Acute cholecystitis is caused by obstruction of the cystic duct that is usually related to impaction in the neck of the gallbladder caused by calculus. Cholecystectomy has been the treatment of choice, occasionally preceded by a temporary procedure such as surgical cholecystostomy in patients who are poor surgical risks. Mortality and complication rates, however, may exceed 20 percent and 42 percent respectively. Percutaneous transhepatic cholecystostomy provides a simple and fast alternative for gallbladder decompression and treatment of infection.

Percutaneous cholecystostomy can be performed under computed tomographic (CT) or ultrasonic guidance after diagnosis without the need for previous gallbladder opacification (Fig. 5.63). Ultrasonic guidance of the procedure requires additional fluroscopic control so that the position of the needle guide within the gallbladder lumen can be confirmed by contrast injection.

Percutaneous cholecystostomy has many advocates, but it is not widely practiced. Currently, this form of treatment competes with medical management of acute cholecystitis, emergency cholecystectomy, and emergency surgical cholecystostomy and interval cholecystectomy. The indications for percutaneous cholecystostomy have not been well established. It has been indicated for diagnostic studies and for the treatment of acute calculous and acalculous cholecystitis, mainly in high-risk patients (Fig. 5.64). With the current use of ESWL, the spectrum of applications of percutaneous cholecystostomy has been enlarged. It can be used to accelerate fragment dissolution with topical agents replacing the oral bile salts (chenodeoxycholate and ursodeoxycholate), and in patients with chronic cholecystitis it can be used to gain access for stone removal and gallbladder ablation.

Several techniques and instruments are used to obtain access to the gallbladder. A 22-gauge removal hub or a Chiba needle can be used to gain initial access to the gallbladder for cholecystography and fluid aspiration. Cholecystostomy can be performed either by the Seldinger technique or the trocar technique. A variety of procedures, including biopsies, diagnostic aspirations, cholecystographies, and therapeutic cholecystostomies, can be performed using percutaneous access. Either a right anterior midclavicular line or a lateral axillary line approach can be used to obtain access to the gallbladder.

Transhepatic needle puncture is thought to be the safest approach, decreasing the likelihood of free intraperitoneal bile leakage. The gallbladder fundus, however, can be entered directly, using a safety system. Different sizes of catheters can be used for gallbladder decompression, including Nos. 6.7, 7.6, and 8.3 French pigtail catheters. The Cope loop monofilament No. 8.3 French catheter or the No. 6.5 French "accordion"

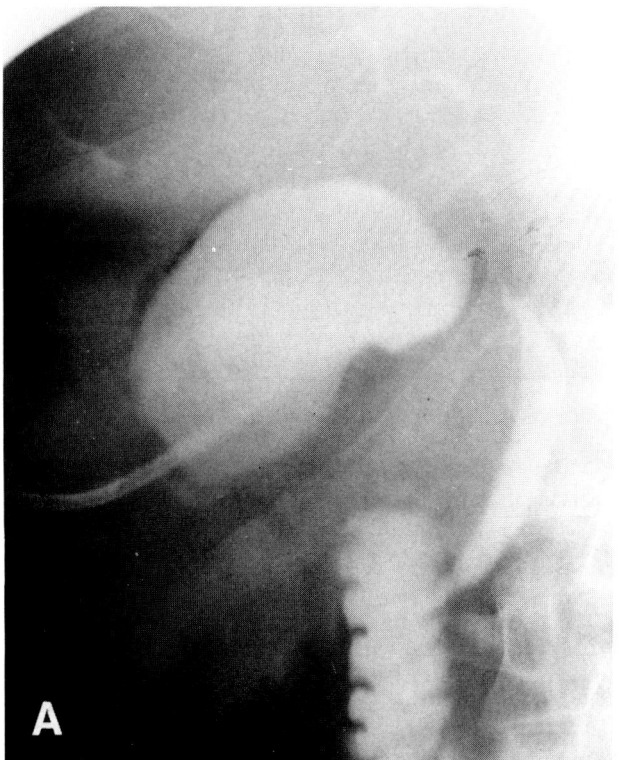

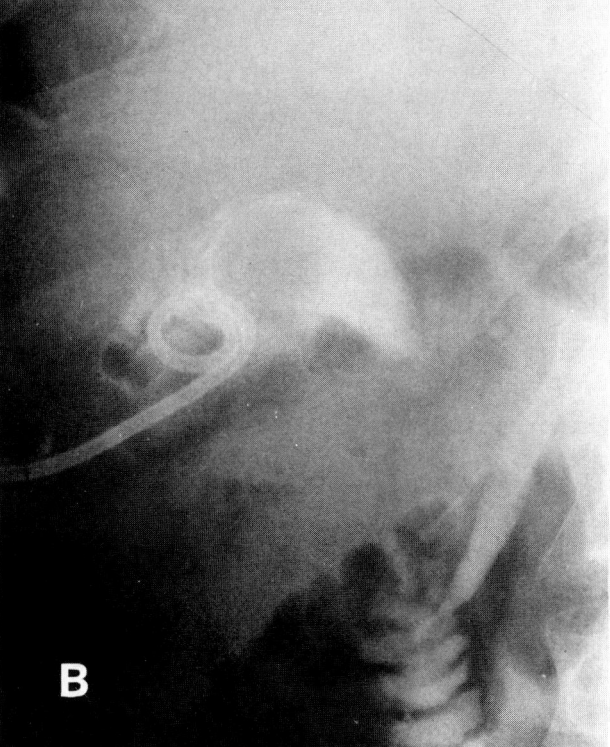

Figure 5.64 (A) Percutaneous cholangiography in a patient with acute cholecystitis. (B) 48 h after drainage with a No. 8.3 French catheter, a type II cholesterol stone was observed. Cholecystectomy was performed after clinical improvement of the infection.

catheter eliminates the need for multiple exchanges of catheters and guidewires and is self-retaining.

Aspirated bile should be sent for culture in all cases. To reduce the risk of sepsis, the catheter should be allowed to drain for 24 h before a diagnostic cholangiography or cholecystography is performed.

Major complications of percutaneous cholecystostomy include catheter dislodgment, septicemia, and life-threatening vagal reactions with severe hypotension and bradycardia. Self-retaining catheters should be used to avoid dislodgement. Intravenous wide-spectrum antibiotics should be administered before the procedure and for at least 48 h afterward to reduce the risk of sepsis. Profound vagal reactions can be treated with minimal intravisceral manipulation and the IV administration of atropine (0.6 mg), fluids, antibiotics, and dopamine. When administered prior to the procedure, atropine appears to reduce the reaction in some patients.

STONE DISSOLUTION AGENTS

There are two main types of gallstones. Seventy-five percent to 80 percent of gallstones are predominantly cholesterol, and 20 to 25 percent are pigment stones, predominantly bilirubin. Most cholesterol gallstones are formed by heterogeneous nucleation and are known as type I stones. These stones are usually multiple, contain more than 60 to 70 percent cholesterol by weight, and range in size from 0.5 to 2.5 cm. Type II stones tend to be solitary, are larger than 2.5 cm in diameter, are 100 percent cholesterol by weight, and are radiolucent. Approximately one-third of type I stones may contain enough calcium to make them radiopaque. Approximately 50 to 70 percent of all gallstones are type I stones, while type II stones account for 5 to 20 percent.

The pathogenesis of cholesterol stones is multifactorial, and several approaches to dissolution are possible using oral bile salts or contact solvents. Expansion of the bile salt pool with oral bile salts has been done successfully. Oral bile salts can dissolve cholesterol gallstones.

Black and brown bilirubinate pigment stones are more frequently radiopaque because of their high content of calcium bilirubinate, calcium phosphate, and calcium carbonate. Bilirubin stones cannot be treated safely and effectively by dissolution techniques at this time.

ORAL BILE SALTS

Cholesterol gallbladder stones can be treated successfully with oral agents. The time required for treatment ranges from 6 months to 4 years. Patient selection criteria for treatment with oral bile salts should include the following.

1. Radiolucent stones. These stones lead to inappropriate treatment in 20 to 33 percent of patients.
2. Analysis of gallbladder bile (bile salts, phospholipids, and cholesterol concentrations).
3. Patient's weight. Obese patients have lower dissolution rates.
4. Degree of gallbladder disease. A functioning gallbladder is necessary for oral drugs to be secreted into the gallbladder.
5. Number and size of stones. A large number of stones or stones larger than 20 mm in diameter have a reduced chance of dissolution.

Chenodeoxycholate and ursodeoxycholate are the currently available oral bile salts that are effective in dissolving gallstones.

Chenodeoxycholic acid is a naturally occurring bile salt that is produced by the liver and accounts for approximately 20 to 30 percent of the bile salt pool. It is administered orally at a dose of 14 to 16 mg/kg/day. The duration of therapy ranges from 6 months to 4 years. Dissolution is usually possible if a significant decrease in the size of the stone is noted within 9 months. Up to 14 percent of patients may have complete dissolution with a dose of 750 mg per day. Recurrence rates, however, may be as high as 25 to 50 percent. Diarrhea and elevation of liver enzymes are the main side effects of chenodeoxycholic acid occurring in approximately 25 percent of patients.

Ursodeoxycholic acid is an epimer of chenodeoxycholic acid that is found in trace amounts in normal humans. The oral dose is 8 to 12 mg/kg/d, with a higher potency than that of chenodeoxycholate. The duration of therapy ranges from 6 to 12 months. Partial or complete dissolution of gallstones occurs in 40 to 55 percent of patients with small floating radiolucent cholesterol stones after 6 to 12 months. The recurrence rate is about 25 percent. Side effects are much less common than are those which accompany chenodeoxycholic acid, but diarrhea and abnormal liver enzymes may occur.

Both chenodeoxycholate and ursodeoxycholate are effective oral agents for the dissolution of cholesterol gallstones. The dosage ursodeoxycholate is approximately half that of chenodeoxycholate. Ursodeoxycholate seems to be more rapid and less hepatotoxic and has fewer side effects. A recent randomized trial comparing the two agents demontrated an increased efficacy of ursodeoxycholate over chenodeoxycholate, with 30 percent versus 7 percent complete dissolution and 30 percent versus 40 percent partial dissolution.

TOPICAL AGENTS

If access to the biliary tree is available through a percutaneous or endoscopic approach, topical agents can be used to dissolve stones in the bile ducts or gallbladder. Most of the topical solutions available are effective in dissolving cholesterol stones. Some agents are more effective than others, and safety also varies. General safety principles should be known before a topical stone dissolution agent is used. The substance cannot be infused under pressure or into the parenchyma of the liver without running the risk of hemolysis. Dissolution agents may be absorbed by the duodenal or intestinal mucosa if they are exposed to it. No peritoneal leaking of the substance should be allowed. To avoid reflux, infusion pressure should not exceed 20 to 30 cmH$_2$O.

A variety of early topical agents have been tried for cholesterol stone dissolution, with different results and side effects. Sulfuric ether is very volatile and has several deleterious side effects that preclude its acceptance even though it is a good cholesterol solvent in vitro. Chloroform is also an excellent solvent, but its use is associated with centrilobular hepatic necrosis, duodenal ulceration, and bleeding. Infusion of saline solutions and heparin has been shown to be as effective as flushing techniques and spontaneous stone passage.

Mono-Octanoin

Mono-octanoin is a normal digestive product of medium-chain triglycerides that has excellent in vitro cholesterol solubility. It is administered percutaneously into the gallbladder or bile duct via a No. 5 French catheter in infusions (3 to 7 mL/h) for several days (average 5 days) to 2 weeks. A 50 to 86 percent rate of complete stone dissolution has been reported when this agent is used for 3 to 7 days. Gallstones with a cholesterol content of 40 percent or more have a 91 percent chance of dissolution within 7 days of treatment. Mono-octanoin is associated with side effects in two-thirds of patients. Local side effects such as gastric and duodenal ulcerations and systemic effects such as nausea, vomiting, diarrhea, abdominal pain, and cramping may be observed. High-pressure infusion into the gallbladder may lead to hemolysis and hemorrhagic pneumonitis with respiratory distress and hypoxia. Infusion should be stopped and reevaluated when side effects are detected. Most of the symptoms can be alleviated by stopping the infusion temporarily and restarting it at a slower rate.

Methyl Tert-Butyl Ether

Methyl tert-butyl ether (MTBE) is an aliphatic ether which is used as an antiknock agent in gasoline. MTBE dissolves cholesterol gallstones in vitro 50 times faster than mono-octanoin does. MTBE is currently the agent of choice for dissolving cholesterol gallstones. Catheters are placed into the gallbladder, using fluoroscopy, sonography, CT, or a combination of guidance techniques. The modified Seldinger technique using a coaxial system is preferred for insertion of the small No. 5 French catheter. The transhepatic route is recommended to prevent leakage of bile and ether. Dissolution with MTBE is applicable only to cholesterol calculi (Fig. 5.65). Manual injections and pumps have been used to improve mixing of the solvent within the gallbladder. Although the time required for dissolution is lengthy (3 to 25 h), MTBE is effective for cholesterol stones of any number and size. This is an advantage compared with ESWL. However, the use of MTBE is restricted by relatively stringent criteria for patient selection.

Patient Selection

Only patients with specific biliary symptoms are considered for therapy with MTBE. To avoid treating patients whose cystic duct has become occluded by fibrosis or an impacted stone, the patency of the duct is verified by means of oral cholecystography or radioisotopic scanning. Patients with evidence of acute inflammation of the gallbladder on physical examination or laboratory tests should not receive this treatment. MTBE can be used for stone dissolution in selected patients with common bile duct stones, provided that an occluding balloon system is used to prevent overflow of the solvent into the duodenum. Endoscopic catheterization and infusion of the agent before sphincterotomy and basket retrieval of stones is a useful alternative in patients with larger stones in the common bile duct (Fig. 5.66). Patients with coagulopathy should be excluded. Abstinence from aspirin and other nonsteroidal anti-inflammatory agents for at least 10 days is required before the procedure.

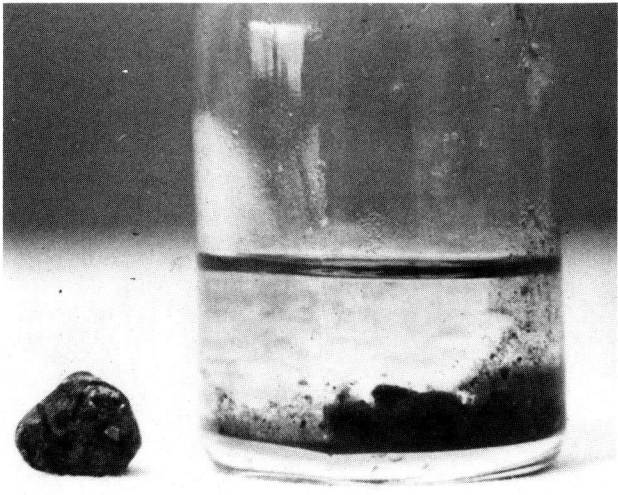

Figure 5.65 In vitro dissolution of cholesterol gallstones with methyl *tert*-butyl ether.

Technique

After percutaneous catheterization in the gallbladder or the common bile duct or endoscopic catheterization in the common bile duct, a small amount of contrast medium (1 to 7 mL) should be injected manually, using a small glass syringe to determine the stone-enveloping volume radiologically before overflow through the cystic duct or Oddi's sphincter. The volume and rapidity of the infusion can be assessed in this manner. Sedation is contraindicated, but analgesia can be used. The solvent is injected in small aliquots, usually in the range of 3 to 7 mL, using a continuous infusion and aspiration technique in which the gallbladder or common bile duct is emptied completely with each aspiration to remove inflowing bile as well as released noncholesterol stone debris and cholesterol-saturated MTBE. A fresh supply of the agent is used every 15 min

Endoscopic placement of a nasobiliary catheter for stones in the common bile duct has some advantages over the percutaneous approach (Fig. 5.67). However, sphincterotomy increases the morbidity of the procedure slightly. Occluding balloon devices that are not soluble in MTBE, such as those made of latex, should be used. The endoscopic approach always requires an occluding system.

Results

Current results of gallbladder stone dissolution using MTBE are encouraging. The Mayo Clinic series reported success in 18 of 19 patients who received MTBE to dissolve gallstones. Approximately half the 19 patients experienced nausea and duodenitis. Hemolysis and sedation occurred in one patient. Recurrence of stones was detected in one patient 6 months after dissolution. The San Diego series included 13 patients with gallstones and 5 with common bile duct stones. Dissolution was

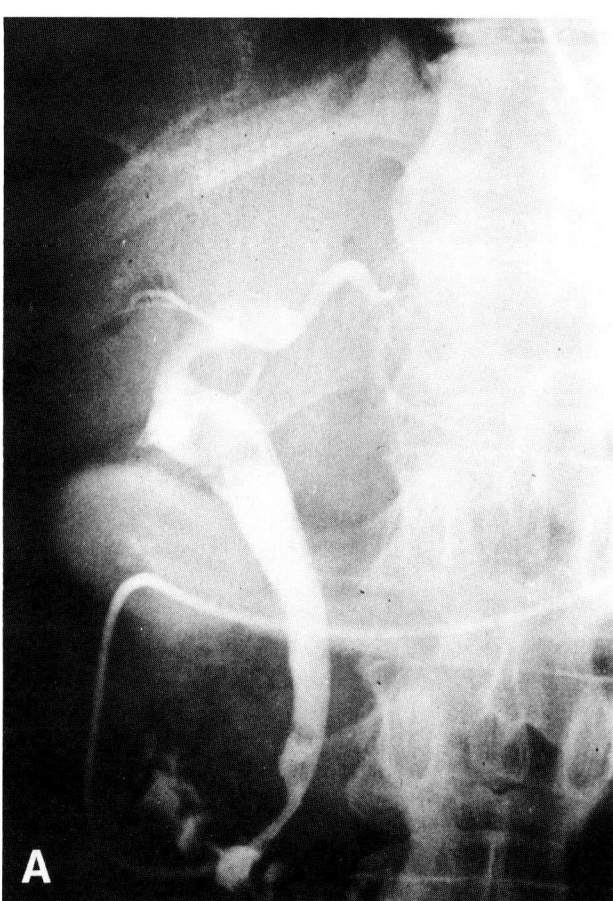
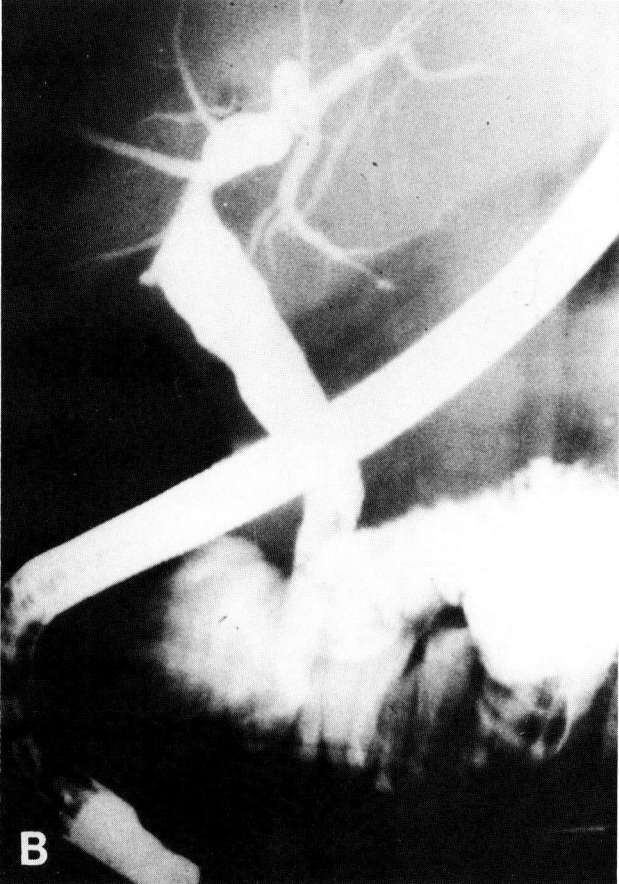

Figure 5.66 (A) Retrograde endoscopic cholangiography with a nasobiliary catheter shows a large radiolucent stone in the common bile duct. Methyl *tert*-butyl ether (MTBE) infusion was started and then maintained for several hours. (B) The bile duct was free of stones after MTBE treatment with dissolution and retrieval of the fragments with a Dormia basket.

successful in 11 of the 13 patients with gallstones and 3 of the 5 patients with common bile duct stones. However, the therapy was mixed, and the results also pertain to MTBE dissolution, basket removal, and mono-octanoin dissolution. Major complications occurred in 2 of the 18 patients. In the Williams series, dissolution of gallstones with MTBE was attempted in 67 patients. Total or nearly total stone dissolution was achieved in 61 patients. In six patients, gallstones were not satisfactorily dissolved. Gallstones recurred in 6 of the 61 patients during the follow-up period of 6 to 54 months (within 12 to 24 months in 2 patients and within 6 to 12 months in 4 patients). In four patients, bile leakage occurred after catheter removal.

The potential for recurrence of gallstones limits the practical utility of therapeutic approaches that leave the gallbladder intact. Initial experience might suggest that gallbladder stones will recur some time after dissolution in a number of patients. If complete stone dissolution has been documented by at least two ultrasound examinations, the risk of recurrence is approximately 20 percent within 2 years. Whether or not oral bile salts are used adjunctively, neither MTBE nor mono-octanoin will ever be the ultimate treatment for cholecystolithiasis. The goal of permanent gallbladder ablation and cystic duct occlusion must be pursued.

PERCUTANEOUS LITHOTRIPSY OF BILIARY CALCULI

Experience with percutaneous lithotripsy of biliary calculi using a variety of techniques is largely experimental. However, some of these techniques have been used in groups of patients with gallstones and common bile duct stones and are well established.

The percutaneous removal of retained common bile duct stones through the T-tube track was described many years ago and is now a standard technique in the armamentarium of the interventional radiologist. Endoscopic sphincterotomy is the treatment of choice for stones in the common bile duct when there is not a percutaneous track, but this technique depends on the skill of the endoscopist.

Direct percutaneous access to either the gallbladder or the bile ducts has been used increasingly to remove or fragment stones in patients who are poor candidates for surgery. A variety of percutaneous methods have been used to treat common bile duct stones and gallstones, including mechanical lithotripsy (basket and grasper stone removal and percutaneous pulverization with a high-speed rotational catheter), ultrasonic lithotripsy, laser lithotripsy, and intracorporeal electrohydraulic lithotripsy.

These techniques require fluoroscopic guidance and/or direct visualization of the biliary tract by means of a choledochoscope. These procedures can be performed through a preexisting T-tube track or a percutaneous puncture, using a No. 18 French sheath. For electrohydraulic lithotripsy, an electrode is connected to a shock wave generator. The electrode is brought into contact with the stone, and the shock wave is delivered for 1 to 2 s. The stone fragments are subsequently irrigated or removed with a basket or forceps. In the percutaneous transhepatic removal technique, a No. 8 French sheath with a check flow valve is placed in a peripheral bile duct and a modified Dormia basket is used to snare the stone, crush it, and advance it into the duodenum. Occasionally larger stones may be reduced in mass with MTBE before being crushed. Balloon dilatation of the sphincter as well as the bile ducts may be necessary in some cases. Sedation with opiates and diazepam is usually needed. This technique has a complication rate of 17 percent, morbidity rate of 13 percent, and a mortality rate of 4 percent. Cholangitis and sepsis are the most serious complications of this procedure. Ultrasonic energy can be used to break up stones after they have been engaged in a stone basket or when they are freed into the biliary duct or gallbladder. This technique can be used for gallstones and common bile duct stones. The ultrasonic probe can be used through a nephroscope under direct visualization or under fluoroscopic guidance for lithotripsy. The stone fragments can be retrieved through the cannula with a basket when they are in the gallbladder or can be advanced in the duodenum when they are in the common bile duct. More recently the tunable dye laser has been used to fragment gallstones of all types. The tunable dye laser can be used with MTBE to accelerate stone fragmentation.

More recently the Kensey catheter, which has a high-speed rotational tip, and the Kensey-Nash device, which has a propeller, have been used to pulverize stones in the bile ducts and gallbladder. The flexibility of the No. 8 French Kensey catheter allows it to be used through a T-tube track. The infusion of saline and contrast material, combined with the rotational cam within a cylinder, creates a vortex (Fig. 5.68). The stones are drawn to the center of the vortex, where the high-speed rotational tip pulverizes them.

GALLBLADDER ABLATION AND CYSTIC DUCT OCCLUSION

Gallbladder ablation and cystic duct occlusion are under intense study in several institutions, and a practical method will probably be developed soon. Gallbladder ablation and cystic duct occlusion are two of the biggest

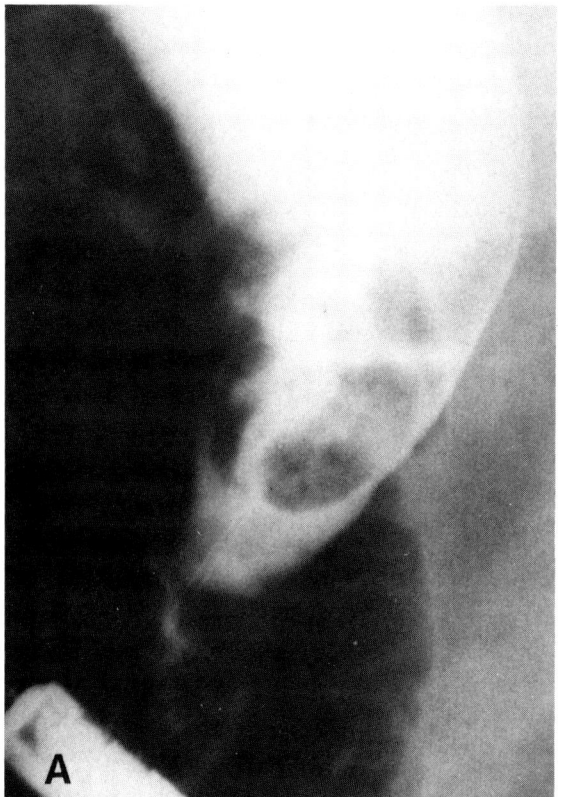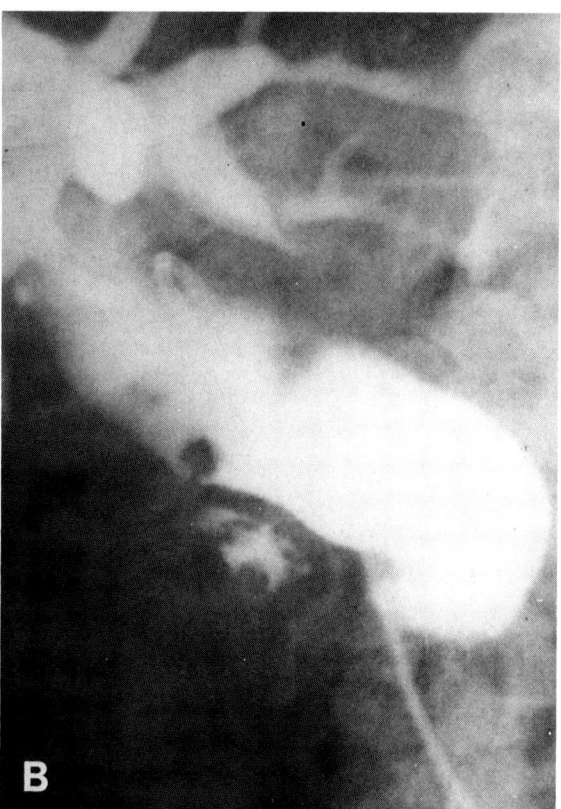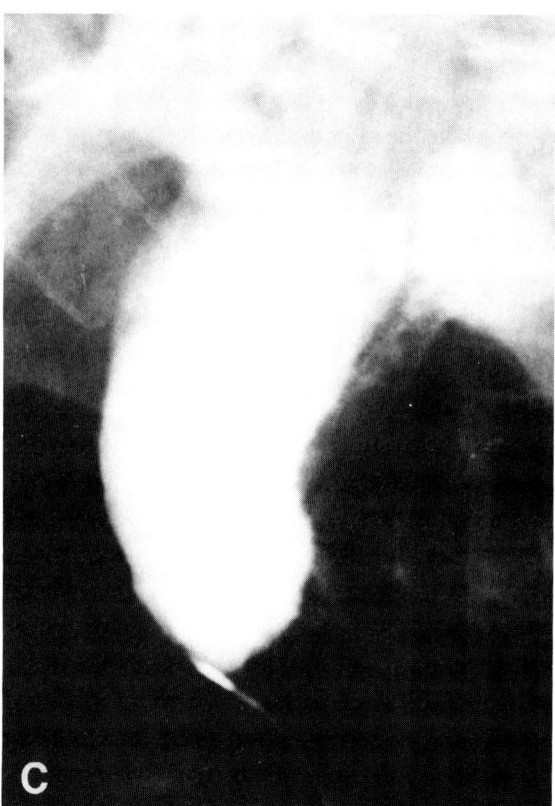

Figure 5.67 (A) Cystic dilatation of the common bile duct associated with choledocholithiasis. (B) Methyl *tert*-butyl ether infusion through a nasobiliary catheter was performed for several hours. Note the reduction in the size of the stones. (C) Cholangiography after dissolution of stones and basket retrieval of the fragments. Sphincterotomy was performed.

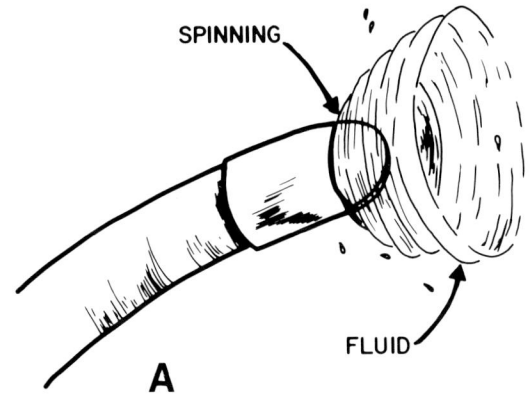
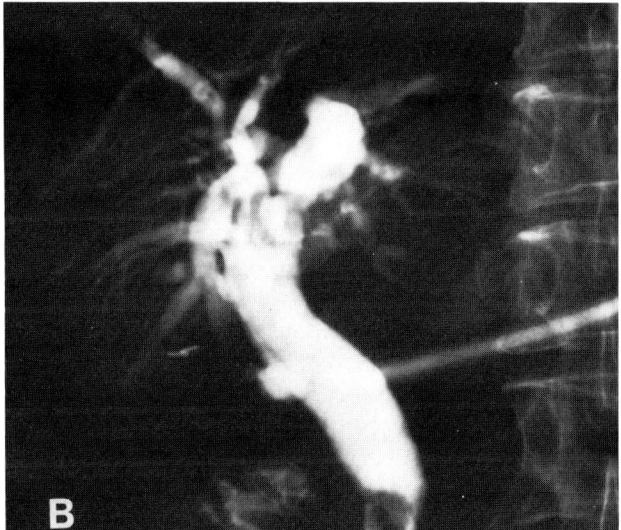
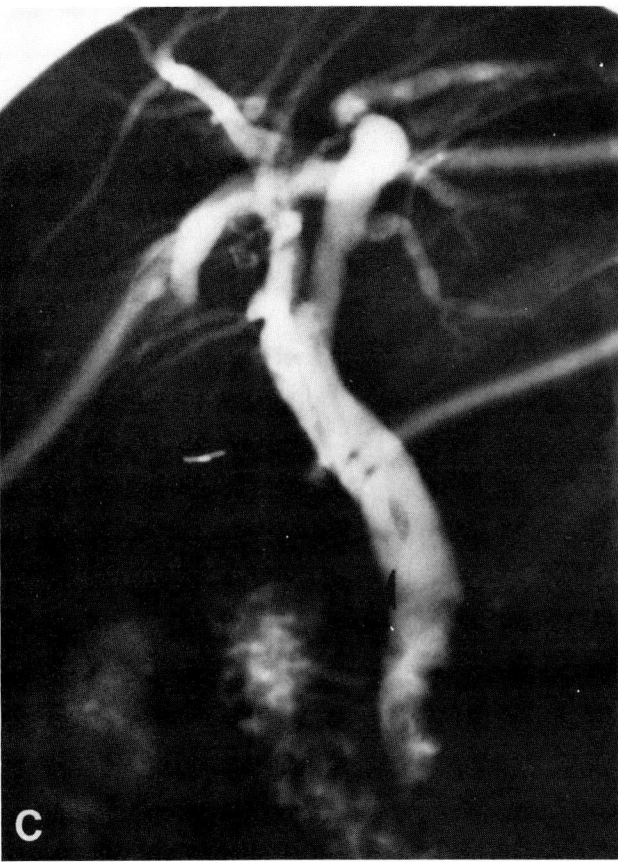
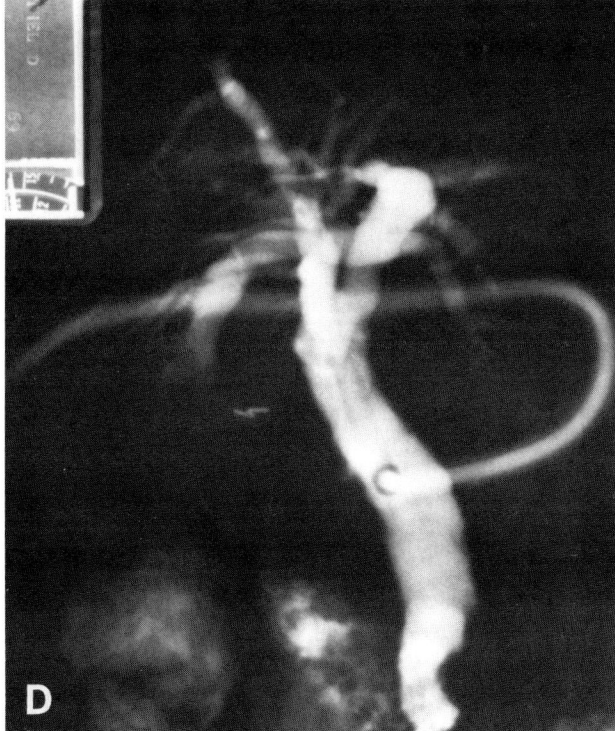

Figure 5.68 (A) Diagram of a Kensey catheter. Note the vortex created by the infusion fluid. Saline and contrast material were used for infusion. (B) A T-tube cholangiogram showing a 2-cm stone at the distal aspect of the common bile duct. (C) Control cholangiography after the use of a Kensey catheter with pulverization of the stone. Residual fragments are still visible (arrow). (D) Follow-up cholangiogram 24 h later shows a normal bile duct.

challenges interventional radiologists have ever faced. Several techniques have been used experimentally for gallbladder sclerosis and fibrosis.

A number of techniques and materials have been evaluated. In a recent study it was found that hot contrast material and sotradecol were both ineffective. Absolute alcohol, however, was effective in the short term, with evidence of regeneration of the gallbladder mucosa due to epithelial growth from the cystic duct inside the gallbladder. The same results were observed with tetracycline, metacrylate, and a mixture of 95% alcohol and 3% trifluoroacetic acid. In a rabbit study that used hot contrast material, chronic cholecystitis with transmural fibrosis was induced. In a recent report, absolute ethanol and 3% sodium tetradecyl sulfate were used successfully in pigs to obtain permanent gallbladder ablation associated with effective occlusion of the cystic duct.

Satisfactory gallbladder ablation or sclerosis seems to be possible only when definitive cystic duct occlusion prevents bile reaccumulation and epithelial ingrowth into the gallbladder. Reliable and permanent cystic duct occlusion can now be done experimentally, using an endoluminal bipolar radiofrequency electrocoagulation technique (RFE) and laser photocoagulation. The RFE technique uses a flow of alternating current in the tissue around the electrode tip to generate heat. A superficial thermal lesion is produced, causing focal cell necrosis, hemorrhage, and peripheral edema. Later histologic findings include a chronic inflammatory and fibrogenic intraluminal reaction (scar tissue). Experimental studies have indicated that cystic duct occlusion with the RFE technique creates an effective barrier that protects the bile ducts from the sclerosants used in the gallbladder. Complete and permanent gallbladder sclerotherapy is possible with ethanol and sodium tetradecyl sulfate without systemic adverse effects, as demonstrated experimentally. Gallbladder sclerotherapy must be followed by effective external drainage to prevent retention of necrotic and inflammatory debris after treatment. Occlusion of the cystic duct and ablation of the gallbladder mucosa through a percutaneous access may become clinically useful in preventing recurrent cholelithiasis after percutaneous or extracorporeal gallstone lithotripsy in the near future.

Mucosal remnants encased by fibrous tissue in the gallbladder wall are unlikely to promote regeneration of the mucosa. The risk of adenocarcinoma, however, cannot be totally ruled out on a long-term basis if epithelial elements remain within a sclerotic gallbladder.

EXTRACORPOREAL SHOCK WAVE LITHOTRIPSY

The medical management of stones changed radically with the report of successful renal lithotripsy by Chaussy et al. in 1982. West German investigators led by Paumgartner at the Grosshadern Hospital in Munich later developed the concept of ESWL for the treatment of gallstones, publishing the first successful results involving nine patients with gallstones and five patients with stones in the common bile duct that could not be removed by endoscopic procedures. A modified MH3 Dornier machine with a water bath tank was used in these patients. The large immersion water tank system has been replaced by a smaller second-generation apparatus without a water tank. This system uses only a compressible membrane-covered water bag housing an electrode ellipsoid assembly that is guided by two real-time diagnostic sonographic transducers that provide bidimensional spatial localization of the stone. The current experience of the Munich group includes over 1,000 patients with gallstones treated by ESWL.

A number of manufacturers have developed second-generation lithotripters with different systems for shock wave generation and different target imaging apparatus. All but two manufacturers (Medstone and Technomed) have replaced the immersion tank with a compressible soft water bag that permits focusing of the shock wave across the body wall and soft tissues through direct contact with a water bag covered by ultrasound gel.

A variety of shock wave generation systems are available for renal and gallbladder lithotripsy (Table 5.3), including electrostatic spark-gap discharge (Dornier, Medstone, Technomed, Northgate), electromagnetic shock wave generation (Siemens), a piezoelectric pulse system (EDAP, R. Wolf, Diasonics), and low-frequency, high-intensity sonography (Labsonics). Most of these systems are marketed primarily as renal devices, but any of them have the potential to treat biliary stones with operational and patient position modifications. A number of clinical trials involving kidney stones or gallstones are under way in the United States; however, gallstones are routinely treated by ESWL in some institutions in Europe. Gallstone lithotripsy probably will be more widely used as a primary treatment technique than will ESWL for stones in the common bile duct.

Principles

Shock waves are high-pressure waves with an extremely short duration of less than 1 msec. The pioneer system of shock wave generation uses a high-voltage generator and underwater electrodes to discharge sparks through a gap that causes sudden evaporation of water between the electrodes, creating a pressure wave of high velocity and energy. The pressure wave is reflected on the walls of the semiellipsoidal metal cavity and directed to a focus 30 mm long and 2 mm wide that has a cigar shape. Pressures of up to 1,000 bar can be generated within nanoseconds. When objects with an accoustic impedance different from that of water are placed in the shock wave focus, they absorb energy. Pressure and tensile forces are created in an object (in this case a stone) when the pressure wave enters and leaves the object. Primary fissures can serve as an interface to liberate shock wave energy within the object, which eventually is fragmented completely. Shock waves cross without damage to tissues with more than 70 percent water content because there is no acoustic impedance. The lungs and bowels, however, may be damaged by shock waves.

Patient Selection

Eligibility criteria for ESWL treatment are very strict, with only symptomatic patients being considered. Gallbladder visualization on oral cholecystography is required to prove cystic duct patency for the elimination of stone fragments. The stone should be a single radiolucent cholesterol stone no larger than 30 mm in diameter or up to three radiolucent stones with a similar total stone mass. These criteria are from the West German protocol. The U.S. protocol differs, especially in regard to the size of stones accepted for treatment (Table 5.4). Patients

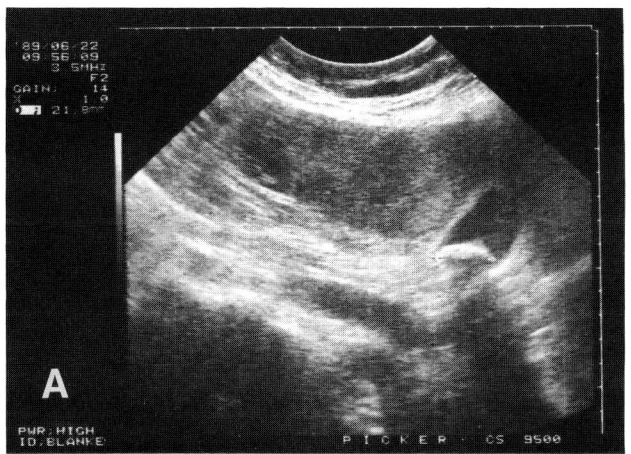

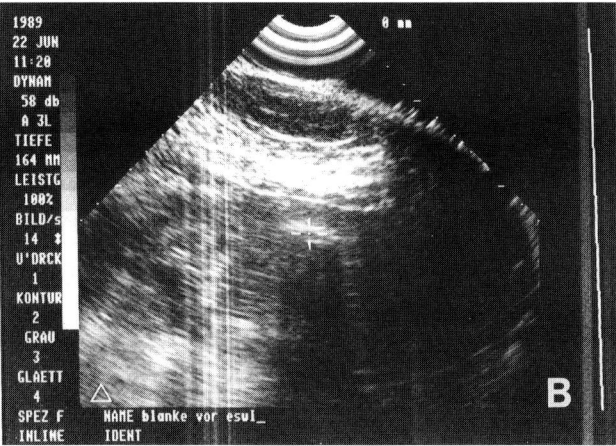

Figure 5.69 (A) Ultrasound examinations showing a 2-cm gallstone. (B) Follow-up ultrasound after extracorporeal shock wave lithotripsy of the cholesterol gallstone shows reduction of the mass to small fragments and sludge. The lithotripter was an MPL-9000 from Dornier (Munich, West Germany).

Table 5.3 – Second-Generation Lithotripters for Treatment of Renal and Gallbladder Stones

Manufacturer	Model	Shock Wave generator	Coupling design	Imaging technique currently available
Dornier Medical Systems Munich, West Germany	MPL-9000	Spark-gap electrode	Water bag	Ultrasound (fluoroscopy in the future)
Medstone Int. Costa Mesa, CA	1050 ST	Spark-gap electrode	Water tank	Ultrasound plus fluoroscopy
Technomed Paris, France	Sonolith 3000	Spark-gap electrode	Water tank	Ultrasound
Northgate	SD-3	Spark-gap electrode	Water bag	Ultrasound
Siemens Erlangen, West Germany	Lithostar Plus	Electromagnetic	Water bag	Fluoroscopy plus ultrasound
R. Wolf Knittlingen, West Germany	Piezolith 2200	Piezoelectric	Water bag	Ultrasound
Diasonics	Therasonic	Piezoelectric	Water bag	Ultrasound plus fluoroscopy
EDAP Marne la Valle, France	LT 01	Piezoelectric	Water bag	Ultrasound
Labsonics Indianapolis, IN	—	Low-frequency, high-intensity sonography	Water bag	Ultrasound

Table 5.4 – Patient Selection Criteria for ESWL

West German Inclusion Criteria
1. History of biliary colic
2. Solitary radiolucent gallbladder stone with a diameter up to 30 mm or up to three radiolucent gallstones with a similar total stone mass
3. Gallbladder visualization on oral cholecystography

United States Inclusion Criteria
1. Up to three gallstones
2. Each gallstone can be up to 30 mm in diameter
3. Noncalcified stones (3-mm rim or central nidus allowed)
4. Functioning gallbladder on oral cholecystography
5. Pretreatment physical class I, II, or III

United States Exclusion Criteria
1. Relevant coagulation problem
2. Pregnancy
3. Cardiac pacemaker or arrhythmia
4. Known common bile duct stones
5. Calcified stone
6. Hepatic cyst or hemangioma in shock wave path
7. Vascular aneurysm in shock wave path
8. Lung in shock wave path
9. Any indication of pigmented stones

with acute cholecystitis, calcified stones, biliary obstruction, or known bile duct stones are not included in the West German protocol. Patients with gastroduodenal ulcer or pancreatitis, patients taking anticoagulant medication, and pregnant patients are also excluded. Clear detection of the stones by ultrasound and positioning in the system must be possible.

In the West German series, all patients received adjuvant litholytic therapy with bile acids 2 weeks before receiving ESWL. A combination of ursodeoxycholic acid and chenodeoxycholic acid is used to desaturate the bile cholesterol, followed by the administration of the same combination of bile salts for several months to achieve dissolution of stone fragments. Multiple randomized clinical trials of the efficacy of adjuvant litholytic therapy are under way in Europe and the United States.

Technique

When a water bath lithotripter is used, the patient, in the prone position, is partially immersed so that the shock waves enter the gallbladder ventrally. In early machines, patients were tied to a cradle suspended from the ceiling. Stone targeting was done by fluoroscopy, and gallbladder opacification with an oral cholecystogram was mandatory. Stones in the common bile duct were treated with the patient in the supine position, and the shock waves entered from the back to avoid bowel interposition in their path. More recent lithotripsy machines have a compressible water bag that allows a wider range of positioning movements and a C-arm that allows either under- or over-the-table positioning of the shock wave generator.

Up to 1600 shock waves are discharged within 30 to 125 min (average, 60 min). Usually the energy level of the shock waves is set around 14 kV at the beginning of the treatment and may reach 22 kV during the treatment, with an average generator voltage of 19 kV. The triggering is monitored continuously by an electrocardiogram. Intravenous analgesia and sedation are generally used. General anesthesia is seldom necessary with the second-generation apparatus.

At this point it is advisable for patients to receive adjuvant litholytic therapy with bile acids to dissolve the stone fragments. Technically adequate lithotripsy should reduce the stones to sand or to fragments up to 2 to 3 mm in diameter to allow the expulsion of the fragments from the gallbladder lumen primarily through the cystic duct, a complex structure that constitutes an anatomic tortuous barrier because of the spiral Heister's valves, and secondarily through the papillae of vater. Although chronic cholecystitis may impair gallbladder contractility, the local trauma of shock wave therapy does not change it. Hospitalization for 2 to 3 days for observation is required in most patients.

About 25 to 30 percent of the population with gallstones may meet the criteria for ESWL. Treatment of larger or multiple stones may require several treatments of ESWL therapy to accomplish adequate fragmentation and fragment expulsion (Fig. 5.70).

Results

Clinical data on ESWL in the treatment of biliary stones up to January 1989 in 5,500 patients treated with 40 Dornier MPL-9000 lithotripters in Germany, Switzerland, Austria, Belgium, Italy, Spain, Yugoslavia, Japan, Malaysia, Pakistan, Singapore, and the United States show the following results.

Average patient age is 45 years, with 30 percent males and 70 percent females. Fifty-five percent of the stones are solitary, while 45 percent are multiple, and average stone size is 17 mm. Ninety percent of the stones are radiolucent, and only 10 percent are calcified. In 27 percent of patients re-ESWL has been necessary. Ninety percent of the patients were treated in the prone position, and 10 percent in the supine position. Forty percent of the patients needed sedation and/or analgesia, and 60 percent did not need medication.

The disintegration rate was 95 percent. Sixty percent of the patients were stone-free at 6 months when the stone was solitary, and 30 percent were stone-free when the stones were multiple. Ninety percent of patients

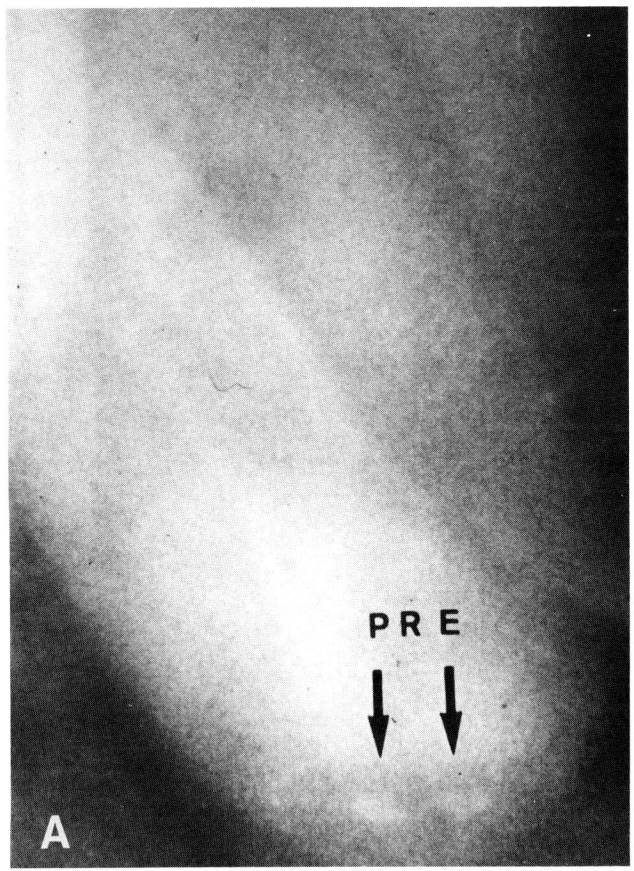
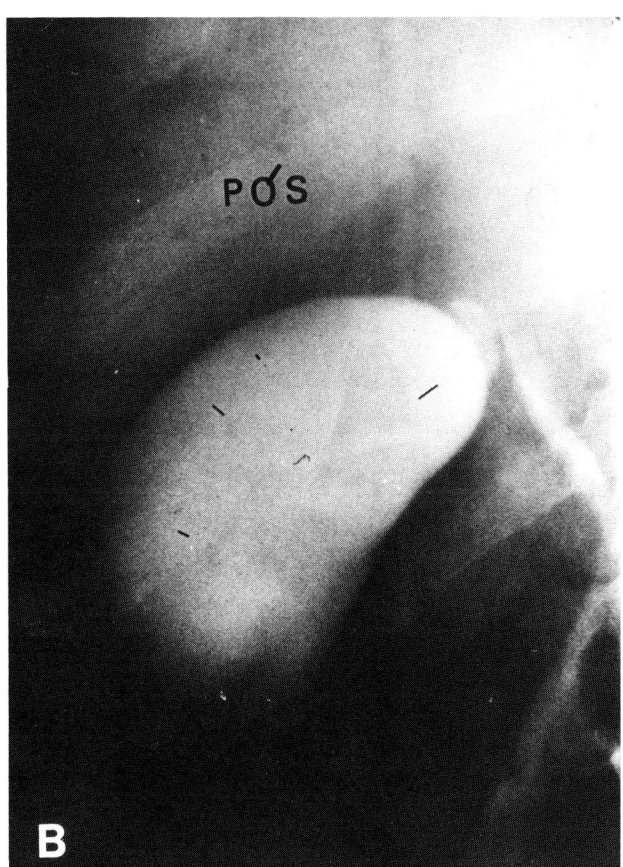

Figure 5.70 (A) Oral cholecystogram showing two gallstones of about 1 cm each with central calcification (arrows). (B) After extracorporeal shock wave lithotripsy with a Lithostar from Siemens (Erlangen, West Germany), the stones were reduced to small fragments. (Case provided by Arnaldo Ganc, MD.)

with single stones and 60 percent of those with multiple stones were stone-free at 12 months. At 18 months, 85 percent of all patients were stone-free. Light biliary pancreatitis was noted in 1 percent of the patients, and less than 1 percent had cholestasis. The probability of stone recurrence was one percent 12 months after treatment and 15 percent 24 months after treatment.

Data on ESWL for biliary stones using a Lithostar Plus (Siemens) with an overhead module and an on-line ultrasound probe recently became available, including information on 106 patients. This series included 28 patients with common bile duct stones and 78 patients with gallstones. The number of shock waves was arbitrarily limited to 4,000 per session. Shock wave generator power was set in the range of 16 to 19 kV, and the average session lasted 60 min. Gallstones were disintegrated by ESWL in 86 percent of all patients, but fragments larger than 4 mm were found after the first treatment in 70 percent of patients (Fig. 5.70). Successful stone fragmentation for bile duct calculi was achieved in 71 percent of patients (Fig. 5.71). The majority of patients who received biliary shock wave therapy developed skin petechiae at the site of the shock head coupling. Serious complications related to ESWL developed in 3.8 percent of the 78 patients with gallstones. One patient had acute cholecystitis, and two had acute pancreatitis.

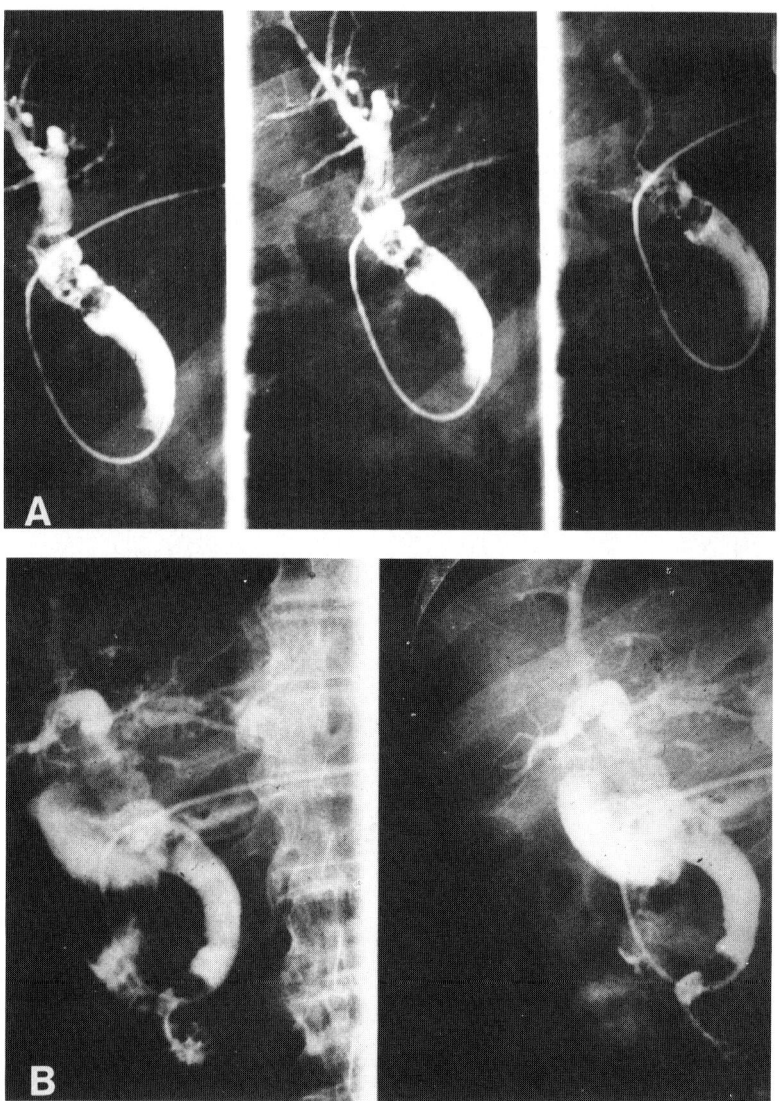

Figure 5.71 (A) Common bile duct stones observed at retrograde cholangiography performed through a nasobiliary catheter. (B) After 2,000 shock waves, the stones were fragmented.

Conclusions

The results reported in the literature on ESWL treatment of gallstones and bile duct stones indicate that it is a useful technique that is successful in 71 to 95 percent of patients. The available data also indicate that to date, the spark-gap system is moderately more effective than are the alternative systems. The adjunctive use of litholytic therapy and percutaneous procedure may enhance the effectiveness of ESWL.

REFERENCES

Allen MJ, Borody TJ, Bugliosi TF, May GR, LaRusso NF, Thistle JL. Cholelithiasis using methyl tertiary butyl ether. *Gastroenterology* 1985;88:122–125.

Allen MJ, Borody TJ, Bugliosi TF, May GR, LaRusso GR, Thistle JL. Rapid dissolution of gallstones by methyl tertiary butyl ether. *N Eng J Med* 1985;312:217–220.

Becker CD, Quenville NF, Burhenne HJ. Gallbladder ablation through radiologic intervention: An experimental alternative to cholecystectomy. *Radiology* 1989;171:235–240.

Becker CD, Quenville NF, Burhenne HJ. Long-term occlusion of the porcine cystic duct by means of endoluminal radio-frequency electrocoagulation. *Radiology* 1988;167:63–68.

Becker GJ, Kopechy KK. Can the newer interventional procedures replace cholecystectomy for cholecystolithiasis? The potential role of percutaneous cystic duct ablation. *Radiology* 1988;167:275–279.

Brendel W, Enders G. Shock waves for gallstones: Animal studies. *Lancet* 1983;i:1054.

Burhenne HJ. The promise of extracorporeal shock wave lithotripsy for the treatment of gallstones. *AJR* 1987;149:233–235.

Burhenne HJ, Becker CD, Malone DE, Rawat B, Fache JS. Biliary lithotripsy: Early observations in 106 patients. *Radiology* 1989;171:363–367.

Chaussy C, Schmiedt E, Jocham D, Brendel W, Forssman B, Walther V. First clinical experience with extracorporeally induced destruction of kidney stones by shock waves. *J Urol* 1982;127:417–420.

Coelho JCU, Moraes LM, Barbara MS, Artigas GV. Colecistectomia no paciente idoso. *Rev Assoc Med Bras* 1988;34:89–92.

Dornier Lithotripter MPL 9000. Clinical data, February 1989.

Faulkner DJ, Kozarek RA. Gallstones: Fragmentation with a tunable dye laser and dissolution with methyl tert-butyl ether in vitro. *Radiology* 1989;170:185–189.

Ferrucci JT. Biliary lithotripsy: What will the issues be? *AJR* 1987;149:227–231.

Gacetta DJ, Cohen MJ, Crummy AB, Joseph DB, Kuglitsch M, Mack E. Ultrasonic lithotripsy of gallstones after cholecystostomy. *AJR* 1984;143:1088–1889.

Gadacz TR. The effect of monoctanoin on retained common duct stones. *Surgery* 1981;89:527–531.

Kerlan RK, LaBerge JM, Ring EJ. Percutaneous cholecystolithotomy: Preliminary experience. *Radiology* 1985;157:653–656.

Martin EC, Getrajdman GI. Does the gallbladder have a future. *Radiology* 1989;170:969–973.

McGahan JP, Walter JP. Diagnostic percutaneous aspiration of the gallbladder. *Radiology* 1985;155:619–622.

Meyer KA, Capos NJ, Mittelpunkt AI. Personal experience with 1261 cases of acute and chronic cholecystitis and cholelithiasis. *Surgery* 1967;61:661–668.

Miller FJ, Kensey KR, Nash JE. Experimental percutaneous gallstones lithotripsy: Results in swine. *Radiology* 1989;170:985–987.

Morrow DJ, Thompson J, Wilson SE. Acute cholecystitis in the elderly. *Arch Surg* 1978;113:149–152.

Pearse DM, Hawkins IF, Shaver R, Vogel S. Percutaneous cholecystostomy in acute cholecystitis and common duct obstruction. *Radiology* 1984;152:365–367.

Picus D, Weyman PJ, Marx MV. Role of percutaneous intracorporeal electrohydraulic lithotripsy in the treatment of biliary tract calculi. *Radiology* 1989;170:989–993.

Pitt HA, McFadden DW, Gadacz TR. Agents for gallstone dissolution. *Am J Surg* 1987;153:233–246.

Sauerbruch T, Delius M, Paumgartner G, Holl J, Wess O, Weber W, Hepp W, Brendel W. Fragmentation of gallstones by extracorporeal shock waves. *N Eng J Med* 1986;314:818–822.

Simeone JF, Mueller PR, Ferrucci JT. Nonsurgical therapy of gallstones: Implications for imaging. *AJR* 1989;152:11–17.

Stokes KR, Falchuk KR, Clouse ME. Biliary duct stones: Update on 54 cases after percutaneous transhepatic removal. *Radiology* 1989;170:999–1001.

Thistle JL. Direct contact dissolution of gallstones. *Semin Liver Dis* 1987;7:311–316.

Thistle JL, Nelson PE, May GR. Dissolution of cholesterol gallbladder stones (CGS) using MTBE. *Gastroenterology* 1986;90:1775.

Van Sonnenberg E, Casola G, Zakko SF, Varney RR, Cox J, Wittich GR, Hoffmann AF. Gallbladder and bile duct stones: Percutaneous therapy with primary MTBE dissolution and mechanical methods. *Radiology* 1988;169:505–509.

Van Sonnenberg E, Hofmann AF. Horizons in gallstone therapy—1988. *AJR* 1988;150:43–46.

Van Sonnenberg E, Hofmann AF, Neoptolemus J, Wittich GR, Princenthal RA, Wilson SW. Gallstone dissolution with methyl-tert-butyl ether via percutaneous cholecystostomy: Success and caveats. *AJR* 1986;146:865–867.

Van Sonnenberg E, Wing VW, Pollgard JW, Casola G. Life threatening vagal reactions associated with percutaneous cholecystostomy. *Radiology* 1984;151:377–380.

Van Sonnenberg E, Wittich GR, Casola G, Princenthal RA, Hoffmann AF, Keightley A, Wing VW. Diagnostic and therapeutic percutaneous gallbladder procedures. *Radiology* 1986;160:23–26.

Wholey MH, Smoot S. Choledocholithiasis: Percutaneous pulverization with a high speed rotational catheter. *AJR* 1988;150:129–130.

Williams HJ. Percutaneous dissolution of gallstones. *Radiology* 1989;170:1105.

Chapter Six

Angioplasty

Introduction

RENAN UFLACKER

Percutaneous transluminal treatment of atherosclerotic lesions with catheters was first introduced in 1964 by Dotter. A coaxial system was used in which a No. 8 French catheter, introduced by guidewire, was used to recanalize the lesion while a No. 12 French catheter was advanced through the lesion to dilate it (Fig. 6.1A). In 1968, Staple modified the approach to percutaneous vascular dilatation by using catheters with diameters varying between No. 7 and No. 12 French, with progressively tapered tips adjusted to a 0.038-in. guidewire. Instruments of this type are known as van Andel catheters (Fig. 6.1B).

The latex balloon catherers used in the 1960s for dilatation of vessels in cases of stenosis were deformed by elongation toward areas of least resistance, resulting in insufficient dilation of narrow areas. Portsmann tried to correct this deficiency by designing a catheter with a balloon inside a "cage" that prevented its deformation, and this type of balloon catheter was first used clinically in the early 1970s.

Gruntzig's work led to the development, in 1974, of double-lumen balloon catheters, made of polyvinyl chloride (PVC), which were designed not to expand beyond predetermined sizes (their diameters ranged from 3 to 9 mm). Because of the deficiencies of PVC (a tendency to expand beyond the predetermined limit and to rupture at pressures over 6 atm), PVC was replaced in 1979 by reinforced polyethylene that is resistant to pressures up to 17 atm (Fig. 6.2). Gruntzig catheters utilizing polyethylene balloons have made possible a revolution in radiologic dilatation procedures and are partially responsible for the increasing popularity of percutaneous techniques for treating vascular lesions.

INDICATIONS AND CONTRAINDICATIONS

Dilatation of arterial stenoses and occlusions through transluminal angioplasty is an alternative to prolonged and costly vascular surgical procedures. Although surgery remains the primary treatment for most patients, the applications of percutaneous angioplasty are increasing rapidly as technology advances and experience grows.

Percutaneous angioplasty can be curative in cases of both stenotic and totally occluded vessels. There are limitations to the use of angioplasty with totally occlusive lesions, although in some of these cases angioplasty may be the definitive treatment.

One major limitation to the use of percutaneous angioplasty involves cases in which the occlusions are longer than 10 to 20 cm (in leg arteries), where it is frequently impossible to pass through the lesion and dilate it properly. Another is the absence of a vascular stump, which may occur in the aorta when there is renal

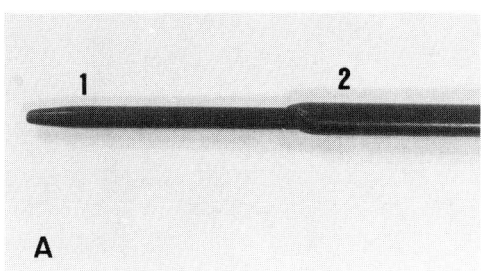
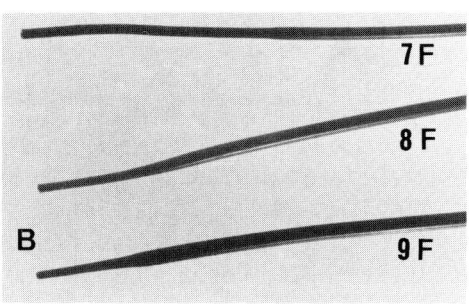

Figure 6.1 (A) Dotter's coaxial system: 1, internal No. 8 French catheter; 2, No. 12 French catheter. Both catheters are Teflon. (B) No. 7, 8, and 9 French Van Andel catheters. Note the progressively tapered tips—5, 3, and 2 cm, respectively.

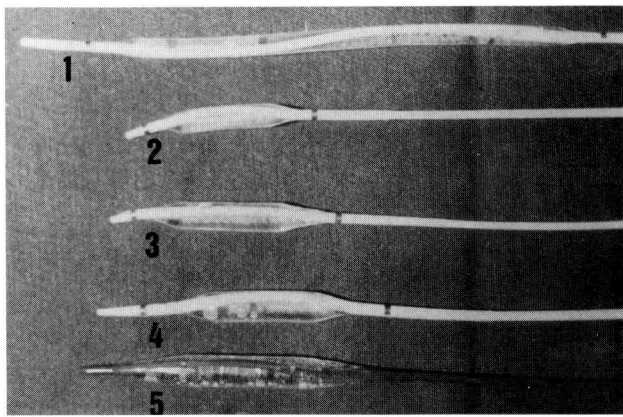

Figure 6.2 Several examples of Gruntzig balloon catheters.
1, No. 7 French Sos balloon catheter, 5 mm in diameter and 10 cm long, used for superficial femoral angioplasty; 2, No. 7 French balloon catheter, 5 mm in diameter and 3 cm long; 3, No. 7 French short-tip renal-type balloon catheter, 6 mm in diameter and 4 cm long; 4, long-tip No. 8 French balloon catheter, 8 mm in diameter and 4 cm long; 5, balloon catheter, 8 mm in diameter and 4 cm long.

artery occlusion or at the origin of the superficial femoral artery at the bifurcation of the common femoral artery or at the origin of the iliac artery at the aortic bifurcation. In these situations, the conventional guidewire cannot be introduced inside the occluded vessels.

The first uses of transluminal angioplasty were in cases involving the lower limb and renal arteries. Applications of the technique were later extended to include the splanchnic arteries (mesenteric, celiac axis), the hypogastric arteries, the abdominal aorta, and the brachiocephalic axis both at its origin and distally. In the venous system, it was used in the vena cava and in subclavian veins, and in arteriovenous fistulas for hemodialysis.

Advances in technology have made possible the use of transluminal angioplasty in vessels supplying functionally critical organs such as the heart and brain. Coronary angioplasty is routinely performed today, and the use of angioplasty for carotid and vertebral arteries is growing.

Applications in the area of congenital cardiopathy, for example, life-saving pulmonary valvuloplasty in neonates and aortic or mitral valvuloplasty in cases of adult stenosis, are growing in popularity. Peripheral pulmonary stenosis is also adequately treated by angioplasty, especially when followed by intravascular stenting. Angioplasty of aortic coarctation is still controversial, due to the risk of rupture. Blalock-Taussig type "shunts" used for treating patients with tetralogy of Fallot may stenose at the anastomosis, causing damage, and these stenoses may also be dilated through the percutaneous route.

Transluminal angioplasty may be used for correcting anastomotic stenosis of arterial grafts in certain areas. In such cases fibrinolysis with streptokinase or urokinase can be used for recanalization of the graft before the dilatation is performed.

Transluminal angioplasty can also be used as a preoperative measure or as a complement to surgery, especially with elderly patients, or those whose health has been affected by multiple organ failure and who will not be able to tolerate extensive vascular reconstructive procedures.

Percutaneous transluminal angioplasty of one or both of the iliac arteries, in cases of stenosis or occlusion, may be used in place of abdominal surgery for insertion of aortoiliac or aortofemoral grafts. This procedure may be accompanied by a femoropopliteal graft performed under peridural anesthesia, thus avoiding the potential trauma of more extensive surgery. Patency of a femoropopliteal graft is often made viable by percutaneous dilatation of an isolated stenosis of the iliac artery. Another angiographic procedure that can be used presurgically is dilatation of a popliteal artery or the tibiofibular axis through a femoropopliteal graft, which makes long-term patency feasible.

Percutaneous angioplasty is definitely indicated in limb salvage procedures for recanalization of the femoral and popliteal arteries in patients who are candidates for amputation due to severe ischemic lesions. Whenever amputation may be necessary, some type of angioplasty should always be considered. In cases in which the limb cannot be saved, it may be possible to reduce the extent of amputation. The future in limb-salvage procedures probably belongs to new, aggressive techniques utilizing laser-beam technology, reperfusion devices, and thrombolytic therapy.

It is important for the interventional radiologist to become acquainted with all aspects of occlusive disease—both clinical and surgical—in order to recommend the best procedure in a given case. One approach is to evaluate the patient in terms of Fontaine's classification of occlusive diseases. In this system patients are assigned to one of four different groups, or stages, according to the severity of symptoms.

Stage I: No symptoms, or atypical symptoms, and normal skin perfusion. (Significant occlusions may be present, but these are supplied by adequate collateral circulation through the deep femoral artery.)

Stage II: Intermittent claudication. Muscle flow is normal during rest, but decreases during exercise. Symptoms are typically fatigue followed by cramps and pain, forcing the patient to stop walking. It is necessary to differentiate symptoms caused by arterial occlusion from symptoms caused by deep venous thrombosis, discopathies, or other foot abnormalities.

Stage III: Pain at rest, particularly in the foot, requiring strong analgesia. Pain becomes more acute during the night due to a reduction in hydrostatic pressure. Marblelike paleness and rigidity are present.

Stage IV: Gangrene. Ulcerating lesions due to trauma or superimposed infection are present. Pain is severe, even at rest, with absence of pulses. Diseases involving small vessels, e.g., diabetes mellitus, are frequent at this stage.

Indications for angioplasty of lower limb arteries in patients in one of the above stages are as follows:

Stage I: These patients do not usually require surgical treatment or angioplasty. Some of them, however, may present with severe stenoses that could easily develop into total occlusions. Dilating stenoses of this type may prevent evolution of the disease to a more advanced stage. This applies particularly to the femoropopliteal region, where chances of occlusion and thrombosis are higher.

Stage II: Patients with intermittent claudication that prevents normal daily or professional activities should be offered some form of treatment. For localized stenoses or segmental occlusions up to 10 cm, percutaneous angioplasty offers excellent chances of success. When the stenosis or occlusion is located at the iliac artery level, angioplasty is always the first choice, particularly with elderly patients or those at high surgical risk.

Stages III and IV: Any recanalization achieved in patients in either of these stages will afford some improvement, even if only incomplete or temporary. When either surgery or angioplasty is a viable option, percutaneous angioplasty should be proposed as a priority. In these cases, it may be useful to combine fibrinolysis, for resolving recent thromboses, and angioplasty, for treating the cause of arterial thrombosis.

TECHNIQUES, MATERIALS, AND HEMODYNAMICS

Basic Techniques of Angioplasty

Balloon catheters for angioplasty should be introduced by percutaneous puncture, according to the Seldinger technique. When the femoral approach is to be used to dilate the aorta or the iliac, renal, mesenteric, or brachiocephalic arteries, the puncture should be retrograde and made at the level of the inguinal fold (Fig. 6.3). When the femoral approach is used for dilating the arteries in the lower limbs, the puncture should be antegrade, and made at a level just below the inguinal ligament, so that a longer arterial segment will be available for manipulation and selection of the superficial or deep femoral artery (Fig. 6.3). When necessary the superficial femoral artery can be punctured directly.

The best known maneuvers used in catheterizing the

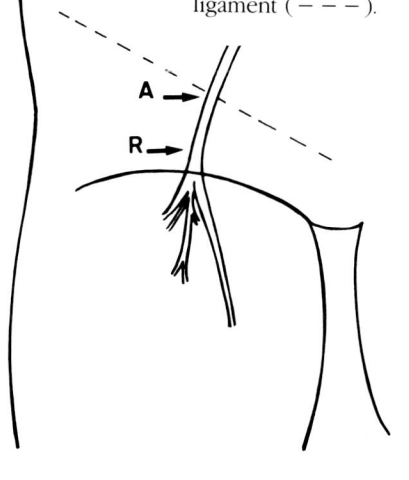

Figure 6.3 Schematic drawing of puncture sites. A, antegrade puncture; R, retrograde puncture. Note the relationship of the puncture to the inguinal fold ($-$) and ligament ($- - -$).

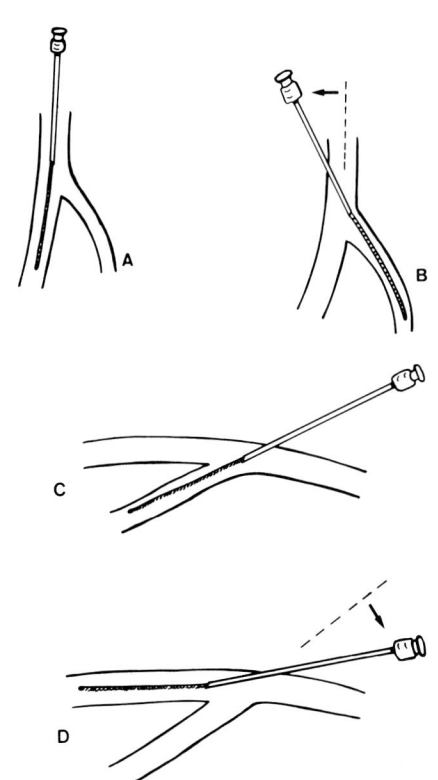

Figure 6.4 Maneuvers used for facilitating entry to superficial femoral artery during antegrade puncture. (A,B) Frontal views in which the needle has been inclined laterally. (C,D) Horizontal inclination of the needle.

superficial femoral artery during antegrade puncture of the common femoral artery are lateral inclination and horizontalization of the needle during introduction of the guidewire (Fig. 6.4).

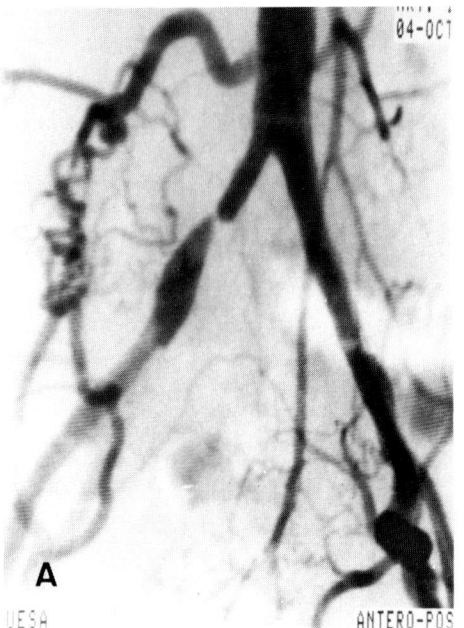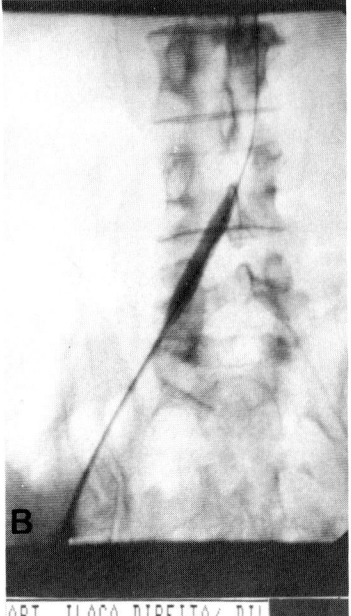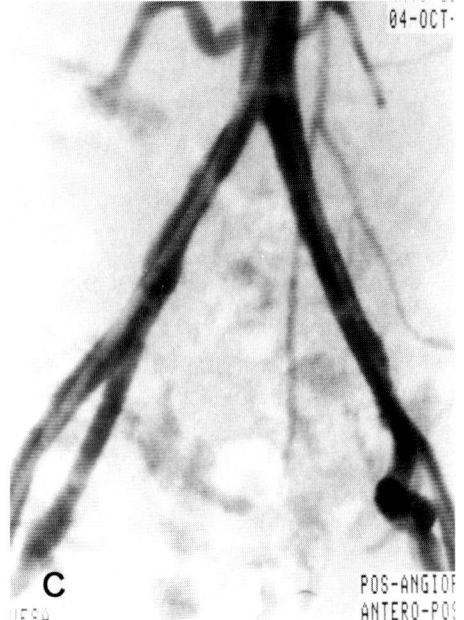

Figure 6.5 (A) Digital angiogram showing a focal stenosis in the right common iliac artery in a 59-year-old patient with 200-m claudication. Note the collateral circulation through the last lumber artery. (B) 8-mm balloon introduced through the ipsilateral artery, dilating the stenosis. (C) Control following dilatation shows that both stenosis and collateral circulation have disappeared using contralateral catheterization for the aortic injection. Systemic pressure before the procedure was 120 mmHg. Predilatation tibial pressure was 70 mmHg; postdilatation tibial pressure, 95 mmHg. The claudication disappeared.

The angioplastic approach, then, may be through the ipsilateral artery, in either the cranial (Fig. 6.5) or caudal direction (Fig. 6.6), or, for iliac and femoral lesions, through the contralateral artery (Fig. 6.7). In the latter case, contralateral catheterization maneuvers are often necessary (see Fig. 6.5, and Chap. 1). The contralateral puncture technique is useful to treat totally occluded iliac and common femoral arteries, with nonpalpable pulse (Fig. 6.8), and in high superficial femoral artery lesions (Fig. 6.9).

When there are no femoral pulses, or when going beyond the lesion with the help of the systems available for the femoral approach is not possible, the axillary route is useful not only for iliac, but also for aortic, renal, or mesenteric, lesions. Using the axillary route preserves the catheter's longitudinal force, making manipulation easier.

When either the contralateral or the axillary approach is used, it is not necessary to perform arterial compression of the treated vessel after the procedure, thus reducing the risk of immediate thrombosis. Contralateral puncture makes possible the simultaneous treatment of stenotic lesions of iliac and femoral arteries on the same side.

The greatest disadvantage of the contralateral puncture is the reduction in linear force that must be applied to the catheter in order to cross the stenosis. The success of any approach maneuver, of course, depends on the tortuosity of the iliac arteries and on the angle of aortic bifurcation. (See Fig. 1.27.) Major difficulties may be encountered in attempting to go beyond the stenosis in vessels to be dilated. Eccentric stenoses are particularly difficult, because it is not possible to advance the guidewire or the catheter beyond them without manipulation techniques appropriate to the situation. For example, when a bent-tip large-radius (7.5-mm) guidewire is advanced, its extremity may stick to the atheromatous plaque (Fig. 6.10). If the guidewire is forced, it may move in the wrong direction, risking intimal dissection and plaque displacement. The correct way to pass beyond the stenosis is to redirect the guidewire by rotating it and advancing it in the appropriate direction (Fig. 6.10). Before performing these maneuvers, arteriography should be carried out. Steerable guidewires have largely replaced those earlier techniques and have greatly increased the chances of success of the catheterization procedure.

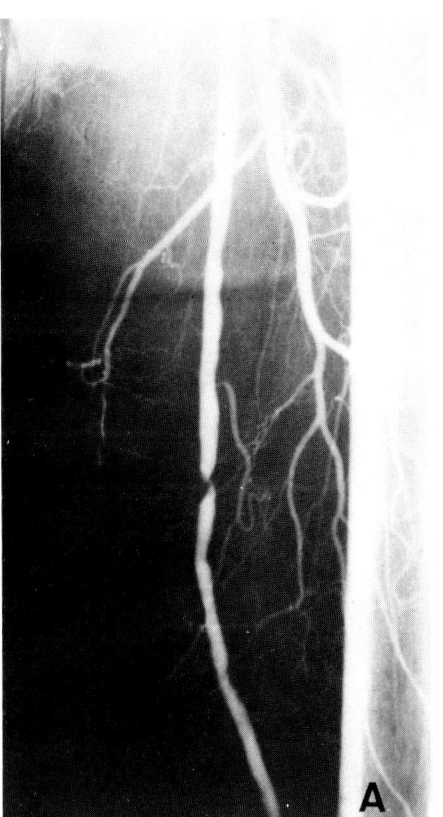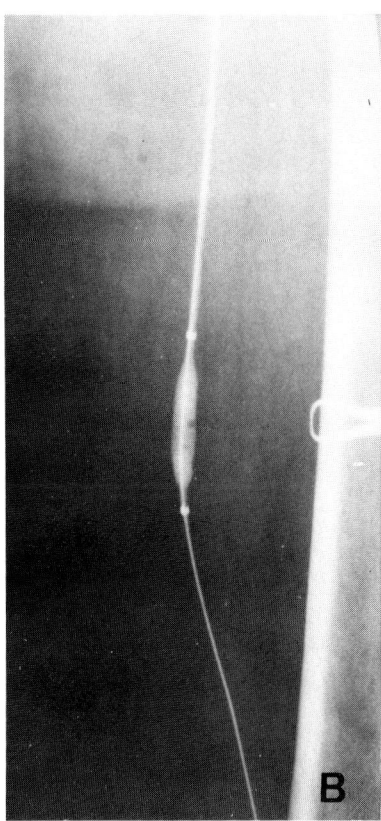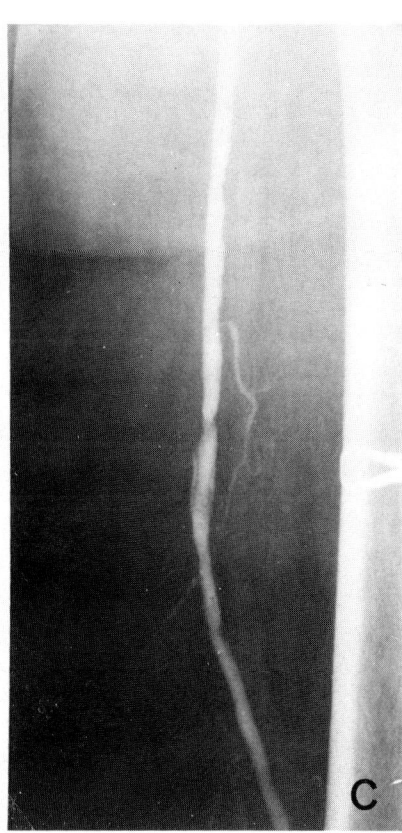

Figure 6.6 (A) Diabetic 69-year-old patient with claudication in the left lower limb and critical stenosis in the middle third of the left superficial femoral artery. (B) Dilatation with 5-mm balloon, using the antegrade approach with caudally oriented catheterization. (C) Control after angioplasty shows patency. There was good evolution, with improvement of symptoms.

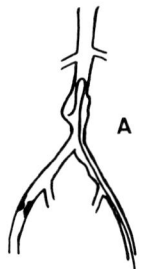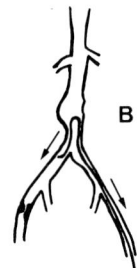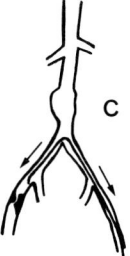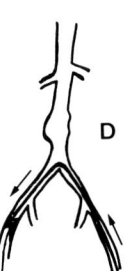

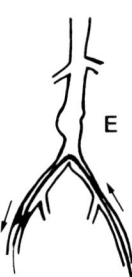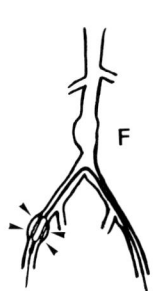

Figure 6.7 Contralateral approach.
(A–F) Schematic drawing showing contralateral puncture by the antegrade route for dilating stenosis of the iliac artery. A Simmons catheter was used.

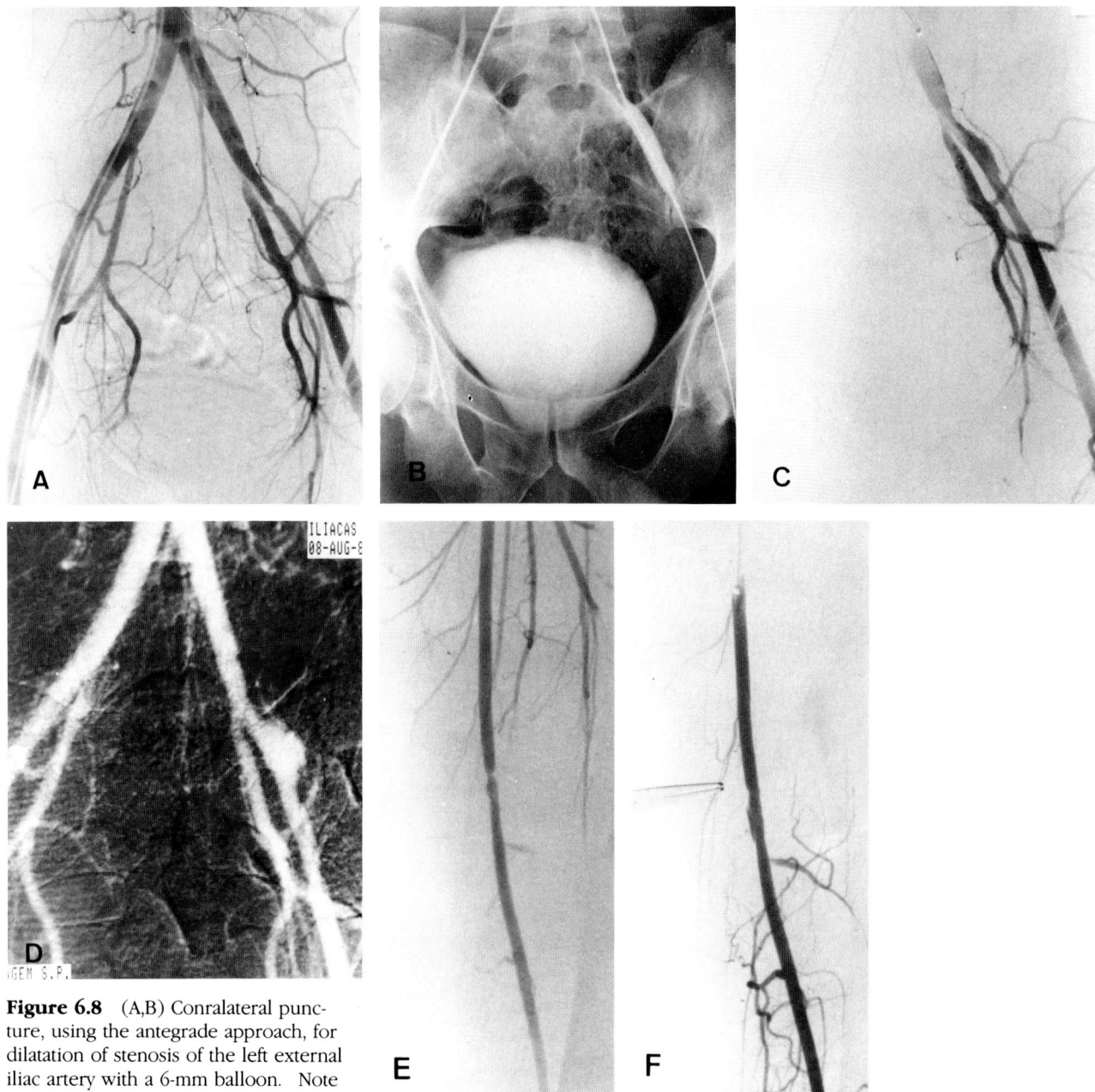

Figure 6.8 (A,B) Conralateral puncture, using the antegrade approach, for dilatation of stenosis of the left external iliac artery with a 6-mm balloon. Note the deformation of the balloon. (C) Control after dilatation shows good results. (D) Later-follow-up (6 months) venous digital control angiogram shows an aneurysmatic image on the site of stenosis. The patient is asymptomatic. (E,F) After changing the balloon, the same antegrade contralateral approach was used for dilating an isolated lesion in the left superficial femoral artery.

One way to advance beyond a complex eccentric stenosis is to use a 150° curved catheter, which allows simultaneous manipulation and contrast injection. Once the orifice of the passage has been identified by small contrast injections, the guidewire is introduced (Fig. 6.11). Although this technique is often less traumatic than blind introduction of a straight guidewire, the contrast injections may cause intimal dissection.

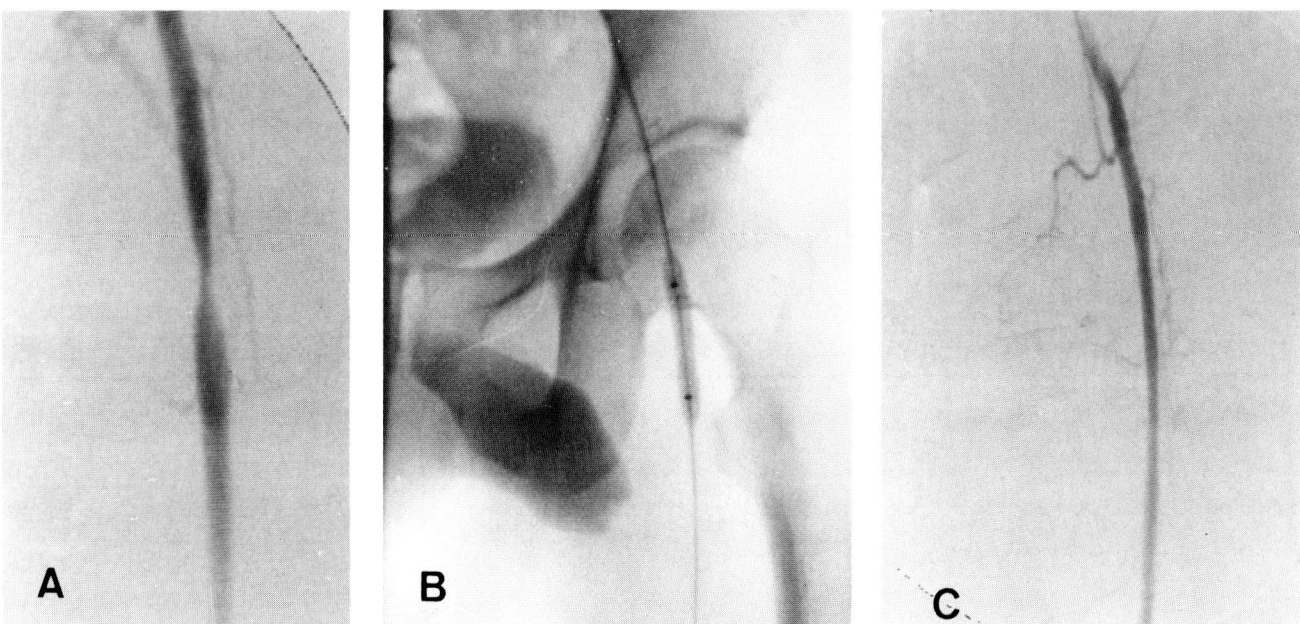

Figure 6.9 (A) 20-m claudication in 28-year-old patient with thromboangiitis obliterans, with occlusion of the deep femoral artery and proximal stenosis of the superficial femoral artery. (B) Adequate indication for using an antegrade contralateral approach, with a 6-mm balloon. (C) Control immediately after dilatation showing excellent results. Clinical control 6 months later showed normal tibial pressure and absence of symptoms.

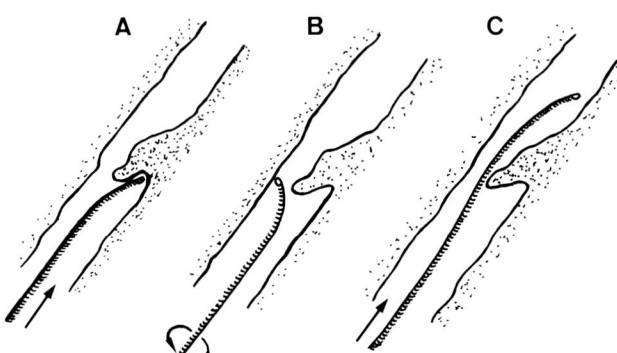

Figure 6.10 **Redirectioning a guidewire. The schematic drawings show how to advance beyond an eccentric arterial stenosis by rotating and redirectioning the guidewire.**
(A) The guidewire, which has an open, curved tip, is stuck at the site of the atheromatous plaque. (B) Rotation has freed the guidewire. (C) After the orifice has been found, the guidewire is advanced. *(Modified from Ring EJ, McLean GK, Interventional Radiology: Principles and Techniques, Boston, Little, Brown, 1981.)*

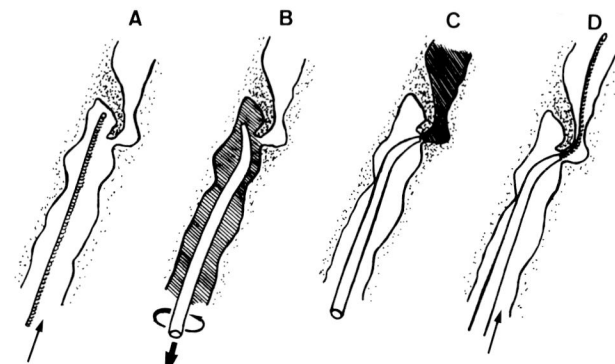

Figure 6.11 **Technique for advancing beyond an eccentric stenosis by using a catheter with an angulated tip (150°).**
(A) The plaque has stopped the advancement of the straight guidewire. (B) Contrast-medium injection with a curved-tip catheter shows the anatomy of the obstruction and the orifice. (C) The catheter is redirectioned through the orifice and a test injection is performed. (D) The guidewire is advanced beyond the stenoses. *(Modified from Ring EJ, McLean GK, Interventional Radiology: Principles and Techniques, Boston, Little, Brown, 1981.)*

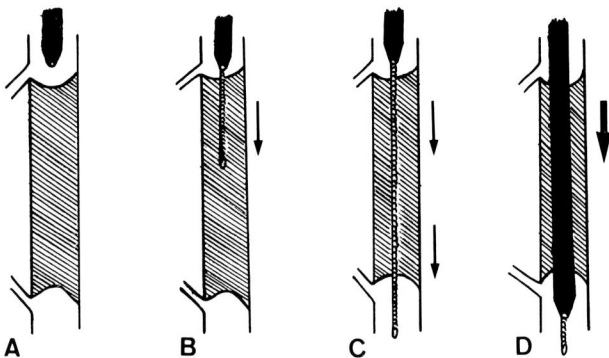

Figure 6.12 Schematic drawing showing how to cross a total occlusion.
(A) The occlusion usually extends from the point of origin of a collateral to the entry point of a collateral. (B,C) The catheter is wedged into the occlusion and the guidewire advanced until it enters the distal recanalized portion.
(D) The catheter is pushed over the guidewire through the occlusion.

It is usually possible to cross total concentric occlusions by a simple maneuver in which a straight catheter is advanced near the occlusion's proximal portion, usually beside the origin of a collateral vessel, and a wedged contrast injection is then performed. It is often possible to outline the virtual lumen inside the occlusion by cavitation with the contrast. A steerable guidewire is then introduced and advanced to the distal arterial lumen, which has been marked on the basis of angiographic studies. The guidewire usually meets some resistance inside the occlusion, due to friction, but this diminishes as soon as the lumen of the recanalized vessel is reached distally. When test injections have demonstrated that the guidewire is inside the lesion's true lumen and that there has been no plaque detachment, the guide catheter (No. 5 or 6 French) is advanced through the occlusion for initial dilatation (Fig. 6.12). Once the catheter has reached the recanalized lumen distally, the guidewire is removed and heparin (5000 IU) is injected. The next step is to replace the guidewire by a more heavy-duty type, and then exchange the No. 5 or 6 French catheter for an angioplasty catheter of the correct size. If resistance is encountered, it may be necessary to introduce one or more van Andel catheters of progressively larger diameters (Nos. 6, 7, 8, and 9 French) before advancing the balloon, in order to adequately dilate the lesion (Fig. 6.13).

Choosing the Axillary or Femoral Approach

The femoral approach, whether antegrade, or retrograde, is successful in the vast majority of cases. However, when there is severe atheromatous disease present in iliac arteries and the infrarenal aorta; when there is an aortoiliac graft; or when the abdominal arteries arise from the aorta in narrow caudal angles, the axillary approach may be used. When the guidewire is in place through the stenosis, the dilatation catheter has a natural tendency to follow the smooth curve formed on the extremity of the guidewire, and will pass through the lesion.

Theoretically, the axillary approach involves a higher risk of arterial lesion at the puncture site, due to the smaller diameter of the axillary artery. However, this risk may be minimized by totally deflating the balloon and wrapping it around the catheter shaft, in association with very gentle manipulation and rotation during introduction and withdrawal of the catheter. There is also the risk of injury to the brachial nervous plexus. Because compression is more effective in the axillary region, the formation of hematomas or pseudoaneurysms in this area seems to be less frequent than in the femoral region. In patients with severe, long-standing hypertension, and in older patients, in whom the aortic arch is elongated and the angle of the left subclavian artery has become more acute, the axillary approach is problematic because of the difficulty of achieving the linear force necessary for proper manipulation of the catheter and penetration through the occlusive lesion.

Dilatation Balloons

Many different balloon catheters are available (Fig. 6.2). Dilatation balloons may be inflated and deflated manually, using disposable syringes with rubber plungers (for visceral or limb angioplasty), or mechanically, with pneumatic guns (for coronary angioplasty). The use of 10-mL syringes is recommended. The use of 3- to 5-mL syringes may generate pressures up to 21 atm, well above the resistance limits of most balloons.

Different authors recommend different inflation times, but 1 to 3 min is common and the prolonged inflation times are becoming more favored. These time periods are short enough not to involve the risk of an ischemic episode or thrombosis, particularly in heparinized patients.

Screw syringes (developed by LeVeen) have recently become available. The screw plunger allows the physician to inflate the balloon, and keep it inflated without additional effort. Because of the risk of rupture, however, a manometer should be used to monitor inflation pressure. (See Figs. 6.14 and 6.15.)

The target lesion should always be located by contrast injection immediately before the procedure is initiated, since it may have progressed since the last diagnostic procedure. The proximal and distal ends of the lesion are marked with metallic clamps or a radiopaque ruler

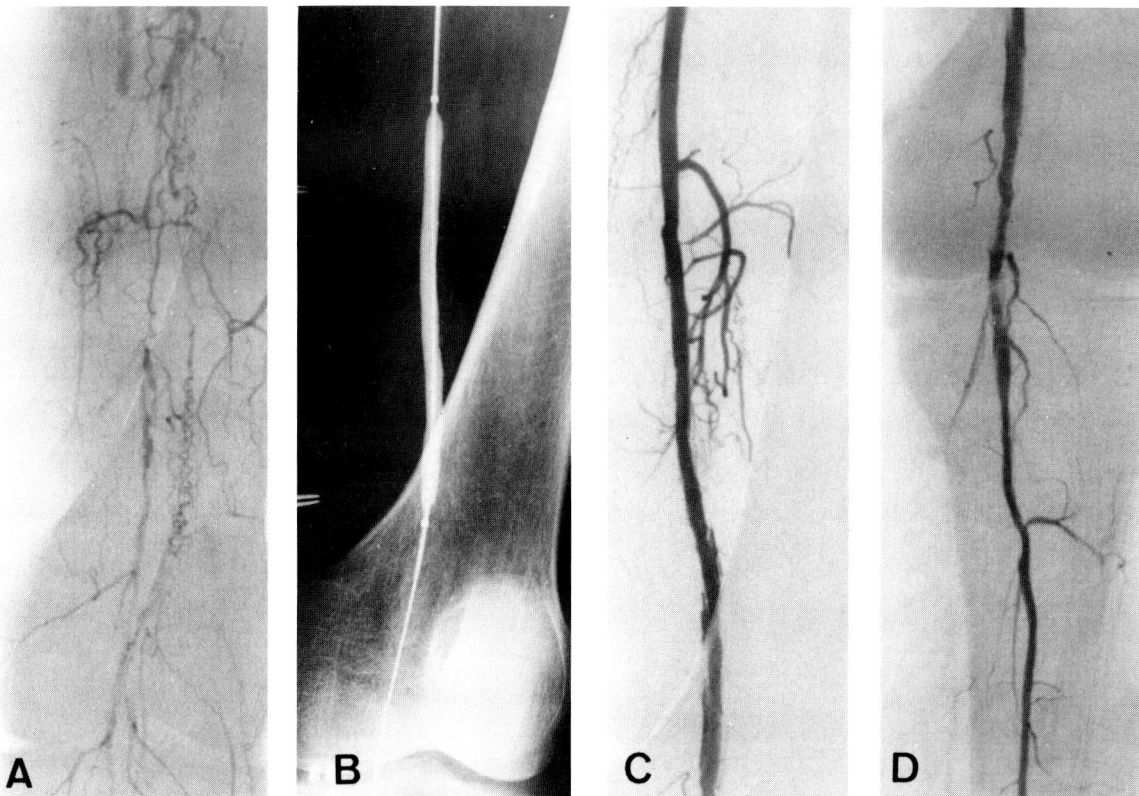

Figure 6.13 (A) Patient with 15-m claudication. Severe occlusive disease of the superficial femoral and popliteal arteries is present. (B) Before passing the 10-cm by 5-mm balloons, it was necessary to recanalize with a No. 8 French Van Andel catheter up to the popliteal and tibiofibular axis. (C) Control taken after recanalization and dilatation of the superficial femoral artery. (D) View of the popliteal and tibiofibular axis following angioplasty. The patient was asymptomatic, and able to walk 3 km.

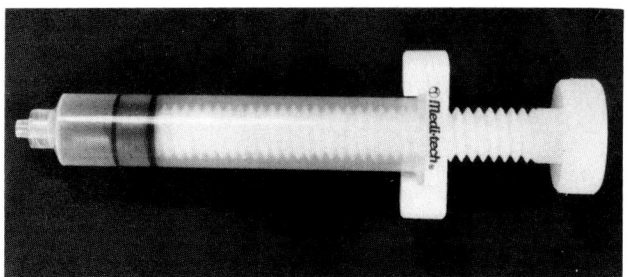

Figure 6.14 A LeVeen syringe allows the technician to keep the balloon inflated without additional effort. Use of a pressure manometer is required, as the risk of balloon rupture exists.

over sterile fields. A digital subtraction angiographic "road map" is quite useful.

When the occlusion is short, the balloon is positioned in the middle of the lesion and dilated twice for 30 s under the recommended pressure limits. If adequate dilatation is not obtained, and an hourglass stricture persists at the site of stenosis, the balloon may be replaced by a high-pressure one. The shape of the balloon is monitored fluoroscopically; an overinflated balloon tends to deform, assuming an oval shape when rupture is imminent.

For long occlusions or stenoses, dilatation begins with the lesions most distal to the puncture site. Dilatation is repeated, with the balloon positioned more proximally each time, until the entire extension has been treated. Long, 8- to 10-cm, balloons are useful for dilating long lesions, obviating displacement and repeated dilatation of the various segments within the lesion. It is not usually necessary to reverse the heparin dose (5000 IU) applied just after going beyond the obstruction because chances of hematoma formation on the puncture site are minimal once the procedure is completed.

Control angiography performed after dilatation should demonstrate any existing residual stenosis or thrombus inside the dilated or recanalized lesion. The catheter is

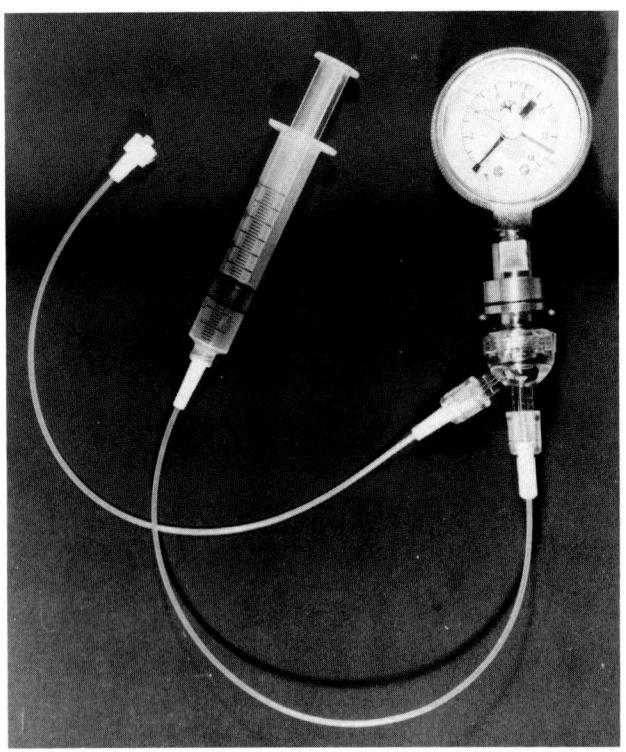

Figure 6.15 A manometer. The syringe is connected to the lower tube, and the balloon catheter is connected to the lateral port.

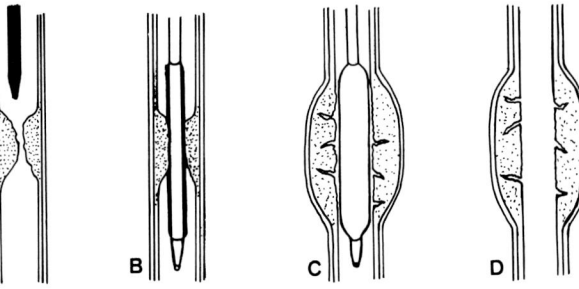

Figure 6.16 Angioplasty.
(A) Approach to the lesion. (B) Advancing beyond the stenosis with the balloon deflated and wrapped around the catheter. (C) Balloon expansion causes dilatation of all elements of the vascular wall, including the adventitia, accompanied by intimal laceration and fracture, primarily longitudinal, of plaque. Laceration and stretching of the medial layer are also present. (D) Postdilatation aspect showing vascular lumen no longer obstructive. Intimal regeneration, with smoothing of the inner surface, has begun.

removed with the balloon deflated while negative pressure is applied to it through a syringe. The puncture site should be compressed for a longer period than is usually necessary in diagnostic angiography, both because the orifice on the vascular wall is larger and because anticoagulants have been used.

In selecting balloon diameter one should take into consideration the fact that conventional angiographic measurement of normal and stenotic arterial diameter results in a 15 to 25 percent distortion due to magnification effects. Thus if one selects an 8-mm balloon for an 8-mm artery the balloon will be about 1 mm larger than the actual diameter of the artery.

THE MECHANISM OF ANGIOPLASTY

Much controversy has been generated over the question of how angioplasty achieves its results. It was initially postulated that enlargement of the vessel lumen was due to compression of atheromatous plaque. Animal studies and human necropsies have shown the presence of endothelial desquamation and fractures of atheromata.

Pathologic studies in humans previously submitted to angioplasty have revealed that there is intimal laceration, longitudinal and tranverse plaque fractures, and stretching or rupture of the medial layer that results in stretching of all elements of the vascular wall, including the most external layer of the adventitia, with an increase in total diameter (Fig. 6.16). Plaque redistribution also occurs to a certain extent, but microscopic studies have failed to reveal any demonstrable compression. It is possible that under compression the plaque becomes partially dehydrated, releasing its fluid content into blood circulation.

The exposure of connective tissue to circulating blood causes platelet deposition and the formation of fibrin mural thrombi.

The linear extravascular images seen in dilated atheromatous plaques are either fractures filled with contrast or spaces filled with atheromatous plaque that has been detached from the vascular wall (Fig. 6.17). Intimal endothelialization will cover the fractured plaque, resulting in healing and smoothing of the plaque surface, keeping the new, enlarged lumen diameter. Angiographic studies a few weeks after angioplasty show regular, smooth vascular surfaces (Fig. 6.18).

Platelet deposition and thrombi formation in injured vessels are inversely proportional to flow around the lesion. It is therefore advisable to maximize flow at the dilatation site, using nonocclusive compression at the puncture site, and to administer vasodilators immediately after the procedure. Aspirin at doses varying from 150 to 300 mg per day is currently being administered, but one pediatric aspirin (150 mg) per day (for a minimum period of 3 months) is usually sufficient. The simultaneous use of Persantin, 75 mg t.i.d., potentiates the antiplatelet action of aspirin significantly.

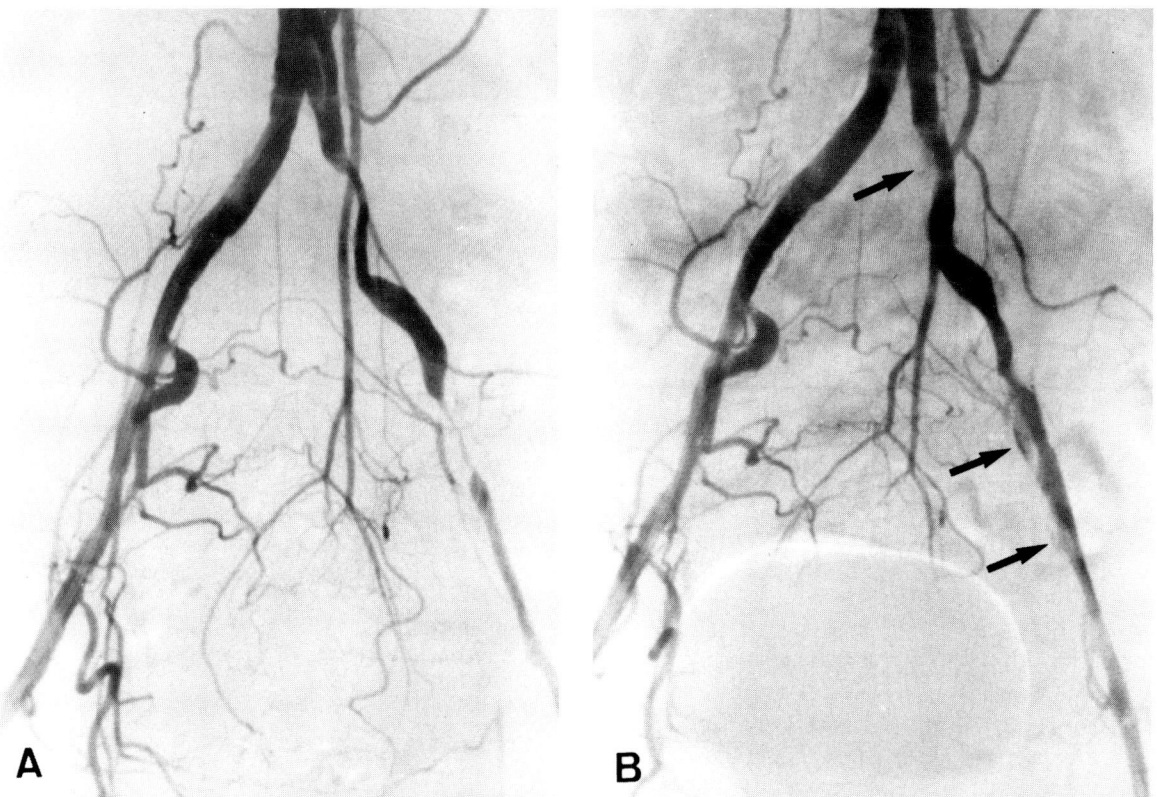

Figure 6.17 Angiogram of left iliac artery with severe lesions, showing contrast-filled longitudinal fractures on the site of stenoses (arrows). The plaque may have been separated from the wall.
(A) Predilatation angiogram. (B) Angiogram after dilatation with an 8-mm balloon. Preangioplasty claudication was 20 m; after angioplasty, it was over 600 m. There was also total occlusion of the superficial femoral arteries.

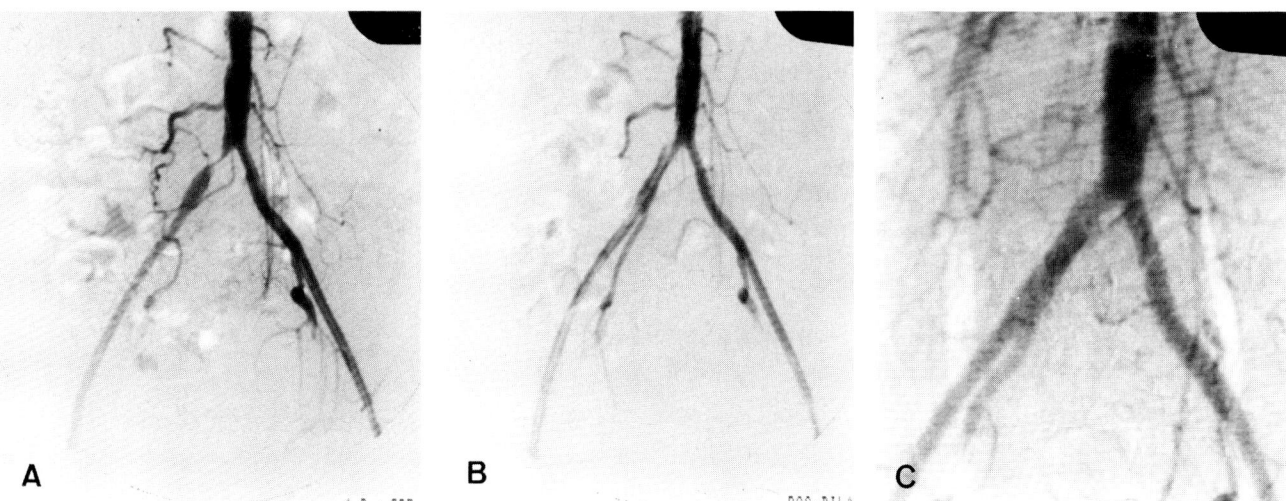

Figure 6.18 (A) 49-year-old patient with severe stenosis of the right common iliac artery caused by atheromatous plaque. (B) Control following dilatation with 8-mm balloon showing patency of the artery and irregularities of outline. (C) Intravenous digital control angiogram after 1 month showing recovery of inner vascular surface. Systemic arterial pressure was 130 mmHg. Before dilatation, the right anterior tibial pressure was 90 mmHg and the right posterior tibial pressure was 100 mmHg. After dilatation, the right anterior tibial pressure was 120 mmHg and the right posterior tibial pressure was 140 mmHg. Systemic pressure was 130 mmHg before and after angioplasty.

Two different experiential criteria are used to determine the effectiveness of dilatation. The first is pain. When arterial dilatation is effective, it causes moderate, short-duration pain which disappears when the balloon is deflated. Acute or shooting pain may be an indication of arterial rupture. If rupture is suspected, it should be confirmed before the catheter is removed from the dilated artery, because the balloon itself may provide adequate hemostasis if it is reinflated inside the ruptured artery. The second is the shape of the balloon. When dilatation is complete, the "waist" formed by plaque on the balloon surface disappears.

TECHNIQUE FOR TRANSLUMINAL ANGIOPLASTY OF RENAL ARTERIES

Transluminal angioplasty of renal arteries should be performed in hypertensive patients when renin values in the renal veins identify the site of the lesion and when cure is a possibility. This procedure is also indicated in cases presenting significant stenosis (larger than 75 percent of the arterial diameter) or a systolic gradient through the lesion that is over 20 percent. Renal artery angioplasty may also be indicated in patients with renal artery stenosis associated with nephrosclerosis, as a possible way to improve flow and function. It may also be used as a therapeutic test for patients with idiopathic hypertension possibly aggravated by renal artery stenosis but in whom the renin assay is inconclusive.

The easiest approach for catheterization of the renal artery is through puncture of the ipsilateral femoral artery. In young patients with a caudally angulated renal artery, the axillary route is an alternative. Before beginning selective catheterization and the attempt to pass through the stenosis, it may be useful to measure the pressure in the aorta and the pressure proximal to the stenosis.

The ostium of the stenosed renal artery is catheterized with a No. 5 French catheter (Fig. 6.19). An attempt is made to pass through the lesion with a steerable, 0.035-

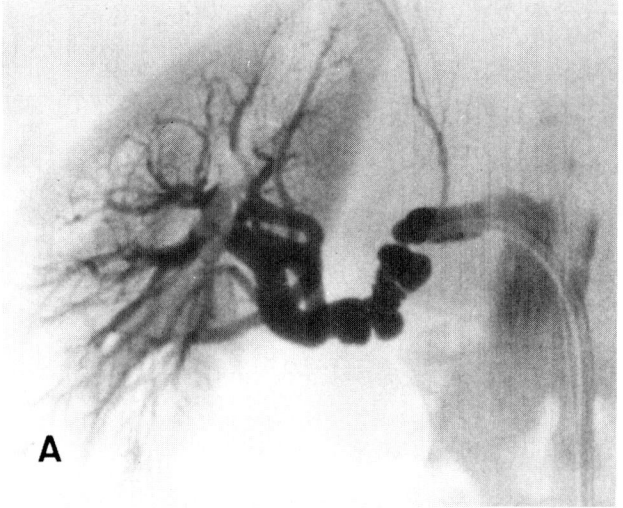

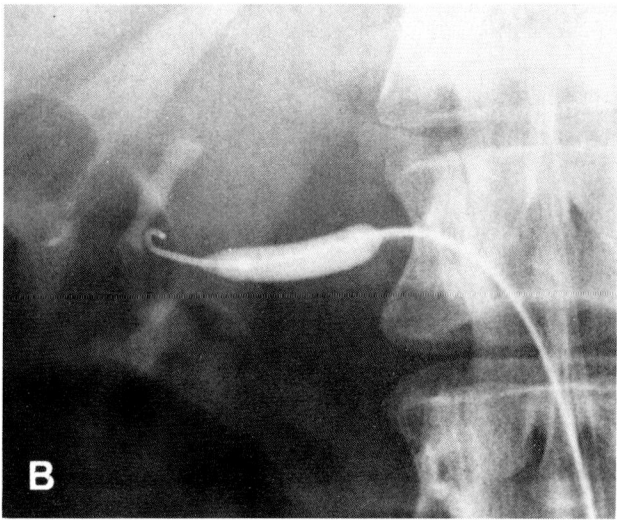

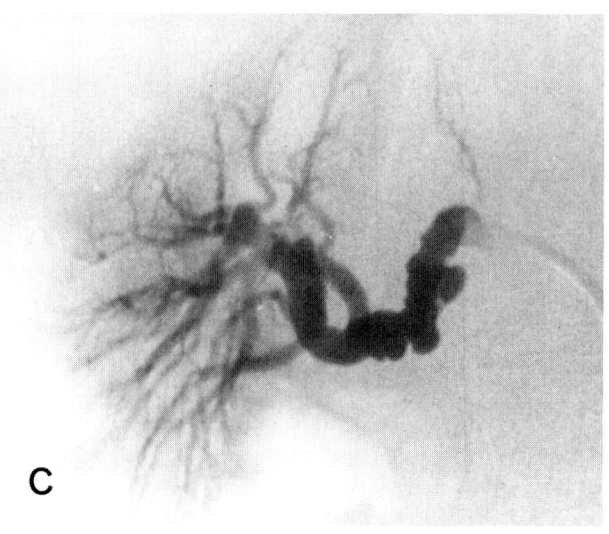

Figure 6.19 (A) Selective diagnostic injection of right renal artery in 45-year-old hypertensive patient with fibromuscular dysplasia and severe stenoses. (B) After the 6-mm balloon has been advanced beyond the lesion using a 1-mm-radius J-guidewire, the balloon is expanded. Note arterial stretching during balloon inflation. (C) Control following dilatation; the stenoses have disappeared while the aneurysmatic lesions remain. Predilatation arterial blood pressure was 190 × 100 mmHg. Postdilatation arterial blood pressure was 140 × 80 mmHg, which was maintained without medication.

or 0.038-in. guidewire. After the guidewire has been placed distally to the stenosis, the catheter is advanced. The guidewire is removed, and pressure is measured beyond the stenosis. A heavy-duty J-guidewire with a 1-mm radius is then introduced and advanced inside the renal circulation (Fig. 6.19). The diagnostic catheter is replaced by a balloon catheter having a diameter compatible with that of the artery, and dilatation is performed. Dilatation pressures must not exceed the safety limits specified for the balloon, and a manometer should always be used to keep track of pressure (Fig. 6.15). The diameter of the inflated balloon should not exceed that of the normal artery, both below and beyond the stenosis. The balloon should be approximately 1 cm longer than the stenotic lesion.

For fibromuscular dysplastic lesions a dilatation time of about 10 to 15 s is enough. For atheromatous lesions, a 1-min dilatation is generally sufficient. Immediately after dilatation has been completed, the balloon catheter is pulled closer to the ostium, with the guidewire being maintained through the lesion, and a control angiogram is taken by using a Y-adapter at the catheter hub. Some authors introduce a second catheter, through the contralateral femoral artery, for taking a control aortogram after catheterization. Although this technique involves a second puncture, it is extremely safe, and is a reliable way to assess the effectiveness of dilatation. When the dilated stenosis is located on the middle third of the renal artery, the dilatation catheter itself is occasionally used for control angiography after angioplasty (Fig. 6.19). However, this technique involves some risk, as it may cause occlusive injury when the injection dissects arterial intima that has already been lacerated by angioplasty. Whatever the technique, control should preferably be made by nonselective injection into the aortic lumen. Another way to pass beyond stenotic lesions is to use a 0.038-in. Sos (open-ended) guidewire, with a 0.018- or 0.021-in. directional-torque guidewire inside it which will eventually allow the catheter to be advanced through the stenosis.

When long segments of the aneurysmal form of fibromuscular dysplasia (medial fibroplasia) are present (Fig. 6.19), it may be difficult to advance the guidewire beyond the lesion. However, forced or prolonged manipulation may cause arterial perforation (Fig. 6.76) and spasm, and in these cases, a 1-mm-radius J-guidewire may be used, which will more easily pass beyond the multiple irregularities (Fig. 6.19). In cases of fibromuscular dysplasia and in caudally oriented arteries (Fig. 6.20), a Simmons-type catheter can be used. The catheter is reshaped in the thoracic aorta, and the caudally oriented tip of the Simmons catheter easily enters difficult arteries and stenoses. A Bentson-type guidewire, with an extremely flexible tip is carefully pushed beyond the stenosis or stenoses, and the catheter is pulled back, with its tip passing beyond the stenosis (Figs. 6.20 and 6.21).

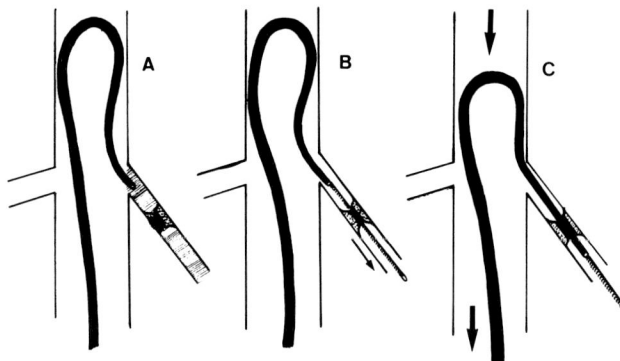

Figure 6.20 Use of the Simmons catheter to advance beyond a very tight or acutely angulated arterial stenosis.
(A) A selectively positioned catheter. (B) A Bentson guidewire passed beyond the lesion. (C) The catheter being pulled inside the aorta, its tip having passed beyond the stenosis.

In cases of renal artery occlusion, the techniques described above are used, although a standard curved catheter usually does not provide sufficient stability to allow the guidewire to pass through, and a Simmons catheter–flexible-tip guidewire set must be used. If that is not effective, a deflecting guidewire and a rigid Teflon catheter may succeed in passing through (see Fig. 6.22).

Figure 6.23 illustrates a successful case of recanalization of renal artery occlusion.

A significant problem in renal angioplasty is the presence of plaque in the arterial ostium, formed as part of the aortic wall atheromatous process. These lesions do not, as a rule, respond to dilatation. Although they often enlarge and break up as the balloon is being inflated, they resume their original position after deflation, and the stenosis remains unchanged (Fig. 6.24). In some cases, the lesions are not displaced even temporarily, and it is impossible to adequately expand the balloon.

MECHANICS AND HEMODYNAMICS

The objectives of vascular dilatation are:

1. To enlarge the vascular lumen, increasing flow
2. To ensure that the vessel remains dilated
3. To smooth the inner surface of the artery
4. To prevent the release of plaque fragments
5. To cause a controlled lesion to the vascular wall

The goals of angioplasty are not achieved unless the balloon catheter reaches the lesion, goes beyond it, and

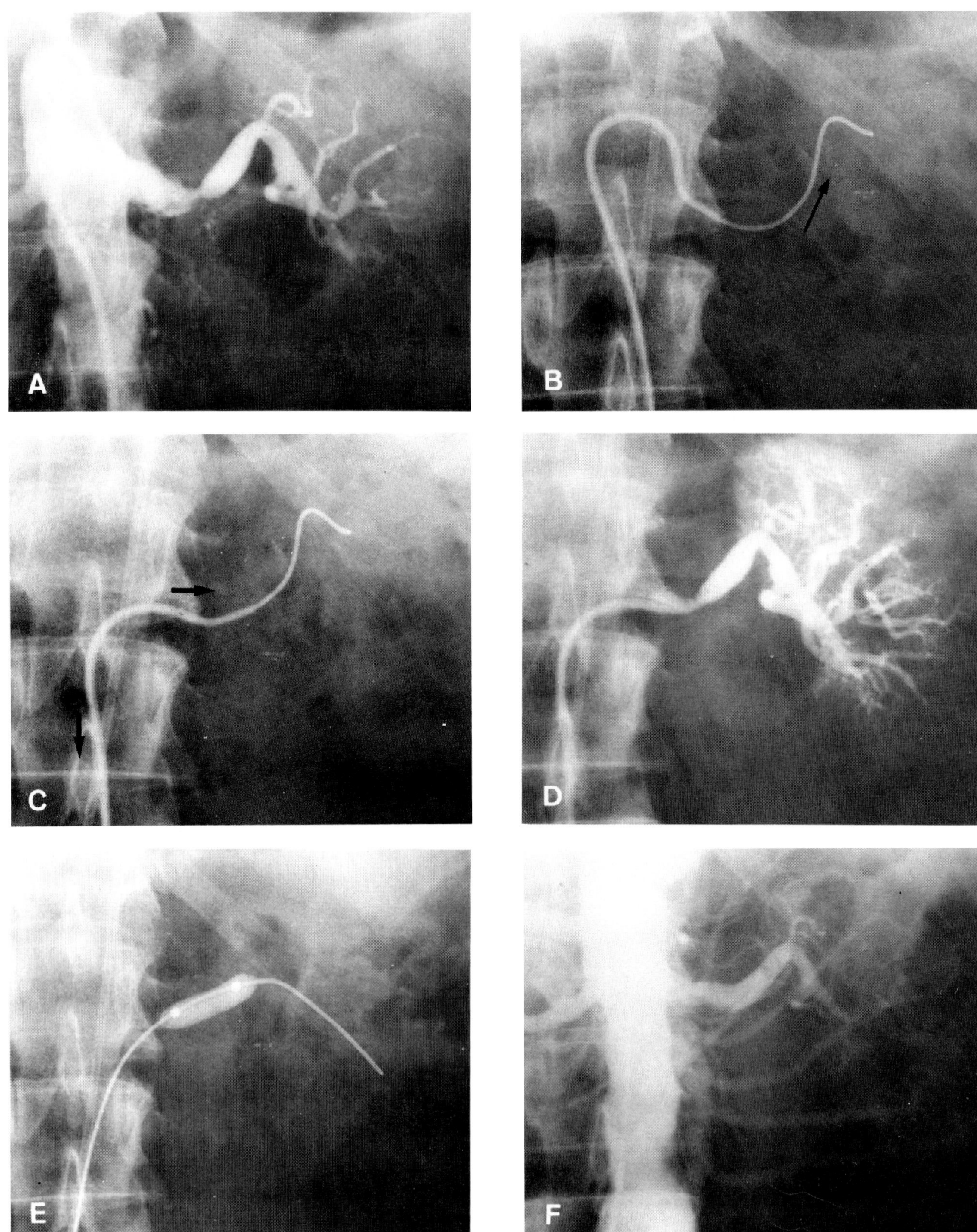

Figure 6.21 Simmons catheter being used to pass beyond a very tight stenosis.
(A) Selective injection into left renal artery showing 90 percent stenosis by atheromatous plaque. The kidney is contracted. (B) A Bentson guidewire (with a long, flexible tip) has passed beyond the stenosis and inside the distal arterial circulation. (C) The catheter has been pulled beyond the stenosis. (D) Selective injection with the tip of the catheter beyond the lesion. (E) After introduction of a Van Andel No. 9 French catheter, an 8-mm-diameter, 2-cm-long balloon was advanced beyond the lesion and dilated. (F) Final control, made with an aortographic catheter, showing a view of the dilated stenosis. The artery is irregular, but patent. Predilation arterial blood pressure was 160 × 100 mmHg. Post dilatation pressure dropped to 140 × 80 mmHg, without medication.

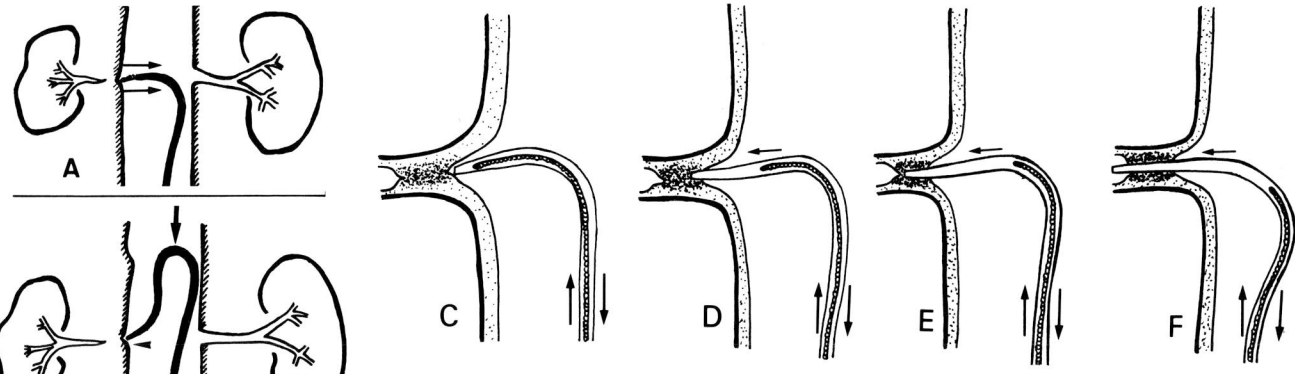

Figure 6.22 Use of deflecting guide were for renal artery occlusions which cannot be passed with a standard straight guidewire (A) or with a Simmons catheter (B). (C) Selective catheter in arterial stump. (D) Angulated deflecting guidewire. The wire is pulled, advancing the catheter. (E) The catheter tip entering the lesion. (F) The catheter tip has passed beyond the occlusion.

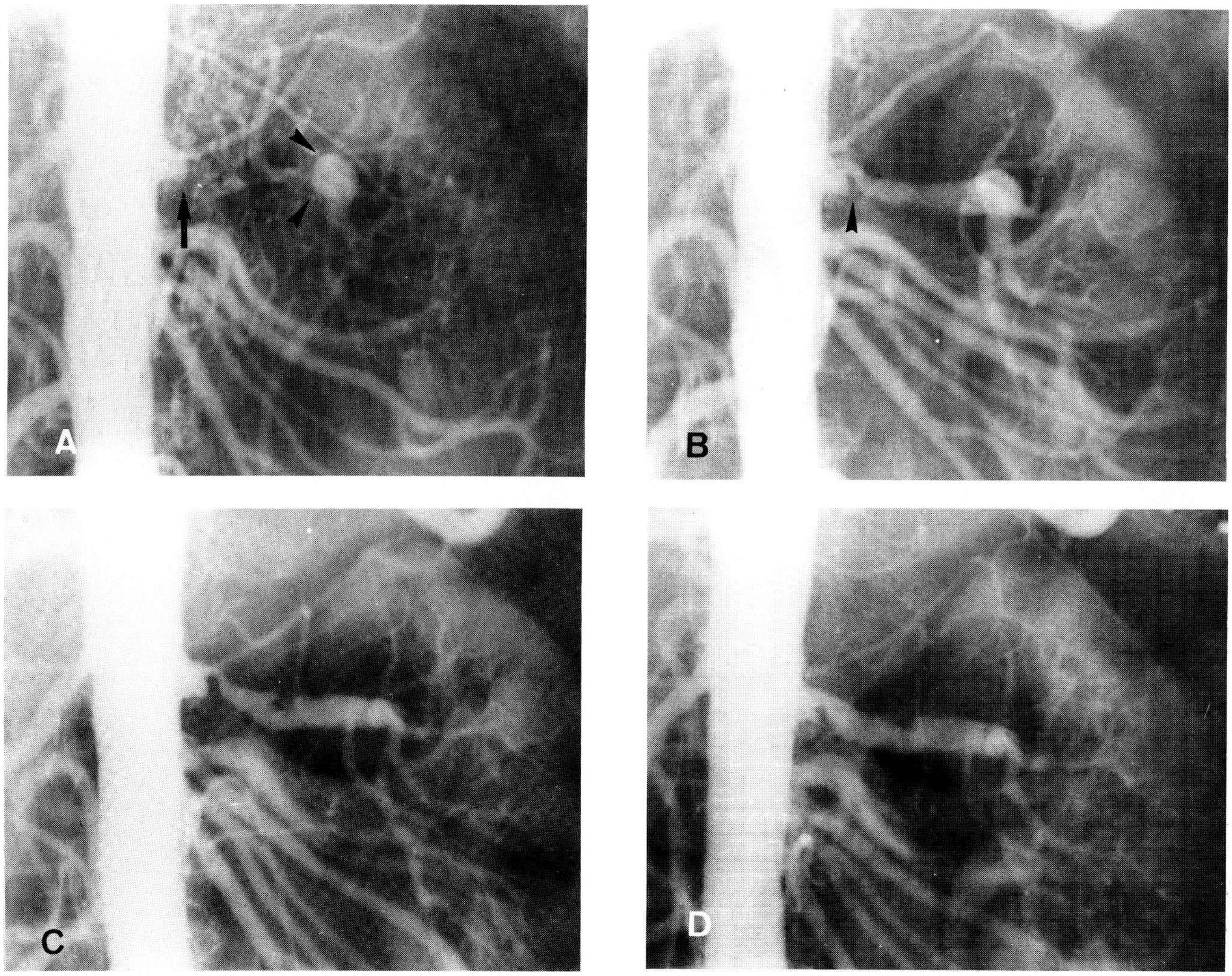

Figure 6.23 Renal artery recanalization using a deflecting guidewire.
(A) Left renal artery occlusion (large arrow). Recanalization of the intrarenal circulation (arrowheads) is evident.
(B) Control following recanalization. Note the intraluminal filling defect, probably caused by intimal flap or detached plaque (arrowhead). Before recanalization, arterial pressure was 180 × 110 mmHg, with medication. After recanalization, pressure dropped to 150 × 80 mmHg. (C) Hypertension has recurred, 1½ years later. Control angiography has shown arterial narrowing, but the artery is still patent.
(D) New dilatation, using a 6-mm balloon, has adequately dilated the lesion, but intimal flap or plaque persists in the arterial lumen. During a 2-year follow-up, hypertension did not recur. It should be noted, however, that intimal dissection persisted unchanged for years after the procedure.

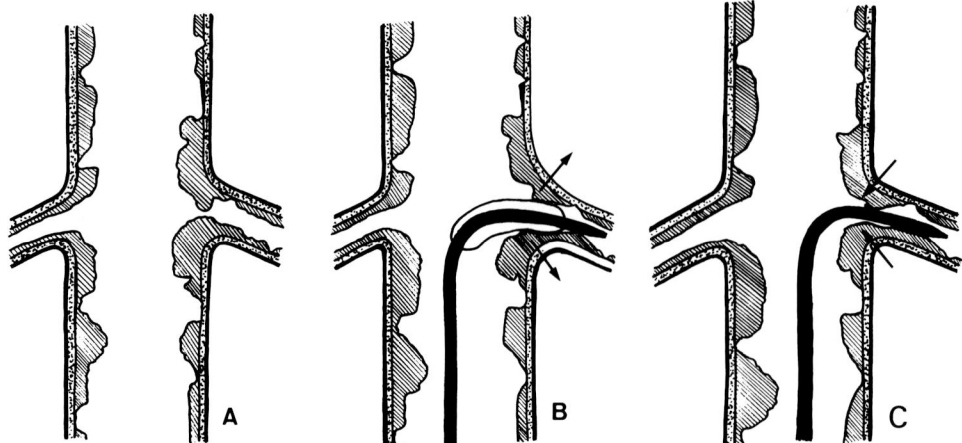

Figure 6.24 (A) Plaque in the arterial ostium has not responded to dilatation. (B) During balloon dilatation, the lesions separate (arrows), but resume their original position when the balloon is deflated [arrows in (C)].

dilates it, and is then immediately removed, having caused minimal local trauma and no trauma to the unaffected part of the artery.

Syringes with a small cross-sectional area are likely to generate high pressures during balloon inflation, and syringe capacity should be at least 10 mL. Larger syringes (with capacities from 20 to 50 mL) may be used for rapid deflation, particularly when large-volume balloons are involved.

Another factor to be considered is the profile, or diameter, of the balloon catheter. For tight lesions or total occlusions, it is more appropriate to use a rigid balloon, with a lower profile at the balloon site. Olbert-type catheters and the new low-profile balloon catheters are designed so that the balloon walls remain adjusted along the axis of the catheter, offering the lowest possible profile.

The dilatation forces exerted by a balloon result from (1) the hydrostatic force produced by the injected fluid and (2) the radial force produced when the balloon tries to resume its original shape under stress. The latter phenomenon, which is an application of Laplace's law, is called circumferential stress and is expressed by

$$CS = P \times D$$

where P is pressure and D is the diameter of the balloon. Thus, large-diameter balloons are subject to higher circumferential stresses than are small-diameter balloons, under the same pressure. This is why, given the same wall thickness, larger-diameter balloons or arteries may rupture under lower pressures than vessels or balloons with smaller diameters (Fig. 6.25).

The relationship between circumferential stress and dilatation force is as follows. When a balloon is deformed at the site of stenosis, radial forces, or force vectors, result in dilatation force. This can be compared to the situation in which one elevates the weight in the center

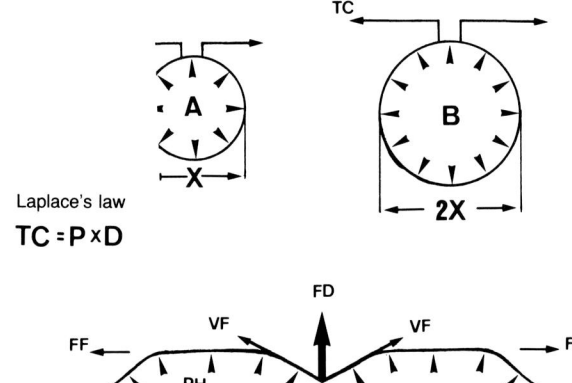

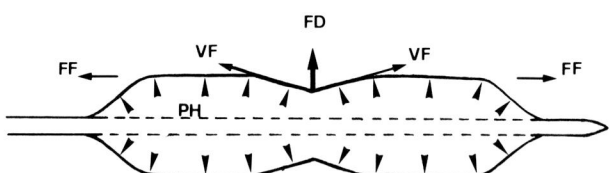

Figure 6.25 (A) An illustration of the LaPlace's effect, showing the effect of increases in pressure and balloon diameter on circumferential stress and dilatation force. CS = circumferential stress; P = pressure; D = diameter. (B) Dilatation force occurs when the balloon, under circumferential stress, exerts radial force against the lesion. This force decreases as the lesion is compressed and the DF-FV angle approaches 90. FD = DF, dilating force; VF, vector force; FF = EF, end force; PH = HP, hydrostatic pressure; TC = CS, circumferential stress.

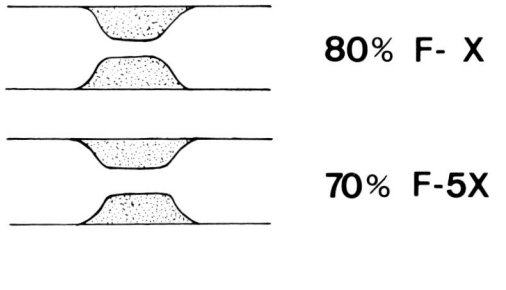

Figure 6.26 Poiseuille's law applied to the analysis of stenoses. If x = flow rate with an 80 percent stenosis, the flow rate with a 70 percent stenosis will be $5x$.

of a clothesline by pulling one of the extremities of the line. The lower the weight the greater the pulling power for the same force, because the force vectors are more perpendicular (Fig. 6.25).

For large-area stenotic lesions, hydrostatic pressure is the most significant factor in achieving adequate dilatation. For focal lesions, the clothesline effect is more significant. More severe stenoses will receive greater dilatation forces.

The following observations can be made about the relationships between balloon size, lesion size, pressure, and dilatation force.

— An elevation in pressure increases dilatation force in a linear fashion, provided that lesion size and balloon diameter remain the same.
— Increasing the pressure to eliminate a small impression produced by the lesion on the balloon will produce a small dilatation force. Chances of balloon rupture will then increase.
— For the same lesion, and at the same pressure, a large balloon will result in a larger dilatation force than a small balloon. Because the lesion will leave a deeper impression on the balloon, the radial vector force will be greater.
— The amount of pressure required to produce a given dilatation force is inversely related to the size of the balloon.
— The force necessary for permanent deformation of a given balloon material is very close to the force that will rupture the balloon.

Balloons which are deformed when dilatation force is applied should not be used in lesions requiring large forces for dilation. It is important to remember that repeated balloon inflations will produce the same initial result.

With balloons made of nondistensible material, dilatation force is independent of length. When the balloon is made of semidistensible material, a short balloon will produce a considerably higher dilatation force than a long balloon.

THE DYNAMICS OF FLOW

Flow through a vessel depends on such hemodynamic factors as peripheral resistance, turbulence, elasticity, and viscosity, as well as specific rheologic factors related to cellular blood elements.

In tight stenoses, small differences in diameter correspond to large differences in flow rate. It should be noted that, unfortunately, angiographic measurements of stenoses are not very accurate, not only due to lack of resolution, but also because the measurement made assumes that the vessel is round in cross section. An adequate idea of the problem may be obtained by considering the following application of Poiseuille's law (Fig. 6.26), where resistance to flow is directly proportional to the length of the stenosis and inversely proportional to the fourth power of the radius:

$$R = \frac{8NL}{\pi r^4}$$

where R = resistance to flow
N = viscosity
L = length of stenosis
π = 3.1416
r^4 = radius of stenosis
(The cross-sectional area of the vessel is πr^4.)

Thus blood flow through a 70 percent stenosis may be 5 times greater than the flow through an 80 percent stenosis. This phenomenon explains why seemingly inadequate angioplasties frequently present spectacular results, increasing arterial flow to the lower limbs and reducing arterial blood pressure in cases of renovascular hypertension. Any dilatation obtained in a tight stenosis can be significant. Just smoothing out the surface of a long, irregular stenosis may change turbulent flow to laminar flow without any increase in vessel diameter.

REFERENCES

Abbott WM. Percutaneous transluminal angioplasty: Surgeon's view. *AJR* 1980;136:917–920.

Abele JE. Balloon catheters and transluminal dilatation: Technical considerations. *AJR* 1980;135:901–906.

Athanasoulis CA. Percutaneous transluminal angioplasty: General principles. *AJR* 1980;135:893–900.

Athanasoulis CA. Therapeutic applications of angiography (second of two parts). *N Engl J Med* 1980;302:1174–1179.

Block PC, Fallon J, Elmer D. Experimental angioplasty: Lessons from the laboratory. *AJR* 1980;135:907–912.

Block PC, Myler RK, Stertzer S, Fallon JT. Morphology after transluminal angioplasty in human beings. *N Engl J Med* 1981;305:382–385.

Fallon JT. Pathology of arterial lesions amenable to percutaneous transluminal angioplasty. *AJR* 1980;135:913–916.

Freiman DB, McClean GK, Oleaga JA, Ring EJ. Percutaneous transluminal angioplasty. In *Interventional Radiology: Principles and Techniques*, edited by Ring EJ, McLean GK. Boston, Little, Brown, 1981:117–244.

Glover JL, Bendichk PJ, Dilley RS, et al. Efficacy of balloon catheter dilatation for lower extremity atherosclerosis. *Surgery* 1982;91:560–656.

Health and Public Policy Committee—ACPH. Percutaneous transluminal angioplasty. *Ann Intern Med* 1983;99:864–869.

Jones EL, Craner JM, Gruntzig AR, et al. Percutaneous transluminal angioplasty. *Ann Thorac Surg* 1982;34:493–503.

Kan JS, White RI, Mitchell SE, Gardner TJ. Percutaneous balloon valvuloplasty: A new method for treating congenital pulmonary valve stenosis. *N Engl J Med* 1982;307:540–542.

Wholey MH. The technology of balloon catheters in interventional angiography. *Radiology* 1977;125:671–676.

Renovascular Hypertension

ROSA MARIA PAOLINI

Knowledge of the relationship between renal artery stenosis and arterial hypertension dates from 1909, when Janeway discovered that reduction of blood supply to the kidney results in an elevation in arterial blood pressure. In 1934, Goldblatt and co-workers showed that hypertension caused by stenosis of the renal artery could be cured by nephrectomy. Since then, specialists have made every effort to identify those individuals whose hypertension may be treated surgically—by nephrectomy, autotransplant, or graft—or, more recently, by percutaneous transluminal angioplasty.

THE PATHOPHYSIOLOGY OF RENAL VASCULAR DISEASE

Renal vascular disease creates a chain reaction: Increase in renin level → angiotensin II level increase → aldosterone increase → salt retention → hypertension.

The mechanism by which this occurs is complex, and not all the factors involved are well understood. It is important to distinguish between the two-kidney model of hypertension and the one-kidney model (Goldblatt's model). In the two-kidney type, three different stages can be identified (Schalekamp, 1976): in the first stage, hypertension results from the vasoconstrictive effect of angiotensin II. In the second stage, usually after a few days, there is a drop in renin level but hypertension persists or even increases. Salt and water retention may be present. The third stage occurs after removal of the abnormal kidney fails to lower arterial blood pressure and the lesion in the contralateral kidney maintains hypertension.

In a patient with hypertension caused by stenosis in one kidney (Goldblatt's sole-kidney model) (Fig. 6.27), peripheral plasma renin is frequently normal, and so normal renin values are not enough to exclude renal vascular disease as the probable cause of hypertension.

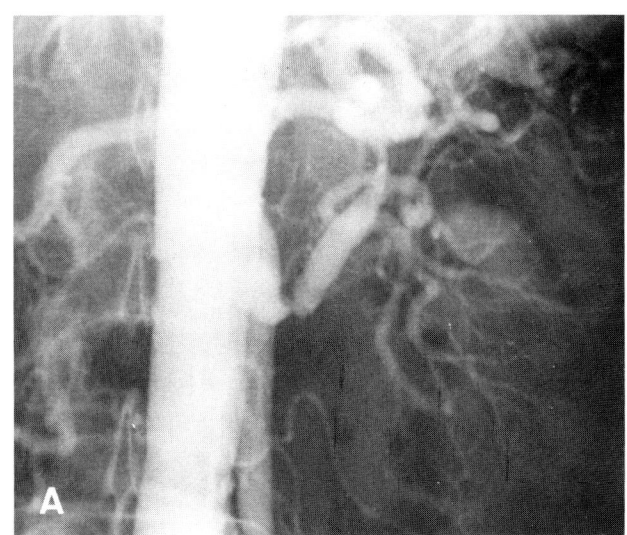
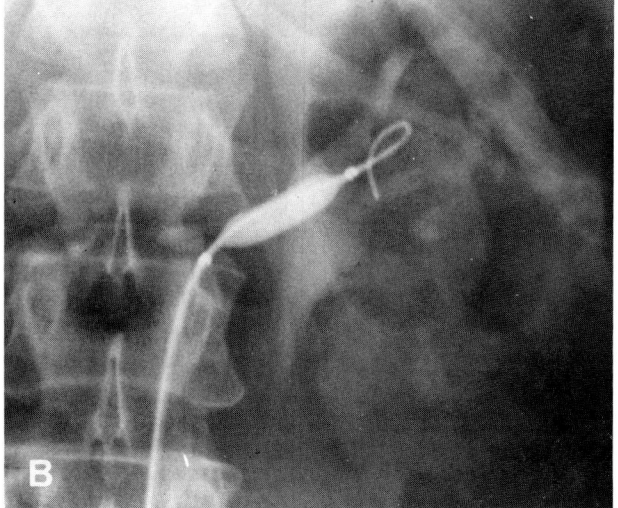
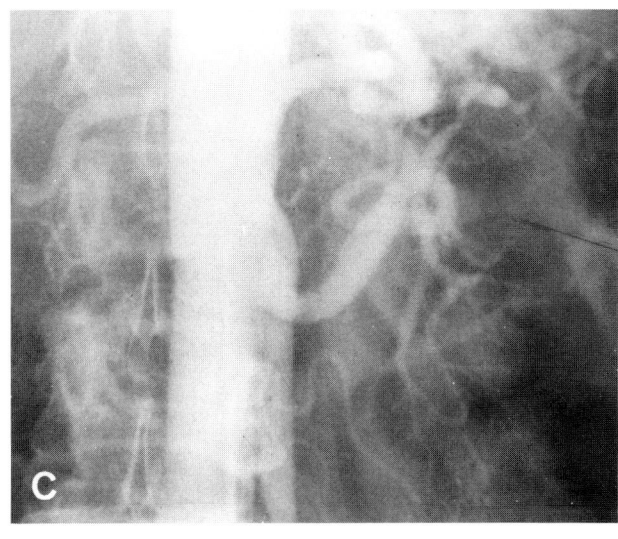

Figure 6.27 (A) 62-year-old patient with right renal artery occlusion and 90 percent arteriosclerotic stenosis in the left renal artery. (B) 6-mm-diameter 3-cm-long angioplasty balloon dilating the artery. (C) Control angiogram following angioplasty shows adequate dilatation of stenosis. Arterial blood pressure before the procedure, with medication, was 240/120. One hour after angioplasty, arterial pressure was 160/90; 24 h later it was 170/90, and 1 week later, it stabilized at 150/90.

The most frequent causes of renal artery stenosis are atherosclerosis and fibromuscular dysplasia. Rarely, it is caused by arteritis (Takayasu's, syphilitic, tubercular, or nonspecific), compression of the renal artery by a renal or extrarenal mass, a dissecting renal artery aneurysm, a lesion to the renal artery caused by irradiation, neurofibromatosis with renal artery dysplasia, Buerger's disease, and retroperitoneal fibrosis.

FREQUENCY

Hypertension in adults is usually idiopathic. Gifford in 1976 reported renovascular hypertension in 4.5 percent and renal hypertension in 5.2 percent of a group of 4939 patients. In 1964 Kaufman et al. established that renal artery stenosis was the original cause of arterial hypertension in 5 to 15 percent of the hypertensive population.

THE HEMODYNAMIC EFFECTS OF RENAL ARTERY STENOSIS

Pemsel et al. and Fissian et al. have identified five factors that affect flow through a stenosed vessel.

1. Diameter of stenosis. Animal studies indicate that beyond a critical level of one-third reduction in normal diameter, a further change of only 0.5 mm will cause a 50 percent reduction in flow volume.
2. Turbulence. Turbulence, which is partially a function of the nature of the inner surface of the vessel, may have a significant effect on flow. The higher the turbulence, the lower the flow rate.
3. Peripheral resistance. When peripheral resistance is high, flow is low, and vice versa.
4. Length of stenosis. The longer the stenosis, the more resistance there will be at the site of stenosis.
5. Blood viscosity. An increase in blood viscosity will reduce flow. However, an increase in viscosity also reduces turbulence, which in turn may increase flow rate.

RENAL ARTERY STENOSIS CAUSED BY ATHEROSCLEROSIS

Renal artery atherosclerotic lesions are more frequently observed in patients above 45 years of age unless predisposing factors are present, such as congenital hypercholesterolemia, diabetes mellitus, smoking, or systemic arterial hypertension. They are more common in men than in women. Renal artery atherosclerosis may produce hemodynamically significant stenosis resulting in diastolic hypertension.

Any arterial atherosclerotic lesion may evolve and become complicated by totally obstructive thrombosis, poststenotic dilatation that assumes aneurysmal proportions, laceration and dissection of the intimal lamina elastica, or formation of a true aneurysm.

Focal atherosclerosis is usually seen on the arteriogram as a concentric or eccentric lesion on the proximal third of the renal artery (Fig. 6.27). Subintimal atheromatous involvement of the abdominal aorta, around the ostium, may extend into the renal arteries. Angioplasty is frequently unsuccessful for treatment of this type of lesion (Fig. 6.24). Involvement of the abdominal aorta by atherosclerosis is usually more severe below the renal arteries, and in such cases may reach to accessory arteries (Fig. 6.77). Atherosclerosis may also involve branches of the renal artery, either on the bifurcation or in small intrarenal branches.

RENAL ARTERY STENOSIS CAUSED BY FIBROMUSCULAR DYSPLASIA

This type of dysplasia, the etiology of which remains unknown, causes arterial stenosing fibrosis, and may involve the intima, the media, or the adventitia. (See Fig. 6.29 and Table 6.1 for a classification of fibromuscular diseases.)

Intimal fibromuscular dysplasia (intimal fibroplasia) is a lesion of the intima and of the inner lamina elastica consisting of localized and circumferential deposition of collagen, with no apparent lipid content. Any arterial segment may be involved (Fig. 6.30).

On the arteriogram, the stenosis may appear as focal or tubular. It is usually symmetrical, with poststenotic dilatation, but a dilated segment may mask the stenotic area. The lumen of the dilated segment is usually irregular, facilitating differential diagnosis with poststenotic dilatation. Intimal fibroplasia may be severe enough to cause luminal occlusion or thrombosis.

Fibromuscular medial dysplasia may be one of two types: multifocal (Fig. 6.31) and focal (Fig. 6.32).

Multifocal medial fibromuscular dysplasia, which occurs mainly in females between 30 and 60 years of age, was formerly described as fibromuscular hyperplasia, but the lesions involved are not actually totally hyperplastic. The renal artery exhibits alternating areas of narrowing and dilatation, presenting a "string of beads" image which is pathognomonic of the multifocal renal arterial process (Fig. 6.31). The narrowed areas represent thickened segments of the media in which muscle and a few fine elastic lamellae have been partially or completely re-

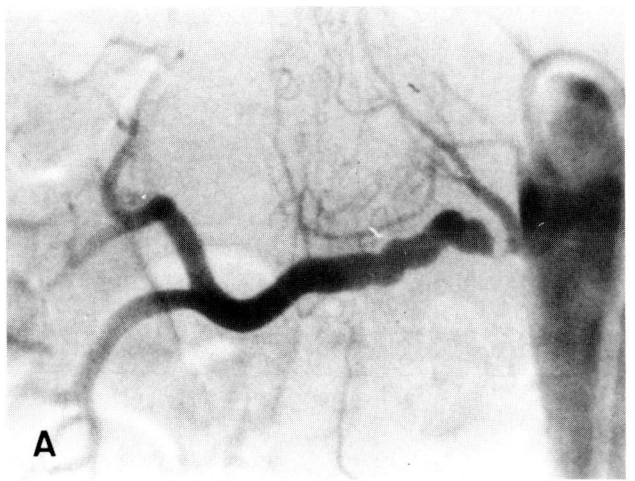 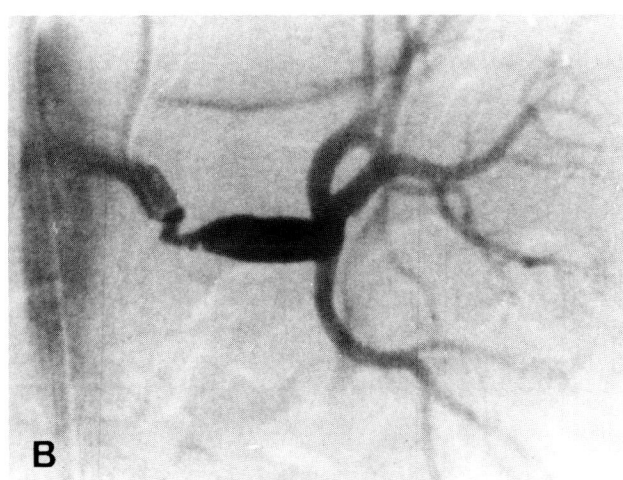

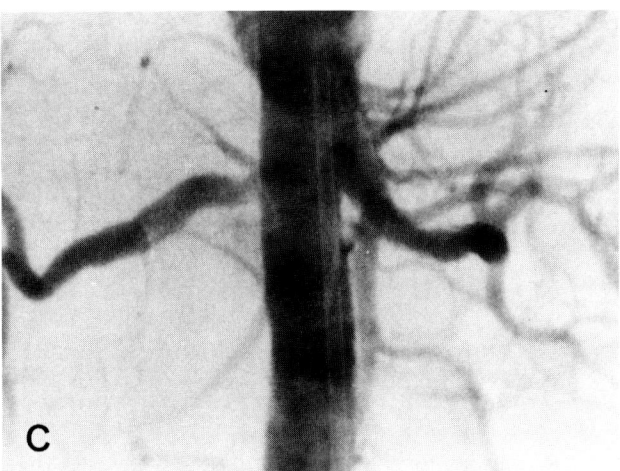 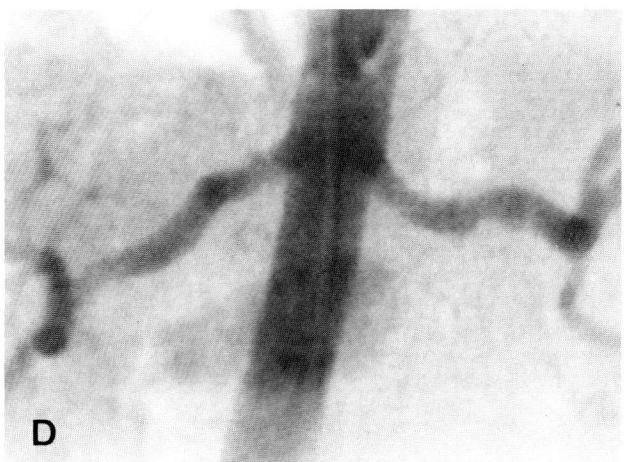

Figure 6.28 35-year-old patient with AH of 5 years' duration. Arterial blood pressure is 220/150, without medication, and 180/100 under medication.

(A) Proximal atherosclerotic stenosis of the right renal artery as a result of fibromuscular dysplasia. (B) Left renal artery stenosis of the proximal third. (C) Using the techniques described in Figs. 6.20 and 6.21, bilateral transluminal percutaneous angioplasty was performed, with a 6-mm balloon. Postdilatation control aortogram shows adequate patency of renal arteries. (D) Routine digital control angiogram 6 months later shows adequate renal circulation. Note that the collateral circulation has disappeared.

Table 6.1 – Classification of muscle fiber lesions and pathologic findings

Type	Pathology
Intimal fibroplasia—middle	Fibrosis Intima
Medial fibromuscular dysplasia	
Medial fibroplasia—distal	Muscle fiber bridges Aneurysm
Medial hyperplasia—middle	Smooth muscle proliferation
Perimedial fibroplasia—middle	External fibroplasia Aneurysm
Medial dissection—middle	Dissection Proliferation
Adventitial fibroplasia—middle	Fibroplasia Adventitia

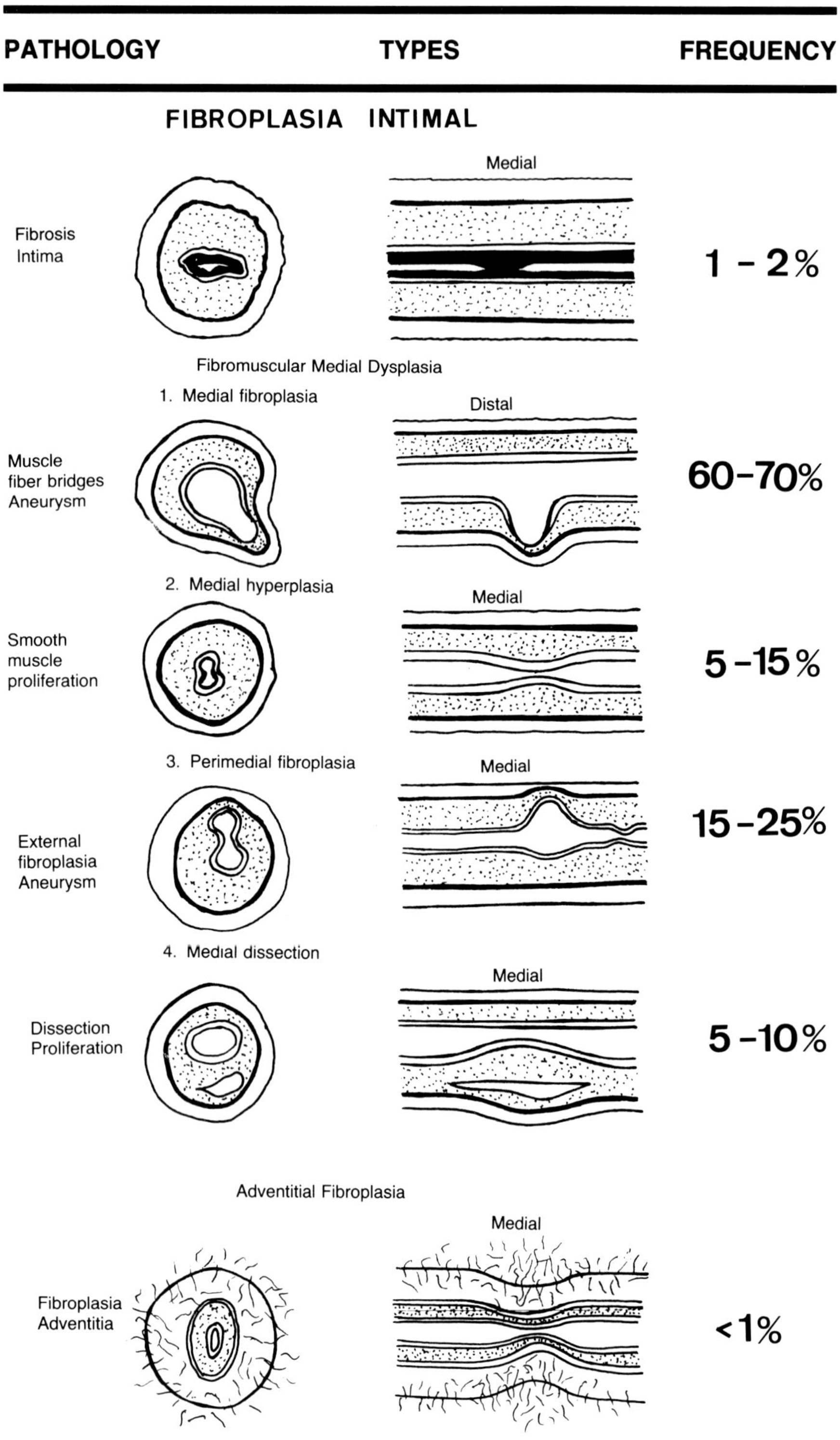
PATHOLOGY
TYPES
FREQUENCY
FIBROPLASIA INTIMAL
Medial
Fibrosis
Intima
1 - 2%
Fibromuscular Medial Dysplasia
1. Medial fibroplasia
Distal
Muscle
fiber bridges
Aneurysm
60-70%
2. Medial hyperplasia
Medial
Smooth
muscle
proliferation
5-15%
3. Perimedial fibroplasia
Medial
External
fibroplasia
Aneurysm
15-25%
4. Medial dissection
Medial
Dissection
Proliferation
5-10%
Adventitial Fibroplasia
Medial
Fibroplasia
Adventitia
<1%

Figure 6.29 Classification of muscle fiber lesions and pathologic findings. (Modified from Sos et al., 1982.)

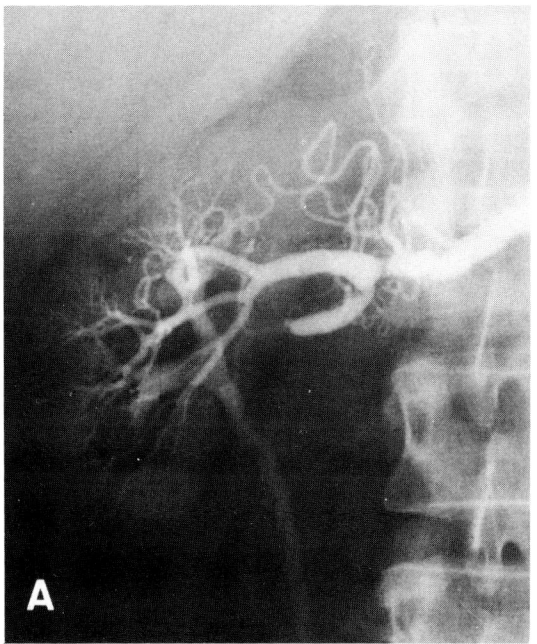
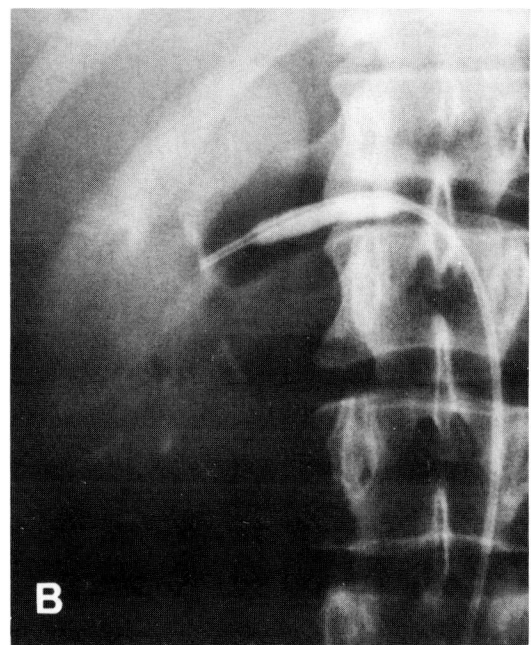
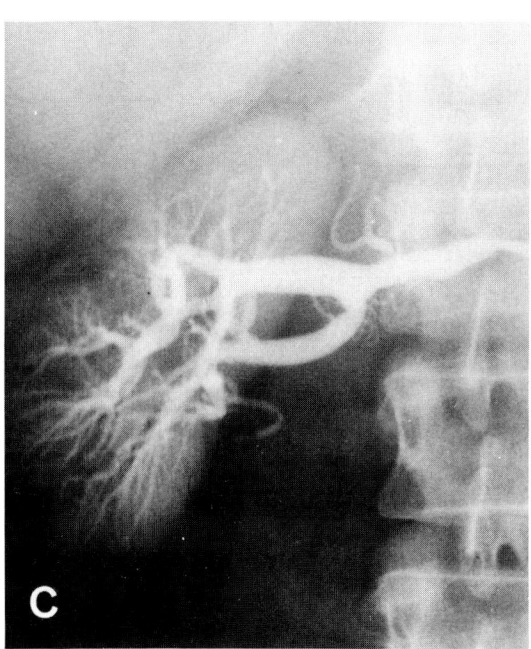

Figure 6.30 (A) 33-year-old patient with arterial hypertension, 220/170, with a stenotic lesion compatible with intimal fibroplasia located in the right renal artery. Note that there is also a lower branch stenosis. (B) Dilatation with 5-mm-diameter balloon. (C) Control following angioplasty shows that intrarenal flow has increased and that collateral circulation has disappeared. This patient presented severe postural hypotension after the procedure, requiring aggressive fluid infusion to restore blood pressure. Pressure later stabilized at 120/90.

placed by collagen. The areas of dilatation represent those sites in which the inner lamina elastica has been partially or totally lost. The media may be totally absent, in which case the arterial wall in the dilated segments is formed only by external lamina elastica and adventitia. Intimal fibroplasia is occasionally associated with a medial lesion. On the arteriogram, this lesion is seen to mainly involve the middle and distal thirds of the renal artery (Fig. 6.33) and/or its branches, but it may also involve the proximal third.

Focal fibromuscular dysplasia of the tunica media, an uncommon disease of the renal artery, occurs primarily in young patients. The stenosis is focal or tubular, and concentric, and consists of a mixture of smooth muscle and fibrotic tissue in variable quantities. Sometimes poststenotic dilatation occurs, and when laceration of the

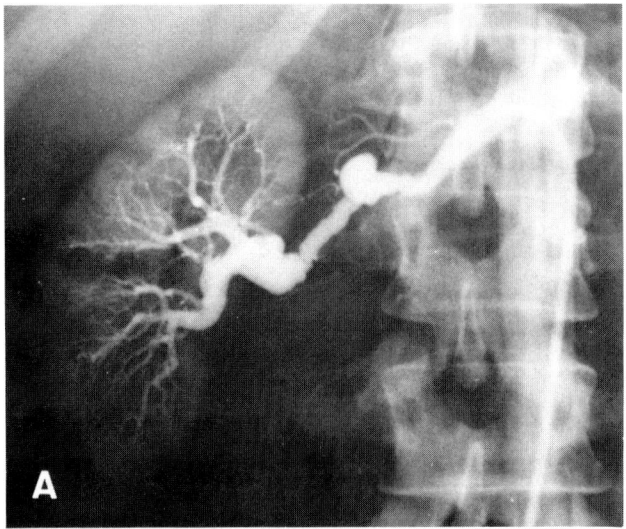
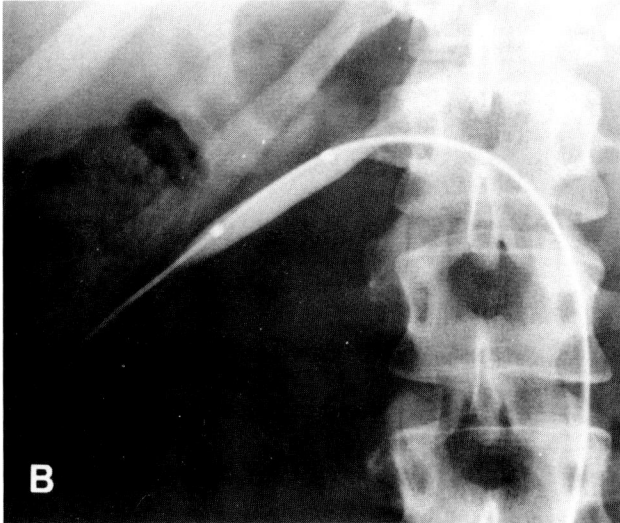
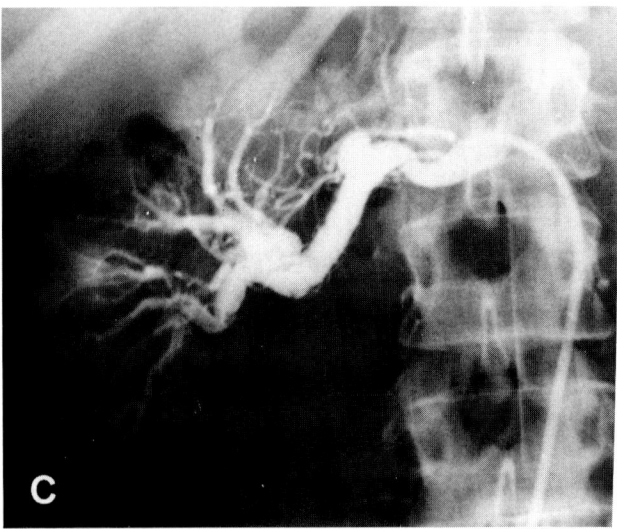
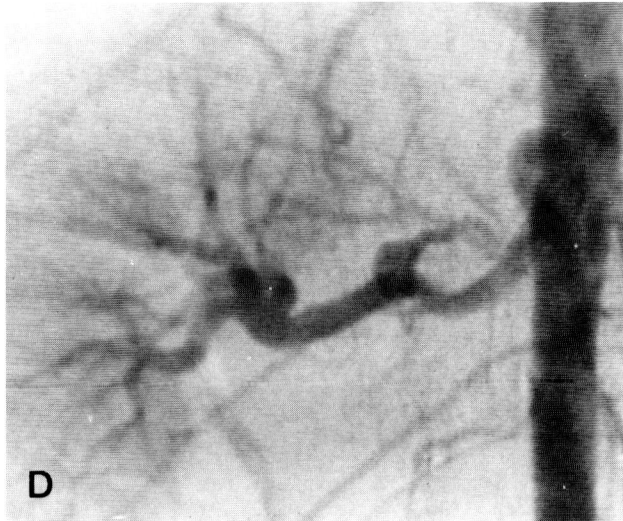

Figure 6.31 (A) 26-year-old patient, with renovascular hypertension, 160/110, as a result of multifocal fibroplastic lesions of the tunica media, with a large aneurysm on the middle third. (B) Dilatation with 6-mm-diameter balloon. (C) Control following angioplasty of long stenotic segment shows that the aneurysm persists. (D) Digital venous angiogram shows adequate arterial patency after 6 months. Pressure stabilized at 120/80 without medication.

inner lamina elastica is present distally to the stenosis, a dissecting aneurysm is formed.

On the arteriogram, it is seen to mainly involve the proximal third of the renal artery (Fig. 6.32).

Subadventitial or perimedial fibroplasia primarily affects females between 20 and 40 years of age, with bilateral involvement in about 25 percent of cases. A circumferential collagen band with variable thickness surrounds the external media and the adjacent external lamina elastica. Collagen fibrils are disposed longitudinally, and the media may be partially or totally replaced in a focal manner by deposition or interdigitation of fibrotic tissue. This type of lesion primarily involves the middle and distal thirds of the main renal artery. The length of the involved portion may range from a 1- to 3-m focal stenosis to a longer, narrower segment. These irregularities in the contour of the artery may appear as a string of beads, or series of waves, both at longitudinal section and on arteriography. This "string," however, differs from the one seen in fibroplasias of the tunica media. In subadventitial fibroplasia, the necklace effect, is related to irregular, microscopic collagen distribution, and larger areas in the lumen do not exceed the original diameter of the artery. Branch stenosis is usually seen as focal, with or without poststenotic dilatation. Occasionally, only one sausage-shaped dilatation is seen (Fig. 6.34).

Adventitial periarterial fibroplasia is restricted to the

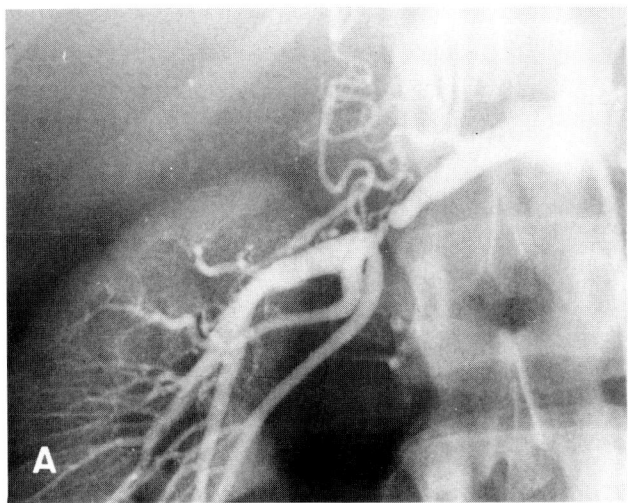
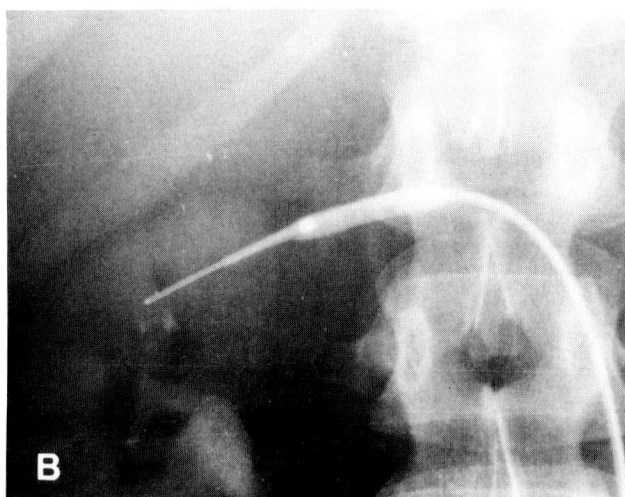
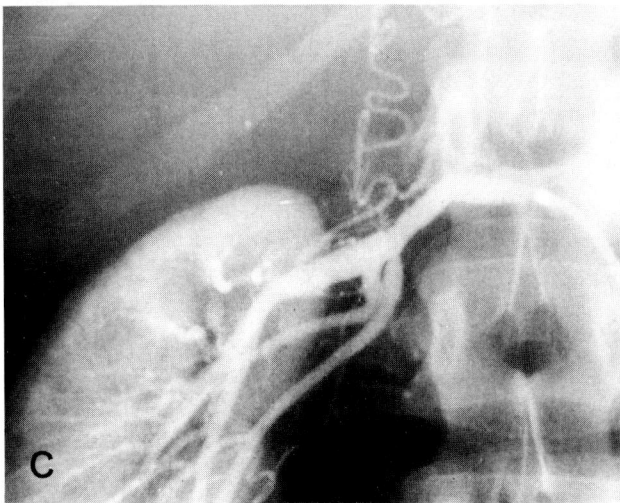

Figure 6.32 (A) 21-year-old patient with a stenotic lesion on the middle third of the right renal artery, compatible with focal fibromuscular dysplasia of the tunica media. Note the capsular collateral circulation. (B) 4-mm-balloon dilating the lesion. (C) Control angiogram showing successful dilatation. During a 5-year follow-up after angioplasty, arterial pressure was normal.

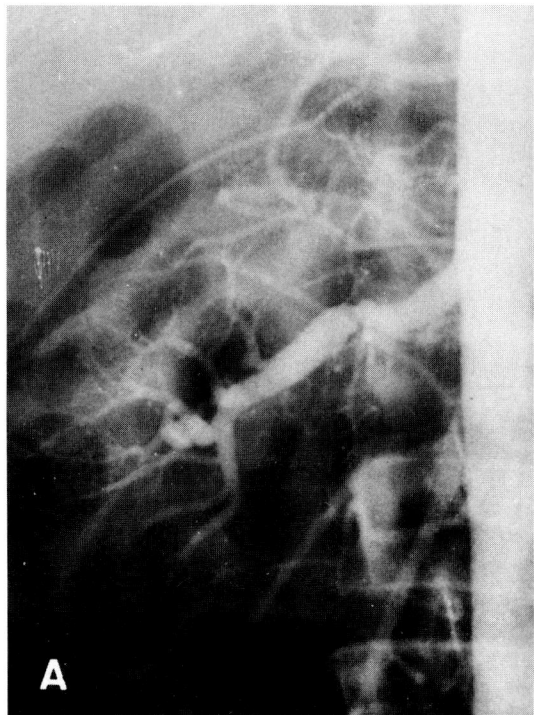
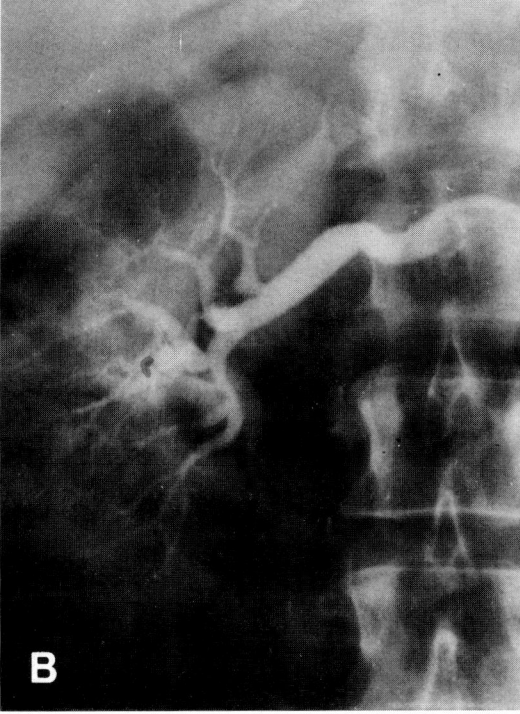

Figure 6.33 (A) 26-year-old patient with severe arterial hypertension, 240/160 under medication, as a result of fibroplastic disease of the tunica media, localized on the middle third of the right renal artery. (B) Control after dilatation with latex balloon catheter for occlusion (not shown) showing adequate dilatation. During an 8-year follow-up, 130/80 blood pressure was maintained.

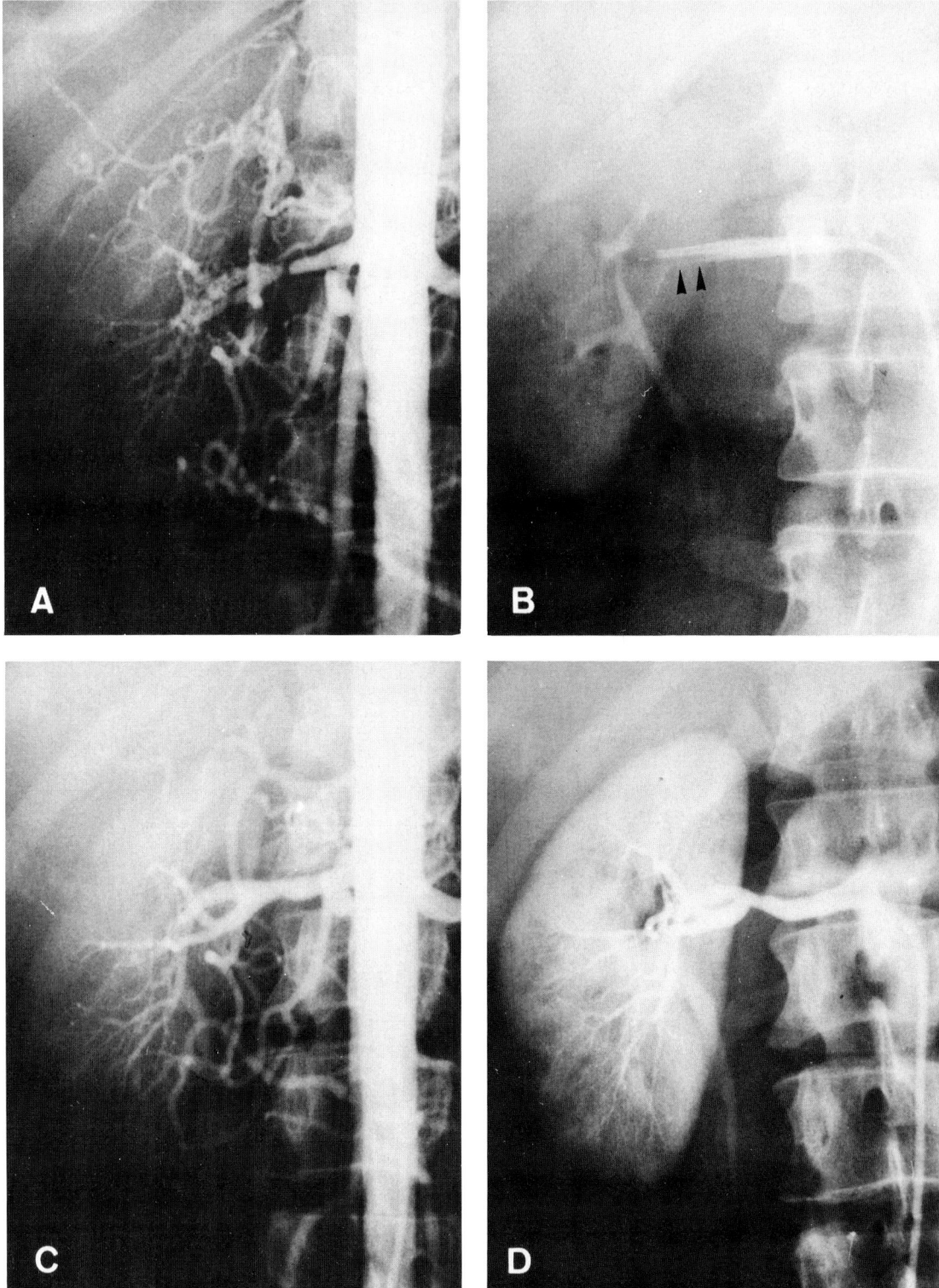

Figure 6.34 (A) 25-year-old patient with isolated septated lesion on the middle third of the right renal artery, compatible with perimedial fibroplasia. Note the presence of capsular and retroperitoneal collateral circulation. (B) Control during inflation showing distal rupture of 4-mm balloon (notice the flow of contrast, arrowheads). (C) Control immediately after angioplasty showing adequate dilatation. (D) Control after 4 months showing that arterial diameter is normal. Blood pressure 12 h after dilatation was 150/80; 4 months later, it was 140/80.

adventitia. It consists of significant hyperplasia and thickening of fibrotic connective tissue, with some duplication of the external lamina elastica. Arteriographically, it is tubular, and it may or may not be associated with poststenotic dilatation (Fig. 6.35).

Branch Involvement

Stenotic involvement of the primary or intrarenal branch of the renal artery is generally caused by muscle fiber dysplasia and may or may not be associated with stenosis of the main renal artery. Other causes of branch lesions are atherosclerosis, arteritis, thrombosis, and embolism. Routine aortograms often do not show branch lesions, and selective renal arteriograms, with one or more oblique projections, may be required to detect them. Study of the nephrographic phase is important, as it may identify ischemic areas. Analysis of blood samples from renal venous branches for renin assay may aid the diagnosis.

RENAL ARTERY STENOSIS CAUSED BY ARTERITIS

The types of arteritis that result in renal artery stenosis involve all three arterial layers with destruction of elastic tissue. The tunica media is replaced by fibrosis, and intimal proliferation and adventitial abnormalities are also present. Progressive arteritis may result in occlusion of the arterial lumen by the disease itself or by thrombosis.

Arteriography shows narrowing and stenosis—usually tubular or focal but sometimes multifocal—on the proximal third of the renal artery, with or without poststenotic dilatation (Figs. 6.36 and 6.37).

Collateralization may occur with any type of stenosis, depending on the evolution of the disease, and on the severity of the stenosis. Occasionally, renal artery stenosis caused by arteritis is accompanied by intrarenal arteriovenous malformation (Fig. 6.37). Atherosclerotic plaque and calcification may develop in arteritic arteries.

MEASUREMENT OF THE STENOSIS

Measuring the extent of renal artery stenosis is very difficult. Stenosis is an asymmetrical process in both atherosclerotic and nonatherosclerotic diseases and lesions may be present on the dorsal and ventral vascular walls, as well as in the ostium of the renal artery. X-ray measurement, which is only a projection, usually causes 15 to 20 percent geometric distortion, overestimating the diameter of the artery and the degree of the stenosis.

COLLATERAL CIRCULATION

When the renal blood supply is reduced by arterial stenosis, small adjacent arteries will dilate in an attempt to maintain normal tissue perfusion. These dilated arteries evolve into collateral circulation channels, the routes of which may be classified as extra- or intrarenal. Extrarenal collateral connections are those arteries communicating with renal arteries before they enter into the renal sinus: the inferior adrenal, renal pelvic, ureteral, capsular, intercostal, subcostal, inferior phrenic, and lumbar arteries.

Small collateral vessels may also originate from the main renal artery or from a branch, bypassing the stenotic area. The intrarenal collateral system consists of vessels communicating with the renal arteries after they enter into the renal parenchyma as interlobar branches.

The perforating capsular arteries, which originate from interlobar branches and communicate with adipocapsular branches on Turner's retroperitoneal arterial plexus, act as a bridge between the intrarenal system and extrarenal collaterals.

CLINICAL AND LABORATORY EVALUATION OF ARTERIAL HYPERTENSION

The initial diagnosis of arterial hypertension is made through measurement of arterial blood pressure. However, there are several possible sources of error, and the clinical and laboratory evaluation of patients who present with high arterial blood pressure must include careful evaluation of etiology, risk factors, and the degree of target-organ involvement.

Etiology

Arterial hypertension of unknown cause, known as *essential, primary,* or *idiopathic hypertension,* accounts for about 90 percent of all cases. The two major causes of *secondary* hypertension are renovascular disease and endocrine disorders (accounting for 90 percent of the remaining cases), including the hormone imbalance caused by taking oral contraceptives.

Risk Factors

Although there is no direct cause-and-effect relationship between risk factors and arterial hypertension, whether primary or secondary, these factors together have a profound effect on the onset and course of the disease, as well as its treatment and the prognosis for recovery. Risk factors are classified as uncontrollable or controllable.

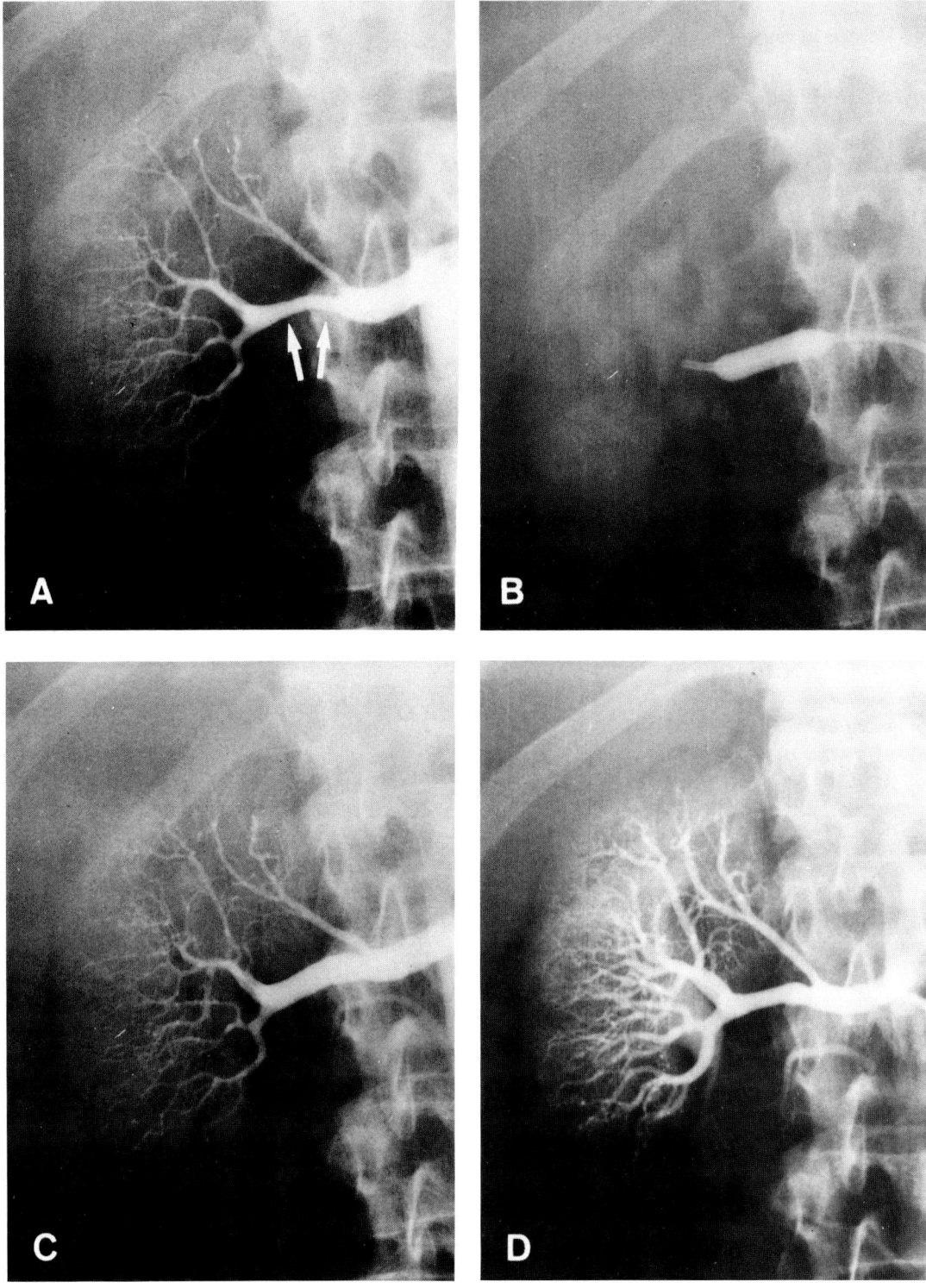

Figure 6.35 33-year-old patient with severe hypertension, 220/110.
(A) Tubular stenosis in distal renal artery (arrows) compatible with adventitial fibroplasia. (B) Dilatation with 5-mm balloon. (C) Control angiogram following dilatation shows patency of the dilated segment. Renin in this patient was increased, but not lateralized. Note the signs of nephrosclerosis. (D) Control angiogram 1 year after angioplasty. The arterial diameter is reduced, and the stenosis remains dilated. 12 h after angioplasty, blood pressure was 150/100; 48 h later it was 140/90. Pressure was stable at 150/100 during angiographic control taken 1 year later.

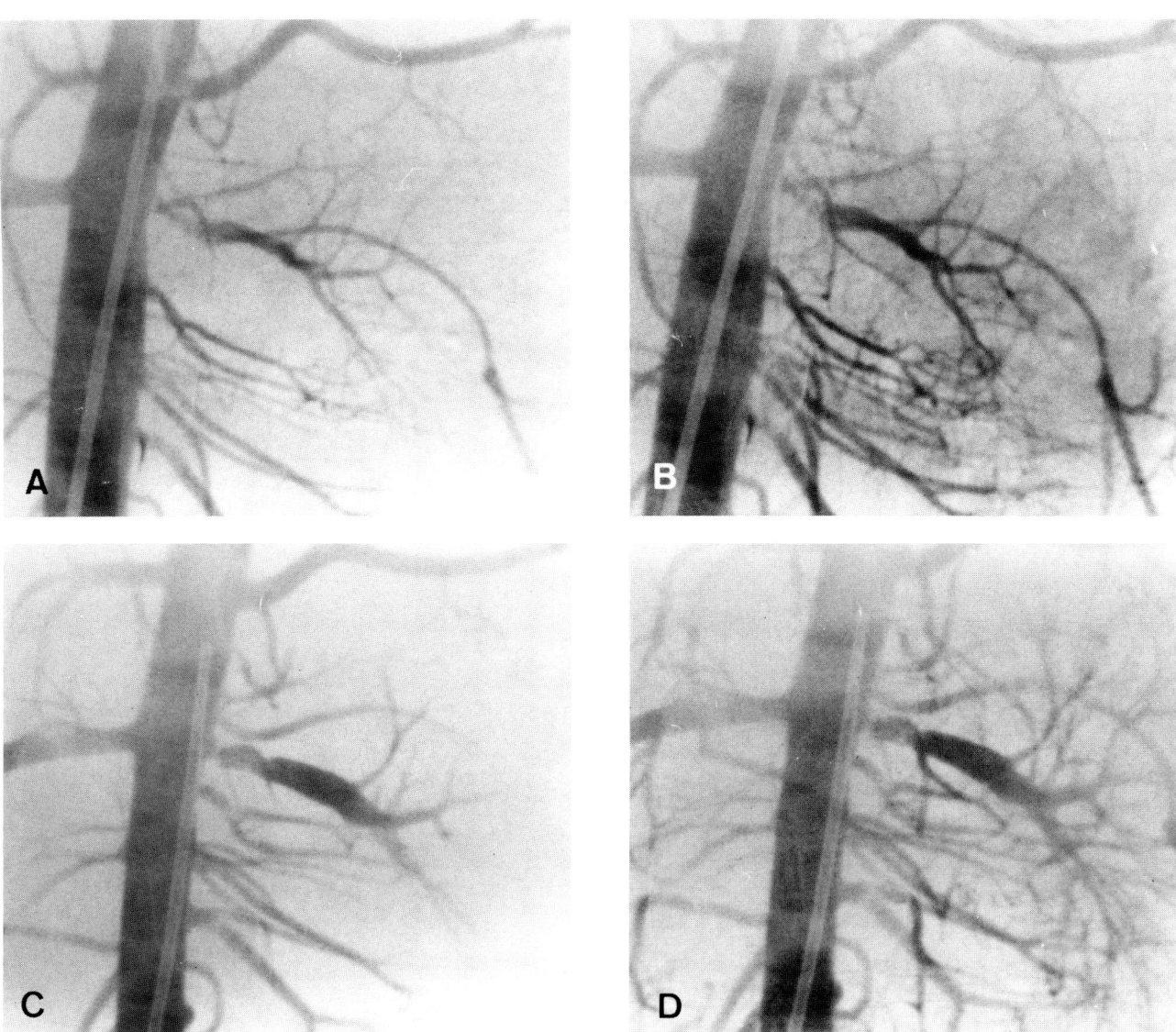

Figure 6.36 (A,B) 8-year-old child, who had been receiving medication for hypertension (160/120) for 1 year. The image is compatible with proximal stenosis as a result of arteritis. (C,D) Angioplasty with 4-mm-diameter high-pressure balloon resulted in adequate dilation of the artery. Pressure stabilized at 130/80.

Uncontrollable Risk Factors

Age: Most studies show that systolic pressure increases with age. In males, diastolic pressure rises until 50 years of age; in females, until 60. In both sexes it tends to decline after that. Younger patients who have arterial hypertension for long periods present higher morbidity and mortality rates than older patients.

Sex: Women over 40 to 50 years old present a higher prevalence of arterial hypertension than men of the same age. However, mortality rates are higher for men.

Genetic factors and race: Many studies demonstrate that heredity plays a role in the development of arterial hypertension. Arterial hypertension is more frequent and presents higher morbidity and mortality rates in blacks. In some populations, for example, in the north of Japan, there is an extremely high prevalence of arterial hypertension, around 35 percent; in others, for example, the Brazilian Indians, no elevation in arterial blood pressure occurs with age, and arterial hypertension is practically nonexistent.

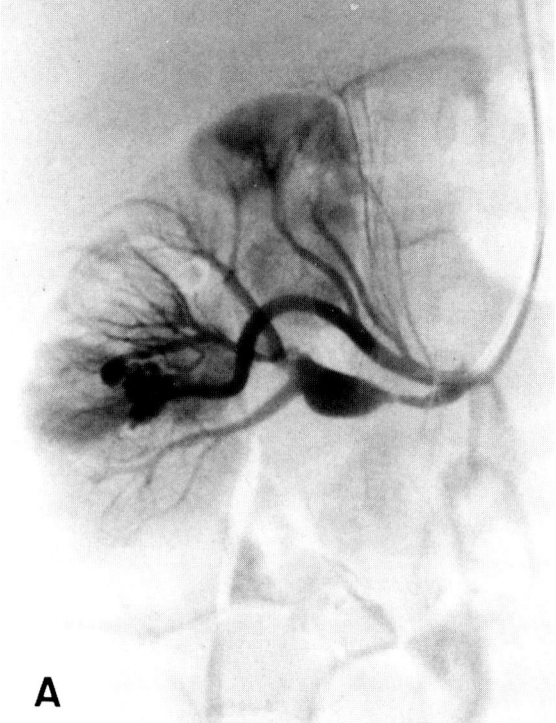 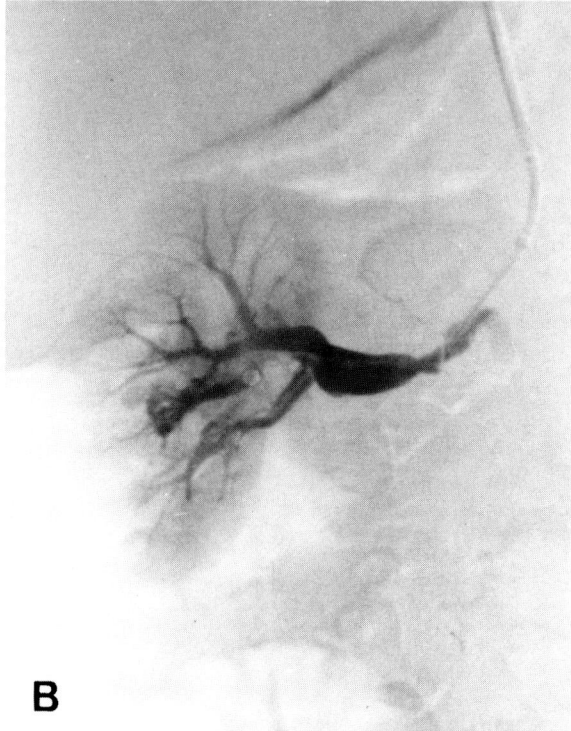

Figure 6.37 23-year-old male with severe arterial hypertension, 170/120.
(A) Severe stenosis of the inferior renal artery, with significant poststenotic dilatation. Note the intrarenal arteriovenous malformation being fed by the renal superior artery and (partially) by the renal inferior artery. (B) After dilatation with high-pressure balloon was attempted (using 17-atm pressure), a slight improvement of stenosis was obtained, but there was no reduction of hypertension. The probable etiology of the vascular lesion was arteritis.

Controllable Risk Factors

Obesity: There is a higher prevalence of arterial hypertension among the obese than among the nonobese, even in those studies in which arm circumference has introduced an error factor in the measurement of arterial blood pressure. Weight gain increases the risk of developing arterial hypertension, and weight loss is associated with a reduction in arterial blood pressure.

Sodium intake: Studies have demonstrated that there is a direct relationship between high salt consumption and the prevalence of arterial hypertension in general populations, but not in individuals.

Stress: Individuals identified as being in a stressful environment (e.g., people living under crowded conditions, or engaged in stressful activities) tend to show a higher prevalence of arterial hypertension.

Alcohol: Several studies have shown a correlation between alcohol intake and arterial hypertension.

Diabetes: Some studies have shown a higher prevalence of arterial hypertension among diabetics.

Hyperuricemia: Arterial hypertension is more frequent among patients with gout.

Smoking: People who smoke are at increased risk of arteriosclerosis.

Hyperlipidemia: Hyperlipidemia is a factor contributing to increased risk of arteriosclerosis.

Target-Organ Involvement

The heart, the brain, and the kidneys are the organs most commonly affected by hypertension. Arteriosclerotic lesions can be the result of hyaline degeneration, hyperplastic thickening, or fibrinoid necrosis; the two latter types are more often found in cases of severe or malignant hypertension. Charcot-Bouchard aneurysms may form in small cerebral arteries. Benign nephrosclerosis is seen in the kidney, where the afferent arterioles are most often involved. In the heart, hypertensive disease is characterized by myocardial ischemic lesions and hypertrophy of the left chambers. Funduscopic evaluation is useful for determining the severity of arterial hypertension.

Clinical Approach

In the search for curable causes of arterial hypertension, the clinical evaluation, including patient history, physical examination, and laboratory tests, should, except in emergencies, precede any administration of drugs.

History

The patient's history will reveal the presence of any of the risk factors discussed above. It should be noted that hypertension that develops before the age of 35 or over the age of 50 is more likely to be renovascular hypertension than essential hypertension. Some findings suggestive of renovascular hypertension are severe hypertension before 40 years of age, especially in females; recent worsening of hypertension; and poor response to previous clinical treatment.

Physical Examination

The physical examination should include the following:

- Evaluation of the patient's general appearance: obesity, signs of edema in the extremities, signs of endocrine disease
- Blood pressure measurement under optimal conditions. A reading of 140/90 mmHg is considered borderline by the World Health Organization. An adult with a diastolic pressure between 85 and 89 is considered high normal; between 90 and 104, mildly hypertensive; between 105 and 114, moderately hypertensive; and over 115, severely hypertensive
- Evaluation and comparison of peripheral pulses
- Pulmonary and cardiac auscultation
- Listening for abdominal murmur (approximately 4 percent of patients with renovascular hypertension will present with abdominal bruit with a diastolic component)
- Examination of the ocular fundi

Laboratory Tests

Serum creatinine: A decrease in serum creatinine clearance is the best clinical indicator of renal disease.

Serum potassium: In the absence of diuretics and with a normal sodium diet, hypokalemia is suggestive of primary or secondary hyperaldosteronism. When the patient is on diuretic therapy, the pretreatment level of potassium should be ascertained.

ECG: The ECG will reveal, at an early stage, the presence of cardiac involvement in arterial hypertension.

Intravenous pyelogram (IVP): An adequately performed IVP will reveal irregularities in around 39 percent of cases of renovascular hypertension and approximately 6 percent of cases of essential hypertension. Two suggestive findings are (1) renal size asymmetry, with a difference in longitudinal length equal to or greater than 1.5 cm (an ischemic kidney is smaller); (2) delayed appearance of contrast.

Captopryl test: This test consists of oral administration of Captopryl, 25 mg, with arterial blood pressure measurements at 60 and 90 min. Captopryl inhibits the conversion of angiotensin I into angiotensin II, and thus causes a drop in the arterial blood pressure of patients with angiotensinogenic hypertension. Patients considered positive are those whose diastolic pressure shows a drop greater than 10 mmHg after 60 to 90 min. At the beginning of the test, positive response is seen in 45 percent of essential hypertension cases and 75 percent of renovascular hypertension patients. Drops of 25 mmHg or greater are seen only in cases of renovascular hypertension and cases of malignant hypertension.

Isotope renogram: Scintigraphic study of the kidney detects renovascular hypertension in approximately 70 to 80 percent of patients.

Plasma renin: Blood samples are obtained by selective catheterization of renal veins and the inferior vena cava below the renals. When the presence of renal artery branch stenosis is suspected, samples should be taken from renal vein branches. Results are given in nanograms per milliliter. The ratio between the affected kidney and the normal kidney should be greater than 1.2.

REFERENCES

Fissian RV, Byar D, Edwards FA. Factors affecting flow through a stenosed vessel. *Arch Surg* 1964;88:105–112.

Gifford RW. Evaluation of specific causes of hypertension: Cost effectiveness considerations. In *Hypertention: A Policy Perspective*, edited by Weinstein MC, Stason WB, et al. Harvard University Press, Cambridge, 1976:198.

Goldblatt H, Lunch J, Hanzal RF, Summerville WW. Studies on experimental hypertension: Production of persistent elevations of systolic blood pressure by means of renal ischemia. *J Exp Med* 1934;59:347–379.

Hunt JC, Harrison EG, Jr., Sheps SG, Bernatz PE, Davis GD. Hypertension caused by fibromuscular dysplasia of the renal arteries. *Post Grad Med* 1965;38:53–55.

Hurley JK, Levy PR. Goldblatt hypertension in a solitary kidney. *J Pediatr* 1977;91:609–611.

Janeway TC. Note on blood pressure changes following reduction of the renal artery circulation. *Proc Soc Exp Biol Med* 1908;6:109–111.

Kaufman JJ, Maxwell MH. Surgery for renovascular hypertension. *JAMA* 1964;190:709–714.

McCormack LJ, Poutasse EF, Meaney TF, Noto TJ, Dustan HP. A pathologic arteriographic correlation of renal arterial disease. *Am Heart J* 1966;72:188–190.

Paul RE, Jr., Ettinger A, Fainsinger MH, Callow AD, Kahn DC, Inker LH. Angiographic visualization of renal collateral circulation as a means of detecting and delineating renal ischemia. *Radiology* 1965;84:1013–1018.

Palubinskas AJ, Ripley HR. Fibromuscular hyperplasia in extrarenal arteries. *Radiology* 1969;82:451–455.

Pemsel HK, Thermann M. Zur hamodynamischen Wirksamkeit der Nieren arterienstenose. ROFO 1978;129:189–192.

Schalekamp MAD. Mechanism of renal hypertension. *Lancet* 1976;5:1219–1221.

Renal Artery Percutaneous Transluminal Angioplasty (RAPTA)

ROSA MARIA RAOLINI

RAPTA is an effective method for treatment of arterial hypertension when the hypertension is exclusively due to renal artery stenosis.

Note that the absence of renin lateralization is not a contraindication; patients who do not show it may still benefit from RAPTA.

INDICATIONS AND CONTRAINDICATIONS

A decision to recommend RAPTA is made on the basis of clinical and anatomic criteria. Clinical criteria are the patient's hemodynamic state, renin lateralization, response to the Captopryl test, blood pressure levels, and response to antihypertensive therapy. Anatomic criteria are isolated stenosis, restenosis, posttransplant stenosis, and graft stenosis.

Anatomic contraindications are the presence of ostial lesions and recent mural thrombus. Total renal artery occlusion, with collateral circulation, is not a contraindication; recanalization is obtained in about 30 percent of such cases.

BASIC TECHNIQUE

The basic technique consists of percutaneous puncture of the femoral or axillary arteries, selective renal artery catheterization, and introduction of a guidewire through the stenosed area. The guidewire is left in position inside one branch of the renal artery, and the diagnostic catheter is removed and a balloon catheter introduced over the guidewire. The balloon is positioned precisely inside the stenosed segment and insufflated several times with contrast medium until the desired dilatation is obtained. Following that, control angiography is performed (Fig. 6.38).

RAPTA has been particularly successful in young patients with fibromuscular dysplasia and a recent history

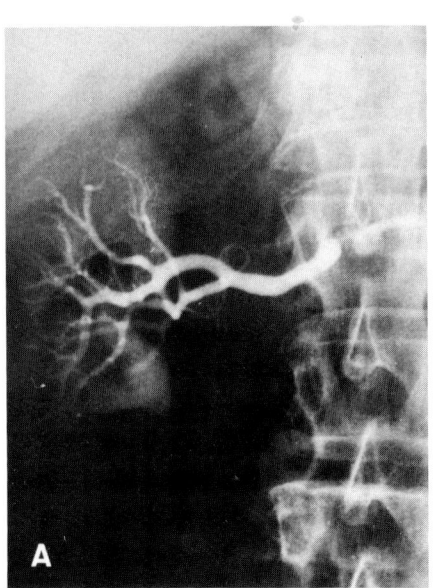
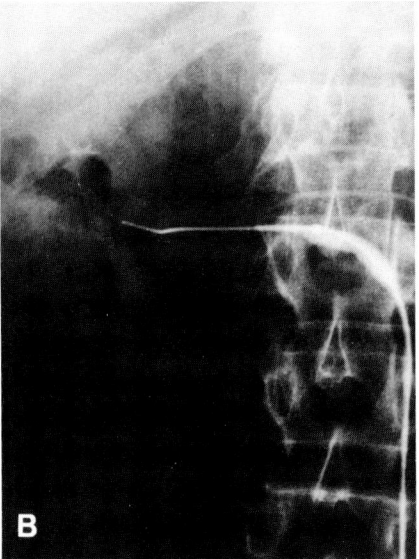
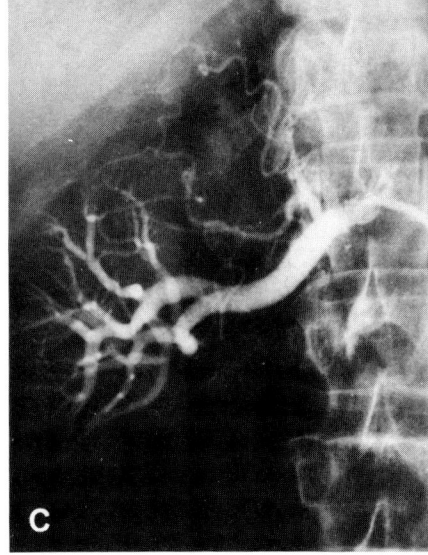

Figure 6.38 (A) 70-year-old patient with almost total arteriosclerotic stenosis at the origin of the right renal artery. (B) Dilatation with 5-mm balloon. (C) Control after dilatation shows recanalization and an increase in diameter of the intrarenal circulation. Before the procedure arterial blood pressure was 220/120; it was 210/120 by the end of the procedure, and 140/80 24 h later.

Table 6.2 – Renal percutaneous transluminal angioplasty: Technical results

	Year	Fibromuscular, %	Total %	Atherosclerotic, %	Restenosis, %
Bussman	1983	...	75	...	20
Lohr	1983	...	81		
Mahler	1983	90	...	79	
Richter	1983	...	92		
Zeitler*	1983	...	90		
Cumberland	1984	...	95		
Paolini	1984	94	...	78	
Obrez	1984	86	...	71	
Sos	1984	93	...	84	
French*					
Joffre	1985	...	82.6		
Puijlaert	1985	81	...	73	8
Schwarten	1985	100	...	94	23
Sorensen	1985	...	85		
Tegtmeyer	1985	...	94	...	13

* Cooperative study.

Table 6.3 – Renal PTA: Clinical findings (six months of follow-up, cured or improved)

	Year	Fibromuscular, %	Total, %	Atherosclerotic, %	Miscellaneous
Colapinto	1982				
Simonetti	1983	86	...	82	
Lohr	1983	...	80		
Mahler	1983	90	...	66	
Richter	1983	...	66		
Zeitler*	1983	78	...	57	
Cumberland	1984	100	...	85	75 trans.
Paolini	1984	90	...	78	
Obrez	1984	86	...	62	20 misc.
Sos	1984	93	...	84	
French*	1985	...	71.3		
Puijlaert	1985	81	...	62	
Schwarten	1985	100	...	94	
Sorensen	1985	89	...	83	
Tegtmeyer	1985	100	...	94	

* Cooperative study.

of short-duration renovascular hypertension, resulting in cure or good control of the disease. Results in patients with arterial stenosis due to atherosclerotic disease are not as good as those obtained in cases of fibromuscular dysplasia, because atherosclerotic patients almost always have a history of long-duration arterial hypertension. They are generally older, and many of them exhibit intrarenal involvement. However, even for these patients ambulatory control of the hypertension may be obtained. (See Tables 6.2 and 6.3.)

Limiting factors are almost always anatomic in nature. The stenosis may be so severe that balloon introduction using standard equipment is impossible; this difficulty is presently being overcome by use of special low-profile catheters. Stenosis may be so calcified or elastic that it resists dilatation, and in some cases it is not possible to reach the stenosis.

RAPTA is a low-cost alternative to surgery. It is generally easy to perform, and complications are rare. Dilatation may be repeated as many times as necessary, and will not prevent surgery from being performed if that becomes necessary.

RAPTA IN KIDNEY TRANSPLANT CASES

Hypertension occurs in 24 to 60 percent of cases of renal transplants. The incidence is higher in patients receiving kidneys from cadavers than in those receiving kidneys from living donors.

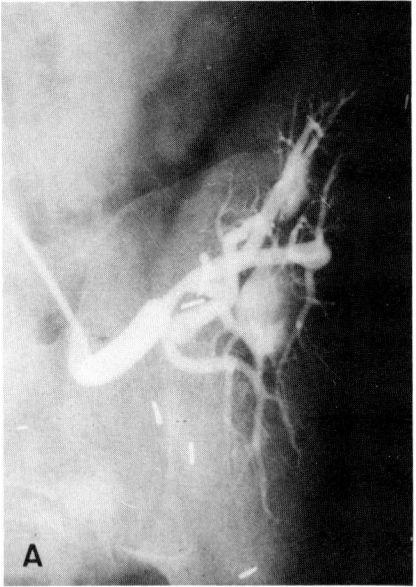 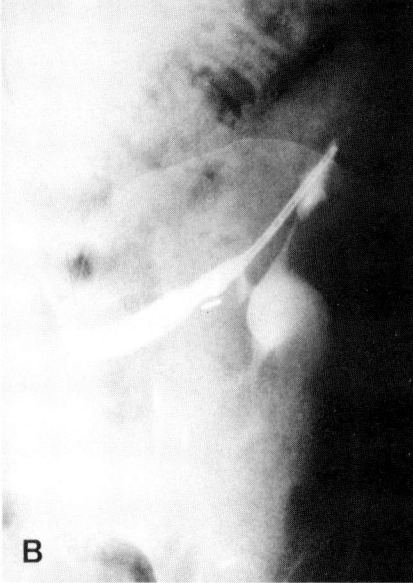 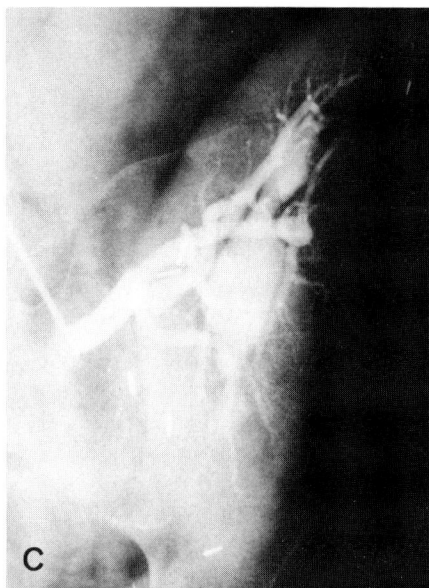

Figure 6.39 (A) 47-year-old patient with transplanted kidney who presented with sudden-onset hypertension, with murmur over the renal graft. Tubular stenosis near the anastomosis was about 70 percent. (B) Dilatation with 6-mm long-tip balloon, inadequate for renal use, using the contralateral approach. (C) Control angiogram after dilatation shows improvement of stenosis. Before dilatation, the systolic pressure gradient was 80 mmHg; after dilatation, only 17 mmHg. Preangiography arterial pressure was 180/120; 24 h after the procedure it was 130/70.

The occurrence of stenosis and occlusions in renal peripheral arterial circulation during the chronic rejection stage is well documented. This causes hyperreninemia, which leads to arterial hypertension. Another cause of hypertension in transplant patients is the chronic use of corticosteroids.

Stenosis of the main artery of the transplanted kidney may lead to hypertension by exactly the same mechanism that occurs in the main artery of the native kidney. The incidence of hypertension as a result of posttransplant arterial stenosis may be 4 to 10 percent; in one series it was 25 percent.

The most common arterial anastomoses in renal transplants are done with the hypogastric artery (end-to-end) and with the external iliac artery (end-to-side). Stenosis seems to be more frequent with end-to-end anastomosis. The causes of stenosis vary. When the stenosis is proximally located in the internal iliac artery, atherosclerosis is the cause. Stenosis located in the anastomosis may be the result of an arterial lesion caused by kidney perfusion, localized reaction to suture, or discrepancies in the arterial diameter between donor and receptor (Fig. 6.39). Rarely, a fibroplastic lesion of the media will develop in the artery of the transplanted kidney (Fig. 6.40).

All transplanted patients, with severe, uncontrollable arterial hypertension which develops after the transplant, with murmur present over the graft, should undergo angiographic evaluation as well as renin assay in the renal veins of both the native and the transplanted kidney. Seventy-five percent reduction in the cross-section area of the transplanted renal artery, and a systolic pressure gradient of at least 20 percent, are indications of significant stenosis, which should be treated.

Technique

The approach to the artery of the transplanted kidney will vary according to the type of anastomosis performed. For end-to-side anastomosis, an ipsilateral femoral puncture is the most appropriate route; end-to-end anastomosis with the internal iliac artery is best approached by contralateral femoral puncture or by the axillary route.

Angiographic identification and assessment of the degree of stenosis are best performed obliquely, with complete dissociation between the internal iliac artery and the renal artery of the graft.

Most stenoses are seen on the site of anastomosis (Fig. 6.39) or are distal to it (Fig. 6.40). To avoid superimposition of the iliac external artery, injection should be selective into the hypogastric artery.

The approach in cases of anastomosis with the hypogastric artery should be contralateral. The catheter is passed through the aortic bifurcation and down into the common iliac until it reaches the hypogastric (Fig. 6.40). After the hypogastric has been catheterized and pressure measured, a guidewire with an extra-flexible straight tip or with a very closed J-tip is advanced through the

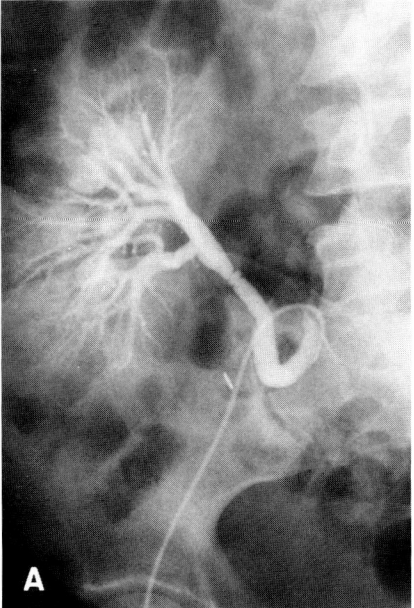 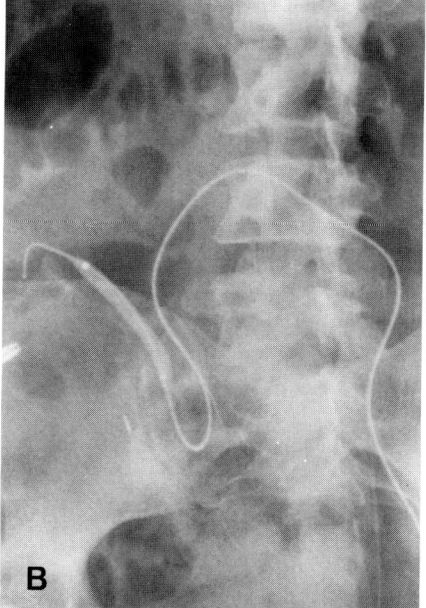 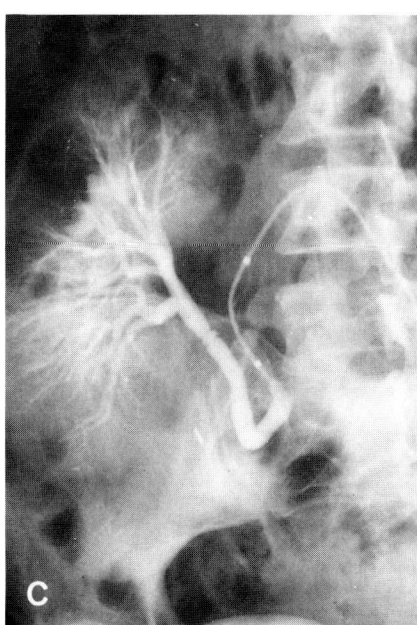

Figure 6.40 (A) Hypertension-producing stenosis due to muscle fiber dysplasia of transplanted kidney artery. Arteriographic study of the living donor had not shown any arterial lesion. (B) Dilatation of very tortuous stenosis using contralateral catheterization with a 6-mm balloon catheter. (C) Control following dilatation shows improvement of the lesion, although constriction rings are still evident. The arterial blood pressure became normal after dilatation.

stenosis. The catheter is then advanced over the guidewire until it reaches the intrarenal circulation, where pressure is again measured. The first guidewire is then replaced by a more rigid guidewire, and the catheter is replaced by a dilatation balloon catheter of the appropriate diameter. A high-pressure balloon catheter should be used when the stenotic lesion is related to an anastomosis in which a fibrotic component predominates.

After angioplasty, intrarenal pressure is measured, and when the catheter is pulled back, hypogastric pressure is once again evaluated. If the systolic pressure gradient is within normal parameters, and a control angiogram shows adequate dilation, the procedure is considered completed.

REFERENCES

Gruntzig A, Kuhlmann V, Vetter W, et al. Treatment of renovascular hypertension with percutaneous transluminal dilatation of a renal artery stenosis. *Lancet* 1978;1:801–802.

Katzen B, Chang J, Lubowsky GH, Abranson EG. Percutaneous transluminal angioplasty for treatment of renovascular hypertension. *Radiology* 1979;131:53–58.

Mahler F, Krenta R, Haertal M. Treatment of renovascular hypertension by transluminal renal artery dilatation. *Ann Intern Med* 1979;90:57–58.

Paolini RM. Clinical and laboratory results of renal artery stenosis percutaneous transluminal angioplasty. *Intervent Radiol 2.* Excerpta Medica 1982;327–331.

Paolini RM, Marcondes M, Widman A, Sabbaga E, Silva HB, Nussensweig I, Magalhaes AA. Percutaneous transluminal angioplasty of renal artery stenosis. *Acta Radiol* 1981;22:571–675.

Saddekni S, Sniderman KW, Hilton S, Sos TA. Percutaneous transluminal angioplasty of nonatherosclerotic lesion. *AJR* 1980;135:975–982.

Schwarten DE. Transluminal angioplasty of renal artery stenosis: 70 experiences. *AJR* 1980;135:969–974.

Sniderman KW, Sprayregen S, Sos TA, et al. Percutaneous transluminal dilatation in renal transplant arterial stenosis. *Transplantation* 1980;30:440–444.

Sos TA, Barbaric ZL, Sniderman KW. Transluminal angioplasty in the management of renovascular hypertension secondary to fibromuscular dysplasia. In *Transluminal Angioplasty,* edited by Castaneda-Zuniga WR. Thieme-Stratton, New York, 1983;70–80.

Sos TA, Pickering TG, Sniderman K, et al. Percutaneous transluminal renal angioplasty in renovascular hypertension due to atheroma or fibromuscular dysplasia. *N Engl J Med* 1983;309:274–279.

Teates CD, Tegtmeyer CJ, Croft BY, Ayers CR. Effects of percutaneous transluminal angioplasty on renal plasma flow. *Semin Nucl Med* 1983;13:245–257.

Tegtmeyer CJ. Percutaneous transluminal renal angioplasty: The evolution of a procedure. *Arch Intern Med* 1982;142:1085–1087.

Tegtmeyer CJ, Ayers CA, Wellons HA. The axillary approach to percutaneous renal artery dilatation. *Radiology* 1980;135:775–776.

Tegtmeyer CJ, Dyer R, Teates CD, et al. Percutaneous transluminal dilatation of the renal arteries. *Radiology* 1980;135:589–599.

Tegtmeyer CJ, Elson J, Glass TA, et al. Percutaneous transluminal angioplasty: The treatment of choice for renovascular hypertension due to fibromuscular dysplasia. *Radiology* 1982;143:631–637.

Tegtmeyer CJ, Kellum CD, Ayers C. Percutaneous transluminal angioplasty of the renal artery: Results and long-term follow-up. *Radiology* 1984;153:77–84.

Tegtmeyer CJ, Kofler TJ, Ayers CA. Renal angioplasty: Current status. *AJR* 1984;142:17–21.

Tegtmeyer CJ, Sos TA, Schwarten DE. Peripheral angioplasty. *Intervention* 1984;1:16–24.

Tegtmeyer CJ, Teates CD, Crigler N, Gandee RW, Ayers CR, Stoddard M, Wallons HA. Percutaneous transluminal angioplasty in patients with renal artery stenosis: Follow-up studies. *Radiology* 1981;140:323–330.

Angioplasty of the Aorta and the Aortic Bifurcation

RENAN UFLACKER

Until relatively recently, angioplasty was not used to treat isolated aortic stenosis or stenosis of the aortic bifurcation, both of which are rare complications of occlusive atheromatous disease. It was believed that inflating the balloon would occlude the contralateral iliac artery and would displace a plaque or cause distal embolization. Advances in materials and technical resources, however, have expanded the indications for angioplasty to include the aorta and the aortic bifurcation (Fig. 6.41).

Transluminal angioplasty of the bifurcation of the aorta is performed using two balloons, which are simultaneously introduced through both femoral arteries and inflated at the same time, to avoid the problem of contralateral occlusion and distal embolism. (This procedure is known as the "kissing balloons" technique; see Figs. 6.42 and 6.43.)

If the bifurcation is not involved and the stenosis is located 1 to 2 cm above the origin of the iliac arteries, two balloons should be used if the normal section of the aorta is not too large (Fig. 6.43). Using catheters with balloons larger than 8 mm is contraindicated due to the risk of thrombotic complications at the site of puncture and the iliac arteries. When the aortic diameter is larger, two large balloons must be used. For example, when the aortic diameter is 13 mm, a 6-mm and a 7-mm balloon should be used, with the smaller one dilating the less stenotic iliac artery or the finer of the iliac arteries. When the aortic diameter is around 16 mm, two 8-mm balloons should be used.

Figure 6.42 illustrates the use of two 8-mm-diameter 8-cm-long balloon catheters.

When there is any doubt regarding success of the angioplasty, a digital venous angiogram may be performed immediately after the procedure in order to demonstrate vascular patency (Fig. 6.42). Diagnostic angiography and angioplasty may be performed at the same time. A 0.035-in. 1.5-mm J-guidewire with a movable core is introduced beyond the lesion. If this is not possible, a No. 5 French catheter with a 150° curve on the tip can be advanced through the stenosis or stenoses. One alternative is to use a guidewire with torque control (Figs. 6.10 and 6.11).

Occasionally, the curved catheter may be maneuvered

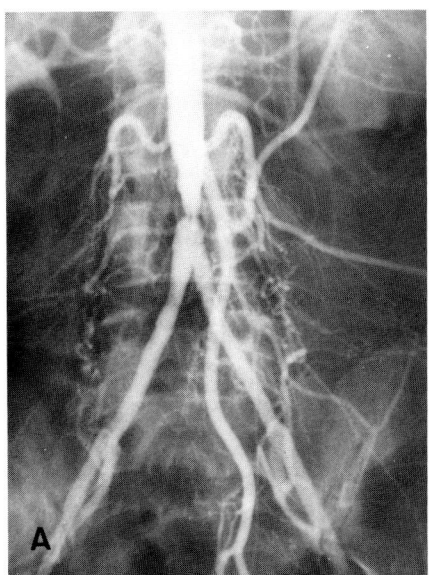
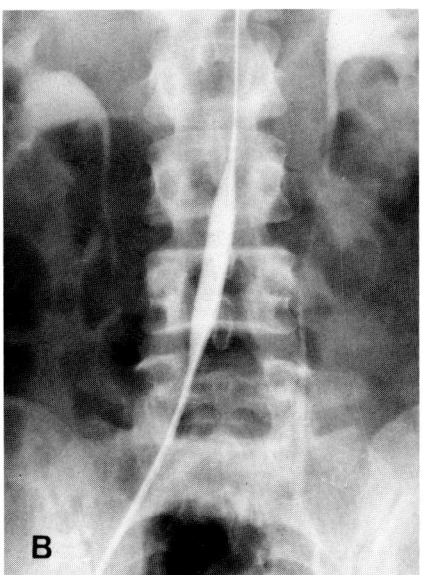
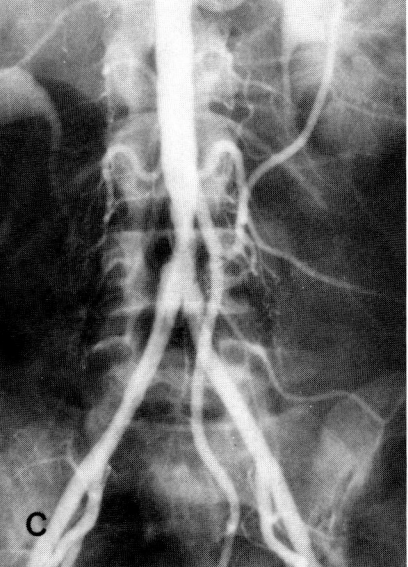

Figure 6.41 (A) 42-year-old patient with lower limb claudication due to 85 percent stenosis in abdominal aorta near the bifurcation. (B) 8-mm catheter dilating the aorta (high-pressure PE-PLUS balloon). (C) Control following dilatation shows dilated segment. Claudication has disappeared, but residual stenosis is present. The thrombosis that occurred on the site of femoral puncture was surgically treated, using local anesthesia.

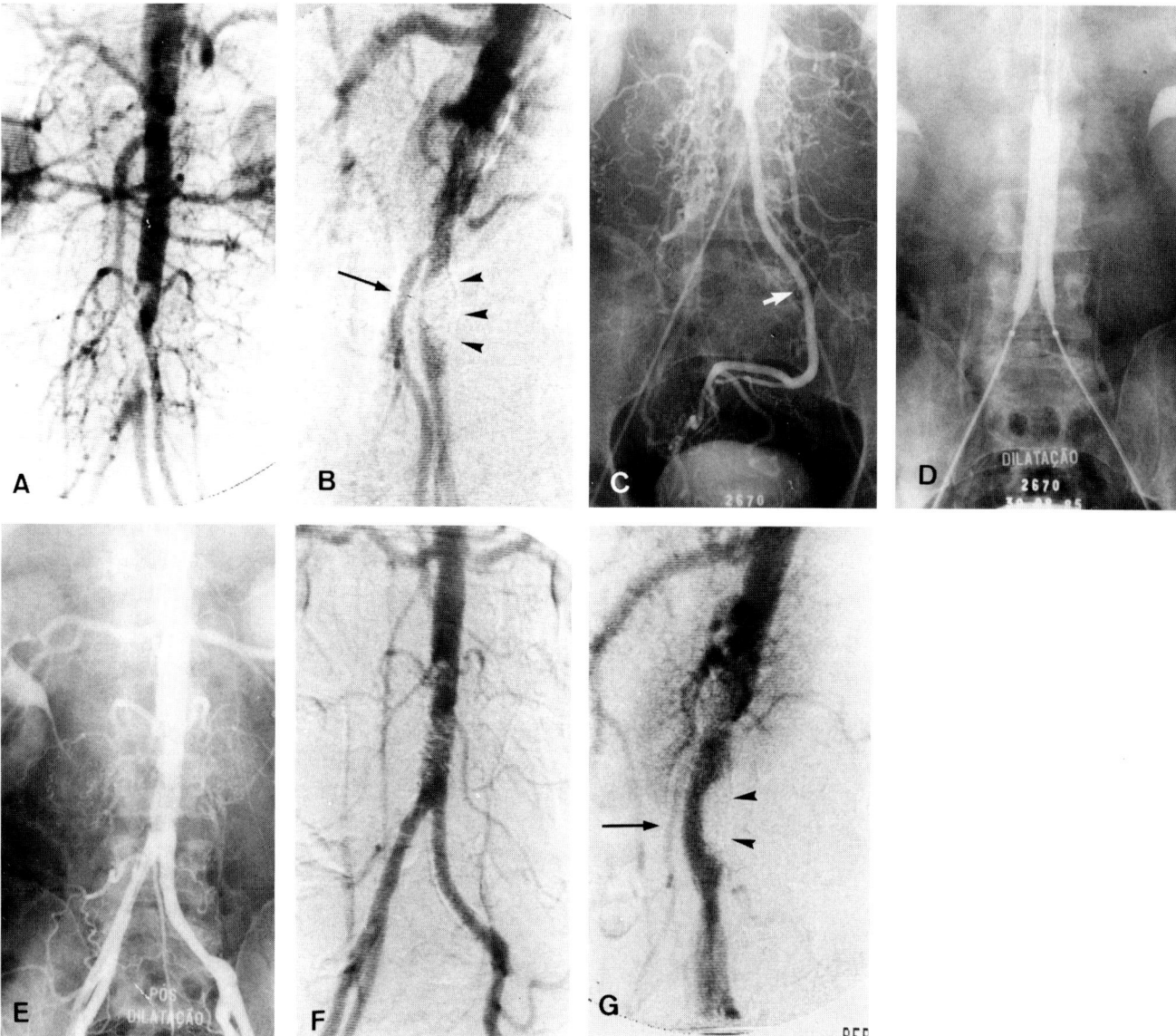

Figure 6.42 (A) 56-year-old patient with lower limb claudication due to aortic occlusion near the bifurcation (anteroposterior). (B) A venous digital angiographic profile of the aorta shows the calcified plaque and severe stenosis (arrowheads). The arrow shows the inferior mesenteric artery. (C) Femoral-route angiogram shows the catheter occluding the stenosis. There is no distal filling of the iliacs. Note the large diameter of the inferior mesenteric artery (arrow). (D) Two 8-mm diameter 8-cm-long catheters dilating the aorta. (E) Control angiogram immediately after dilatation shows aortic recanalization. (F) Venous digital angiogram (anteroposterior view) about 1 month after angioplasty shows reasonable smoothness of the dilated segment and occlusion of the left external iliac, which was treated with femoral iliac graft. (G) Aortic lateral view shows the dilated segment and the remaining plaque (arrowheads). The inferior mesenteric artery (arrow) was reduced in size.

under fluoroscopic guidance, with simultaneous contrast injection. The patient should be heparinized with 5000 IU directly into the aorta after the lesions have been passed. If the use of two balloons is necessary, the same procedure is performed on the other side.

When the kissing balloons technique is used, the distal tips of the balloons should remain in the aorta, slightly above the aortic plaque, and the proximal tips inside the iliac arteries (Fig. 6.42). With this method, 10- to 12-atm pressures may be needed for effective dilatation. In a recent series, in which follow-up varied from 1 to 53 months after dilatation (average, 14 months), the procedure was successful in 94 percent of the cases. Redilatation was required in 10 percent of those cases due to lesion recurrence.

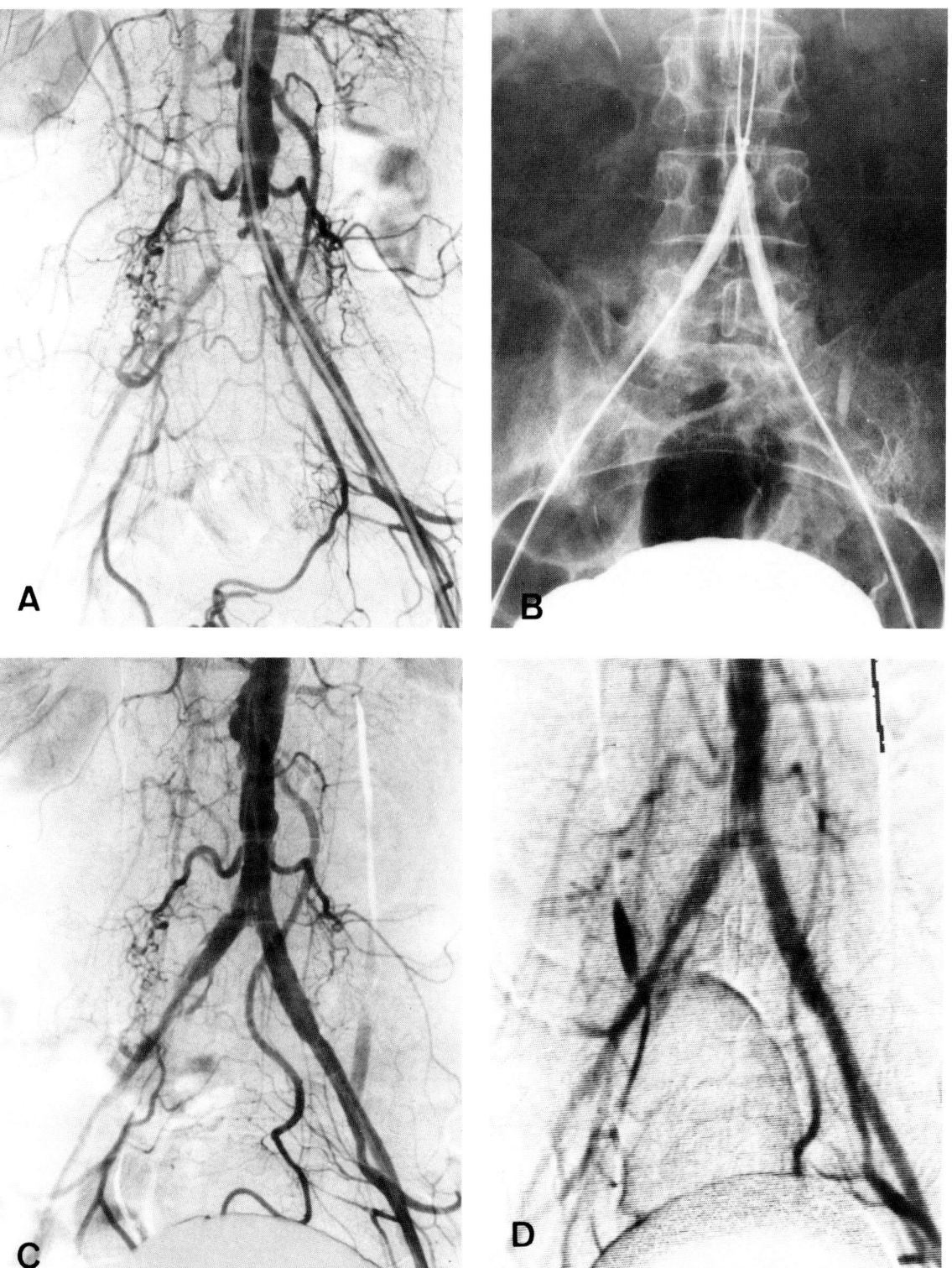

Figure 6.43 (A) 59-year-old patient with aortoiliac occlusion on the right and aortoiliac stenosis on the left. (B) Femoral-route dilatation with two 6-mm ("kissing") balloons. (C) Angiogram immediately after angioplasty showing adequate recanalization of the dilated segment. (D) Venous digital angiogram taken immediately after compression for "absence" of pulse on the right, which actually turned out to be only a spasm. Before dilatation, for 130 mmHg systemic pressure, tibial pressures on the right were 50 mmHg before dilatation. 24 h following dilatation, for 120 mmHg systemic pressure, tibial pressures on the right were 110 mmHg.

REFERENCES

Castaneda-Zuniga WR, Amplatz K. Transluminal angioplasty of the abdominal aorta. In *Transluminal Angioplasty,* edited by Castaneda-Zuniga WR. Thieme-Stratton, New York, 1983;195–200.

Feldman CJ, Genro CH, Vitola D, et al. Angioplastia transluminal percutanea da aorta abdominal: Relato de caso. Rev AMRIGS 1986;30:36–38.

Groilman JH, Delvicario M, Mittal AK. Percutaneous transluminal abdominal aortic angioplasty. *AJR* 1980;134:1053–1054.

Ingrish H, Seyferth W, Kuffer G. Percutaneous transluminal angioplasty in cases of stenosis in the region of the infrarenal abdominal aorta and the aortoiliac bifurcation. In *Percutaneous Transluminal Angioplasty,* edited by Dotter CT, Gruntzig AR, Schoop W, Zeitler E. Springer-Verlag, Berlin, 1984:127–130.

Tegtmeyer CJ, Kellum CD, Kron IL, et al. Percutaneous transluminal angioplasty in the region of the aortic bifurcation: The two-balloon technique with results and long-term follow-up study. *Radiology* 1985;157:661–665.

Tegtmeyer CJ, Wellons HA, Thompson RN. Balloon dilatation of the abdominal aorta. *JAMA* 1980;244:2636–2637.

Velasquez G, Castaneda-Zuniga WR, Formaneck AG, et al. Nonsurgical aortoplasty in the Leriche syndrome. *Radiology* 1980;134:359–360.

Angioplasty of the Iliac Arteries

RENAN UFLACKER

ILIAC STENOSIS

The "ideal" lesion for angioplasty in the iliac arteries is the atherosclerotic plaque localized in one segment of a straight artery, without any other type of lesion (Fig. 6.44). Dilatation of this type of plaque is completely successful in a vast majority of cases (Fig. 6.44). Occasionally, the follow-up study will show a residual although broadly patent, lesion (Fig. 6.44) in oblique or profile view.

Either the retrograde (ipsilateral) or antegrade (axillary or contralateral) approach may be used. For lesions in the common iliac and proximal external iliac arteries, the retrograde approach is a better choice. For lesions in the external iliac artery, close to the inguinal ligament, the antegrade approach should be used. When it is not possible to advance beyond the lesion using a retrograde approach, the antegrade approach may be tried.

There are two reasons for preferring the retrograde approach. First, a catheter introduced retrogradely may be maintained in position after pressure measurement, making it unnecessary to change the balloon catheter before performing control angiography (Fig. 6.45). Second, in case of intimal dissection or plaque separation, there is minimal chance of flow occlusion. With the axillary approach, in contrast, intimal dissection acts as a valve and may occlude the artery.

Although bilateral femoral puncture involves two arterial punctures, it is quite safe, because manipulation through the lesion is minimal and there is a low risk of hematoma formation on the puncture site. The selection of balloon diameter and length is made by taking cross-sectional measurements of the normal artery above and below the lesion. For a common iliac artery in a patient of average size, an 8-mm-diameter 4-cm-long balloon will be adequate in most cases. In young women and patients whose body weight is below average, a 6-mm-diameter balloon will be adequate. Occasionally, when the affected artery is occluded or extremely reduced in diameter due to low flow, the diameter of the contralateral artery may be used as the baseline for balloon selection.

The ipsilateral retrograde approach involves puncturing an impalpable vessel, and thus anatomic landmarks or ultrasound must be used to locate the vessel. After puncture, particularly when the occlusion is total, low-pressure flow will be obtained. A straight No. 5 French catheter is then introduced for measuring the pressure. If the artery is rectilinear and the stenosis concentric, a straight guidewire may be gently advanced beyond the lesion to reach the abdominal aorta. If the stenosis is eccentric and/or the artery is tortuous, a J-guidewire and a Tegtmeyer catheter with an angulated tip should be used. Techniques for advancing the catheter-guidewire set were described earlier in this chapter (see Figs. 6.10 and 6.11).

After the catheter has been advanced, a control injection may be performed, pressure measurements taken, and anticoagulants administered. The catheter is then removed, the guidewire being maintained in position for introduction of the balloon catheter. It is seldom necessary to dilate the track with Teflon dilators. The force applied to the balloon catheter is linear, so it is easy to advance the catheter into the virtual lumen of the artery. Generally, pressure should not exceed 4 atm, and a manometer should always be used during dilatation. Complete insufflation of the balloon means that maximum dilation has been achieved.

An 8-mm balloon that has been used in the common iliac artery should not be pulled down and used to dilate the external iliac artery, as the risk of rupture is very high. There is even the possibility that a pseudoaneurysm could be formed (Fig. 6.8). The same balloon may, however, be used to dilate the contralateral iliac artery using the antegrade approach (Fig. 6.46).

Some authors advise that the balloon be pulled down below the stenosis (distally) after dilatation, and a new pressure measurement taken while a small-diameter (0.021-in.) guidewire is kept in position through the dilated lesion. Reintroduction of a guidewire through a dilated iliac lesion may cause trauma, raising intimal flaps and leading to thrombosis. The balloon catheter is then replaced by an angiographic catheter in order to perform the control. Generally, a large-diameter catheter is used, to prevent bleeding at the puncture site due to arterial hole enlargement when the balloon is removed. Frequently, the angiographic catheter is introduced through the contralateral femoral route, which prevents this exchange, and care must be taken to advance the balloon to the aorta over the guidewire. With postsurgical arterial lesions, in which a fibrotic component predominates,

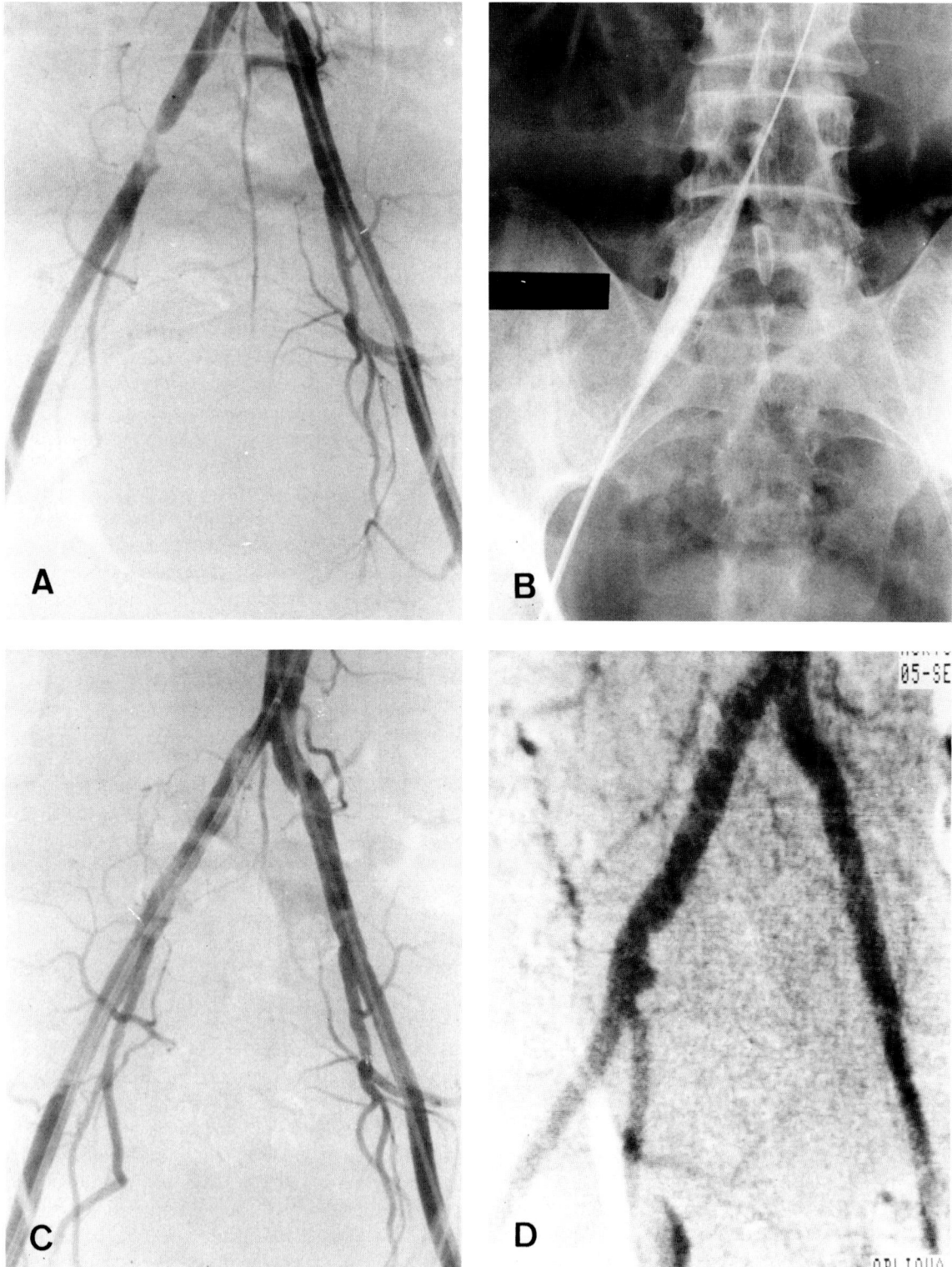

Figure 6.44 (A) 59-year-old patient with focal stenosis on the right iliac common artery, and severe claudication. (B) Dilatation with 8-mm balloon catheter. (C) Control after dilatation shows smooth arterial surface. (D) Digital venous control, right anterior oblique view, 2 months later, shows posterior residual plaque. The patient was asymptomatic. Pretreatment systemic pressure was 150 mmHg; tibial pressures were both 90 mmHg. Posttreatment systemic pressure was 135 mmHg; tibial pressures were both 135 mmHg.

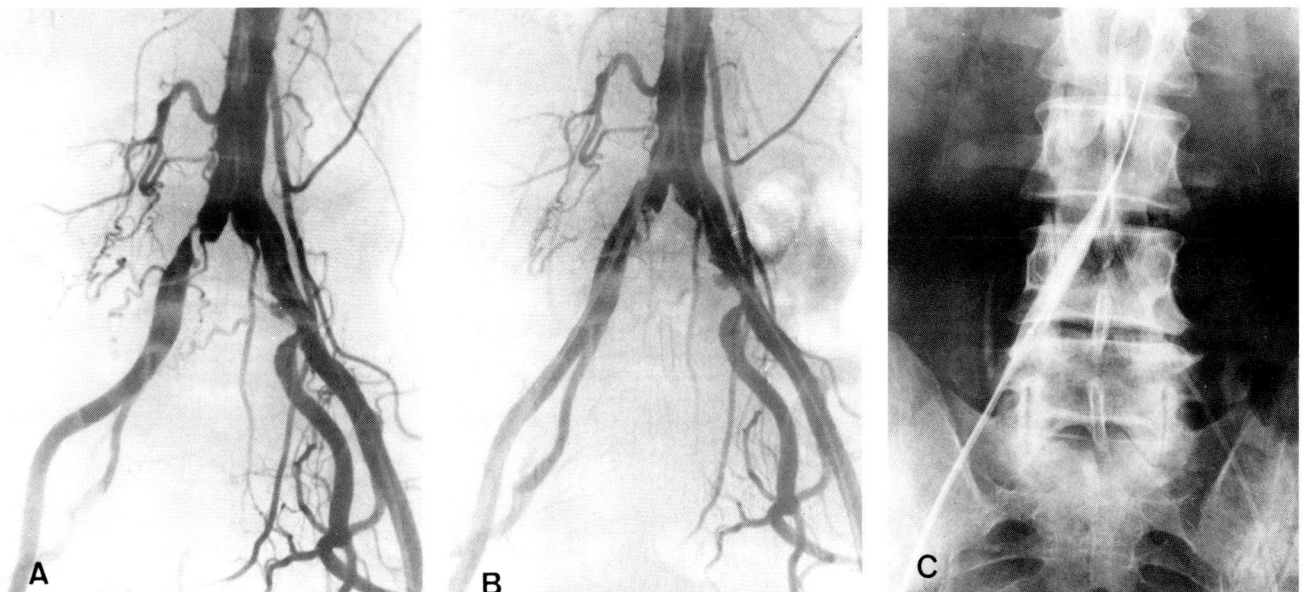

Figure 6.45 (A) 57-year-old patient with preocclusive stenosis of the right iliac common artery, and claudication. Systemic pressure was 140 mmHg. Right anterior tibial pressure was 90 mmHg; right posterior tibial pressure was 120 mmHg. (B) Control after dilatation shows residual stenosis. Postdilatation systemic pressure was 140 mmHg; tibial pressures were both 140 mmHg. (C) 8-mm balloon in position for dilatation. Patient was asymptomatic following the angioplasty.

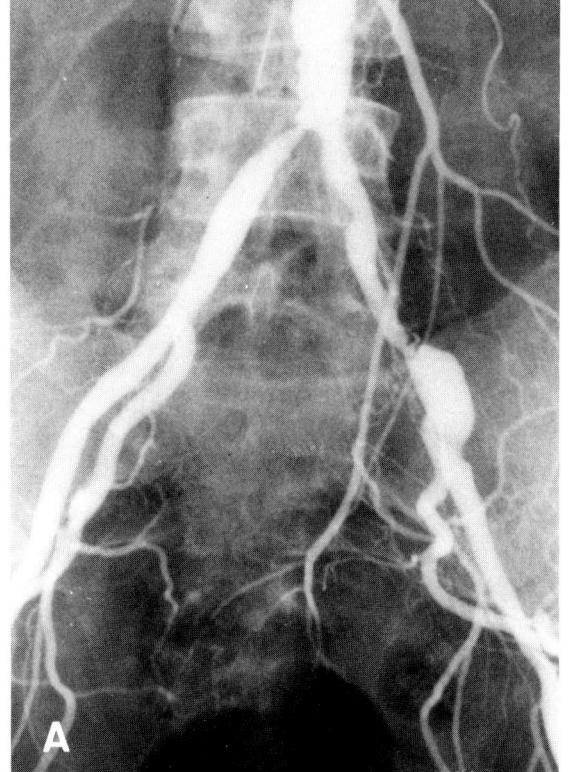
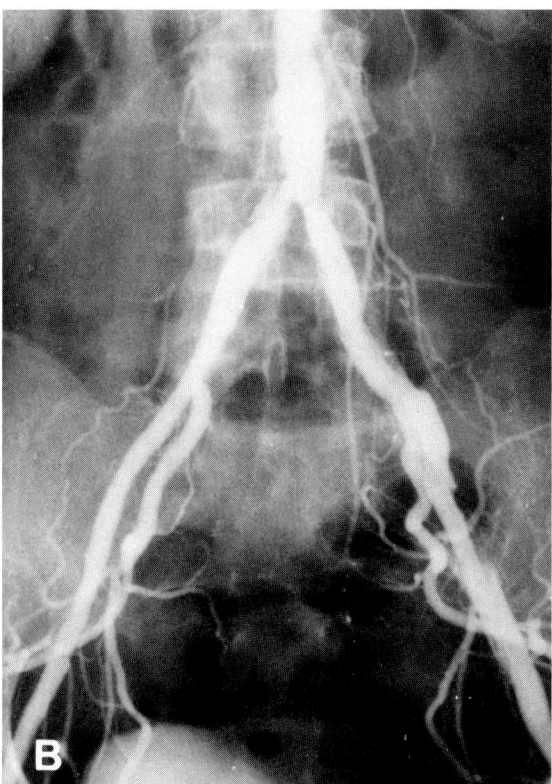

Figure 6.46 (A) 54-year-old patient with multiple stenoses in both iliac arteries, including poststenotic dilatation on the left, and 50-m claudication. (B) Control following bilateral angioplasty using unifemoral puncture. Note the fractures in the atheromatous plaques. The symptoms were resolved, and claudication disappeared.

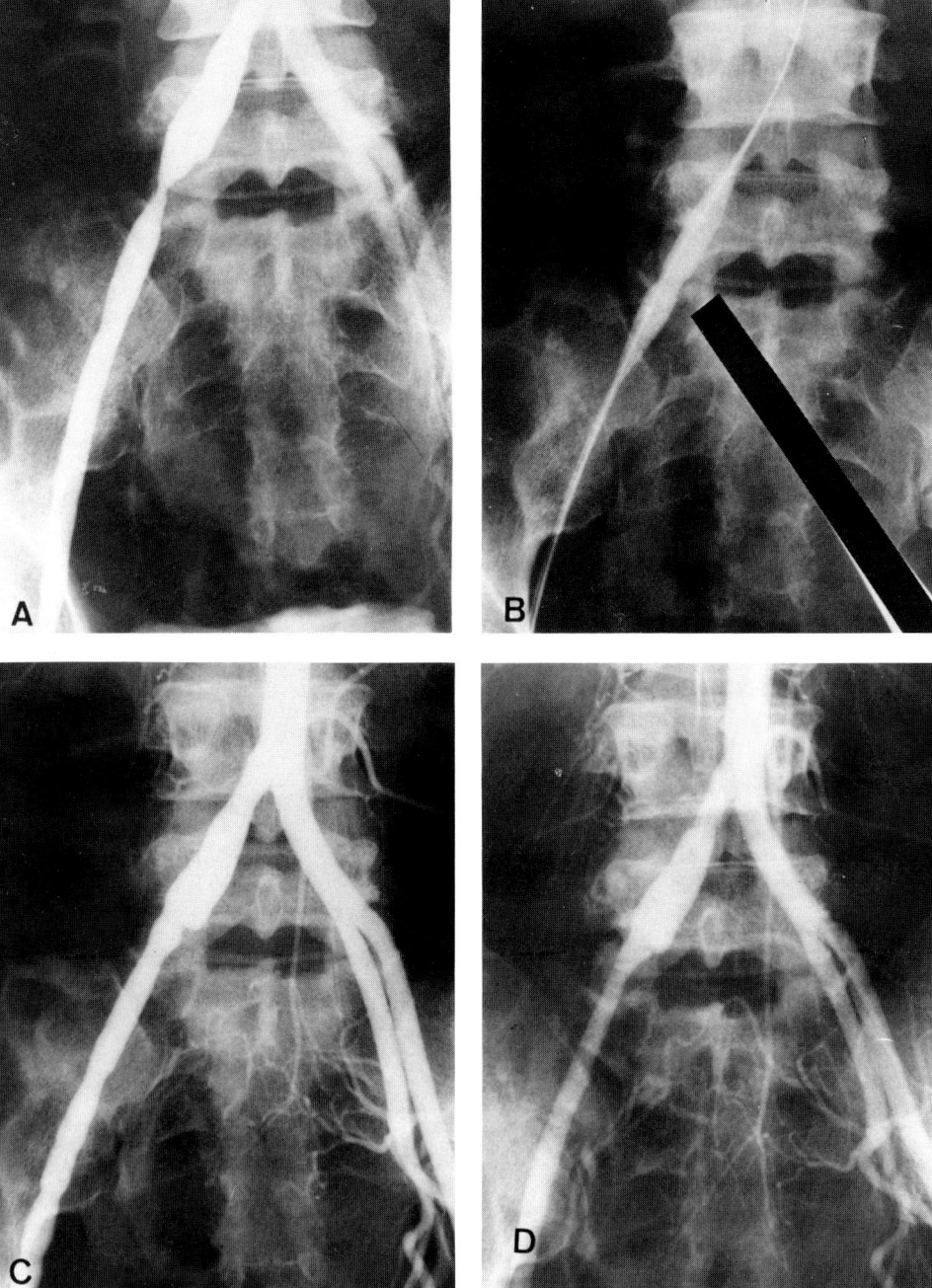

Figure 6.47 (A) Residual stenosis following thromboendarterectomy of the right common iliac artery. 100-m claudication due to ischemic ulcerating lesions in toes. (B) 8-mm balloon dilating the lesion. Notice the hourglass shape of the high-pressure balloon. (C) Control angiogram immediately after dilatation showing good results. (C) Claudication recurred 1 month later due to distal occlusive lesions (thromboangiitis obliterans); however, the femoral pulse was good, and the artery was patent.

complete dilation of the balloon may not be possible, even under high pressure (Fig. 6.47). The dilatation that is obtained, however, is effective and permanent.

In aortoiliac or femoroiliac grafts with stenosis on the anastomosis, it is advisable to use the contralateral approach, so as to prevent direct puncture of the graft. Here, also, complete dilatation may not be possible (Fig. 6.48). The contralateral antegrade approach is also recommended if the retrograde method has not been successful, the pulse is not palpable, or the stenosis is too close to the puncture site. Note, however, that if the pulse is not palpable, fluoroscopically guided puncture is successful in most cases. The technique of contralateral iliac artery catheterization was discussed in Chap. 1; it is shown schematically in Fig. 6.7. When the axillary approach is used, it is generally necessary to use catheters at least 100 cm in length. With the antegrade approach, practically all vessels of the treated limb, from the iliac to the popliteal artery, may be reached (Fig. 6.8).

Manipulation of dilatation catheters around the aortic bifurcation may cause the catheters to bend inside the

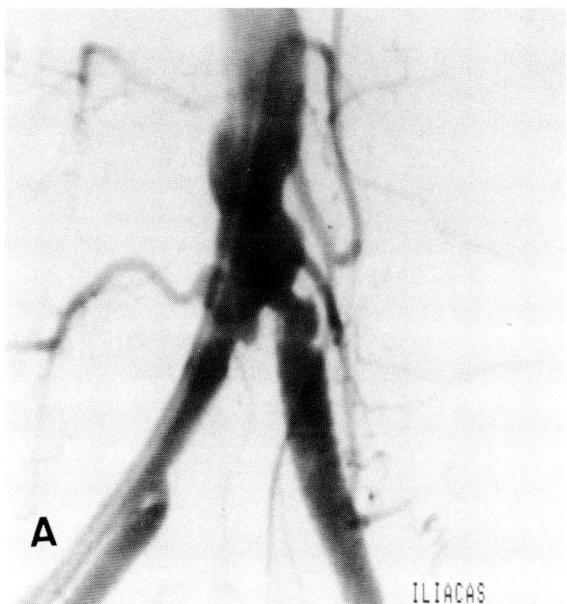

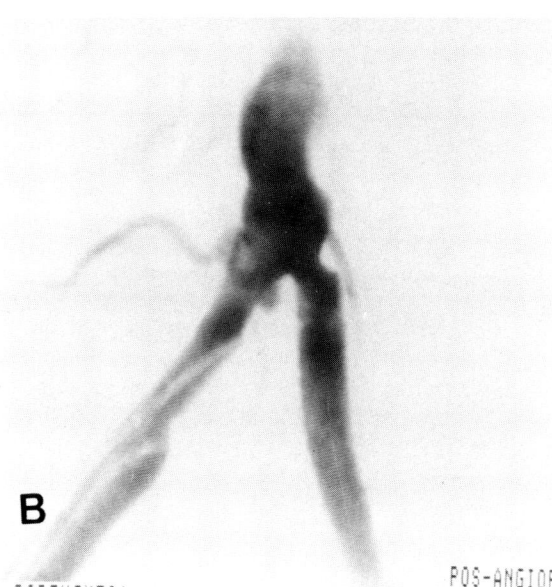

Figure 6.48 (A) 52-year-old patient with stenosis in femoroiliac graft. Predilatation left anterior tibial pressure index was 0.3. (B) After dilatation with an 8-mm balloon, the left anterior tibial pressure index went up to 0.5. Claudication improved, as did the digital ischemic lesions.

abdominal aorta, such that they do not have the necessary force to pass beyond the lesion. The use of more rigid guidewires may prevent this problem. Compressing the femoral artery on the treated side and holding the guidewire while the catheter is being advanced is generally a successful maneuver. The guidewire tip should not be moved up-and-down randomly inside the femoral artery; this may cause intimal lesion and spasm, which are risk factors for thrombosis.

Patency rates for angioplasty of iliac arteries are 93 percent after 1 year, 87 percent after 2 years, and 79 percent after 3 years.

ILIAC OCCLUSION

The proper angioplastic techniques for use at all stages in the development of atheromatous stenoses are well understood. It is more difficult, however, to understand the process by which an artery with a diameter as large as that of the iliac artery becomes totally occluded and how to achieve lasting recanalization of such an artery. The amorphous mass occluding the artery is the result of thrombosis and stagnation associated with the presence of occlusive plaques. There is no doubt that the obstruction is initiated by plaque growth, both by deposition of thrombi on the surface of the lesion and by hemorrhage into the space underneath it. In the aortoiliac axis, atheromatous plaques tend to accumulate on the aortic bifurcation and on the iliac bifurcation. After occlusion at plaque level, the flow stagnates and thrombosis results.

The thrombus tends to extend itself, both proximally and distally, as far as the origin of the vessel and up to the point of confluence with collateral vessels. Such thrombi are not well organized, and the occlusive mass is composed mainly of pasty, acellular fibrotic tissue which may remain unchanged for months or even years (Fig. 6.49). When the occlusion is of recent onset, fresh thrombi may also be identified in the occlusive mass. This mass may, of course, be dilated, compressed, and redistributed according to established angioplastic principles. Increased flow in the area may in turn lead to compression and resolution of recent thrombi.

Technically, however, angioplasty of an iliac occlusion presents difficulties not generally found in femoral arteries with the same level of occlusion. First of all, the iliac arteries tend to be more tortuous, making it difficult to advance guidewires and catheters inside them. Secondly, iliac stenoses are often extremely eccentric, making location of the entry point more difficult.

A straight catheter, or one with a 150° curve, can be used to enter the lumen, under fluoroscopic guidance. More recently, steerable guidewires with torque control have been added to the angiographic armamentarium, making it easier to advance inside tortuous or eccentric lesions.

The most difficult point to advance beyond is the origin of the common iliac artery on the aortoiliac junction, as this is where the largest atheromatous plaques are usually found. Here, guidewire and catheter may deviate from the lumen, penetrating the aortic wall and, very often, dissecting the plaque and the intima.

Once the aorta has been reached, the patient is

heparinized. The guidewire and catheter are then advanced to a higher point and a balloon catheter of the proper diameter is introduced.

Even if perfect final results are not obtained, and the iliac artery walls are irregular, the walls will smooth out due to the high flow in that artery and the final flow will be increased as compared with the immediate postangioplasty flow (Fig. 6.47).

Postangioplasty control angiography should always be performed using a catheter introduced into the contralateral artery, so as not to interfere with the dilated site (Figs. 6.49 and 6.50).

Following the angioplasty, thrombi are frequently identified inside the artery. In fact, one risk involved in this procedure is ipsilateral or contralateral distal embolism due to displacement of occlusive clots by the balloon. These clots may be repositioned, aspirated, or lysed with fibrinolytic agents (Fig. 6.50). These potential complications have led some authors to classify iliac occlusion as a disease treatable only by surgery. Overall results have, however, been quite good, the primary success rate varying between 75 and 80 percent. The patency rate after 2 years has been about 83 percent.

Angioplastic treatment of combined occlusions of the common and external iliac arteries has an extremely low success rate, below 30 percent in the small series that have been published, and therefore should not be considered as a routine procedure.

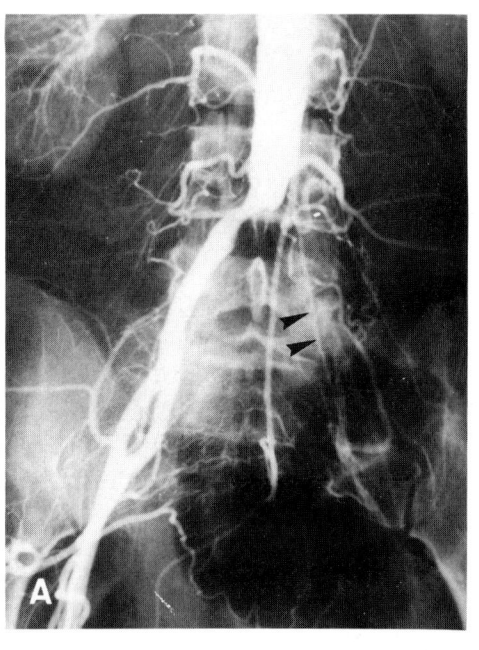
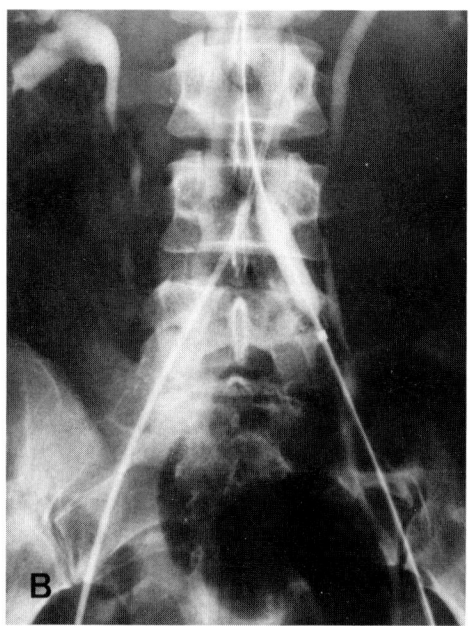
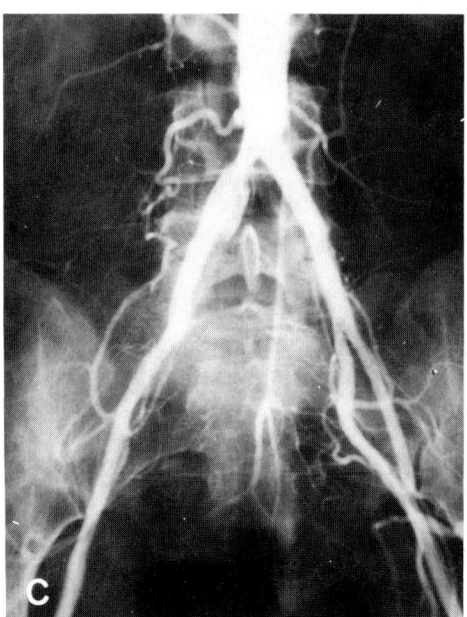
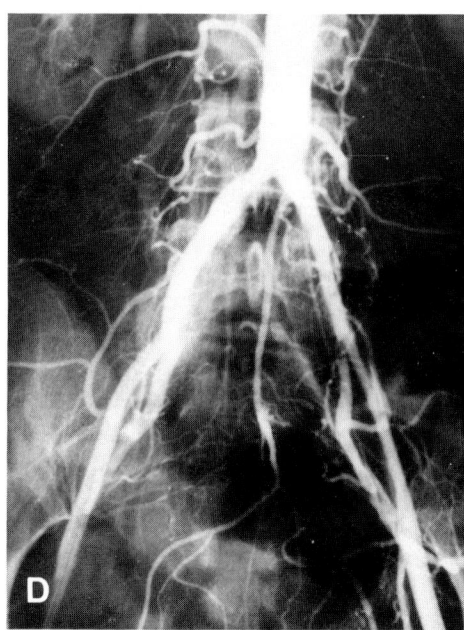

Figure 6.49 (A) Complete occlusion of the left common iliac artery, with recanalization at the external iliac level (arrowheads), in addition to stenosis of the right common iliac. (B) 8-mm balloon, introduced by the retrograde route, positioned inside the occlusion. Note the angiographic catheter on the right. (C) Control following bilateral angioplasty showing fractured plaque on the right. (D) Control 12 months later showing adequate patency of the dilated arteries, with flattening of the lesions seen in (C).

Figure 6.50 (A) 52-year-old patient, with total occlusion of the left common iliac artery, with distal recanalization. (B) 8-mm-balloon in position for dilatation. (C) Control immediately after angioplasty. Note the thrombus inside the recanalized common iliac artery (arrow). (D) The clot was manipulated and partially aspirated, remaining on the aortic bifurcation (arrow). Angioplasty was successful. Symptoms, were corrected, and no complications were caused by the thrombus.

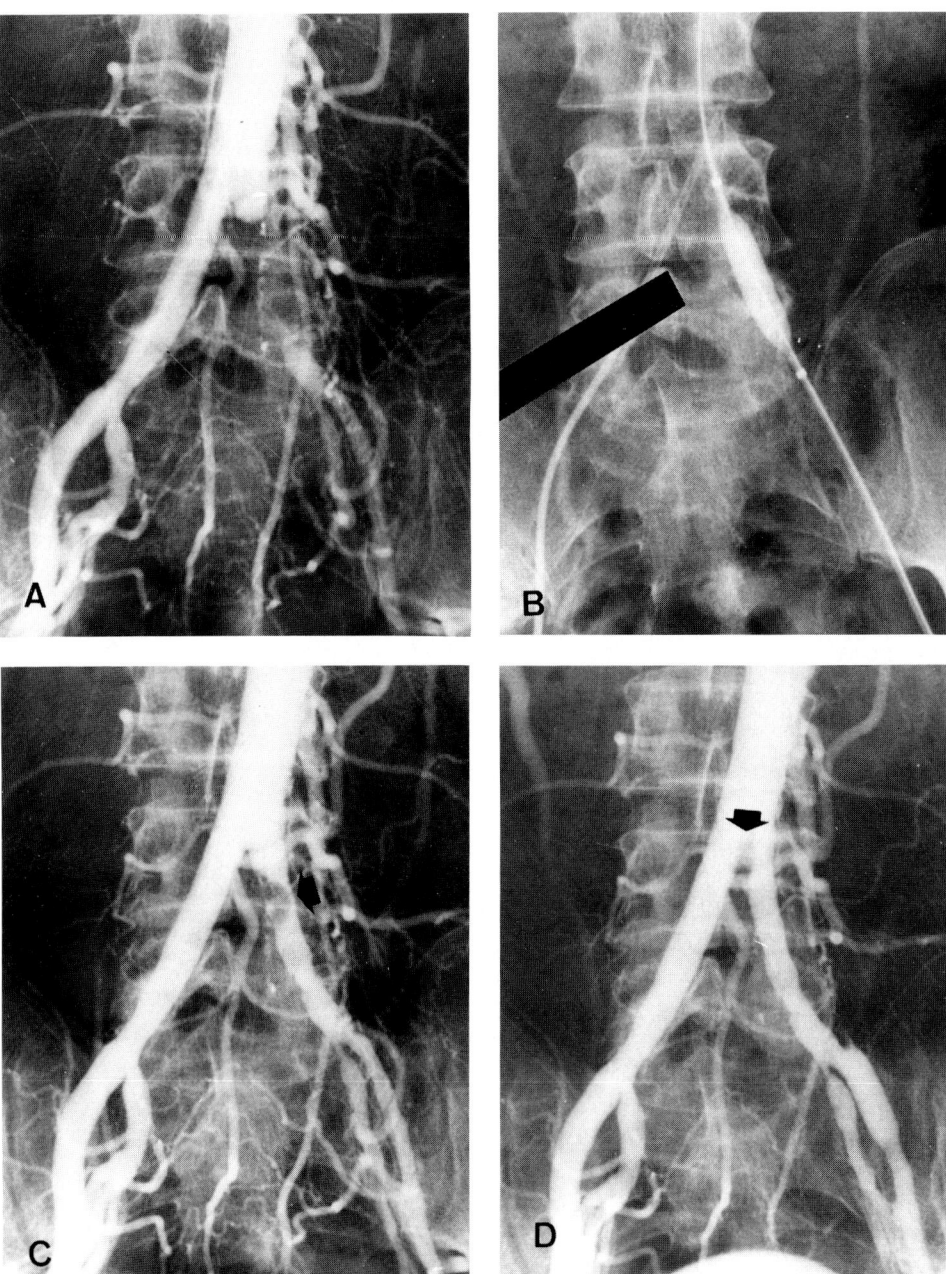

SIMULTANEOUS TREATMENT OF ILIAC AND DISTAL ARTERIES

A few alternatives for simultaneous treatment of iliac and distal arterial stenotic lesions should also be included in the angioplasty armamentarium.

It happens with relative frequency that severe claudication of the lower limb is the result of the association of a critical iliac arterial lesion with a severe lesion in one of the distal arteries. Both lesions may be treated percutaneously. If they are both located on the same side, they should be treated at different stages, due to high risks associated with performing both retrograde and antegrade punctures on the same artery at the same time. The iliac artery should be treated first in order to increase the blood supply to the limb; a few days later, the femoral artery, or the tibiofibular axis and its branches, can be treated. An iliac lesion accompanied by a contralateral distal lesion can be treated simultaneously (Fig. 6.51).

There are techniques available for inverting the direction of puncture, using a Cobra catheter forming a Waltman loop (Figs. 1.26 and 1.27), and selectively catheterizing the superficial femoral artery.

It is quite common to use a retrograde puncture for treating the iliac artery on one side and an antegrade puncture for treating the femoropopliteal distal lesions on the other (Fig. 6.52).

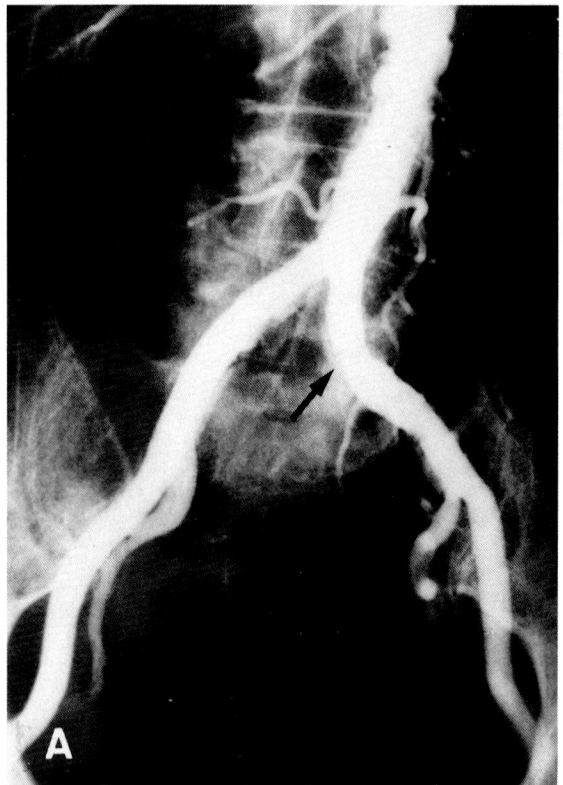
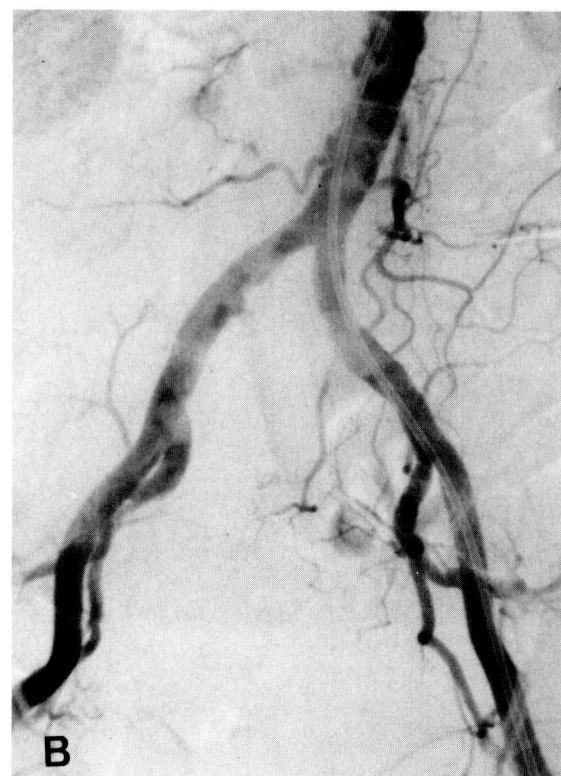
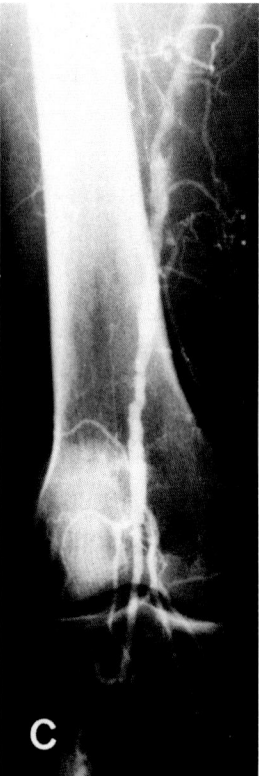
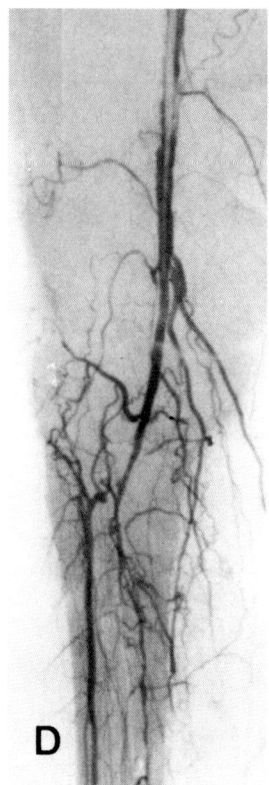

Figure 6.51 79-year-old diabetic patient with pain at rest. The preangioplasty right anterior tibial index was 0.4.
(A) Left iliac stenosis and occlusive lesion of the right tibiofibular axis (C). (B) Control following iliac angioplasty. (C) Severely involved popliteal artery and tibiofibular truncus. (D) Control after recanalization of the tibiofibular axis and distal branches. The pressure index went up to 0.8 after angioplasty. However, 5 months after the procedure was performed, acute occlusion of the right superficial femoral artery was surgically treated with a femoropopliteal graft.

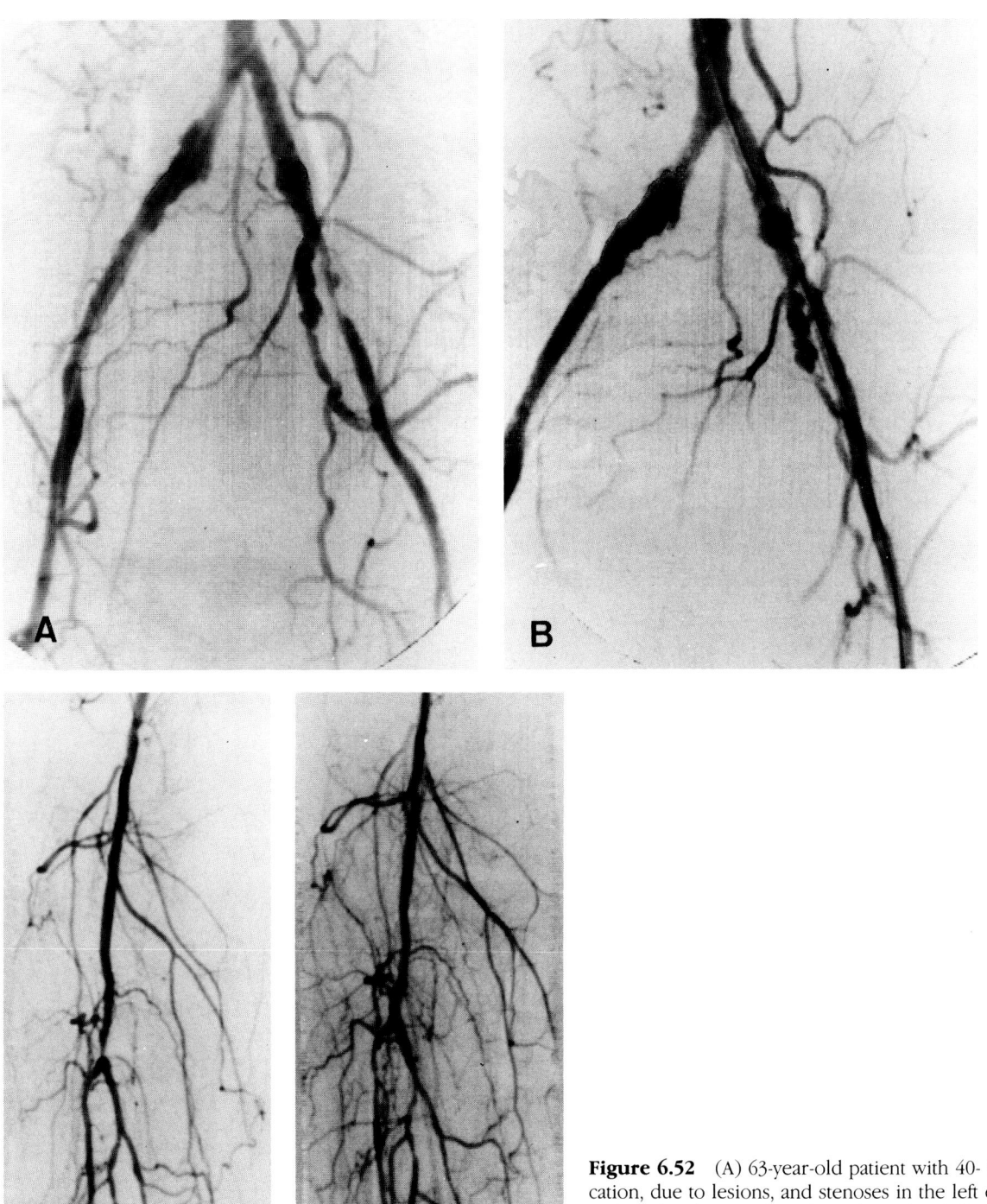

Figure 6.52 (A) 63-year-old patient with 40- to 50-m claudication, due to lesions, and stenoses in the left external iliac and popliteal artery (not shown). (B) Left iliac postangioplasty view. (C) 90 percent stenosis of the right tibiofibular truncus. (D) Postangioplasty control of tibiofibular truncus showing good response. 1-year follow-up showed no recurrence of claudication. All lesions had been treated at the same time.

REFERENCES

Katzen BT. Percutaneous transluminal angioplasty for arterial disease of the lower extremities. *AJR* 1984;142:23–25.

Motarjeme A, Keifer JW, Zuska AJ. Percutaneous transluminal angioplasty of the iliac arteries: 66 experiences. *AJR* 1980;135:937–944.

Pilla TJ, Peterson GJ, Tantana S, et al. Percutaneous recanalization of iliac artery occlusions: An alternative to surgery in the high-risk patient. *AJR* 1984;143:313–316.

Schwarten DE. Percutaneous transluminal angioplasty of the iliac arteries: Intravenous digital subtraction angiography for follow-up. *Radiology* 1984;150:363–367.

Spence RK, Freiman DB, Gatenly JG, et al. Long term results of transluminal angioplasty of the iliac and femoral arteries. *Arch Surg* 1981;116:1377–1386.

Tegtmeyer CJ, Moore TS, Chander R, et al. Percutaneous transluminal dilatation of a complete block in the right iliac artery. *AJR* 1979;122:532–535.

Uflacker R. Angioplastia transluminar das arterias dos membros inferiores. *Radiol Bras* 1985;1:1–8.

Van Andel GJ, Van Erp WFM, Krepel VM, Breslau PF. Percutaneous transluminal dilatation of the iliac artery: Long-term results. *Radiology* 1985;156:321–323.

Waltman AC. Percutaneous transluminal angioplasty: Iliac and deep femoral arteries. *AJR* 1980;135:921–925.

Zeitler E, Richter EI, Roth FJ, Schoop W. Results of percutaneous transluminal angioplasty. *Radiology* 1983;146:57–60.

Femoral, Popliteal, and Distal Branch Angioplasty

RENAN UFLACKER

FEMORAL ANGIOPLASTY

The standard method for performing angioplasty in the femoropopliteal axis is through antegrade puncture into the common femoral artery. Puncture of the common femoral artery is made as high as possible; an attempt is made to keep the entry site into the artery below the inguinal ligament, even if the small skin incision is above it (Figs. 6.3 and 6.4). Puncturing the femoral common artery above the inguinal ligament may cause life-threatening bleeding and severe pelvic hematomas. The contralateral antegrade route is only used for proximal superficial femoral lesions (Fig. 6.8).

After the puncture has been performed, care must be taken to position and advance the guidewire horizontally, so that it will penetrate the femoral superficial artery and not the deep femoral, which is the easiest way (Fig. 6.4). If in spite of all efforts, the guidewire does not advance into the superficial femoral artery, contrast medium should be injected in order to ascertain which vessel has been punctured and the level of puncture. If the puncture has been made into the deep femoral and the objective is the superficial femoral, the needle should be removed and a new puncture performed. If the needle is adequately positioned in the common femoral but the guidewire will not advance inside the superficial femoral, a guidewire with an open, curved, steerable tip should be tried. Steerable guidewires with torque control are particularly useful for this maneuver. A short, curved-tip catheter may also be useful.

After the guidewire has been positioned inside the superficial femoral artery, usually above the lesions to be treated, the needle is replaced by a straight polyethylene No. 5 French catheter.

At this stage, contrast injections should always be used to locate the stenoses, which should be marked with some type of radiopaque marker—needle, forceps, or ruler—on the sterile towel. To prevent the occurrence of spasm and pain, diluted or low-osmolarity contrast should be used.

The straight, flexible-tip, steerable guidewire is advanced to the level of the obstructive lesion together with the catheter. Localized, concentric stenoses are usually easily passed through on the first attempt (Fig. 6.53). In cases where eccentric stenoses are present (Fig. 6.53), it is more difficult to introduce the guidewire, but passage should never be forced. In such cases, steerable guidewires are especially useful.

The tip of the guidewire should be advanced up to the proximal popliteal artery in order to avoid distal spasm and spasm of the tibiofibular arteries.

In cases of femoral artery occlusion, the guidewire should be carefully advanced, with moderate force. It feels as if the guidewire is being advanced through a substance with the same consistency as butter, although somewhat greater resistance is encountered at the site of stenosis due to the atheromatous plaque. As soon as the guidewire goes beyond the occlusion, it should move more freely (Fig. 6.12). If, after the distal limit of the occlusion has been passed, advancement is still difficult, changes of subintimal involvement are high and the procedure should probably be ended at that point.

If the guidewire tip curves outside of the arterial line, it may have entered into a collateral branch or dissected the vascular wall. There is a risk of perforation in such situations, and the position of the guidewire should be checked, either using an open-ended guidewire or exchanging the steerable device for a small catheter for contrast injection. A 1-mm radius J-guidewire may, surprisingly, "find" its way inside a lesion such as this.

Contrast injection within the virtual path inside the plaque, with the tip of th catheter wedged, will quite often open the virtual path into a track for guidewire penetration.

After pasing beyond the lesion, it is advisable to maintain the tip of the guidewire in the proximal portion of the popliteal artery while starting heparinization with 5000 IU and injecting papaverine or nitroglycerin and 50 mg of lidocaine, in order to prevent distal spasm.

Once the guidewire has been positioned, the puncture site is dilated with a No. 5 to No. 7 French dilator and the balloon catheter inserted over the guidewire through the previously marked stenosis or occlusion.

As in all angioplastic procedures, balloon selection will depend on measurement of the cross section of the normal vessel, above and below the stenosis or occlusion or their extensions. For focal lesions, a balloon 2 to 4 cm long and with a 4- to 6-mm diameter is commonly

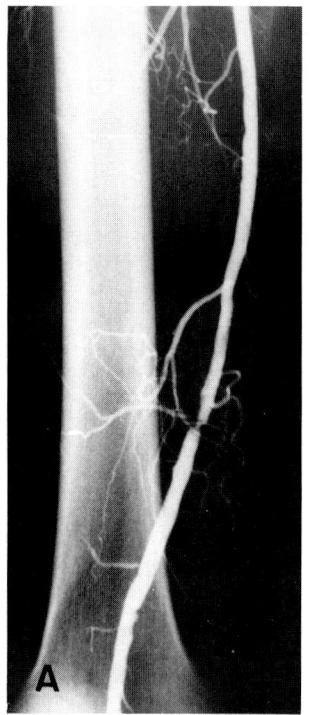 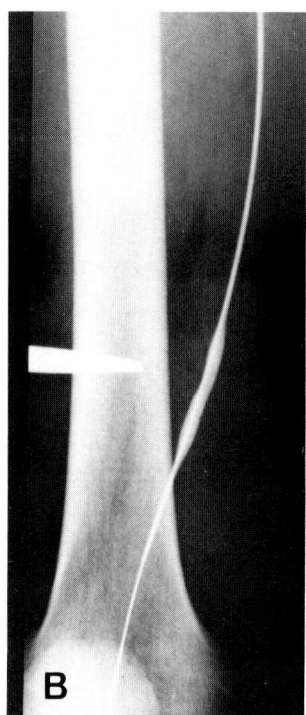 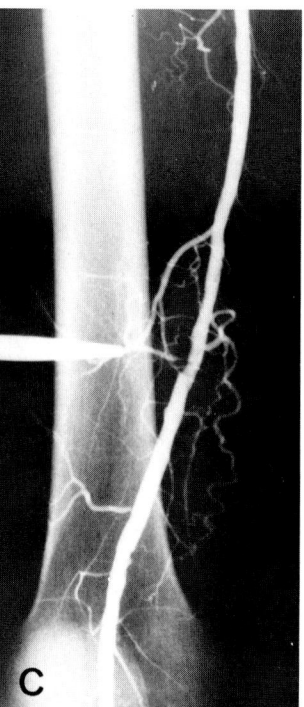

Figure 6.53 (A) 61-year-old heavy smoker, with 100-m claudication and severe stenotic lesion located in the right superficial femoral artery. (B) Dilatation with 5-mm balloon. (C) Control after angioplasty showing lesion patency.

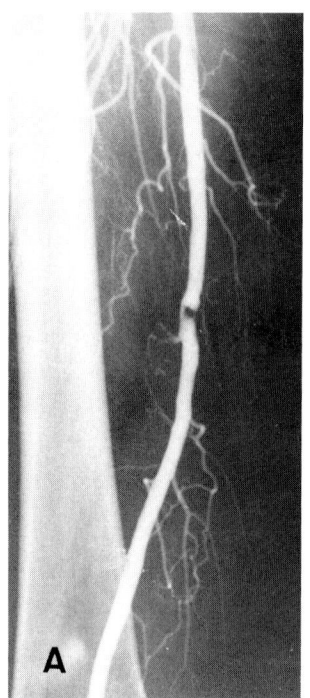 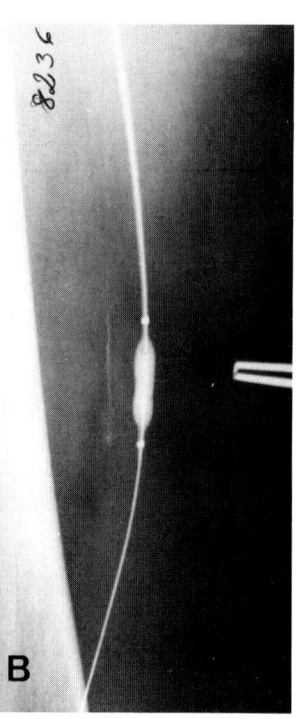 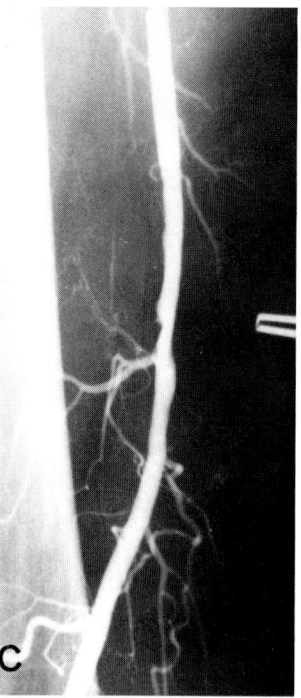

Figure 6.54 (A) 50-year-old patient with 100-m claudication and eccentric stenotic lesion in the right superficial femoral artery. (B) Dilatation with 5-mm balloon. (C) Control after dilatation showing adequate patency. Before treatment, there was digital cyanosis and no tibial pulses. In the postangioplasty period, tibial pulses became symmetrical, without digital cyanosis.

Figure 6.55 (A) 48-year-old patient with segmental left superficial femoral occlusion. (B) Recanalization with 10-cm-long 5-mm-diameter balloon. (C) Control following dilatation showing good patency. However, one month later, claudication recurred. (D) Proximal occlusion of superficial femoral artery. (E) Distal recanalization of superficial femoral artery. The patient underwent a femoropopliteal graft.

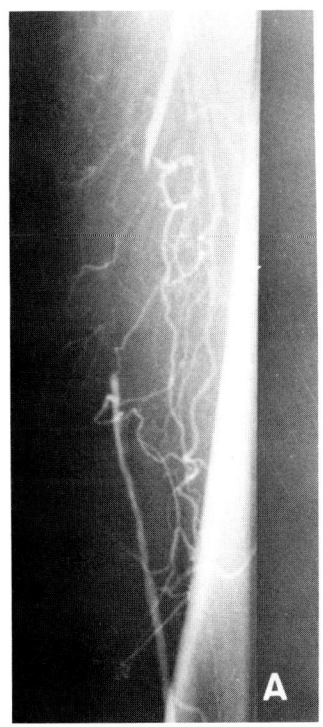
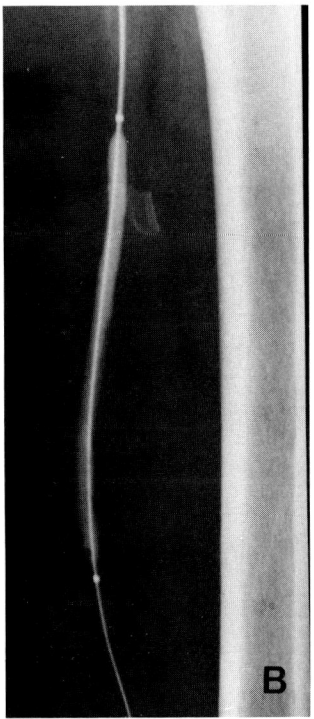
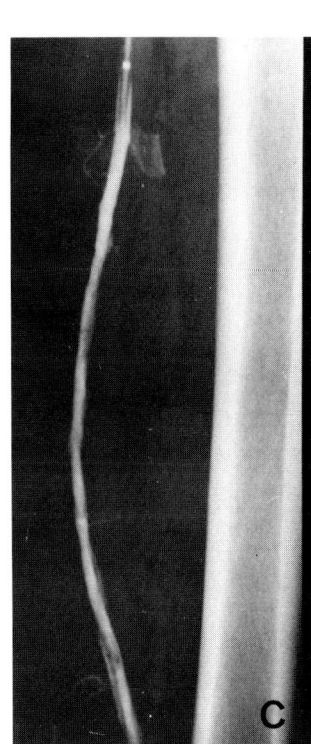
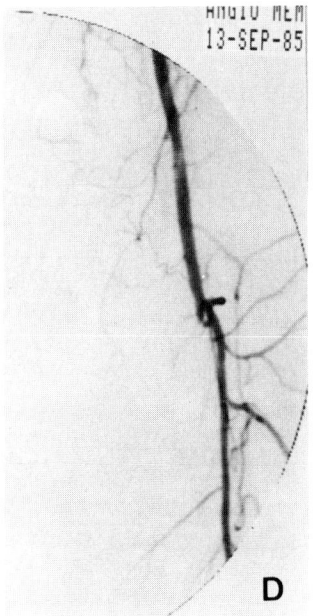
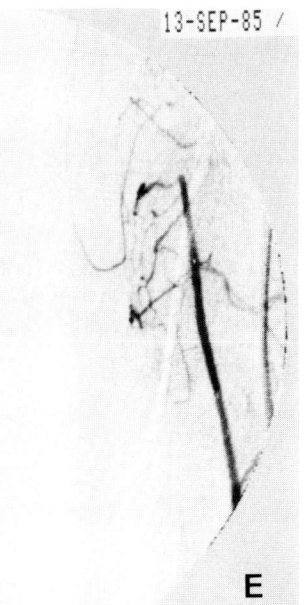

used; for long occlusions, or with multiple stenoses, longer (8- to 10-cm) balloons are used, with the same diameter (Fig. 6.55).

In the presence of multiple severe stenoses, the distal segment should be dilated first, in order to ensure an adequate increase in distal flow during manipulation of the proximal lesion (Fig. 6.56).

In some cases, the atheromatous plaques may be so rigid and calcified that it is impossible to pass the balloon through. In those cases, a van Andel catheter [Nos. 6, 7, 8, or 9 French (Fig. 6.1)], may be used to dilate the lesion, with a higher longitudinally transmitted force, before introducing the baloon. Longer balloons—8 or 10 cm—are the most difficult to introduce. However, recanalizations performed with a No. 9 French Teflon van Andel catheter may be adequate (Fig. 6.57). Some currently available recanalization devices are particularly useful for superficial femoral artery treatment. After arterial recanalization with one of those devices, balloon angioplasty is still often required to achieve adequate luminal dilatation.

Dilatation is generally performed with a 10-mL syringe. The same syringe provides rapid deflation. Syringes smaller than 10 mL should under no circumstances be used. Twenty-mL syringes are useful only for deflation. It takes 30 to 60 s to completely inflate the balloon. Some lesions require more than one inflation, and, depending on the severity of the stenosis or occlusion, higher-pressure balloons may be necessary.

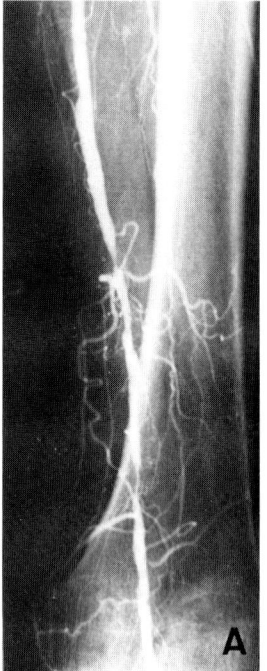 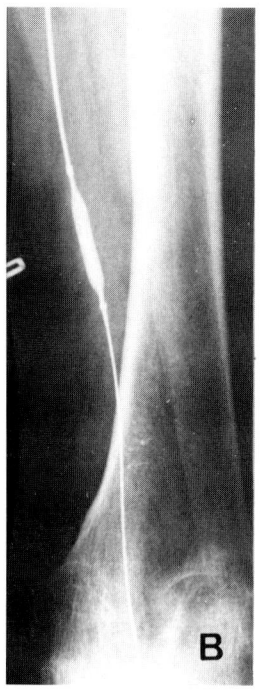 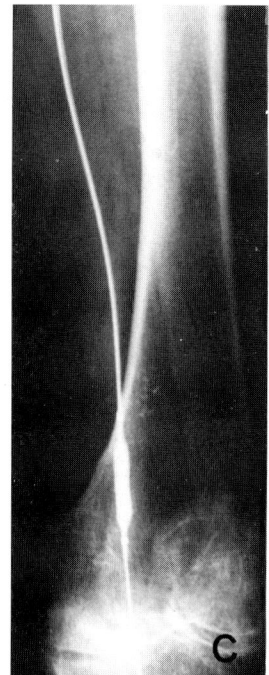 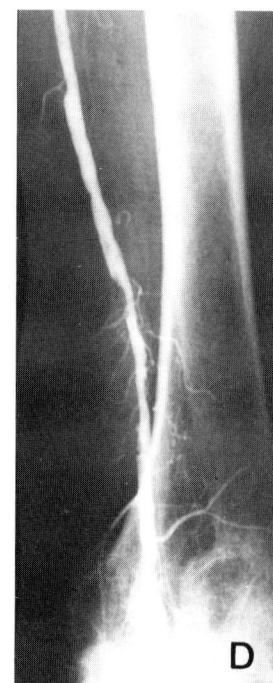

Figure 6.56 (A) 69-year-old patient with infected ischemic ulcer of the left ankle and multiple stenoses in the superficial femoral and popliteal. (B) Dilatation of the proximal lesion. (C) Dilatation of the distal lesion. (D) Control following angioplasty. Tibial pulses returned, and the ulceration had healed after 4 weeks.

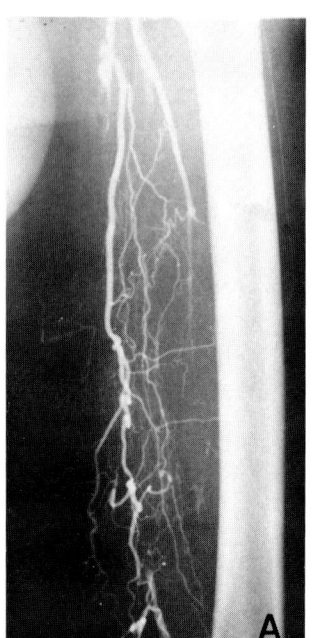 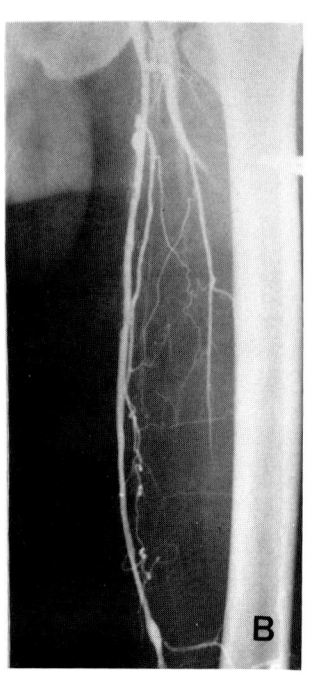 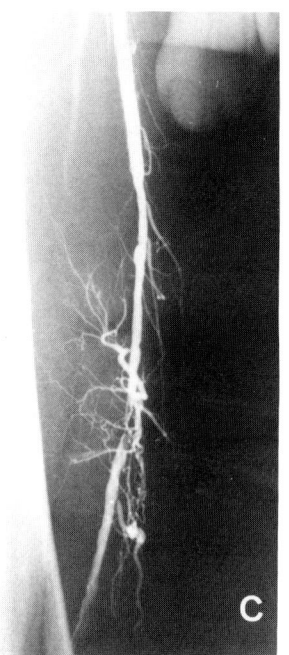 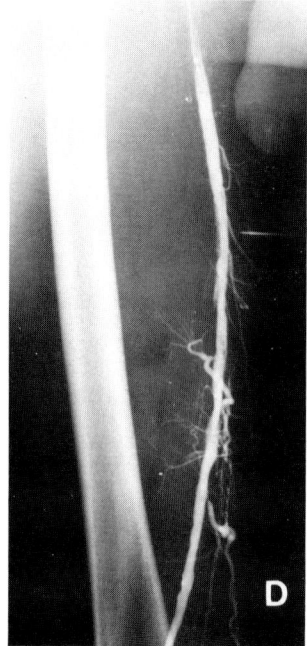

Figure 6.57 (A,C) 52-year-old patient with 100-m claudication in both legs, 23-cm left superficial femoral occlusion (A), and highly localized right superficial femoral occlusion (C). (B,D) Controls after angioplasty of left (B) and right (D) superficial femoral arteries. For the left femoral, only one van Andel No. 9 French catheter was used in the recanalization; on the right, a 5-mm balloon was used. Claudication disappeared, but tibial pulse did not return on the left side.

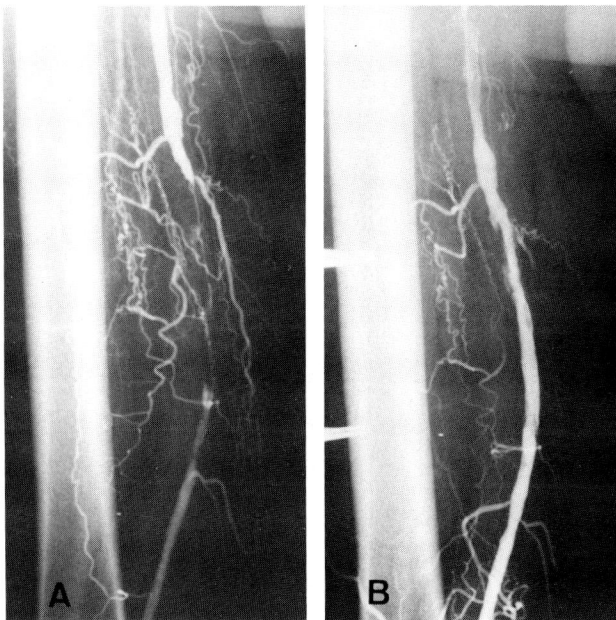

Figure 6.58 56-year-old patient with 50-m claudication in the right leg.
(A) Angiographic control showing recent segmental occlusion of the superficial femoral. Examination 2 weeks earlier had shown only stenosis. (B) Control after recanalization with 6-mm balloon. Note the filling defects and irregularities. The tibial pulse became palpable, and pressures returned to normal.

After dilatation, the balloon is totally deflated, and the catheter pulled up above the point at which the lesion begins. Serial angiography can then be performed, with the dilatation catheter itself, for purposes of postangioplasty documentation (Fig. 6.58).

Pressure measurements are not indispensable in most cases. Frequently, the cosmetic results after angioplasty will be unsatisfactory and the lesion will have an irregular appearance, with filling defects, and there will be no pressure gradient. This should not be a cause for concern, because wall reshaping and healing will take place over time, not only improving the appearance of the lesion but also allowing a higher flow to pass through.

After the deflated balloon is removed, heparin reversal is not required. Conventional compression should be applied to the puncture site.

Results obtained with transluminal angioplasty in femoral arteries compare favorably with surgical results. After 1 year, patency remains in 77 to 79.5 percent of cases, compared with 81 percent obtained with femoropopliteal grafts. After 3 years, about 73 percent of the angioplasty cases are still patent, compared with about 78 percent of the reconstructive surgery cases. One-, two-, and three-year results in limb-salvage procedures are also similar to those obtained by surgery, although figures are slightly lower for both methods.

Angioplasty of the deep femoral artery can be performed using the same technique described for the superficial artery. Note, however, that the stenoses of this artery are usually more proximally located (Fig. 6.59). A 3- to 5-mm balloon is usually effective in these lesions. Occasionally, when an iliac stenosis is treated by the contralateral route, and the superficial femoral is occluded, it is convenient to extend the dilatation to the deep femoral. The deep femoral is the most important collateral route for the lower limbs, and remarkable improvement of tibial pressure can be obtained merely by dilating that artery (Fig. 6.60).

ANGIOPLASTY OF THE POPLITEAL AND DISTAL BRANCH ARTERIES

Until the late 1970s and early 1980s angioplasty of the popliteal artery and distal arteries was reserved for limb-salvage procedures. The main reason for this was the high number of failures due to severe spasm in the popliteotibial truncus, involving the risk of proximal and distal thrombosis and even jeopardizing previously successful dilatations of the femoral superficial artery. In addition, lesions in the popliteal and tibial arteries are seldom isolated findings (Figs. 6.13, 6.59, 6.60, and 6.61). Changes in procedures and technique, however, have resulted in success rates comparable to those obtained by angioplasty in other arteries.

The diagnostic study should be retrogradely performed, through the contralateral femoral artery of the diseased limb. The puncture for the therapeutic procedure should be antegrade, as previously described (Figs. 6.3 and 6.4) for angioplasty of the superficial femoral artery. A No. 5 French catheter is advanced up to the popliteal artery, near the lesion; following that, a localized angiographic study is made using a low-osmolarity or diluted contrast medium. When the level of the popliteal artery is reached, about 5000 IU of heparin is injected into the arterial lumen, without the need of later reversal. For this type of arterial segment, immediately before attempting to advance beyond the lesion, it is appropriate to use spasmolytic agents in the following sequence: lidocaine (Xylocaine) 30 mg, Papaverine (50 mg), or nitroglycerin.

Fibrinolytic therapy can be a valuable pre- and postangioplasty procedure for thrombotic occlusions of the popliteal artery.

The straight tip of the guidewire is advanced 2 to 3 cm beyond the catheter tip, and the whole set is taken inside the lesion using gentle longitudinal force to advance beyond obstacles. If the 0.035- or 0.038-inch straight guidewire cannot be advanced beyond the lesion, the guidewire tip may be slightly bent, by pulling it

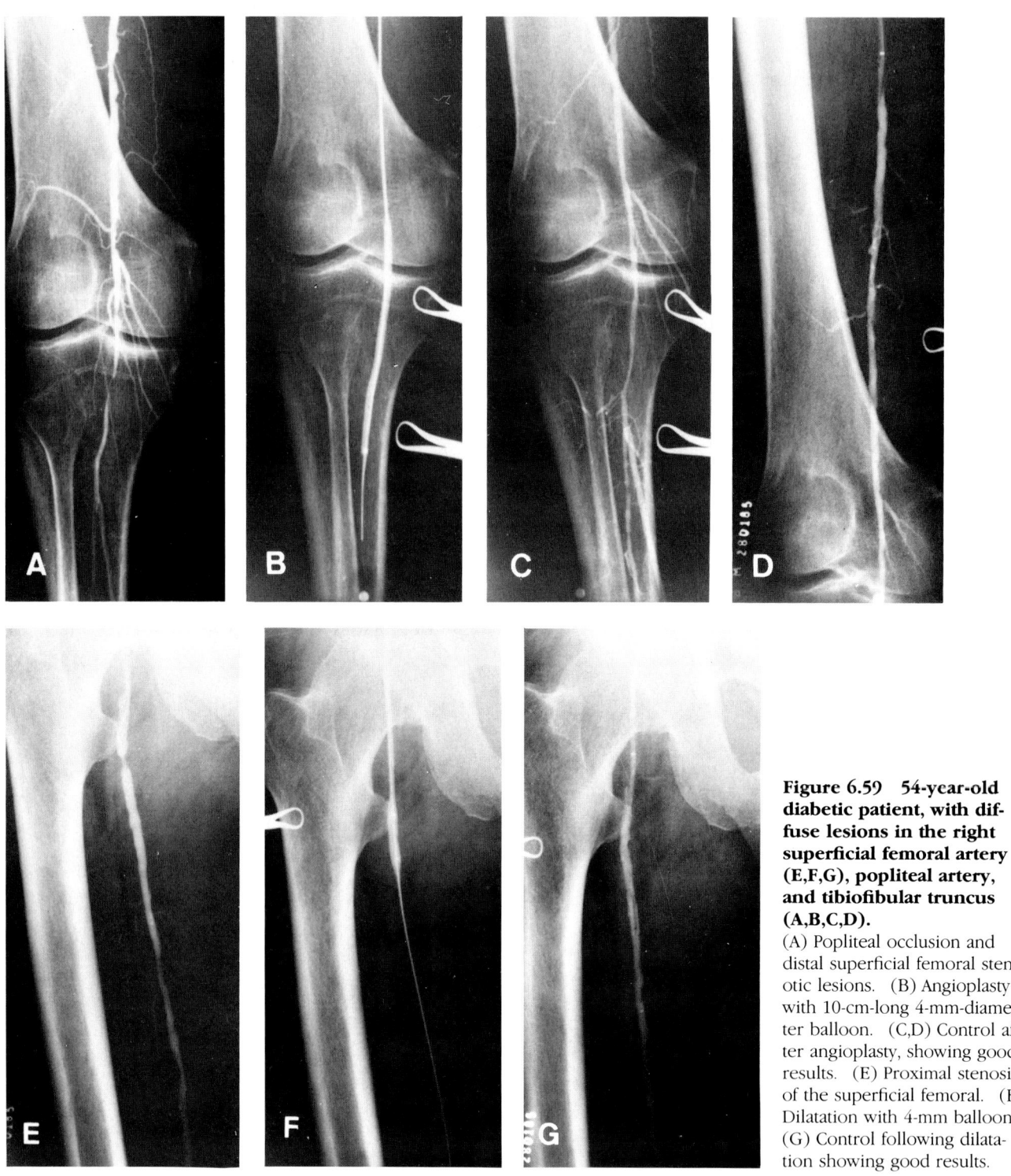

Figure 6.59 54-year-old diabetic patient, with diffuse lesions in the right superficial femoral artery (E,F,G), popliteal artery, and tibiofibular truncus (A,B,C,D).
(A) Popliteal occlusion and distal superficial femoral stenotic lesions. (B) Angioplasty with 10-cm-long 4-mm-diameter balloon. (C,D) Control after angioplasty, showing good results. (E) Proximal stenosis of the superficial femoral. (F) Dilatation with 4-mm balloon. (G) Control following dilatation showing good results.

between the thumbnail and the tip of the second finger, and then gently rotated and maneuvered through the lesion using small longitudinal advances. Another option is to use a No. 5 French Teflon catheter with a slightly bent tip, handling it as just described. Extreme care must be taken at all times. As discussed above, a contrast injection with a catheter the tip of which is wedged in the lesion may be helpful in finding the right track.

Dilatation of the popliteal artery (Fig. 6.62) may be performed with a 4- to 6-mm balloon. For the tibiofibular truncus and the distal arteries (Fig. 6.63), a van Andel-type Teflon catheter [No. 5 French (1.67 mm) to No. 9

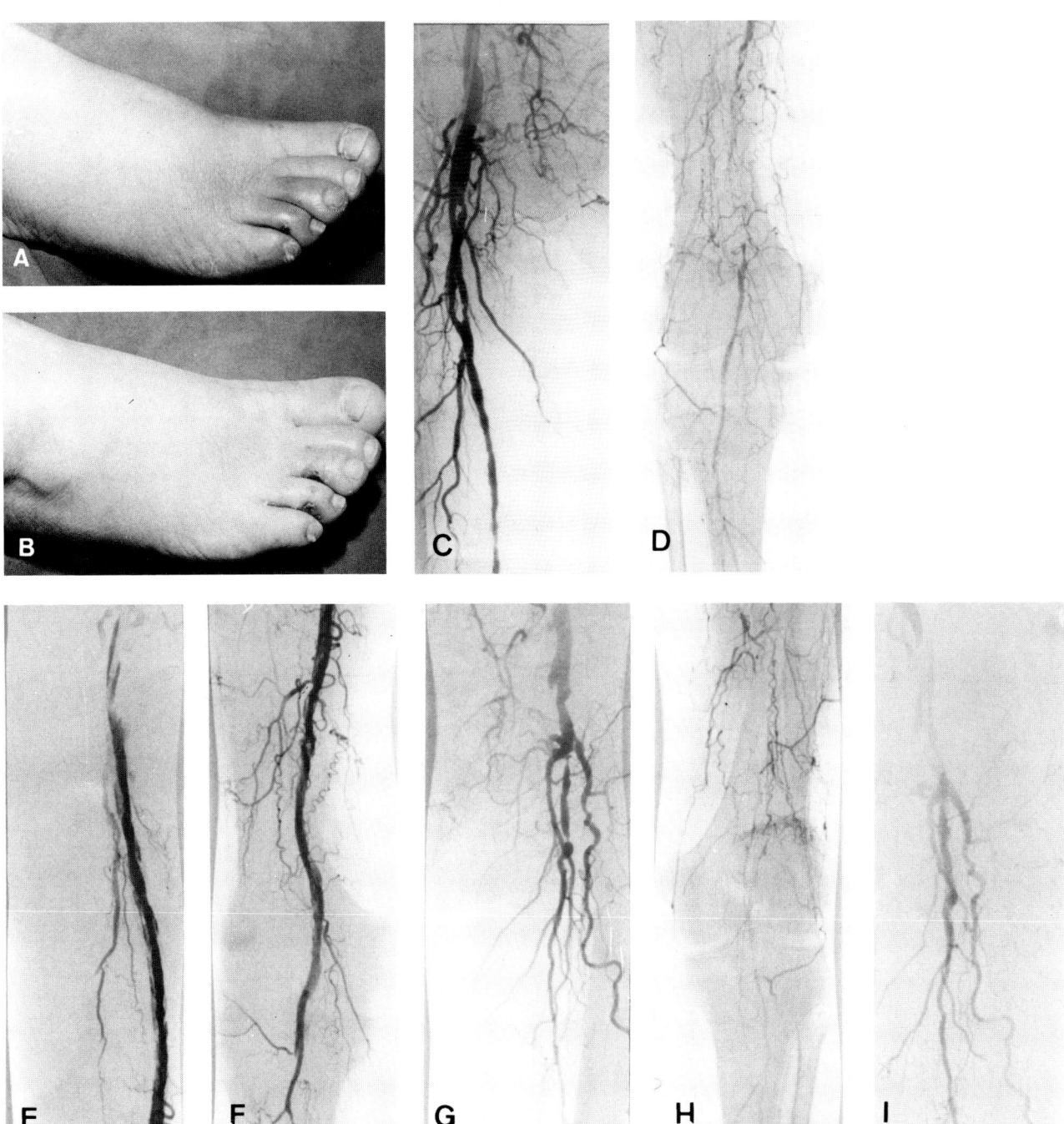

Figure 6.60 (A) 72-year-old diabetic patient with pain at rest and digital ischemic lesions. (B) Patient 4 weeks after angioplasty of the right limb. Notice that edema has disappeared, and the lesions, although still ulcerated, are dry and in the process of healing. Pain disappeared, and walking became possible. (C) Right proximal superficial femoral artery with diffuse lesions. (D) Distal midthird occlusion of the right superficial femoral with popliteal recanalization. (E,F) Result of angioplasty in the right superficial femoral, with distal recanalization and popliteal dilatation, with 10-cm-long 4-mm-diameter balloon. (G) Severe diffuse stenoses in the left deep femoral artery. (H) Occlusion of the superficial femoral, with poor distal recanalization. (I) Control following angioplasty of the left deep femoral performed by the antegrade route. Preangioplasty systemic pressure was 180 mmHg; RPT, 50 mmHg; LPT 50 mmHg; RAT, 0; LAT, 0. Immediately after angioplasty, systemic pressure was 140 mmHg; RPT, 52 mmHg; LPT, 76 mmHg; RAT, 50 mmHg; LAT, 60 mmHg. 2 months later, systemic pressure was 130 mmHg; RPT, 90 mmHg; LPT, 76 mmHg; RAT, 66 mmHg; LAT, 64 mmHg. Note that angioplasty of the left deep femoral alone resulted in significant improvement in tibial pressures.

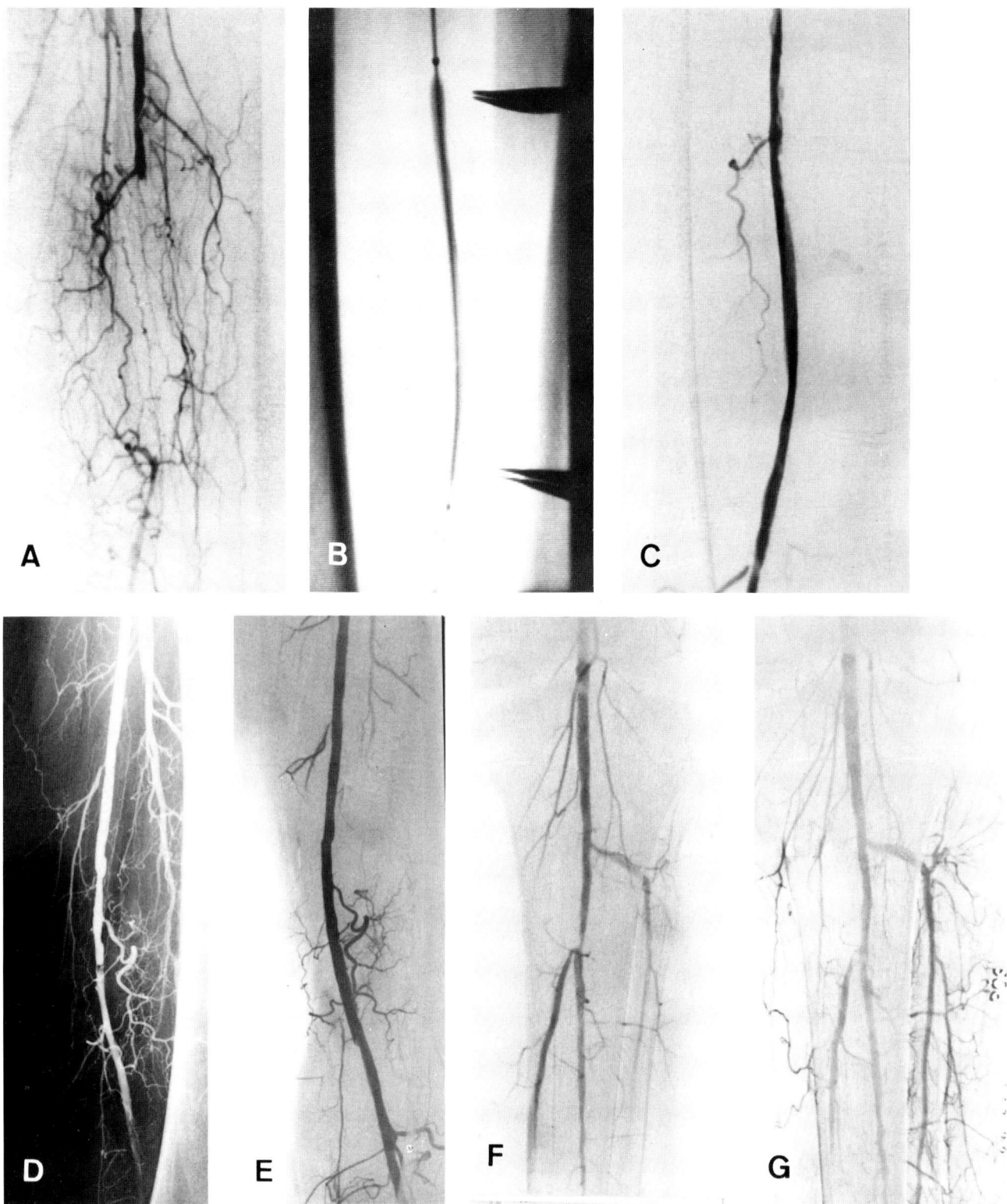

Figure 6.61 54-year-old insulin-dependent diabetic patient with 50-m claudication on the right.
(A) Right superficial femoral occlusion. (B) Recanalization with long balloon. (C) Postdilatation control showing adequate patency. (D,E,F,G) After angioplasty, the patient remained without symptoms on the right side, but symptoms due to 150-m claudication on the left side appeared. Two days after the first treatment, angioplasty of the superficial femoral and the tibiofibular truncus was performed, with complete success. The patient became asymptomatic, walking many miles every day.

Figure 6.62 (A) 72-year-old patient with pain at rest due to 20-m claudication of the right lower limb and severe stenosis of the popliteal artery. (B) Dilatation with 5-mm balloon. (C) Control following angioplasty. The patient became asymptomatic.

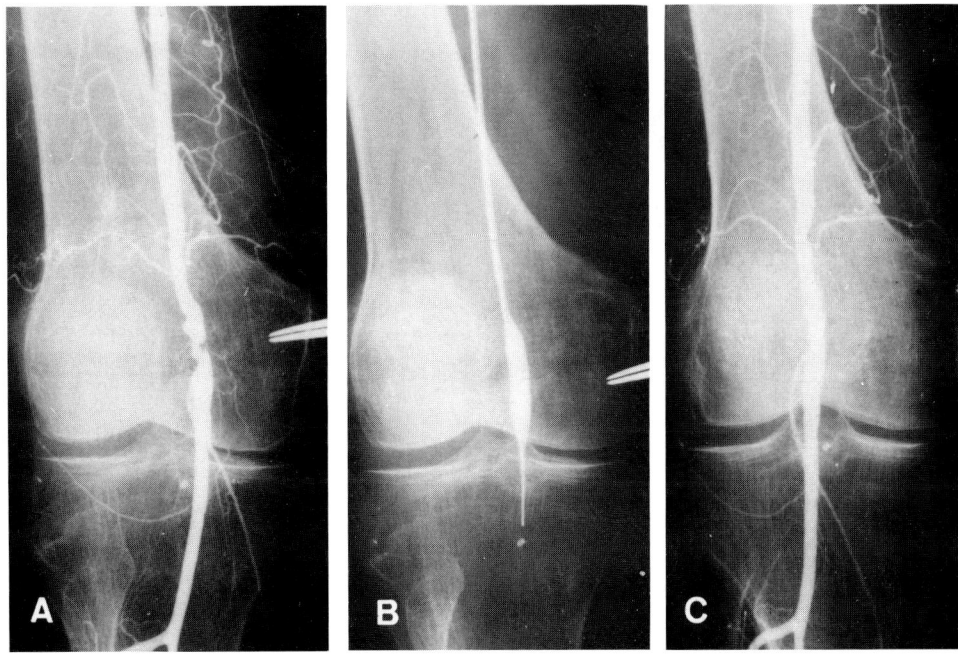

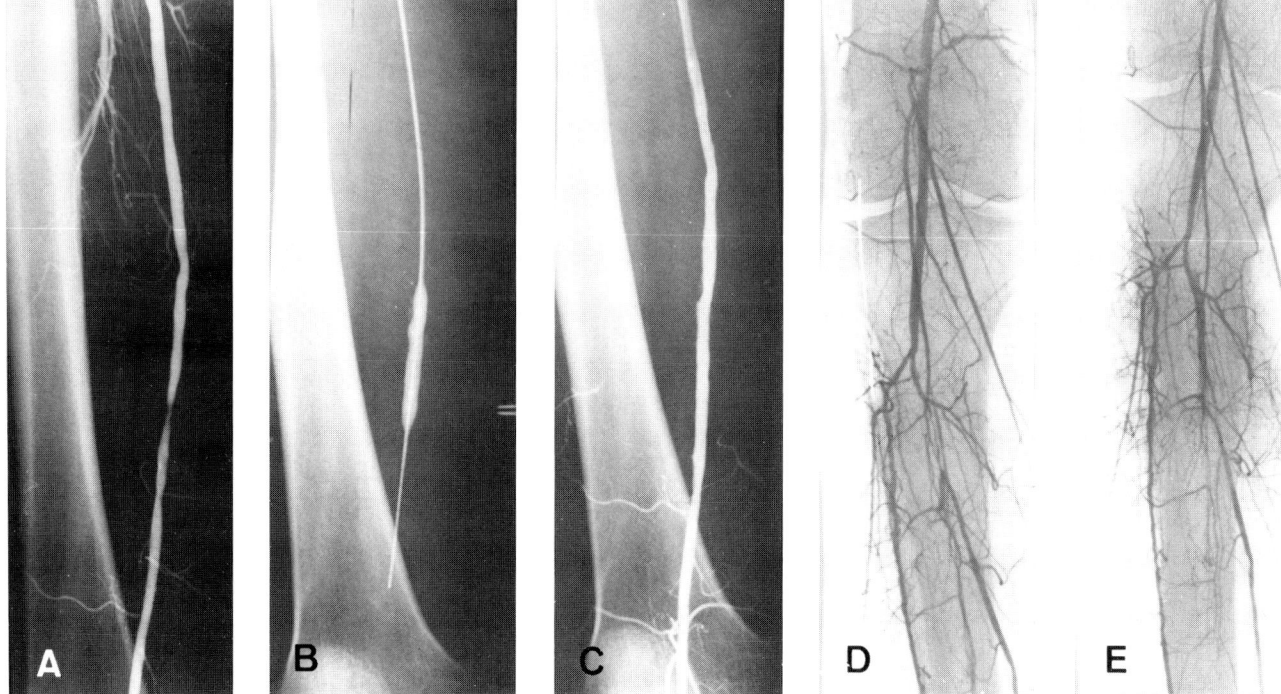

Figure 6.63 36-year-old diabetic patient with advanced gangrene of the right foot.
(A) Multiple superficial femoral lesions. (B) Dilatation with 6-mm balloon. (C) Postangioplasty control. (D) Occlusion of the tibiofibular truncus on the same side. (E) Recanalization of the truncus was performed with a No. 8 French van Andel catheter. Pain improved. The borders of the gangrene were much more clearly delineated after angioplasty, and only the front part of the foot had to be amputated.

French (3 mm)] or a small coronary angioplasty balloon catheter (1.5 to 3 mm in diameter) may be useful. In the popliteal artery, to achieve effective dilatation it is quite often necessary to first introduce a No. 7 or No. 8 French van Andel catheter and then introduce a balloon catheter (Figs. 6.13, 6.59, 6.60, and 6.62).

It is important to remember that small changes in the luminal diameter of these small arteries may have dramatic effects on flow and distal pressure. Therefore, moderate dilatation of the tibial arteries or the tibiofibular truncus may significantly increase the flow to an already painful foot or one with ulcerating ischemic lesions (Fig. 6.63). A higher level of dilatation, however, may be necessary to improve intermittent claudication.

Recently there have been significant improvements in the techniques for small-vessel angioplasty. The use of such devices as 0.018- and 0.014-in. steerable guidewires with torque control, and 2- to 4-mm-diameter balloons with No. 3 to No. 5 French catheters, which were developed for use with coronary arteries, has led to an increased success rate.

The results are also encouraging in larger series, although they are much less significant than for all other arterial segments. The initial success rate is about 89 percent, but the reocclusion rate 2 to 10 months following the procedure is approximately 20 percent. In one series of 29 patients, arterial patency after 1 and 2 years was about 57 percent.

REFERENCES

Freiman DB, Spence R, Gatenby HD, et al. Transluminal angioplasty of the iliac and femoral arteries: Follow-up results without anticoagulation. *Radiology* 1981;141:347–350

Krepel VM, Van Andel GJ, Van Erp WFM, Breslan PJ. Percutaneous transluminal angioplasty on the femoropopliteal artery: Initial and long-term results. *Radiology* 1985;156:325–328.

Lu CT, Zarins CK, Yang CF, Turcotte JK. Percutaneous transluminal angioplasty for limb salvage. *Radiology* 1982;142:337–341.

Martin EC, Fankenchen EI, Karlson KB, et al. Angioplasty for femoral artery occlusion: Comparison with surgery. *AJR* 1981;137:915–919.

Probst P, Cerny P, Owens A, et al. Patency after femoral angioplasty: Correlation of angiographic appearance with clinical findings. *AJR* 1983;140:1227–1232.

Sos TA, Snideman KW, Beinart C. Gruntzig catheter with a 10 cm long balloon. *Radiology* 1981;141:825–826.

Tamura S, Snideman KW, Beinart C, Sos TA. Percutaneous transluminal angioplasty of the popliteal artery and its branches. *Radiology* 1982;143:645–648.

Angioplasty of Other Arteries

RENAN UFLACKER

BRANCHES OF THE THORACIC AORTA

Subclavian and Brachial Arteries

Stenosis of the subclavian arteries often remains untreated. Sometimes it is asymptomatic, presumably because abundant collateral circulation supplies the upper limbs with sufficient blood flow. If symptoms do appear, affected individuals often simply avoid physical activity that puts strain on the upper limbs. However, for those whose professions require significant upper-limb exercise, claudication may be incapacitating.

Stenosis or occlusion of the subclavian artery proximal to the origin of the vertebral artery also result in a drop in blood flow sufficient to cause the subclavian steal syndrome. The blood flow to the upper limbs originates from the contralateral vertebral artery, passing through the circle of Willis, with reversal of ipsilateral vertebral arterial blood flow. In cases of subclavian stenosis, exercise of the involved upper limb will cause demand to increase to the point at which blood will be diverted from the brain, causing cerebral ischemia. This in turn may produce vertebobasilar failure, causing loss of coordination and imbalance, as well as cortical blindness (Fig. 6.64).

Subclavian arterial stenosis or occlusion may also be associated with digital ischemia, usually as a result of reduction in collateral circulation caused by fibrosis or by a therapeutic procedure that affects the supraclavicular region, for example, radiotherapy (Fig. 6.65). This occurs rarely; however, more distal occlusions, at the levels of

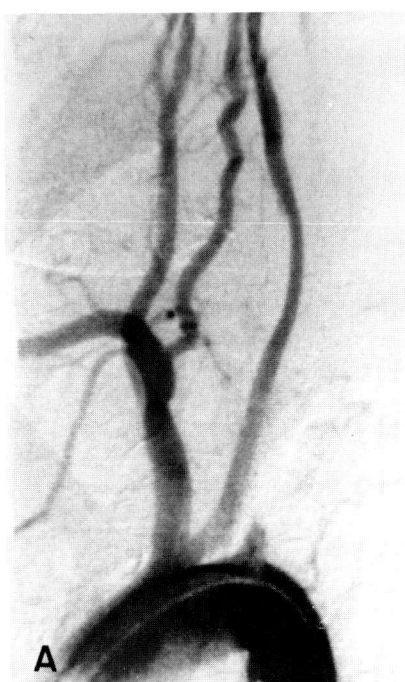 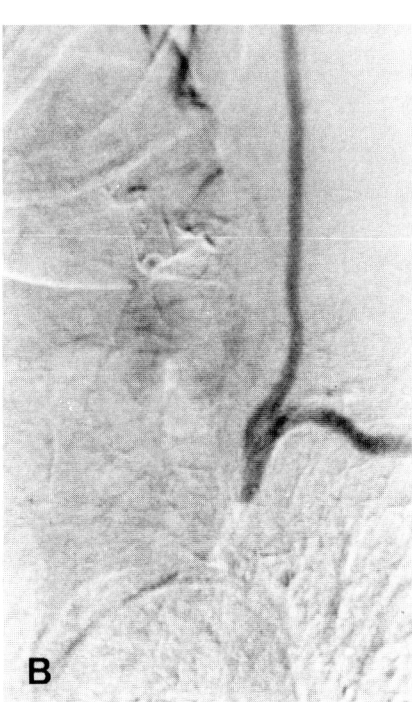 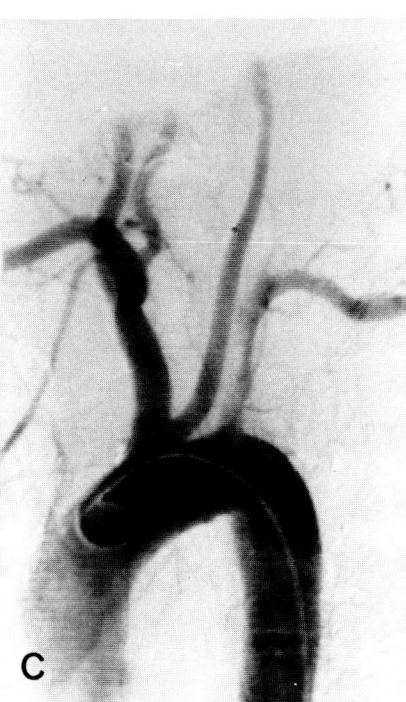

Figure 6.64 52-year-old patient with symptoms of the subclavian steal syndrome, including vertebrobasilary problems and ischemic attacks. The patient also had carotid stenosis due to fibromuscular dysplasia (Fig. 6.67).
(A) Left subclavian occlusion. (B) Antegrade flow in the left vertebral, filling the subclavian on the same side (stealing through the vertebral artery). (C) Control following angioplasty with 6-mm balloon. The patient's arm pressures became symmetrical. Notice that the left vertebral did not opacify. Control 6 months after angioplasty showed normal vertebral circulation and left subclavian patency.

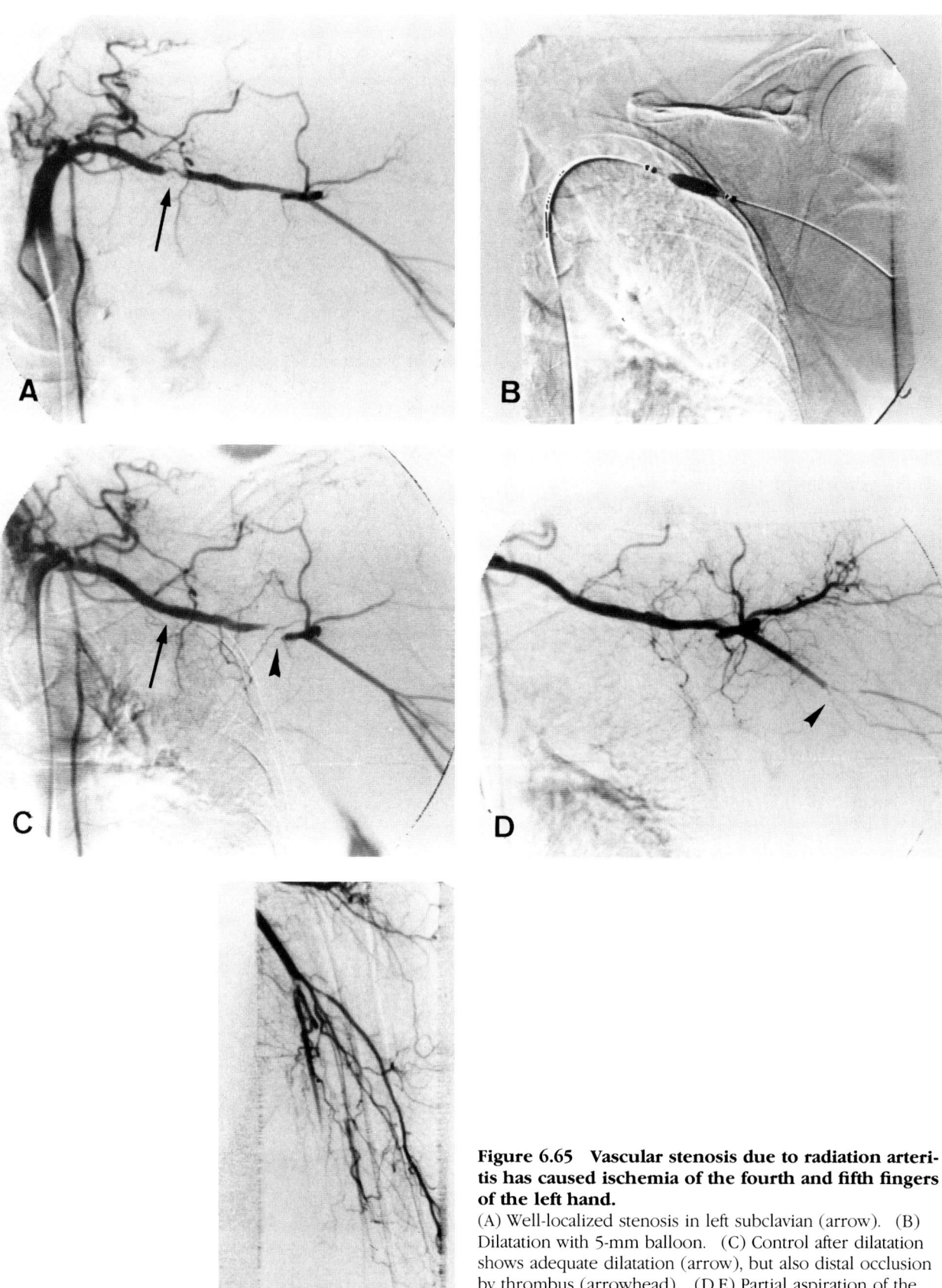

Figure 6.65 Vascular stenosis due to radiation arteritis has caused ischemia of the fourth and fifth fingers of the left hand.
(A) Well-localized stenosis in left subclavian (arrow). (B) Dilatation with 5-mm balloon. (C) Control after dilatation shows adequate dilatation (arrow), but also distal occlusion by thrombus (arrowhead). (D,E) Partial aspiration of the thrombus caused it to migrate to a more distal position (arrowhead). The brachial artery was recanalized by Fogarty balloon embolectomy, and the ischemia improved.

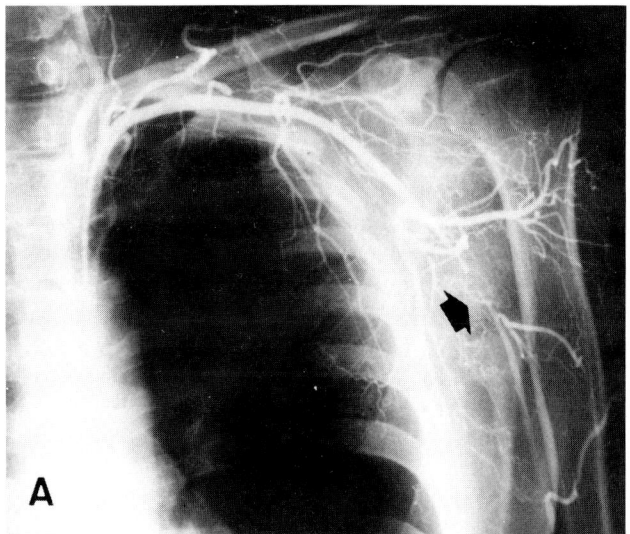
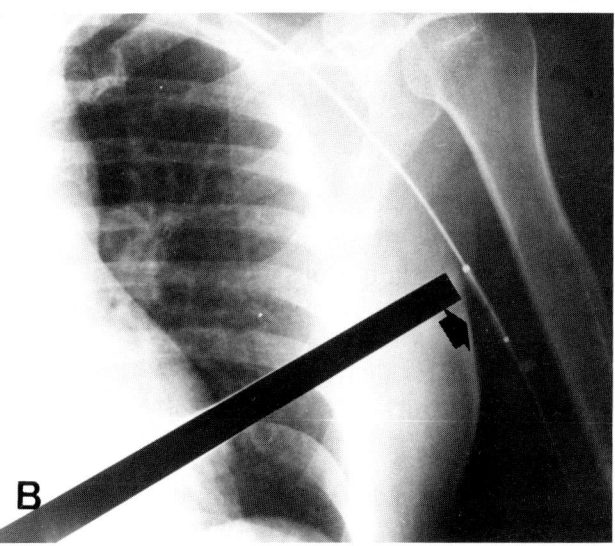
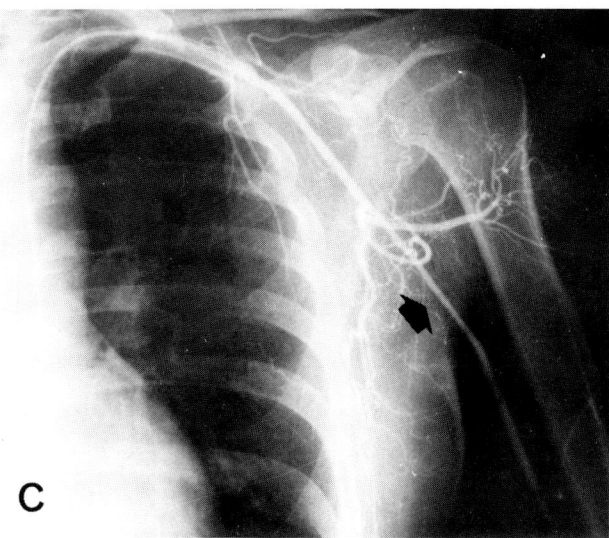

the brachial artery, will cause digital ischemic symptoms more frequently due to the reduced collateral circulation at this level (Fig. 6.66).

The four basic etiologies for stenotic lesions in supraaortic vessels according to frequency are:

1. Atherosclerotic lesions. These are the most frequent; they vary in type, but are generally segmental, and hence respond well to angioplasty (Figs. 6.64 and 6.66).
2. Takayasu's arteritis. This may either be localized or involve long arterial segments.
3. Arteritis caused by radium therapy most often for treatment of breast carcinoma.
4. Fibromuscular disease. Usually of the medial fibroplasia type, this involves both narrowed areas and aneurysmal areas. In the carotids, it more frequently involves the mid and distal portions of the internal carotid arteries (see following item). Vascular compression due to the so-called thoracic outlet syndrome is untreatable by angioplasty because it is caused by external factors.

It should be noted that although the risk of peripheral embolism during angioplasty is very low, if it does occur in cases involving the upper limbs it can be extremely serious. If the embolic occlusion reaches the trifurcation of the brachial artery, it requires embolectomy (see Fig. 6.65). There is also a high risk of spasm caused by manipulation of the brachial artery and its branches, and pharmacologic precautions against spasm are necessary. There is a still greater risk of cerebral embolism when dilatation is performed below the point where the vertebral artery emerges from the subclavian artery, as in Fig. 6.64. Fortunately, some 30 to 45 s elapse before flow is reversed in the vertebral artery, which, in theory, protects this vessel from embolism.

Most lesions in the subclavian arteries may be approached by the femoral route, using a "head hunter" type catheter for selective catheterization and introduction of the guidewire through the stenosis. The use of a long exchange guidewire (1.8 to 2 m long) is recommended. Long catheters, 1 to 1.1 m long, and 6- to 8-mm-diameter balloons, should be selected, their dimensions depending on the normal arterial diameter. The brachiocephalic artery may require a 10-mm-diameter balloon catheter.

Figure 6.66 (A) 42-year-old patient with well-segmented high brachial arterial occlusion (arrow), without pulses in the left upper limb. (B) Dilatation was performed by the femoral route, with a 4-mm Olbert-type balloon (arrow). (C) Angiogram showing recanalization. Radial pulses were good. However, spasm occurred, causing fluctuations in the radial pulse.

In some cases, the approach may be done by the axillary route, which offers greater maneuverability and a more rectilinear track, facilitating advancement beyond the subclavian stenoses and occlusions.

When brachial arterial lesions are approached by the femoral route (Fig. 6.66), the long guidewire should be introduced up to the elbow region. It should then be compressed inside the artery, keeping it stationary and allowing the balloon to be advanced through the stenosis without any back-and-forth movement of the guidewire tip, which could cause spasm (Fig. 6.66).

The published results regarding angioplasty performed on subclavian and brachial arteries are not conclusive, although so far the success rate is comparable to that obtained with angioplasty on the femoral arteries.

Carotid and Vertebral Arteries

There has been understandable reluctance to use modern angioplastic techniques in treating lesions involving the internal or external carotid arteries due to the risk of embolic episodes, with potentially serious neurologic consequences. There is, however, already a reasonable amount of literature regarding the dilatation of lesions in these arteries and in the vertebral arteries. The most frequently dilated lesions are those caused by fibromuscular dysplasia. Small differences in luminal diameter may account for the difference between normal and reduced flow, this being valid both for the carotids and the vertebral arteries.

Doubt still persists both in the literature and in medical practice on which is more significant in the development of transient ischemic vascular attacks (TIA): the occasional reduction of carotid flow, or repetitive microembolism originating from ulcerated atheromatous plaques or in areas of stasis in fibromuscular dysplastic lesions. Angiologists and vascular surgeons tend to think that repetitive embolism is responsible for TIAs. However, many TIA patients are found without any evidence of infarction, and the TIA episodes in these cases are probably related to transient drops in cerebral flow.

A few techniques have been used to minimize the risks of cerebral embolism during angioplasty of the internal carotid arteries. The simplest involves compressing the internal carotid while dilating the common carotid or its bifurcation. Another method uses what is known as the "washout" technique, in which arteriotomy is performed above the stenotic site in order to wash the carotid with the patient's own blood, in a controlled manner, by opening the ligation after dilatation with the balloon. A variation of this technique is temporary surgical ligation of the carotid below the balloon during angioplasty (with intraoperatively introduced catheter), which creates a retrograde blood flow that washes the angioplasty site, after which the arterial ligation is opened.

A newer technique involves occluding the carotid artery with a latex balloon or a filter above the stenosis, while performing dilatation with the angioplasty balloon. Active washing of the occluded segment with saline, and successive aspirations, are necessary. Only then will the flow be released when the occlusion balloon is deflated.

Recently, stenotic lesions caused either by atheromatous plaques or by fibromuscular dysplasia (Fig. 6.67), have been adequately treated with conventional balloon angioplasty systems. The balloon is rapidly inflated inside the internal carotid, under intraarterial heparinization (5000 IU). The patient takes 300 mg of aspirin for 6 days before the procedure, and is given dipyridamole (Persantine), 75 mg tid for at least 3 days. Postangioplasty transient ischemic complications occurred in only 3 to 10 percent of cases.

MESENTERIC VESSELS

Transluminal angioplasty in the mesenteric circulation has been used primarily to treat abdominal angina, described as a postoperative syndrome, with colic and diarrhea followed by significant weight loss and reduction in D-xylose absorption due to changes in the intestinal mucosa.

Until 1980, when the first studies were published on mesenteric arterial angioplasty, mesenteric revascularization was the preferred method for correcting stenoses of the mesenteric circulation. Since then angioplasty has been gaining increasing popularity as a viable alternative to surgery, which offers less than ideal results and is associated with significant morbidity and mortality rates.

The symptoms of mesenteric angina are, however, complex, and it is difficult to obtain a precise diagnosis. Quite often, for example, a lesion is found only in one vessel. For this reason, it is worthwhile to use transluminal angioplasty as a therapeutic trial, instead of automatically recommending a surgical procedure. There are in the literature reports of resolution of symptoms after dilatation of a single vessel (Fig. 6.68).

It should be noted that there is no indication for angioplasty in cases of median arcuate ligament compression syndrome, the pathologic significance of which remains in doubt.

The most common causes of mesenteric arterial stenosis are atheromatosis and, less frequently, fibromuscular dysplasia. Transluminal angioplasty is effective in both cases (Figs. 6.68 and 6.69). Atheromatous lesions are most often located near the ostium or on the first few centimeters of the superior and inferior mesenteric arteries, although they are not infrequently found in the mid-third and distal branches of these branches reducing the chance of collateralization and producing symptoms

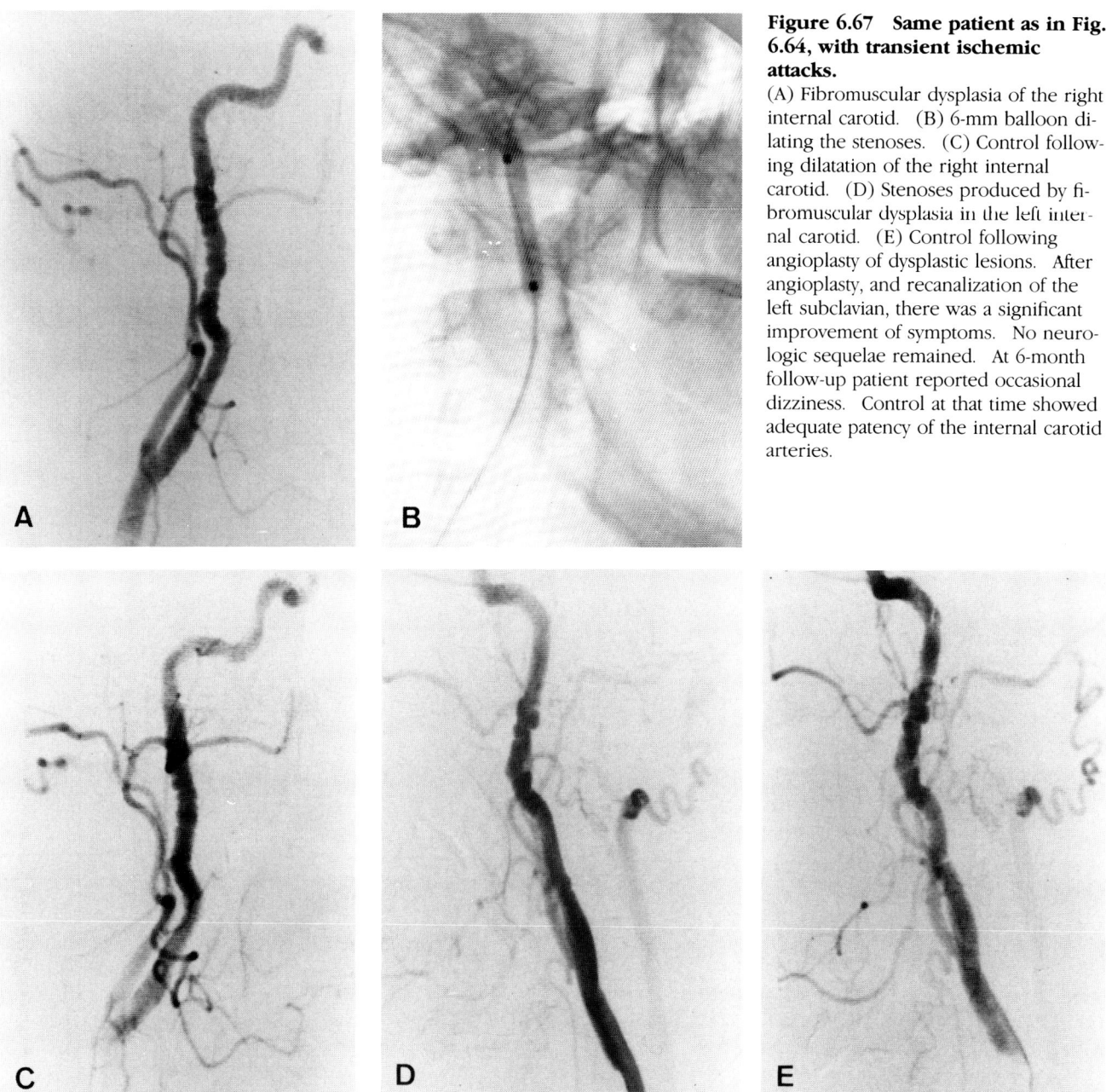

Figure 6.67 Same patient as in Fig. 6.64, with transient ischemic attacks.
(A) Fibromuscular dysplasia of the right internal carotid. (B) 6-mm balloon dilating the stenoses. (C) Control following dilatation of the right internal carotid. (D) Stenoses produced by fibromuscular dysplasia in the left internal carotid. (E) Control following angioplasty of dysplastic lesions. After angioplasty, and recanalization of the left subclavian, there was a significant improvement of symptoms. No neurologic sequelae remained. At 6-month follow-up patient reported occasional dizziness. Control at that time showed adequate patency of the internal carotid arteries.

(Fig. 6.69). Stenoses due to fibromuscular dysplasia occur predominantly in the mid-third of the mesenteric arteries.

It is important to examine each case of mesenteric angina by both anteroposterior and lateral aortograms, in order to visualize the ostia of the mesenteric arteries. Lateral inspiration and expiration images should be obtained to establish a diagnosis of the median arcuate ligament compression syndrome.

If the angle of the origin of the superior mesenteric artery is open, the approach may be done by the femoral route (Figs. 6.68 and 6.69). The stenosis is passed with a Cobra or Simmons-type catheter (Figs. 6.20 and 6.21), a heavy-duty guidewire being then introduced deeply into the superior mesenteric artery, after heparinization with (2000 to 5000 IU). The 6- to 8-mm-diameter balloon catheter, selected on the basis of the diameter of the normal artery, is introduced up to the level of the lesion and dilated for 30 to 60 s.

The axillary approach is a good alternative for arteries with a very acute angle as related to the aorta, even making possible the use of van Andel catheters. The femoral approach, however, is useful in distal dilatations of the mesenteric circulation, particularly when PVC

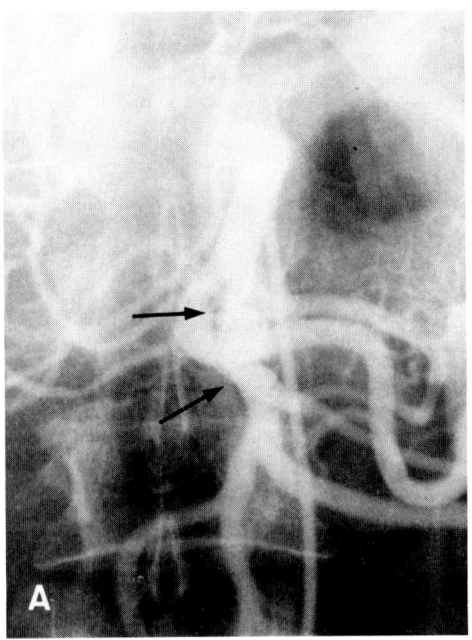
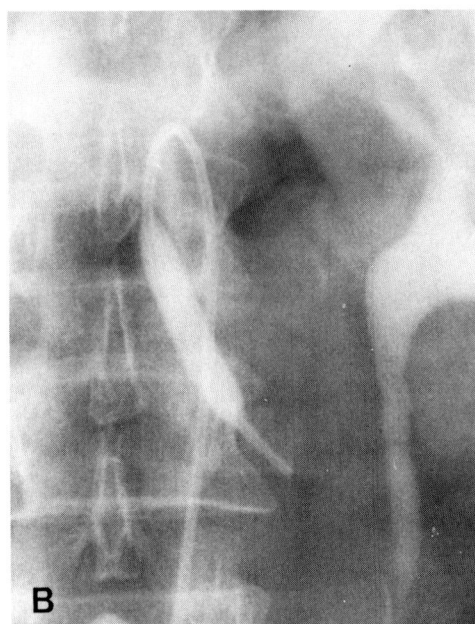
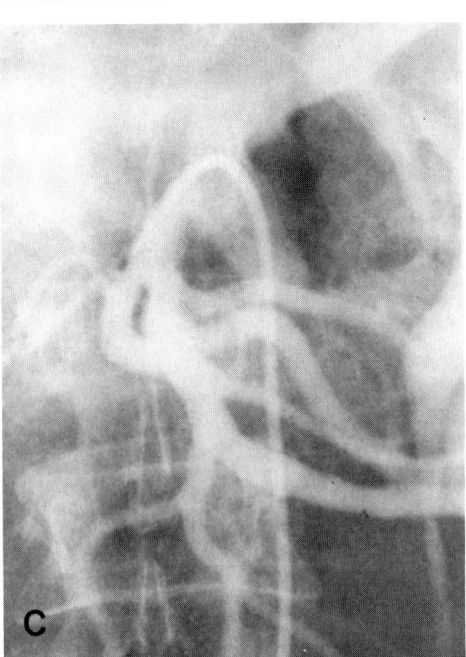

Figure 6.68 (A) 50-year-old patient with mesenteric angina. Selective injection into the superior mesenteric artery shows stenoses due to fibromuscular dysplasia, with a ringlike appearance (arrows). Note filling of the duodenopancreatic arcades through arteries leaving the inferior pancreatic artery, originating on the site of stenosis, and extending beyond the level of collateral circulation to the mesenteric arteries, through the celiac axis. (B) 6-mm balloon at the site of dilatation. (C) Angiographic control following dilatation showing smoothing of stenoses. At 4-year follow-up patient was asymptomatic.

balloons are used, which are more flexible than those made of polyethylene (Fig. 6.69).

The resolution of symptoms is uniform in most patients (over 80 percent), with pain reversal and improvement in D-xylose absorption.

HYPOGASTRIC ARTERIES

In 1923 Leriche described the association between sexual impotence and lesions causing vascular occlusion. In 1969 May found that almost 70 percent of patients with aortoiliac occlusive disease also showed penile erection dysfunction, but it was not until the 1970s that the relationship between sexual impotence and vascular occlusive dysfunctions became clearly understood.

Evaluation of patients whose sexual impotence is suspected to be of vascular origin should start with noninvasive studies, such as plethysmography and ultrasound. Only after those studies have demonstrated that vascular abnormality exists should angiography be performed.

Aortoiliac vascular problems are easily identified, but more distal changes require more selective, more detailed studies. When the occlusive change is limited to the aortoiliac segment, percutaneous angioplasty may be performed as described in the section "Angioplasty of the Aorta and Its Bifurcation" in this chapter. If the

Figure 6.69 80-year-old patient with gynecologic neoplasia and postoperative abdominal pain of mesenteric angina type.
(A) Injection into the mesenteric superior, showing stenoses in the main artery (arrowheads) and in the ileocolic branch (arrow). (B) 5-mm balloon expanded into the main artery. (C) Same balloon expanded inside the ileocolic branch. (D) Control following angioplasty shows good arterial patency in both areas. Note that the two stenotic sites prevent the development of any collateral circulation to the distal mesenteric territory. Postprandial pain disappeared.

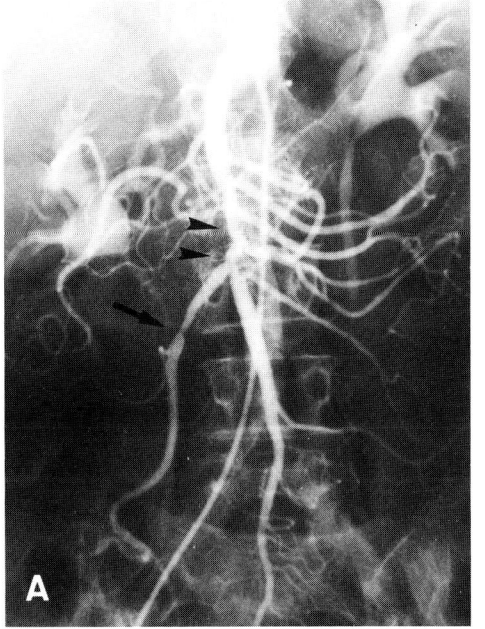
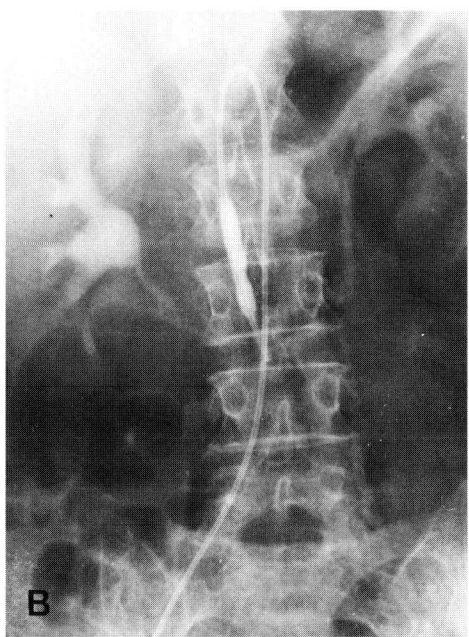
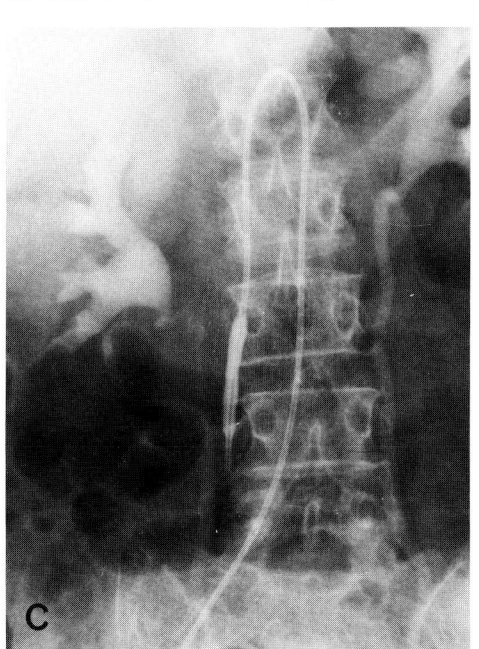
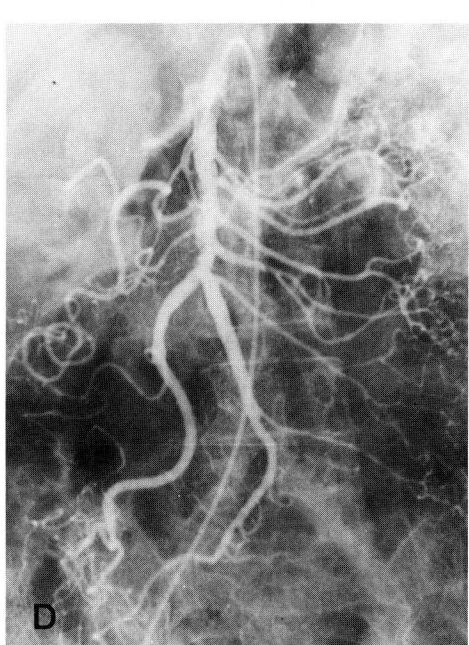

occlusive lesion is located in the hypogastric artery, percutaneous angioplasty, associated or not associated with dilatation of the iliacs, may be performed (Fig. 6.70) The approach to these vessels for dilatation should preferably be through the axillary route, because it is extremely difficult to follow the hypogastric bend through the ipsilateral femoral artery. The contralateral approach is sometimes appropriate, although it cannot be used in cases where occlusion of the contralateral iliac is present, as shown in Fig. 6.70.

When the procedure is successful, significant improvement is obtained in penile arterial flow, with a good chance of returning to sexual activity if the cause is strictly the occlusive arterial disease (Fig. 6.70).

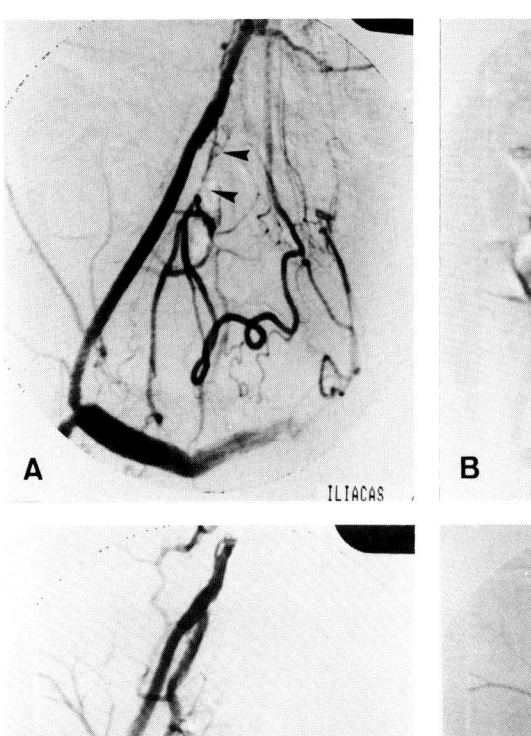
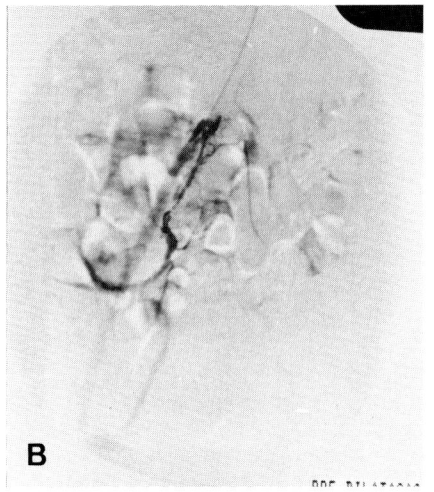
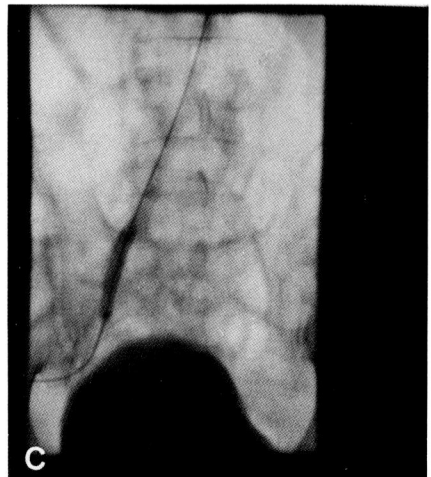
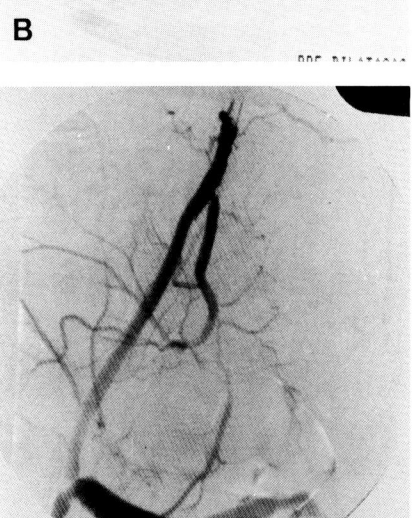

Figure 6.70 Treatment of sexual impotence by dilation of hypogastric artery.
(A) 60-year-old patient with diffuse atheromatous disease involving the aorta and the iliac, hypogastric (arrowheads), and femoral arteries. Angioplasty of the right iliac had previously been performed twice, and patient had undergone a femorofemoral graft. Erection impotence recently had developed. (B) Selective injection into almost occluded right hypogastric. (C) Dilatation of hypogastric artery with a 4-mm balloon. (D,E) Control following dilatation, anteroposterior and oblique views, showing recanalized hypogastric artery. The anterior distal circulation showed some degree of spasm; however, there was excellent functional response with regard to erection.

REFERENCES

Backman DM, Kim RM. Transluminal dilatation for subclavian steal syndrome. *AJR* 1980;135:995–996.

Bird CR, Hasso AN. Percutaneous transluminal angioplasty of the carotid artery. In *Transluminal Angioplasty,* edited by Castaneda-Zuniga WR. Thieme-Stratton, New York 1983:154–161.

Bockenheimer S, Mathias K. Percutaneous transluminal angioplasty in arteriosclerotic internal carotid artery stenosis. *AJNR* 1983;4:791–792.

Castaneda-Zuniga WR, Amplatz KA. Transluminal angioplasty of pelvic arteries in the management of vasculogenic erectile impotence. In *Transluminal Angioplasty,* edited by Castaneda-Zuniga WR. New York, Thieme-Stratton, New York, 1983:192–295.

Castaneda-Zuniga WR, Smith AD, Kaye K, et al. Transluminal angioplasty for treatment of vasculogenic impotence. *AJR* 1982;139:371.

Derauf BJ, Erickson DL, Castaneda-Zuniga WR, Cardella JF, Amplatz K. "Washout" technique for brachiocephalic angioplasty. *AJR* 1986;146:849.851.

Furrer J, Gruntzig A, Kugelmeier J, Goebel N. Treatment of abdominal angina with percutaneous dilatation of an arteria mesenterica superior stenosis. *Cardiovasc Intervent Radiol* 1980;3:43–44.

Garrido E, Montoya J. Transluminal dilatation of internal carotid artery in fibromuscular dysplasia. *Surg Neurol* 1981;16:469–471.

Golden DA, Ring EJ, McLean GK, Feiman DB. Percutaneous transluminal angioplasty in the treatment of abdominal angina. *AJR* 1982;139:247–249.

Guthaner DF, Schmitz L. Percutaneous transluminal angioplasty of radiation-induced arterial stenoses. *Radiology* 1982;133:77–78.

Hasso AN, Bird CR, Rinke DE, Thompson JR. Fibromuscular dysplasia of the internal carotid artery: Percutaneous transluminal angioplasty. *AJR* 2981;136:955–960.

Kerber CW, Cromwell LD, Loehden BL. Catheter dilatation of proximal carotid stenosis during distal bifurcation endarterectomy. *AJNR* 1980;1:348–349.

Kachel R, Endert G, Basche S, et al. Percutaneous transluminal angioplasty (dilatation) of carotid, vertebral and innominate artery stenoses. *Cardiovasc Intervent Radiol* 1986;10:142–146.

Leriche R. Des obliterations arterialles hautes comme cause d'insuffisance circulatoire des membres inferieures. *Bull Mem Soc Chir Paris* 1923;49:1404–1406.

Martin EC. Percutaneous transluminal angioplasty of various categories of vascular disease. In *Angioplasty*, edited by Jang GD. McGraw-Hill, New York, 1986:83–103.

Mathias K, Seeman W, VonRurtern S. Dilatation treatment of supra-aortic artery disease. Presented at the 71st Scientific Assembly and Annual Meeting of the RSNA. Chicago, November 17–22, 1985.

May AG, DeWeese JA, Robb CG. Changes in sexual function following operation on the abdominal aorta. *Surgery* 1969;65:41–47.

Motarjeme A, Keifer JW, Zuska AJ. Percutaneous transluminal angioplasty of the vertebral arteries. *Radiology* 1981;139:715–717.

Motarjeme A, Keifer JW, Zuska AJ. Percutaneous transluminal angioplasty of the brachiocephalic arteries. *AJR* 1982;138:457–462.

Novelline RA. Percutaneous transluminal angioplasty: Newer applications. *AJR* 1980;135:983–988.

O'Leary DH, Clouse ME. Percutaneous transluminal angioplasty of the cavernous carotid artery for recurrent ischemia. *AJNR* 1984;5:644–645.

Ring EJ, McLean GK, Freiman DB. Selected techniques in percutaneous transluminal angioplasty. *AJR* 1982;139:767–773.

Ringelstein EB, Zeuner H. Delayed reversal of vertebral artery blood flow following percutaneous transluminal angioplasty for subclavian steal syndrome. *Neuroradiology* 1984;26:189–198.

Roberts L, Wertman DA, Mills SR, Moore AV, Heaston DK. Transluminal angioplasty of the superior mesenteric artery: An alternative to surgical revascularization. *AJR* 1983;31:117–134.

Schutz H, Yeung HP, Chiu MC, Terbeugge K, Ginsberg R. Dilatation of vertebral artery stenosis. *N Engl J Med* 1981;304:732–733.

Smith RB, Moore T, Russel W. Transluminal angioplasty of the cerebral circulation. *Clin Neurosurg* 1983;31:117–134.

Theron J, Courtheoux P, Henriet JP, Pelouze G, Derlon JM, Maiza D. Angioplasty of supraaortic arteries. *J Neuroradiol* 1984;11:187–200.

Uflacker R, Goldany MA, Constant S. Resolution of mesenteric angina with percutaneous transluminal angioplasty of a superior mesenteric artery stenosis using a balloon catheter. *Gastrointest Radiol* 1980;5:367–369.

Vitek JJ. Percutaneous transluminal angioplasty of the external carotid artery. *AJNR* 1983;4:796–799.

Vitek JJ, Keller FS, Duvall ER, Gupta KL, Chandar-Sehar B. Brachiocephalic artery dilatation by percutaneous transluminal angioplasty. *Radiology* 1986;158:779–785.

Venous Angioplasty

RENAN UFLACKER

Veins are subject to occlusions due to persistent pressure, blunt traumas, heavy exercise, adjacent inflammatory processes, phlebitis (with various etiologies, including the presence of indwelling catheters), neoplasms, and other, less obvious, causes. Thrombosis may be incomplete or recanalized, and in either case venous stenosis may result. A wide range of venous lesions have been successfully treated by transluminal angioplastic procedures.

The creation of arteriovenous fistulas for dialysis, either by direct anastomosis (Brescia-Cimino fistula), or by using synthetic or biological grafts, will produce a high-flow situation in a system designed to operate under low flow. In these cases, venous stenosis results from flow turbulence and wall damage caused by constant pressure; atheromatous plaques may also develop. Intimal fibrosis may be present in venous valvular regions (Fig. 6.71). Direct arteriovenous fistulas may cause the development of postsurgical fibrosis on the site of anastomosis, the shunt thus becoming inadequate for dialysis due to its low flow (Fig. 6.72). Angioplasty using a high-pressure balloon can adequately dilate both the fibrotic and stenosed vein (Fig. 6.71), as well as fibrotic and almost occluded anastomoses (Fig. 6.72). When the Brescia-Cimino fistula is located on the wrist, either the high radial or brachial artery may be punctured in order to reach the shunt (Fig. 6.72). When the fistula is located on the elbow fold, the femoral approach may be used.

In actual venous stenosis, the vein itself may be punctured through the arm (Fig. 6.71).

Subclavian venous occlusions, which are usually due to uncommon physical effort, can, in most cases, be recanalized and adequately dilated by large (8- to 12-mm-diameter) balloon catheters.

Two conditions that are strong indications for angioplasty are superior vena cava syndrome and Budd-Chiari syndrome. The superior or inferior vena cava may be dilated by using a balloon with a diameter of 12 to 16 mm. For treating Budd-Chiari cases, the Yamada technique, which makes use of three or four 8-mm balloons, can be used. Venous percutaneous angioplasty is also highly successful in treating some types of hepatic vein occlusion that may eventually cause Budd-Chiari syndrome (see Fig. 3.78).

Caval stenosis secondary to neoplasm and radiotherapy will not respond to angioplasty because of the elastic properties of the tumor (Fig. 6.73), and in these cases a Gianturco Z-stent is usually placed.

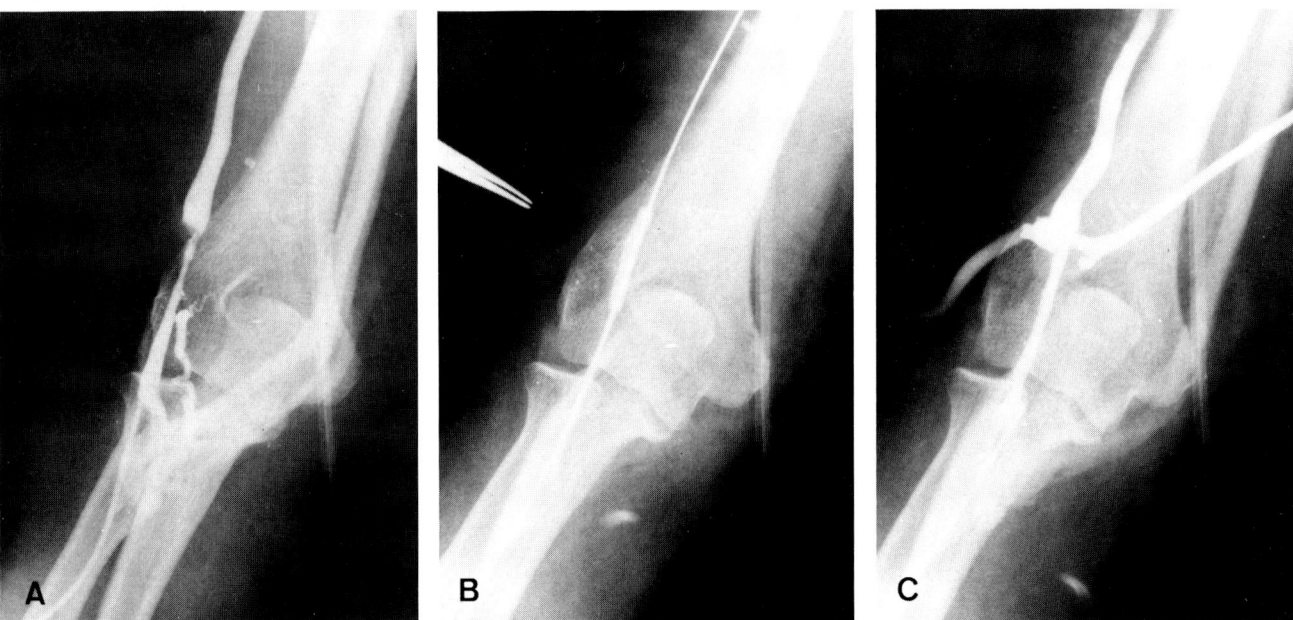

Figure 6.71 (A) Drainage vein stenosis in hemodialysis shunt. (B) Dilatation with 4-mm balloon. (C) Final venous angiogram showing improvement of the vein caliber allowing hemodialysis.

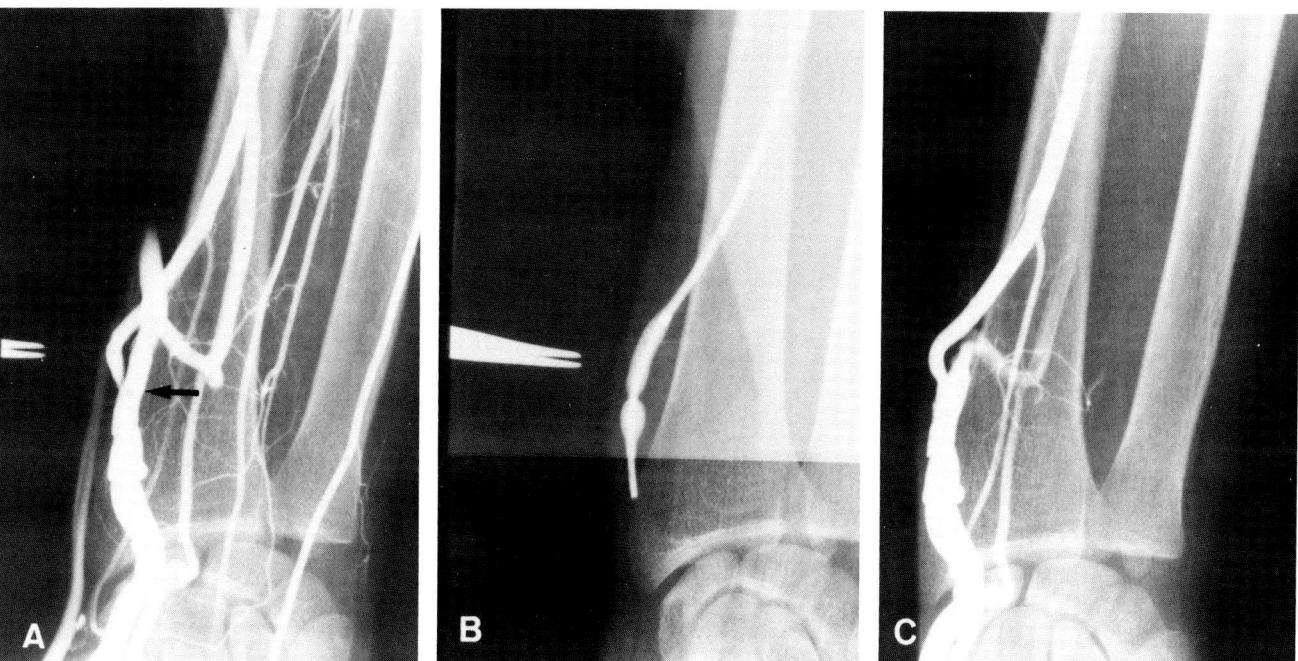

Figure 6.72 (A) Stenosis in radial Brescia-Cimino-type arteriovenous fistula. Note the thrombus (arrow). (B) Transluminal angioplasty with 4-mm balloon by puncture into the brachial artery. (C) Control following angioplasty shows a reasonable amount of flow passing through the anastomosis. The same fistula was used for hemodialysis for an additional 1½ years.

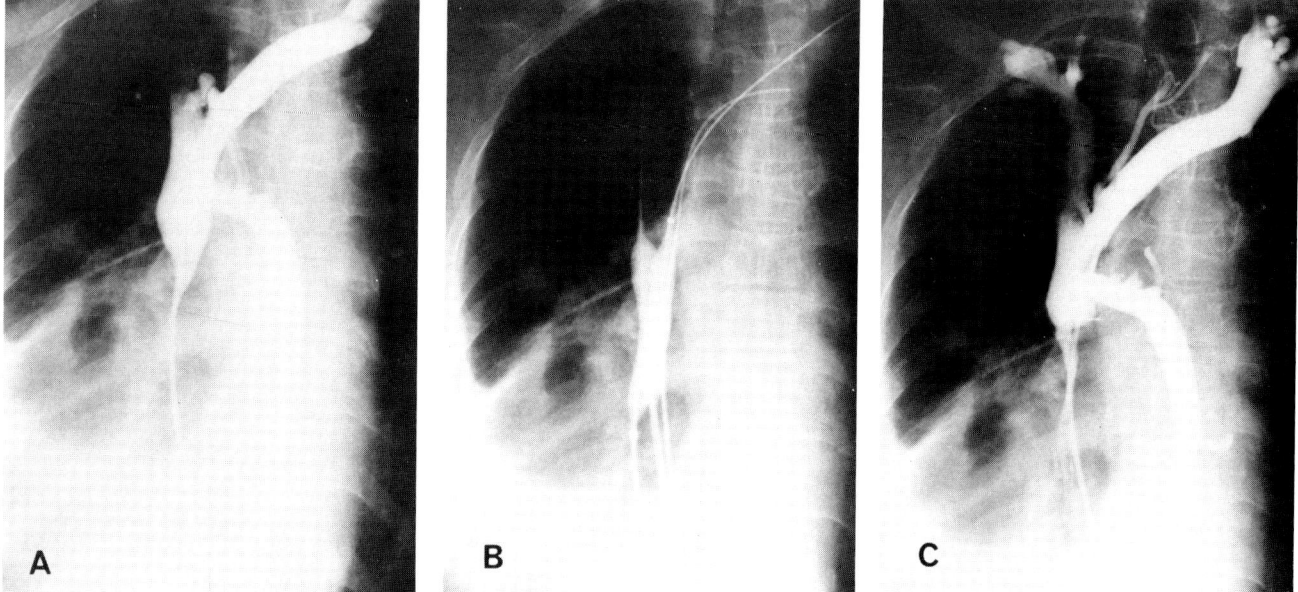

Figure 6.73 Attempted angioplasty in the superior vena cava of a patient with superior vena cava syndrome. The vein was occluded by a lung neoplasm, which had been operated on and irradiated.
(A) Severe superior caval stenosis just before the right atrium. (B) Three 8-mm balloons dilated at the same time in the stenosis. (C) Control showing poor results, with inadequate dilatation. The tumor recurred, this being the most likely cause of caval occlusion. A Gianturco Z-stent was indicated.

Portal vein occlusion causing portal hypertension and bleeding varices may, in selected cases, be treated by transhepatic angioplasty when patency of the main portohepatic radicules (see Fig. 3.60) allows catheterization.

REFERENCES

Alpert JR, Ring EJ, Berkowitz HD, et al. Treatment of vein graft stenosis by balloon catheter dilatation. *JAMA* 1979;242:2769–2771.

Gardiner GA, Meyerovitz MF. Dissection complicating angioplasty. *AJR* 1985;145:627–631.

Glanz S, Gordon D, Butt KMH, Hong J, Adamson R, Sclafani SJA. Dialysis access fistulas: Treatment of stenoses by transluminal angioplasty. *Radiology* 1984;152:637–642.

Gordon DH, Glanz S, Butt KM, Adamsons RJ, Koenig MA. Treatment of stenotic lesions in dialysis access fistulas and shunts by transluminal angioplasty. *Radiology* 1982;143:53–58.

Sherry CS, Diamond NG, Meyers TP, Martin RI. Successful treatment of superior vena cava syndrome by venous angioplasty. *AJR* 1986;147:834–835.

Trerotolo SO, McLean GK, Burke DR, Merange SG. Treatment of subclavian venous stenoses by percutaneous transluminal angioplasty. *J Intervent Radiol* 1986;1:15–18.

Uflacker R, Alves MA, Cantisani GG, Souza HP, Wagner J, Moraes LF. Treatment of portal vein obstruction by percutaneous transhepatic angioplasty. *Gastroenterology* 1985;88:176–180.

Uflacker R, Francisconi CF, Rodriguez MP, Amaral NM. Percutaneous transluminal angioplasty of the hepatic veins for treatment of Budd-Chiari syndrome. *Radiology* 1984;153:641–642.

Yamada R, Sato M, Kawaterba M, Nakatsuka, Nakamura K, Kobayshi N. Segmental obstruction of the hepatic inferior vena cava treated by transluminal angioplasty. *Radiology* 1983;149:91–96.

Complications of Angioplasty

RENAN UFLACKER

The complications that may arise from transluminal angioplasty (Table 6.4) may be broken down into four categories according to their origin and evolution (Laerum, 1983):

1. Reactions associated with arterial puncture
2. Local reactions
3. Hemodynamic effects at dilatation site
4. Effects produced by contrast medium and other active substances

Reactions Associated with Arterial Puncture

The most frequent minor complication of angioplasty is hematoma formation. At least three factors have a bearing on the development of hematoma:

— The size of the arterial orifice after the balloon has been passed (even if folded and empty)
— The use of heparin
— The presence of arterial hypertension

Table 6.4 – Complications of angioplasty

Type	Incidence, %
Arterial rupture	0.4
Hypotension	
Occlusion of stenosis	
Renal failure	
Distal embolization	5.7
Vascular perforation by guidewire	2.8
Bacterial endoarteritis	
Hematoma on puncture site	5.7
Pseudoaneurysm on puncture site	
Vascular spasm	10
Intimal dissection	5.5
Transverse rupture of balloon	
Deformation of balloon (PVC)	

Hematoma formation is more frequent when the axillary route has been used, as is the occurrence of pseudoaneurysms (Fig. 6.74).

The presence of thrombi at the puncture site may cause vessel occlusion or distal embolism.

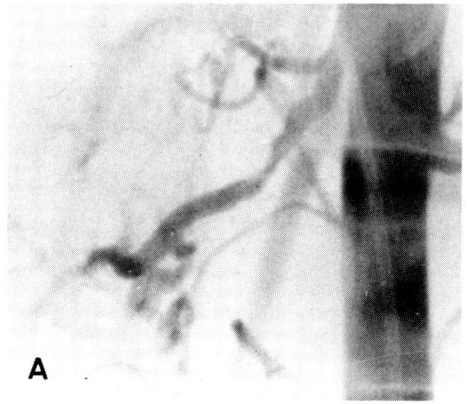
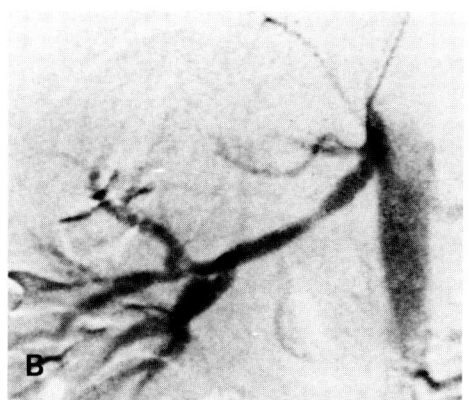
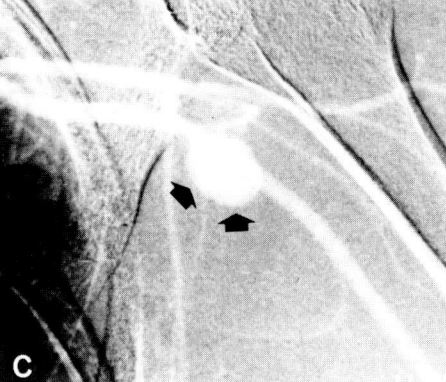

Figure 6.74 Pseudoaneurysm of axillary artery which appeared after the axillary approach was used for renal angioplasty. (A) Right renal artery stenosis in caudally angulated artery. (B) Control after angioplasty with 6-mm balloon, showing no significant results. (C) The pseudoaneurysm on the axillary puncture site was treated by surgery.

Local Reactions

Guidewire manipulation, catheter introduction, and balloon inflation can cause a number of local reactions. Manipulation of the guidewire–catheter set will cause spasm in about 10 percent of cases, more if the peripheral circulation is involved. The displacement of atheromatous plaques and the distal embolism that are seen in diagnostic angiographic procedures may also occur with angioplasty, since its action principle includes plaque fracture, intimal rupture, and release of fragments.

Dissection of the intima by the guidewire or by contrast injection is the second most frequent complication of angioplasty (after hematoma) (Fig. 6.75), and emergency surgery may be necessary to clear the involved artery. Spontaneous recanalization may occur in a few cases.

Another local complication, one which is related to guidewire introduction at the subintimal level, is arterial perforation. This has no major consequences for lower limb circulation, but may be quite severe in the iliac arteries, the aorta, and the renal arteries. Two ways to avoid arterial perforation are local compression of the limbs and balloon inflation in the renal arteries, both of which act to prevent the formation of hematoma.

Rupture of the intima or of the tunica media is a common occurrence in angioplastic procedures; the adventitia is usually not affected. However, when advantitial laceration does occur, a lesion of the pseudoaneurysmic type may develop, or hemorrhage may occur in the perivascular space. Such hemorrhage, although rare, is the most serious complication of angioplasty, and is associated with high mortality rates (Fig. 6.76). It may involve larger arteries, such as the iliac and renal arteries especially when multiple renal arteries are being treated (Fig. 6.77).

Hemorrhage due to arterial laceration, which causes severe pain and hypotension, may even be a late manifestation after angioplasty. Once the diagnosis of arterial rupture has been established, the balloon should be kept inflated inside the artery until definitive action is taken, either surgery or embolotherapy. Embolization of a renal artery feeding a kidney with multiple arteries will

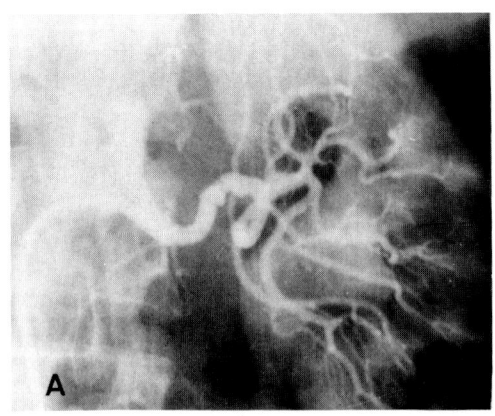
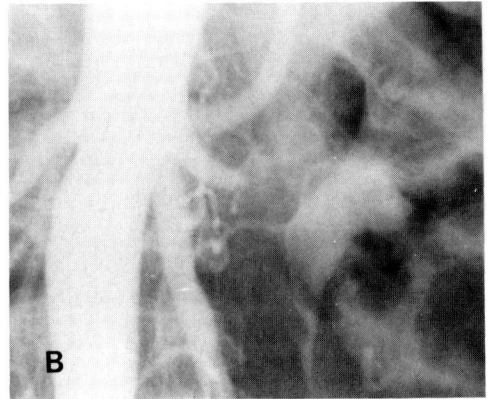
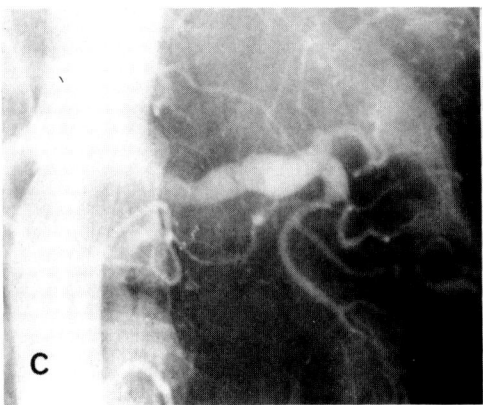

Figure 6.75 Occlusion of the left renal artery during an angioplasty attempt.
(A) Fibromuscular dysplasia in the left renal artery. (B) After an attempt to use the Simmons-catheter technique, both intimal dissection and arterial occlusion have occurred. There was no worsening of hypertension.
(C) Partial recanalization has occurred after 1 month, with aneurysmal dilatation of the renal artery, which was traumatized during the procedure. The patient's clinical status remained unchanged.

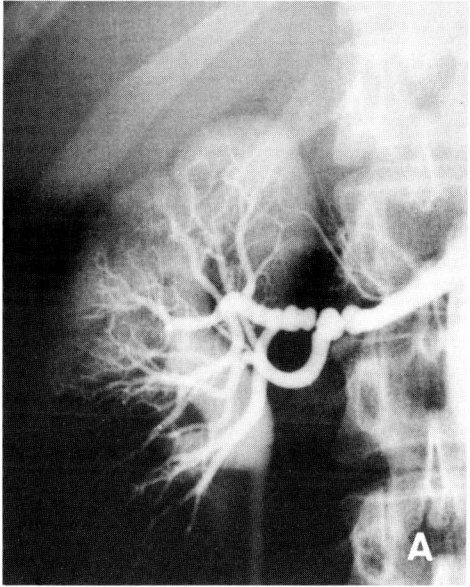
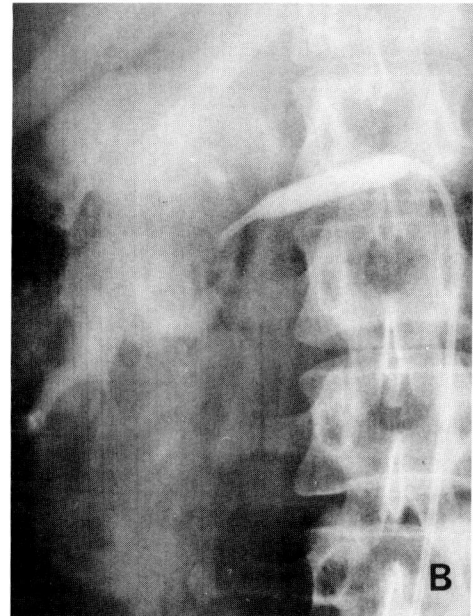
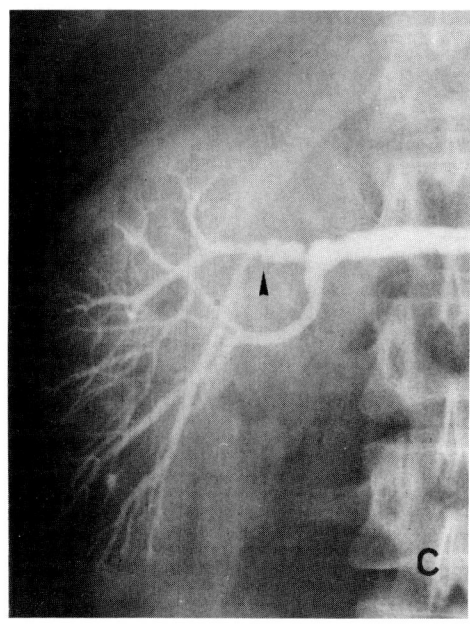

Figure 6.76 (A) 32-year-old patient with renovascular arterial hypertension (180/130) as a result of fibromuscular dysplasia in the right renal artery. (B) Manipulation of the catheter guidewire set caused renal artery perforation and the formation of a retroperitoneal hematoma. A balloon catheter was inflated for hemostasis. Note the presence of contrast medium in the retroperitoneum. (C) Angiographic control following hemostasis showing with visible improvement of stenoses, one of which persisted. The umbilication present most probably corresponds to the perforation (arrowhead). Treatment was conservative. Pressure under medication was 140/100.

not cause any problem in terms of viability of the kidney, even if solitary (Fig. 6.78). When the kidney is fed by a single artery, the solution is more difficult. In cases involving a single artery, the artery may be occluded by balloon and operated on or embolized with coils, proximally. When there is a solitary kidney, surgery is the only alternative, and the balloon should be kept inflated until the renal pedicle has been surgically dissected (Fig. 6.78).

The development of periarterial fibrosis may lead to occlusion, both secondary to puncture and as a direct result of puncture, and contrast extrasavation into the periarterial space (Fig. 6.79). Other local complications are related to thrombosis on the dilated site, when

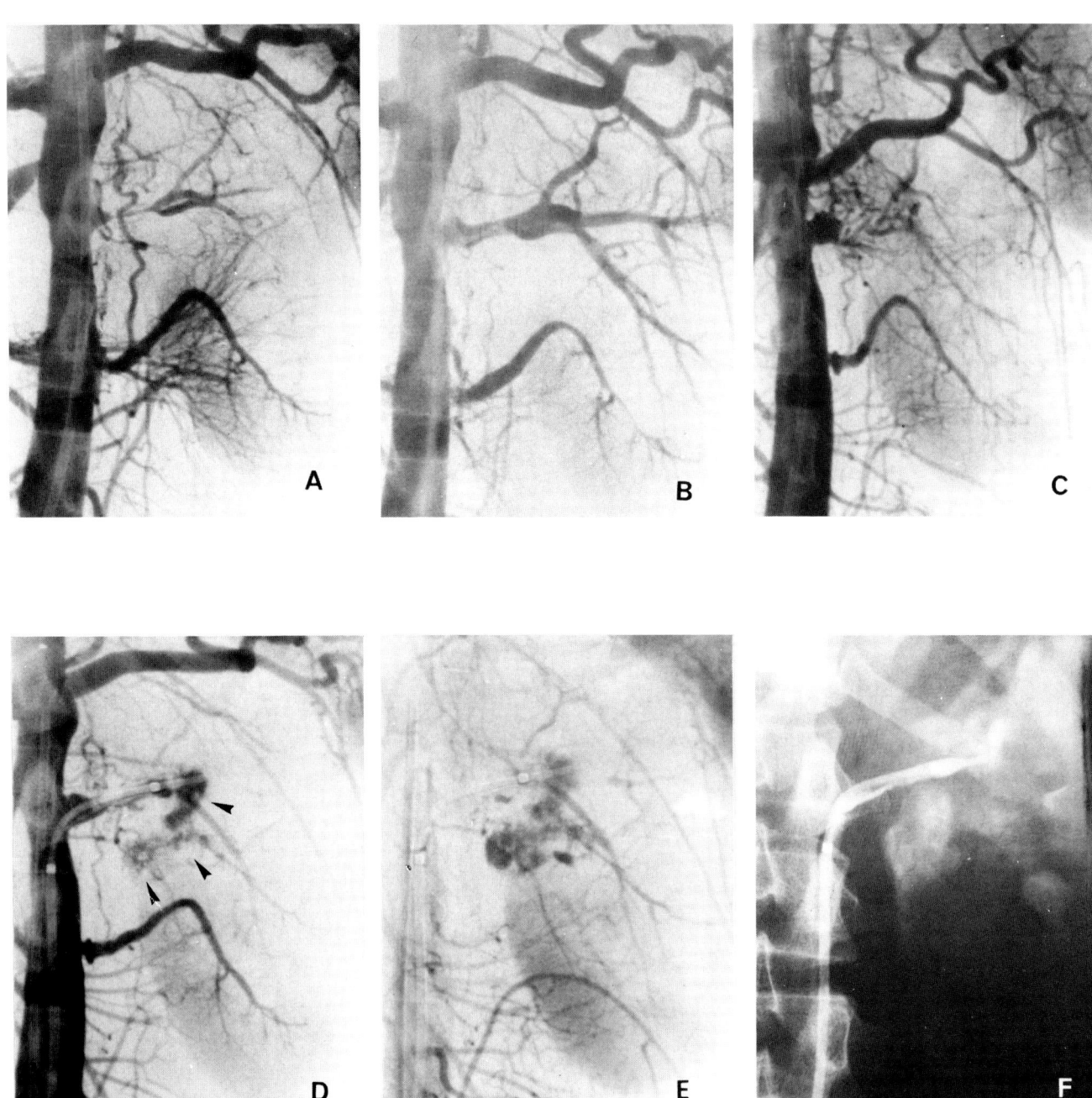

Figure 6.77 A 21-year-old patient with a solitary kidney who presented with renal failure. Arterial pressure was 180/120 without medication and 140/100 with medication.

(A) Severe stenosis of the left main renal artery and stenosis of the polar artery at its origin. Note the lesions in the aorta and the superior mesenteric artery, which are compatible with Takayasu's disease. There was also occlusion of the left pulmonary artery. (B) Postangioplasty control showing excellent response in both vessels. Pressure dropped to 140/90 without medication. (C) After 1 month, arterial hypertension recurred, accompanied by occlusion of the left main renal artery and renal failure. (D,E) New transluminal angioplasty has caused arterial laceration with retroperitoneal hemorrhage (arrowheads). (F) The balloon was kept inflated for hemostasis, and the patient was taken to surgery in good clinical condition. After arteriorrhaphy, the patient remained comatose for 3 days. Blood pressure was normal or moderately elevated and renal failure persisted. The patient died 24 h after fever and pneumonia occurred on the fifth postoperative day, in the only functional lung.

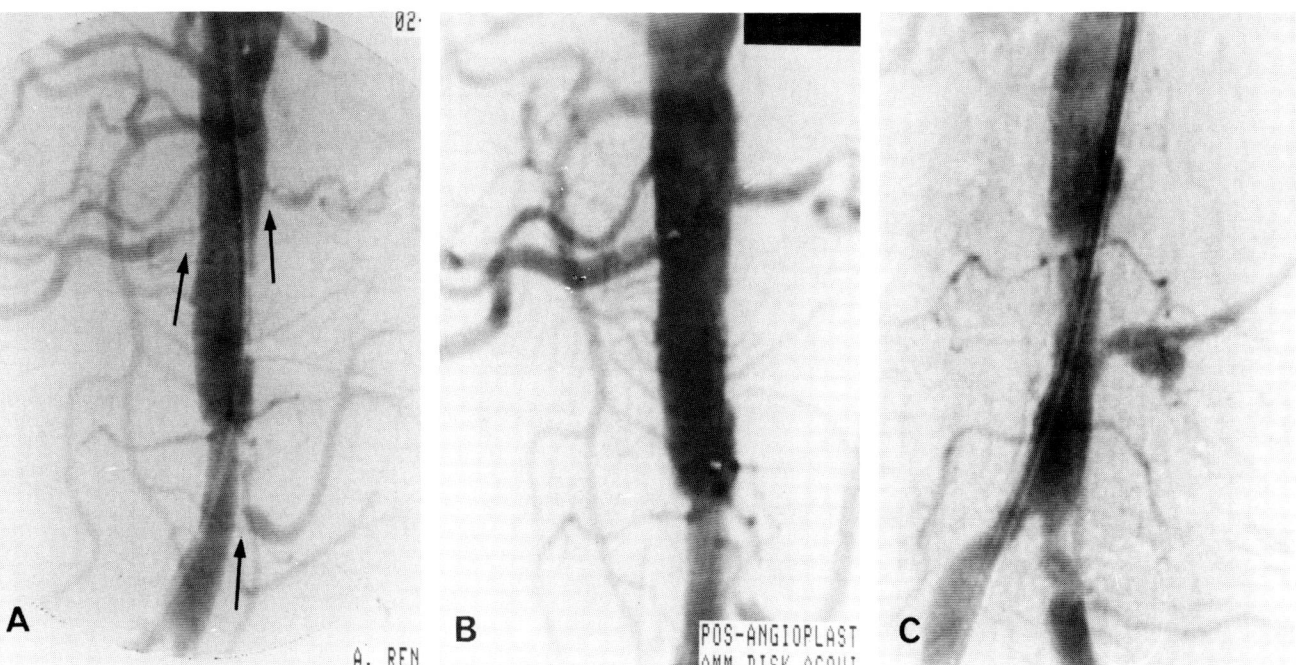

Figure 6.78 (A) 56-year-old patient with severe and uncontrollable arterial hypertension, and severe stenosis of all renal arteries. Note the presence of aortic and renal ostial lesions. (B) Control following angioplasty of the main renal arteries, showing good patency. (C) Because the left inferior polar artery, the last artery to be dilated, had not responded to a 5-mm balloon, a 6-mm balloon was used, resulting in arterial rupture with retroperitoneal hematoma. Surgery consisted of arteriorrhaphy. The patient developed ventricular fibrillation upon wall closure, and did not recover.

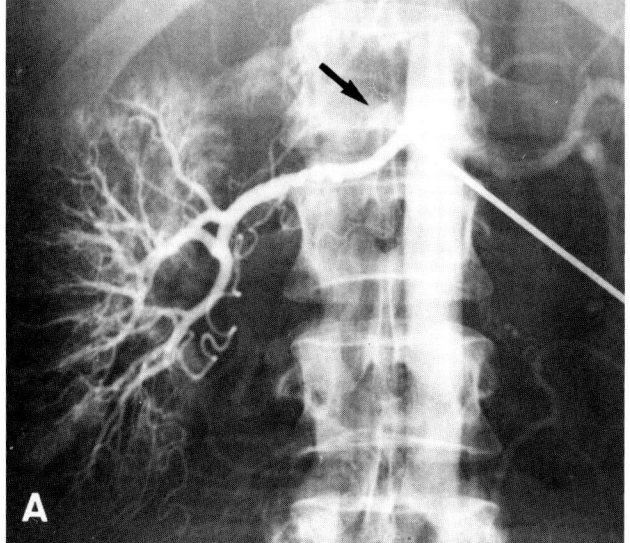
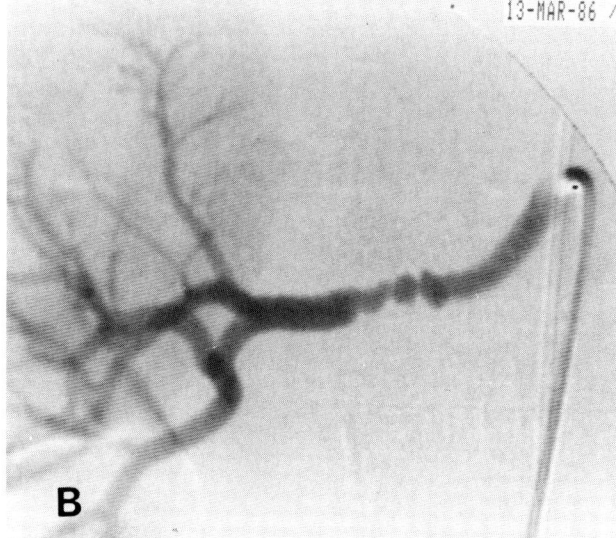

Figure 6.79 38-year-old patient with arterial hypertension of 170/100.
(A) Translumbar aortogram performed elsewhere showing fibromuscular dysplastic lesion and perivascular extravasation of contrast medium (arrow). (B) Selective preangioplasty angiogram of the right renal artery. (C) Postangioplasty control showing excellent results, but with spasm of the intrarenal branches. Postprocedure pressure was 140/80. (D) Occlusion of the right renal artery. Five months after angioplasty, hypertension was again 170/100. An earlier angiogram (not shown) demonstrated intact angioplasty results, but showed a tubular stenosis at the ostium, probably related to the extravasation seen in (A). A few days later this was occluded, preventing a new attempt at angioplasty. The segment dilated in (C) was intact. The most likely cause of occlusion was the development of perivascular fibrosis due to extravascular injection, or (less likely) to manipulation during angioplasty. A right nephrectomy was performed.

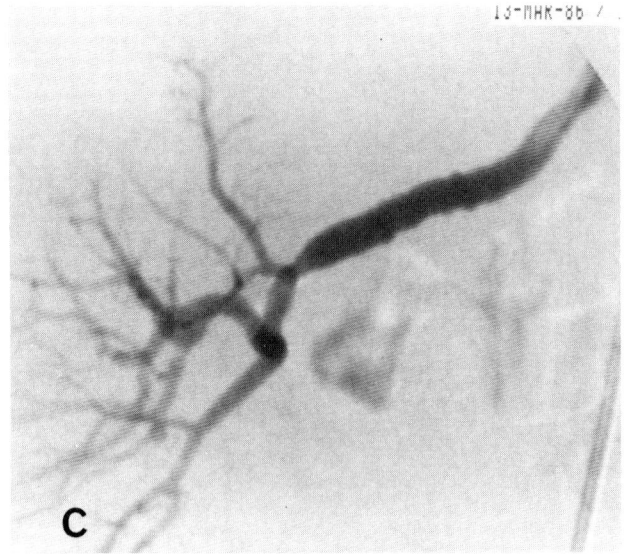
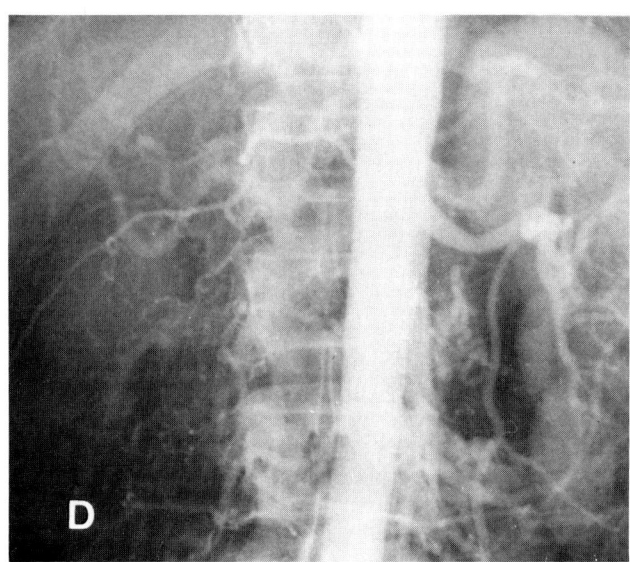

Figure 6.79 *Continued*

arterial flow is low or when hypotension occurs after the procedure.

Balloon abnormalities may lead to "explosive" rupture (bursting) of the balloon or to formation of an "aneurysm" on the balloon wall (Fig. 6.80). This may cause sudden overdilatation of the artery and rupture or intimal laceration. In cases where transverse rupture of the balloon prevents it from being removed through the puncture orifice, a vascular sheath may be used to retrieve the balloon, thereby protecting the artery from damage.

Hemodynamic Problems

Hemodynamic problems following successful renal artery angioplasty are usually secondary to the development of excessive diuresis and hypotention. Dehydration and hypotension may lead to thrombosis of the dilated artery at any level, as well as to myocardial infarction and cerebral ischemic vascular problems. Hypotension may be related to hemorrhage with retroperitoneal hematoma originating from the femoral artery puncture, and not simply due to the reduction in blood pressure resulting from the angioplasty.

When successful angioplasty of the lower limbs allows a patient who formerly suffered from severe claudication to walk much more than was previously possible, acute myocadial infarction may develop, followed by death.

Reaction to Contrast Media or Medication

The use of large volumes of contrast medium may cause acute tubular necrosis and transient renal failure. Drugs commonly used in angioplastic procedures as preventive or adjuvant medication, such as heparin and fibrinolytic agents (streptokinase, urokinase) may cause acute hemorrhagic episodes in recent surgical incisions and at puncture sites, as well as hemorrhagic strokes, which may complicate even further existing problems of blood crasis.

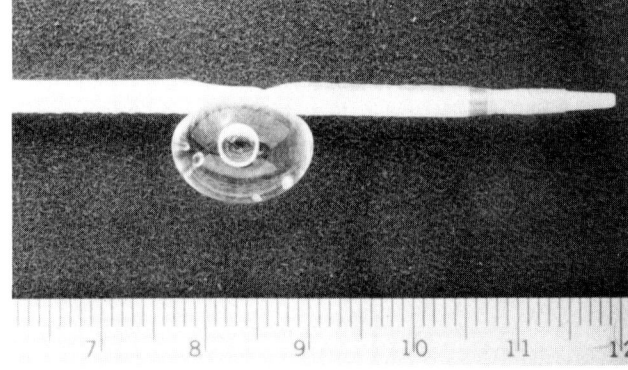

Figure 6.80 "Aneurysmal" deformity of Olbert balloon.

REFERENCES

Connolly JE, Kwann JHM, McCart PM. Complications after percutaneous transluminal angioplasty. *Am J Surg* 1981;142:60–66.

Gardiner GA, Meyerovitz MF, Stokes KR, Clouse ME, Harrington DP, Bettmann MA. Complications of transluminal angioplasty. *Radiology* 1986;159:201–208.

Jensen SR, Voegeli DR, Crummy AG, et al. Iliac artery rupture during transluminal angioplasty: Treatment by embolization and surgical bypass. *AJR* 1985;145:381–382.

Laerum F, Castaneda-Zuniga WR, Amplatz KA. Complications of transluminal angioplasty. In *Transluminal Angioplasty,* edited by Castaneda-Zuniga WR. Thieme-Stratton, New York, 1983:41–44.

Puijlaert CBAJ, Mali WPTM, Rosenbusch G, Van Straalen AM, Klinge J, Feldberg MAM. Delayed rupture of renal artery after renal percutaneous transluminal angioplasty. *Radiology* 1986;159:635–637.

Ring EJ, Freiman DB, McLean GK, et al. Percutaneous recanalization of common iliac artery occlusions: An unacceptable complication rate? *AJR* 1982;139:587–589.

Samson RH, Sprayregen S, Veith FJ, Scher LA, Gupta SK, Ascer E. Management of angioplasty complications: Unsuccessful procedures and early and late failures. *Ann Surg* 1984;199:234–240.

Simonetti G, Rossi P, Passariello R, Faraglia V, Spartera C, Pistolesk R, Florani P. Iliac artery rupture: A complication of transluminal angioplasty. *AJR* 1983;140:989–990.

Tegtmeyer CJ, Beziridijian DR. Removing the stuck, ruptured angioplasty balloon catheter. *Radiology* 1981;139:231–232.

Uflacker R, Mourao GS, Piske Rl. Renal artery rupture during transluminal angioplasty. *J Intervent Radiol* 1988; 3:99–103.

Intravascular Stents

JULIO C. PALMAZ

INTRODUCTION

Charles Dotter's first paper on percutaneous stenting was published 20 years ago, at a time when percutaneous angioplasty itself was at an early stage of development. The skepticism which his visionary ideas aroused was due to the fact that the available data did not support the theoretical notion that mechanical scaffolding of a stenotic lumen could result in long-term vessel patency. Extrapolation from classical surgical concepts suggested that vascular stents could not work. Foreign bodies tend to migrate, cause perforation, and create chronic inflammatory reactions, and it was assumed that an intravascular metallic stent would cause rupture, the formation of fistulas or aneurysms, or other serious complications. Compliance mismatch between the arterial wall and the unyielding stent could create intimal hyperplasia similar to that occurring at anastomotic sites. By serving as a nidus for thrombus formation, prosthetic material could lead to occlusion or distal embolization. Furthermore, hemodynamic alterations induced by stenting could potentially create accelerated atherosclerosis, stenosis, and, ultimately, occlusion. Instead, experiments in laboratory animals yielded unexpected results. Both medium- and large-sized vessels demonstrated remarkably good tissue tolerance to metal stents. Stents of various designs became covered with endothelialized intimal tissue within days or weeks, providing protection against low-flow thrombosis, the main complication affecting surgical synthetic grafts.

The rapid incorporation of stents into the thickness of the arterial wall may explain the relatively mild intimal hyperplasia that covers the lumen of most stents. Stents placed in atherosclerotic rabbit arteries were incorporated in the vessel wall as quickly as in normal vessels, and the tissue covering the stents did not undergo atherosclerotic changes despite the continuation of atherogenic diets. The stable inner surface of the stented vessels allowed new tissue growth, preventing the surface irregularity, turbulence, platelet deposition, and fibromuscular proliferation that result in vessel restenosis and occlusion.

The recent development of new percutaneous vascular techniques has been driven by the need for safer, less costly alternatives to surgery. Despite their potential, some of these techniques, such as balloon angioplasty, have remained underutilized in the peripheral vasculature. In contrast, percutaneous transluminal coronary angioplasty (PTCA) has been used extensively. However, PTCA has a restenosis rate of 30 percent and an abrupt closure rate of about 3 percent, and percutaneous stenting has the potential for improving the results of these procedures by preventing both acute and delayed failures.

TYPES OF VASCULAR STENTS

Regardless of type, all intravascular stents are introduced through a small arteriotomy and are expanded to a larger diameter at the intravascular target site. The expanded stent is initially fixed in place through the action of frictional force resulting from the expansile strength of the stent and the elastic recoil of the vessel wall. Intravascular stents are classified according to their mechanism of action as one of three types:

1. Thermal-memory stents
2. Spring-loaded stents
3. Plastic-deformation stents

Thermal-Memory Stents

These are made of a nickel-titanium alloy known as nitinol. They change their shape when placed in contact with warm blood or saline, adopting a coiled configuration of predetermined diameter. Although U.S. experience with thermal-memory stents is limited to laboratory animals, the Soviet Union, which has surprisingly extensive clinical experience with nitinol coils, reports good results.

Spring-Loaded Stents

Spring-loaded stents are made of tempered stainless steel alloy wire arranged in a tubular fashion and compressed inside a small-diameter delivery catheter for introduction into the vascular lumen. At the target site, the device is freed from the constraining sleeve, where it expands. The final diameter represents the point of equilibrium between the residual elasticity of the stent and the elastic recoil of the vessel wall. Examples of spring-loaded

Figure 6.81 Zigzag (Gianturco) stent. Its elastic properties allow the device to spring open to a larger diameter after extrusion from a sleeve container. This particular stent is composed of two portions joined by a bridge.

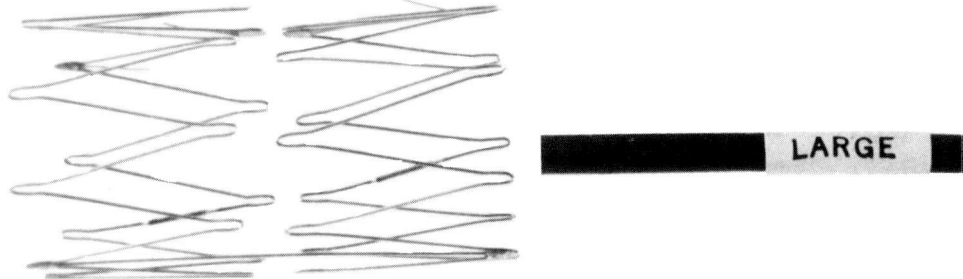

stents are the zigzag, or Gianturco, stent (Fig. 6.81) and the Medinvent stent.

Plastic-Deformation Stents

Plastic-deformation stents are made of malleable metal, usually annealed stainless steel. They are expanded to their elastic limit by the inflation of a coaxial balloon. The balloon expands the arterial wall and the stent simultaneously, and the device is pressed flush against the dilated vascular surface. The balloon-expandable intravascular stent, a continuous slotted metal tube that opens into a mesh, works according to the mode of action shown in Fig. 6.82. Other stents fabricated of malleable metal that operate on plastic-deformation principles include one stent with interdigitating, alternating wire windings or a woven metal mesh.

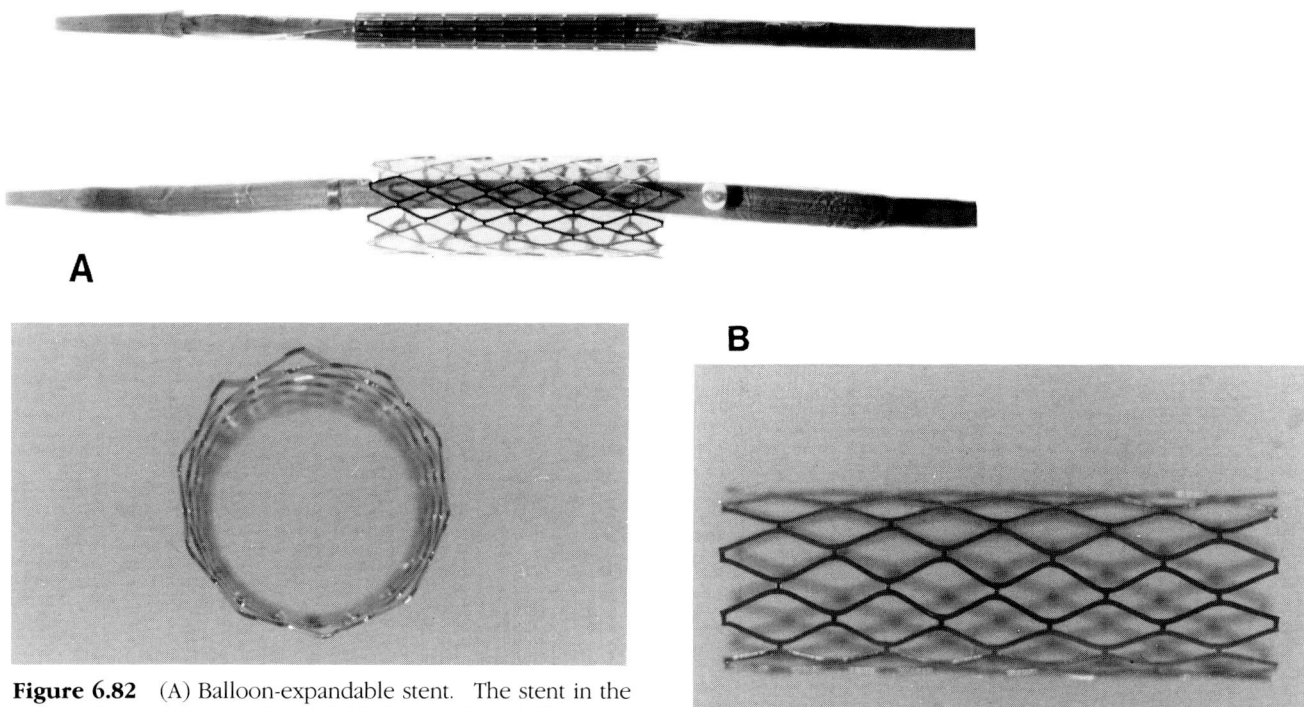

Figure 6.82 (A) Balloon-expandable stent. The stent in the collapsed state is crimped on a folded angioplasty balloon. After balloon inflation, each slot of the tubular mesh opens to a diamond shape, causing an increase in diameter. (B) End-on and lateral views of an expanded stent. The stent lumen remains cylindrical and regular, without an increase in wall thickness.

CURRENT USE AND PROSPECTIVE CLINICAL APPLICATION

Stents have been successfully used in a small series of patients with superior vena cava stenosis. The early human experimental application of stents in patients with iliofemoral or coronary artery stenosis proved the feasibility of clinical application and stimulated further interest in the subject. Emerging data from multicenter trials using balloon-expandable intravascular stents in human iliac and coronary arteries are very promising (Fig. 6.83A and B). However, it will be several years before the safety and efficacy of these devices are firmly established

Elastic recoil is the major limitation of vascular dilatation methods using balloons. Thus any method which overcomes this difficulty and achieves a permanently cylindrical lumen without overdilatation, provided that it can be safely and effectively accomplished, has enormous appeal (Fig. 6.84). The use of stents in the prevention of postangioplasty restenosis in the coronary arteries and in the ostia of stenotic renal arteries is also promising, and stents may become the primary therapy in cases of pulmonary artery branch stenosis, where angioplasty is largely ineffective.

Dilatation of growing vessels, for example, in children with pulmonary artery stenosis or aortic coarctation, with stents that can be redilated at a later date, after they have been incorporated into the vascular wall, has great potential, and the use of stents in cases of acute aortic dissection has also been suggested.

Theoretical vascular applications of stents embedded in a thin webbing of elastomers or absorbable materials include the bridging of fusiform or saccular aneurysms and arteriovenous fistulas. Coated stents may also be tailored to function as flow restrictors or occluders of large vessels. Stents, lasers, atherectomy devices, and other equipment still in the developmental stage are

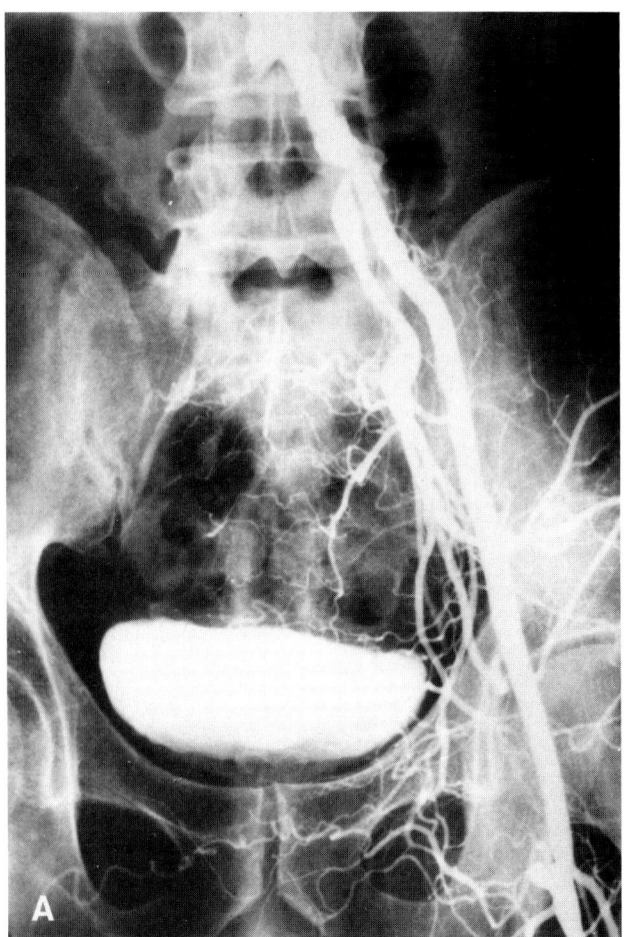
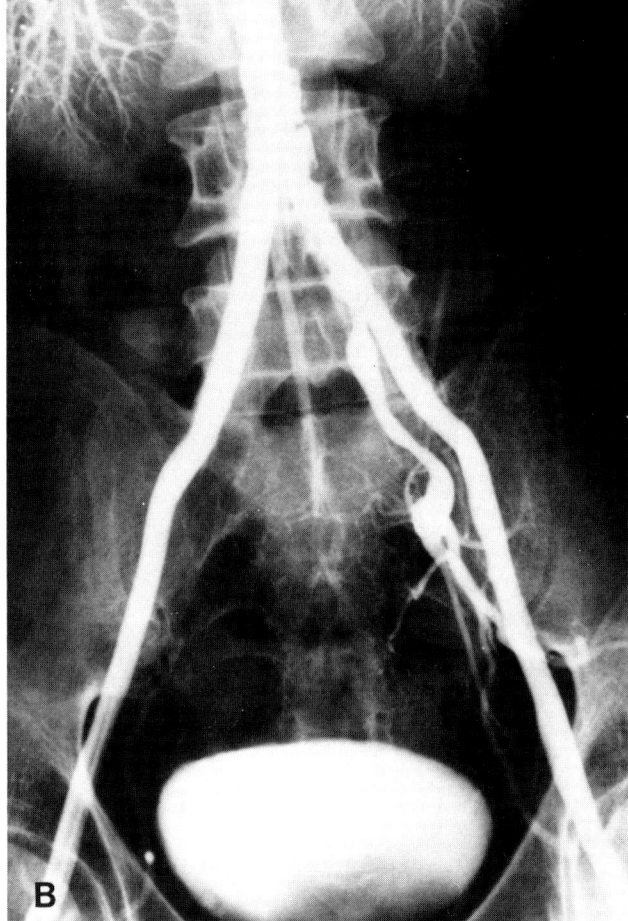

Figure 6.83 (A) 52-year-old male with nonhealing ulcer in the right heel and a right ankle-arm index of 0.48. The abdominal aortogram shows complete occlusion of the right common iliac artery. (B) Two stents were placed in the right common iliac artery following a 3-h infusion of urokinase and balloon dilatation.

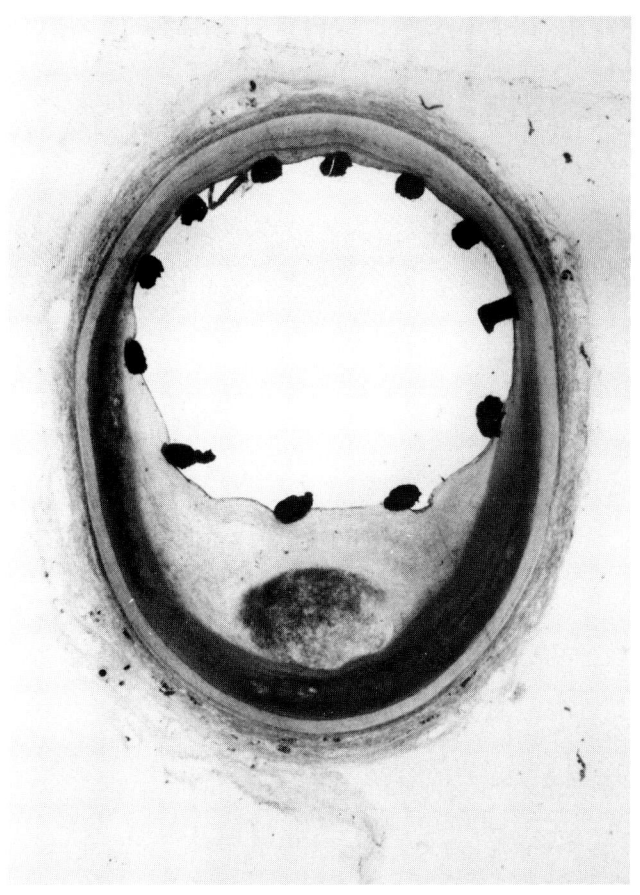

likely to be used in association with one another to improve the results of vascular intervention procedures. However, as stents and other invasive techniques develop, some serious territorial conflicts may develop between specialists currently involved in vascular therapy. Undoubtedly, for example, the effective use of stenting requires expertise in a number of areas: the clinical aspects of vascular disease, noninvasive hemodynamic assessment, dexterity in catheter manipulation, and knowledge of x-ray equipment and radiation in terms of both physics and safety.

In addition, placing an endovascular stent or performing some of the more advanced vascular therapeutic techniques requires a long-term commitment to continued involvement in follow-up. Such commitment may require profound changes in the patterns of current interventional radiology practice to allow for a better physician-patient relationship.

Figure 6.84 Cross section of a human cadaver coronary artery after placement of an intraluminal stent. The partially calcified atherosclerotic plaque (bottom) is displaced outwardly, producing an oval deformity of the contour of the artery. The enlarged lumen is attained by stretching the disease-free arterial wall.

REFERENCES

Becker GJ, Katzen BT. Peripheral angioplasty and the newer circulatory interventions: Whose responsibility? *AJR* 1988;150:1235–1240.

Charsangavej C, Carrasco CH, Wallace S, et al. Stenosis of the vena cava: Preliminary assessment of treatment with expandable metallic stents. *Radiology* 1986;161:295–298.

Charsangavej C, Wallace S, Wright KC, Carrasco CH, Gianturco C. Endovascular stent for use in aortic dissection: An in vitro experiment. *Radiology* 1985;157:323–324.

Cragg A, Lund G, Rysavy J, Castaneda F, Castaneda-Zuniga W, Amplatz K. Non-surgical placement of arterial endoprostheses: A new technique using nitinol wire. *Radiology* 1983;147:261–263.

Dotter CT. Transluminally placed coilspring endarterial tube grafts: Long-term patency in canine popliteal artery. *Invest Radiol* 1969;4:327–332.

Dotter CT, Buschmann RW, McKinney MK, Rosch J. Transluminally expandable nitinol coil stent grafting: Preliminary report. *Radiology* 1983;147:259–260.

Doubilet P, Abrams HL. The cost of underutilization: Percutaneous transluminal angioplasty for peripheral vascular disease. *N Engl J Med* 1984;310:95–102.

Duprat G, Wright KC, Charsangavej C, Wallace S, Gianturco C. Flexible balloon-expanded stent for small vessels. *Radiology* 1987;162:276–278.

Holmes DR, Vliestra RE, Smith HC, et al. Restenosis after percutaneous transluminal coronary angioplasty (PTCA): A report from the PTCA Registry of the National Heart, Lung and Blood Institute. *Am J Cardiol* 1984;53:77c–81c.

Kouchoukos N. Percutaneous transluminal coronary angioplasty: A surgeon's view. *Circulation* 1985;72:114–1147.

Morrow J, Palmaz JC, Tio FO, et al. Paper presented at the annual Meeting of the American Heart Association, Washington, November 1988.

Mullins CE, O'Laughlin M, Vick W, et al. Implantation of balloon-expandable intravascular grafts by catheterization in pulmonary arteries and systemic veins. *Circulation* 1988;77:188–199.

Palmaz JC, Richter GM, Noeldge G, et al. Intraluminal stents in atherosclerotic iliac artery stenosis: Preliminary report of a multicenter study. *Radiology* 1988;168:727–731.

Palmaz JC, Sibbitt RR, Reuter SR, Tio FO, Rice WJ. Expandable intraluminal graft: A preliminary study. *Radiology* 1985;156:73–77.

Palmaz JC, Windeler SA, Garcia F, Tio FO, Sibbitt RR, Reuter SR. Atherosclerotic rabbit aortas: Expandable intraluminal grafting. *Radiology* 1986;160:723–726.

Rabkin J. Revascularization par implantation d'une prosthese Radioendovasculaire. *Radiologie Interventionelle en Pathologie Cardiovasculaire*. Interventional Congress, Toulouse, France, February 1988.

Rousseau H, Puel J, Joffre F, et al. Self expanding endovascular prosthesis: An experimental evaluation. *Radiology* 1987;164:709–714.

Schatz RA, Palmaz JC, Tio FO, Garcia O, Reuter SR. Balloon-expandable intracoronary stents in the adult dog. *Circulation* 1987;76:450–457.

Sigwart V, Puel J, Mirkovitch V, Joffre F, Kappenberger L. Intravascular stents to prevent occlusion and restenosis after transluminal angioplasty. *N Engl J Med* 1987;316:701–706.

Strandness DE. Angioplasty devices will not prevent restenosis. *Cardiology* 1987;4:116–120.

Strecker EP, Berg G, Weber H, Bohl J, Dietrich B. Experimentele Untersuchungen mit einer neven perkutan ein fuhrboren und aufdehnbaren Gefabendoprosthese. *Fortschr Rontgenstr* 1987;147:669–672.

Sugita Y, Shimomitsu T, Oku T, et al. Non-surgical implantation of a vascular ring prosthesis using thermal shape memory Ti/Ni alloy (nitinol wire). *ASAIO Trans* 1986;32:30–34.

Wright KC, Wallace S, Charsangavej C, Carrasco CH, Gianturco C. Percutaneous endovascular stents: An experimental evaluation. *Radiology* 1985;156:69–72.

Percutaneous Mechanical Recanalization Techniques

MARK H. WHOLEY

INTRODUCTION

The appeal of percutaneous mechanical recanalization is rapidly increasing as more experience is gained with various recanalization devices. The recanalization of native vessels seems a more reasonable alternative than performing peripheral bypass surgery, especially when autogenous saphenous vein is unavailable and prosthetic graft material must be used. These methods also reduce hospital costs, since they can frequently be performed on an outpatient basis. Furthermore, unsuccessful attempts to recanalize occluded native vessels rarely worsen patients' symptoms, and patients undergoing the procedure for intermittent claudication are still candidates for peripheral bypass surgery if that proves necessary. Limb salvage cases are always an indication for percutaneous mechanical recanlization, as the only alternative is amputation.

A current wave of interest has developed in devices and techniques for reperfusion of occluded arterial segments. In cases of slowly progressive atherosclerosis in the superficial femoral artery, claudication worsens and the profunda femoris artery becomes an important collateral for perfusing outflow beyond the diseased artery. (This is in contrast to an abrupt occlusion of the artery, which does not allow sufficient time for the development of profunda collateralis.) Traditionally, vascular surgeons have encouraged patients with reconstituted popliteal segments to endure the symptoms of intermittent claudication unless their condition limits the ability to function in society or results in limb-threatening ischemia. This approach is now being challenged, since percutaneous mechanical recanalization offers a viable alternative to extensive vascular reconstruction.

NEW RECANALIZATION DEVICES

The Kensey Dynamic Angioplasty Catheter

A device recently approved for peripheral mechanical recanalization is the Kensey dynamic angioplasty catheter. The body of the catheter is made of flexible polyurethane in No. 5 and No. 8 French sizes. At the distal tip is a rotating cam which is driven at speeds of 5000 to 100,000 rpm by a bedside direct current motor. Contrast solution injected through the catheter during the rotation of the cam allows the procedure to be conducted under fluoroscopic guidance. A vortex is created at the catheter tip that takes advantage of the physiologic ability of a normal arterial wall to expand and contract. However, in a diseased arterial segment, expansion does not occur in a physiologic manner, and the atheromatous material is exposed to the rotating cam. Pulverization of the plaque occurs due to the proximity of the rotating cam to the diseased segment (Fig. 6.85A and B). A negative

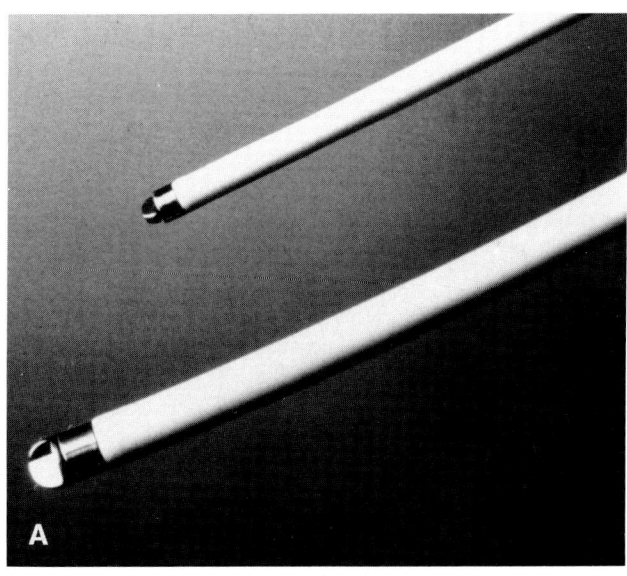

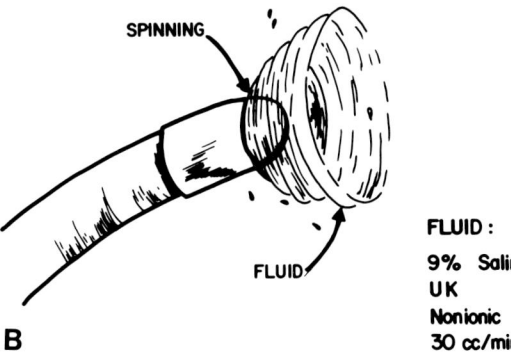

Figure 6.85 (A) No. 5 French and No. 8 French Kensey catheters at the distal end of the catheter is a high-speed rotational metallic cam. (B) Diagrammatic illustration showing the high-energy vortex created by the infusate and the cam.

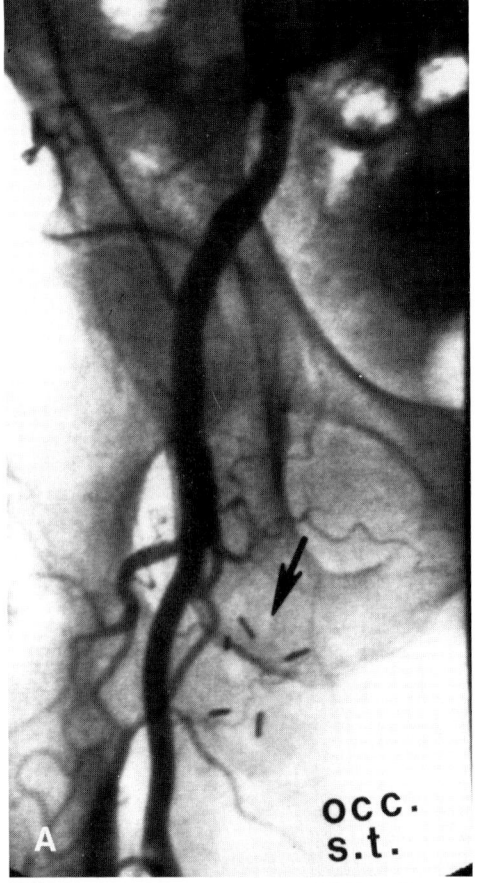

pressure effect in the fluid vortex causes recirculation and further pulverization of the plaque to a size of 5 to 10 μm. These particles are small enough to pass through the capillary network, and they have not been associated with clinically important peripheral embolization.

Indications for use of the Kensey catheter include patients with symptoms of rest ischemia or intermittent claudication. Short segmental occlusions or diffusely diseased arterial segments are treated providing there is at least one vessel outflow beyond the diseased segment. The No. 5 French Kensey catheter creates a vessel lumen 1.67 mm in diameter, while the No. 8 French catheter creates a lumen 2.7 mm in diameter. This enables the technician to easily traverse the diseased segment with a conventional guidewire and an angioplasty balloon of appropriate size. Thus the Kensey catheter can be used to open the lumen of totally occluding vessels, making them amenable to conventional balloon angioplasty (Fig. 6.86).

Figure 6.86 (A) Femoral arteriogram demonstrating total occlusion of the right superficial femoral artery at its origin and occlusion of a prior femoral popliteal saphenous vein bypass graft. (B) Reconstitution of the popliteal artery from occasional deep femoral collateralization. The entire superficial femoral artery is occluded. (C) Follow-up angiogram 24 h after effective recanalization of the entire superficial femoral artery utilizing the Kensey catheter. (D) The popliteal tibial outflow is intact, no distal embolization is evident.

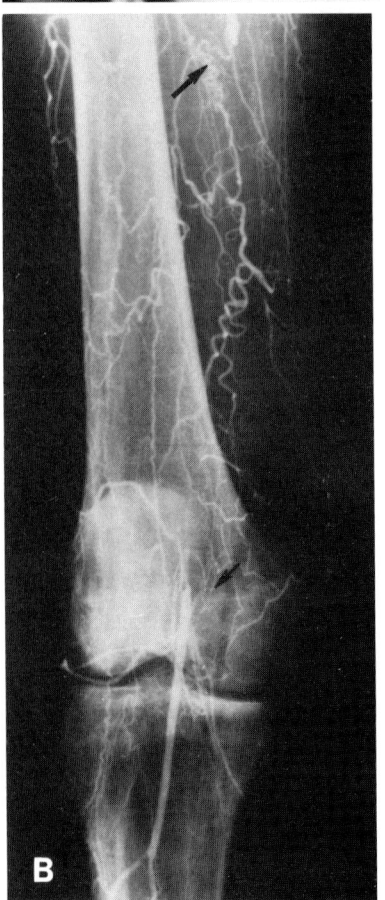
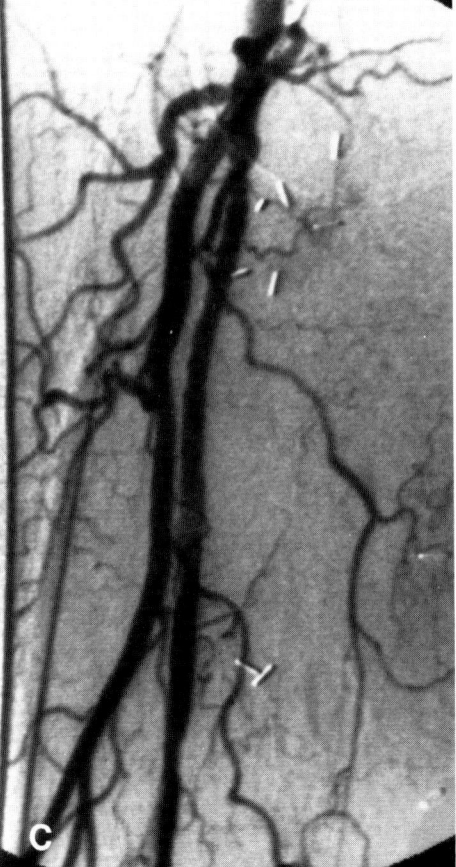
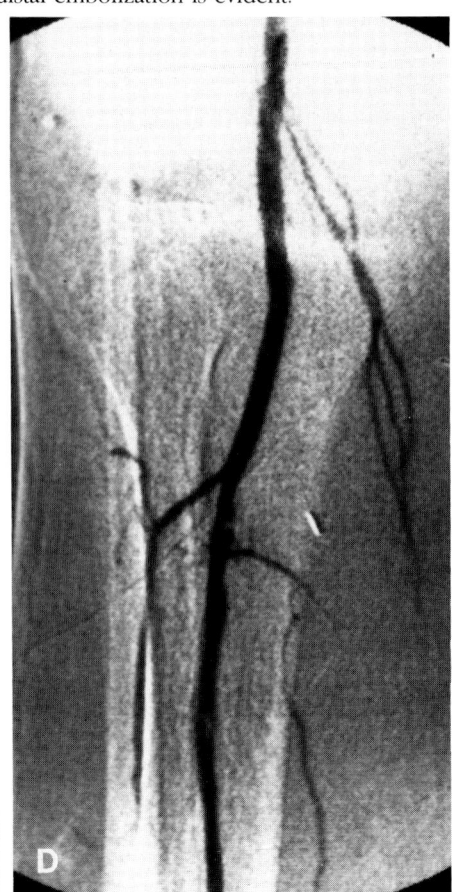

Clinical experience with the Kensey catheter is limited. Eight investigating sites in the United States and four European centers were used to evaluate the procedure for Food and Drug Administration approval. One hundred and ten procedures were evaluated prior to approval of the device. Since approval, 69 superficial femoral artery lesions, and 28 distal superficial femoral and popliteal lesions, have been treated. Experience with the iliac arteries is similarly limited. Thirty-eight procedures were reported using the phase II Kensey catheter, which has subsequently been modified. In 72 procedures performed using Kensey catheters that closely resemble the current device, the catheter demonstrated an excellent ability to cross stenotic lesions and effectively establish a pilot hole. It was less successful in traversing total occlusions; 68 percent of the treated vessels were considered a technical success (Fig. 6.87). The overall clinical success in this group of patients was 52 percent, while the clinical failure rate was 48 percent in patients followed for 2 months.

Minor complications associated with use of the Kensey catheter included, in order of decreasing frequency, perforation, intimal dissection, extensive extravasation of contrast material, and hematoma formation at the insertion site. None of these complications required further medical or surgical intervention. Embolization occurred in one patient; this was considered a major complication and necessitated surgical intervention (Fig. 6.88).

Atherolytic Reperfusion Wires

As mentioned, recanalization of an occluded arterial segment requires that a pilot hole be established through the occlusion itself before conventional balloon angioplasty is performed. Establishing the pilot hole, which is of vital importance, can be accomplished by various means: simple advancement of a steerable guidewire, laser recanalization, recanalization with a thermal radio frequency probe, or recanalization with a Kensey catheter. An additional option is the atherolytic reperfusion wire (Fig. 6.89). The optimal device penetrates the occlusion in a plane which does not disrupt the integrity of the atheroma or detach the plaque from the vessel wall. Although intraoperative angioscopy and endovascular ultrasound show promise, they are cumbersome, and steering through the central lumen with the aid of these

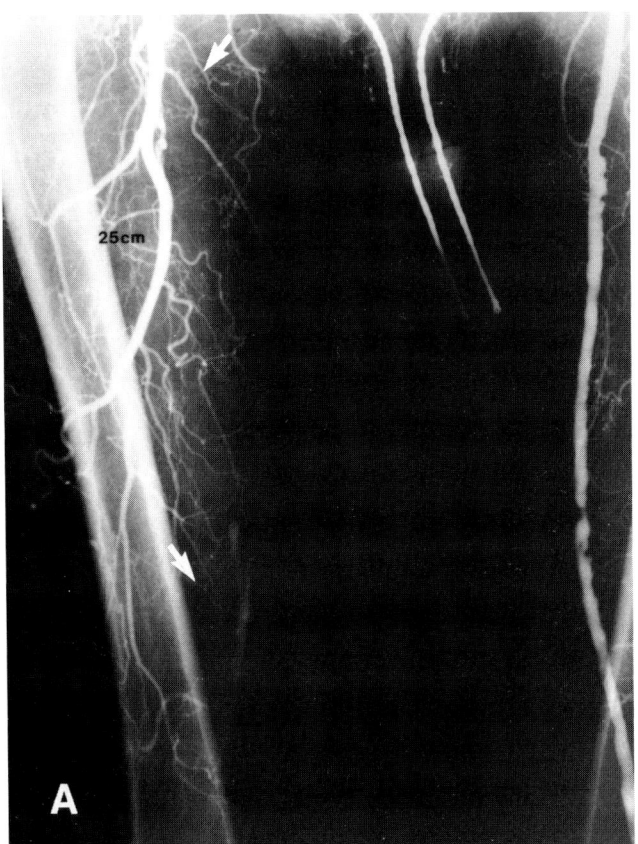
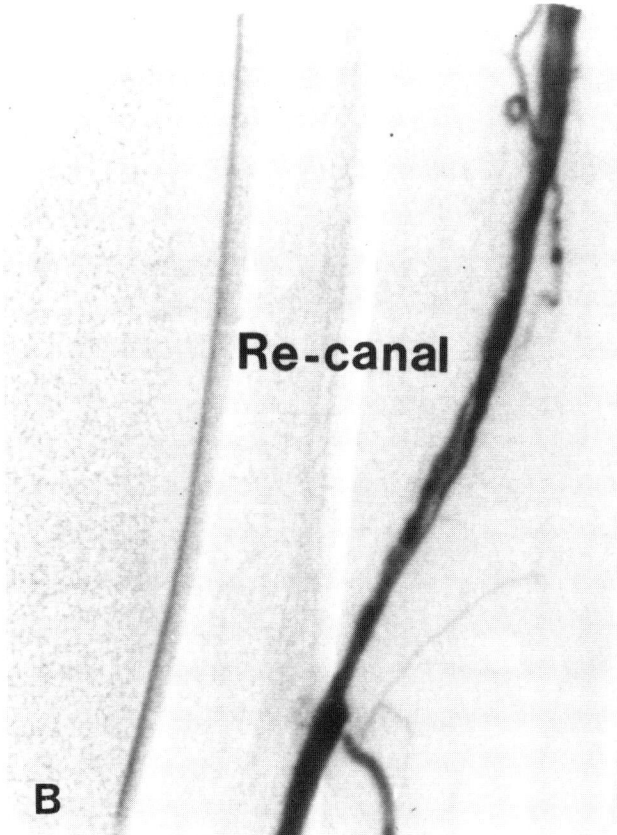

Figure 6.87 (A) Bilateral femoral arteriogram showing a 25-cm occlusion of the right superficial femoral artery. (B) Visible patency of the superficial femoral artery following effective recanalization with the Kensey catheter. Note, however, the irregular intimal fragmentation at the recanalization site.

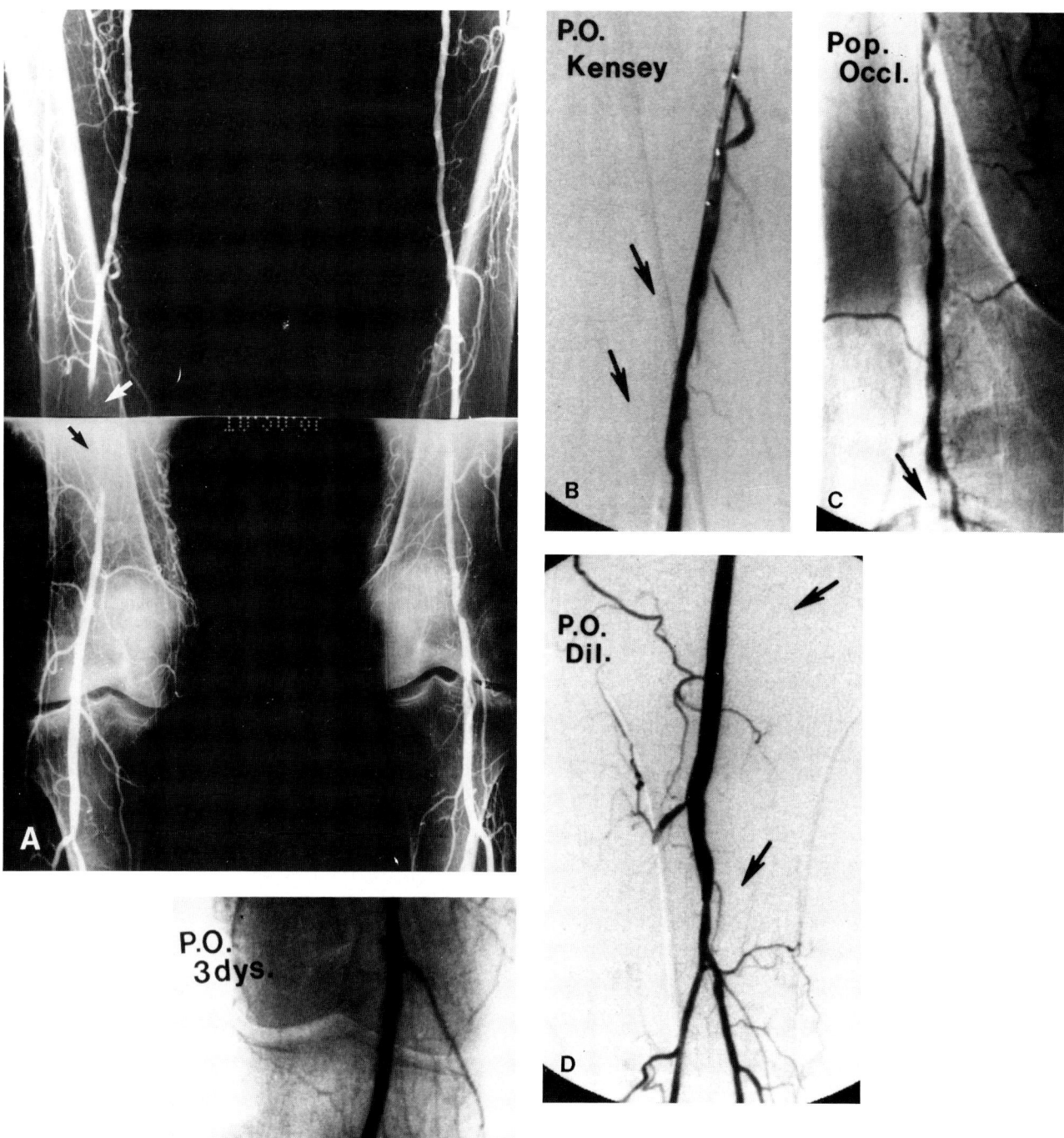

Figure 6.88 (A) Bilateral femoral arteriogram showing an 8-cm occlusion involving the distal right superficial femoral artery and extending into the popliteal artery. (B) Angiogram showing satisfactory patency following effective Kensey recanalization of the occluded segment. (C) Post-Kensey recanalization demonstrating total occlusion of the politeal artery. (D) Reestablished patency following regional thrombolytic therapy (300,000 IU urokinase). (E) Reocclusion of the tibio-fibular trunk 3 days after the original recanalization.

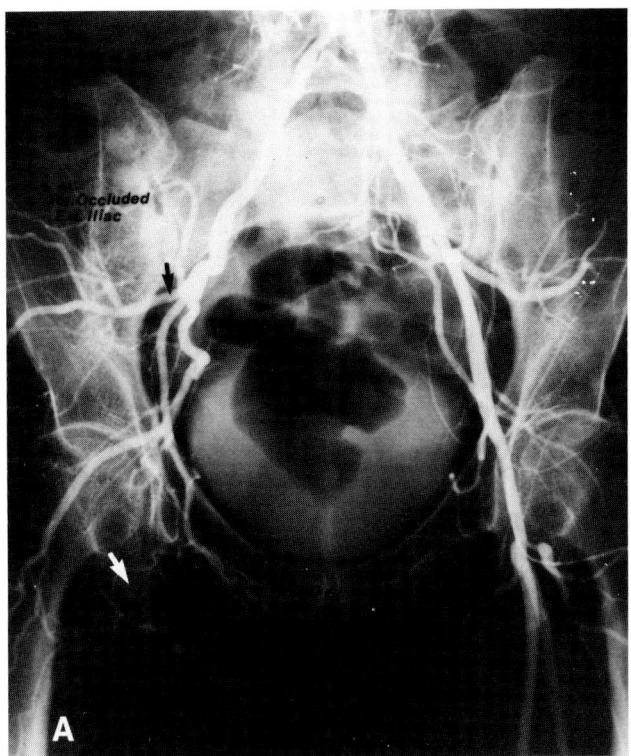 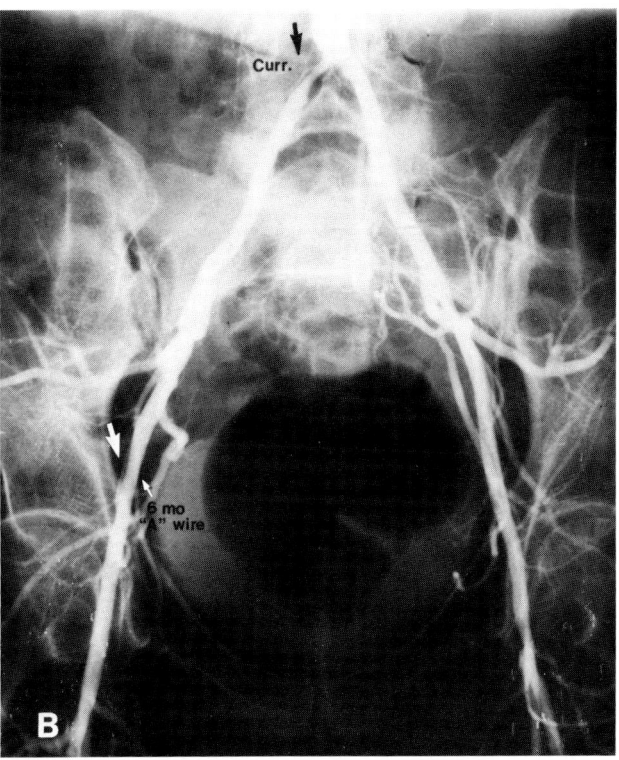

Figure 6.89 (A) Pelvic arteriogram demonstrating total occlusion of the entire right external iliac artery. Reconstitution and collateralization have reestablished the common femoral (note arrow). (B) Follow-up pelvic arteriogram 6 months after effective recanalization utilizing an atherolytic wire and supplemental balloon angioplasty. The external iliac artery is now widely patent (lower arrows). Note the newly developing stenosis at the right common iliac artery, which was effectively dilated during this procedure.

devices is currently not practical. Thus, practitioners are dependent on fluoroscopic guidance, which can be deceiving and does not always indicate when the intima has been penetrated. For these reasons, the atherolytic reperfusion wire offers certain benefits. The prototype consists of a 0.035-in. wire with a distal cutting edge at the tip of the wire (Fig. 6.90). Flexibility of the wire tip varies from 2 to 3 cm depending on how hard the lesion is to penetrate. The wire is attached proximally to a hand-held battery-powered motor-driver unit that is easily activated by pressure on the central piston. The wire may be used through conventionl angioplasty balloons or through any conventional catheter with an 0.035-in. internal diameter. Advancing the angioplasty balloon catheter gives additional support for the atherolytic reperfusion wire, which is rotated at 700 rpm by the hand-held device. Once the lesion is crossed, the angioplasty balloon is tracked over the wire, which is used to stabilize the balloon for the dilatation procedure. If a different catheter is utilized, the catheter is positioned over the wire once it has crossed the lesion and a conventional guidewire is exchanged for the appropriately sized angioplasty balloon.

Atherolytic reperfusion wires are used to recanalize total arterial occlusions which cannot be crossed using conventional guidewires (Fig. 6.91). They are most useful in relatively straight vessels, i.e., iliac, superficial femoral, or popliteal arterial segments. However, current efforts are focused on developing a 0.014-in. wire, with properties similar to the 0.035-in. wire, which can be used for recanalization of totally occluded coronary vessels.

Clinical experience with the wire is limited. Our experience in 12 patients with lesions from 2 to 8 cm in length resulted in technical success in 8 of the lesions treated. Four patients had rigid lesions which were calcified and could not be crossed with the rotational wire. One patient, with a short common iliac occlusion, could not be treated using a contralateral approach due to lack of flexibility across the aortic bifurcation. All of the technically successful lesions were subsequently treated with conventional angioplasty. (See Fig. 6.92.)

The potential complications of using the atherolytic reperfusion wire include vessel perforation. However, since the wire is only 0.035 in. in diameter, clinically significant hemorrhage is unlikely and has not occurred in vessels below the inguinal ligament. Nor have we experienced any perforations in the iliac vessels treated. Other potential complications include embolization of atherosclerotic material and hematoma formation at the puncture site. Neither complication has been encountered in clinical trials on these 12 patients.

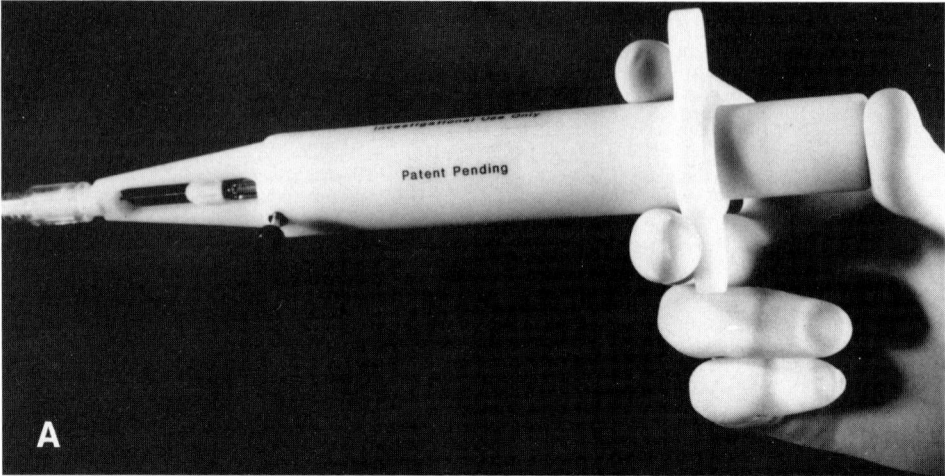

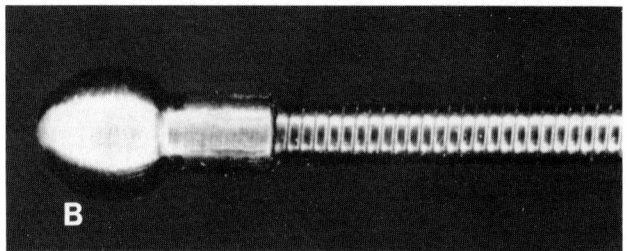

Figure 6.90 (A) Power-pack and other components for use with atherolytic wires. The Luer-lok attachment for the wire is distal. Proximal thumb pressure on the piston activates the rotational drive. (B) The distal tip of the wire is available in several configurations. The one shown is an elipsoid.

Transluminal Extraction Catheters

A group of atherectomy catheters designed to remove arthcromatous debris during the recanalization process are presently being investigated. One of these instruments, the transluminal extraction catheter (TEC), consists of a flexible, torque-controlled tube incorporating a cutter device at the distal tip (Fig. 6.93). During rotational cutting, continuous aspiration is occurring through the tube to the aspiration bottle. The value of this approach is that while the cutter and aspiration unit are functioning, distal embolization cannot occur. Furthermore, the unit functions over a steerable 0.014-in. wire. For these reasons, the device can be efficiently utilized in total obstructions. Initially, the total obstruction is recanalized with a steerable 0.035-in. Wholey wire followed by a conventional No. 5 French catheter. The 0.035-in. wire is replaced by the 0.014-in. wire, the No. 5 French catheter is removed, and the TEC is passed over the wire to the proximal obstruction site. The torque-controlled tube-cutter set is then activated by a hand-held power-pack unit. TECs can also be used for high-grade stenotic lesions (Fig. 6.94). The cutter is presently available in Nos. 5, 7, and 9 French sizes.

Clinical experience in a multicenter trial currently underway involves both the peripheral and coronary circulation. In a recent series of 100 patients with stenosis in the peripheral circulation who were treated with the TEC, restenosis rates were 14 percent when the atherectomy catheter was used independently of the balloon.

In a group of our patients with lengthy (8 to 20 cm) total occlusions in the superficial femoral artery, the rate of recurrence of stenosis was about 33 percent, requiring supplemental balloon angioplasty (Fig. 6.95).

The TEC is presently our method of choice when recanalizing total obstructions (Fig. 6.96). The excised tissue is withdrawn from the obstruction site through the torque-driven catheter unit by means of the attached vacuum source.

Distal embolization has not been observed in any of our patients or the 100 patients in the multicenter trial. Technical success was achieved in 92 percent of cases and clinical success in 90 percent.

In most situations, the No. 7 or No. 9 French catheter provides an adequate lumen through the high-grade stenosis or obstruction. When there is total obstruction in more distal vessels at the popliteal and tibial level, the No. 5 French catheter can be utilized to establish an adequate lumen. For larger vessels at the superficial femoral or iliac level, we use the No. 7 or No. 9 French cutter. When residual stenotic changes are present following TEC recanalization, supplemental balloon angioplasty can be performed. When the TEC is used to debulk the lesion in lengthy total occlusions prior to supplemental angioplasty, postangioplasty results show

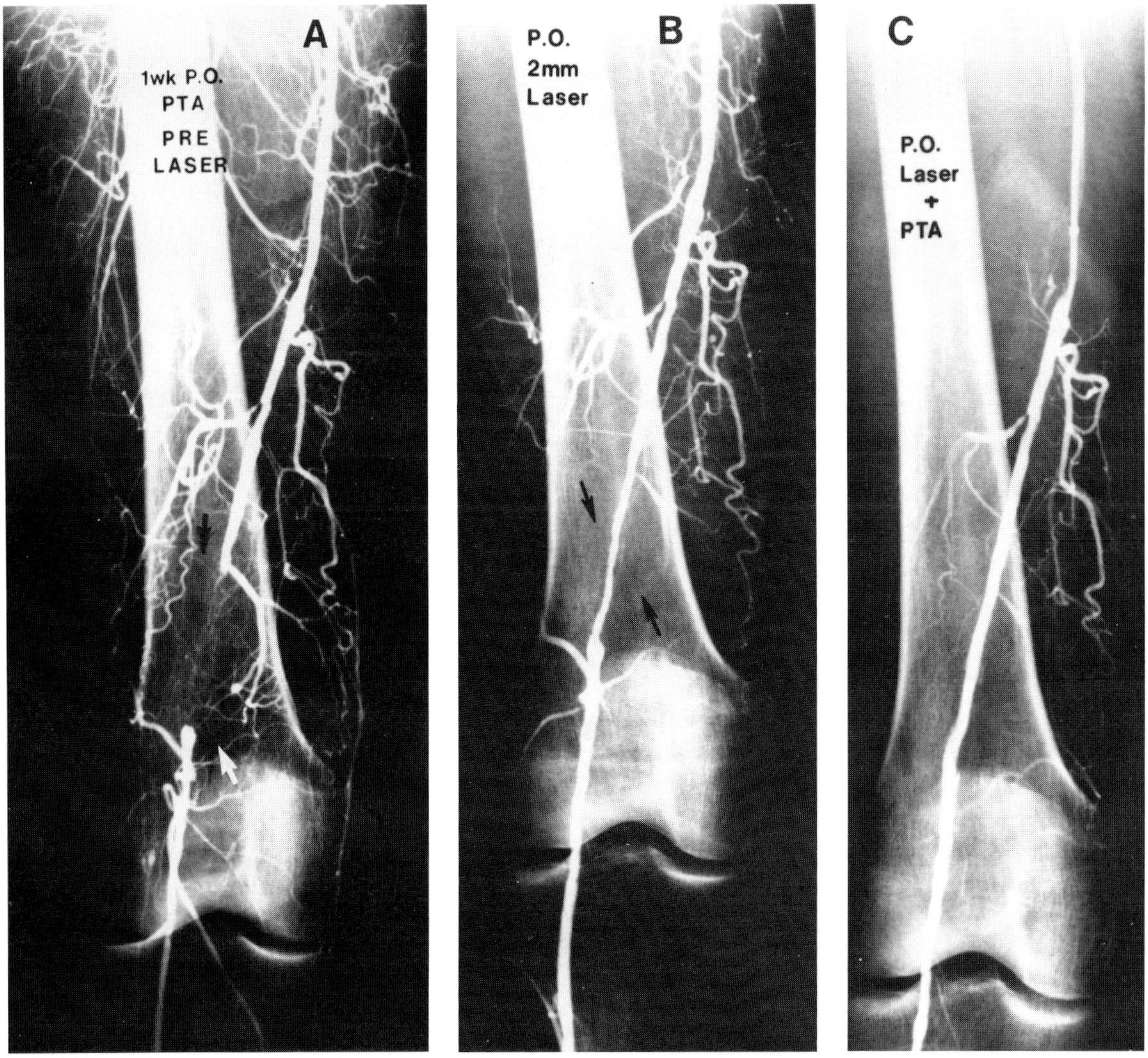

Figure 6.91 (A) Recurrent occlusion in the proximal popliteal artery 3 weeks after atherolytic wire recanalization and balloon angioplasty. (B) Recanalization with a 2-mm laser probe with a hot-tip system. (C) Balloon angioplasty, following initial recanalization with the laser probe, has resulted in effective dilatation.

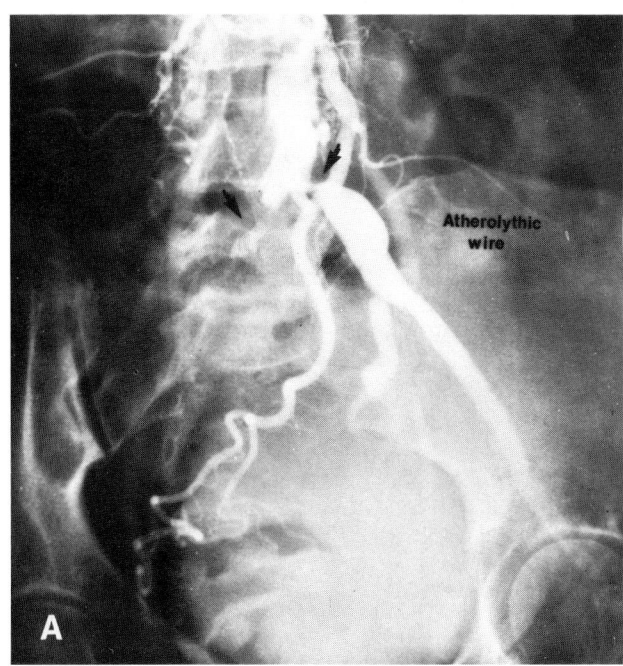

Figure 6.92 (A) Pelvic arteriogram demonstrating total occlusion of the right common iliac artery and high-grade stenosis at the origin of the left common iliac artery. (B) Delayed phase demonstrating collateralization and reconstitution of the right external iliac artery. Note, however, that total occlusion of the common iliac artery persists. (C) Digital map from the ipsilateral side showing the occlusion site. (D) Effective recanalization of the common iliac artery on the right utilizing an atherolytic wire and supplemental balloon angioplasty.

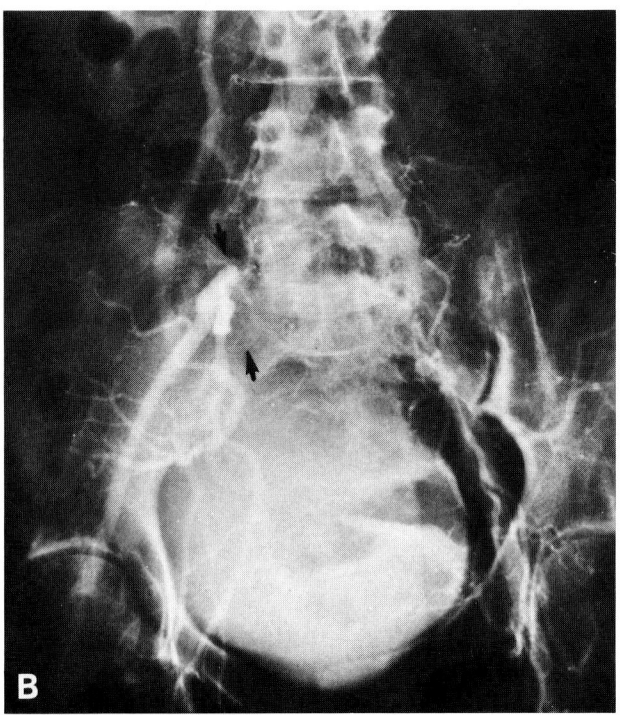
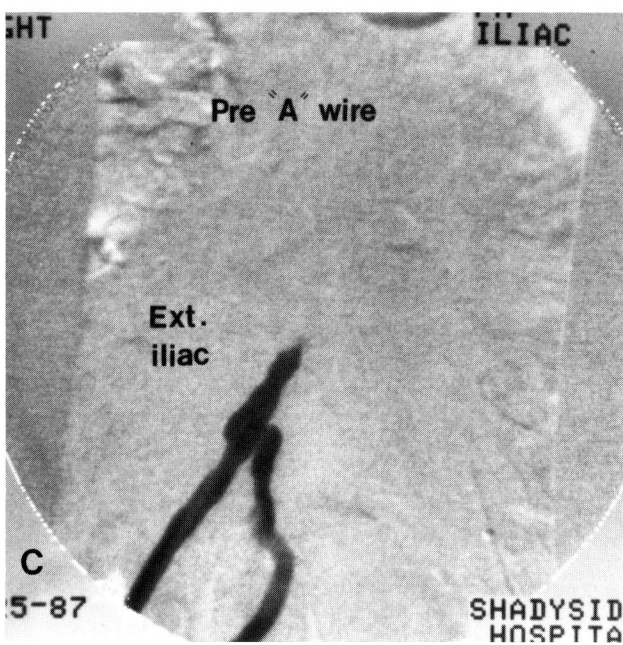
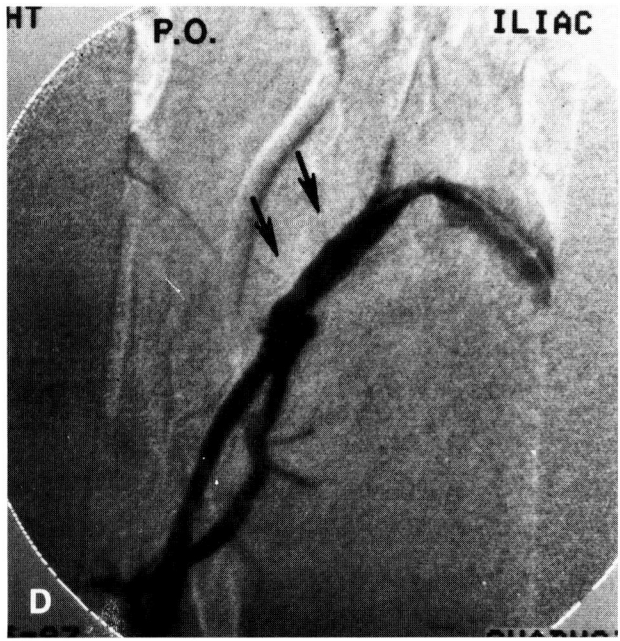
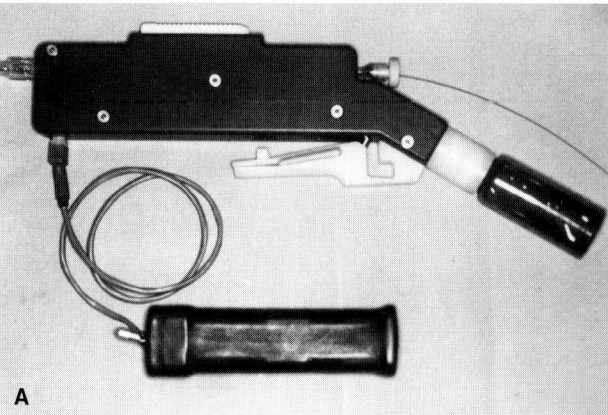
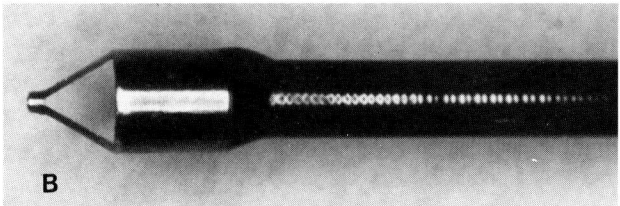

Figure 6.92 *Continued*

Figure 6.93 (A) Operational unit for the transluminal extraction catheter incorporating a vacuum bottle, a battery power pack, and a 0.014-in. steerable wire. (B) Torque-controlled tube-cutter unit for the transluminal extraction catheter. During rotational cutting, continuous aspiration occurs through the tube.

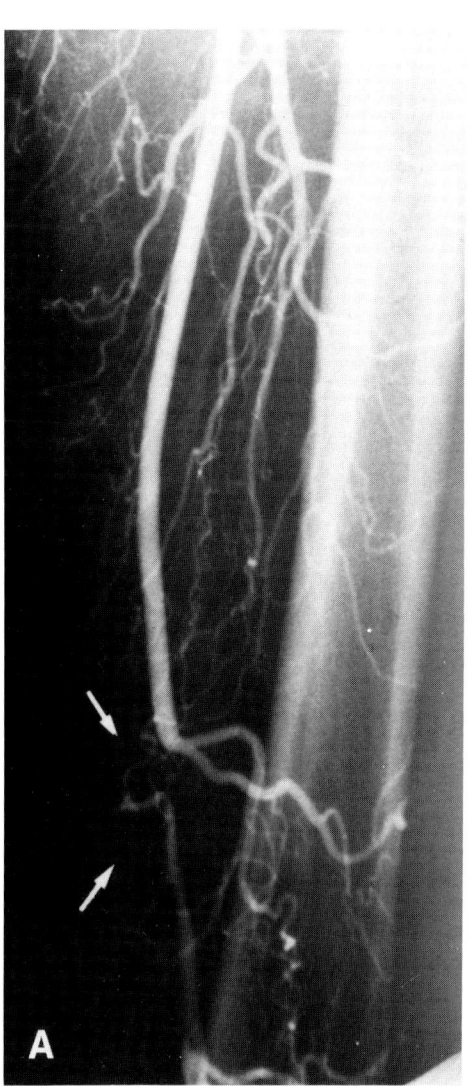 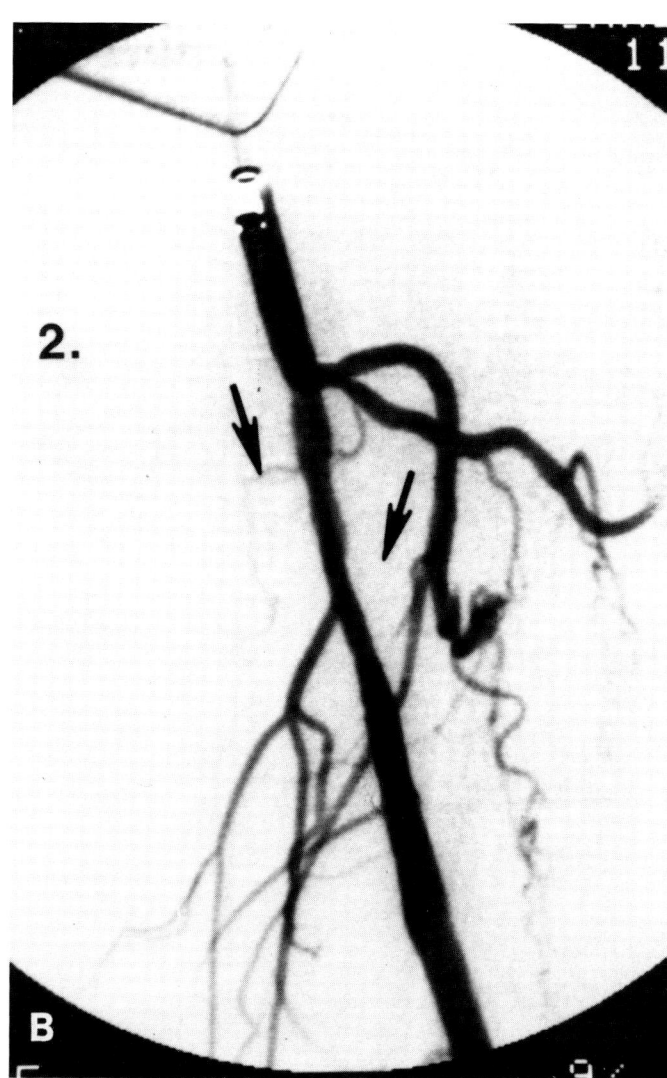

Figure 6.94 (A) Femoral arteriogram demonstrating a 2-cm segment of total occlusion in the superficial femoral artery with retrocollateralization over an additional 4-cm segment that is totally occluded. (B) A digital subtraction arteriogram demonstrates satisfactory dimensions following effective recanalization utilizing the transluminal extraction atherectomy catheter. Note that there is less intimal fragmentation than ordinarily seen with conventional balloon angioplasty.

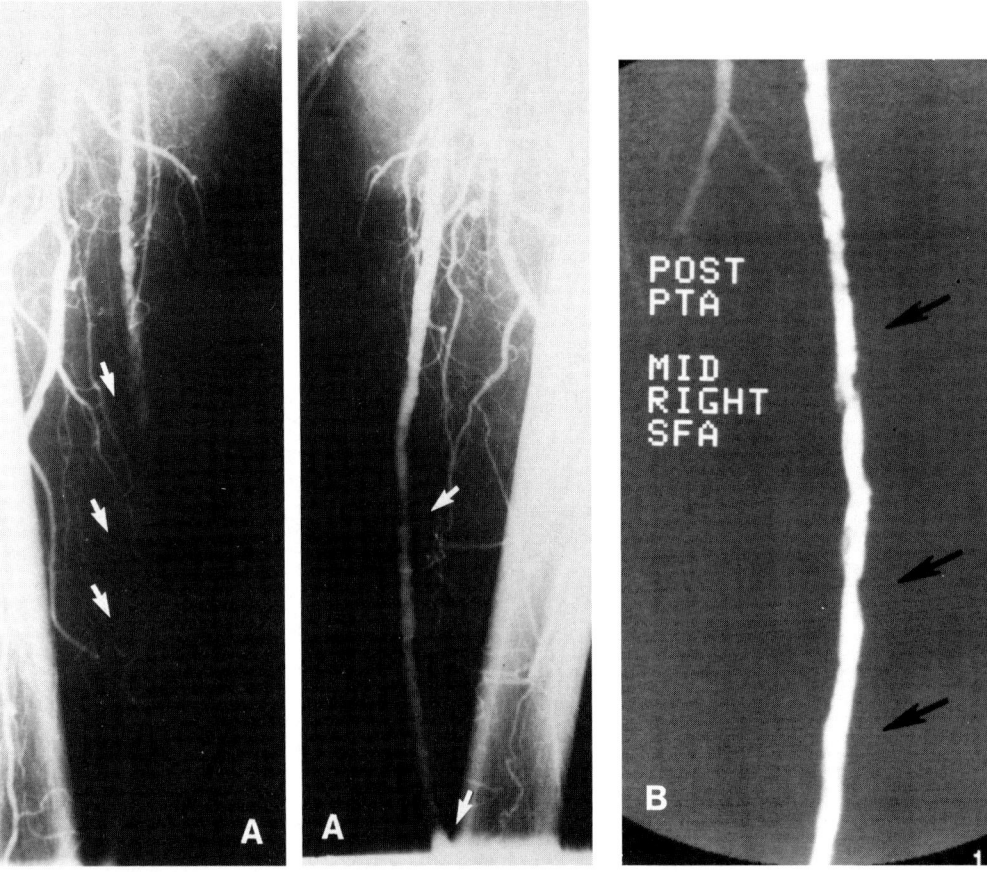
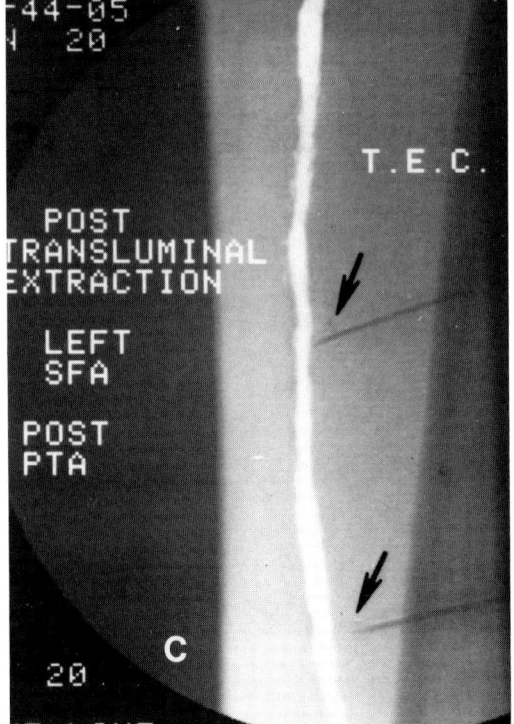

Figure 6.95 (A) Bilateral femoral arteriogram demonstrating calcific atherosclerotic occlusion over a lengthy segment in the left superficial femoral artery and diffuse stenotic disease involving multiple segments in the right superficial femoral artery. (B) Arteriogram following diffuse angioplasty procedure on the right superficial femoral artery. (C) Arteriogram following transluminal extraction catheter recanalization on the previously obstructed left superficial femoral artery. Note the considerable intimal fragmentation in the right superficial femoral artery and the relatively smooth surface in the left superficial femoral artery.

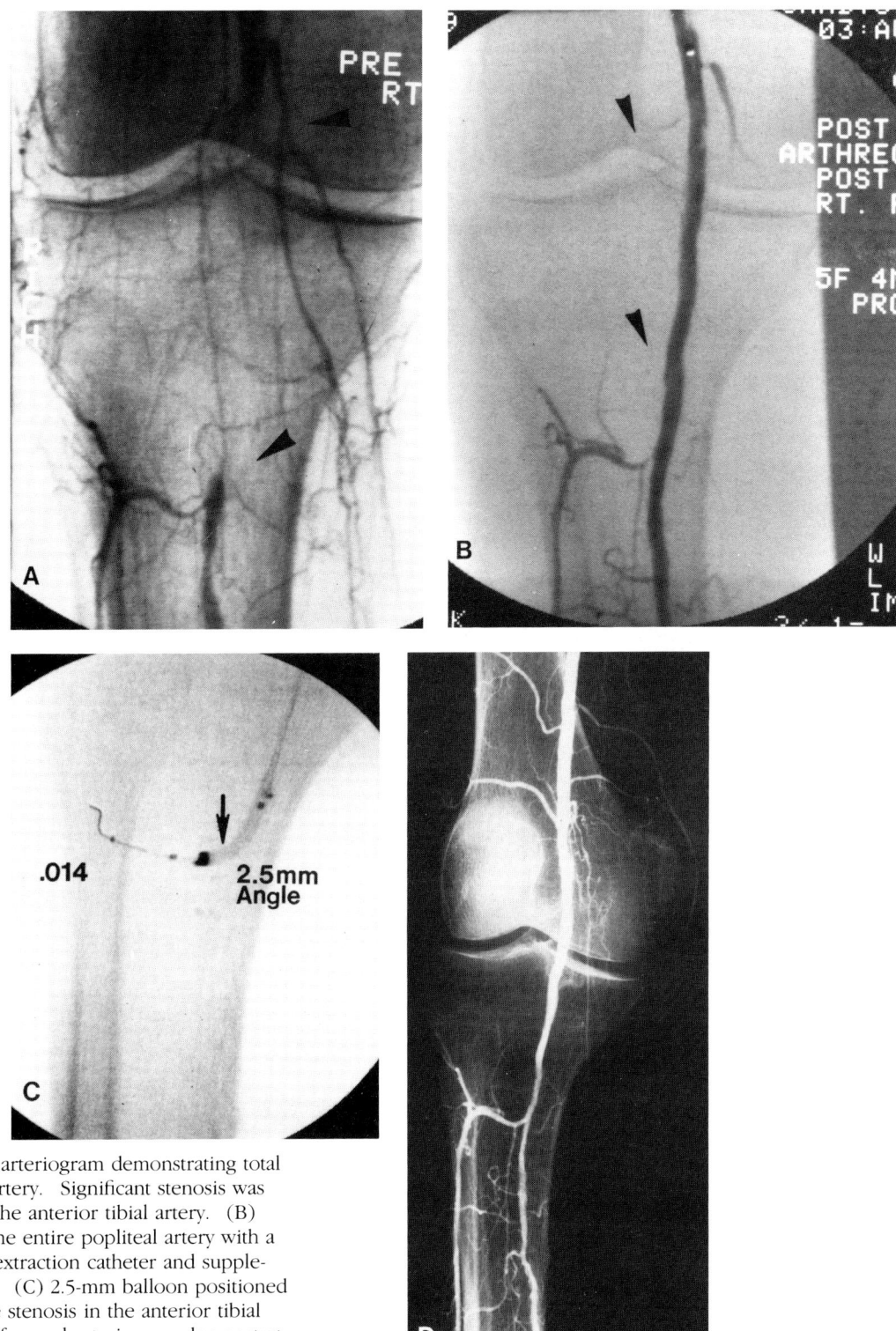

Figure 6.96 (A) Femoral arteriogram demonstrating total occlusion of the popliteal artery. Significant stenosis was also noted at the origin of the anterior tibial artery. (B) Effective recanalization of the entire popliteal artery with a No. 5 French transluminal extraction catheter and supplemental balloon angioplasty. (C) 2.5-mm balloon positioned at the site of the high-grade stenosis in the anterior tibial artery. (D) Postprocedure femoral arteriogram demonstrating satisfactory patency through the popliteal artery and effective dilatation of the anterior tibial artery.

considerably less intimal fragmentation and improved lumen dimensions in comparison with results using conventional balloon angioplasty alone.

In the future, improvements in cutter design will allow eccentric cutting within the lumen, thus enabling the cutter to create a reperfused lumen with dimensions larger than its own. Externally controlled expandable cutters, which would allow, say, a No. 7 French cutter to create a No. 9 French lumen or a No. 5 French cutter to create No. 7 French dimensions, are presently in the development stage.

CONCLUSION

Intense efforts are currently being focused on mechanical recanalization techniques. Few individuals would argue against the use of balloon angioplasty as a safe, cost-effective, alternative to vascular surgery for patients suffering from intermittent claudication or limb-threatening ischemia. As our ability to mechanically cross total arterial occlusions increases, so do the indications for angioplasty. Currently several devices are available that create a sufficient lumen to permit conventional angioplasty in cases in which it would otherwise be difficult or impossible. It is our hope that these devices, in conjunction with improved balloon technology, will lead to a steady increase in the number of vascular problems that can be treated percutaneously.

REFERENCES

Diethrich EB, Timbadia E, Bahadir I, et al. Applications and limitations of laser-assisted angioplasty. *Eur J Vasc Surg* 1989;3.

Diethrich EB, Timbadia E, Bahadir I, et al. Argon laser assisted peripheral angioplasty. *Vasc Surg* 1988;22:77–87.

Doubilet P, Abrams H. The cost of under utilization: Percutaneous transluminal angioplasty for peripheral vascular disease. *N Engl J Med* 1984;310:95–102.

Gruntzig A, Hopff H. Perkutane rekanalisation chronischer arterieller verschlusse mit einem neuen: Dilatationskatheter-Modifikation der Dotter-Technik. *Dtsch Med Wochenschr* 1984;99:2502–2505.

Kensey KR, Nash JE, Abrahams C, Zarins CK. Recanalization of obstructed arteries with a flexible, rotating tip catheter. *Radiology* 1987;165:387–389.

Snyder SO, Wheeler JR, Gregory RT, Gayle RG, Mariner DR. The Kensey Catheter: Preliminary results with a transluminal atherectomy tool. *J Vasc Surg* 1988;4:541–543.

Uflacker R, Wholey MH. Technical note: A new low-speed, rotational atherolytic device for ureteral recanalization. *AJR* 1988;151:1157–1158.

Wholey MH, Jarmolowski CR. An introduction to new reperfusion devices: The Kensey catheter; the atherolytic reperfusion wire device; and the Transluminal Extraction Catheter. *Radiology*. In press.

Wholey MH, Smith JAM, Godlewski P, Nagurka M. Recanlization of total arterial occlusions with the Kensey Dynamic Angioplasty catheter. *Radiology*. In press.

Wholey MH. Advances in balloon technology and reperfusion devices for peripheral circulation. *Am J Cardiol* 1988;61:87G–95G.

Wholey MH. The "TEC" atherectomy catheter: Results in the first 100 patients (abstract). Program of the International Symposium on Peripheral Vascular Intervention, presented by the Miami Vascular Institute, Baptist Hospital, Miami, February 10, 1990.

Fibrinolytic Therapy for Peripheral Vascular Disease

MARK H. WHOLEY

INTRODUCTION

The superiority of regional arterial infusion of thrombolytic agents over conventional systemic intravenous techniques has been established in both experimental animals and humans. Clot lysis appears to occur more rapidly when a catheter is in close contact with the thrombus. In addition, this technique offers the advantage of higher concentrations of the agents at the thrombotic site, permitting a smaller total dosage to be utilized. Interval angiographic observations and pressure measurements can both be obtained through the perfusion catheter. The regional approach, however, requires specially trained teams with modern angiographic laboratories at institutions where occasional surgical intervention can be performed if necessary.

TYPES OF FIBRINOLYTIC AGENTS

At present, controversy exists over the choice of a specific fibrinolytic agent. Our experience has been limited entirely to three agents: streptokinase, urokinase, and tissue plasminogen activator (t-PA). Originally, intraarterial urokinase was primarily used in those patients who had previously demonstrated a resistance to streptokinase; now, however, urokinase is routinely used in most of our fibrinolytic applications. Tissue plasminogen activators have been successfully used for clot lysis in various centers in both Europe and the United States. This type of agent, however, has generally been used for cases of acute myocardial infarction where the fibrinolytic agent was to be given in a peripheral systemic vein. Its intraarterial application has been less frequently described.

The mechanism of action of streptokinase involves the formation of an activator complex combining streptokinase with serum plasminogen. This complex then activates the conversion of circulating plasminogen to plasmin. In contrast, urokinase acts directly on plasminogen, and plasmin is formed as a direct conversion product. Streptokinase is obtained from cultures of group C β-hemolytic streptococcal bacteria; consequently, it can occasionally be antigenic and has, rarely, been associated with pyrogenic reactions. Urokinase, which is obtained from cultures of fetal renal parenchymal cells, is almost never antigenic but unfortunately is considerably more expensive than streptokinase. Both agents have brief half-lives: the $T_{1/2}$ of urokinase approaches 20 min, and the two forms of streptokinase have half-lives of 20 and 8 min. Tissue plasminogen activators convert the inactive plasminogen molecule directly to plasmin on the surface of the thrombus by combining with the fibrin in the clot itself, thereby producing in situ fibrinolysis. Because the tissue plasminogen activator is tissue–fibrin-clot specific, it can be introduced intravenously, and may ultimately eliminate the need for selective regional catheterization.

CLINICAL INDICATIONS

Our early experimental studies demonstrated that an induced thrombus within the renal artery of a rabbit could be effectively recanalized with a dose of 1000 IU/min of streptokinase administered over a 10-min period. After 20 min, essentially all of the existing thrombus had been recanalized and renal function was satisfactory. Follow-up studies 2 weeks after the procedure subsequently demonstrated continued patency and normal renal function. From these studies evolved a group of patients in whom selective regional intraarterial thrombolytic therapy was applied in a group of patients who presented with arterial thrombosis and

—underlying atherosclerotic occlusive disease
—prior arteriotomy
—abrupt postangioplasty occlusion
—bypass-graft anastomotic stenoses
—occlusion following conventional arteriography

Past experience and data suggest that emboli and thrombi that have been present for less than 72 h are associated with considerably more complete lysis than those lesions that have been present for more than 2 weeks (Fig. 6.97). This, however, does not preclude the successful recanalization of the chronically organized thrombus or the chronically occluded graft, and fibrinolysis has been successful as long as 3 months after known occlusion (Fig. 6.98).

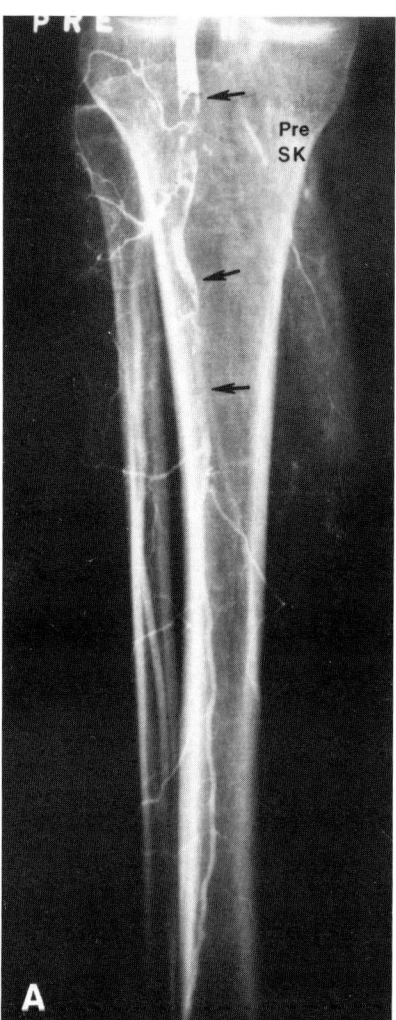 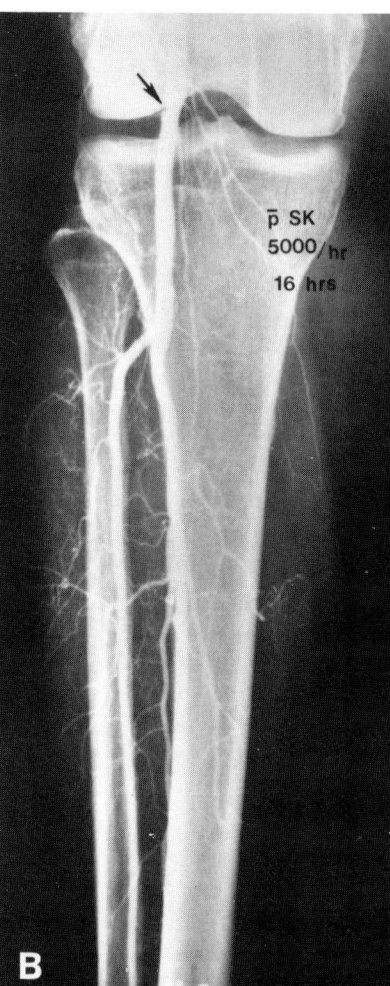

Figure 6.97 (A) Diffuse recent thrombotic changes involving the distal popliteal artery with extension into the anterior tibial as well as the posterior tibial trunk. (B) Effective recanalization with no further evidence of residual thrombi following regional intraarterial urokinase with the catheter positioned just proximal to the thrombus and infusion continued for 16 h at 1000 IU/h preceded by a loading dose of 250,000 units in the first hour.

The available literature and our own series indicate that when vessel outflow is limited, although successful reperfusion may occur, the reocclusion rate is high. These poor results are most apparent at the popliteal level, and can occur even when the stenotic segment responsible for the thrombosis has been restored to satisfactory dimensions by t-PA. In contrast, one can anticipate a more successful result and longer vessel patency in the larger, high-flow vessels at the aortic bifurcation, the iliac circulation, the renal artery, or other sites with vessel dimensions of 7 mm or greater (Fig. 6.99). Absolute contraindications to fibrinolytic therapy have been confined to patients with active internal bleeding, a recent cerebrovascular accident, or gastrointestinal bleeding, as well as the immediate postoperative patient. Relative contraindications, where benefits versus risks must be weighed, include the following: the first postoperative week, post organ biopsy, postpartum, recent skeletal fractures, uncontrolled coagulation disorders, severe hypertension, pregnancy, and any general condition that might present a major hemorrhagic risk (Fig. 6.100).

Figure 6.98 (A) Thrombotic occlusion of the distal popliteal artery of 2 weeks' duration. An intraaterial digital subtraction angiogram was obtained after 30 min. of urokinase at 4000 IU/min with only minimal improvement in the popliteal flow. (B) Intraarterial digital subtraction angiogram following 20 h of urokinase infusion demonstrates effective recanalization of the entire popliteal artery as well as a widely patent posterior tibial trunk and anterior tibial division.

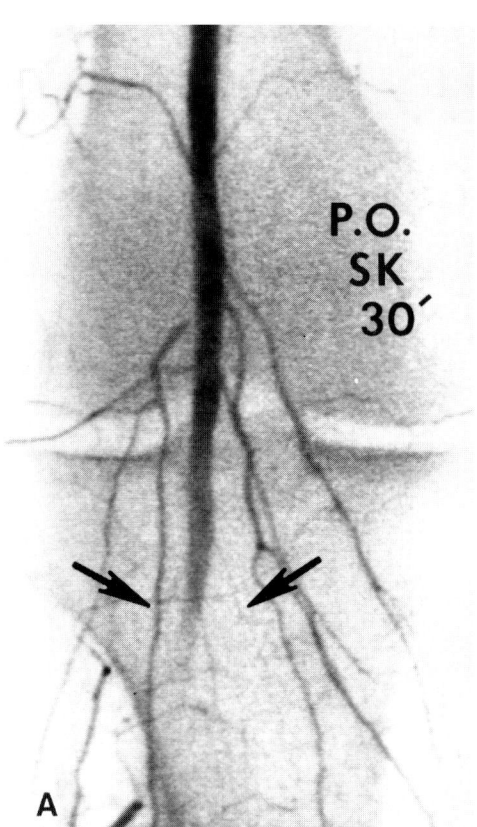
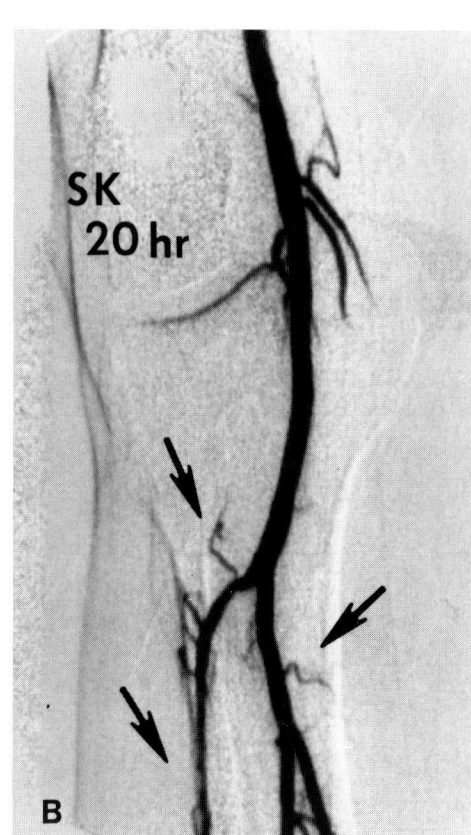

TREATMENT

With the onset of acute ischemia and angiographically demonstrated occlusion, embolectomy or thrombectomy is the treatment of choice, particularly when limb viability is immediately threatened. In chronic cases, when occlusive changes have occurred following initial thrombectomy, and when there are contraindications to surgery, fibrinolytic therapy provides a valuable treatment option. High-quality conventional diagnostic arteriography should be used to indicate the precise location of the occlusion, its extent, and the status of the vascular supply distal to the occlusion. Coagulation parameters are established prior to therapy, and these are monitored regularly throughout the period of infusion. We presently include a hematocrit, thrombin time, partial thromboplastin time, fibrinogen level, and fibrinogen degradation products titer. Occasionally a streptococcal antibody titer and/or streptokinase resistance testing are useful.

When thrombi of the superficial femoral or popliteal arteries are treated, an ipsilateral antegrade approach is preferred. After skin preparation and local anesthesia, the antegrade puncture is performed with a thin-walled 18-gauge needle; if possible, an anterior wall puncture should be used. A 0.035-in. steerable wire is then passed through the needle, and a No. 5 French sheath positioned within the superficial femoral artery. The steerable wire is manipulated to a position directly adjacent to the occlusion site. Subsequently, either a 0.035-in. or a 0.018-in. directionally controlled steerable wire is manipulated through the occluded vessel. A thrombolytic infusion catheter is then positioned over the wire, in close contact with the clot. Thrombolytic infusion catheters are available in dimensions approximating a No. 4.7 French catheter and accept a 0.018-in. steerable wire. The multiple side holes within the infusion catheter allow equal distribution of the thrombolytic agent along the length of the clot.

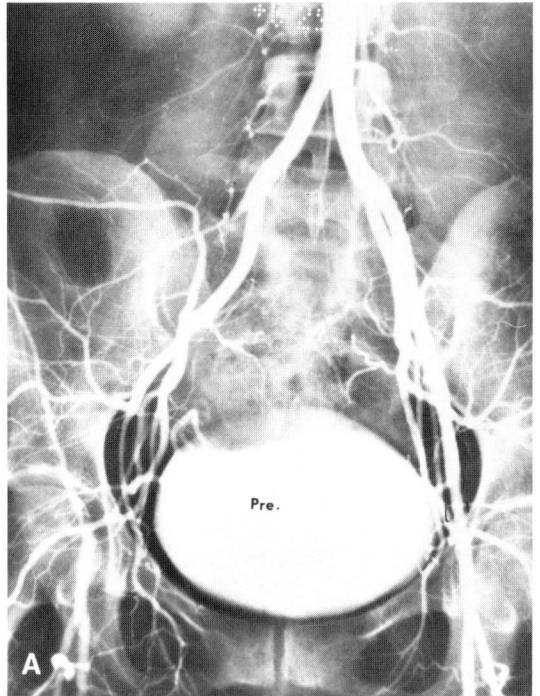
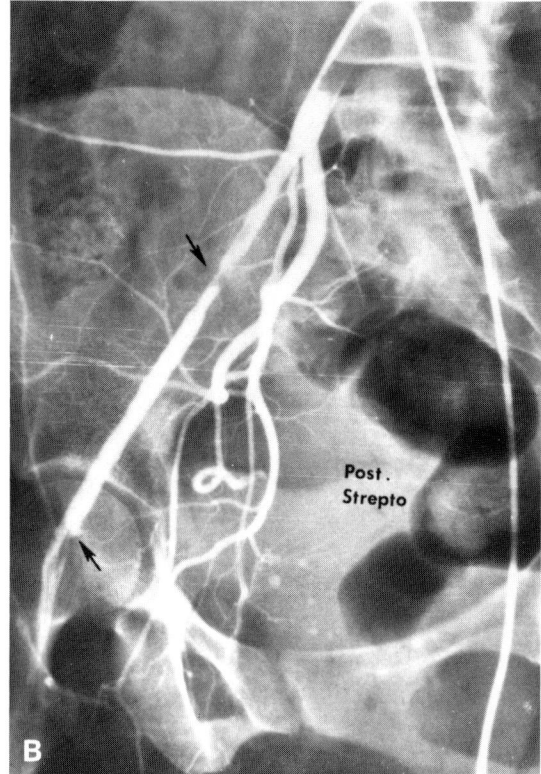
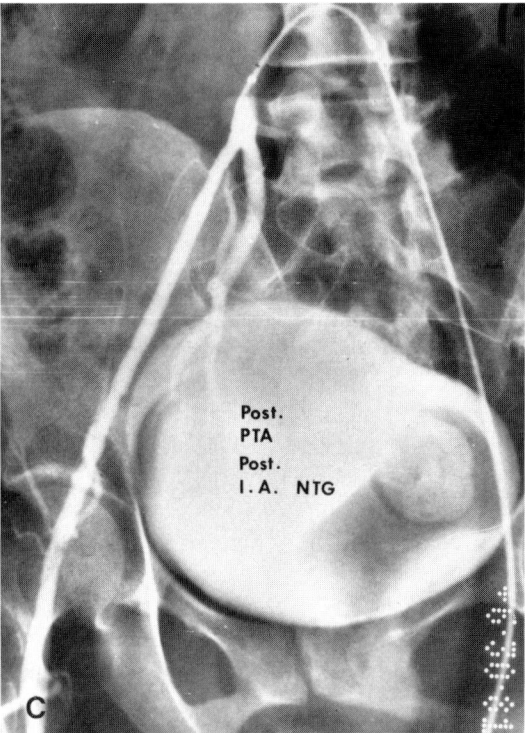

Figure 6.99 (A) Total occlusion of the entire right external iliac artery with progressive ischemic changes developing in the lower extremity 2 weeks after coronary arteriography. (B) A No. 4.7 French thrombolytic infusion catheter, with multiple side holes, was positioned from the contralateral femoral artery just proximal to the thrombotic occlusion. After 24 h of urokinase recanalization is adequate, but with residual stenosis at the puncture site and in the mid right external iliac artery. (C) Following effective recanalization with urokinase and balloon angioplasty at the stenotic site, the dimensions of the right external iliac and the common femoral artery are now within normal limits.

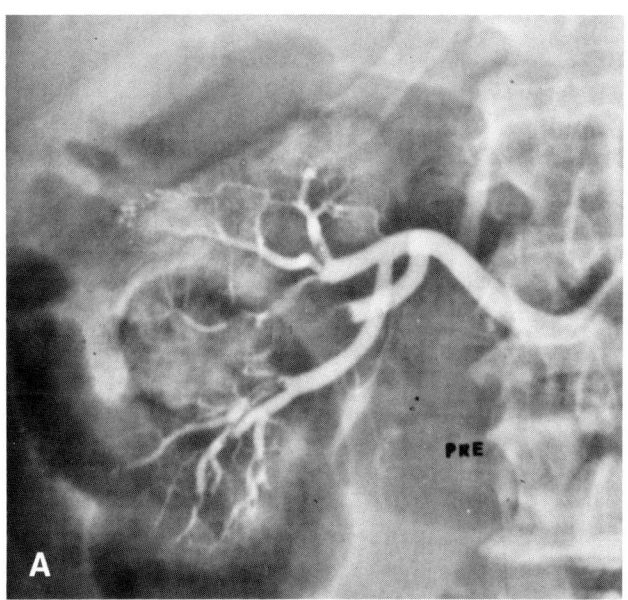

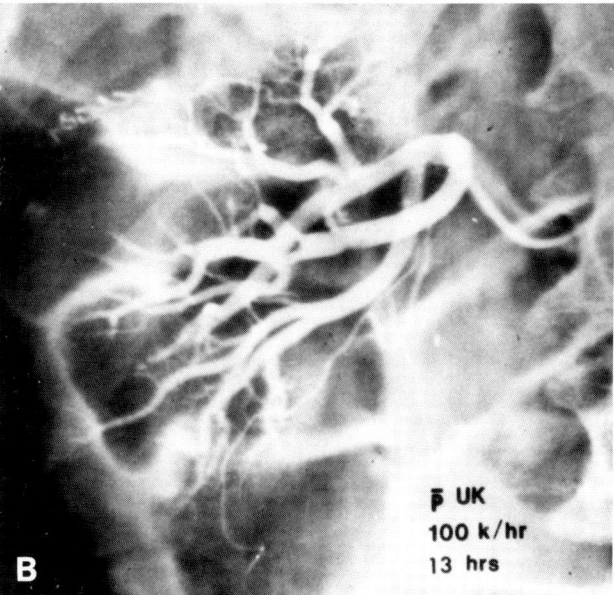

Figure 6.100 (A) Acute embolic occlusion of a principal ventral division of the right renal artery. (B) Following infusion of 100,000 IU of urokinase for 13 h, a minimal residual clot exists and there has been significant improvement in flow through the ventral division of the right renal artery with visualization to the arcuate level.

When the ischemia is relatively acute and viability is in question, we initiate a high-dose routine similar to that which is ordinarily used in our coronary occlusion program (Fig. 6.101). Urokinase, approximately 4000 IU/min, is given for 60 min. Arteriography is then performed and, if significant improvement is evident, the dose regimen is continued at approximately 100,000 IU/h for 16 to 20 h. When recanalization is complete, the patient is returned to the ICU and the thrombolytic agent is gradually tapered off. The catheter is then removed, and the patient continued on intravenous heparin (15–20,000 IU/24 h). If the thrombosis is not significantly resolved at the end of a 24-h period, the procedure is terminated. When there is improvement but reperfusion is incomplete, we may continue the urokinase for an additional 24 h, although this has rarely resulted in additional improvement. When streptokinase must be used, the dosage is approximately 3000 IU/min over a 30-min period. When repeat arteriography shows some degree of improvement, the high-dose regimen is continued for approximately 1 h, after which 5000 IU/h is given for an additional 5 to 6 h. Our experience with t-PA suggests that a dose of approximately 3 mg/h for 5 to 6 h is usually sufficient. Rarely have we exceeded a total dose of 18 mg. Coagulation parameters are routinely checked at 6- and 20-h intervals.

In cases in which a high-dose regimen is not indicated, the thrombolytic agent is usually given at approximately 50 mL/h in a 5% dextrose and water or normal saline solution. Simultaneous heparinization via continuous IV infusion of 15,000 to 20,000 IU per day is also begun. The patient is returned to the angiographic suite after 18 to 24 h for repeat arteriography for evaluation of therapeutic results. If the recheck examination shows fibrinolysis, the urokinase may be continued for an additional 24 h. Observation of coagulation parameters is continued. If the thrombosis is not resolved within 48 h, it is unlikely that improvement will occur and the procedure is usually terminated. Those patients whose treatment has been extended to 72 h have had the highest incidence of thrombotic and hemorrhagic complications.

When it is not possible to perform an antegrade puncture on the ipsilateral side, the contralateral approach with a retrograde puncture is performed. The catheter is manipulated across the aortic bifurcation and appropriately positioned at the occlusion site. This is the preferred approach for patients with iliac artery thrombosis. Thromboembolic changes within the renal and abdominal visceral circulation are best approached using a femoral technique. Upper-extremity thrombotic changes following arteriotomy or brachial arteriography are also best treated via the femoral route. Heparin therapy, to protect either the uninvolved contralateral iliac vessels or the smaller visceral or upper-extremity vessels, is routine in these cases. When neither femoral

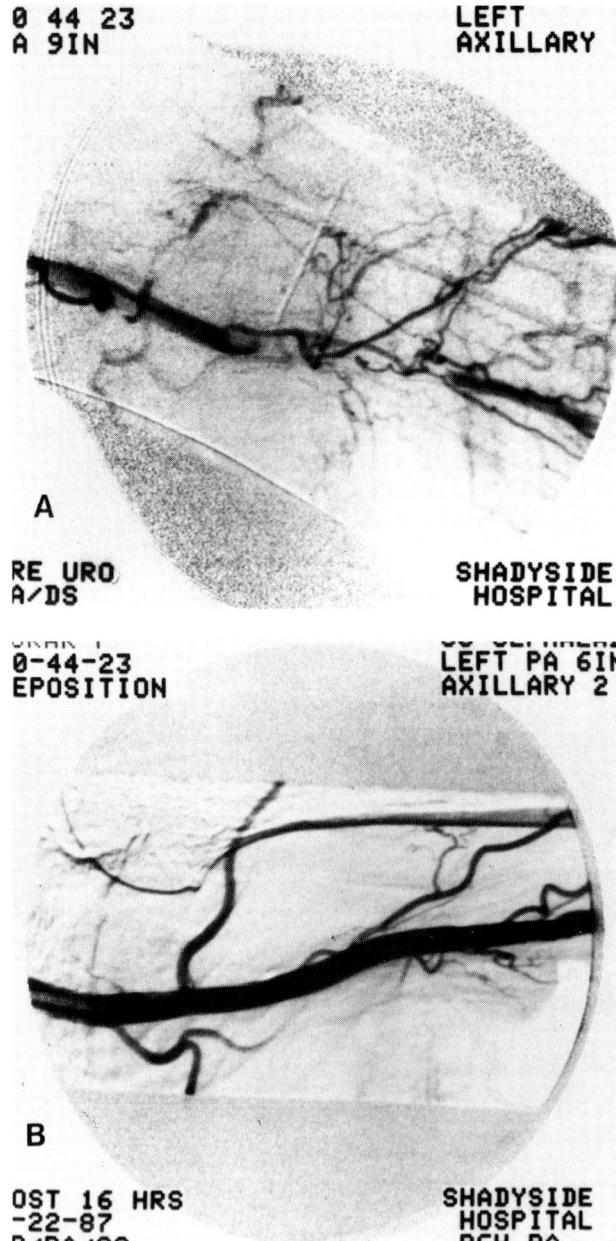

Figure 6.101 (A) Selective left subclavian digital subtraction arteriogram demonstrating acute thrombotic changes in the distal left axillary–brachial artery segment. (B) Following a 16-h regional infusion of urokinase, the left axillary artery and brachial artery are now widely patent.

puncture site is available, the axillary artery remains an option, although potential bleeding complications at this site pose a much higher risk to the patient because of possible injury to the brachial plexus.

An underlying stenosis due either to intrinsic atherosclerotic involvement or anastomotic narrowing of a bypass graft is frequently treated by postangioplasty dilatation in order to maintain effective outflow and prevent abrupt reocclusion. Patients whose underlying lesions are not treatable generally do not have satisfactory long-term results, as this indicates that the underlying causes that produced the initial thrombosis have not been relieved.

During the infusion, all puncture procedures should be avoided and careful observation for external and internal bleeding sources carried out. Streptokinase and t-PA, more so than urokinase, will unmask occult gastrointestinal bleeding or spontaneous hematuria (Fig. 6.102). However, it has been our experience that bleeding complications are most often related to heparin, and thus heparin should be terminated first. If bleeding continues, whatever agent is being used should be discontinued. Distal embolization with fragmentation of the thrombus is occasionally observed during thrombolytic therapy with any of the agents, and continued therapy will ordinarily lyse even the most distal fragments.

CONCLUSIONS

A significant renewal in interest in the application of fibrinolytic agents has occurred since Dotter recommended selective intraarterial regional therapy in 1974. Hemorrhagic complications in earlier series, in which 100,000 IU/h IV were administered for major pulmonary thromboembolic disease, were as high as 40 percent. With the regional approach, hemorrhagic complications were controlled at acceptable levels of approximately 10 percent, and frequently these were heparin-related when a combined approach had been used. From our experiences, it is apparent that the size of the thrombus is also of critical importance: small clots present considerably less difficulty than extensive, organized clots. Effective recanalization is also related to the duration of the thrombus; clots 7 days old or less are more effectively lysed than the long-standing chronic organized thrombis. It is also apparent that thrombotic changes within prostheses are more easily managed than in thrombotic involvement of autogenous saphenous vein grafts. In addition, thrombi in small, totally occluded vessels with essentially no runoff are much more difficult to manage than thrombi in larger vessels with visible outflow.

Unfortunately, there is no single criterion for pre-

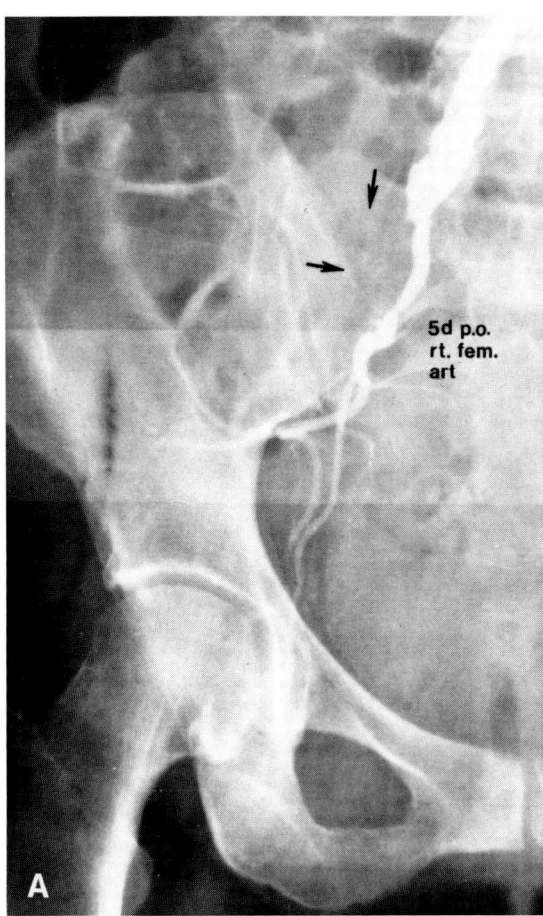
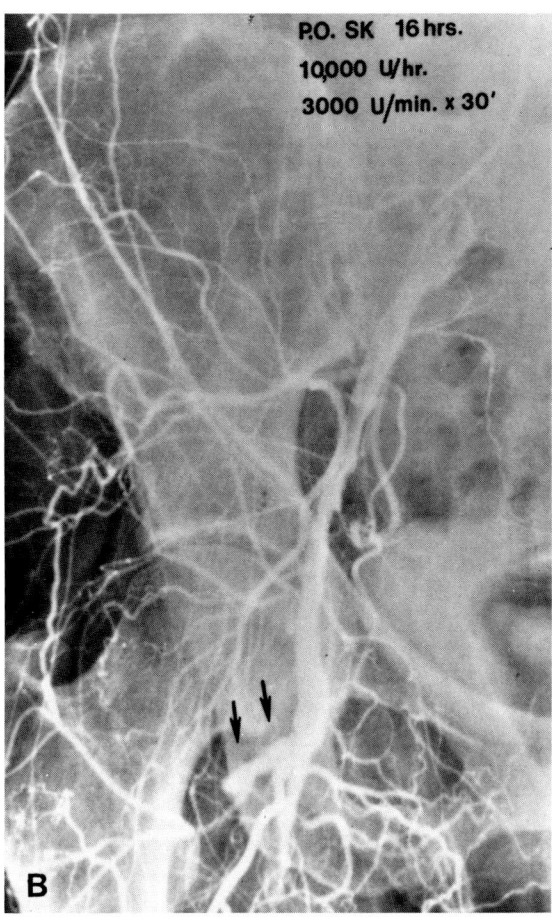

Figure 6.102 (A) Total occlusion of the right external iliac artery and right common femoral artery following right femoral artery puncture and conventional arteriography. (B) A No. 5 French opaque catheter was positioned from a contralateral approach just proximal to the thrombotic occlusion site in the right external iliac artery. The angiogram demonstrates effective recanalization following urokinase for 16 h: 4000 IU/min was given for 30 min followed by 100,000 IU/h. Although the entire iliac artery is recanalized, the arrows indicate the extravasation site and subsequent hematoma that developed from the arterial puncture 5 days earlier.

dicting effective clot lysis. Although the age, size, and location are relevant, the single most important factor is the degree of ischemia. In the acutely ischemic patient threatened with amputation, surgery, if at all feasible, remains the method of choice. If a surgical contraindication exists, selective regional fibrinolytic therapy is a promising alternative. Variations in protocol still exist, and there is no firmly established dose regimen. In the acute ischemic situation, initial intensive regional intraarterial therapy should be followed by a low-dose approach (Figs. 6.103 and 6.104). Chronic lesions are managed most effectively and safely with a low-dose regimen. If local bleeding complications occur, they are usually well managed by manual compression. When this approach is not effective, infusion should be discontinued, and it may be necessary to administer fresh frozen plasma or whole blood. Unfortunately, when hemorrhagic complications, including intracerebral hemorrhage do occur, they are difficult to control and occasionally fatal (Figs. 6.105 and 6.106).

In carefully selected patients, results with regional fibrinolytic therapy can be impressive. Scrupulous monitoring of coagulation parameters during infusion and avoidance of additional punctures are critical if bleeding complications are to be minimized. The most favorable outcomes have been in patients with recent-onset symptoms, relatively small clot size, and favorable distal vessel outflow. With few exceptions, combined heparinization is required. Successful results are rarely obtained when infusions are continued beyond a 48-h period.

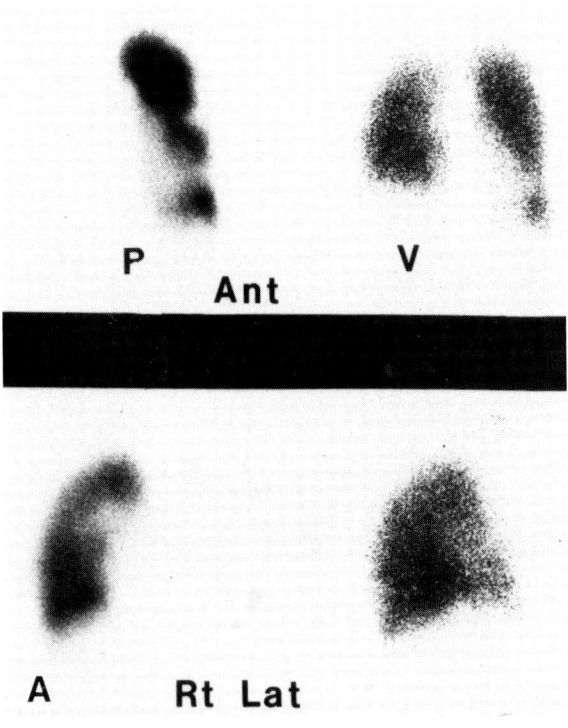
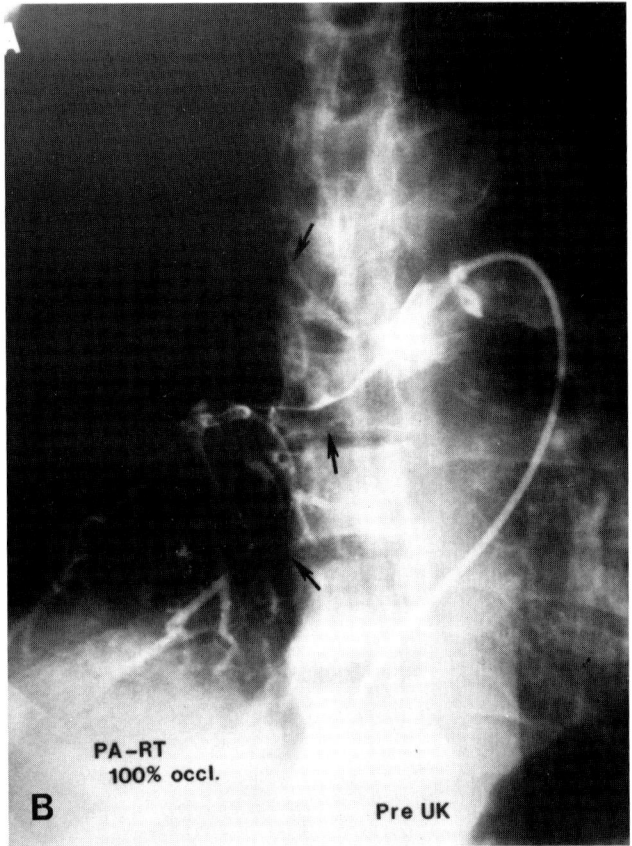
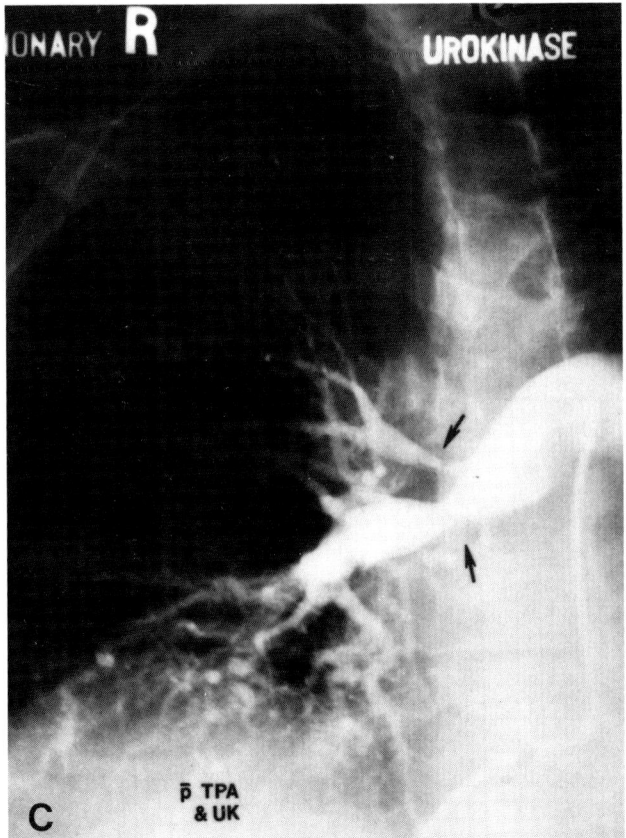

Figure 6.103 (A) Ventilation perfusion scan demonstrating an absence of perfusion in the entire right lung in addition to segmental perfusion defects in the left lung consistent with massive thromboembolic involvement. (B) Selective pulmonary arteriography demonstrating total thrombotic occlusion of essentially the entire right pulmonary circulation. (C) Following 5 mg/h of tissue plasminogen activator for 1 h, and 100,000 IU/h of urokinase for 16 h, significant improvement in the perfusion pattern now exists through the right upper lobe and right lower lobe pulmonary circulation.

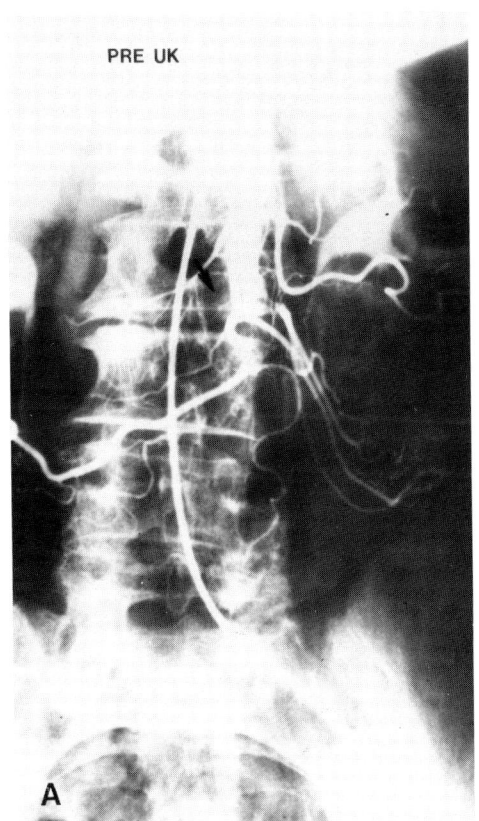
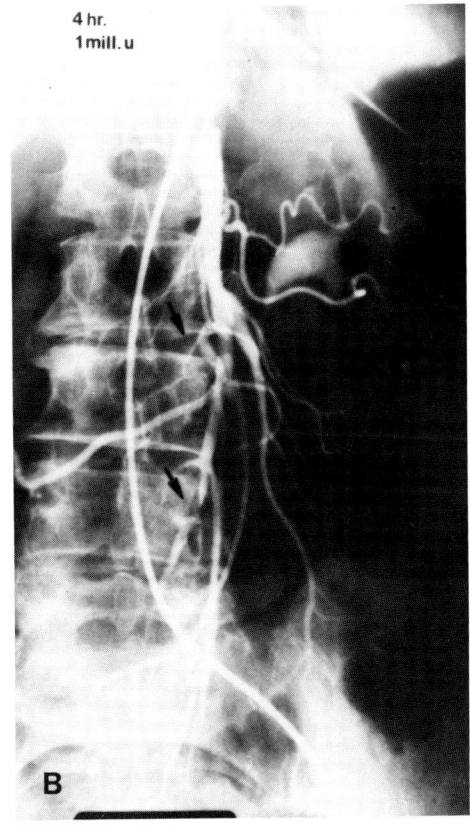
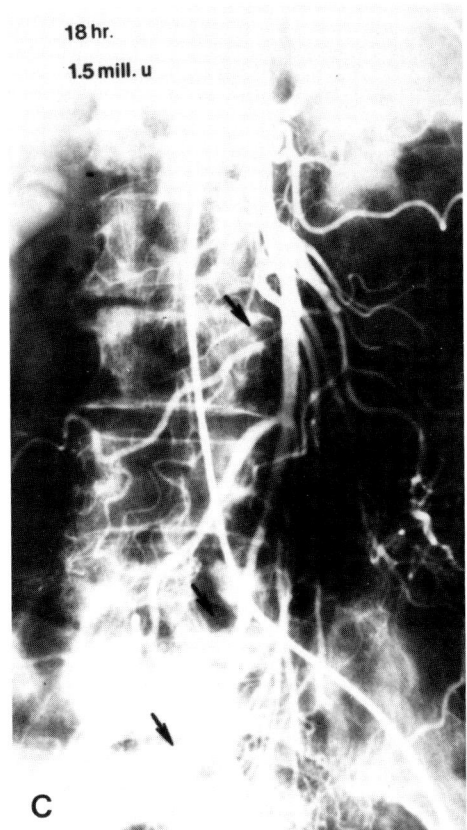

Figure 6.104 (A) Selective mesenteric arteriogram demonstrating acute embolic occlusion of the superior mesenteric artery with little or no distal arterial visualization beyond the proximal jejunal vessels. (B) Following 1 million IU of urokinase given over a 4-h period there is now marked improvement in the superior mesenteric circulation. (C) After 18 h and 1.5 million IU of urokinase, the perfusion pattern to the superior mesenteric circulation is essentially normal.

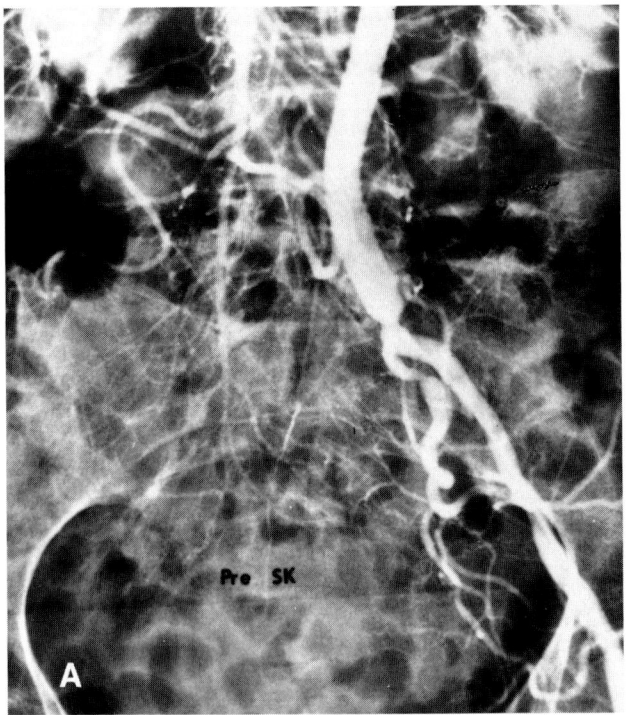
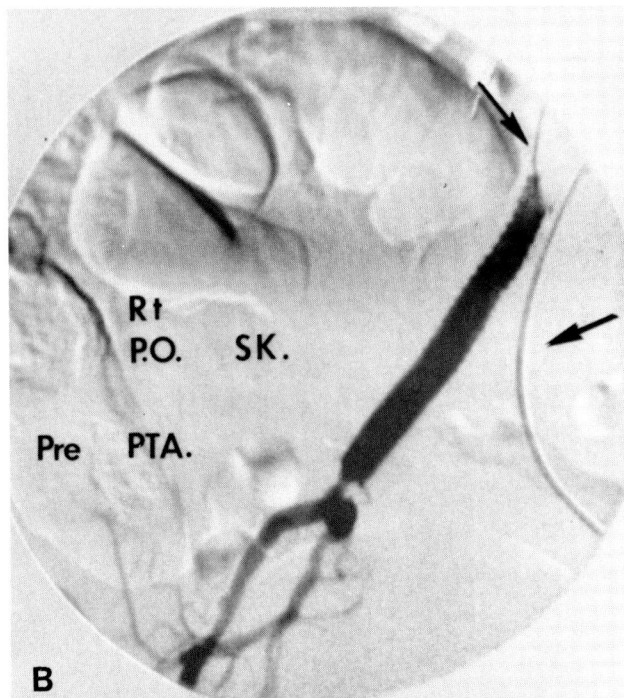
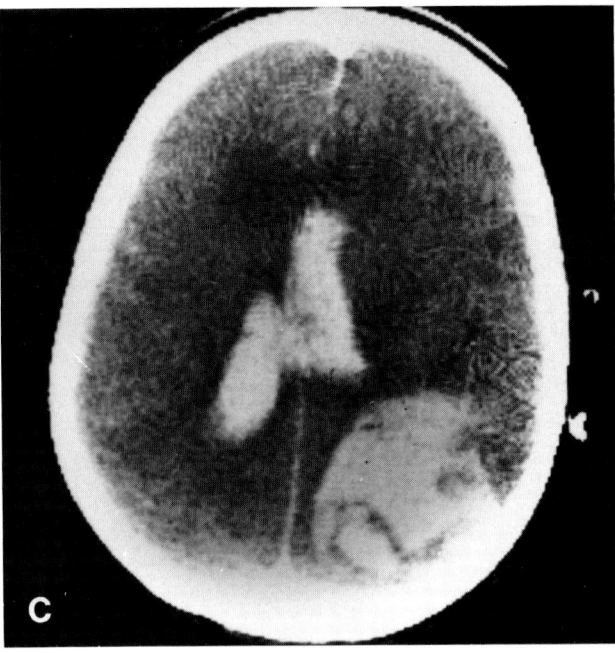

Figure 6.105 (A) Total occlusion of the right limb of an aortoiliac graft. Prestreptokinase angiogram done from a left femoral approach. (B) Effective recanalization with satisfactory patency of the right limb of the aortoiliac graft. Note the stenotic site at the distal anastomosis. The stenosis would account for the thrombotic changes in the graft and would also be amenable to poststreptokinase angioplasty. (C) Following 12 h of streptokinase, and prior to angioplasty, the patient developed hemiplegia of the right side with deteriorating CNS changes that necessitated computed tomography. The unenhanced scan demonstrates dense posterior left parietooccipital hemorrhage with associated intraventricular hemorrhage and displacement of the ventricular structures.

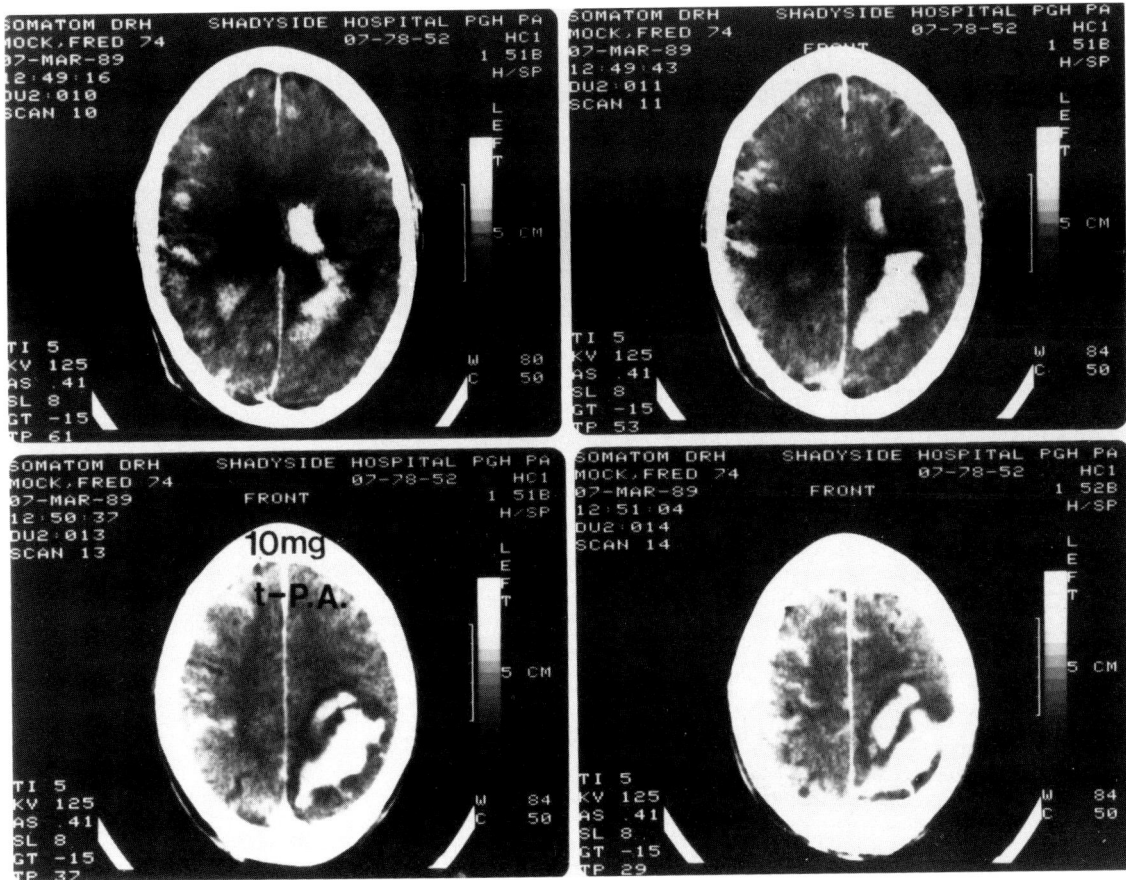

Figure 6.106 Unenhanced computed tomographic examination of the head demonstrating intracranial hemorrhage in the left posterior parietal occipital lobes in addition to subarachnoid bleeding secondary to infusion of tissue plasminogen activator for left iliac artery thrombotic occlusion.

REFERENCES

Eskridge JM, Becker GJ, Rabe FE, et al. Catheter-related thrombosis and fibrinolytic therapy. *Radiology* 1983;149:429–432.

Hirshberg A, Schneiderman J, Garnick A, et al. Error and pitfalls in intraarterial thrombolytic therapy. *J Vasc Surg* 1989;10:612–616.

Holden RW. Plasminogen activators: Pharmacology and therapy. *Radiology* 1990;174:993–1001.

Katzen BT, van Breda A. Low dose streptokinase in the treatment of arterial occlusions. *AJR* 1981;136:1171–1178.

Lammer J, Pilger E, Justich E, et al. Fibrinolysis in chronic arteriosclerotic occlusions: Intrathrombotic injections of streptokinase. *Radiology* 1985;157:45–50.

Marder VJ, Sherry S. Thrombolytic therapy: Current status (1st part). *N Engl J Med* 1988;318:1512–1520.

Marder VJ, Sherry S. Thrombolytic therapy: Current status (2nd part). *N Engl J Med* 1988;318:1585–1595.

McNamara TO, Fischer JR. Thrombolysis of peripheral arterial and graft occlusions: Improved results using high-dose urokinase. *AJR* 1985;144:769–775.

McNamara TO. Technique and results of "higher-dose" infusion. *Cardiovasc Intervent Radiol* 1988;11:S48–S57.

Ricotta JJ, Green RM, DeWeese JA. Use and limitations of thrombolytic therapy in the treatment of peripheral arterial ischemia: Results of a multi-institutional questionnaire. *J Vasc Surg* 1987;6:45–50.

Risius B, Graor RA, Geisinger MA, et al. Thrombolytic therapy with recombinant human tissue-type plasminogen activator: A comparison of two doses. *Radiology* 1987;164:465–468.

Sasahara AA. Fundamentals of fibrinolytic therapy. *Cardiovasc Intervent Radiol* 1988;11:S3–S5.

Sullivan KL, Gardiner GA, Shapiro MJ, et al. Acceleration of thrombolysis with a high-dose transthrombus bolus technique. *Radiology* 1989;173:805–808.

van Breda A, Katzen BT, Deutsch AS. Urokinase versus streptokinase in local thrombolysis. *Radiology* 1987;165:109–111.

Chapter Seven

Percutaneous Retrieval of Intravascular Foreign Bodies

RENAN UFLACKER

INTRODUCTION

Percutaneous retrieval of a foreign body from the cardiovascular system is the treatment of choice for patients with a foreign body lost inside the vascular system. Surgical treatment in these patients usually involves extensive procedures including thoracotomy and the opening of large vessels or cardiac chambers. These surgical interventions can be avoided through the use of a percutaneous technique.

Nonsurgical removal of an embolized foreign body was first performed in 1964 by Thomas and coworkers. Most cases of intravascular foreign bodies that must be removed involve fragments of venous infusion catheters that have fractured within the subclavian vein or the jugular vein. The most frequent sites where foreign bodies are found are the superior vena cava, the right side of the heart, and the pulmonary artery; intraarterial foreign bodies have been reported less frequently.

A progressive increase in the use of indwelling intravascular catheters, parenteral feeding catheters, and angiographic and hemodynamic diagnosis catheters has led to a higher frequency of displacement, fracture, and embolization of tube fragments within the cardiovascular system. Aside from these medical materials, trauma produced by firearms, knives, and fragmented objects can also cause embolization in the cardiovascular system. The development of therapeutic angiographic techniques for vessel occlusion and prosthesis placement has created yet another type of material which can be lost inside the cardiovascular system.

CAUSES

The most frequent cause of fracturing of intravascular material is the degeneration of the plastic used in the manufacture of catheters, along with problems related to the handling, removal, or introduction of catheters.

The use of disposable materials and more resistant and durable plastics should reduce the incidence of foreign body embolisms.

The most common problems involving catheter rupture and embolism include tube fracture on the cutting bevel of a puncture needle in the subclavian vein, catheter detachment from the connection system, and accidental rupture of a tube when skin fixation stitches or dressings that adhere strongly to the tube are cut. Fracture during catheter manipulation may occur during angiographic procedures; catheters and guidewires are involved in these cases.

Most intravascular foreign bodies embolize to the superior vena cava, the right ventricle and atrium, the pulmonary artery, or a combination of these sites. Foreign bodies are less frequently found in the aorta and in arterial branches.

The position of a foreign body inside the cardiovascular system depends on the entry route and, if the foreign body migrates inside the vascular system, on gravity and the patient's position when the accident occurs. The final position of the fragment depends on the length and rigidity of the material and the type of flow in the vessel or cardiac chamber that contains the foreign body.

Long catheters introduced through the subclavian vein usually locate themselves with the distal tip somewhere on the wall of the right ventricle. The proximal tip usually remains in the superior vena cava. Long fragments, if they are flexible and have curved distal tips, sometimes penetrate into the lumen of the pulmonary artery, with the distal tip localized inside the left pulmonary artery and the proximal tip inside the right cardiac chambers. If the fragment is short, its distal tip usually remains stuck to irregularities in the wall of the right ventricle and its proximal tip remains in the right atrium. Occasionally, small fragments migrate directly to the pulmonary artery, where they are even more difficult to retrieve.

Fragments rarely migrate from the lower extremities, but in these cases, they are preferentially located in the right atrium or ventricle and the inferior vena cava. They may also be found in the superior vena cava and the hepatic veins.

Heavier materials, such as guidewire fragments, tend to migrate shorter distances but can be more thrombogenic because they become fixed onto vascular walls. Heavy foreign bodies, such as bullets, can travel extraordinarily long distances.

Surgical retrieval of foreign bodies may be associated with high morbidity rates in these patients, who as a rule are severely ill and under intensive care. Percutaneous retrieval of foreign bodies is an extremely attractive option for these patients.

Today many different approaches and techniques are used for foreign body retrieval. In our experience, the most useful and safest way of removing a foreign body is the so-called snare technique, which consists of a guidewire loop and an adequate catheter. The next most favorable method utilizes a flexible "basket" assembly similar to the biliary stone retrieval system.

MATERIALS AND RESULTS

Our series included 20 patients (10 men and 10 women) ranging in age from 5 months to 65 years. In 16 of these patients the foreign bodies were "intracath" fragments. Four patients had fragments of diagnostic angiographic catheters, two had fractured ventricular valves, and one had a bullet in the pulmonary circulation. Eight of the catheters were inside the superior vena cava, six were in the pulmonary arteries, and two were in the right side of the heart. One fragment was in the subclavian vein, one was in the thoracic aorta, and two were in the aortoiliac segment (Fig. 7.1).

Percutaneous retrieval should always be preceded by localization x-rays. After the foreign body has been found, an angiographic series should be performed to reveal any clots around the foreign body.

In our experience, approximately 95 percent of these procedures have been successful in removing foreign bodies (19 of 20 patients). No significant complication has resulted from these procedures, except for transient cardiac arrhythmias during catheterization and catheter fragmentation in two patients.

TECHNICAL ASPECTS OF FOREIGN BODY RETRIEVAL

Snare Technique

The snare technique is the most versatile, useful, and successful method for retrieving an intravascular foreign body. Once the intravascular foreign body has been

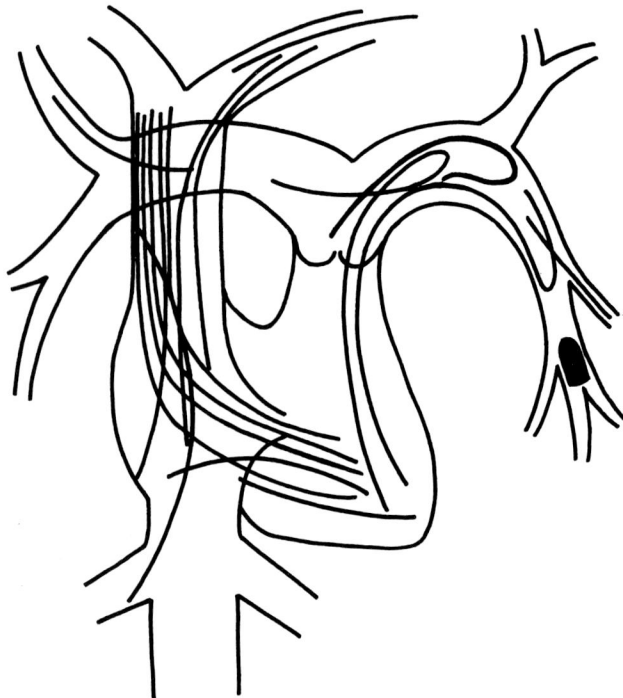

Figure 7.1 Schematic drawing showing the position of 17 of 20 foreign bodies within the cardiovascular system in our series. Foreign bodies within the arterial system are not shown.

found, the guidewire loop is opened near the free tip of the catheter fragment. Several attempts usually must be made before the catheter fragment is encircled, after which the loop is firmly closed around the fragment. Once the fragment is firmly held inside the loop, it can be pulled through the vascular system up to a Desilet-Hoffman–type angiographic sheath, which should always be available for this procedure (Figs. 7.2 and 7.3).

The femoral route approach with a Seldinger-type puncture and the use of a sheath with a diameter larger than that of the catheter is a prerequisite for success and for minimizing risk.

A venotomy or arteriotomy may occasionally be necessary to remove a foreign body, depending on its size. A venotomy is always required to extract a bullet from within the venous system (Fig. 7.4).

Foreign bodies can be retrieved in most angiography laboratories. The instrument used for this purpose is a Teflon or polyethylene No. 8 French catheter with a wide lumen and thin walls. This catheter has a tip curved 30°. A 0.018- or 0.20-in. pediatric guidewire without the movable core at least 1.45 m long is used to form the loop.

To form the loop, both guidewire extremities are introduced retrogradely into the catheter. The tips are asymmetrically visible at the catheter's proximal extrem-

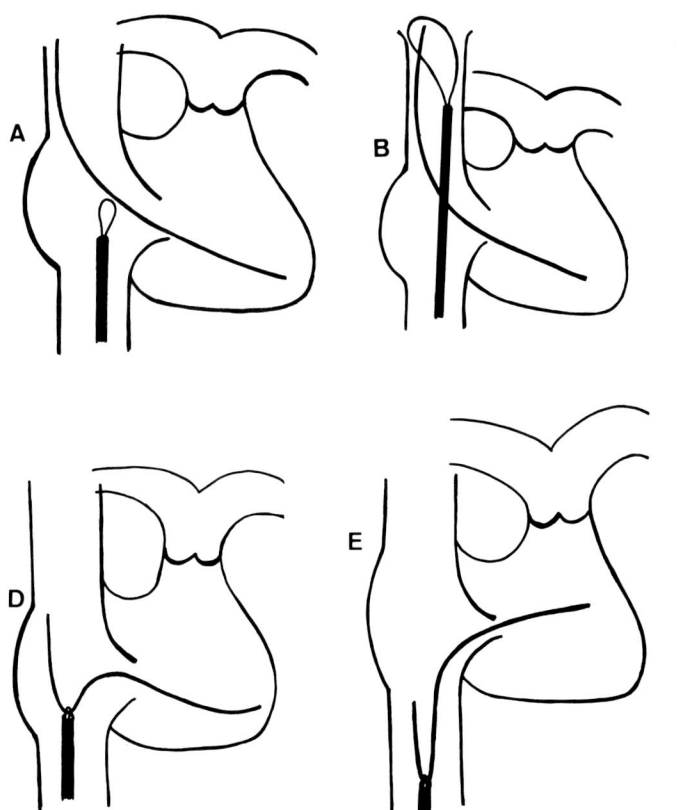

Figure 7.2 Snare technique.
(A) A foreign body in the most common position, within the superior vena cava and right ventricle. (B) The removal loop is positioned around the free tip of the catheter fragment in the superior vena cava. (C) The snare is fastened firmly around the fragment. (D) The catheter fragment is pulled out of the heart. (E) The fragment is removed from the vascular system through a sheath in the femoral vein.

ity; i.e., one tip should be shorter than the other. Only one tip should be pushed forward to open the loop and then pulled back to close it. The set as a whole usually has enough torque to enter the superior vena cava and the right side of the heart. A snare-type device for foreign body retrieval is commercially available.

Frequently, the foreign body is wedged into a vessel or a cardiac chamber, with no free extremities on which the snare technique can be used. In such cases it has to be displaced with the help of a catheter and placed in a more favorable position, with at least one extremity free (Fig. 7.5). The use of a pigtail catheter for fragment displacement in inaccessible vessels by means of rotation and traction is another method which can be utilized to reposition a foreign body when the snare technique is to be used subsequently. Variants of this technique include using a hook-tip catheter or a controllable-tip guidewire to displace the catheter fragment, along with rotation and repositioning of the foreign body.

Dormia Basket

A variant of the snare technique makes use of a Dormia-type wire basket to capture and retrieve a foreign body from the cardiovascular system. This method is highly efficient technically, although its use is limited when a very tortuous pathway or sharp curves must be traversed before the foreign body is reached.

Forceps Technique

The forceps technique utilizes endoscopy equipment for use in the digestive tract or respiratory tract. This is sometimes an appropriate alternative; the method is identical to that used in the bronchi, esophagus, and urinary tract. The fragment is caught by the "alligator jaws" and then pulled out through an angiographic catheter and sheath. Curves and angularity limit the use of rigid or semirigid forceps.

Modified Snare Technique

The snare technique had to be modified to extract cardiac pacemaker electrodes. The difficulty in these cases is related to the absence of free extremities that can be snared. These extremities are firmly attached proximally on the wall of the subclavian vein and distally on the wall of the right ventricle.

A Judkins-type left coronary catheter is introduced around the electrode and snared on its tip by the loop used for foreign body removal. When the left coronary catheter has been firmly engaged by the loop, the whole

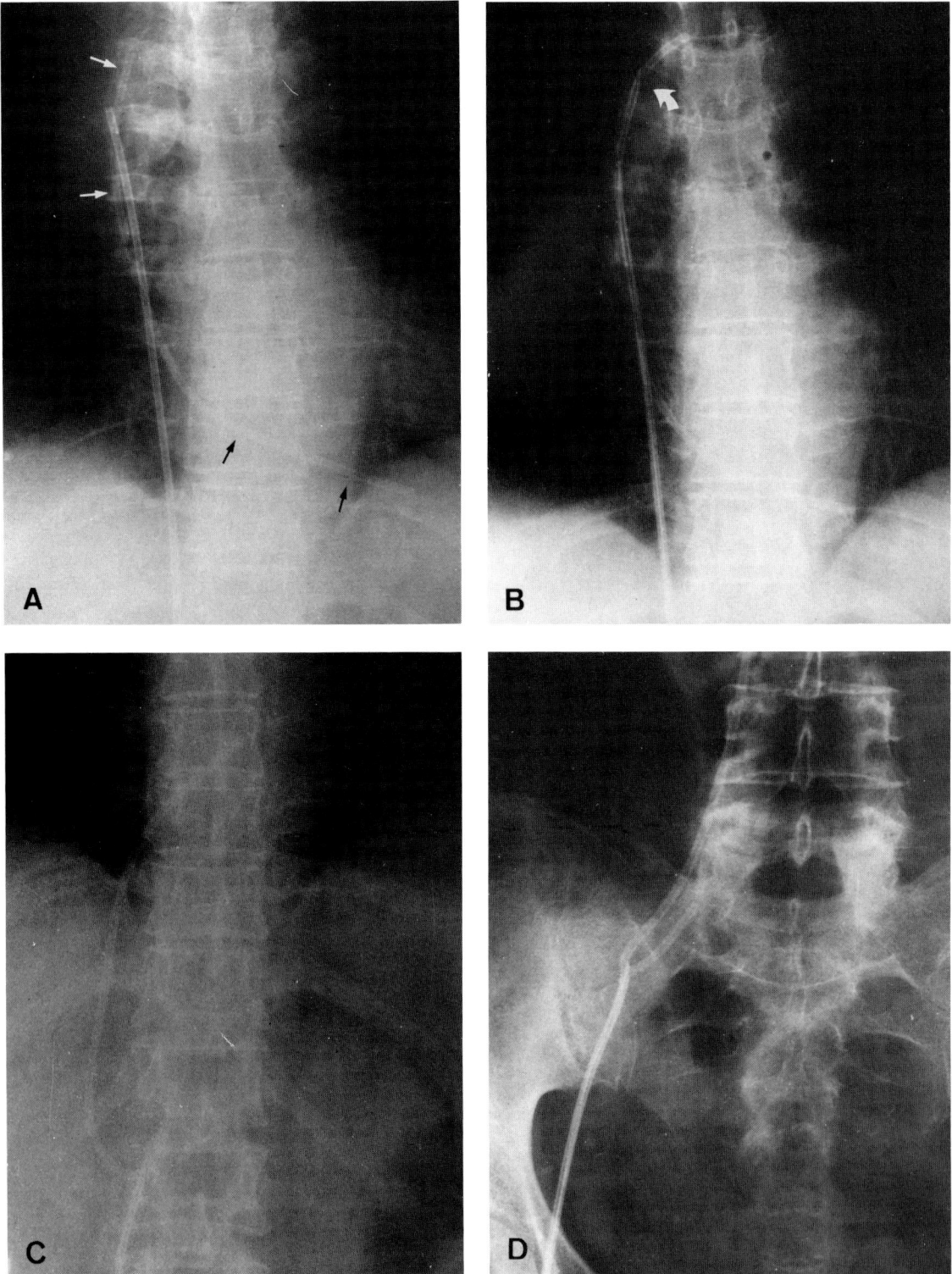

Figure 7.3 Snare technique.
(A) A long catheter fragment in the superior vena cava, right atrium, and right ventricle (arrows). The snaring catheter is in position. (B) The loop is firmly fastened around the foreign body (arrow). (C) A catheter fragment inside the inferior vena cava during removal. (D) A catheter fragment during removal through the right iliac vein.

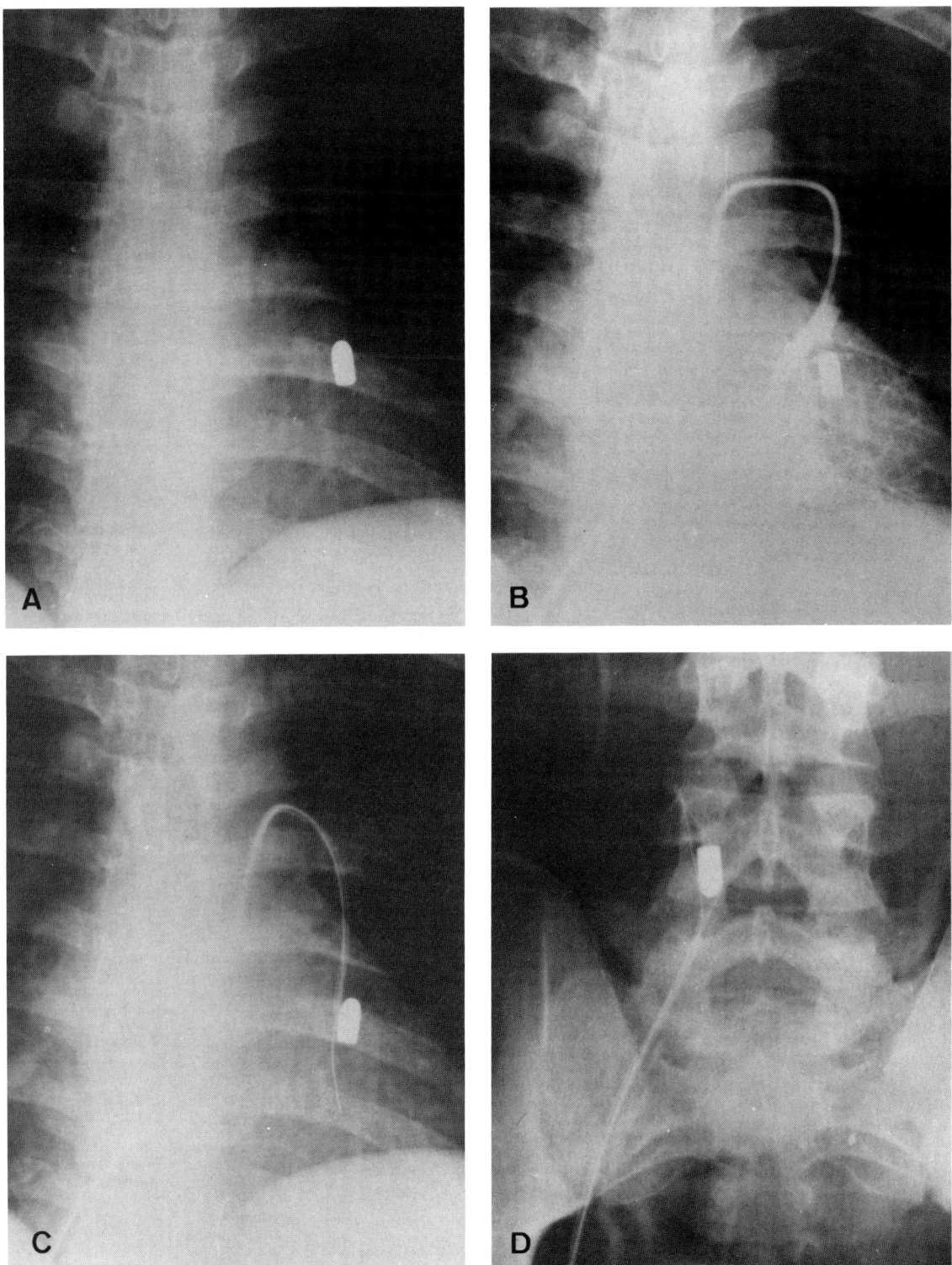

Figure 7.4 Snare technique.
(A) A patient was shot in the right iliac fossa, and the bullet was finally lodged in the left pulmonary arterial circulation after migrating through the entire cardiovascular system. (B) Contrast injection shows a projectile inside the left pulmonary circulation. (C) A metal loop is passed downstream from the bullet and fastened firmly around the foreign body. (D) The bullet was extracted through a right femoral venotomy after being snared.

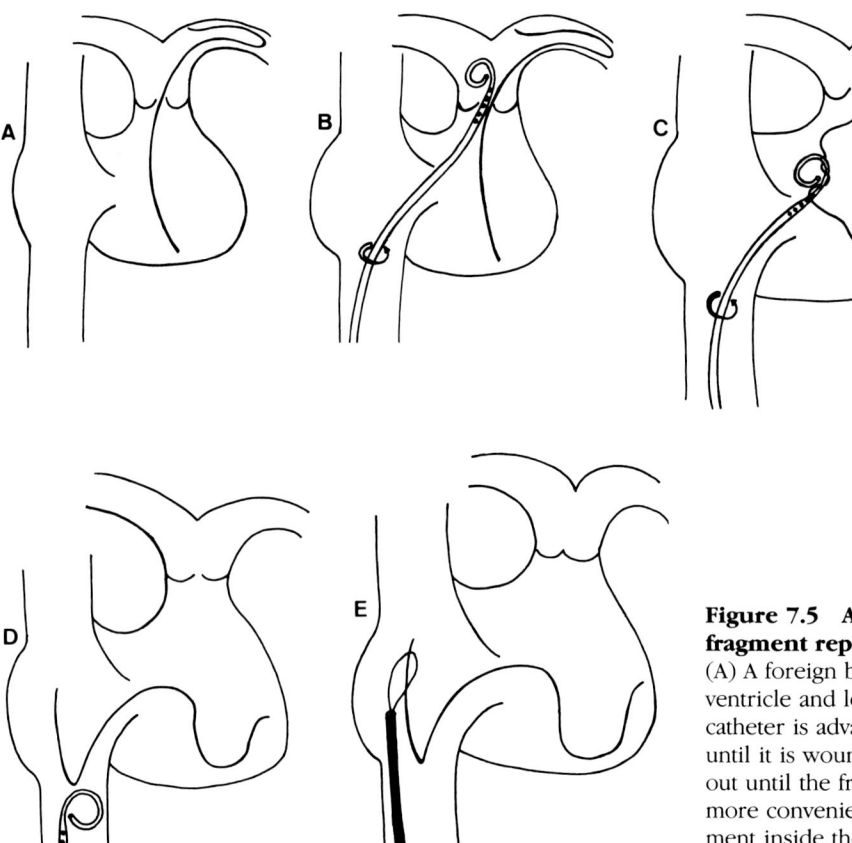

Figure 7.5 Alternative use of a pigtail catheter for fragment repositioning.
(A) A foreign body without free tips inside the right ventricle and left pulmonary artery. (B,C) A pigtail-type catheter is advanced close to the fragment and rotated until it is wound around the fragment. Then it is pulled out until the fragment is repositioned with a free tip in a more convenient location. (D) Repositioning of a fragment inside the heart. (E) The snare loop is finally fastened around the fragment, which is then removed.

system is pulled back until one extremity of the electrode is released. The free tip of the electrode is then snared by the loop and removed by conventional means (Fig. 7.6). Retrieval of electrodes that are firmly attached to the vascular walls or endocardium usually requires a reasonable amount of force and may cause severe arrhythmia as a consequence of myocardial pulling.

Coaxial (Pass-Over) Technique

When a small catheter fragment is wedged into the pulmonary circulation, one of two techniques can be employed. The first technique involves the use of a balloon catheter which is positioned beyond the foreign body and is then inflated and pulled back so that it can be repositioned and the removal system can be used. The second technique makes use of a larger-diameter catheter which is introduced coaxially above the fragment simultaneously with the introduction of a guidewire through the lumen of the catheter fragment. Once the system has been properly positioned, the whole system is removed, with the larger catheter (No. 12 French) covering the foreign body inside it (Fig. 7.7). This technique was used successfully in only one patient in our series (Fig. 7.8).

DIFFICULTIES

The major difficulty encountered in some of these procedures is additional fragmentation of the embolized fragment, which can turn an uncomplicated problem into a dangerous embolization episode. This is particularly dangerous when the procedure is performed via the arterial tree (Fig. 7.9). Polyurethane diagnostic catheters can suffer deleterious effects as a result of aging of the material or the action of ionizing radiation. This in turn may result in layer splitting and fragmentation, with a high probability of iatrogenic accidents if the catheters are reused or held in stock for long periods.

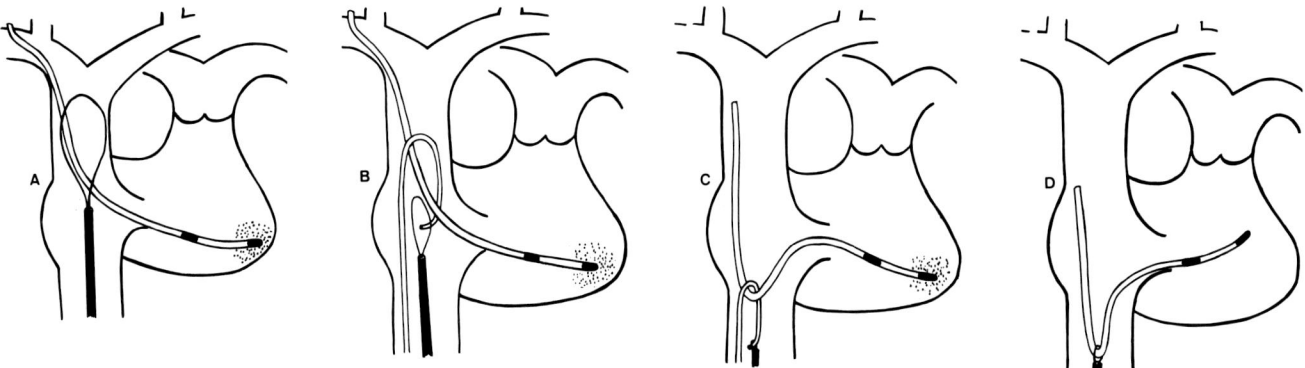

Figure 7.6 Technique for removing broken pacemaker electrodes from inside the vascular system.
(A) An electrode fragment is firmly attached to the wall of the subclavian vein and the endocardium of the right ventricle. The loop cannot be fastened to either tip of the electrode. (B) A Judkins left coronary catheter is passed around the electrode, and its tip is caught in the snare. The system is then pulled out till one of the electrode tips is released from the vascular wall or ventricle. (C) Once one of the tips has been released, the snare loop is used for conventional retrieval, as shown in Fig. 7.2.

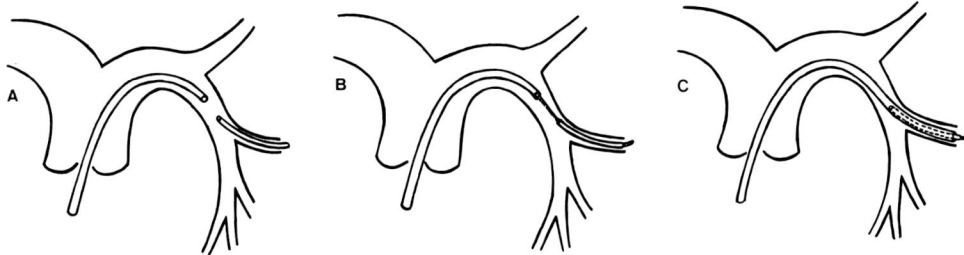

Figure 7.7 Schematic drawing of the pass-over technique for retrieval of small fragments in the peripheral pulmonary circulation.
(A) The catheter fragment is wedged within the peripheral pulmonary artery. (B) A straight guidewire is introduced through a larger catheter into the catheter fragment. (C) After the wire is inside the fragment, the larger catheter is advanced coaxially until it encircles the fragment. The entire system is then removed.

CONTRAINDICATIONS

There are only a few contraindications to intravascular foreign body retrieval, including the following:

1. Large thrombi close to the foreign body
2. Perforation of the vascular wall or cardiac chamber
3. Fixation of a foreign body to a vascular wall for a long period
4. Extravascular location of a foreign body

CONCLUSION

Percutaneous procedures for foreign body retrieval are highly effective and relatively simple compared with surgical procedures. Percutaneous procedures are safe, with only a small number of possible complications. Percutaneous retrieval of a foreign body should always be attempted prior to exploratory surgery.

Among all the techniques used for this purpose, the metal snare technique is the most important because of its simplicity and effectiveness (Fig. 7.10). This technique can be used by any experienced angiographer, at any angiography laboratory, for patients of any age.

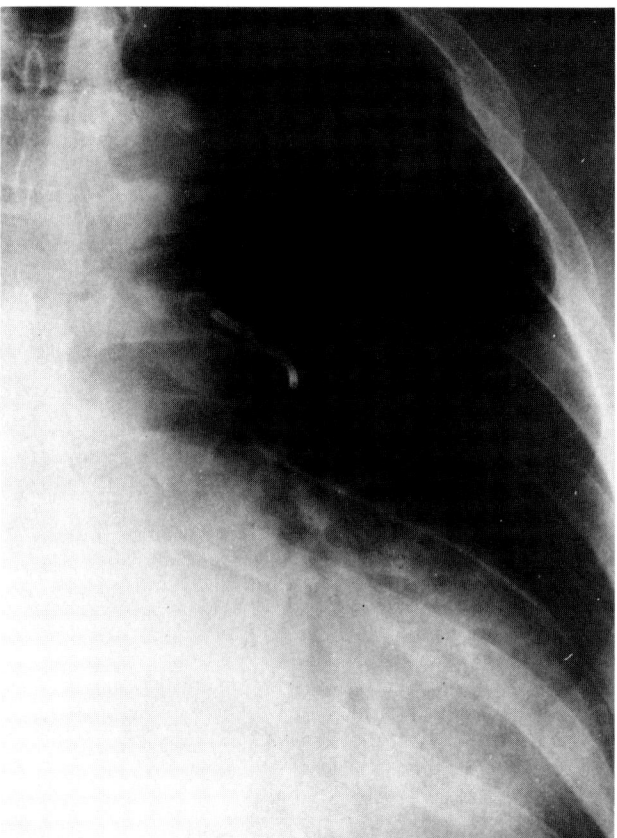

Figure 7.8 A small fragment of an angiographic catheter retrieved by means of the coaxial technique described in Fig. 7.7

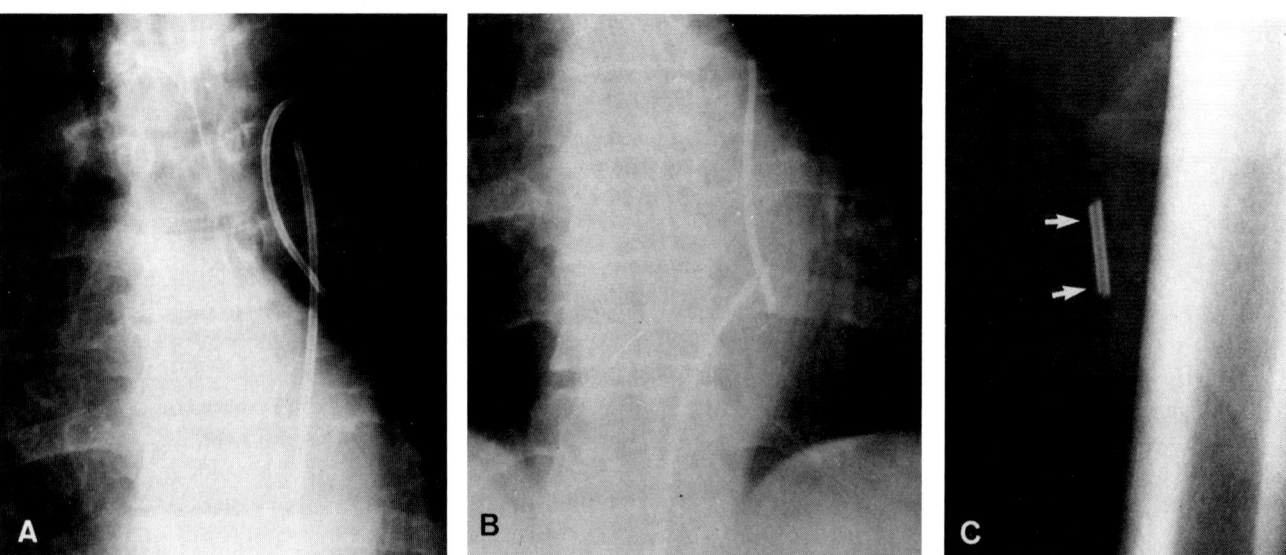

Figure 7.9 (A) Fracture of a polyurethane catheter in the thoracic aorta. (B) The fragment was removed by means of the snare technique in spite of fragmentation during the procedure which led to embolization to the left deep femoral artery, as shown in (C) (arrows).

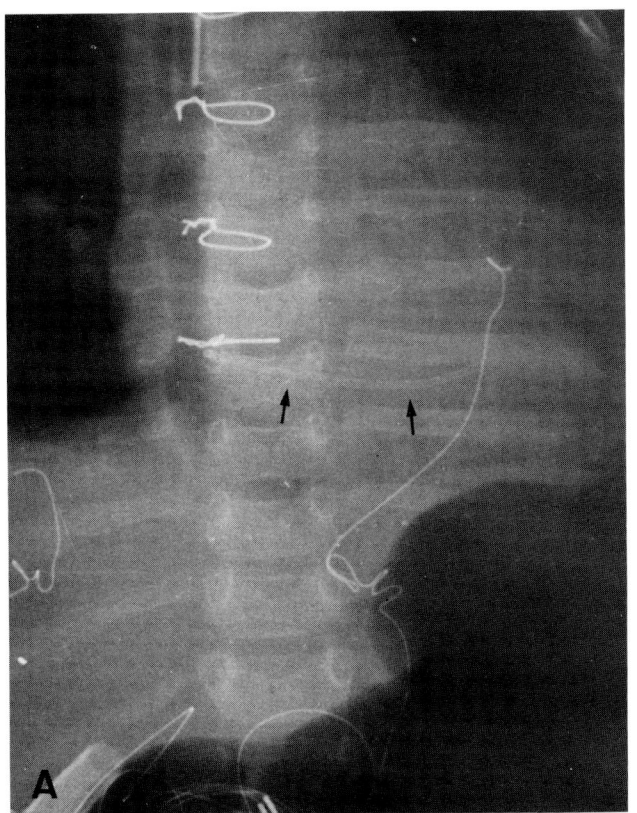
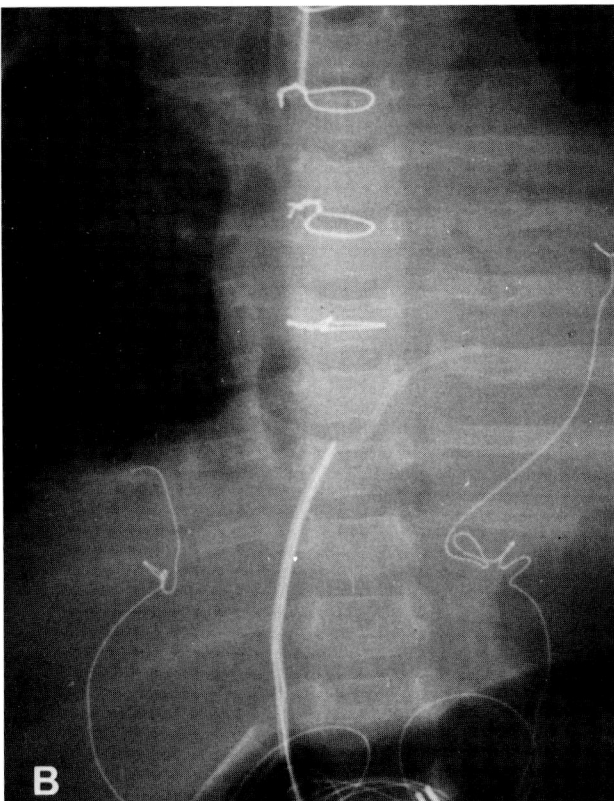
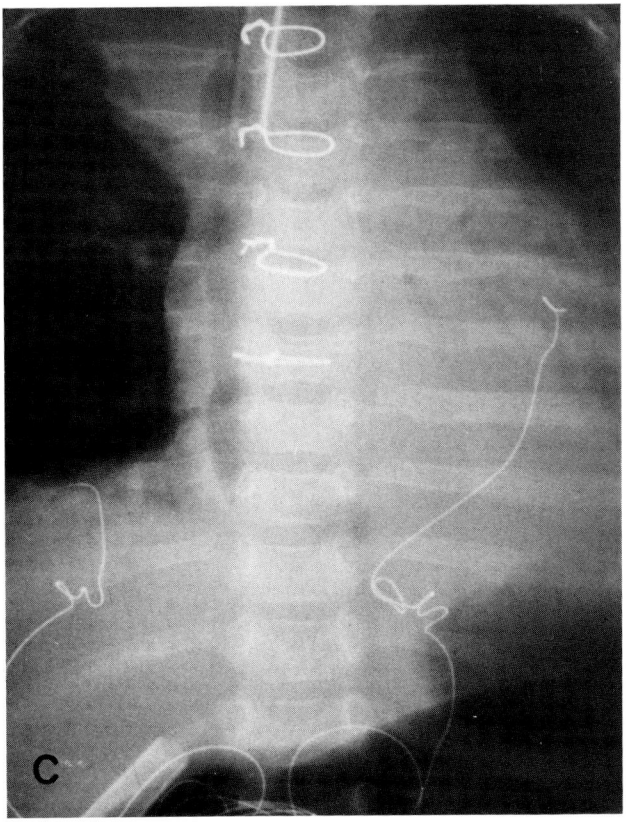

Figure 7.10 (A) A small catheter fragment inside the right side of the heart of a 5-month-old child after surgery for congenital heart disease (arrows). (B) A catheter fragment being retrieved with a loop. (C) Chest x-ray after retrieval of the foreign body.

REFERENCES

Bloomfield DA. Techniques of nonsurgical retrieval of iatrogenic foreign bodies from the heart. *Am J Cardiol* 1971;27:538–545.

Curry JL. Recovery of detached intravascular catheter or guidewire fragments: A proposed method. *AJR* 1969;105:894–896.

Dotter CT, Rosch J, Bilbao MC. Transluminal extraction of catheter and guidewire fragments from heart and great vessels: 29 collected cases. *AJR* 1971;111:467–472.

Enge I, Flatmark A. Percutaneous removal of intravascular foreign bodies by the snare technique. *Acta Radiol [Diagn] (Stockh)* 1973;14:747–752.

Fischer RG, Ferreyro R. Evaluation of current techniques for nonsurgical removal of intravascular iatrogenic foreign bodies. *AJR* 1978;120:541–548.

Fjalling M, List AR. Transvascular retrieval of an accidentally ejected tip occluder and wire. *Cardiovasc Intervent Radiol* 1982;5:34–36.

Kadir S, Athanasoulis CA. Percutaneous retrieval of intravascular foreign bodies. In *Interventional Radiology,* edited by Athanasoulis CA, Greene RE, Pfister RC, Roberson GH. Saunders, Philadelphia, 1982:379–390.

Rossi P. Hook catheter technique for transfemoral removal of foreign body from right side of the heart. *AJR* 1970;108:101–106.

Rubinstein ZJ, Morag B, Itzchak Y. Percutaneous removal of intravascular foreign bodies. *Cardiovasc Intervent Radiol* 1982;5:64–68.

Thomas J, Smith BS, Bloomfield D, et al. Nonsurgical retrieval of a broken segment of steel spring guide from the right atrium and inferior vena cava. *Circulation* 1964;30:106–108.

Uflacker R, Lima S, Melichar AC. Intravascular foreign bodies: Percutaneous retrieval. *Radiology* 1986;160:731–735.

Chapter Eight
Uroradiologic Procedures

Percutaneous Nephrostomy

João Rubião Hoefel Filho

INTRODUCTION

Endoscopic procedures were first used in urology in 1876, when Nitze devised a rigid apparatus with features which made direct viewing of the urethra and bladder possible. Since that time there has been continuous development of new apparatuses and accessory equipment as well as improvement in the technical performance of these procedures. However, until the 1950s, access to the upper urinary tract remained limited.

In 1955 Goodwin suggested the use of percutaneous drainage in hydronephrotic kidneys, stressing the good results he had obtained with this technique. In 1965 Bartley reported his experience with applying percutaneous drainage as had been proposed by Goodwin 10 years earlier. After 1967, different papers analyzed previous statistical results in 516 patients and reported the successful use of this technique in 18 new patients.

In 1976 Fernstrom and Johnson, in a paper titled "Percutaneous Pyelolithotomy," described a new technique for extracting renal stones.

In 1979 Smith and associates described their technique, using the term *endourology* for the first time. In 1981 Aiken defined techniques and procedures for accessing the renal collecting system and recommended the use of endoscopic devices for the removal of stones and tumors from the excretory system.

These reports contributed to an increased interest in the use of percutaneous nephrostomy. This procedure was defined as a technical procedure through which percutaneous access to renal collecting tubes could be obtained by means of translumbar puncture with a 18 × 15 needle coupled to a guidewire to direct a catheter into the renal pelvis or ureter.

This technique is not difficult for an experienced radiologist. Indications for its use have been extended both in less complex situations—for instance, alleviating pain from nephretic colic—and in more serious cases and emergencies, such as pyonephrosis. Accessing the kidney through percutaneous nephrostomy has created new possibilities for handling high-incidence urologic diseases, such as renal-ureteral obstruction by stones.

Percutaneous nephrostomy was first performed by inserting a trocar at the level of the posterior hemiaxillary line, close to the 12th rib, through which a fine needle and a catheter were introduced. A major disadvantage was catheter obstruction by blood clots or pus clumps. As the Seldinger technique, adapted to renal procedures, was used more frequently, it became possible to gradually increase the size of catheters introduced into the collecting system with the assistance of guidewires.

With the development of x-ray equipment and the accessory materials required for the procedure, all the difficulties of the method were gradually solved. Good-quality x-ray images obtained through the use of image intensifiers made it easier to locate the renal pelvis, allowing the radiologist to handle the renal collecting system more efficiently. This has contributed to more frequent use of antegrade pyelography and has made percutaneous nephrostomy possible.

Utilization of an adequate access route for exploring the urinary tract has allowed radiologists and urologists working in conjunction to safely and successfully extract renal stones, perform biopsies, and reestablish a normal flow of urine through fistulized or stenosed ureters. The entire range of methods and techniques necessary for the performance of this joint work has created a new specialty: interventional uroradiology.

These developments and the relative simplicity and lower morbidity rate of this procedure compared with other surgical procedures explain why percutaneous nephrostomy for both diagnostic and therapeutic purposes has become the procedure of choice for accessing the renal collecting system.

RENAL ANATOMY

Position and Location of Kidneys

The kidneys are classically located beside the vertebral spine, with their respective pelvises close to L2 on the right and a few centimeters above it on the left (Fig. 8.1).

In the embryo, at the beginning of its development, the kidney is in the small pelvis; later it migrates toward the lumbar region. Blood is supplied by the middle sacral artery, continuing through the iliac and lumbar arteries and finally reaching the proper renal arteries. For this reason, changes in kidney location and position are commonly accompanied by vascular changes.

The coronal plane divides the body, and thus the kidney, into anterior and posterior halves. During the migratory process resulting from the presence of the psoas muscle, the kidneys rotate anteriorly, with their coronal planes in a 30 to 50° angle in relation to the coronal plane of the body. As a consequence of the psoas muscle's pyramidal shape, the kidneys, besides being rotated anteriorly, have their larger axis frontally and laterally displaced, causing the upper pole to be more medially and posteriorly located than is the lower pole.

Renal Beds, Fasciae, and Renal Spaces

Four different anatomic structures envelop and demarcate the kidney and are thus of special interest to the radiologist: the renal capsule, perirenal fat with the fascia of Gerota, the posterior reflection of the peritoneum with anterior pararenal fat, and the posterior pararenal space. These structures are all anatomically well demarcated spaces; depending on their involvement and the eventual pathologic process, they produce many different radiologic images (Fig. 8.2). A perfect understanding of the configuration of these spaces and of the fascia of Gerota is essential for the correct performance of a percutaneous nephrostomy.

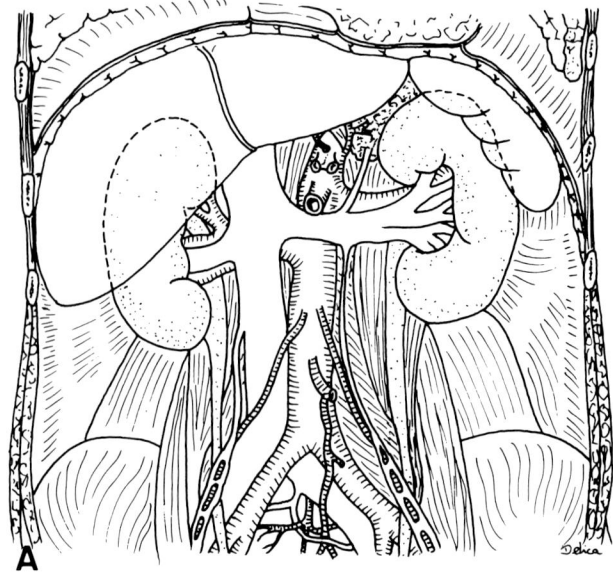

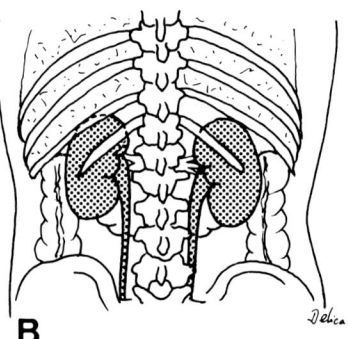

Figure 8.1 (A) Schematic drawing shows the relationhship of the kidneys to adjacent structures and large vessels in an anterior view. (B) The relationship of the kidneys to the vertebrae and lower ribs as seen from behind.

After the skin and subcutaneous cellular tissue have been penetrated, the needle should meet two points of resistance: the dorsal lumbar fascia and the true capsule formed by a fibrotic membrane which adheres firmly to the kidney and is rich in nerve endings. When conductive anesthesia instead of general anesthesia is used, extreme sensitivity of the renal capsule should be taken into account, along with the need to have anesthetization at an adequate level during its transfixion.

The fascia of Gerota is formed by fibroelastic tissue and perirenal fat. Its most anterior layer is less developed and is called Toldt's fascia. It originates next to the tunica adventitia of the great vessels and fuses itself to the posterior leaflet laterally to the kidney. The posterior fascia (fascia of Zuckerchandl) is more developed and

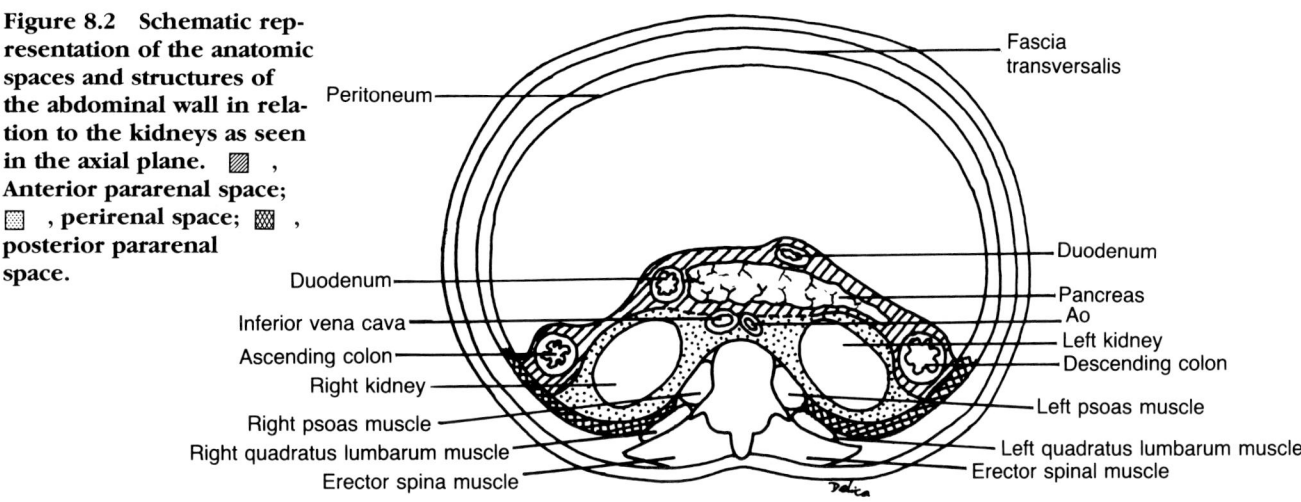

Figure 8.2 Schematic representation of the anatomic spaces and structures of the abdominal wall in relation to the kidneys as seen in the axial plane. ▨, Anterior pararenal space; ▦, perirenal space; ▩, posterior pararenal space.

originates from prevertebral tissues forming the fascia transversalis and the anterior leaflet. These structures are not fused caudally, allowing for continuity with the extraperitoneal tissues of the small pelvis but fusing themselves cranially to the infradiaphragmatic fascia (Fig. 8.3).

Technical precision resulting from anatomic detailing is significant not only in regard to the performance of percutaneous nephrostomy but also in regard to punctures for renal aspiration because of the capacity of the perirenal space to accumulate considerable volumes of blood, urine, or pus.

In such a case, without any discontinuity present in the fascia transversalis, the fluid volume will accumulate next to the kidney. As a consequence of anatomic caudal continuity, this may cause "freezing" of tissues in the small pelvis.

Anatomic relationships between the renal pelvis and

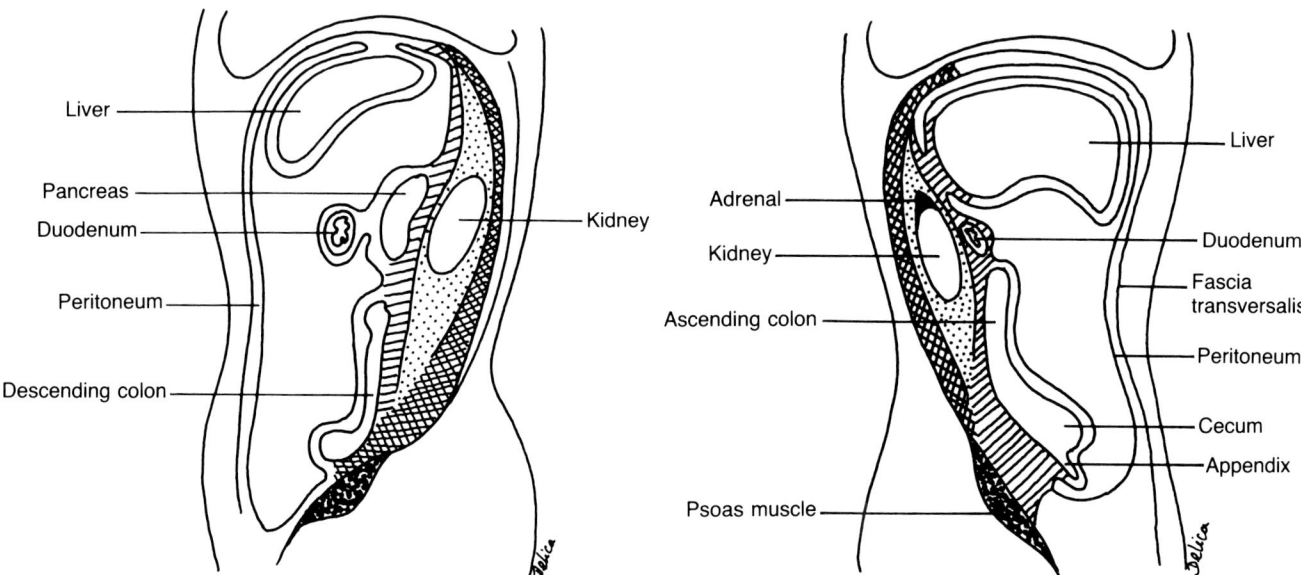

Figure 8.3 Schematic representation of the perirenal anatomic spaces in the paramedial sagittal plane, showing nonfusion of the fascia of Gerota caudally, allowing the continuity of the perirenal spaces and extraperitoneal spaces of the small pelvis, on the left (A) and the right (B). ▨, Anterior pararenal space; ▦, parirenal space; ▩, posterior pararenal space. (Modified from Meyers, 1982.)

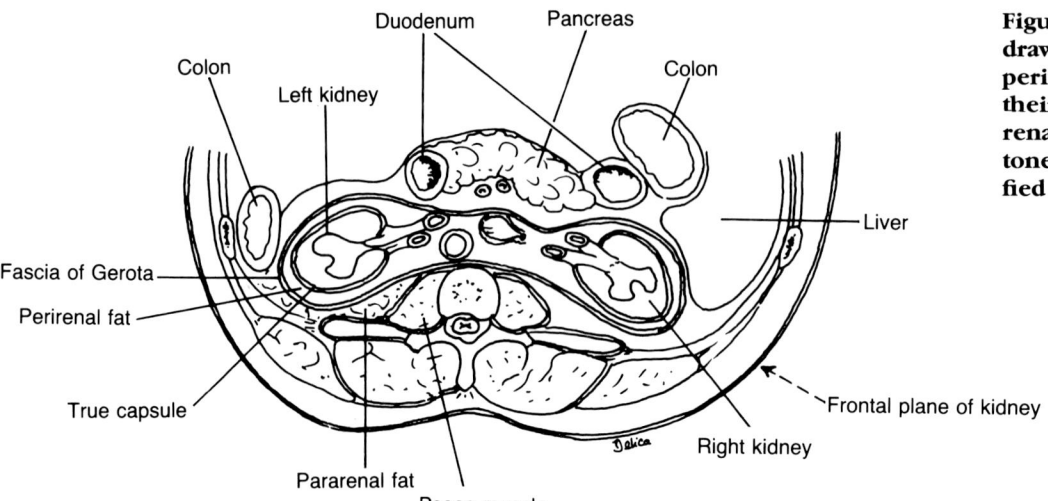

Figure 8.4 Schematic drawing of the posterior peritoneal reflections and their relation to the perirenal spaces and retroperitoneal structures. (Modified from Meyers, 1982.)

the posterior reflection of the peritoneum are significant. If the pelvis is anteriorly transfixed, blood, pus, or urine will extravasate to the peritoneal cavity, which will have to be opened anteriorly for surgical exploration (Fig. 8.4).

It is not likely for the posterior pararenal space to be involved as a consequence of the dissection of oblique muscles. However, if this occurs, an accumulation of blood, pus, or urine may cause hematomas or cellulitis on the anterior wall of the abdomen (Fig. 8.4).

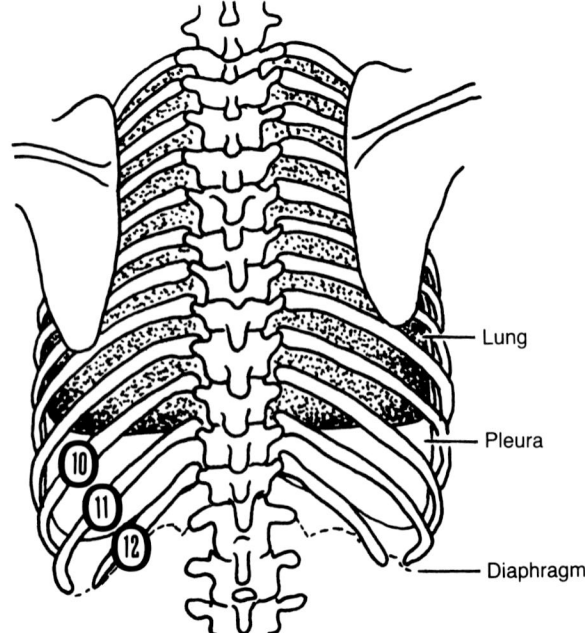

Figure 8.5 Schematic representation of the relation of the posterior pleural space to the ribs and the position of the kidneys. Compare with Fig. 8.1B.

Topographic Relationships of the Kidney

The kidney's closet relationship is with the pleura, which is separated from the upper pole by a thin fatty layer and by the diaphragm. The pleural caudal portion usually extends beyond the 12th rib in its posterior dorsal course (Fig. 8.5). In some instances the pleural posterior recess is next to the renal upper pole. This is why intercostal punctures directed toward the upper pole can cause a pneumothorax.

The right kidney is related to the 12th rib, and the left kidney to the 11th and 12th ribs. Other posterior relationships exist to muscles and ligaments: the psoas, quadratus lumborum, and transversus abdominis (Fig. 8.6).

Lateral to the right kidney, before the hepatic flexure, are the liver and the ascending colon, which is usually in the anterior lateral position, on the right parietocolic gutter. Rarely, as a consequence of anatomic variation, the colon may be in a posterolateral location and therefore may be transfixed accidentally during percutaneous nephrostomy (Fig. 8.7). The spleen and descending colon are located lateral to the left kidney. Therefore, when splenomegaly is present, special care should be taken because of an increased possibility of spleen transfixation (Fig. 8.7).

Anterior to the left kidney are the adrenal gland, spleen, stomach, pancreas, and descending colon; anterior to the right kidney are the adrenal gland, liver, colon, and duodenum (Figs. 8.6 and 8.7). Medial to both kidneys are the greater vessels and spine.

Renal Calices

The development of percutaneous nephrostomy stimulated interest in the anatomy of the kidney and the renal collecting system. The growing number of papers and dynamic findings has created a conflict with morphologic

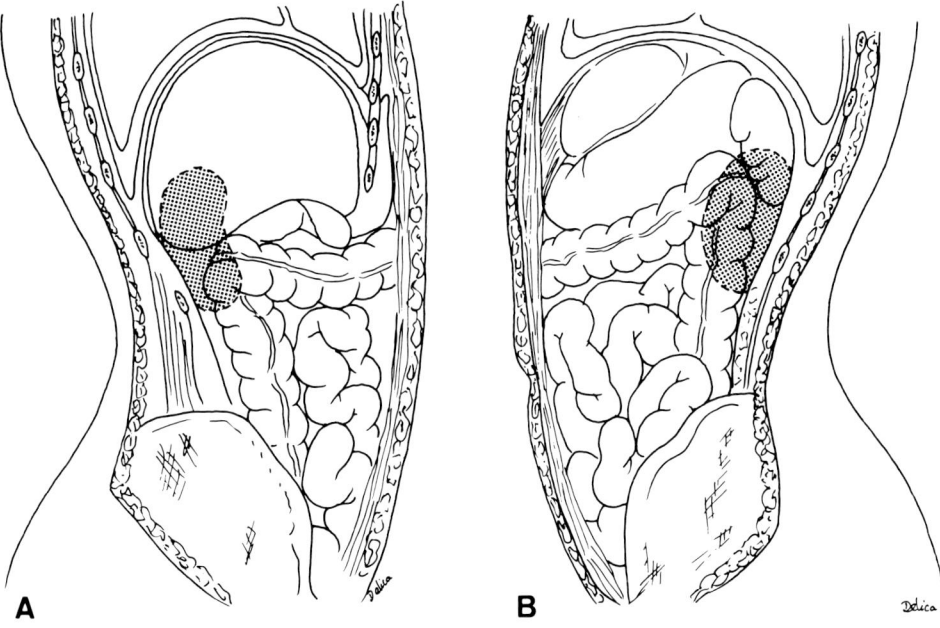

Figure 8.6 Representation in the right oblique lateral view (A) and left oblique lateral view (B) of the kidneys in relation to the neighboring structures.

descriptions based on postmortem anatomic dissection. It was soon understood that significant differences existed between these two sources. This realization not only led to dynamic and functional findings but also gradually reduced interest in classic and conventional studies.

Proper performance of percutaneous nephrostomy requires exact knowledge not only of the anatomy of the renal calices and infundibula but of caliceal space orientation in relation to the coronal planes of the kidney and the body.

Compound calices are oriented in different angles in renal poles, while in medial areas they are distributed only posteriorly and anteriorly (Fig. 8.8). In a classic study published in 1901, Brodel established the fact that the anterior calices deviate 70° to the front in relation to the coronal plane and that the posterior, longer calices deviate 20° backward in relation to the same plane. He also stated that renal convexity is greater anteriorly than posteriorly.

In opposition to Brodel's study, Hodson stated that

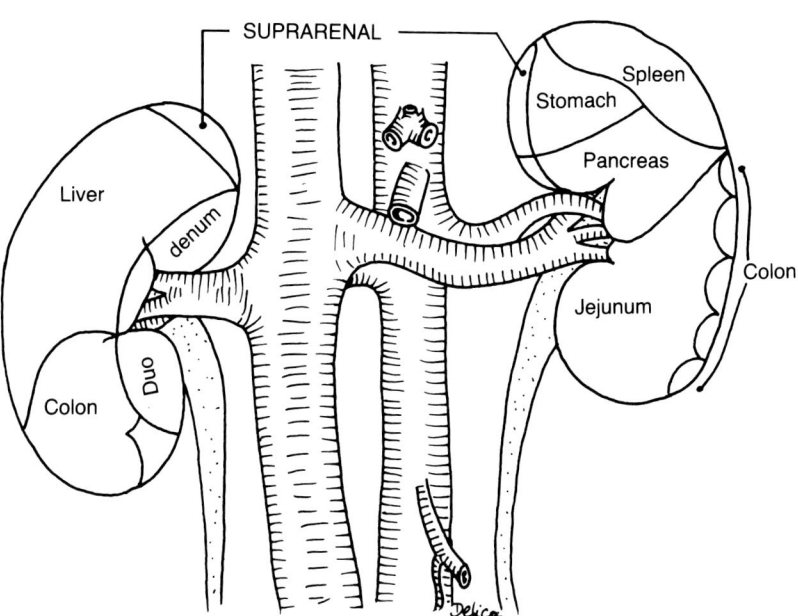

Figure 8.7 Schematic drawing shows the relation between the surface of both kidneys and the adjacent abdominal organs. The division shown here is approximate, and small individual variations may occur.

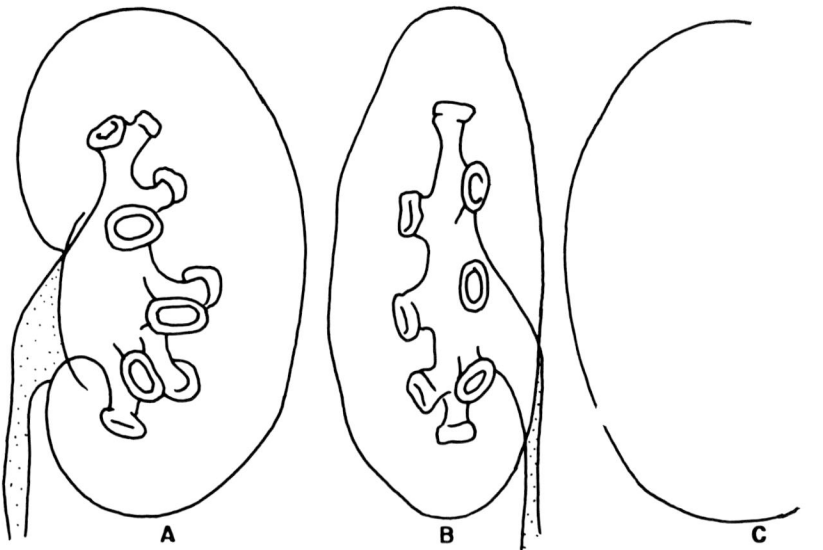

Figure 8.8 Distribution of calices in the collecting system of the kidney from different angles.
(A) anterior view; (B) oblique view; (C) posterior view. Calices in the medial zones are anteriorly and posteriorly distributed, while on the poles, orientation angles may vary. (Modified from Clayman and Castaneda-Zuniga, 1984.)

the anterior calices are longer, deviating 20° in relation to the renal frontal plane, and that posterior calices are smaller, with a 70° backward deviation (Fig. 8.9). On the basis of results obtained from dynamic studies, Kaye stated that Hodson-type kidneys are found 75 percent more frequently than are those described by Brodel.

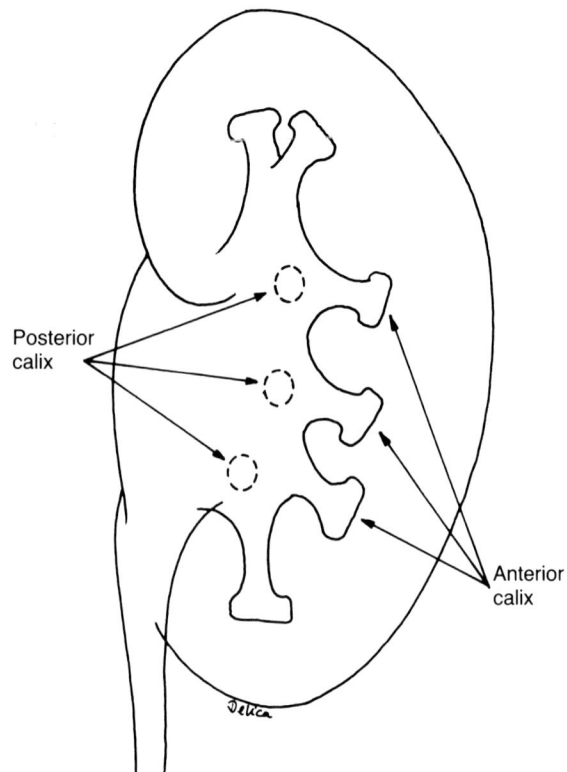

Figure 8.9 An easy rule for identifying anterolateral and posteromedial calices. The latter are seen in an axial view. (Modified from Clayman and Castaneda-Zuniga, 1984.)

By the time the kidney has completed its cranial migration, the hilum is displaced forward and the renal lateral border is displaced backward. Kaye therefore was able to identify anterior and posterior calices through intravenous urography. The anterior calices were visualized in their full extension next to the lateral border of kidney, and the posterior calices were seen as small, circular contrasted formations close to the renal pelvis.

Kaye also found out that lateral projection of the anterior calices occurs in 74 percent of patients and that superimposition to posterior calices occurs in 22 percent; in the remaining 4 percent of patients, the posterior calices are in a more lateral position (Fig. 8.9). It has traditionally been assumed that the kidney has 14 lobes, each represented by a cone of medullary tissue surrounded by a layer of cortical tissue.

One or more lobes may drain into each calix, depending on the presence or absence of lobes fused through the medullary layer of the papilla itself (Fig. 8.10). When fusion occurs next to the papilla, the tissue band separating the two lobes is formed by the cortical layer, which penetrates deeply to the innermost medullary layer (Fig. 8.11). This portion of the parenchyma, known as the column of Bertin, is richly vascularized; therefore, accidental puncture of this area can cause undesirable complications (Fig. 8.11).

The 14 classic lobes of the kidney drain into their respective calices, with a varying incidence of fusion. Fusion of lobes through the medullary layer is observed more frequently in the lower pole and through the papillae in the upper pole.

Fusion through the papilla, especially when it occurs in the upper pole, may also present as an anatomic variation in which the ostia of collecting tubules have larger diameters that facilitate intrarenal reflux. Therefore, when a technical procedure is performed with

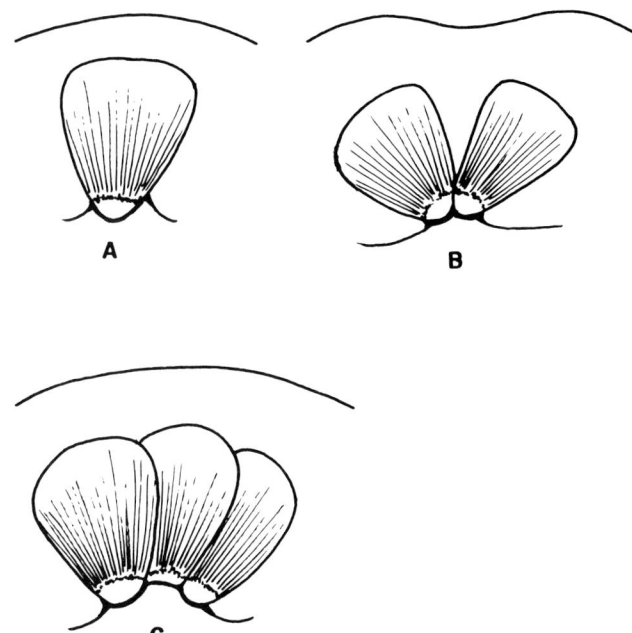

Figure 8.10 Schematic illustration of the different degrees of lobular fusion.
(A) A single lobule draining into a calix, without fusion and with a single papilla. (B) A simple pyramid with compound papilla and without lobular fusion. (C) A compound pyramid with a compound papilla.

optical devices, in which case irrigation is indispensable, diuresis should be induced until the procedure has been completed. Intravenous furosemide is generally used at 2 mL every 30 min without exceeding a maximum dose of 10 mL. An irrigation vial containing 0.9% simple saline should be maintained no more than 40 cm above the table level.

Renal Vascular Supply

Because the kidney is a richly vascularized organ, percutaneous procedures should be performed carefully and precisely, and the radiologist should have good knowledge of the spatial distribution of blood vessels. The renal arteries originate from the aorta just below the superior mesenteric artery; they are located between the renal pelvis posteriorly and the renal vein anteriorly. These arteries bifurcate close to the kidney, giving rise to the anterior and posterior branches. The anterior renal artery divides into the superior, middle, inferior, and apical segments (Fig. 8.12). The posterior renal artery irrigates the posterior area, which corresponds to the superior and middle segments (Fig. 8.13).

Arterial irrigation of the renal posterior portion is supplied by the first branch of the renal artery, which follows the posterior pelvis perpendicularly to the infundibula of the renal calices, describing an archlike path (Fig. 8.14). Arterial injury can result from mishandling of the nephroscope used to extract stones from the upper calices.

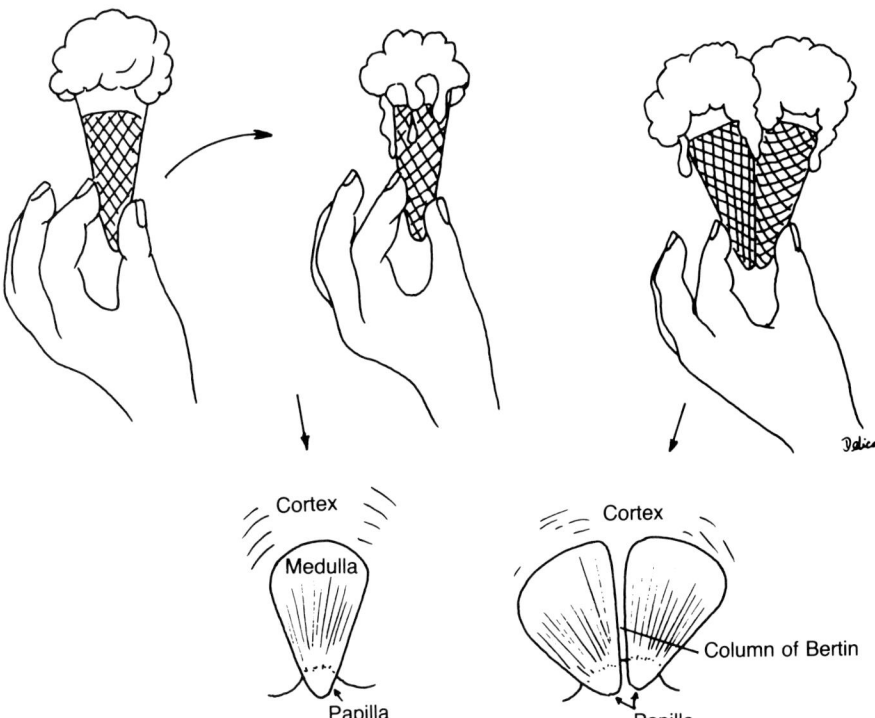

Figure 8.11 The cone concept according to Kaye.
The ice cream cone is related to the medulla, the scoop to the renal cortex, and the cone tip to the papilla. Melted ice cream covers the lateral portions of the cone (medulla), except for the tip (papilla). A large portion of the renal cortex surrounds the medulla, except for the papilla. (Modified from Clayman and Castaneda-Zuniga, 1984.)

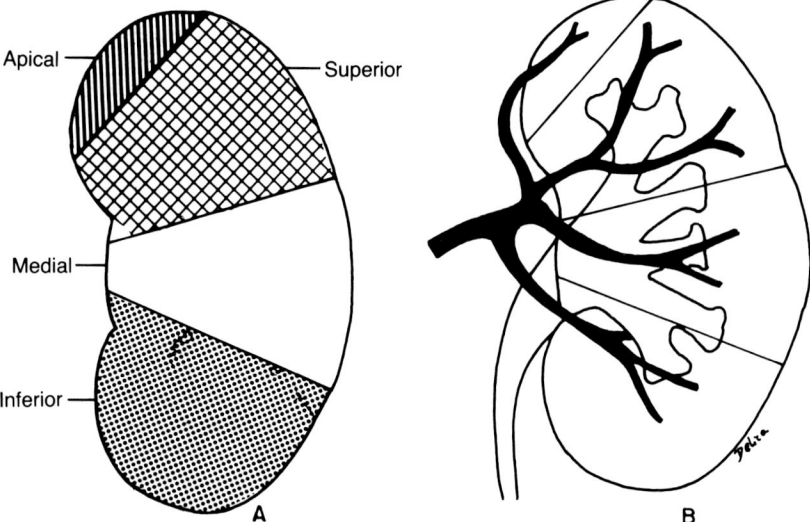

Figure 8.12 Schematic illustration of the posterior renal artery.
(A) Segmental branches; (B) arterial branches.

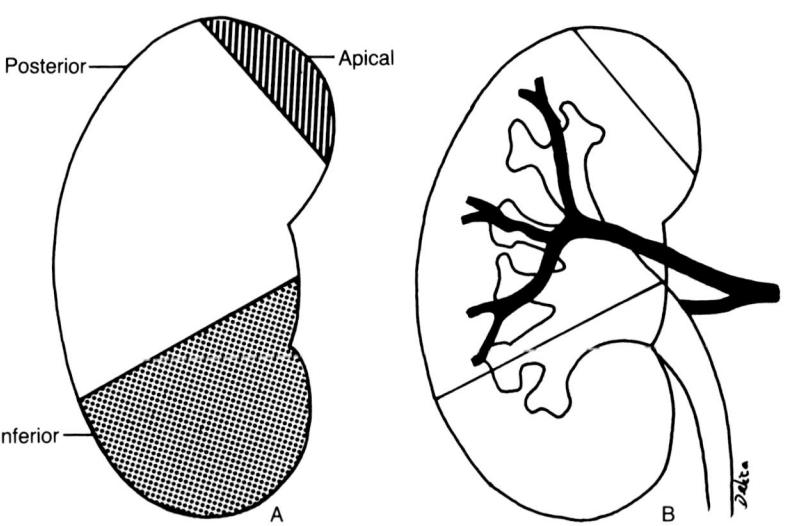

Figure 8.13 Schematic drawing of the distribution of the posterior renal artery.
(A) Segmental branches; (B) arterial branches.

At the junction of the kidney's anterior and posterior halves is Brödel's avascular plane (Figs. 8.14 and 8.15). This plane is not represented on the external renal surface. It is located 1 to 2 cm posterior to the kidney's lateral margin and is the plane one attempts to reach when performing a puncture in order to reduce the chances of bleeding. This plane should not be mistaken for Brödel's white line, which is richly vascularized and corresponds to the fusion of the anterior and posterior cortical layers (Fig. 8.16).

The calix chosen for puncture should be one of the most posteriorly located ones, since this is the usual location of renal stones. This choice will facilitate catheterization of the ureter and reduce the chances of puncturing the pleura, which lies below the 12th rib (Fig. 8.17). If the physician reaches Brödel's avascular plane or moves along its space, the puncture needle can be kept away from the posterior segmental artery (Fig. 8.18).

Because there is no collateral circulation between the renal segments, injury to any artery will cause the whole segment to become ischemic.

TECHNICAL PROCEDURE

General Considerations

The abandonment of the use of the trocar and the application of the Seldinger technique in percutaneous handling of the kidney made it possible to dilate the

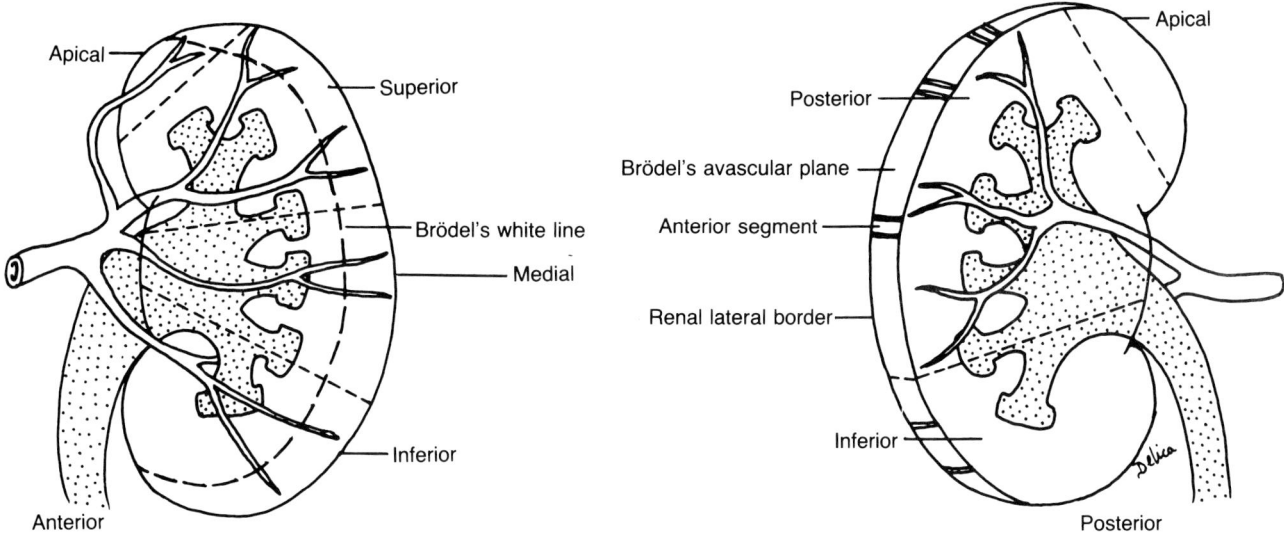

Figure 8.14 Arterial supply to the kidney, with five segmental branches to the anterior and posterior faces. Note the lateral and posterior faces supplied by anterior branches. (Modified from Clayman and Castaneda-Zuniga, 1984.)

nephrostomy path and to use catheters with sizes appropriate for the objectives to be attained. This made it possible to remove renal stones, dilate stenoses of the ureter, and drain pyonephrosis.

Despite the variety of techniques that have been proposed for performing percutaneous nephrostomy and the use of different materials and equipment, all these techniques are based on an adaptation of the Seldinger technique to urologic procedures. This modification consists basically of the introducion of a guidewire through a needle into the collecting system.

Percutaneous access to the kidney involves two stages: creating a percutaneous tract and introducing the nephroscope for visualization of the collecting system.

The ideal nephrocutaneous tract should be as shallow as possible, rectilinear, and just long enough to introduce the nephroscope. Access to the kidney is facilitated by the use of x-ray or ultrasonic devices.

Patients should routinely be admitted 24 h before the procedure and should receive conventional clinical examination and radiologic study as well as additional tests, including prothrombin time (PT), partial throm-

Figure 8.15 (A) Medial posterior calices (arrows). (B) Schematic drawing shows the relation of the posteromedial calices to Brödel's line and the coronal plane of the body. The arrow shows the access path to the collecting system.

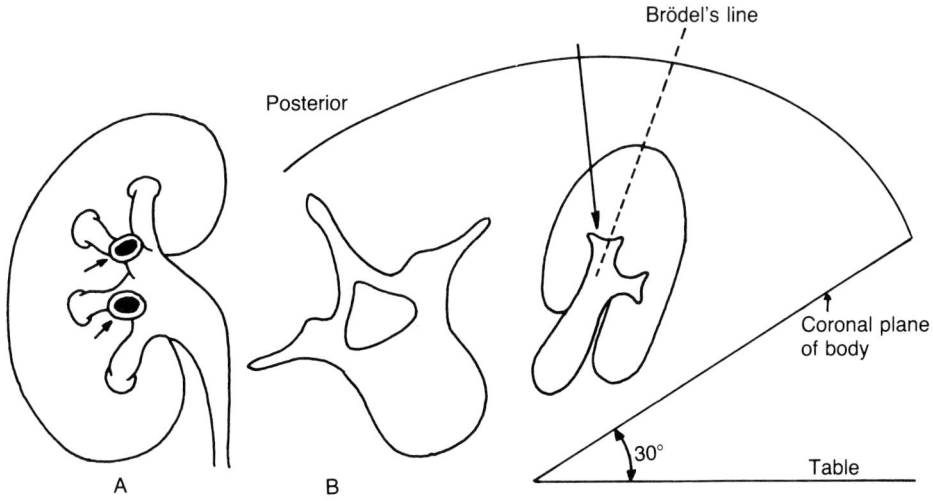

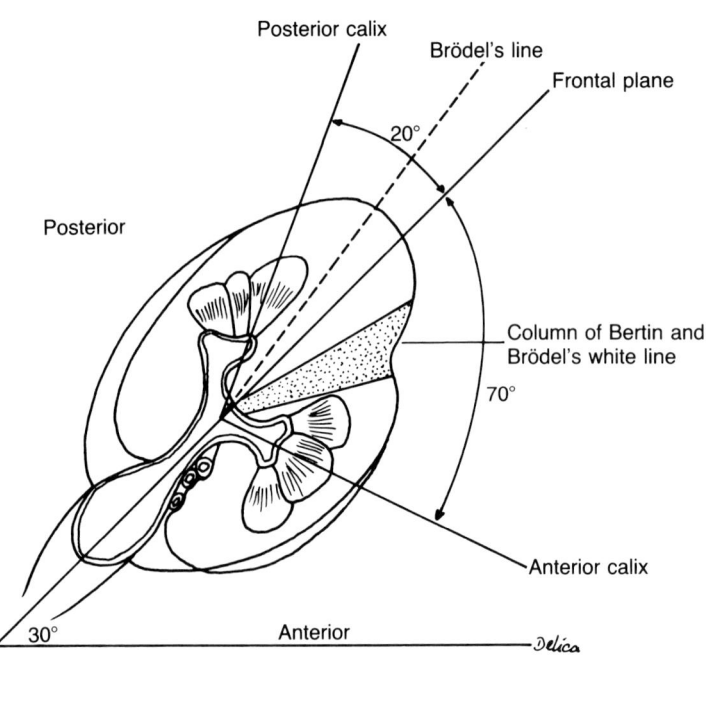

Figure 8.16 View from above (axial plane) of the left kidney showing the anterior projection of the anterior calices 70° in relation to the frontal plane and the posterior projection 20° in relation to the frontal plane. (Modified from Clayman and Castaneda-Zuniga, 1984.)

Figure 8.17 Puncture of the collecting system in the left kidney, with 25 to 30° elevation on the involved side to facilitate vertical puncture of the posterior calix. (Modified from Clayman and Castaneda-Zuniga, 1984.)

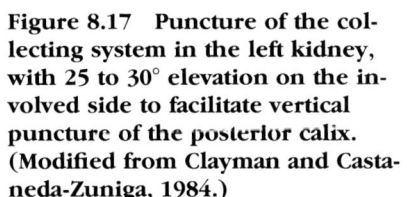

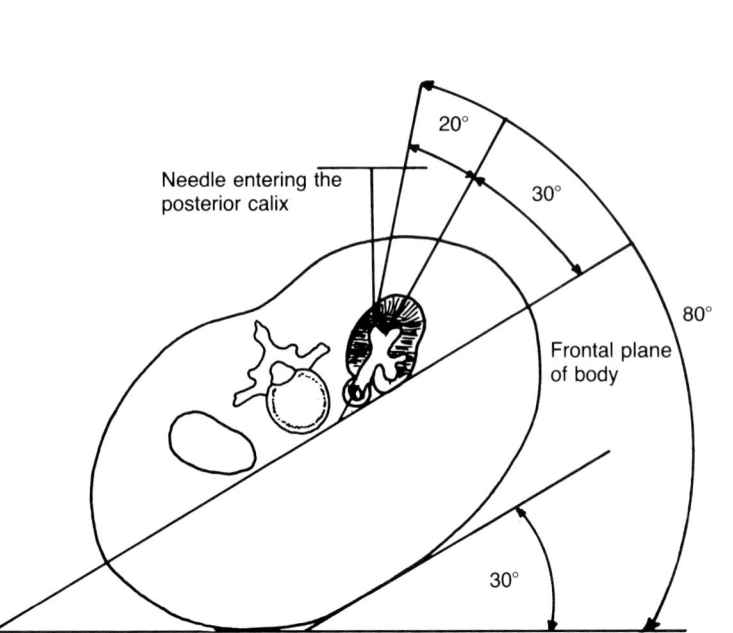

Figure 8.18 Oblique pronation with a 30° angle to the table.
The needle enters vertically. If the patient is not placed in an oblique position, the inclination of the needle should be 30° in relation to the kidney's frontal plane and 50° in relation to the body's frontal plane. (Adapted from Clayman and Castaneda-Zuniga, 1984.)

boplastin time (PTT), and a urine sample with culture.

The blood tests suggested here are of the utmost importance. As major causes of renal and perirenal hemorrhage, blood dyscrasias represent a contraindication to this procedure.

As part of the routine, a cleansing enema should be performed to eliminate residues and gases, which may cause colonic distension, increasing the risk of bowel perforation. Fasting should be prescribed for at least 6 h before the procedure. This will prevent the occurrence of nausea and vomiting, with all the consequent inconveniences and hazards.

The patient should be put under sedation with either meperidine (1.5 mg/kg body weight) or fentanyl chlorhydrate (0.02 to 0.05 mg/kg body weight), administered intravenously.

Regardless of whether signs or symptoms of urinary infection are present, antibiotics should be given before the procedure. Intravenous cefoxitin (1 g every 8 h) and intramuscular gentamycin (Garamycin) (80 mg) have been shown to be effective. In the vast majority of cases, percutaneous nephrostomy can be performed under local anesthesia, always in the presence of an anesthesiologist. During the procedure and at the radiologist's and anesthesiologist's discretion, additional doses of meperidine, fentanyl chlorhydrate, or equivalent drugs may be given intravenously. The use of diazepam should be restricted to agitated or anxious patients.

The site of choice for a percutaneous nephrostomy is the posterior hemiaxillary line, below the 12th rib (Fig. 8.18). Infiltration of skin, subcutaneous cell tissue, and deep muscle planes should be done with a 2% lidocaine solution without a vasoconstricting agent, never exceeding a volume above 4 mL/kg body weight.

After infiltration of the skin and subcutaneous cell tissue, a small incision of about 0.5 cm is made on the skin, with the tissues being exposed with the help of a Kocher clamp. A fine 15-cm-long needle, e.g., a Chiba needle, is then introduced to achieve infiltration of the subcutaneous cell tissue and the subsequent muscle planes until the extremely innervated, and consequently sensitive, renal capsule is reached (Fig. 8.19).

After the collecting system has been punctured, an anesthetic should be injected. Bupivacaine hydrochlorate is used for this purpose in a 0.25% solution, with a total volume up to 20 mL. For extremely sensitive patients and in procedures involving ureteral dilation and the removal of small residual fragments, general anesthesia is the method of choice.

Finally, although percutaneous nephrostomy is characterized as a simple procedure, it still must be performed in an adequate surgical environment. ECG monitoring and measurement of the patient's blood pressure and body temperature are also recommended.

Opacifying the Collecting System

Clear visualization of the collecting system is indispensable in radiologic manipulation. Any of the techniques described below can be used for this purpose. In patients whose renal function has been preserved, opacity of the collecting system is obtained 10 min after the intravenous injection of 40 to 80 mL of iodized contrast.

In cases of loss of renal function or obstruction of the collecting system and when greater distension of the collecting system is necessary, opacity of the collecting system can be achieved by means of posterior puncture of the renal pelvis with a fine, long needle such as a

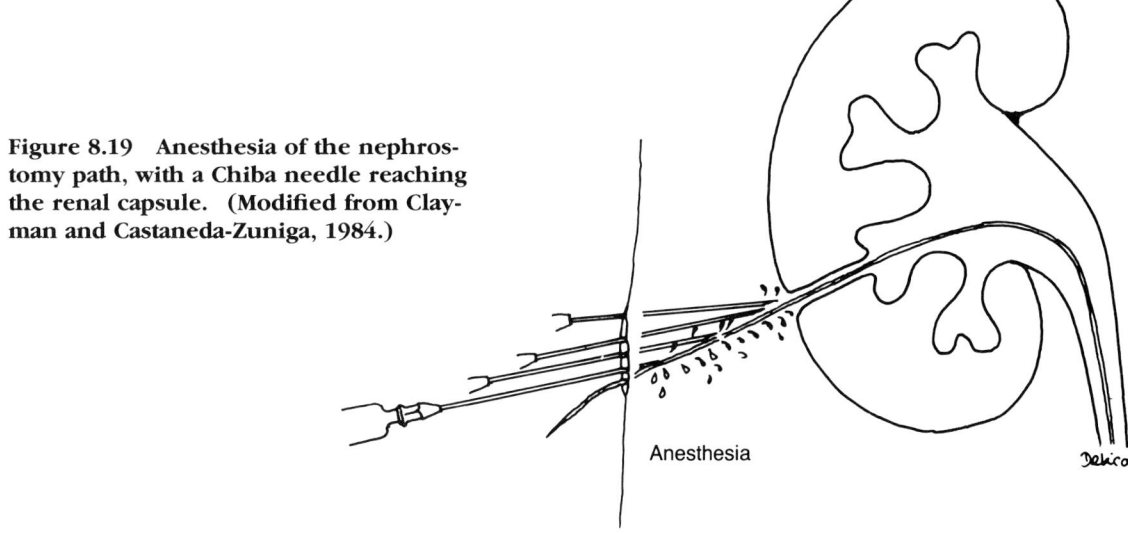

Figure 8.19 Anesthesia of the nephrostomy path, with a Chiba needle reaching the renal capsule. (Modified from Clayman and Castaneda-Zuniga, 1984.)

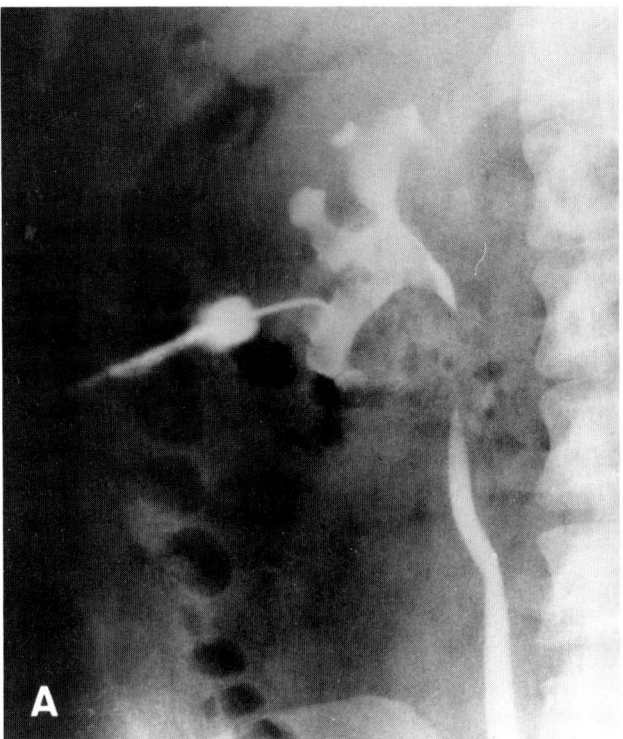
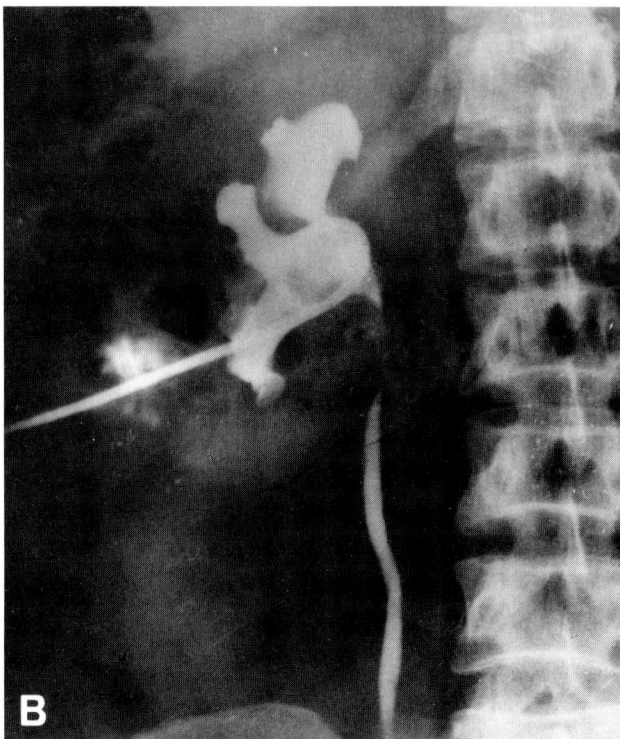

Figure 8.20 (A) Antegrade pyelography of the right kidney done with direct puncture of the collecting system in the vertical position, performed on the patient's dorsum with the patient in a prone position. Puncture was performed with a 22-gauge Chiba needle. Note the intrapelvic filling defect caused by a low-density calculus. (B) Nephrostomy in the same patient done by puncture of the posterior axillary line and penetration into the infundibulum of the lower caliceal group. Note the catheter curving around a pelvic stone.

Chiba needle (Fig. 8.20). It is recommended that the puncture be performed next to L1 and L2, about 8 cm lateral to the midline, perpendicularly, with the needle maintained in position till the end of the procedure; this will prevent perirenal extravasation.

In patients with atrophic kidneys or with a poorly distensible collecting system, the introduction of the needle into the collecting system should be guided by ultrasound. When nephrolithotripsy is indicated, the collecting system can be opacified through a catheter introduced into the ureter by means of cystoscopy.

Renal Puncture

In most patients the reference point for renal puncture is the middle portion of the infundibulum, which lies between the fornix and the neck of the calix, or the fornix itself. This procedure reduces the risk of vascular injury but increases the risk of papillary injury.

The renal pelvis should not be punctured or dilated, since after its dilation lateral displacement of catheters or nephroscope sheaths may occur. Such displacement increases the risk of formation of perirenal collections (Fig. 8.21).

The possibility of renal vascular injury is increased in transpelvic medial puncture. It is important not to advance the needle beyond the renal pelvis in order to prevent injuries to the pleural and peritoneal cavities.

The patient can be placed in a prone position (Fig. 8.22) or with a 30° inclination of the coronal plane in relation to the plane of the table (Fig. 8.23). This can be achieved by placing one or more cushions (Fig. 8.24) under the patient's abdomen. This inclined position will make the x-ray beam parallel to the plane in which the posterior calices are oriented. This is important, as most stones are located in this area. The needle is oriented parallel to the x-ray beam and, consequently, parallel to the plane of orientation of the posterior calices.

The problem here is the radiation level to which the operator is exposed. Two solutions have been proposed: using a modified Amplatz needle (Fig. 8.25) and placing the patient in a prone position without any inclination. The second option requires that the needle be introduced from the posterior hemiaxillary line at a 30° angle anteriorly.

A diamond-tip needle is usually used, generally without a bevel tip; this makes it possible for the needle to follow a practically straight-line path between the skin

Figure 8.21 Direct puncture of the renal pelvis.
Direct poterior puncture may lead to the posterior segmental artery. If the puncture goes beyond the anterior wall, the anterior arteries may be injured. The lower margin of the ribs should be avoided to prevent injury to the vascular nevous bundle. (Modified from Clayman and Castaneda-Zuniga, 1984.)

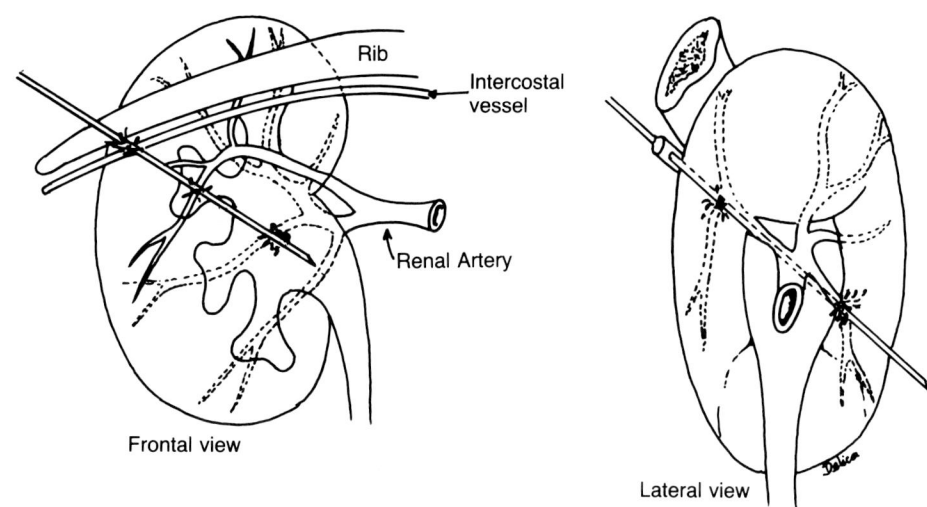

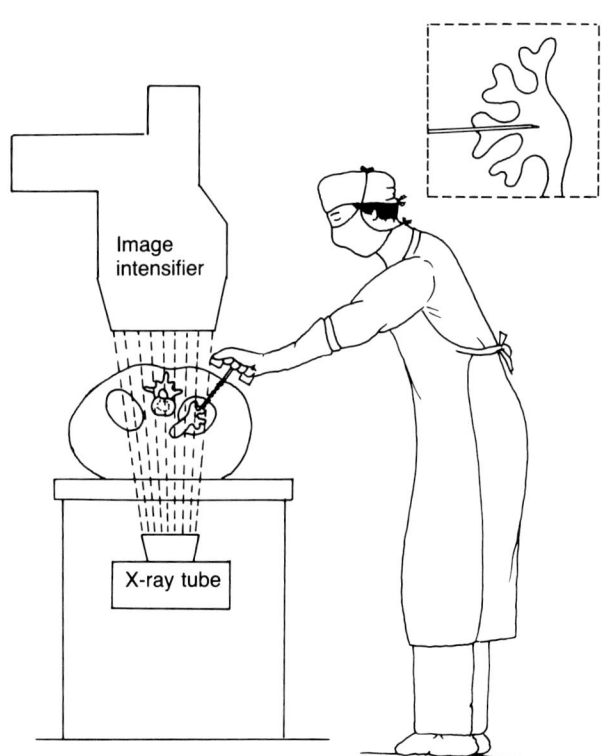

Figure 8.22 Patient being punctured in pronation.
Note needle angulation and hand position with regard to the central beam. (Modified from Clayman and Castaneda-Zuniga, 1984.)

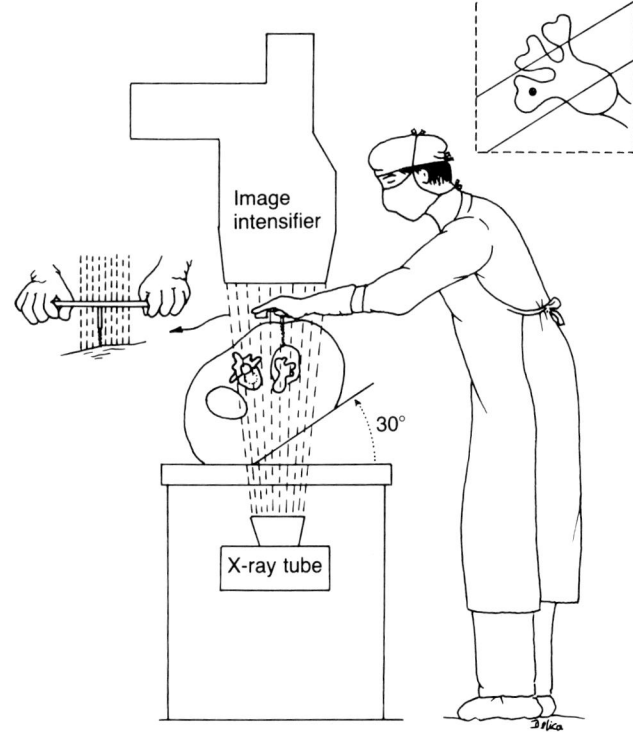

Figure 8.23 A patient receiving a puncture in pronation with oblique inclination.
The needle enters vertically, parallel to the main beam. Note the use of an Amplatz needle support to keep the operator's hand from being on the main beam path under continuous fluoroscopic view. (Modified from Clayman and Castaneda-Zuniga, 1984.)

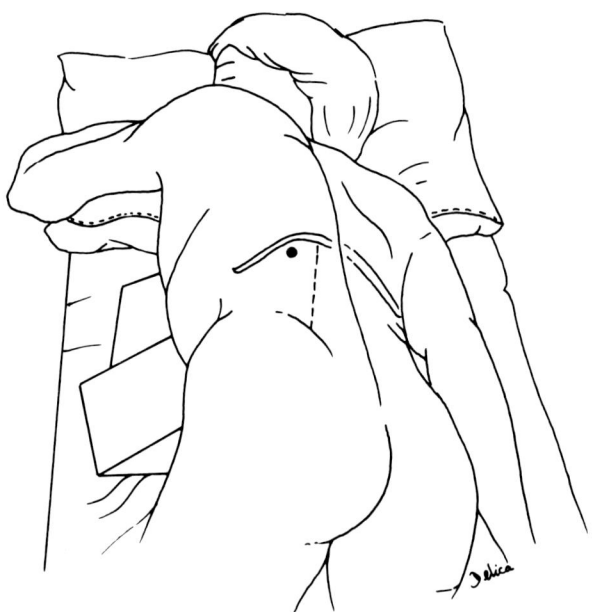

Figure 8.24 Patient's position with 30° inclination, with cushions under the abdomen.

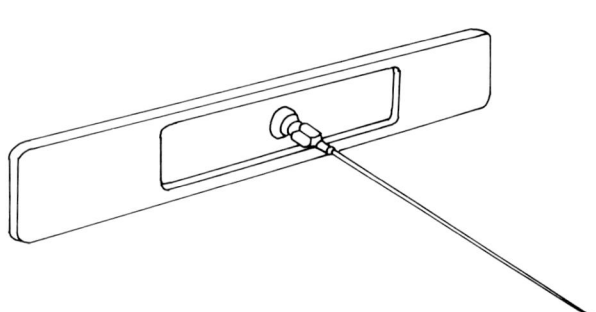

Figure 8.25 Detailed drawing of an Amplatz needle support. (Modified from Clayman and Castaneda-Zuniga, 1984.)

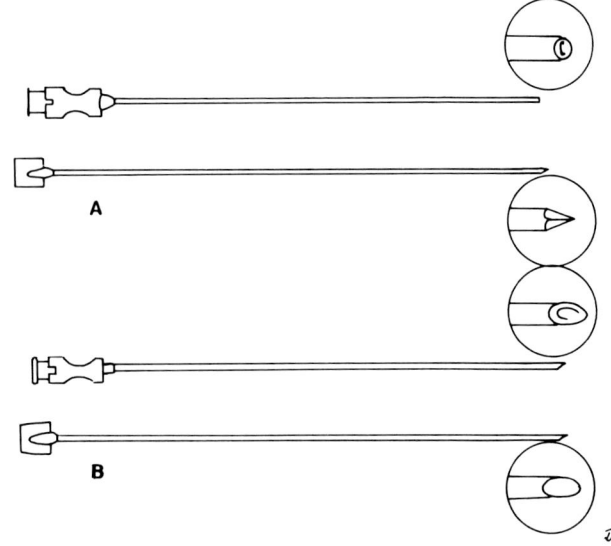

Figure 8.26 Needles for puncture in nephrostomy.
(A) Diamond-tip needle without bevel; (B) beveled needle. (Modified from Clayman and Castaneda-Zuniga, 1984.)

and the urinary tract. Conversely, conventional beveled needles may deviate from the desired path when going through a muscle or fat tissue plane (Fig. 8.26).

When a puncture below the 12th rib is indicated, the patient should hold the breath during inspiration. At this moment the needle should be introduced. In the intercostal approach, the puncture should be performed during expiration in order to reduce the incidence of pleural injuries.

Evidence that the collecting system has been reached is provided when urine, contrast, or both appear in the needle. Opacity of the system, which is caused by contrast injection or by CO_2 insufflated through the same needle can also provide such evidence (Fig. 8.27). Upon confirmation, a Teflon J-guidewire (0.035 or 0.038 in.) should be introduced and, under fluoroscopy, be directed toward the ureter. Progressive dilation of the nephrostomy track follows, with No. 7, 8, and 9 French dilators utilized sequentially.

When an anterior calix is punctured, the guidewire should reach the pelvis. A major difficulty during this

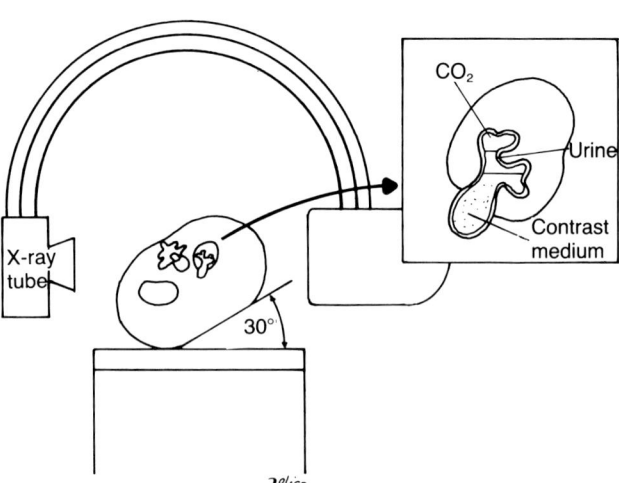

Figure 8.27 Opacification of the renal collecting system with the patient in pronation and with a 30° inclination.
Contrast settles on the bottom; the entry calix is not opacified. Urine stays at the intermediate level. If CO_2 is injected, there is adequate opacification of the entry calix with gas. (Modified from Clayman and Castaneda-Zuniga, 1984.)

Figure 8.28 Technique used for entering the ureter with a Cobra catheter or torque guidewire (Lunderquist).

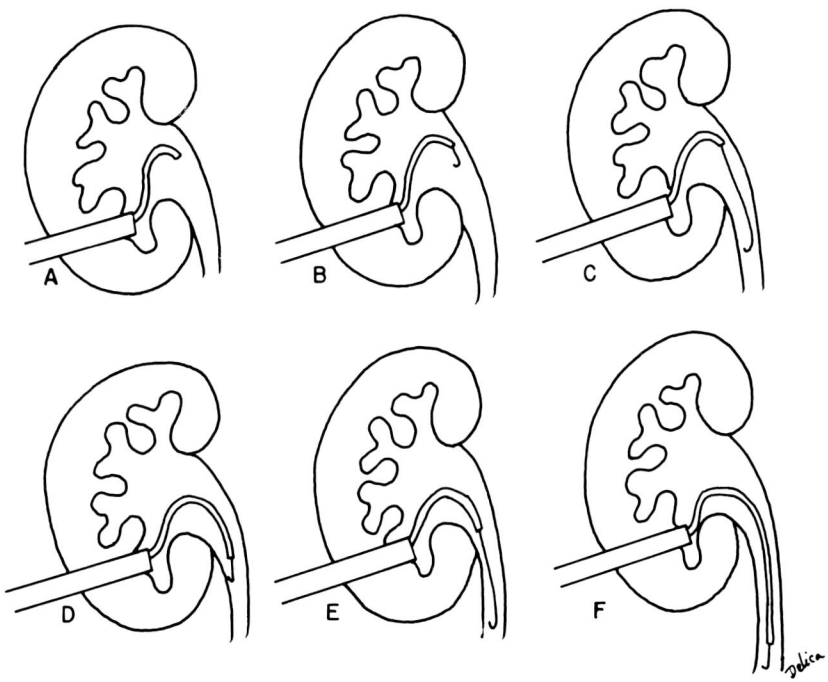

maneuver is bypassing of the angle formed by the calix and the pelvis. This can be overcome by utilizing a Lunderquist-type torque guidewire with a shapable tip.

If it is difficult to advance the guidewire to the ureter, a Cobra-type model C2 visceral catheter or a right coronary catheter should be used, because both types have high torque and "memory." Using either of these catheters plus a Lunderquist-type guidewire, most anatomic accidents within the collecting systems can be prevented and the guidewire, inserted through the pelvis, can complete its course to the urinary bladder (Figs. 8.28 and 8.29).

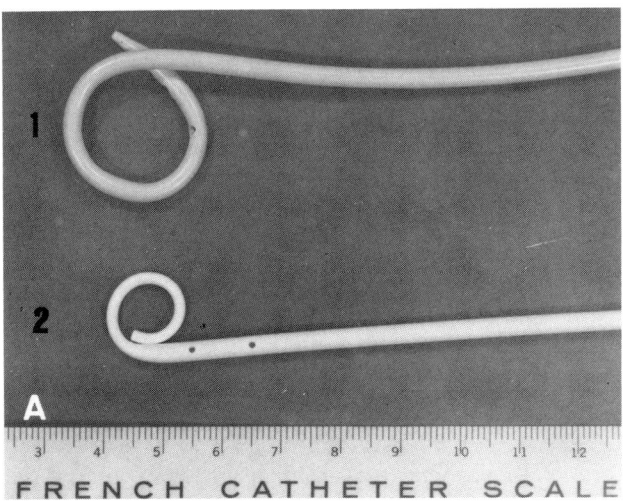
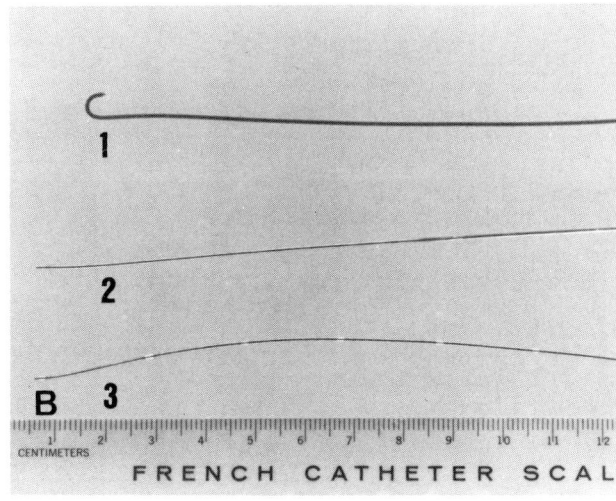

Figure 8.29 Catheters and guidewires used for nephrostomy and to gain access to the collecting system of the kidney.
(A) A Cope-type No. 10 French nephrostomy catheter (1). A pigtail No. 10 French catheter for nephrostomy (2). (B) A 1.5-mm J-guidewire for catheterization of the collecting system (1). A Lunderquist-type catheter exchange guidewire, also used to change catheters in the collecting system and tortuous ureters (2). A Lunderquist torque guidewire with a shapable tip for catheterization of the collecting system and tortuous ureters (3).

Diagnostic Pyelography

Pyelography is one of the methods that have been proposed for opacifying the collecting system. With this technique, contrast is injected through the excretory route and thus is not eliminated by the kidney, as occurs in intravenous urography.

Pyelography is done retrogradely when the ureter is catheterized and the contrast is injected into it. It is done antegradely when performed by puncture or by the placement of a catheter in the renal pelvis for contrast injection. Pyelography makes it possible to map the renal collecting system by illustrating its anatomic variations and thus to identify diseases that are specific to the excretory system.

The volume of contrast should be proportional to the size of the pelvis and calices to avoid intrarenal reflux. If reflux occurs, germs and contrast material may penetrate into the collecting tubes and the renal interstitium may be involved. As a consequence, bacteremia becomes practically unavoidable, frequently followed by bacteremic shock.

The contrast material should be diluted from 30 to 50% so that outline drawings of the pyelocaliceal cavities and ureter can be obtained. This allows the identification of stones or tumors that otherwise could be interpreted as filling defects in excretory system on x-ray films.

By using this technique and paying attention to details indispensable for a successful outcome, it is possible to establish the location, amplitude, and extension of renoureteral obstructions and gather information that will help in selecting the right type of therapy. Locating urinary fistulas and determining their output helps one determine the indication or contraindication for any specific form of percutaneous therapy. In patients with pyonephrosis, data obtained from pyelography are usually inconclusive.

Pus in the collecting system will restrict the use of contrast medium to a minimum volume, as in these patients intrarenal reflux and the resulting bacteremia are undesirable and serious side effects. Outline drawing of the cavities is sufficient for guiding both puncture and catheter placement.

Specific Procedures

Pyonephrosis

Pyonephrosis is characterized by the presence of purulent urine in the renal collecting system. This is an extremely serious clinical condition, which requires emergency therapeutic measures because of the possibility of bacteremia and subsequent bacteremic shock. The highest incidence of pyonephrosis occurs in patients with obstruction from renal and ureteral stones (Fig. 8.30).

Patients who have been clinically and radiologically diagnosed as having nephretic colic are usually controlled by comparing hemograms and axillary temperature values that are measured successively and at regular intervals. When signs of infection are detected, the patient is immediately admitted to the hospital with an indication for surgery for removal of stones and decompression of the urinary system. Sometimes the clinical condition progresses rapidly to pyonephrosis, increasing the surgical morbidity and mortality rates.

The use of percutaneous nephrostomy in patients who present with a clinical, laboratory, and radiologic condition suggestive of pyonephrosis has created new perspectives in the prognosis of these patients. Percutaneous drainage has prevented nephrectomy and in most cases has allowed a recovery of renal function. Any procedure should, however, be performed with great care, strictly observing all the technical details, which may vary from patient to patient (Fig. 8.31). The reduced volume of contrast that can be used in pyelography usually is not sufficient to establish the etiology of pyonephrosis precisely. Translumbar lateral puncture, as described earlier, permits the introduction of a larger catheter into the renal pelvis; this facilitates drainage of the usually very thick material that is collected.

Notwithstanding the use of antibiotics, most patients present with signs of bacteremia which vary according to each case, with an unavoidable risk of septic shock. The most probable cause of septic shock is communication between the infected collecting system and the richly vascularized renal parenchyma. After needle puncture of the collecting system and placement of a guidewire, angiographic dilators are introduced. As the collecting system is usually hypertensive, purulent urine will reach the skin surface through the track created by the guidewire. When this occurs, a portion of the material contaminated by contact with the renal parenchyma enters the bloodstream, making it possible for bacteremia to develop.

After the catheter has been introduced and fixed onto the skin, diuresis should be induced by means of adequate medication. If the obstruction is recent and renal function has been maintained, the response will be satisfactory. This will in turn help restore the collecting system to a normal condition (Fig. 8.32).

Usually 48 h after the procedure, urine drained through the catheter will no longer be purulent, and the kidney will no longer need diuretic stimulation. On the third day, a new pyelogram should be performed to establish a final diagnosis and direct the course of management, which usually consists of open surgery or a percutaneous procedure.

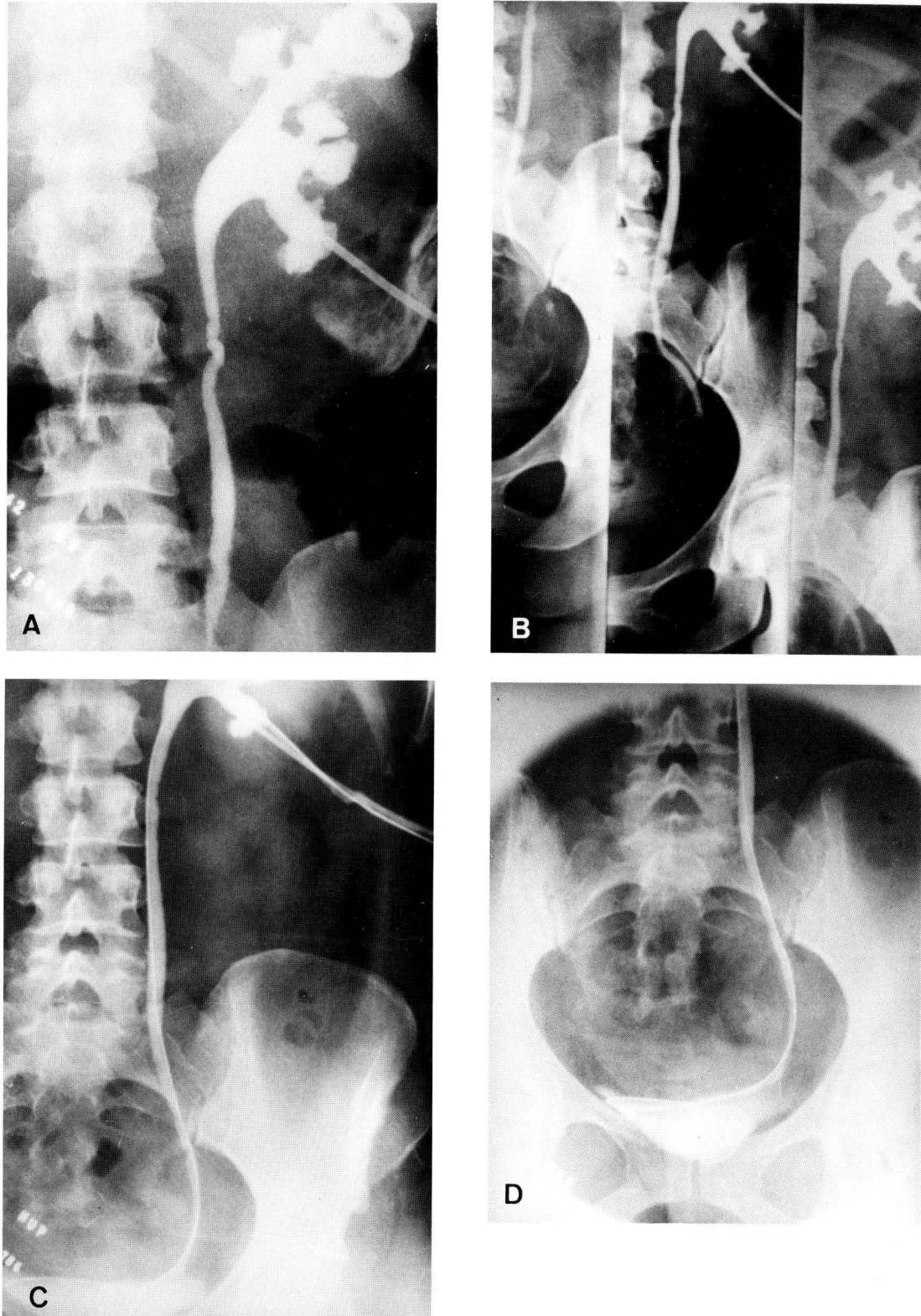

Figure 8.30 A patient with pyonephrosis resulting from ureteral obstruction by a stone.
(A) Relief nephrostomy for pyonephrosis. Note the irregular aspect of the dilated collecting cavities and the cavity on the upper pole of the left kidney. (B) Control pyelography 1 week after nephrostomy, with resolution of the inflammatory process. The ureter remains obstructed by a stone. There was spontaneous migration of the stone away from the ureteral stenosis. (C,D) Control pyelography after ureter dilation with No. 6, 7, and 8 French catheters for 3 weeks, showing resolution of stenosis just before removal of the catheters.

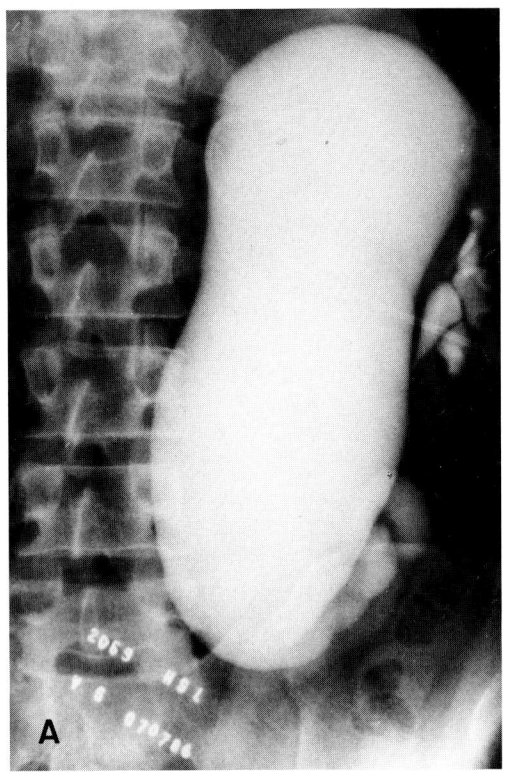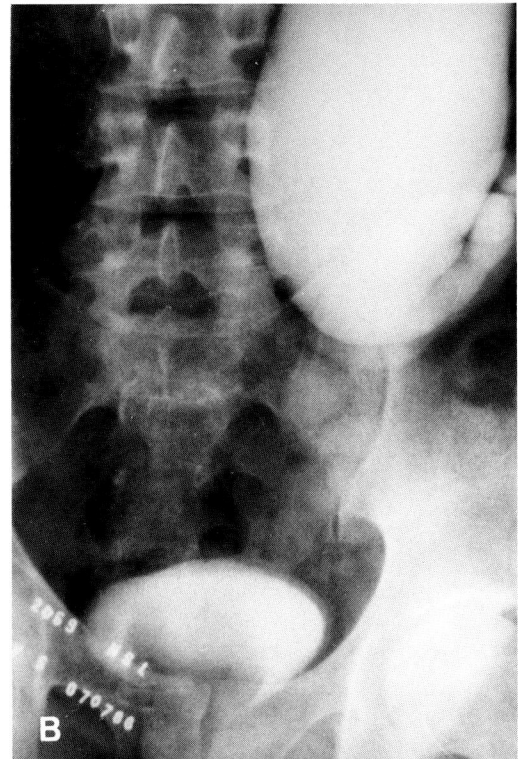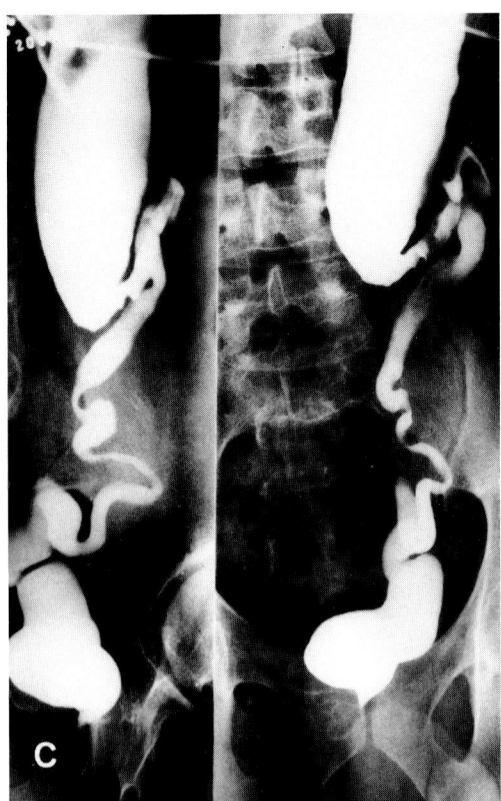

Figure 8.31 (A, B) Pieloureteral complete duplication with anomalous ureteral implantation causing piohydronephrosis in the superior caliceal group. (C) Control after percutaneous nephrostomy shows reduction in size of the renal cavities. After improvement of the piohydronephrosis, a left heminephrectomy was performed.

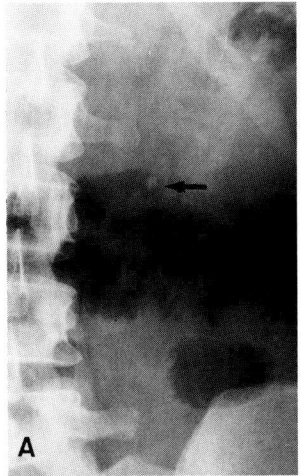 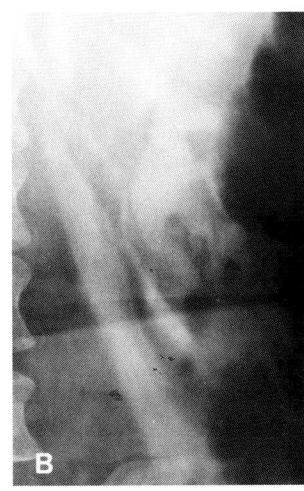 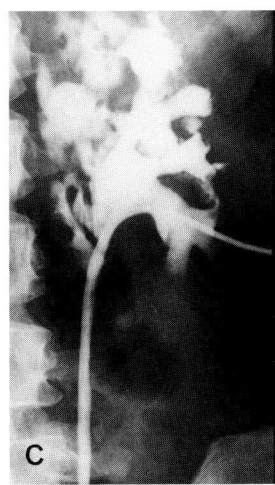 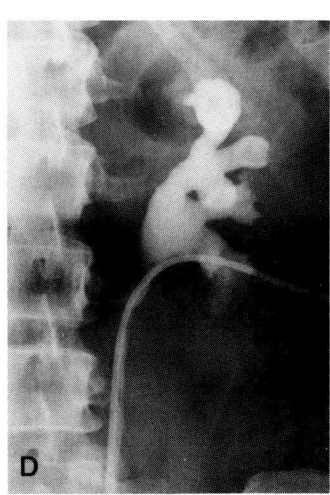

Figure 8.32 (A) Spontaneous rupture of the renal pelvis due to the obstruction by a ureteral stone (arrow). (B) Intravenous pielography showing contrast medium extravasation in the retroperitoneal tissues. (C) Percutaneous pielography and nephrostomy show the massive extravasation of contrast medium. The ureteral stone passed spontaneously to the urinary bladder. (D) Catheter pielography shows complete resolution of the pelvic laceration after 15 days of drainage. Note the catheter inside the ureter.

Neoplastic Obstructions

Obstructive anuria from a tumor is a frequent complication in advanced stages of pelvic neoplasms (Fig. 8.33). Prostate, bladder, cervicouterine, colonic, and lymphatic system neoplasms are usually the source of ureteral obstruction by compression or invasion. The management of these tumors, which requires high-dose radiotherapy, may cause actinic stenosis of the ureter, which occurs in approximately 30 percent of patients (Fig. 8.34).

The presence of tumoral anuria as a clinical condition is an indication for simple nephrostomy and the introduction of a pigtail-type catheter into the renal pelvis. This procedure leads to a reduction in the patient's blood creatinine and potassium levels, thus controlling uremia.

After this procedure, the results obtained from diagnostic pyelography, in association with other clinical and laboratory findings, enable the physician to choose an appropriate therapeutic procedure with greater precision. Biopsy is particularly important in this regard, since it provides a histologic definition of the type of neoplasm that is present. The most significant aspect to be considered, however, should be the average survival time expected on the basis of the evolution of the type of neoplasm present in the individual patient.

Depending on the degree of involvement of the excretory system, the following alternatives are available: performing a nephrostomy for the introduction of a catheter into the renal pelvis (Fig. 8.35), introduction of

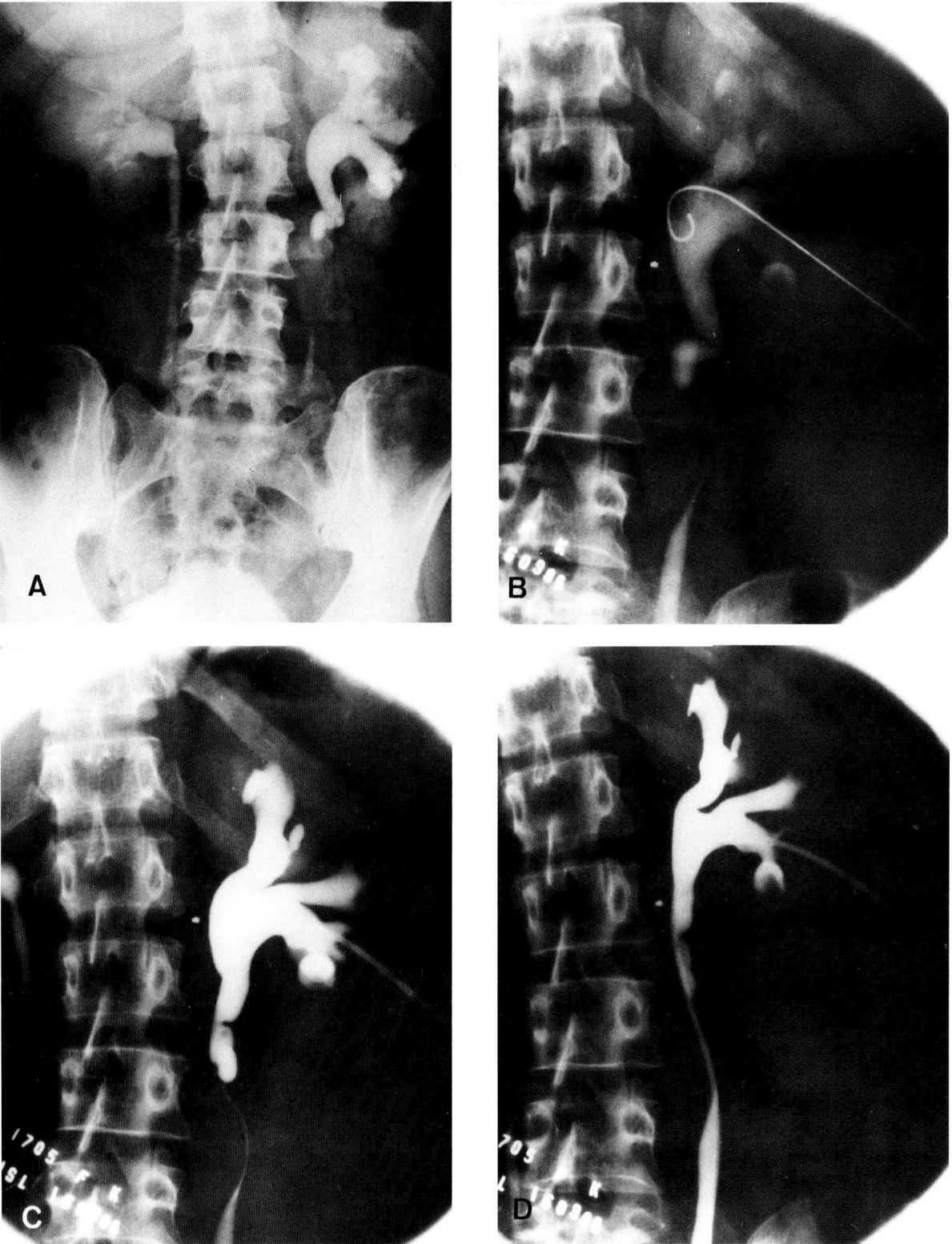

Figure 8.33 (A) Left ureteral obstruction by retroperitoneal metastasis of an ovarian adenocarcinoma, causing dilation of the renal collecting cavities with pyonephrosis. (B) Percutaneous puncture and catheterization for nephrostomy. (C) Temporary nephrostomy for alleviating the left kidney. (D) Collecting cavities have normal size after drainage for 3 weeks. Note the tutor across the stenosis. The left ureter was surgically released after cure of the infectious process.

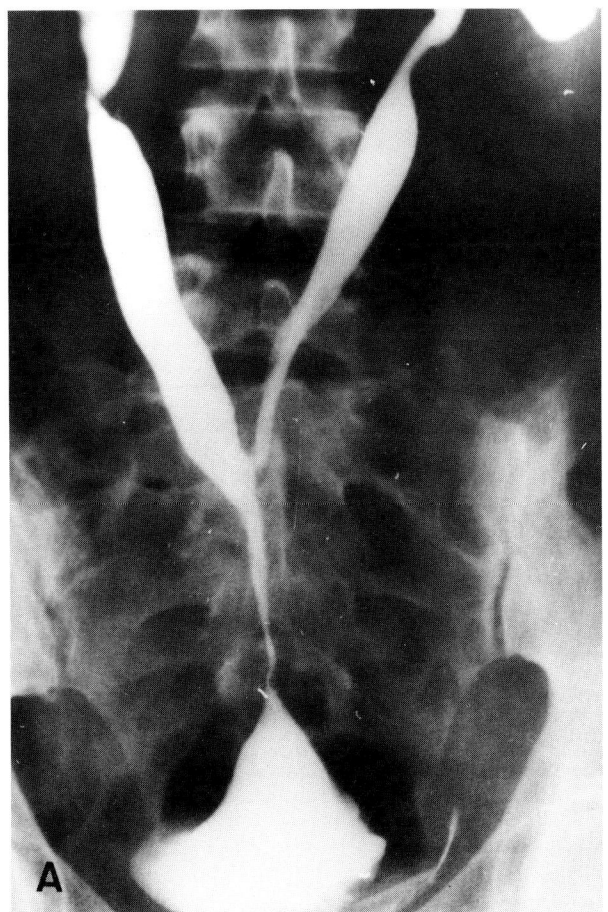
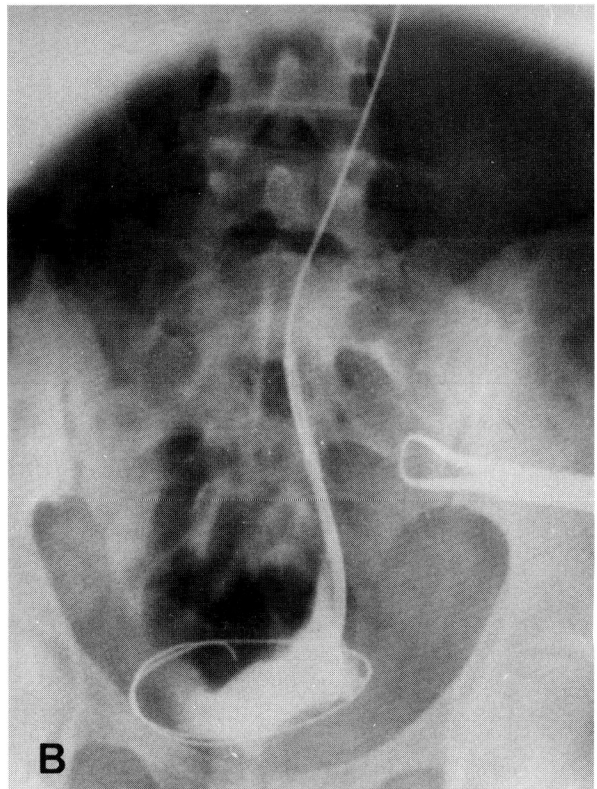
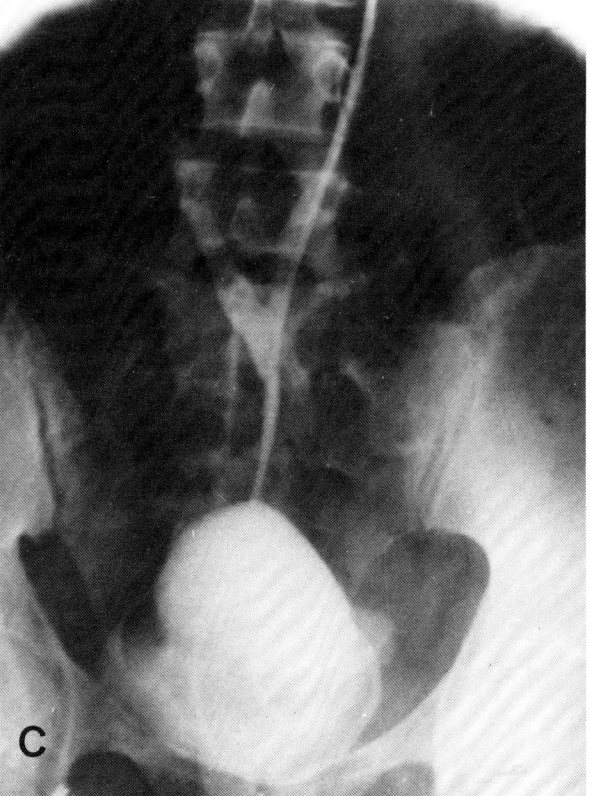

Figure 8.34 (A) Bilateral hydronephrosis in the postoperative period of a transureteral anastomosis, with a bladder flap for ureteral stenosis at the level of the anastomosis. The original obstruction of the ureters was caused by a uterine neoplasm, which was treated with radiotherapy. (B) Dilatation with a 5-mm-diameter balloon. (C) Control after dilation shows the catheter (tutor) still through the stenosis, with significant improvement as a result of resolution of hydronephrosis.

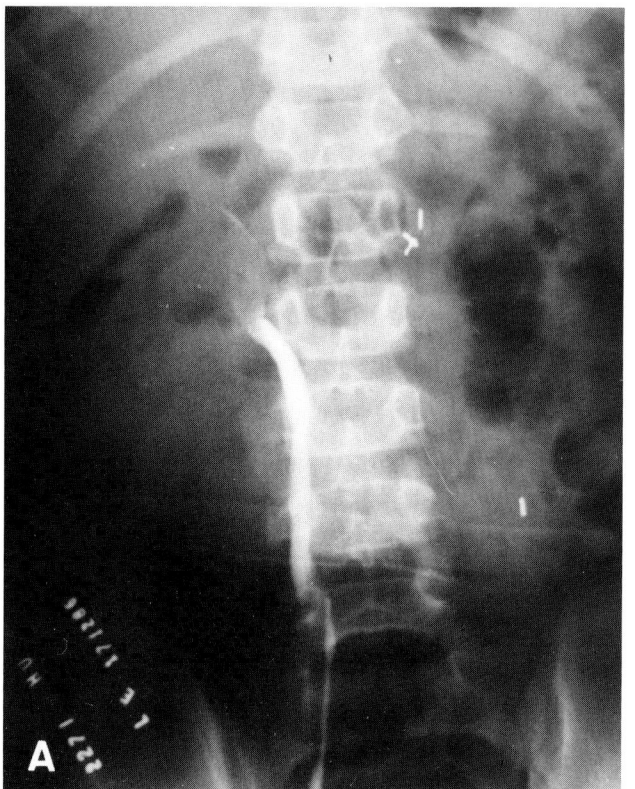
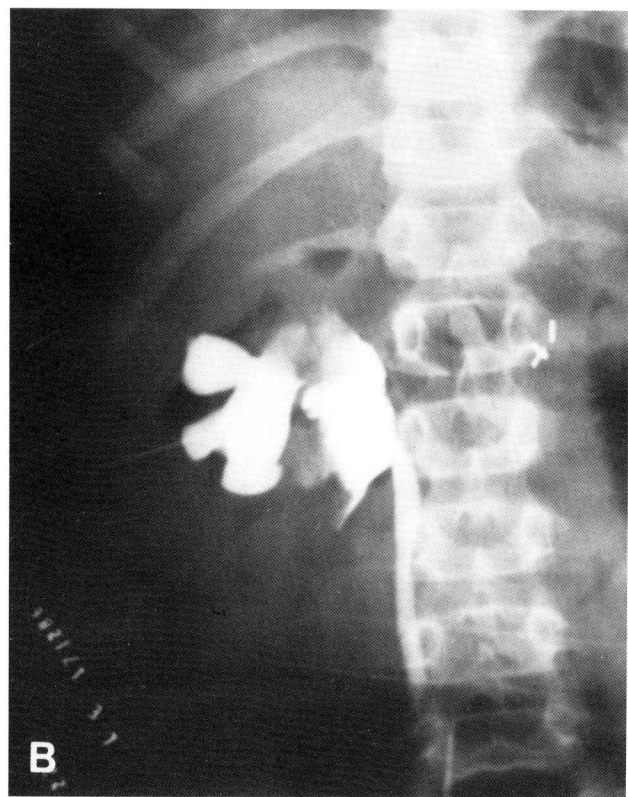
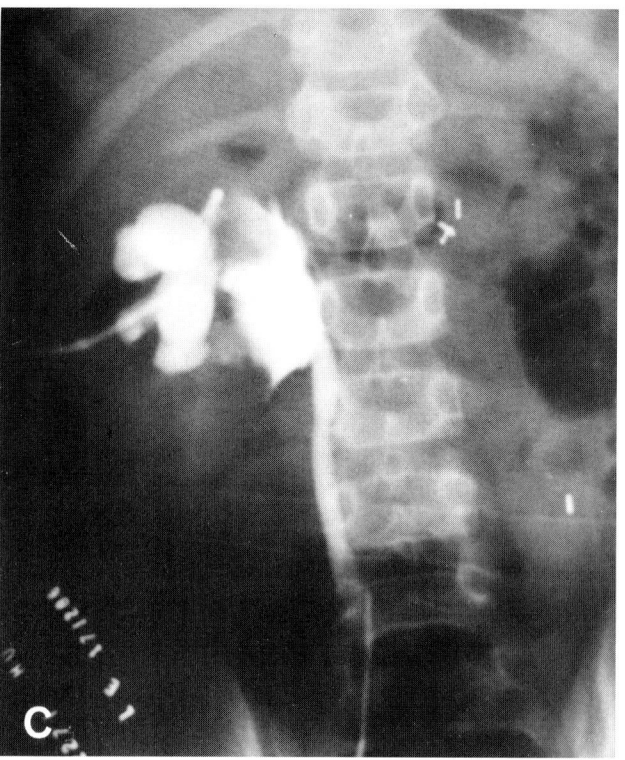

Figure 8.35 (A) Retrograde pyelogram in a patient with a solitary kidney and anuria due to ureteral obstruction for recurrence of a previously operated Wilms' tumor (left nephrectomy and partial right nephrectomy). (B) Percutaneous puncture with a Chiba needle. (C) Relief nephrostomy with recovery of diuresis.

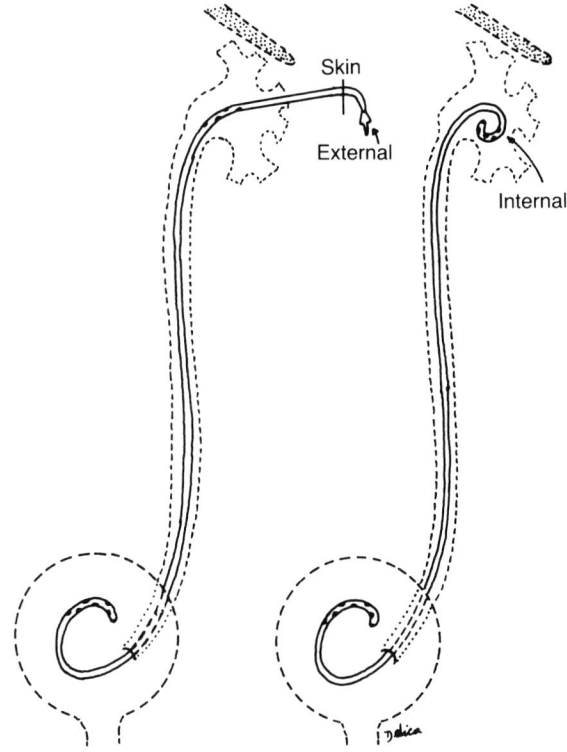

Figure 8.36 Schematic drawing shows the catheter (tutor) system with internal-external drainage on the left and internal drainage with a ureteral prosthesis (double J-catheter) on the right.

Figure 8.37 Schematic drawing shows an internal-external drainage catheter used to resolve a ureteral obstruction. A catheter which is exteriorized on the skin can be useful for performing the necessary changes during patient evolution.

a ureteral double J-type prosthesis until the urinary bladder is reached (Fig. 8.36), and placement of a long pigtail-type catheter so that one extremity remains inside the bladder and the other is fixed onto the skin (Fig. 8.37).

Depending on the patient's clinical condition, the second alternative will involve difficulties inherent in the replacement of the prosthesis itself as a consequence of its obstruction by the accumulation of calcium salt deposits. The use of a long pigtail-type catheter, always on the basis of the patient's clinical condition, will allow discontinuation of external drainage and the placement of a less painful catheter.

Irritating cystitis and trigonitis are frequently observed as a consequence of the long dwelling time of the catheter inside the bladder in the second and third procedures. These effects can be minimized with the use of the newer, extremely soft catheters made of Silastic or silicone. In this case it is still possible for the patient to receive a simple nephrostomy and then be sent for conventional surgery and a urinary shunt. As a rule, most patients are referred for conventional surgery, usually as a result of their failure to take good care of catheters and nephrostomy collectors.

Correction of Fistulas and Stenoses

Urinary fistulas frequently result from trauma or complications of previous surgery, such as ureterolithotomy (Fig. 8.38).

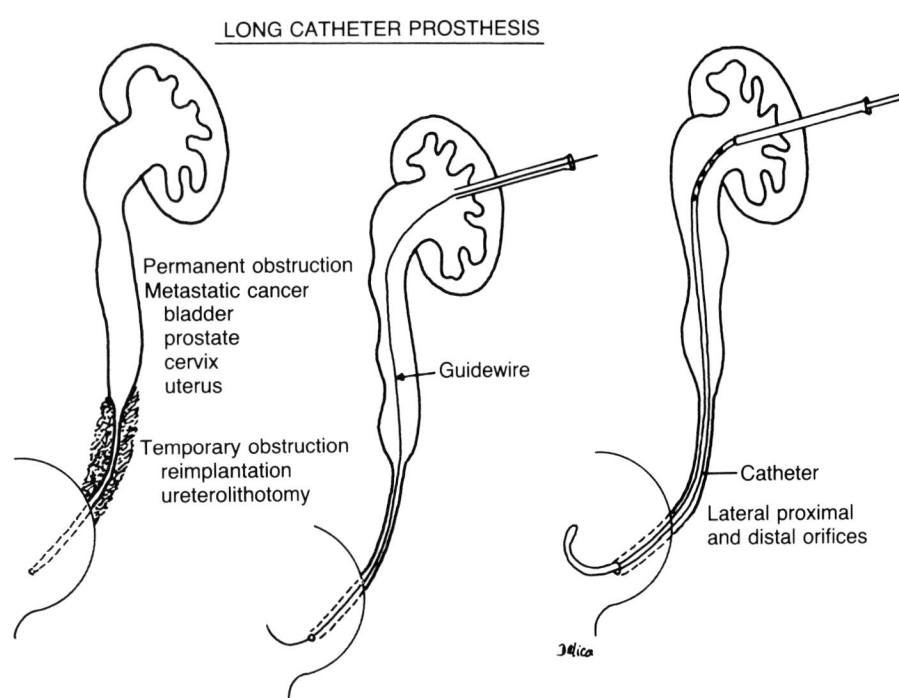

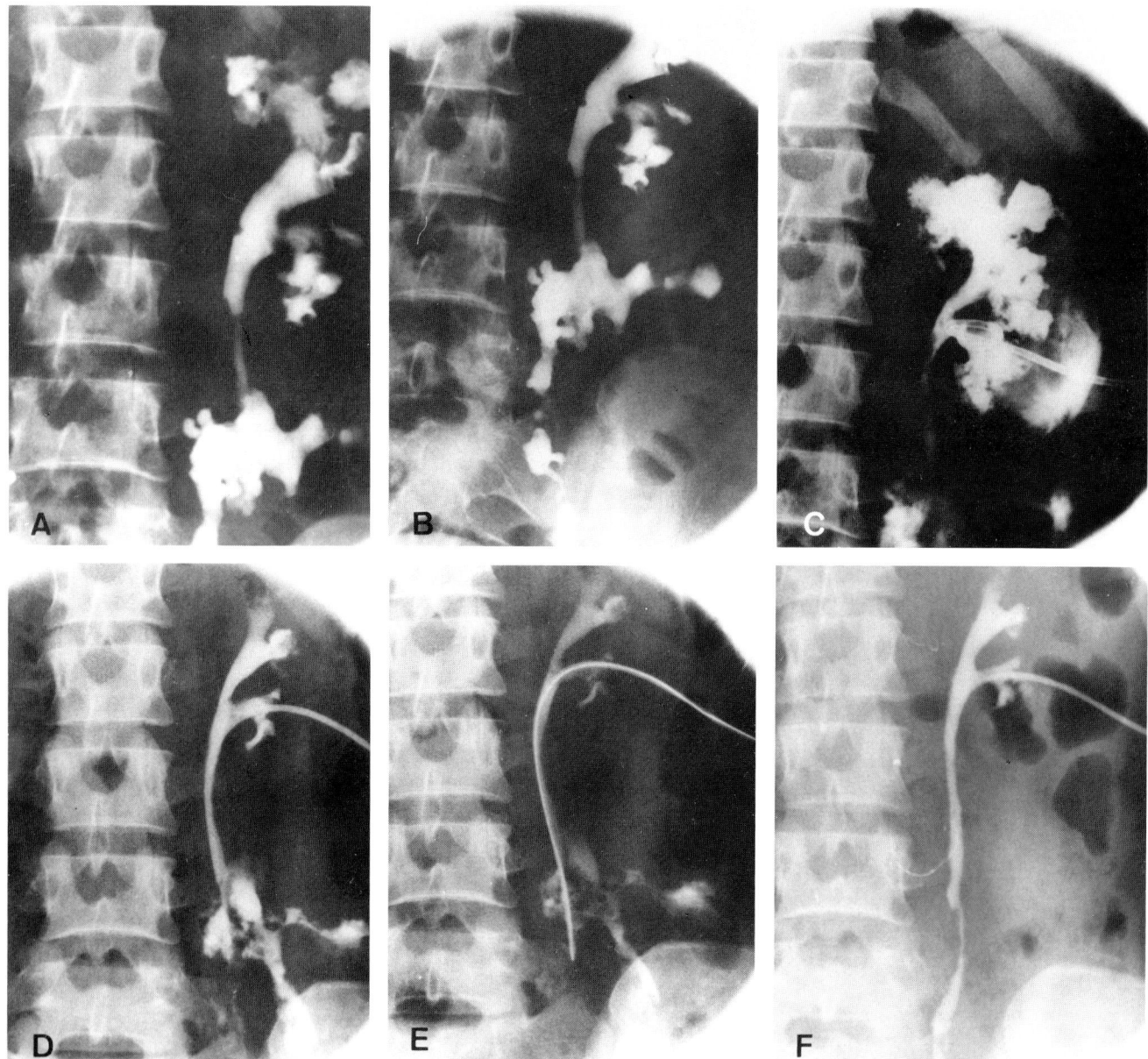

Figure 8.38 Ureteral fistula after ureterolithotomy with the development of pyonephrosis.
(A) Antegrade pyelography shows dilation of collecting cavities with ill-defined borders and a large ureteral fistula. (B) Ureteral fistula without identification of the distal ureter. (C,D) After percutaneous nephrostomy was performed, there was regression of pyonephrosis and extravasation (D). The distal ureter is already seen in control (D) after 1 week. (E) Catheterization through the stenosis and fistula. (F) Control pyelography shows ureteral patency and closure of the fistula after the use of a No. 9 French tube for 3 weeks.

The presence of urine outside the collecting system can cause infection and a large inflammatory reaction, precluding any possibility of spontaneous cure (Fig. 8.39). It is therefore necessary to perform the drainage by conventional surgery or by the percutaneous route. The use of percutaneous nephrostomy with the introduction of a pigtail-type catheter has proved to be effective when the purpose is to interrupt the flow of urine through a fistulous track.

Pyelography sometimes shows significant urinary output through a fistula and large volumes of urine accumulating in the retroperitoneum. In this case, a guidewire should be advanced beyond the fistula. Under its directional guidance, a straight, large-diameter, multi-perforated catheter should be introduced to allow urine to deviate externally and thus not perpetuate the urinary fistula (Fig. 8.39).

In a patient with a urinoma, which is characterized

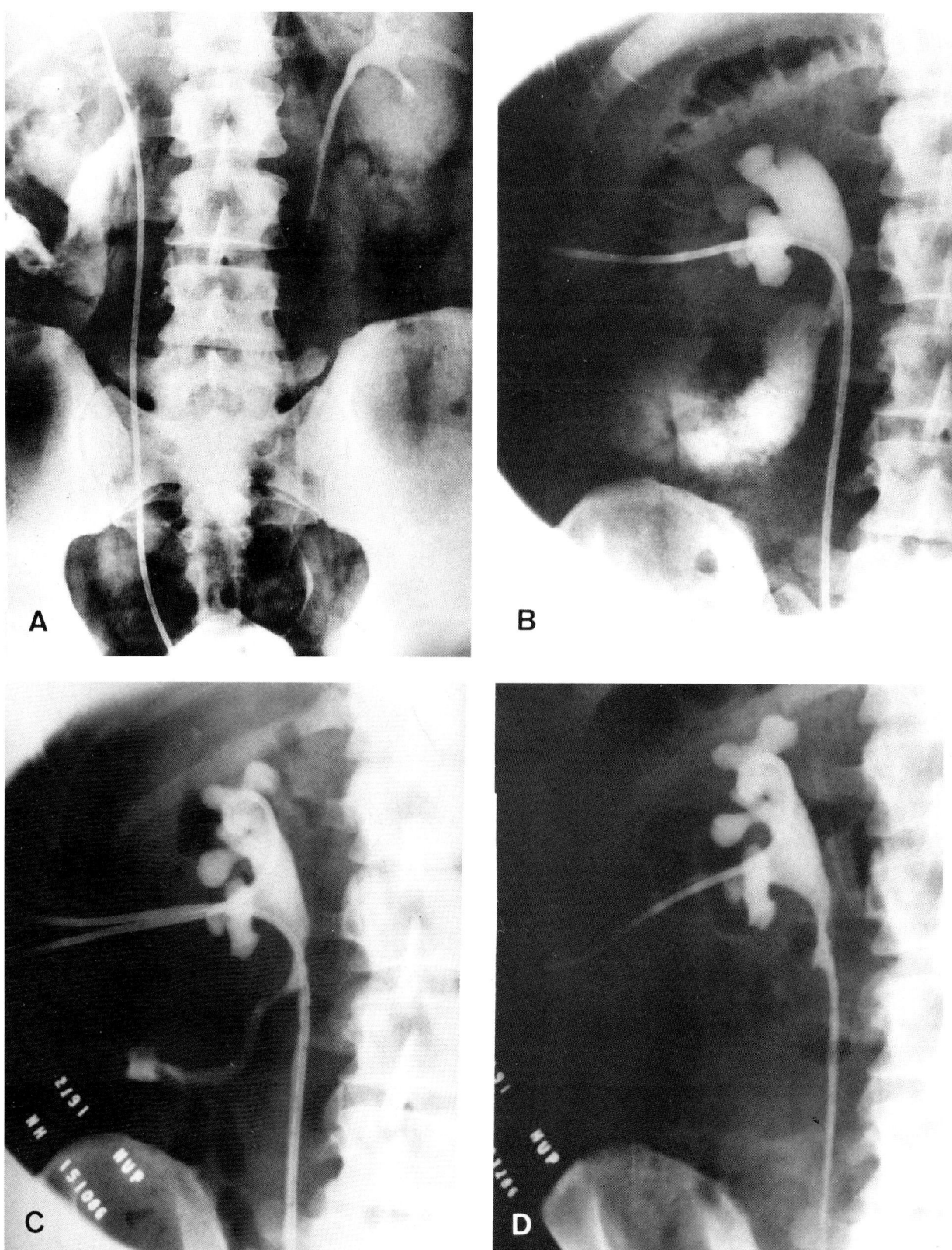

Figure 8.39 Control of a ureteral fistula with two catheters.
(A) A large right ureteral fistula after ureterolithotomy treated with a ureteral prosthesis, which was not sufficient to drain the collecting system. (B) Introduction of an internal-external drainage catheter still showing the fistula, followed by the introduction of a second nephrostomy catheter. (C) Control after 1 week with double drainage, showing reduction of the fistula. (D) Control after drainage for 21 days shows fistula occlusion without ureteral stenosis.

by the collection of volumes of urine outside the urinary tract, another catheter should be introduced into the collection for emptying purposes in order to obtain subsequent drainage and prevent infection.

Success in curing a fistula depends on changes related to the ureteral or pyelic walls. Thus, the earlier the drainage, the lower the degree of periureteral fibrosis; in most cases the fistula will close completely after 3 weeks.

Ureteral stenosis and some types of fistulas may appear as a consequence of the removal of long-standing ureteral stones, which cause edema and a periureteral inflammatory response. Stenosis and ureteral fistula are common findings in these patients (Fig. 8.40).

Treatment of ureteral stenosis was first proposed by Keley in 1890, but the percutaneous route was not used until almost 100 years later, when it was proposed by Witherington in a paper published in 1980. The use of a percutaneous route for treating ureteral stenoses is based on Dotter and Judkins's experience in utilizing the percutaneous technique for artery dilation (Fig. 8.41). In 1964 dilating angiographic catheters were utilized. In 1974 they were replaced with balloon catheters by Gruntzig (Fig. 8.42).

In ureteral stenosis, access to the renal pelvis is facilitated by the degree of dilation which is commonly found throughout the collecting system. Partial drainage of the system makes it possible to perform a pyelogram, which will determine the exact location of the stenosis. The next step is to gain access to the ureter; as described earlier, this should be done with a Cobra visceral catheter.

After the ureter has been reached, an attempt should be made to advance the guidewire beyond the stenosis. In most cases, a straight catheter with straight or curved guidewires varying between 0.035 and 0.038 in. has been shown to be useful for this purpose. The guidewire tip should get as close as possble to the bladder or be advanced into it, increasing the safety of the procedure and favoring the dilatation process. To obtain proper dilatation, long angiographic dilators similar to those used by Dotter and Judkins should be employed. The dilator diameter should be increased progressively as resistance to catheter introduction decreases. When the diameter of the tube corresponds to No. 7 or 8 French,

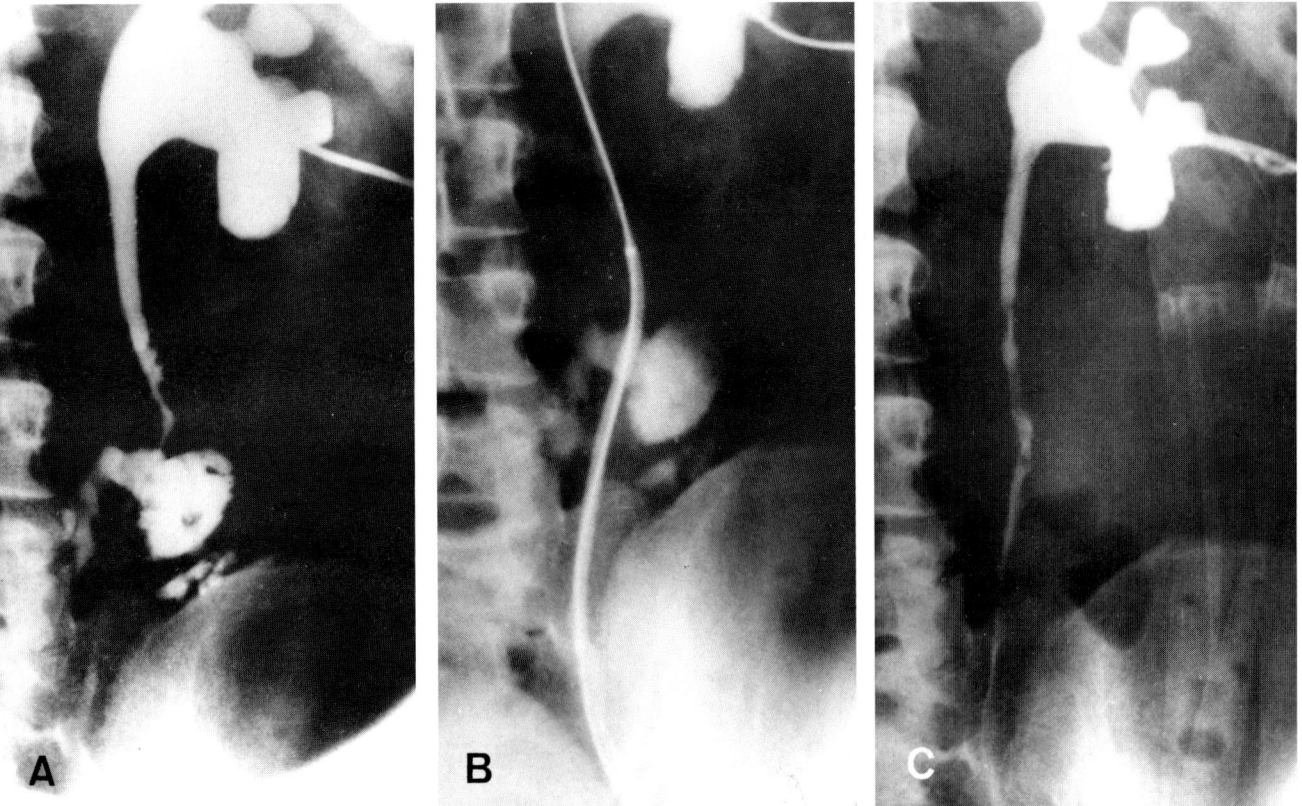

Figure 8.40 (A) Ureteral fistula and stenosis after ureterolithotomy. (B) Dilation of the ureteral stenosis with a balloon 4 mm in diameter and 20 cm long. (C) Control pyelography 22 days after internal-external drainage with a tutor through the stenosis, showing resolution of the fistula and ureteral patency.

Figure 8.41 Schematic drawing shows the use of catheters with progressively larger diameters for ureter dilation and drainage of the collecting cavities.
Dilation is increased progressively at 2-week intervals. The largest catheters should be No. 9 or 10 French.

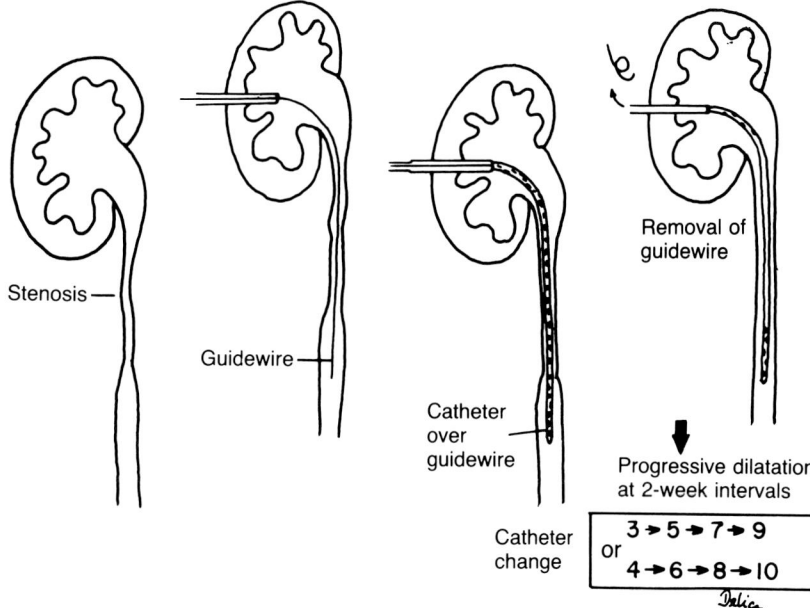

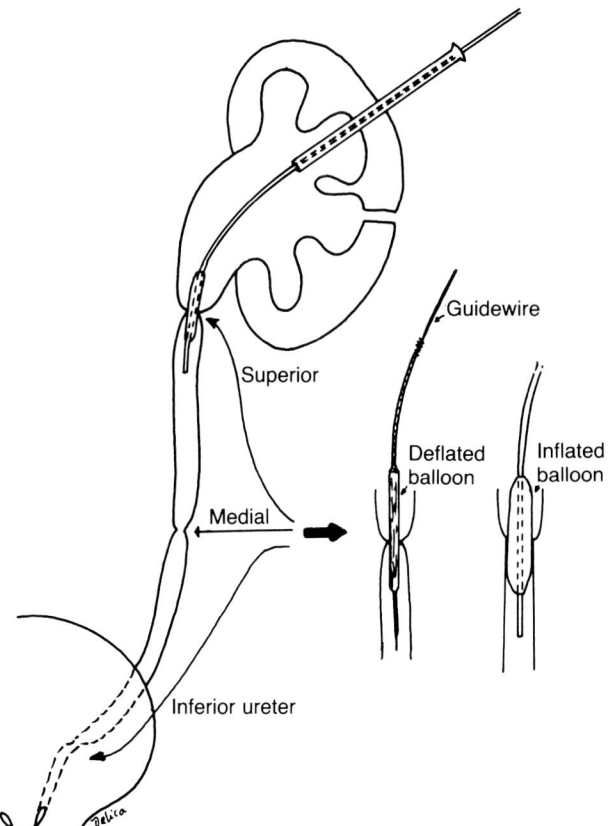

Figure 8.42 Schematic illustration of ureteral dilation with a Gruntzig-type balloon catheter.
Stenoses can be superiorly, medially, or inferiorly located. The balloon system should be introduced through a sheath. When inflated, the balloon promotes laceration of the ureteral wall and permanent dilation.

it should be replaced by a Gruntzig balloon catheter (Fig. 8.43).

Balloon diameters vary, and those between 4 and 10 mm are recommended. The balloon selected should be appropriate for the diameter of the ureter (Fig. 8.44). When the balloon is distended by the injection of iodized contrast medium diluted to 50%, it will be possible to visualize and define the outline of the stenosed segment. This image will disappear as soon as dilatation of the segment is obtained. The balloon should be distended at least three times during a period of 3 to 5 min, after which the ureter should be dilated.

After dilatation is achieved, No. 8 or 9 French multiperforated catheter should be introduced as a guide. It will remain in place for 3 weeks, acting as a "mold."

Stenosis also occurs in ureters that are reimplanted into the bladder (Fig. 8.45) and in intestinal loops; in the latter case, the technical procedure should be identical to the one described above. Long dwelling times of "mold" catheters in the urinary bladder in patients with dilatation of reimplanted ureters frequently cause irritating cystitis and trigonitis. Ureteral stenosis and a urinary fistula are often present simultaneously. This occurs more frequently during the postoperative period in patients who receive plastic surgery in the pyeloureteral junction. In these cases, placing a pigtail catheter into the renal pelvis is the most frequently adopted and effective solution. Handling the pyeloureteral junction and dilating it with a balloon catheter are seldom necessary.

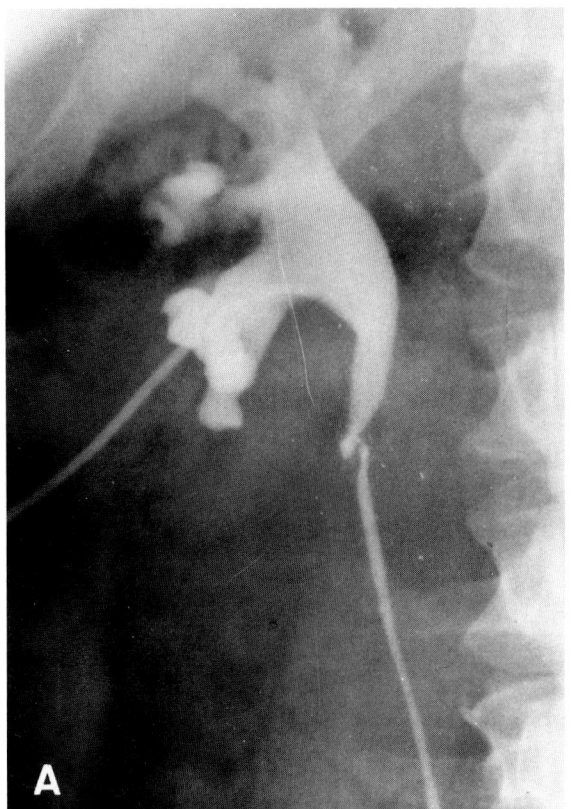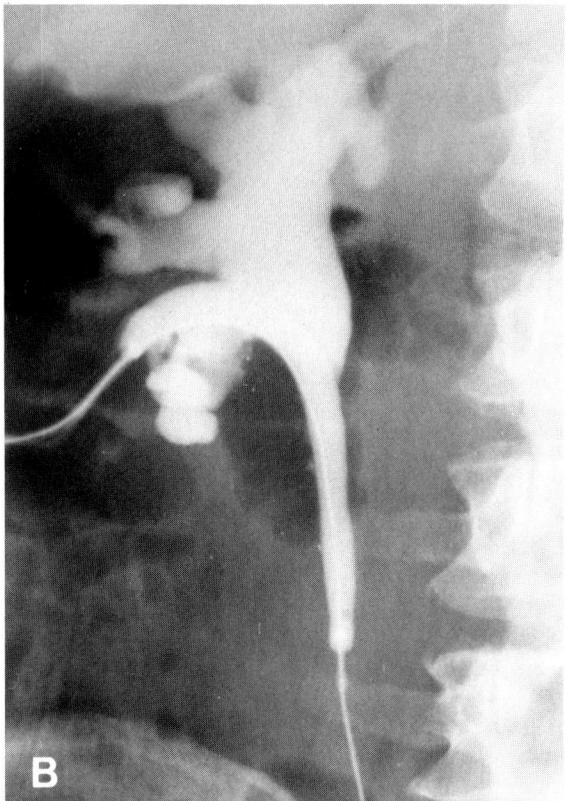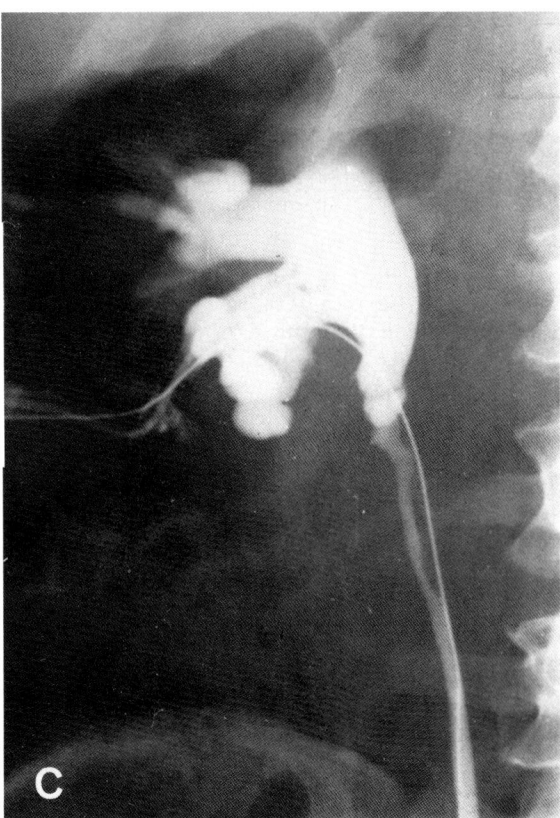

Figure 8.43 (A) Stenosis after ureterolithotomy on the right side. (B) Stenosis dilation with an Olbert-type 10-mm-diameter balloon. (C) Control 21 days after dilation of the ureter shows patency, even though there is laceration and the guidewire seems to be outside the ureteral lumen.

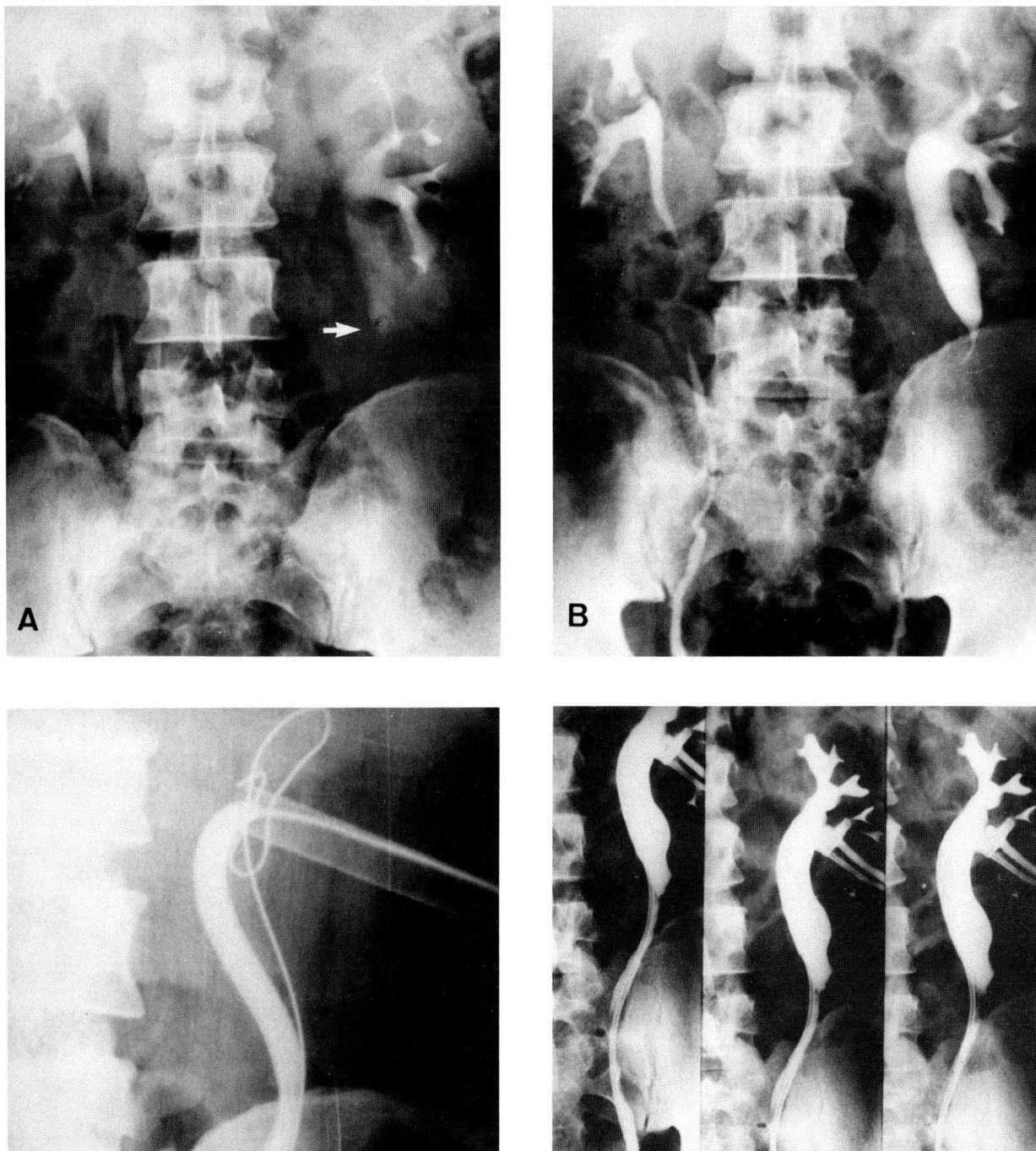

Figure 8.44 (A,B) Lithiasis in the proximal ureter (arrow) causing stenosis and hydronephrosis. (C) Percutaneous lithotripsy followed by ureteral dilation with an Olbert-type 10-mm balloon. (D) Control 21 days after ureteral dilation shows patency, with a No. 9 French tutor still inside.

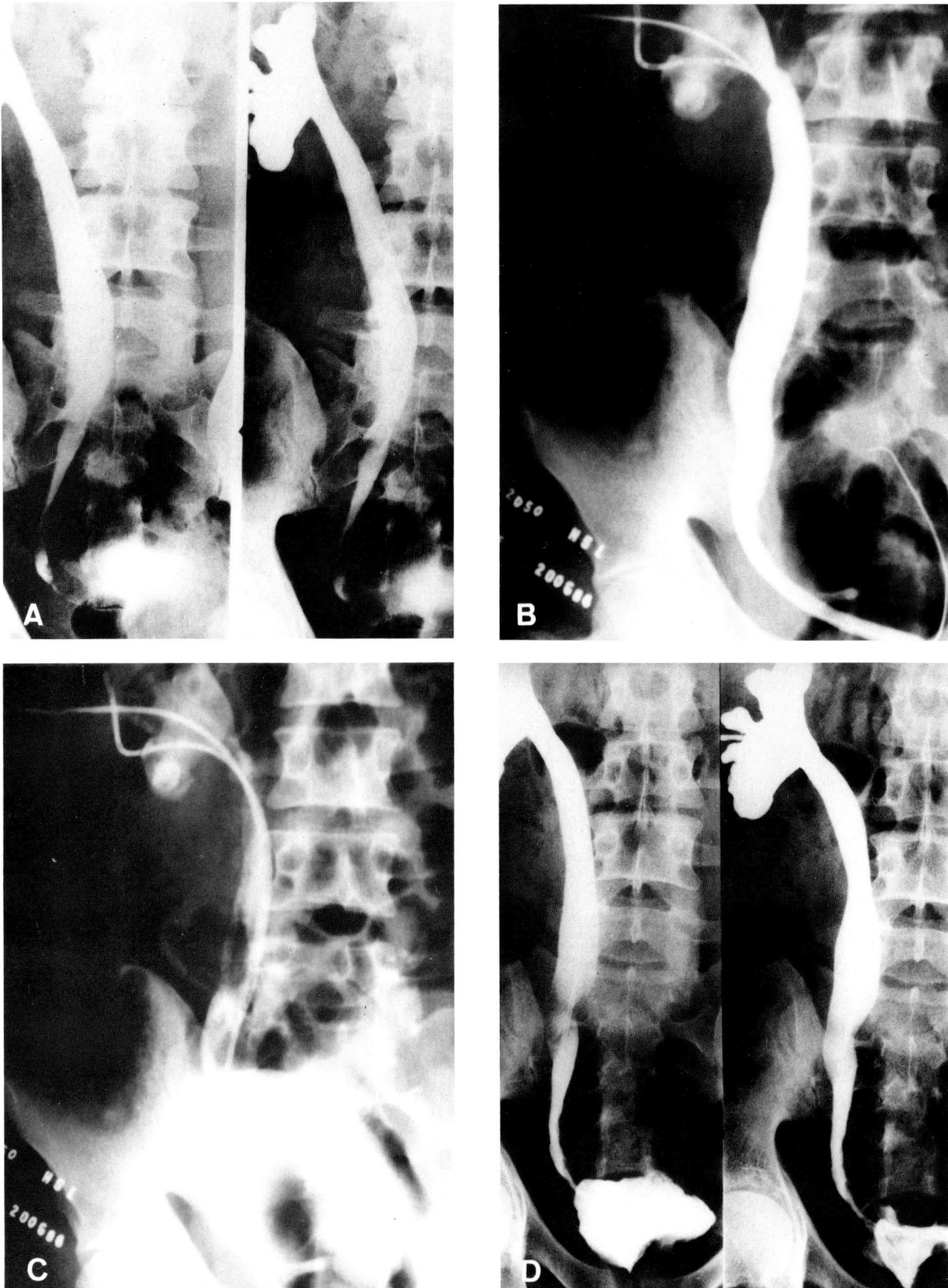

Figure 8.45 (A) Ureteral stenosis after reimplantation on the right side. (B) Dilation of the terminal ureter with an Olbert-type 10-mm balloon catheter. (C) Control pyelography with the tutor still inside the dilated area. (D) Control after dilation and tutor removal shows ureteral patency.

Urinary Lithiasis

The indication for percutaneous nephrostomy in patients with renal colic should result from careful clinical evaluation based on the interaction of symptoms. Priority is determined according to the significance of these symptoms, which include the frequency, intensity, and type of pain and the location, shape, size, and evolution time of the stones (Figs. 8.30 and 8.32).

When the stone is less than 1 cm and is located in the ureteral segment between its two distal thirds, retrograde catheterization is the preferred method. When stones are larger than 1 cm and are located in the proximal third of the ureter, percutaneous nephrostomy, which also alleviates the symptoms, should be the therapeutic method of choice. The use of a nephroscope or Dormia-type catheter will make it possible to extract the stones (Fig. 8.44). With a proximally located ureteral stone smaller than 1 cm, nephrostomy should offer pain relief and decrease the ureteral edema surrounding the stone, affording an opportunity for its migration toward the urinary bladder.

Ureteral obstruction should be considered an emergency procedure in patients with only one kidney. In this situation percutaneous nephrostomy is the treatment of choice (Fig. 8.46).

Apart from extraction, the percutaneous route also makes it possible to dissolve stones by litholysis, provided that the nature of the different constituents of the stone has been established previously (Fig. 8.46).

In this technique two different catheters are used. One should be introduced through the ureter until it reaches the stone, and the other should be placed inside the renal pelvis. Specific solutions are injected through the catheter into the ureter to cause litholysis of the different types of stones: 2 M sodium bicarbonate for uric acid stones, renascedine for struvite stones, and a 2% solution of diacetylcysteine acid for cystine stones. Authors have expressed optimism about the results that can be achieved with this technique, and in practice considerable success has been obtained.

Intrarenal and Extrarenal Collections

Intrarenal collections are usually of infectious origin, with cortical and medullary renal abscesses being the most common causes. Cortical renal abscesses are generally of hematogenous origin; staphylococcus is the causal organism in most cases. The original foci may be almost anywhere in the body but should be looked for first in the teeth and on the skin. There have been published reports about the growing participation of *Escherichia coli* in the development of these processes. *E. coli* is commonly found in the urinary tract, and it is believed that it is taken to the renal cortical layer through lymphatic drainage. Medullary renal abscesses are usually associated with changes in the urinary tract resulting from the presence of calculi or vesicoureteral reflux; the germs responsible for the infection are those which usually are present there.

The diagnosis of an intrarenal collection almost always implies a previous involvement of both the medullary and cortical renal layers. It is almost impossible to distinguish between the two possibilities.

An intrarenal abscess is characterized by an insidious onset of the clinical condition, accompanied by fever, changes in the hemogram suggesting the presence of infection, changes in urine test results, and negative urine culture in most cases.

Intravenous urography may identify displacement of the renal calices or the renal pelvis. Ultrasound may establish the characteristics of the lesion and its precise location as well as indicate the best site for performing a diagnostic puncture.

The puncture should be performed with a long, fine needle, similar to a Chiba needle, in an area that has been demarcated with ultrasound or computed tomography. The purpose of this procedure is to define the nature of the contents of the abscess.

Through partial aspiration of the abscess material, it is possible to inject a small volume of contrast medium, which will demarcate the limits of the cavity to be drained.

Utilizing the translumbar technique suggested here for percutaneous nephrostomy, from the posterior hemiaxillary line below the 12th rib, a second puncture should be performed through which a catheter will be introduced. The catheter should preferably have No. 8 or 9 French diameter; this will facilitate drainage of the collection, which usually consists of purulent, thick, and viscous material. This so-called definitive drainage, in combination with antibiotic therapy, has been shown to be effective in treating these patients. The symptoms usually disappear after 6 to 48 h (Fig. 8.47).

Control of regression of the process should be done with the aid of ultrasonography, which can also identify any septations inside the cavity. The presence of septations is always an indication for introducing two or more catheters to maintain effective drainage.

The catheter should have its lumen washed with 0.9% simple saline at regular intervals over a 12-h period, using an average of 20 mL each time. This procedure will help keep the drainage material reasonably liquefied, a condition indispensable for maintaining its efficacy.

When the ultrasonographic study can supply information on regression and disappearance of the process, the catheter can simply be pulled out, with its orifice protected by a compression dressing. When ultrasound is not available, the scheme proposed by Ferruci will indicate the proper time for catheter removal.

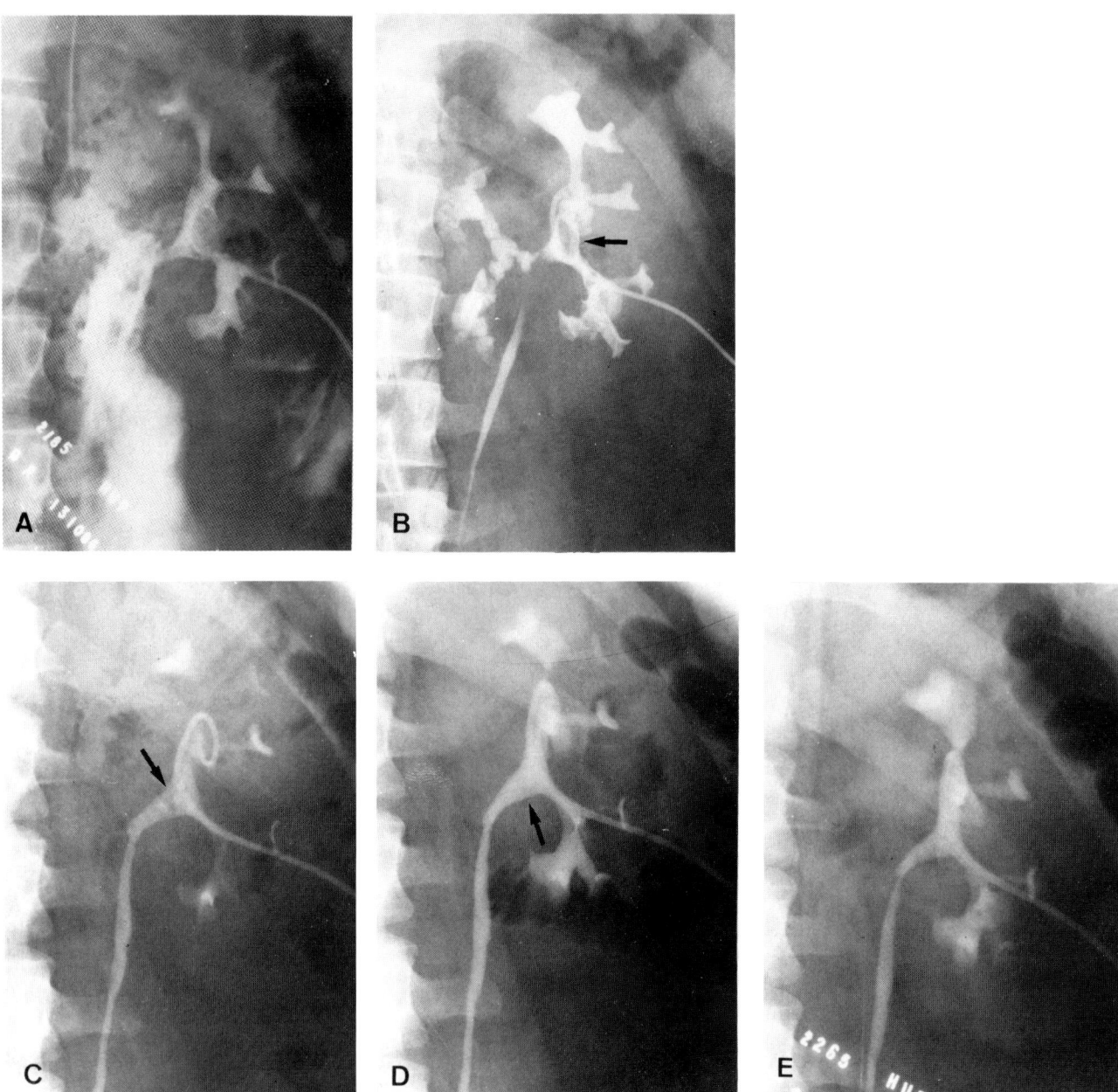

Figure 8.46 (A) A uric acid stone in the pelvis of a solitary kidney on the left. The renal pelvis was lacerated during nephrostomy performed 2 weeks earlier in another center. Note the copious extravasation of contrast medium after nephrostomy. (B) Control pyelography 1 week later shows reduction of the fistula and the radiolucent stone (arrow). (C) Closure of pelvic fistula after 3 weeks, with the beginning of sodium bicarbonate litholysis, which was maintained for 1 month (20 mL twice a day). The calculus is still visible (arrow). (D) Control after 2 weeks shows stone reduction (arrow). (E) Control after 1 month shows stone resolution with completely successful litholysis.

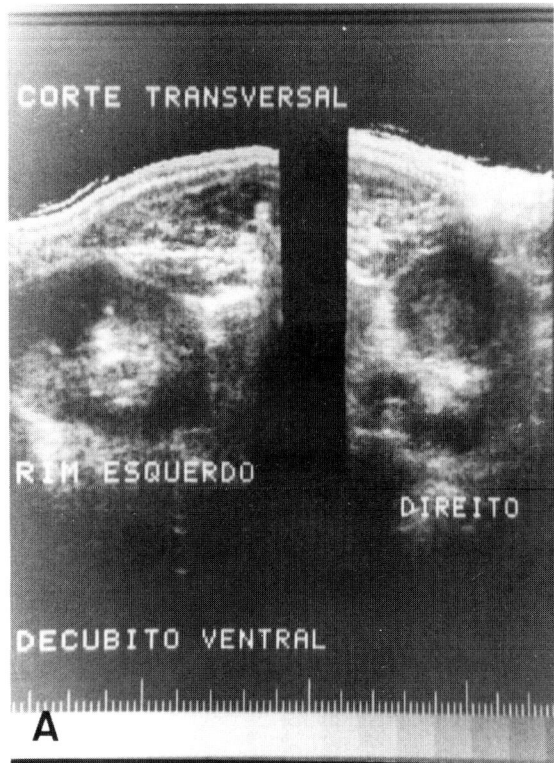
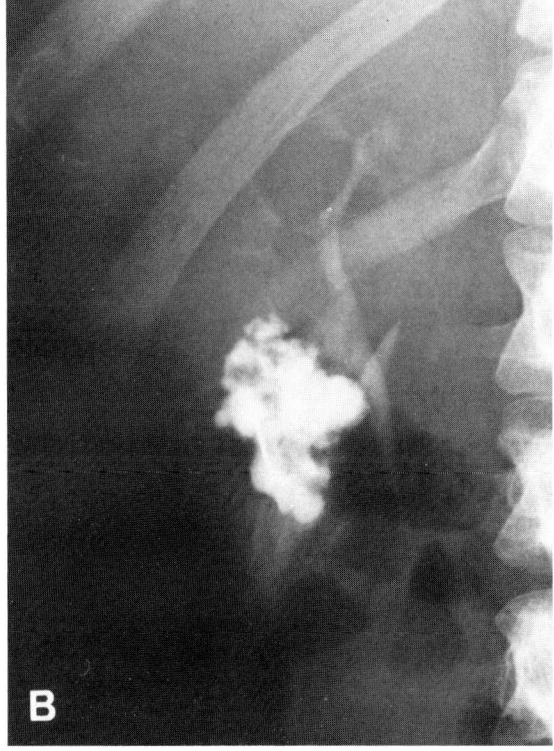
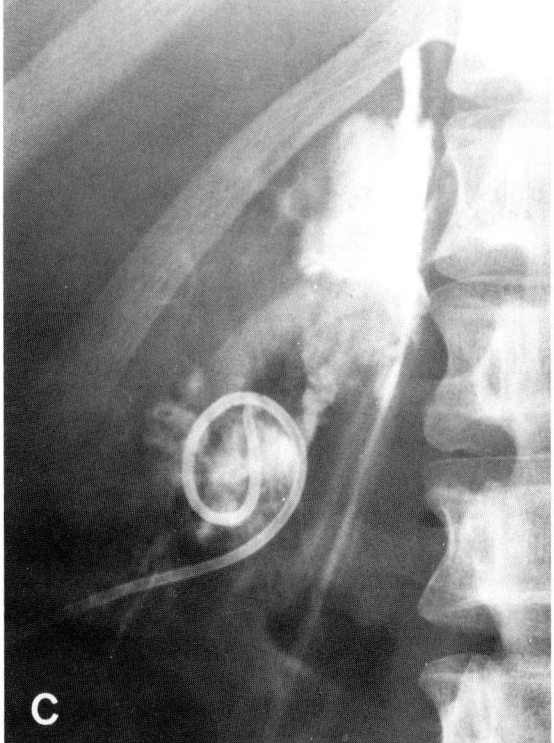

Figure 8.47 (A) Ultrasound shows a collection compatible with a right kidney parenchymal abscess in a patient with sepsis and a poor general condition. (B) Percutaneous puncture with a Chiba needle opacifying the collection. (C) Percutaneous drainage with a pigtail No. 8 French catheter shows a fistula in the retroperitoneum. The process resolved in 5 days, and the patient's general condition improved within 10 to 12 h.

A perirenal abscess is a fluid collection of infectious origin that is located in the perirenal space and is usually secondary to previous renal injury (Fig. 8.48).

Involvement of the cortical layer and later capsule rupture will allow germ and pus extravasation into the perirenal space, which may also be involved when there is injury to the collecting system. This occurs in patients with pyonephrosis when purulent material leaks from the excretory canal. It should be emphasized that from a physiopathogenic standpoint both forms of perirenal space involvement are similar to infrarenal lesions.

A urinoma is a collection of encapsulated urine that extravasates from the collecting system into the retroperitoneal space. Outside the excretory canal, urine is a chemical irritant and produces a significant inflammatory response in the tissues with which it is in contact. An infected urinoma is thus a natural consequence of the presence of urine outside the collecting system.

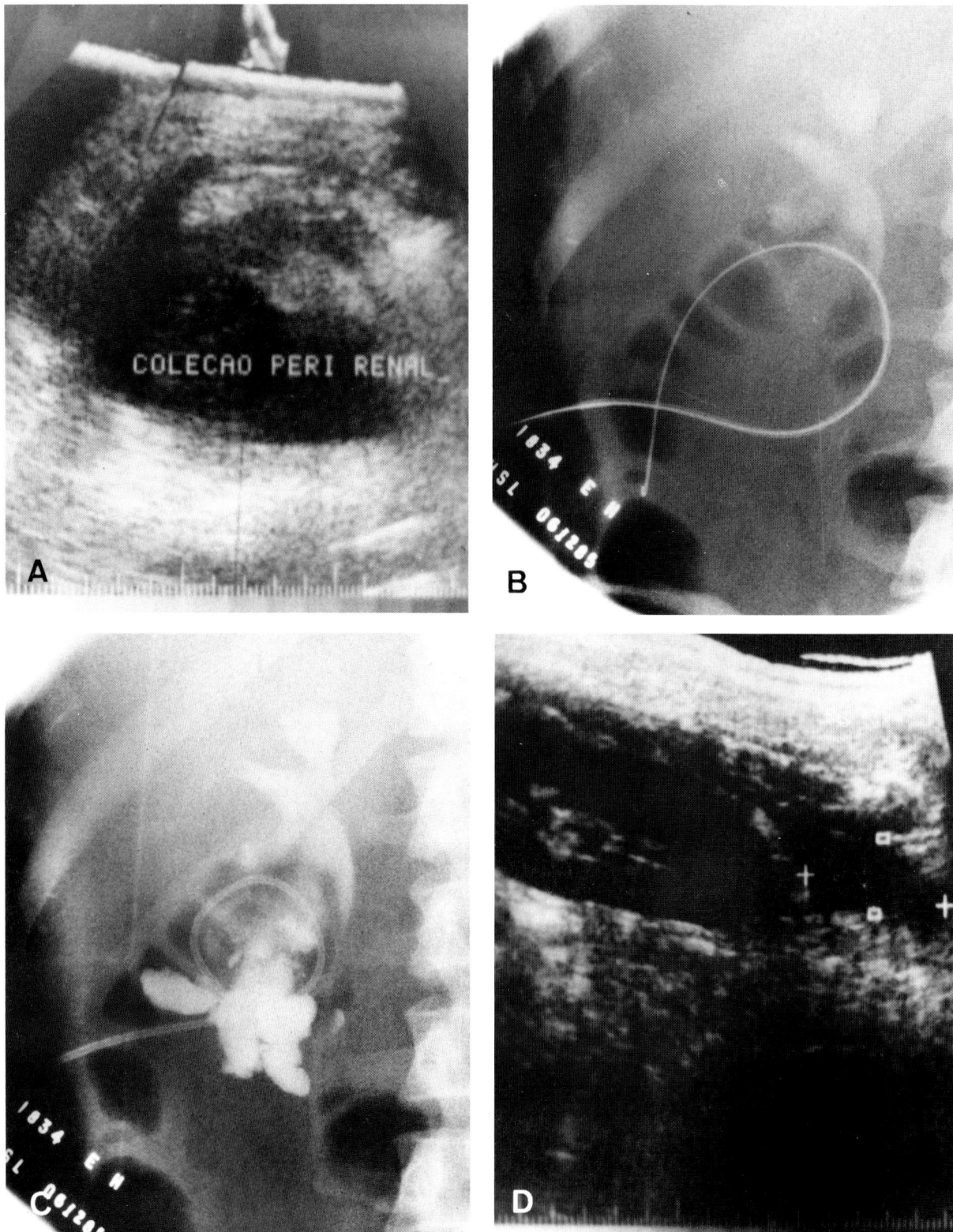

Figure 8.48 Drainage of perirenal collection.
(A) Ultrasound shows a right perirenal collection. (B) Percutaneous puncture with a guidewire inside the perirenal abscess. (C) No. 8 French drainage catheter inside the collection with contrast injection opacifying several different loculations. (D) Ultrasound shows that the collection disappeared after drainage for 15 days. Note the single small cavity, which disappeared spontaneously in follow-up.

The most common causes of urinoma are trauma to the excretory system; postoperative complications, especially in patients who receive ureterolithotomy; and urine extravasation due to fornix rupture during the course of nephretic colic.

Perirenal abscesses and urinomas should both be treated by the percutaneous route. The treatment is identical to that for pyonephrosis and intrarenal collections.

When there is involvement of the excretory system, the possibility and indication exist for introducing two catheters: one in the encapsulated urinoma and the other into the renal pelvis.

Nephroscopy

For diagnostic purposes, nephroscopy is performed with the aid of a rigid or flexible optical device, which is introduced into the collecting system to allow internal visualization of calices, the renal pelvis, and the ureter.

The applications of nephroscopy are broad and diversified. It can be used for calculi removal with special forceps under direct view or disintegration of calculi by ultrasound; for the identification of bleeding and for cauterization; in needle biopsies and punctures under direct view; when the use of a uretrotome (Sacks knife) becomes necessary for dilating caliceal infundibula; and for performing a pyeloplasty (Figs. 8.49 and 8.50).

INDICATIONS AND CONTRAINDICATIONS

Percutaneous nephrostomy can be indicated as a surgical alternative and a general form of temporary treatment, allowing the percutaneous route to serve as a basis for the subsequent of a more convenient and definitive treatment.

Because it allows decompression of the collecting system, percutaneous nephrostomy has made it possible for conventional surgeries which often were considered emergency measures to be classified as elective interventions which can be performed at the most convenient time. This has resulted in lower surgical morbidity and mortality rates.

Percutaneous nephrostomy is indicated for patients with pyonephrosis, neoplastic obstructions, fistulas, and ureteral stenosis. It also can be used in specific technical procedures, including litholysis, drainage of intrarenal and extrarenal collections, extraction of calculi, and nephroscopy.

Because of the broad variety of etiologic causes for which percutaneous nephrostomy may be indicated, these patients as a rule present with a clinical picture which may include pain, fever, bacteremia, and uremia, all at the same time or in different combinations. The most frequent indications for bilateral percutaneous nephrostomy are bladder and prostate neoplasms. In cases of lithotripsy, pyonephrosis, and urinary fistula, a unilateral procedure is generally indicated.

Even though there are no absolute contraindications for performing percutaneous nephrostomy, relative contraindications should always be considered. Among those requiring special attention are blood dyscrasias, in which there is a possibility of causing prolonged hematuria or perirenal hematoma, and the presence of polycystic kidneys, which present a risk of an infectious process, resulting in nephrectomy.

Finally, it should be remembered that the nature and clinical results of the procedure have progressively reduced the number of clinical conditions that preclude its application.

COMPLICATIONS

The most frequent complications of percutaneous nephrostomy are related to the anatomic features of the kidney itself, the neighboring organs and structures, and the presence or absence of infected urine.

After a catheter has been introduced, the urine drained is frequently hematuric, because the renal parenchyma is highly vascular. Hematuria usually disappears completely during the first 24 h, and this period can be shortened by the use of diuretics.

If hematuria does not disappear within the first 48 h, the possibility of a vascular lesion must be considered; the most frequent causes are arteriovenous fistula and pseudoaneurysm. Selective renal arteriography is indicated in these patients for diagnostic purposes and posterior embolization (Fig. 8.51).

Neighboring organs may be inadvertently punctured; the most common example is pleural puncture. Pneumothorax and pleural effusion result from this complication, and simple drainage of the pleural cavity has been shown to be effective in most cases. The spleen and colon also may be punctured.

Besides obstruction of the catheter lumen by blood clots, pus clumps, or small calculi, collections, which are usually caused by catheter displacement, occur frequently.

The clinical manifestations of bacteremia are common in patients with purulent urine. The clinical picture, however, is less intense and is less frequently observed when an antibiotic is given 24 h prior to the procedure and the volume and pressure of the iodized contrast injected during pyelography are kept to the minimum necessary.

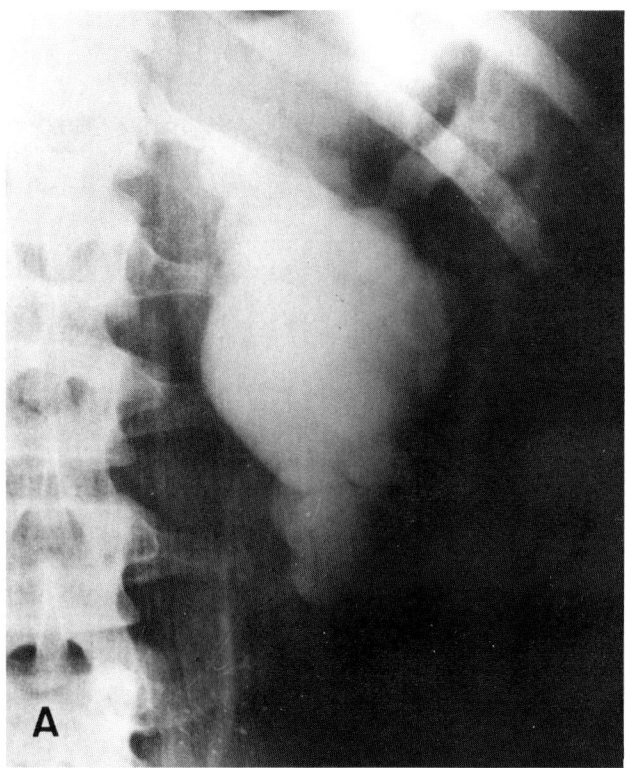
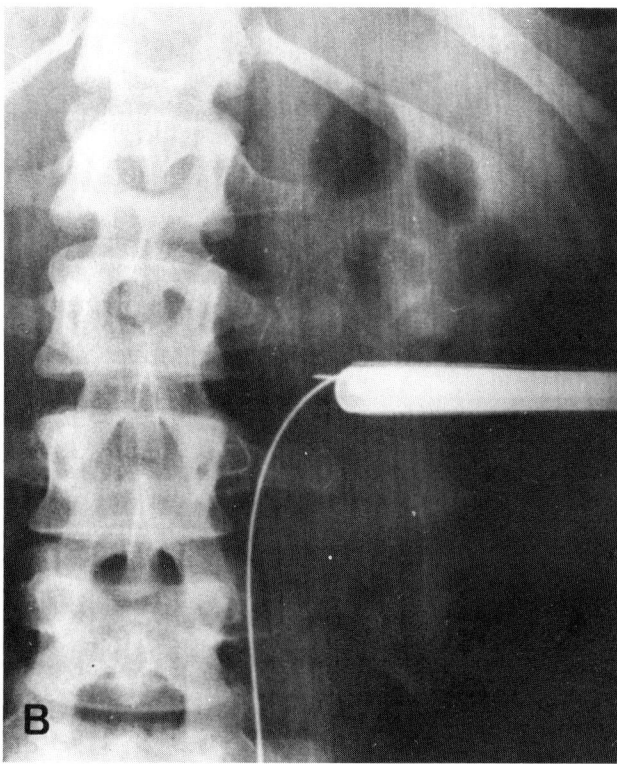
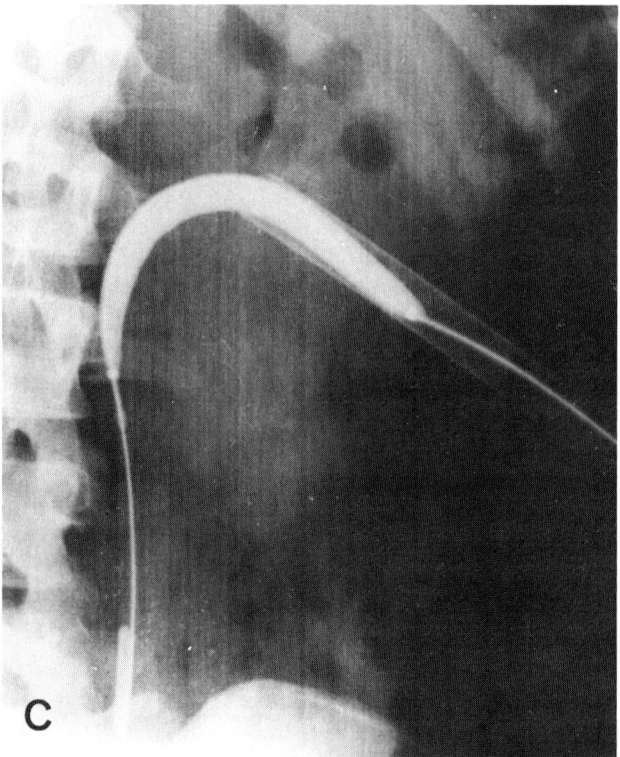
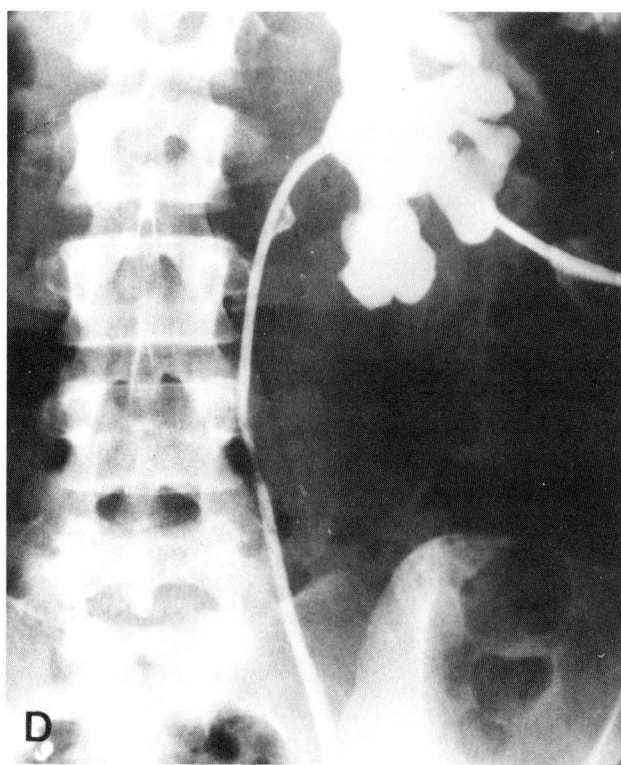

Figure 8.49 (A) Congenital stenosis of the pyeloureteral junction with a large hydronephrosis. (B) Creation of the nephrostomy track and introduction of a No. 26 French sheath, with ureteral catheterization and a Sacks knife utilized for nephroscope-guided ureterotomy. (C) Junction dilation with an Obert-type 10-mm balloon. (D) Control after dilation, with the tutor catheter maintained through the junction. There was a good evolution, with the hydronephrosis resolving (not shown).

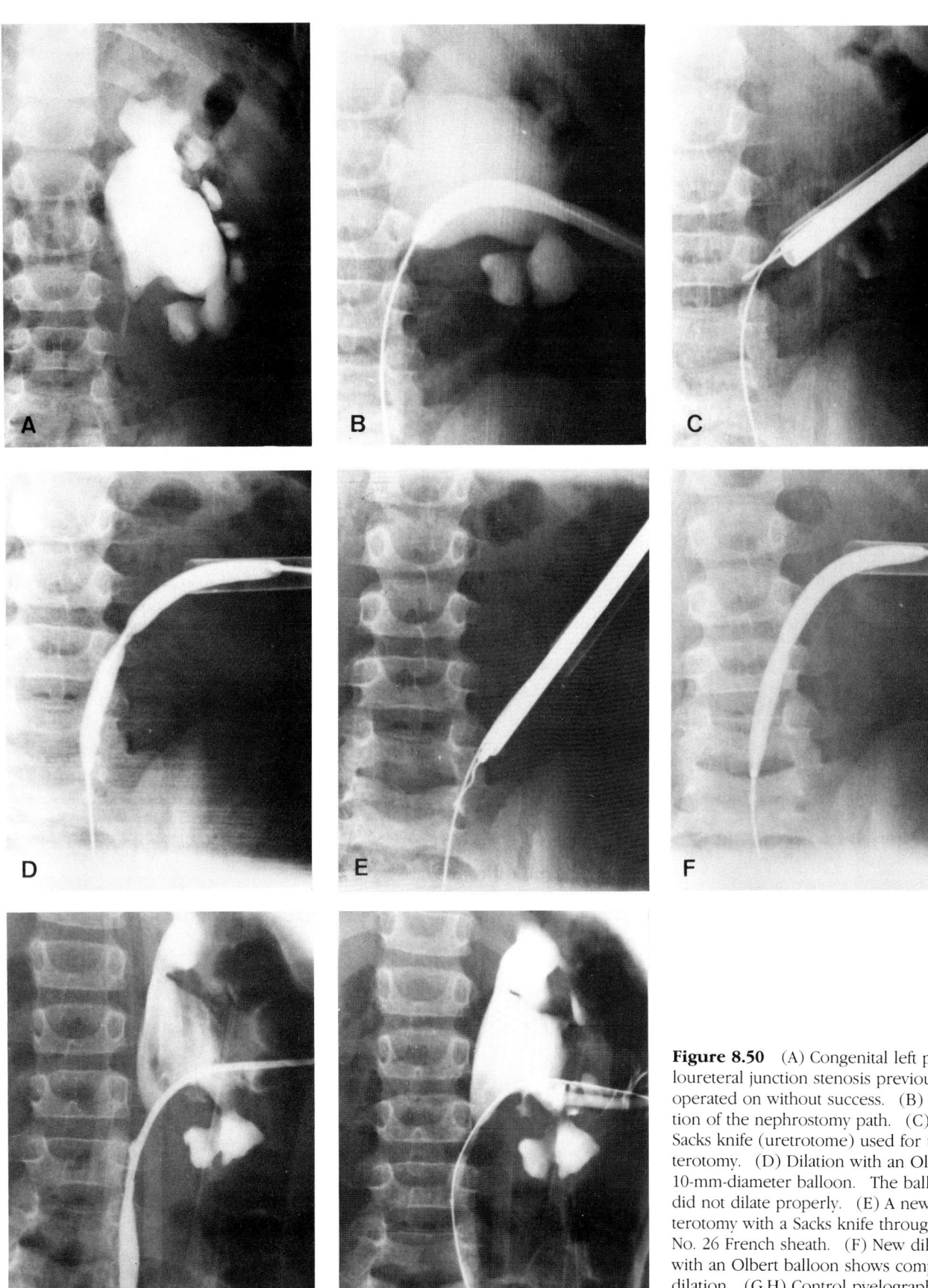

Figure 8.50 (A) Congenital left pyeloureteral junction stenosis previously operated on without success. (B) Dilation of the nephrostomy path. (C) A Sacks knife (uretrotome) used for ureterotomy. (D) Dilation with an Olbert 10-mm-diameter balloon. The balloon did not dilate properly. (E) A new ureterotomy with a Sacks knife through a No. 26 French sheath. (F) New dilation with an Olbert balloon shows complete dilation. (G,H) Control pyelography 21 days after surgery shows patency of the pyeloureteral junction.

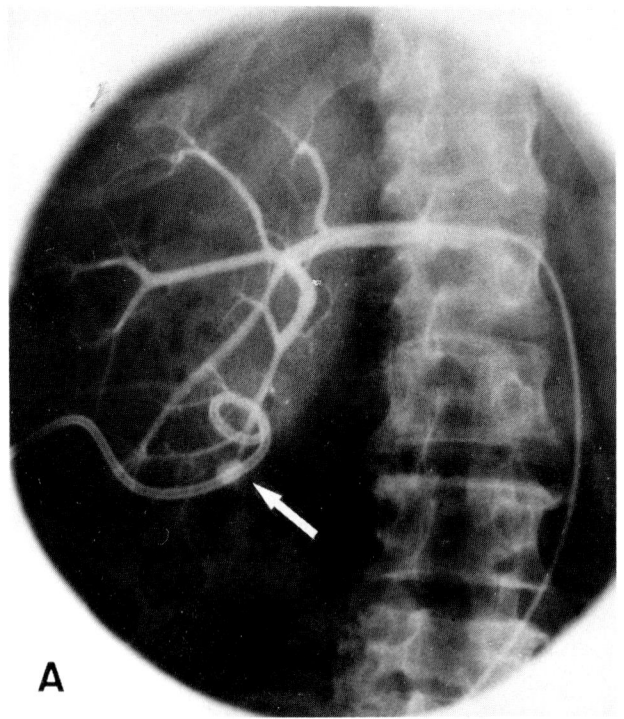 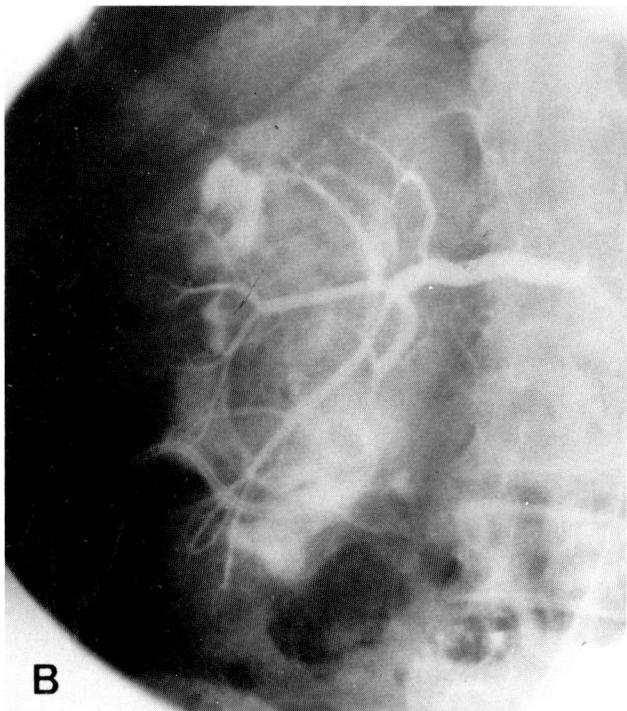

Figure 8.51 Massive hematuria after nephrostomy for hydronephrosis caused by tumoral obstruction of the distal ureter (uterine carcinoma).
(A) A nephrostomy catheter in the lower position associated with arterial trauma and the formation of a pseudoaneurysm (arrow). (B) Control after embolization of the lower pole branch with Gelfoam particles, which achieved permanent control of hematuria.

REFERENCES

Alken P, Huttschenreiter G, Gunter R, Marberger M. Percutaneous stone manipulation. *J Urol* 1981;125:463–466.

Almgard LE, Fernstrom I. Percutaneous nephropyelostomy. *Acta Radiol [Diagn] (Stockh)* 1974;15:288–294.

Bartley O, Chidekel N, Rabderg C. Percutaneous drainage of the renal pelvis for uraemia due to obstructed urinary outflow. *Acta Chir Scand* 1975;129:443.

Brodel M. The intrinsic blood vessels of the kidney and their significance in nephrotomy. *Johns Hopkins Hosp Bull* 1901;118:10–13.

Bush WH, Brannen GE, Lewis GP, Burnett LL. Upper ureteral calculi: Extraction via percutaneous nephrostomy. *AJR* 1985;144:795–799.

Caldamone AA, Frank IN. Percutaneous aspiration in the treatment of renal abscess. *J Urol* 1980;123:92–93.

Clayman RV, Castaneda-Zuniga WR. *Techniques in Endourology: A Guide to Percutaneous Removal of Renal and Ureteral Calculi.* Year Book, Chicago, 1984.

Dehesa MT, Castellano F, Cuerpo E, Revilla BJ, Pavon E. Nefrostomia percutania: Tecnica y resultados. Simposium sobre Endourologia, Zaragoza, 1985.

Dotter CT, Judkins MP. Transluminal treatment of arteriosclerotic obstruction. *Circulation* 1964;30:654–656.

Druy EM. A dilating introducer sheath for the antegrade insertion of ureteral stents. *AJR* 1985;145:1274–1276.

Ferruci JT, Wittenberg J. *Interventional Radiology of the Abdomen.* Williams & Wilkins, Baltimore, 1982.

Fernstrom I, Johnson B. Percutaneous pyelolithotomy: A new extraction technique. *Scand J Nephrol* 1976;10:257–259.

Gerber WL, Brown RC, Culp DA. Percutaneous nephrostomy with immediate dilation. *J Urol* 1981;125:169–171.

Goodwin WE, Kasey WC, Woolf W. Percutaneous trocar nephrostomy in hydronephrosis. *JAMA* 1955;157:981–984.

Gruntzig A, Hollf H. Perkutane rekanalisation chronischer arterieller: Verschlussmit einem neuem dilatationskatheter: Modifikation der dotterteqhnik. *Dtsch Med Wochenschr* 1974;99:502–505.

Haetinger RG, Bica VP. Adenocarcinoma de célula renal—revisão da literatura a propósito de dois casos de apresentação não usual. *Radiol Brasil* 1985;18:9–16.

Haetinger RG, Bica VP. Formas de apresentação e abordagem diagnóstica por imagem. Absc Retrod XVII Jornada de Radiologia do Rio de Janeiro, 1986.

Hodson J, Maling MJ, McManamon PJ, Lewis MG. Reflux nephropathy. *Kidney Int* 1975;8:50–58.

Kaye KW, Reinke DB. Detailed caliceal anatomy for endourology. *J Urol* 1984;132:1085–1088.

Leal JL. A new technique for the transurethral or percutaneous removal of renal stones. *J Urol* 1985;134:936–939.

Le Roy AJ, May GR, Bender CE, Williams HJ Jr, McGough PF, Segura JW, Patterson DE. Percutaneous nephrostomy for stone removal. *Radiology* 1984;151:607–612.

Lunderquist A, Lunderquist M. Guidewire for percutaneous transhepatic cholangiography. *Radiology* 1979;132:228–232.

Marberger M, Stackl W, Hrudy W, Kroise A. Late sequelae of ultrasonic lithotripsy of renal calculi. *J Urol* 1985;133:170–173.

Mauren W, Muller P, Ferruci J, Butch R, Simeone J, Neff C, Yoder I, Coladu N, Pfister R. Percutaneous drainage of postoperative abdominal and pelvic lymphoceles. *AJR* 1985;145:1065–1069.

Mayo ME, Krieger NJ, Rudo TG. Effect of percutaneous nephrostolithotomy on renal function. *J Urol* 1985;133:167–169.

Mercado S, Hawkins J, Herrera MA, Caridi JC, Hawkins IF. Simplified method of introducing double-J stent catheters using a coaxial sheath system. *AJR* 1985;145:1271–1273.

Meyers MA. *Dynamic Radiology of the Abdomen: Normal and Pathologic Anatomy.* Springer-Verlag, New York, 1982.

Neashore F, Andrew N, Lowell K, Diondu P. Balloon dilation of upper ureteral strictures in primatas. *J Urol* 1986;136:342–343.

Okuda K, Tanikawa K, Emura T, Kuratomi S, et al. Nonsurgical percutaneous transhepatic cholangiography, diagnostic significance in medical problems of the liver. *Dig Dis Sci* 1974;19:21–36.

Pedersen JF, Hancke SH, Kristensen JK. Renal carbuncle: Antibiotic therapy governed by ultrasonically guided aspiration. *J Urol* 1973;109:777–778.

Picus D, Weyman PJ, Clayman RV, McClennam BL. Intercostal space nephrostomy for percutaneous stone removal. *AJR* 1985;147:393–397.

Quinn SFQ, Dyer R, Smathers R, Glass T, Wright E, Roberts C, Argenhright RT. Balloon dilatation of prostatic urethra. *Radiology* 1985;157:57–59.

Reddy PK, Hulbert JC, Lange PH, Clayman RV, Marcuse A, Steven L, Muller RP, Hunter DW, Castaneda-Zuniga WR, Amplatz K. Percutaneous removal of renal and urethral calculi: Experience with 400 cases. *J Urol* 1985;134:662–665.

Rhasidy LR, Smith AD. The reentry nefrotomy catheter for endourological applications. *J Urol* 1985;133:165–166.

Rives RK, Harty JI, Amin M. Renal abscess: Emerging concepts of diagnosis and treatment. *J Urol* 1980;124:446–447.

Scales FE, Katzen BTK, VanBreda A, Alperstein J, Abramson E, Rhame R. Impassable urethral strictures: Percutaneous transvesical catheterization and balloon dilatation. *Radiology* 1985;157:59–61.

Scott JES. The role of surgery in the management of vesico-ureteric reflux. *Kidney Int* 1975;8:73–79.

Segura JW. Endourology. *J Urol* 1984;132:1079–1084.

Seldinger S. Catheter Replacement of the needle in percutaneous arteriography: A new technique. *Acta Radiol [Diagn] (Stockh)* 1953;139:368–372.

Smellie J, Edwards D, Hunter N, Normand ICS, Prescod N. Vesicouteteric reflux and renal scarring. *Kidney Int* 1975;8:65–71.

Smith AD, Reinke DB, Miller RP, Lange PH. Percutaneous nephrostomy in the management of ureteral renal calculi. *Radiology* 1979;133:49–54.

Smith PK. Glomerular lesions in atrophic pyelonephritis and reflux nephropathy. *Kidney Int* 1975;8:81–84.

Torres LJM, Ruiz SS, Gonzales HJ, Sanz RC. Nefrostomia percutanea: III. Fin de semana urologico. Simposium sobre Endourologia, October 1985.

Webb DR, Payne SR, Wickhan JEA. Extracorporeal shockwave lithotripsy and percutaneous renal surgery. *Br J Urol* 1986;58:1–5.

Witherington R, Shelor WC. Treatment of postoperative ureteral stricture by catheter diltation: A forgotten procedure. *Urology* 1980;16:592.

Young AT, Hunter DW, Lange P et al. The CO_2 flush: A new technique for percutaneous extraction of ureteral calculi. *Radiology* 1985;154:828–829.

Ureteral Procedures

RENAN UFLACKER

A range of different percutaneous procedures are currently performed to treat ureteral obstructive lesions. The procedure chosen varies in accordance with the nature of the obstructive process. Lithiasis is the most common cause of ureteral obstruction, followed by pelvic and retroperitoneal neoplastic lesions, congenital stenoses, changes related to surgical procedures, and ureteral occlusive abnormalities due to a retroperitoneal fibrotic process.

Overlapping of and associations between these etiologies occur frequently. The possibility of developing serious infectious processes occurs simultaneously with obstruction. The percutaneous therapeutic approach to these abnormalities depends in most cases on the access route created through percutaneous nephrostomy. The methodology, the different options, and the processes treated with percutaneous nephrostomy are discussed in the section on percutaneous nephrostomy. The anatomic aspects involved in this process of puncture and drainage were discussed earlier in this book.

UROLITHIASIS

Urolithiasis involving the urinary tract is a multifactorial disease which represents a significant public health problem. A variety of intrinsic and extrinsic factors influence the incidence of this disease in both individuals and populations.

About 16.4 of 10,000 people in the United States will develop urinary lithiasis (around 12 percent of the population). Stones in the upper urinary tract are found predominantly in the ureter in two-thirds to three-fourths of patients, and only one-fourth to one-third of stones are found in the kidney. Distal ureteral calculi are found in 70 to 80 percent of these patients; spontaneous displacement of stones occurs in over 62 percent.

Renal stones are solid and are formed by crystalline aggregates with small organic and inorganic noncrystalline portions. There are four main types of renal calculi, classified according to the predominant component: calcium (70 to 80 percent), with phosphate (5 to 10 percent), oxylate (35 to 50 percent), or both (20 to 30 percent); struvite (15 to 20 percent); cystine (1 to 3 percent); and uric acid (5 to 10 percent).

Struvite stones are invariably associated with urease-producing microorganisms, most frequently *Proteus* sp. This is the component which predominates in staghorn calculi.

Many intrinsic and extrinsic risk factors are associated with urolithiasis, but extrinsic factors seem to play a more significant role in calcium stones.

EXTRACTION OF URETERAL CALCULI

Proximal and medial ureteral calculi are better approached through percutaneous nephrolithotomy (nephrostomy, dilation, and instrumentation) than through the use of an ureterorenoscope. The opposite is true of distal calculi. Calculi in the middle third, however, may be better approached endoscopically.

Some authors suggest that before the procedure is started in the upper ureter, an angioplasty-type balloon catheter with a 6-mm diameter should be introduced in a retrograde fashion.

Puncture of the collecting system should be made into the middle caliceal group at the infundibular level to create a relatively straight track. Intercostal puncture into the renal upper pole provides an even more direct and rectilinear path, but there is a much greater chance of developing complications related to violation of the pleural space. The objective of this procedure is to displace the stone from the ureter into the pelvis. Several different methods can be used for this purpose. Retrograde introduction of a catheter into the ureter by itself may displace a stone into the pelvis, where it can be more easily removed.

A balloon catheter can also be used retrogradely for releasing the stone, displacing it, or washing it away. A saline jet or diluted contrast medium injected retrogradely at 10 to 15 mL/s will displace the calculus in most cases. A sheath or large nephrostomy tube should be kept open throughout the procedure. Forced injections of carbonic gas can be used as an alternative.

According to some authors, irrigation procedures should always precede direct instrumentation of the ureter with baskets, guides, catheters, and nephroscopes. Without irrigation, trauma may occur, causing edema and preventing displacement. This type of technique was successful in about 87 percent of cases in a recent series. Other authors consider the flushing technique dispensable and proceed directly to antegrade instrumentation.

Antegrade manipulation of ureteral calculi should be attempted only when the stones have been lodged in the

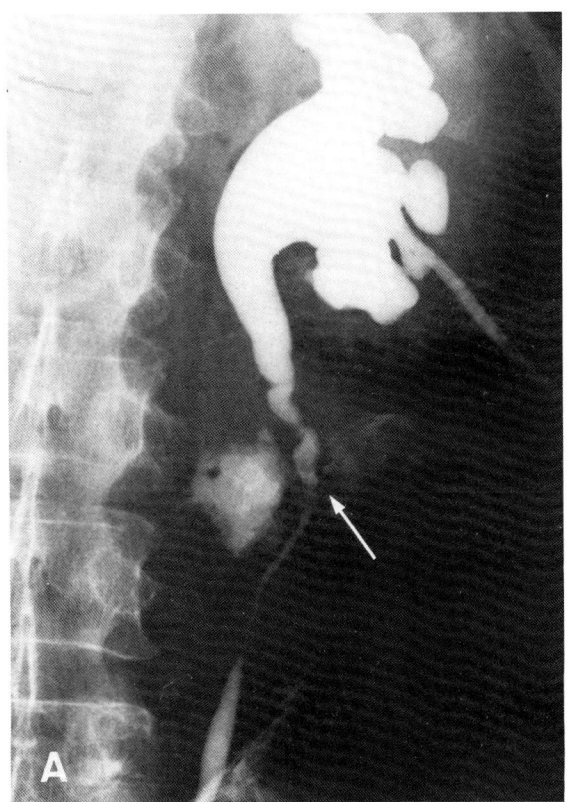 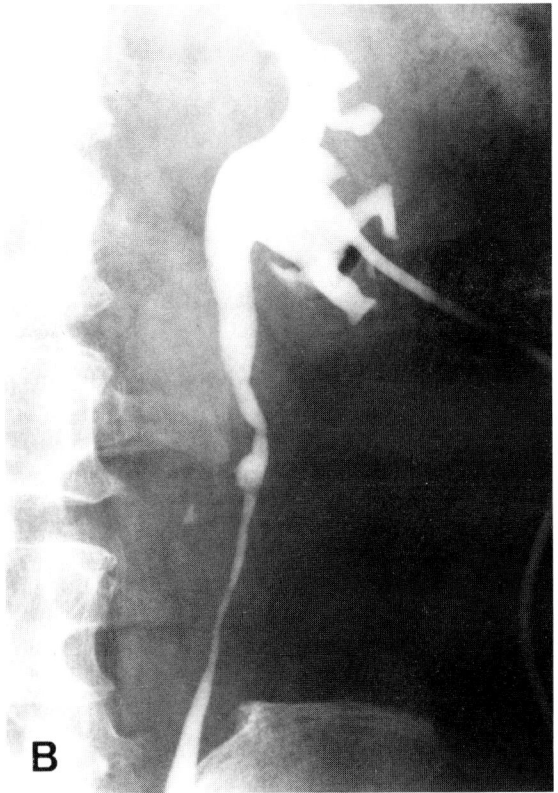

Figure 8.52 (A) A 53-year-old patient with sepsis caused by pyonephrosis after unsuccessful surgical ureterolithotomy caused an ureterocutaneous fistula. The stone remained in the ureter (arrow) for 6 weeks. (B) Nephrostomy was kept open for 22 days, closing the fistula and resolving the infection. The stone adhered to the ureteral wall for a total of 9 weeks. Removal by the percutaneous route was contraindicated. A new surgical ureterolithotomy was successful.

ureter for less than 3 to 4 weeks. After that, the calculus remains firmly fixed to the ureteral walls, and its percutaneous removal becomes difficult or even impossible (Fig. 8.52), with a higher risk of developing a ureteral lesion.

Manipulation of ureteral calculi is usually technically easy but the results obtained may sometimes be disappointing. In a recent paper, LeRoy reported a 93.8 percent success rate with antegrade percutaneous removal of calculi 3 to 6 mm in diameter from the proximal ureter.

After dilation of the nephrostomy track, with a safety guidewire maintained all the way outside the sheath, a Dormia basket may be introduced down the ureter to grasp the stone under fluoroscopic view only (Fig. 8.53). This is frequently unsatisfactory, and it may be necessary to handle the stone basket with direct viewing through a flexible nephroscope. This technique may also be insufficient; in that case a rigid nephroscope may be used to grasp the calculus with a forceps or rigid clamp.

In handling ureteral calculi, it is advisable to use a modified stone basket with a filiform and flexible distal tip, similar to a guidewire. This will allow repeated advances of the sheath and basket beyond the calculus. The safety guidewire should remain above the ureteral stone to prevent interference with the basket and to decrease the number of instruments near the calculus.

The basket can be steered with a Cobra-type catheter or through a steerable-tip catheter manufactured by Medi-Tech (Fig. 8.53). Antegrade removal of ureteral stones is more frequently successful in acute obstructions when the ureter is dilated. Chronic ureteral calculi are more common and are usually trapped between edematous folds of ureteral mucosa, which prevent stone grasping by the basket. If the ureter is dilated with an angioplasty balloon, it is possible to obtain full opening of the basket.

Even in acute occlusions, a catheter should be maintained across the site where the stone was previously lodged in order to prevent the formation of synechias and ureteral occlusion after the procedure (Fig. 8.53). If handling results in trauma and obstruction by a synechia, the obstruction usually can be reopened and dilated with a No. 8 or 9 French catheter, which is kept inside the ureter for 3 weeks to resolve the obstruction (Fig. 8.53).

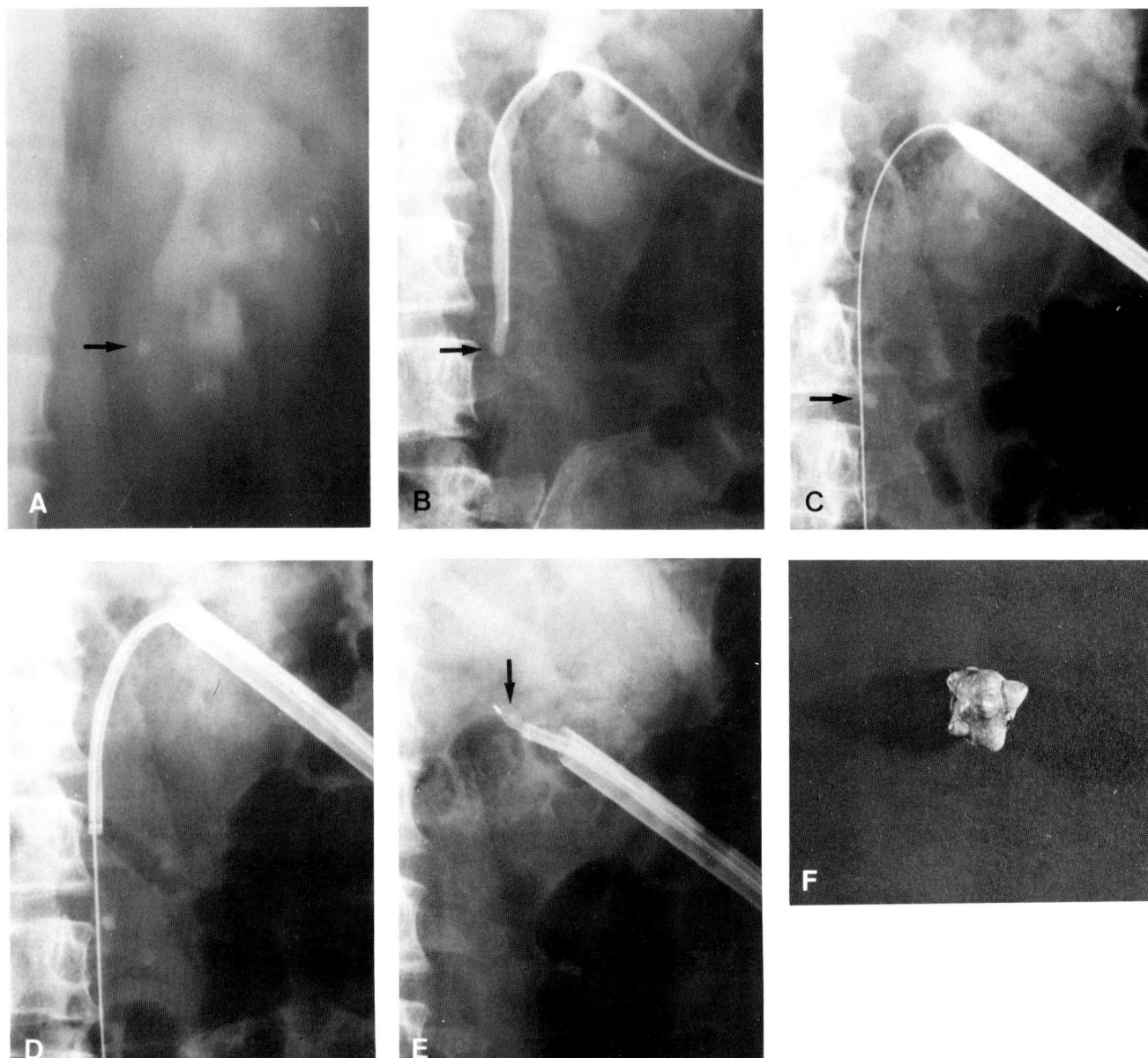

Figure 8.53

DILATATION, URETERAL RECANALIZATION, AND STENTS

Nonlithiasic ureteral obstructions are most frequently caused by a tumor or a surgical or percutaneous procedure. They can also be congenital (at the level of the ureteropelvic junction) or can result from retroperitoneal processes (retroperitoneal fibrosis).

Different solutions are indicated for different types of ureteral occlusion. The use of ureteral chronic double J-stents provides adequate palliation for obstructions caused by malignant lesions, but this is not the proper way to deal with benign postsurgical obstruction. Balloon dilation is useless in malignant lesions, except in making the introduction of drainage catheters easier. It is appropriate, however, for postsurgical and other benign lesions, such as retroperitoneal fibrosis. Dilation of a benign lesion may nonetheless be followed by the placement of a ureteral prosthesis for a fixed period to "mold" the ureter. Congenital lesions also require combined procedures, with the use of a balloon, a Sacks knife, and ureteral stents for several weeks.

Ureteral dilatation can be obtained by using straight catheters; balloons are not necessary in some cases. The normal diameter of a ureter varies from No. 5 French (1.67 mm) to No. 9 French (3.00 mm), and it is necessary to dilate the ureter above these limits.

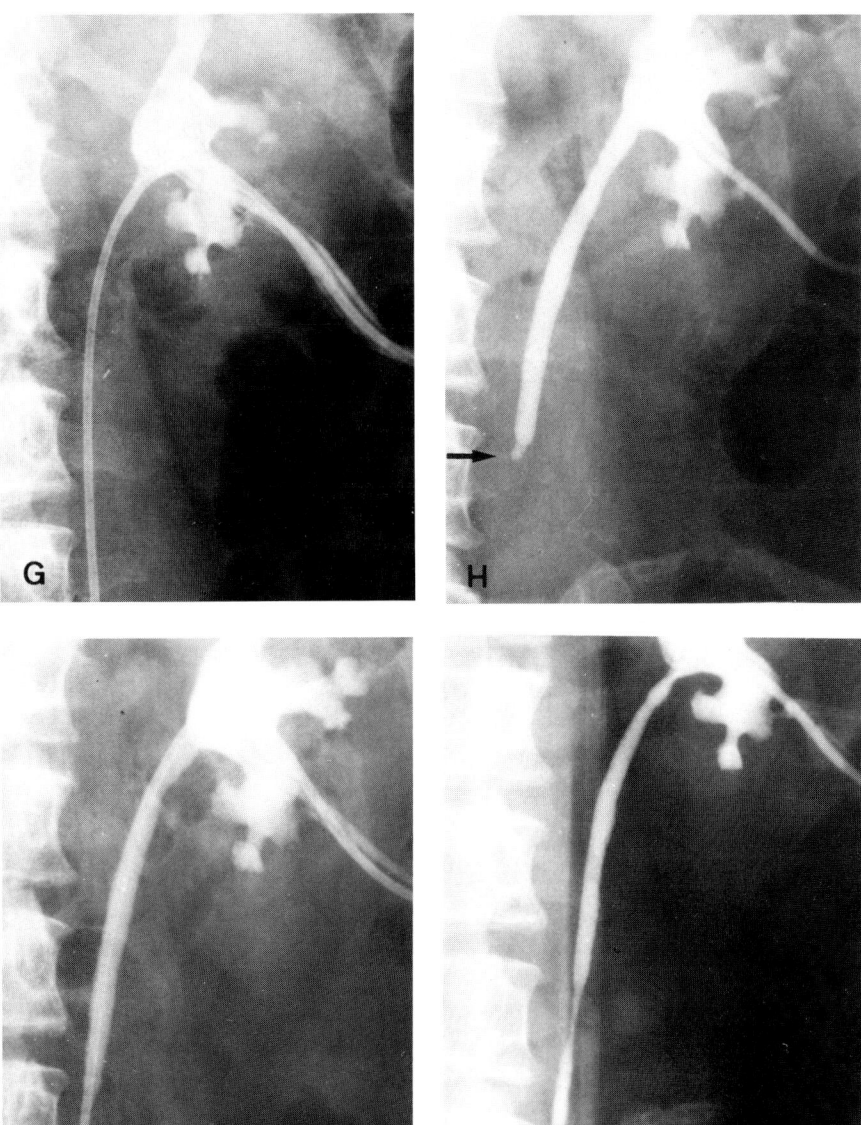

Figure 8.53 Percutaneous extraction of a ureteral calculus.
(A) Urographic study with a tomogram shows the calculus in the proximal ureter (arrow). The patient was scheduled for percutaneous lithotripsy. (B) By the time nephrostomy was performed, the stone had migrated to the middle third of the ureter (arrow). A decision was made to dilate the track at the same time, using a Dormia basket for extraction. (C) A guidewire passing beyond the ureteral calculus (arrow) and dilation with Amplatz system. (D) A No. 24 French sheath inside the track and a steerable-tip catheter (Medi-Tech) entering the ureter. (E) The stone already trapped inside the Dormia basket (arrow) and being removed. (F) A spiked ureteral calculus with a diameter of 5 mm. (G) A Malecot probe for nephrostomy was placed and a ureteral tube was introduced through the stone site. (H) The ureteral tube was accidentally removed on the third day, and a ureteral obstruction developed because of a synechia (arrow). (I) After 2 weeks, a new ureteral tube was passed and remained in position for 3 additional weeks. (J) After treatment, the ureter was kept permanently patent.

Dilatation with a Balloon

As in all other cases of percutaneous renal manipulation, the procedure should start with a nephrostomy, which can be performed in one or more sessions. When nephrostomy has been performed previously, renal function tests can be obtained and the track becomes mature, favoring posterior manipulation. When nephrostomy is used only to gain access to the collecting system, the tube should be dilated to No. 9 or 10 French to minimize resistance to its introduction in the flank and kidney. Access to an interpolar calix makes manipulation easier, as it creates a more rectilinear track than can be obtained when a lower calix is punctured.

The ureter is cannulized according to a previously described technique (Fig. 8.28), and a straight catheter with a distal orifice and No. 6 French diameter is introduced through the stenosis. The neoplastic or benign nature of the lesion should be defined before dilation is performed. Computed tomography, tumor smear, and/or puncture biopsy can be used if the diagnosis was not known previously. When the catheter is near the obstruction, contrast medium is injected to document the stenosis and its extension.

A Lunderquist torque guidewire or a Terumo guidewire is manipulated through the stenosis, and the No. 6 French catheter is advanced over the guidewire. After passing beyond the stenosis, the guidewire can be replaced by a more rigid Lunderquist exchange type or an extra-stiff Amplatz type. A dilatation balloon with a diameter from 4 to 10 mm (most frequently 6 to 8 mm) and a length of 4 cm is then introduced over the guidewire (Fig. 8.54).

Radiopaque markings on the balloon are centralized at the level of the stenosis, and the balloon is then inflated with contrast diluted to 50% until it reaches its maximum diameter (Fig. 8.42). In treating these ureteral lesions, it is advisable to use high-pressure balloons (up to 12 to 17 atm) (Fig. 8.44). Distension is maintained up to 60 s and repeated three to four times in accordance with the response observed in the formation of the balloon's central waist. Common polyethylene and polyvinyl chloride balloons deform when used in rigid ureteral stenoses and may even be ruptured (Fig. 8.55).

After dilation with a balloon, a No. 9 or 10 French tube is introduced and then kept in place for 3 weeks. After the ureteral tube is pulled, a nephrostomy tube is placed for at least 48 h. If control pyelography shows patency and if intrapelvic pressure is below 12 to 15 cm H_2O, the nephrostomy tube can be removed. If dilation is not successful, the procedure should be repeated two or three more times until optimum results are obtained. Some lesions restenose a few days, months, or years after treatment.

The duration of dilation with a balloon is controversial. Some authors initially advocated prolonged dilations up to 6 h instead of a few minutes. Today it is believed that dilations lasting for hours can cause ischemia in the ureteral wall, with potentially irreversible lesions. Therefore, it is much safer to repeat the dilation as many times as necessary but not for such long periods.

Dilatation with a Catheter

When catheters alone are used, it may not be possible to dilate the ureter to the desired diameter in the first session. The catheter size is increased to No. 10 French. The first No. 6 to 7 French catheter should remain through the stenosis site for 4 to 8 weeks; subsequent changes can be made every 2 weeks. Van Andel–type catheters may be useful, but their high linear progression force can cause ureteral injury, including total rupture, and so their use should be restricted to experienced hands.

Retrograde dilatations with a catheter are more useful in females because of the ease of catheterization under cystoscopy.

After the desired ureteral dilatation has been achieved, an internal-external catheter or a ureteral stent (double J-catheter) may be maintained for several weeks. The ureteral prosthesis can be handled by the urethral route and can even be replaced if occlusion occurs (Fig. 8.56).

The literature suggests the following schedule for maintaining stents and ureteral tubes in place:

1. 3 to 5 days after ureteral manipulation for edema
2. 10 to 15 days after the operative period for surgical ureteral anastomosis
3. 25 to 30 days for ureteral anastomosis with a risk due to stress, infection, or fibrosis
4. 35 to 45 days for maintaining the diameter to allow regeneration of injured or fistulous sites

The experience of some authors has shown that 3 to 5 days is too short a period for removing a ureteral catheter after manipulation because of the high risk of forming synechias. It is therefore suggested that the catheter be maintained in place for 1 or 2 weeks in these patients.

Thirty-five to 45 days is usually too long for treating fistulas; 21 to 25 days is usually sufficient. With a nephrostomy alone, ureteral or junctional fistulas may close without stenotic sequelae in 3 weeks (Fig. 8.57).

The use of ureteral stents requires additional information. Very soft silicone ureteral stents are preferable, although they are more difficult to introduce. One of the most recently developed types is the universal-length ureteral Druy stent (Fig. 8.58), which requires the use of

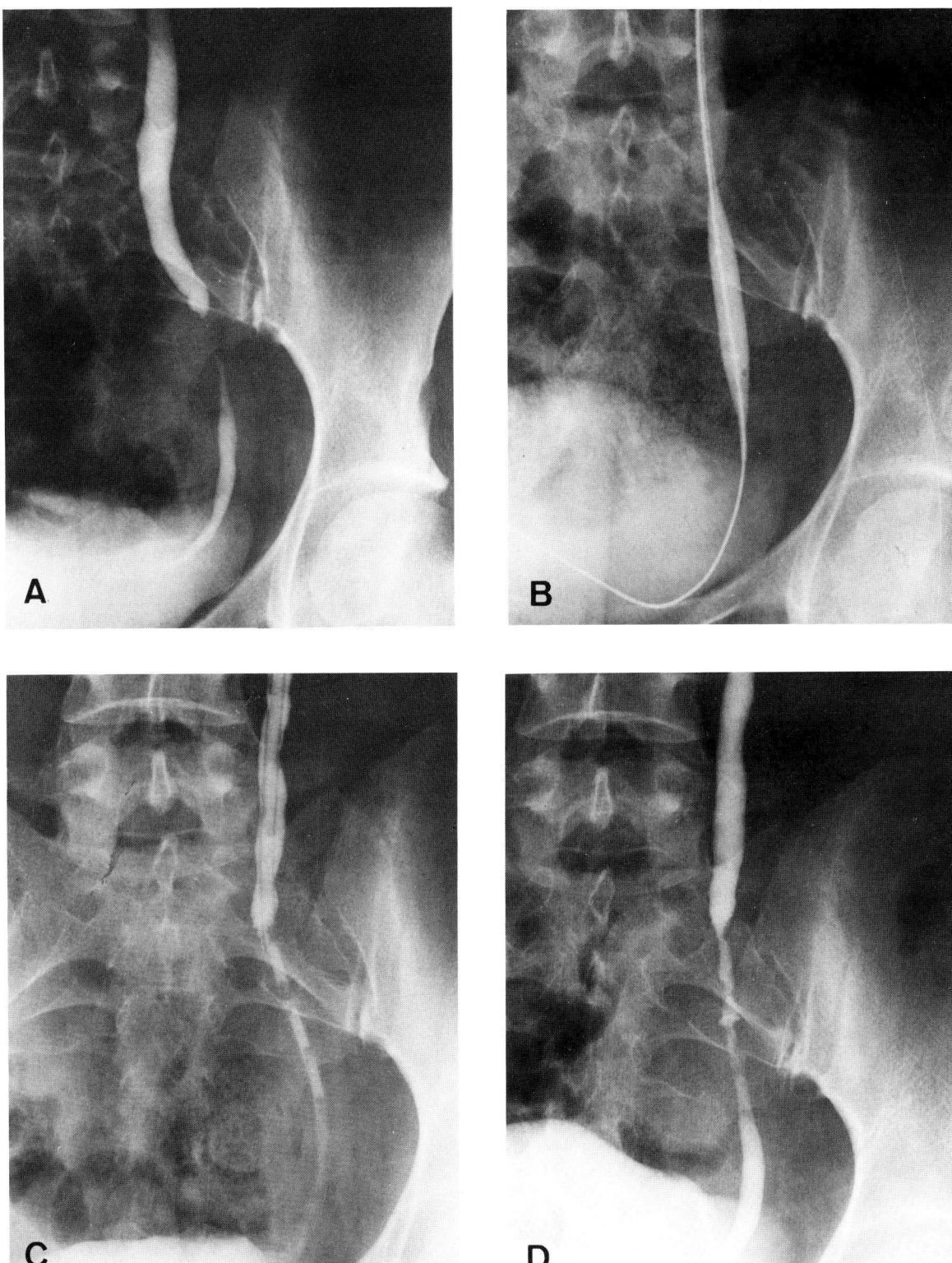

Figure 8.54 (A) A ureteral stenosis probably due to fibrosi after urinary bladder surgery for endometriosis that caused left hydronephrosis. (B) Nephrostomy was performed, and after 48 h the ureter was manipulated and dilated with an 8-mm balloon. Urethral catheterization had to be used to stretch the guidewire and pass the balloon through the stenosis (not shown). (C) After dilation, a No. 10 French catheter was maintained as a tutor through the stenosis for 3 weeks. (D) Final result of ureteral dilation shows patency, but with irregular margins.

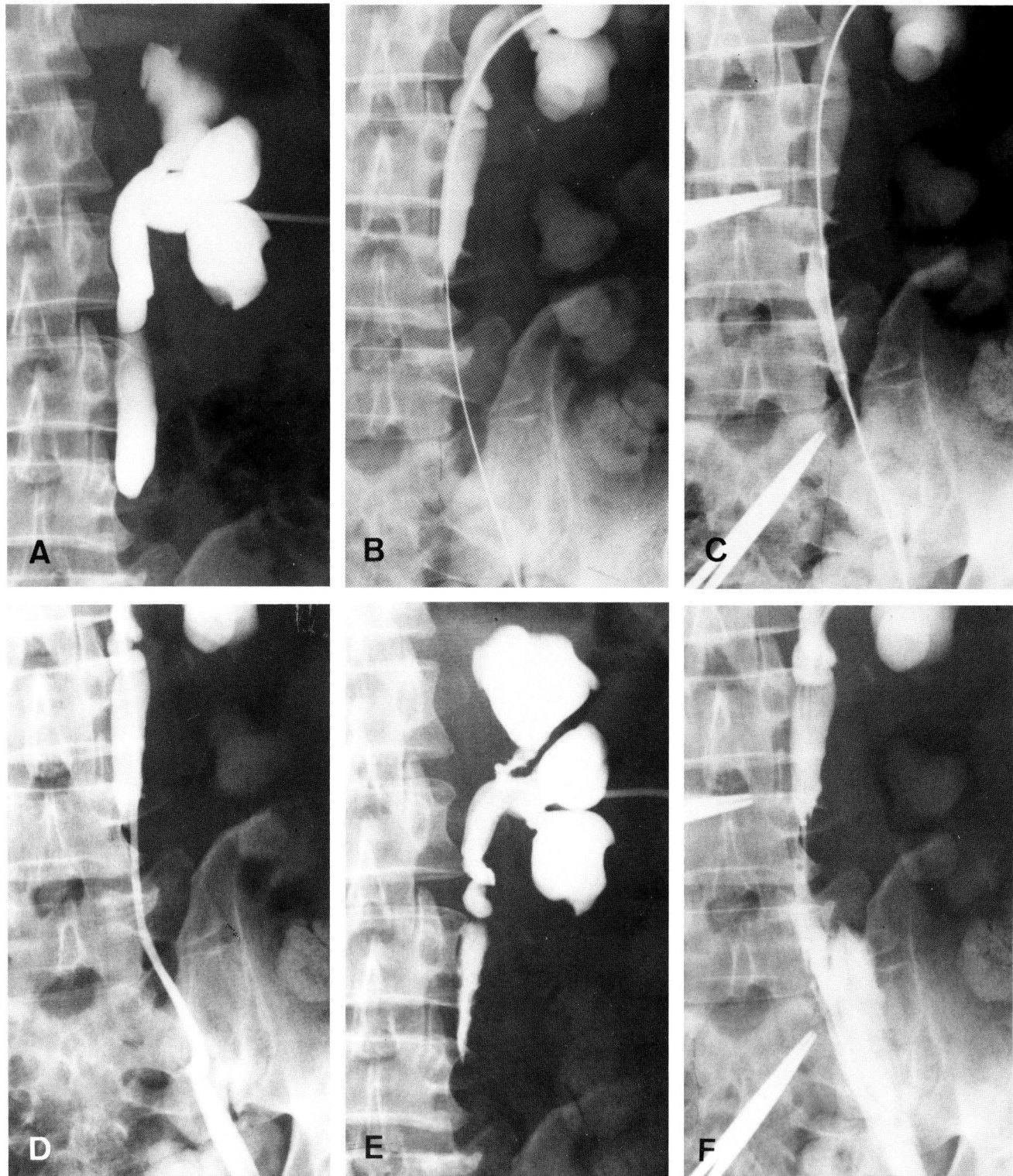

Figure 8.55 A patient with retroperitoneal fibrosis and bilateral ureteral obstruction.
(A) Left nephrostomy showing dilatation of the collecting system and ureteral obstruction. Nephrostomy was performed bilaterally and provided relief for 3 weeks. (B) After 3 weeks, the left ureter was manipulated and the obstruction was passed. (C) The site of stenosis was dilated with a 6-mm balloon. Note the deformity of the polyethylene balloon caused by rupture. (D) A No. 8 French tutor catheter maintained for 3 weeks through the stenosis. (E) Control after tutor removal showing ureteral occlusion. (F) A new dilation was performed with a 10-mm balloon, which caused ureteral laceration with extravasation. (G) Control after 2 weeks showing ureteral patency, with normal diuresis having resumed. (H) Control after right nephrostomy shows right ureteral obstruction. (I) Ureteral manipulation with the introduction of a guidewire into the bladder. (J) Dilatation with an 8-mm balloon. (K) A No. 8 French tutor catheter crossing the dilated lesion. A good evolution was obtained with removal of the nephrostomies after 3 weeks, with normal diuresis.

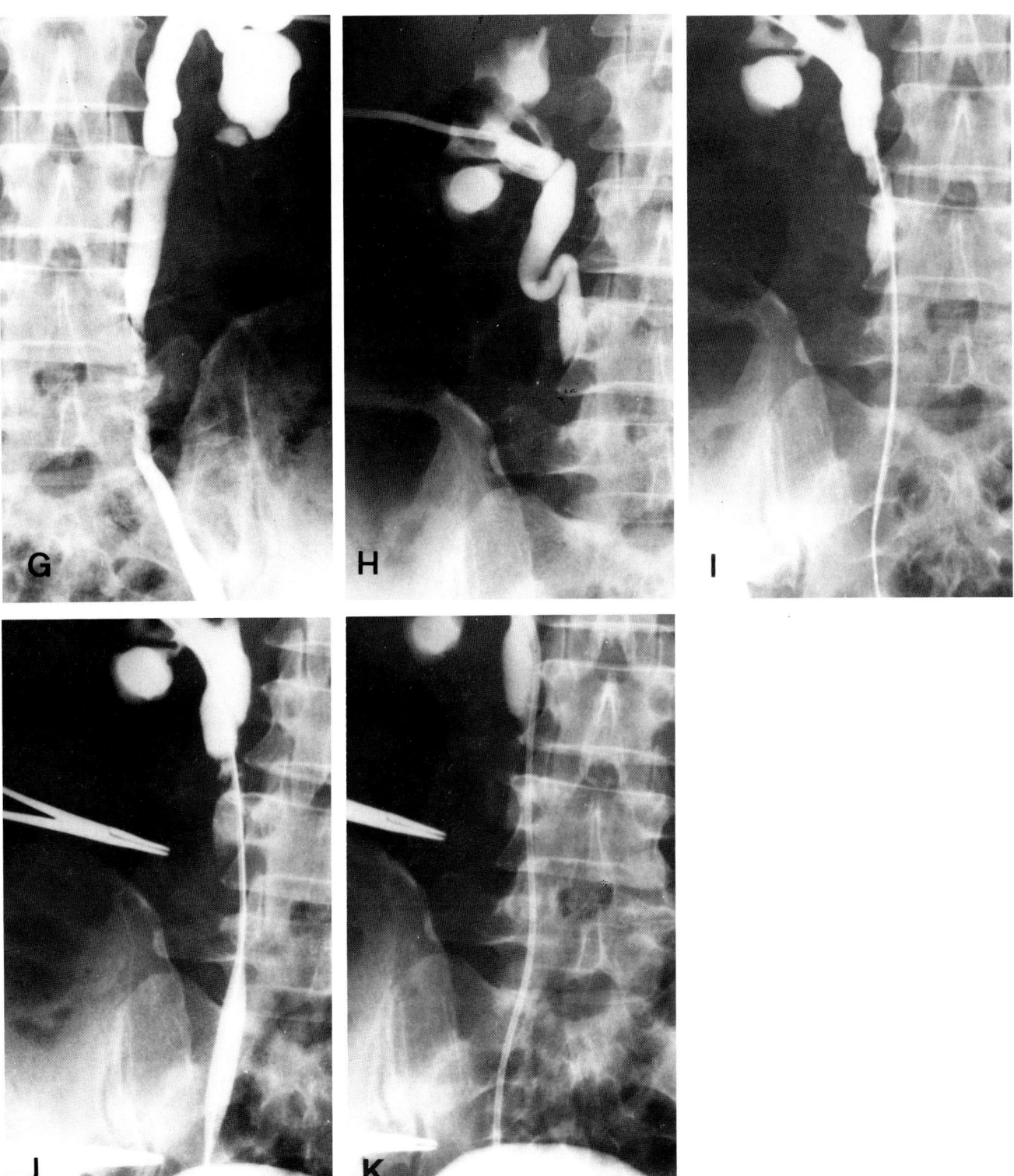

Figure 8.55 *Continued*

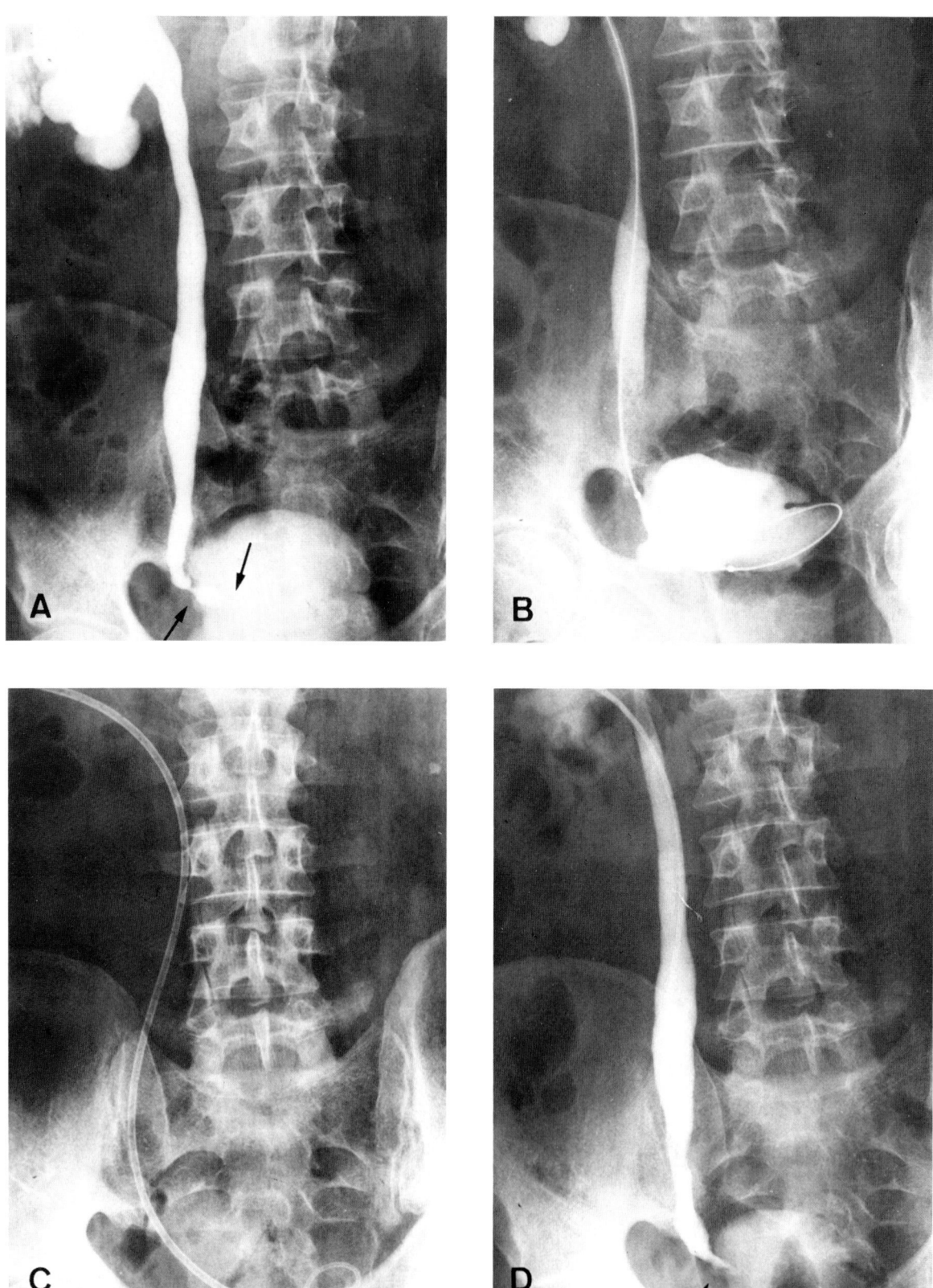

Figure 8.56 (A) A right ureteral stenosis after a vesicoureteral anastomosis (arrows). (B) Dilation with an 8-mm balloon in the ureterovesical junction. (C) A No. 9 French internal-external drainage catheter which remained in place for 3 weeks after dilation. (D) Control after 3 weeks shows some residual stenosis (arrow). (E) A double J-catheter was placed as a ureteral stent on the right. (F) Control shows tube patency. (G) A Druy stent in an adequate position during control after removal of the nephrostomy. (H) Excretory urography showing patency of the ureteral stent. The stent was removed after 6 months.

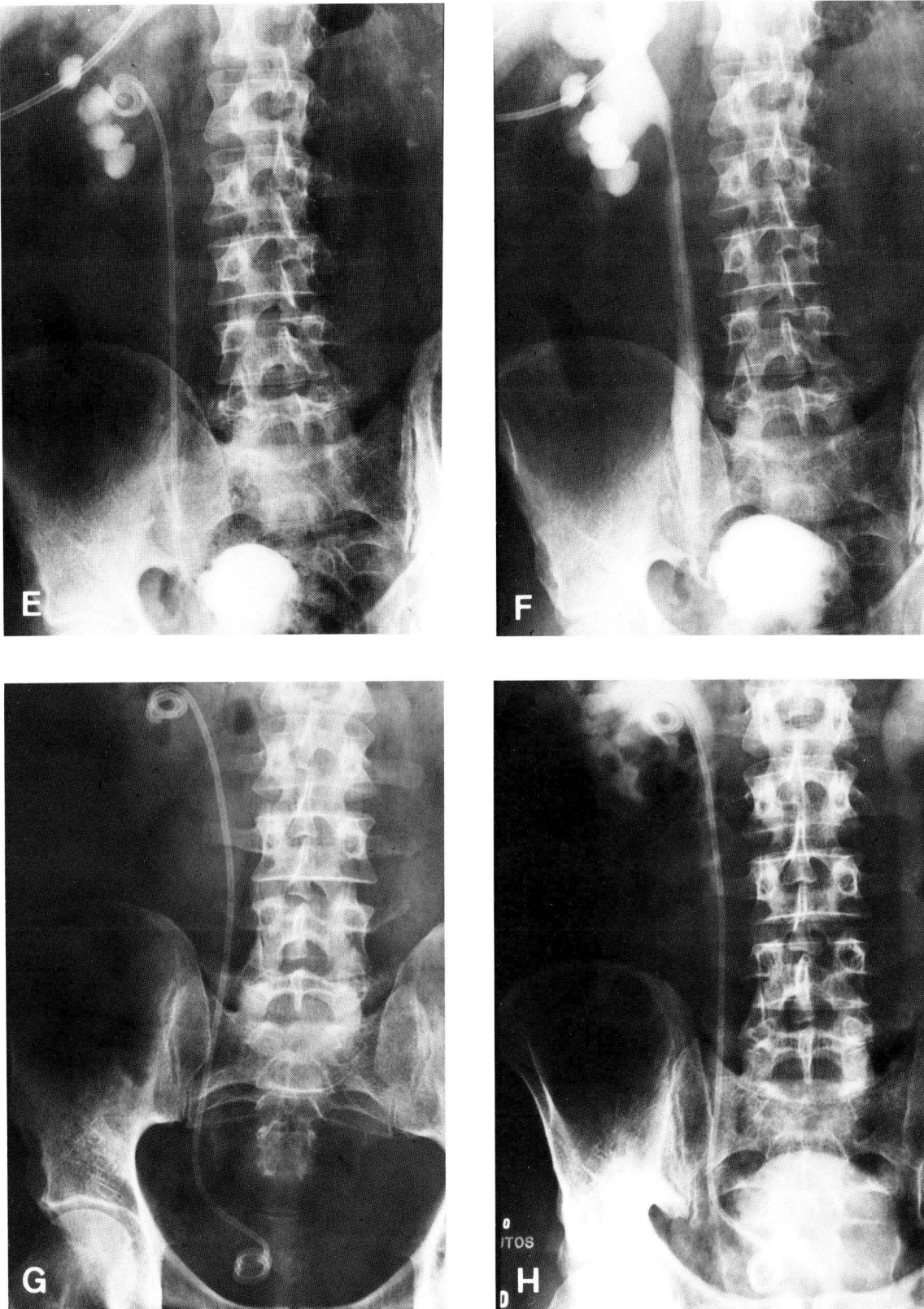

Figure 8.56 *Continued*

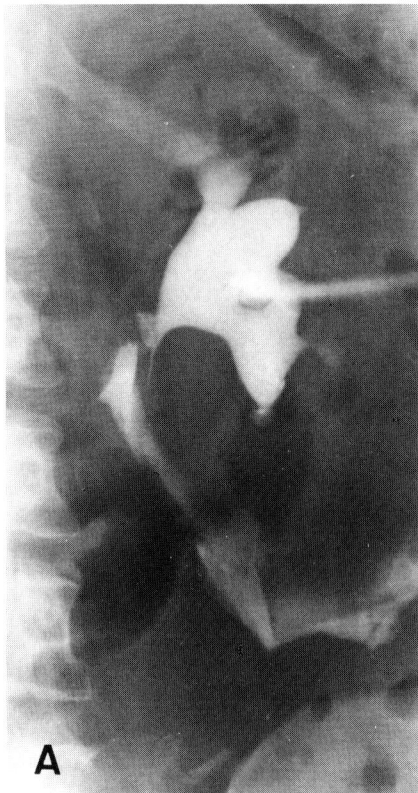 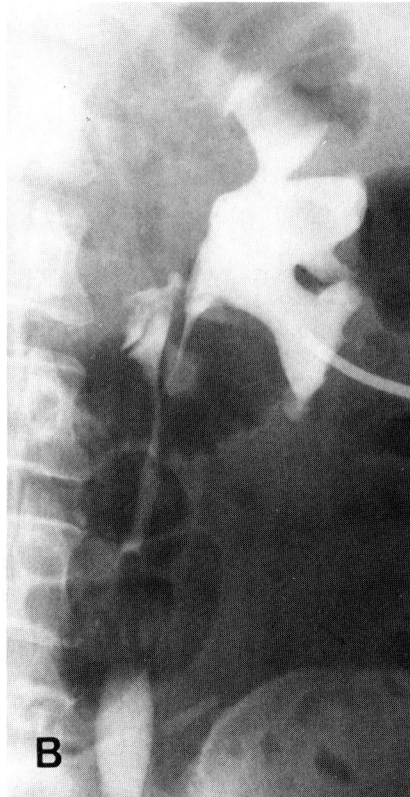 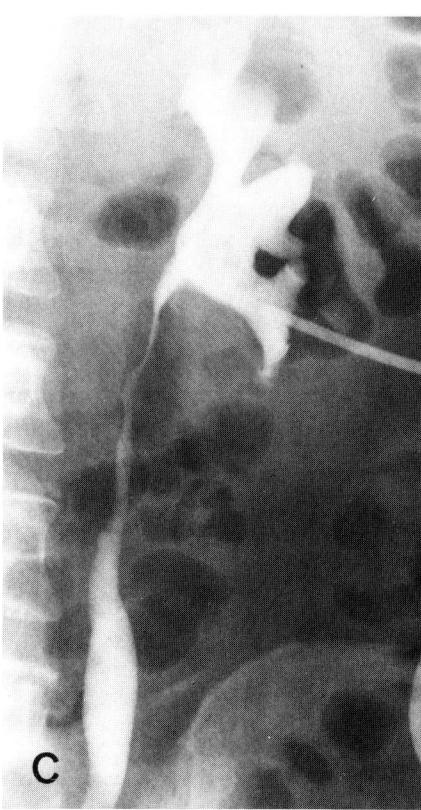

Figure 8.57 (A) A fistula at the pyeloureteral junction after ureterolithotomy. (B) The fistula became dry within 2 days after nephrostomy was performed. Extravasation of contrast medium was present after 1 week. (C) Control after 3 weeks showing a completely occluded fistula; the nephrostomy catheter was then removed. There was no residual ureteral stenosis.

a peel-away sheath that should be torn when the stent is removed. The placement technique is as follows:

1. Nephrostomy is performed as previously described.
2. A guidewire is introduced into the bladder. A Cobra No. 6.5 French catheter can be used for this manipulation.
3. The sheath is introduced into the bladder with a Teflon introducer inside, coaxially, over the guidewire. The introducer is then removed (Fig. 8.58).
4. The ureteral prosthesis is lubricated with silicone and advanced through the sheath and over the guidewire. When it is totally inside the sheath, a special insertion catheter is used to push it through until its tip reaches the renal pelvis.
5. With the introducer and the guidewire kept stationary, the peel-away sheath is slowly removed and torn in two by pulling both white knobs (Fig. 8.58) until it is removed completely.
6. While the introducer is kept stationary with the ureteral prosthesis, the guidewire is pulled until it is free in the renal pelvis so that a nephrostomy tube can be introduced. Removal of the guidewire will allow the extremities of the prosthesis to be coiled to take the whole length of the ureter (Fig. 8.56). One of the two anchoring suture slings is then cut and pulled until the stent is released. This suture sling can be used for stent repositioning if necessary.
7. A nephrostomy catheter is placed for 1 or 2 days.
8. The nephrostomy tube is removed after control of the patency of the ureteral prosthesis has been obtained.

Occasionally it is necessary to use a more rigid guidewire to pass beyond the stenosis or even to use a small 4-mm balloon to facilitate the introduction of the large-diameter sheath. In more difficult cases, a torque guidewire that is available with the Druy stent set can be passed through the urethra and exteriorized to achieve traction and track rectification, making the introduction of the sheath and introducer easier.

Figure 8.58 (A) A Druy ureteral stent with universal length. Note the wire used for stent repositioning. (B) A peel-away sheath and system introducer for stent placement.

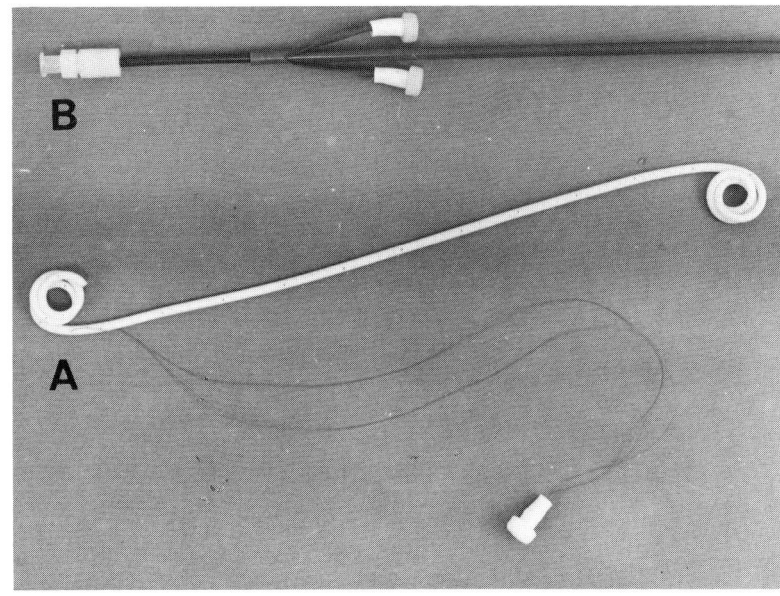

Congenital Obstructions

Congenital obstructions have a few unique features. These obstructions are almost exclusively limited to the pyeloureteral junction and cause extensive unilateral or bilateral congenital hydronephrosis, which usually is not diagnosed before adolescence or early adulthood. This type of occlusion is generally treated by means of pyeloplasty.

These obstructions may be related to a congenital abnormality caused by the presence of an adynamic ureteral segment or aberrant vessel. Postsurgical obstructions with the formation of a fibrotic scar and stenosis occasionally occur after a pyeloplasty for correction of a congenital lesion.

The approach in these cases can be either antegrade or retrograde. Finding the orifice by the percutaneous antegrade route may be impossible because of occlusion and dilation of the collecting system. In these cases retrograde manipulation by cystoscopy is advisable.

Nephrostomy should be the initial procedure for two reasons. First, the kidney should be relieved of its obstruction and its functional capacity should be assessed before any therapeutic procedure. If renal function is absent or minimal, nephrectomy is the best treatment. Second, a viable percutaneous access to the collecting system should be created for eventual manipulation through this route.

Dilation of these stenoses with balloon catheters has recently been performed successfully (Fig. 8.59), even in patients with a solitary kidney or when a urethrotome (Sacks knife) is used as an aid in rupturing the mucosa and submucosa. This procedure is associated with dilation with a large-diameter balloon (Figs. 8.49 and 8.50).

As in any other renal procedure, after nephrostomy, the track is dilated and a sheath compatible with the balloon or with a nephroscope combined with a Sacks knife should be utilized.

The results obtained with this type of procedure are reasonably good. However, aggressive intervention with large-diameter balloons and laceration with a Sacks knife are necessary. These congenital obstructions do not respond to balloons smaller than 4 to 5 mm, and so balloons with diameters larger than 6 mm should be used, along with No. 9 to 10 French tutor catheters, which are maintained through the obstruction for at least 30 days (Fig. 8.59).

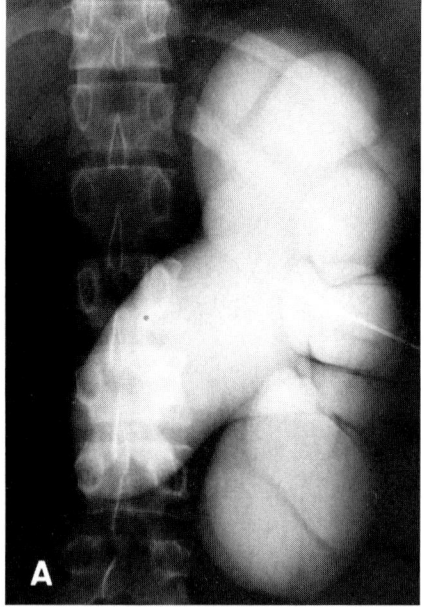
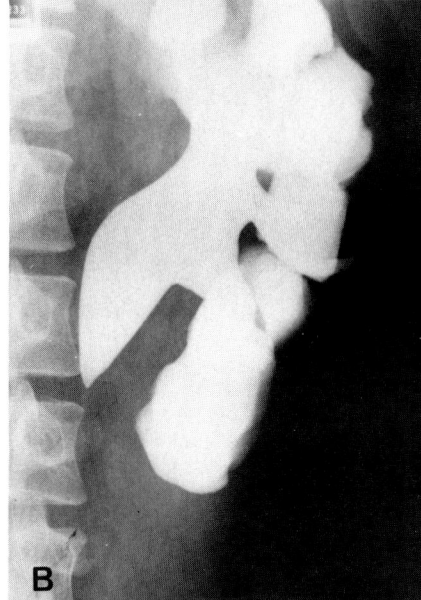
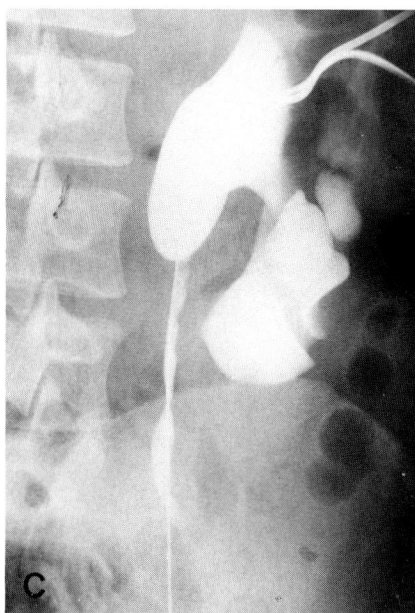
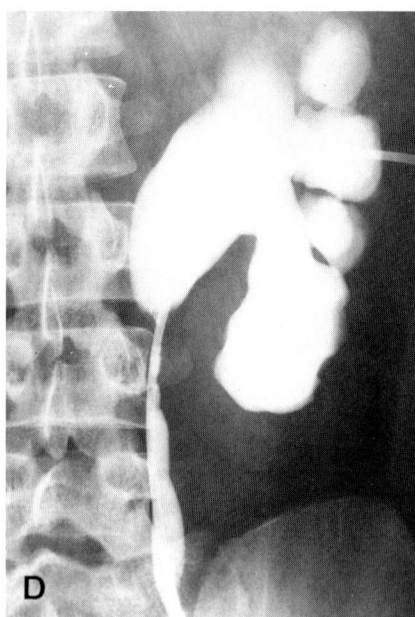
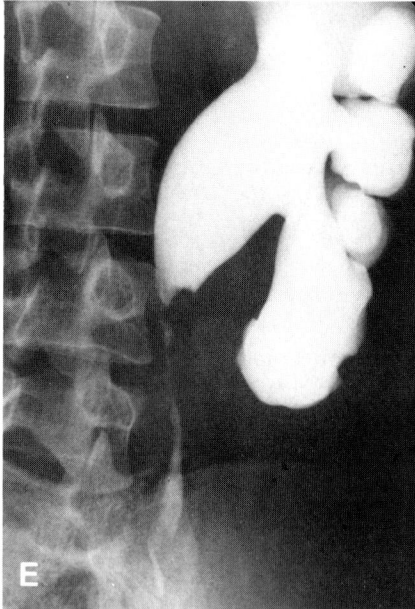

Figure 8.59 (A) A 24-year-old patient with a solitary kidney and congenital stenosis at the pyeloureteral junction, which caused hydronephrosis. (B) Nephrostomy with external drainage for 1 week shows significant reduction of the collecting system and obstruction at the junction. (C) Control pyelography after junction dilation with a 6-mm balloon catheter, with the guidewire maintained through an already well dilated stenosis. (D) A tutor catheter maintained for 3 weeks through the dilated spot. (E) Control 4 weeks after dilation shows ureteral patency in spite of irregular borders.

REFERENCES

Banner MP, Pollack HM. Percutaneous extraction of renal and ureteral calculi. *Radiology* 1982;144:753–758.

Banner MP, Pollack HM. Dilatation of ureteral stenoses: Techniques and experience in 44 patients. *AJR* 1984;143:789–793.

Banner MP, Stein EJ, Pollack HM. Technical refinements in percutaneous nephroureterolithotomy. *AJR* 1985;145:101–107.

Bettman MA, Permutt L, Kinhelstein J, et al. Percutaneous placement of soft, indwelling ureteral stent. *Radiology* 1985;157:817–818.

Clayman RV, Castaneda-Zuniga WR. *Techniques in Endourology: A Guide to the Percutaneous Removal of Renal and Ureteral Calculi.* Year Book, Chicago, 1984.

Jenkins AD, Tegtmeyer CJ. Percutaneous transrenal placement of indwelling ureteral catheters. *J Urol* 1981;126:730–733.

Kadir S, White RI, Engel R. Balloon dilatation of a ureteropelvic junction obstruction. *Radiology* 1982;143:263–264.

Lang EK. Antegrade ureteral stenting for dehiscence, strictures and fistulae. *AJR* 1984;143:795–801.

LeRoy AJ, Williams HJ, Bender CE, et al. Percutaneous removal of small ureteral calculi. *AJR* 1985;145:109–112.

Mitty HA, Train JS, Dan SJ. Antegrade ureteral stenting in the management of fistulas, strictures and calculi. *Radiology* 1983;149:433–438.

Mitty HA. Ureteral stenting facilitated by antegrade transurethral passage of guidewire. *AJR* 1984;142:831–832.

Reimer DE, Oswalt GC. Iatrogenic ureteral obstruction treated with balloon dilatation. *J Urol* 1981;126:689–690.

Rozenblit G, Tarasov E, Skur MF, et al. Druy ureteral stent set: Clinical experience in 25 patients. *Radiology* 1986;160:737–740.

Percutaneous Lithotripsy

Renan Uflacker

Surgery has been the traditional therapy for renal lithiasis, with removal of symptomatic stones whenever necessary. In the last few years, percutaneous techniques have become available, changing the approach to renal calculi and even replacing surgical procedures. A large number of smaller calculi (below 1 cm) can be removed intact with forceps, while calculi above 1 cm should be fragmented first.

In 1978 Alken and Guthaner developed the concept of percutaneous removal of renal calculi, and in 1981 they performed percutaneous nephrolithotripsy with ultrasound. The procedure gained worldwide acceptance quickly and became the method of choice for treating renal stones.

This procedure combines the methods of the radiologic percutaneous renal approach with nephroscopy-guided stone disintegration. This has promoted a joint effort by radiologists and urologists for treating these patients. As the technique evolved, countless variations were developed regarding the details of the approach and the availability of equipment.

INDICATIONS FOR THE PROCEDURE

Currently almost all renal stones, from caliceal stones to staghorn calculi, should be considered for treatment with percutaneous lithotripsy. Originally the percutaneous technique was indicated almost exclusively for small, movable, and recurrent calculi. As experience with the method grew, the range of indications was broadened significantly. Renal stone patients who can be treated clinically (those with uric acid and cystine stones) are candidates for percutaneous intervention only if the clinical treatment fails.

Patients with small, asymptomatic stones with no indication for surgery should not be considered for the percutaneous technique. Contraindications to the procedure include uncorrectable hemorrhagic diathesis, active infection, anatomic abnormalities requiring sugical correction, a calculus coexisting with a neoplasm, and renal tuberculosis. Classical cases of percutaneous removal are shown in Figs. 8.60 and 8.61.

Previous Examinations

A complete recent urographic study, including tomographic evaluation, is necessary for defining the anatomy of the renal collecting system and the number, size, and location of renal stones. It is also convenient to have clinical and laboratory evaluation data on renal function available.

The percutaneous procedure is planned on the basis of the anatomy of the collecting system and the location of the stone just before the procedure. It is common to find radical changes in the position of the stone between the examination and the beginning of the procedure.

Access

As with all other renal percutaneous procedures, percutaneous nephrostomy is the initial stage. This involves the establishment of a track to the renal collecting system, and this track can be manipulated, dilated, and maintained as long as necessary for treatment purposes. Actually, the whole procedure depends on the access supplied by nephrostomy. A range of different materials and techniques are available for performing percutaneous nephrostomy.

Nephrostomy is performed exclusively under fluoroscopy. Selection of the calix to be punctured and its relation to the stone can be better assessed under fluoroscopic view. Manipulation with guidewires and catheters is also done under fluoroscopy.

In many patients the puncture is performed in the nondilated collecting system, and this can make puncture and catheterization difficult. Unlike relief nephrostomies for acute or chronic obstruction with infection or a fistula present, where the collecting system is dilated, pelvic calculi frequently do not cause dilation.

The puncture is made with an 18-gauge diamond-tip needle, although some authors prefer a finer needle (21-gauge) and a more complex catheterization system, with the patient in pronation. Occasionally, several needle passes are necessary before one is able to puncture the infundibulum of the selected calix, usually in the lower group.

Antibiotics should be instituted before the procedure, even if active infection is not present. It is necessary to maintain an infusion route for mild sedation with diazepam as well as analgesia with fentanyl or another opiate. About 50 to 80 mL of urographic contrast medium is injected intravenously for kidney opacification 10 min before puncture is started. If there is obstruction or functional exclusion, direct posterior puncture of the collecting system may be necessary.

The puncture route selected should be short and

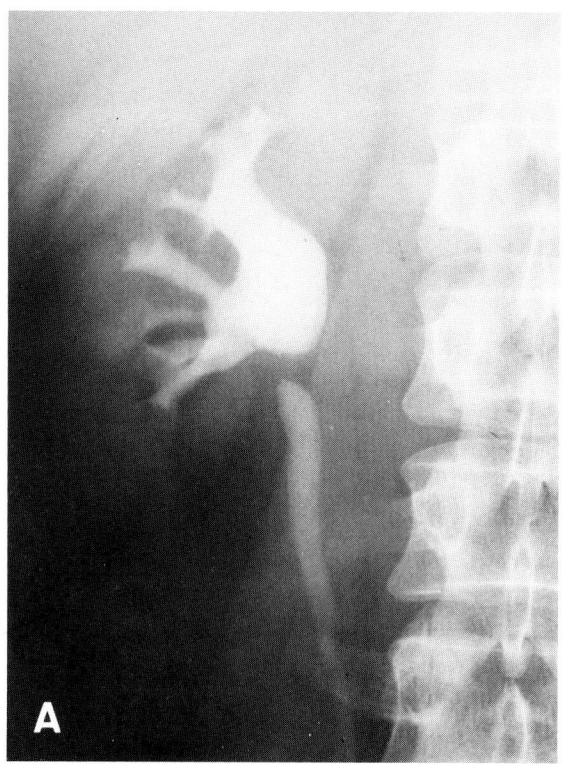
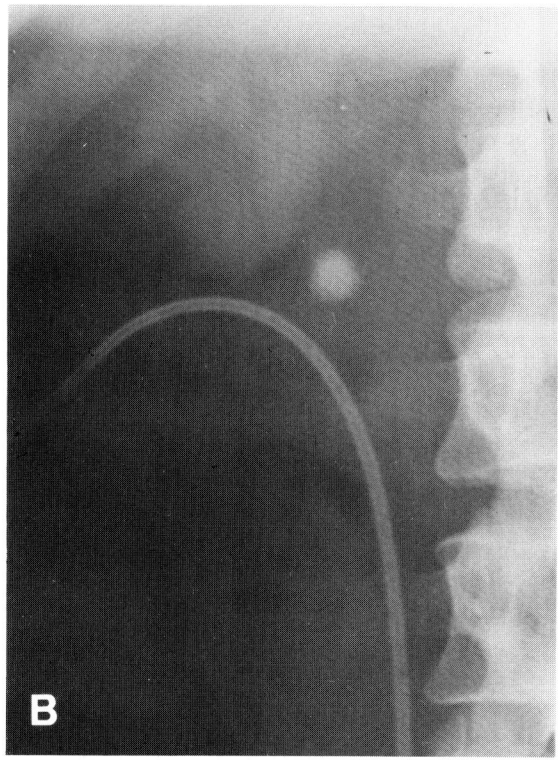
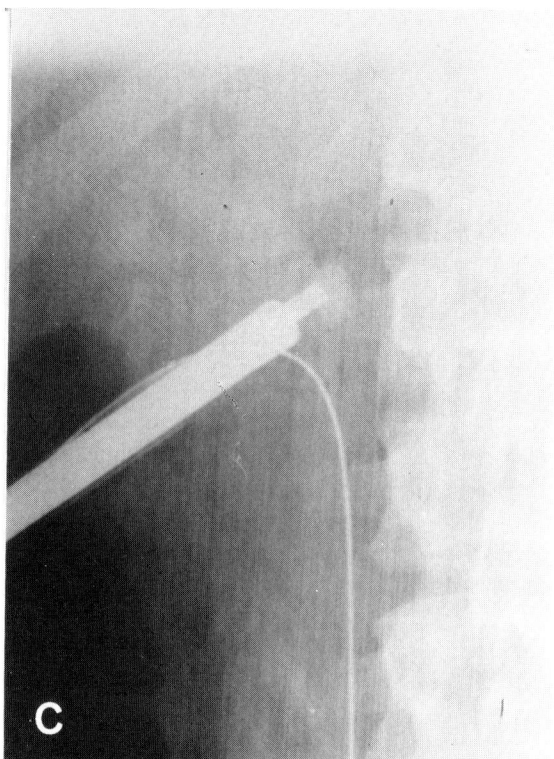
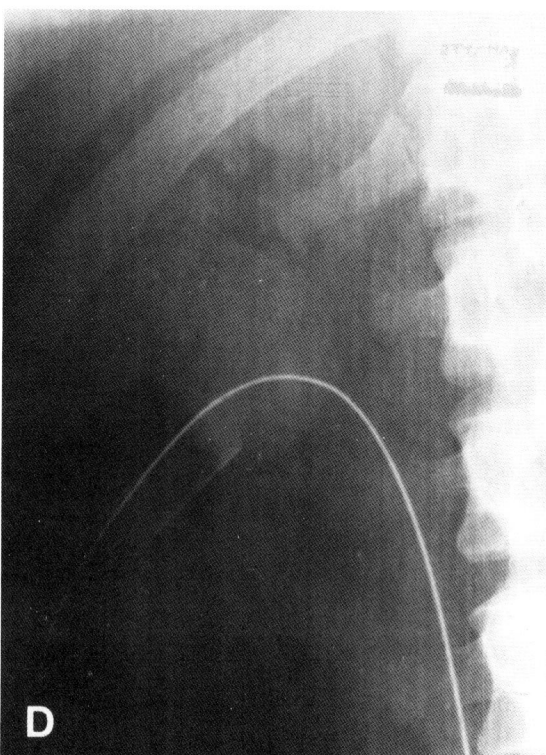

Figure 8.60 Percutaneous lithotripsy with ultrasound.
(A) Moderate dilation of the renal pelvis by a calculus and junction narrowing. (B) Nephrostomy with a straight tube positioned in the ureter. Note the radiopaque stone in the renal pelvis. (C) An ultrasonic lithotripter acting on the calculus through the nephroscope and an Amplatz No. 26 French sheath. Note the safety guidewire outside the sheath, descending into the ureter. (D) Control after fragmentation and total removal of the stone. Note that the safety guidewire and sheath are still in position.

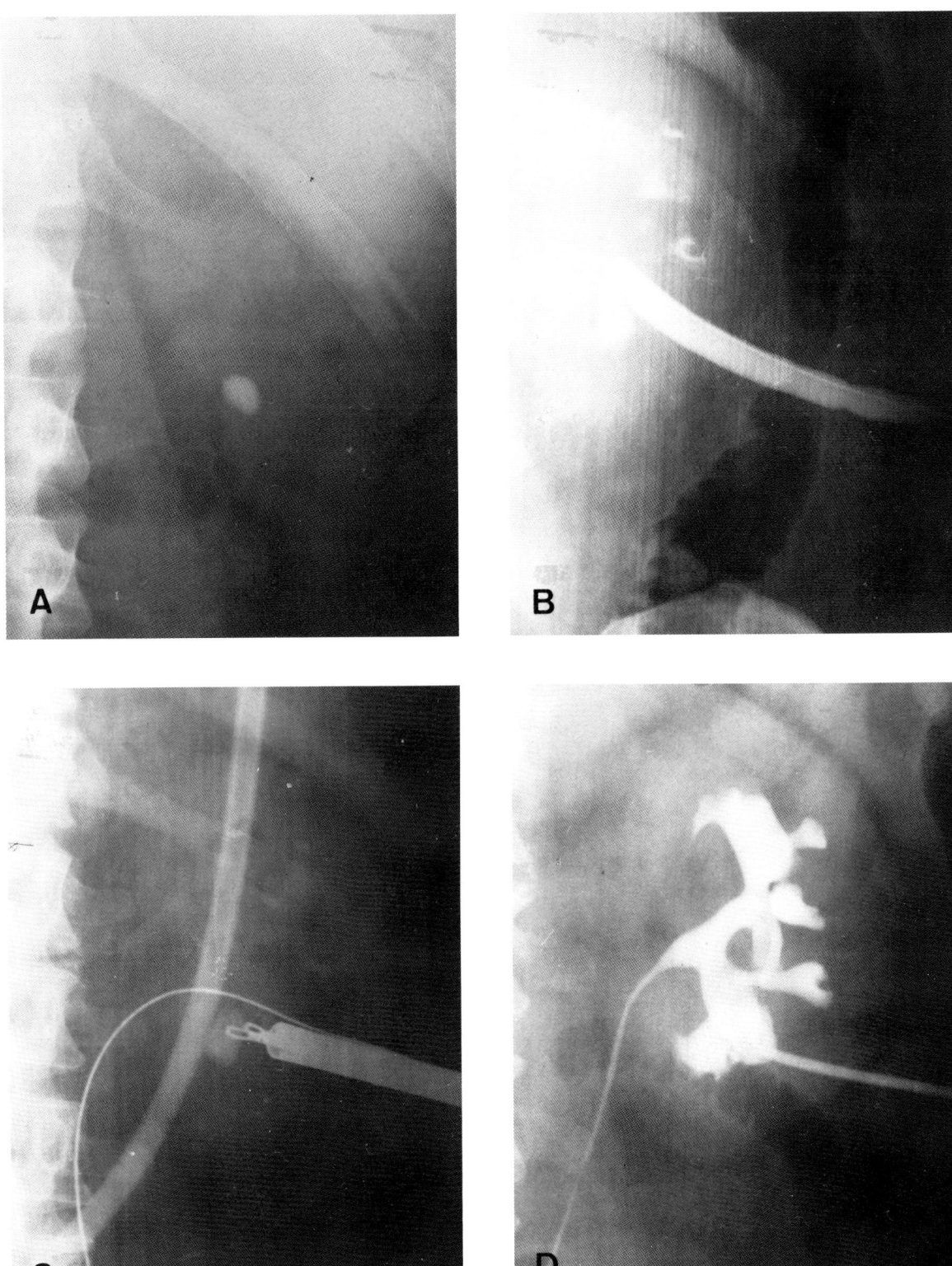

Figure 8.61 Percutaneous lithotripsy.
(A) A calculus about 1 cm in diameter in the pelvis. (B) Nephrostomy track dilation with a 10-cm-long and 10-mm-diameter Olbert balloon. (C) Stone removal without fragmentation by forceps. (D) Control nephrostomy after removal of a pelvic calculus.

straight from skin to stone, with the track being a straight line, since the system used for most types of stones is rigid and rectilinear. The ideal puncture site lies below the last rib on the posterior axillary line, bypassing the pleura, colon, liver, spleen, and intercostal or subcostal vessels. The entry point should always be through one calix (on its infundibulum), never directly into the renal pelvis.

Intracaliceal stones should be approached by means of direct puncture into the involved calix. If one of the upper calices is involved, a lower puncture can still reach it in most cases, even when a nonflexible instrument is used.

After the calix has been punctured, a guidewire is advanced inside the collecting system and positioned in the proximal ureter through the pyeloureteral junction (Fig. 8.60). After dilation to No. 8 or 9 French, a multiperforated No. 8 French catheter is introduced into the ureter, across the renal pelvis, and sutured to the skin. It is kept open into a drainage flask until the following day, when the procedure is continued.

In selected cases, dilation of the collecting system may have to be done through contrast injection into a catheter that is retrogradely introduced into the ureter of the target kidney. This procedure, however, is usually unnecessary.

Track Dilatation

The track should be dilated to allow the introduction of a No. 26 or 30 French sheath through which instrumentation can be carried out. There are two alternatives with regard to the stages of the procedure. The procedure can be performed in only one session or in two stages, with nephrostomy done on the first day and dilation and stone removal on the second.

The two-stage approach appears to be easier. It involves less bleeding, pelvic clots can be removed easily on the second day, there is an opportunity for hydration of the patient, and it is well accepted by patients.

Initially, track dilatation was done gradually, with progressive increases in the diameter of the catheters over several days or weeks. Today, however, this procedure is not used.

Fast track dilatation is safe and effective in most cases. A system of dilators and sheaths with diameters varying from No. 8 to 36 French and two-point increments can be used to dilate the nephrostomy track (Fig. 9.7A). More recently, a special Olbert-type balloon catheter 10 cm long and 10 mm in diameter that is resistant to high pressure became available (Fig. 8.62). This balloon is currently preferred by radiologists and urologists, as it has made dilation of access routes to the renal collecting system extremely simple and rapid.

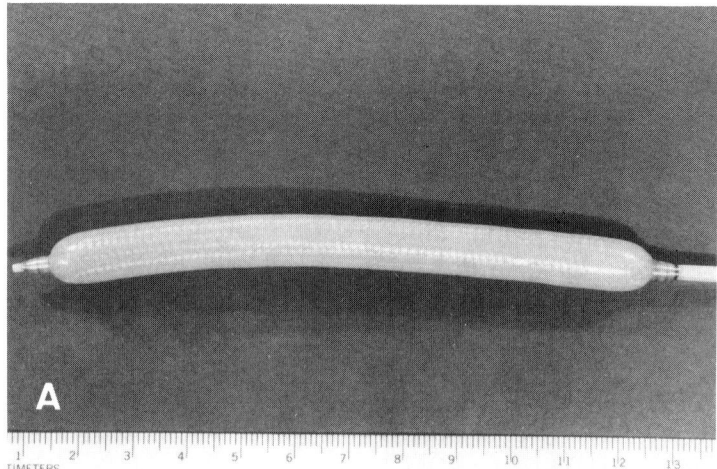
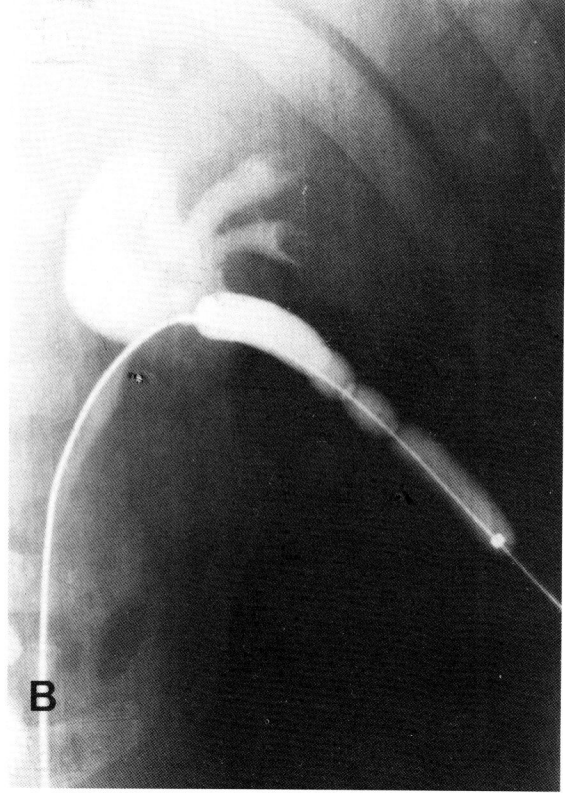

Figure 8.62 (A) An Olbert-type balloon catheter for dilation of a nephrostomy track. This is a high-pressure balloon 10 cm long and 10 mm in its maximum diameter. (B) An Olbert catheter dilating a nephrostomy track. Note the constriction of the balloon at the renal capsule and the fascia of Gerota. The dilator and No. 26 French sheath are mounted on the catheter, behind the balloon, and are advanced in a progressive and rotational mode over the deflated balloon after track dilation. The Olbert catheter is removed as soon as the sheath is in position.

Balloon dilatation is sometimes incomplete because of the presence of scar tissue or the resistance of the different fasciae surrounding the kidney (Fig. 8.62). The track dilatation systems supplied by Wolf and Stortz, the manufacturers of nephroscopes available in the market, are neither appropriate nor safe, and their use is being discontinued. The Wolf system utilizes metal dilators with progressively increasing diameters as fascial dilators. The Stortz system includes coaxial tubes of the radio antenna type, which are also difficult to handle and are not very safe.

The dilatation and subsequent handling of the nephrostomy track are painful and should be performed under local anesthesia with strong sedation, with peridural anesthesia and sedation, or, preferably, under general anesthesia.

A total procedure may be very time-consuming, lasting as long as a few hours when extensive use of ultrasound in multiple large stones is necessary. Therefore, because of stress, it becomes very difficult for the patient to remain in the same position under local or peridural anesthesia and sedation alone. As increasing doses of sedatives will be necessary, this will involve unnecessary risks when the patient is not intubated and is placed in a prone position.

For all these reasons, it seems more reasonable and safe for the second half of the procedure to be performed with the patient intubated and under general anesthesia, even if the anesthesia is only superficial.

At the start of the process, it is advisable to introduce a second safety guidewire, which will remain beside the work guidewire and outside the sheath, just after dilation (Fig. 8.61). The safety guidewire makes it possible to reestablish the track in case of sheath displacement or damage to the work guidewire. The safety wire placed in the ureter is a technical standby resource which should be removed only after completion of the procedure, following the placement of a nephrostomy.

Nephrostomy and Stone Extraction

With a No. 26 or 30 French sheath in place (in accordance with stone size), a rigid No. 24 French nephroscope is introduced into the collecting system through the dilated track. The nephroscope includes a high-quality optical system and irrigation and aspiration ducts in addition to a manipulation channel.

Stones smaller than 1 cm can be removed with special forceps (Fig. 8.61) or with a Dormia basket or a trident forceps. Larger stones should be pulverized, using an ultrasonic lithotriptor with waves that have a frequency between 23,000 and 27,000 Hz. After visual inspection of the collecting system, the device is directed with the stone under frontal view. Some clots may have to be removed to obtain a better view of the calculus. The lithotripter is advanced toward the stone and activated when it establishes contact with the stone. The calculus is then fragmented into small, 1- to 2-mm-diameter particles (sand), which are quickly aspirated by the suction system (Fig. 8.60).

Stones disintegrate at different velocities, depending on their composition. After disintegration, the resulting pieces can be aspirated or removed with a forceps. After disintegration, an x-ray should be taken for control of residual fragments. If there are stones in the proximal ureter, they can be removed by the same method.

After one is sure that no residual fragments are left, the nephroscope is removed and a Foley catheter with the tip cut off or a Malecot catheter is introduced through the sheath until it reaches the renal pelvis. This catheter is maintained in open nephrostomy.

It is not necessary to maintain a catheter in the ureter. The position of a probe in a nephrostomy is controlled by x-ray, and the catheter is stitched onto the skin. Two days after the procedure, when hematuria has disappeared, the nephrostomy catheter is closed for 24 h and then removed, with the track obliterated spontaneously.

If any residual calculus is found in the kidney after a percutaneous intervention, manipulation can be performed a few days later through the same dilated route. In patients with staghorn calculi, multiple procedures are frequently necessary. The procedure is successful in 96 percent of patients, according to the literature.

Complications are uncommon but are often associated with perforation of the collecting system as a result of careless handling of instruments. These complications are treated with a nephrostomy that is open to a flask for a few days. Bleeding occurs in less than 2 percent of patients and may be related to a vascular lesion with the formation of a pseudoaneurysm (Fig. 4.31). The treatment for this type of problem consists of catheter embolization.

The application of percutaneous lithotripsy with ultrasound is undergoing rapid change, with increasingly frequent use of extracorporeal shock wave lithotripsy. This procedure is noninvasive and can disintegrate 90 percent of all renal stones.

The new role of percutaneous lithotripsy remains limited to patients in whom extracorporeal lithotripsy is ineffective and those in whom spontaneous migration of renal stone fragments through the ureter proves difficult. Several different types of equipment are available for performing extracorporeal lithotripsy. The ideal type, however, remains to be identified.

REFERENCES

Alken P, et al. Percutaneous stone manipulation. *J Urol* 1981;125:463–466.

Brannen GE. Endourology: Perspectives in percutaneous stone removal. *J Intervent Radiol* 1986;1:9–14.

Chaussy C, Schmiedt E. Extracorporeal shock wave lithotripsy (ESWL) for kidney stones: An alternative to surgery? *Urol Radiol* 1984;6:80–87.

Clayman RV, Castaneda-Zuniga W. Nephrolithotomy: Percutaneous removal of renal calculi. *Urol Radiol* 1984;6:95–112.

Kaye KW. Renal anatomy for endourologic stone removal. *J Urol* 1983;130:647–648.

Kerlan RK, Kahn RI, Ring EJ. Percutaneous renal and ureteral stone removal. *Urol Radiol* 1984;6:113–123.

LeRoy AJ, Segura JW. Percutaneous ultrasonic lithotripsy. *Urol Radiol* 1984;6:88–94.

Mayo ME, Krieger JN, Rudd TG. Effect of percutaneous nephrolithotomy on renal function. *J Urol* 1985;133:167–173.

Segura JW. Endourology. *J Urol* 1984;132:1079–1084.

Van Arsdalen KN. Pathogenesis of renal calculi. *Urol Radiol* 1984;6:65–73.

Wickhan JEA, Kellet MJ. Percutaneous nephrolithotomy. *J Urol* 1981;53:297–299.

Chapter Nine

Pulmonary Thromboembolism and Interruption of the Inferior Vena Cava

RENAN UFLACKER

PULMONARY EMBOLISM

Basic information on pulmonary thromboembolism and its natural history is still unavailable. This has led to the difficulties commonly encountered in the diagnosis and treatment of pulmonary embolism.

The total incidence of pulmonary embolism among different populations and the annual death rate from this disease are unknown. Available data are misleading about the number of patients who suffer from pulmonary embolism. The pathologic findings are even more difficult to explain, showing an incidence ranging from 6 to 64 percent. The wide range of the findings apparently results from the pathologist's commitment while researching pulmonary embolism during necropsy.

The death rate from this disease is about 30 percent in symptomatic patients, and this reveals the importance of establishing an accurate diagnosis. It is difficult, however, to establish a technical diagnosis of this disease. Frequent symptoms such as dyspnea, chest pain (thoracalgia), and cough are usual complaints, but these symptoms can have different etiologies. Because physical and laboratory examinations are nonspecific, radiologic assessment of these patients is essential.

RADIOLOGY OF THE THORAX

Several radiologic findings of pulmonary embolism have been reported in patients with thromboembolism. Ninety percent or more of patients who undergo chest x-ray have abnormal results. Nonetheless, a significant number of patients with clinical symptoms have a normal thorax on radiography.

The usual radiologic findings are generally nonspecific and include elevation of the hemidiaphragm, pleural effusion, and pulmonary consolidations. When these consolidations are in the costophrenic angle of the lung, they present a round aspect directed at the pulmonary hilum. These features constitute the so-called Hampton sign. The most specific finding in standard thorax radiography is a sign described by Westermark as dilatation of the pulmonary artery (Fig. 9.1).

In a recent prospective study, less than 50 percent of diagnoses of pulmonary embolism were correct. The low specificity and sensitivity can be accounted for by the high percentage of cases which could not be diagnosed. Consequently, thorax radiography is insufficient to establish a diagnosis of pulmonary embolism. Its basic function is to exclude clinically similar diseases such as pneumothorax, costal fracture, and acute pleural effusion and to compare them with data from pulmonary scintigraphy obtained either on ventilation or on perfusion.

PULMONARY SCINTIGRAPHY

Pulmonary scintigraphy has high sensitivity in detecting abnormal pulmonary perfusion despite its low specificity in detecting pulmonary embolism. It is always important to correlate pulmonary perfusion scintigraphy with pulmonary ventilation scintigraphy and thorax radiography.

Two scintigraphic patterns are diagnostic:

1. Up-to-date evidence proves that normal scintigraphy can exclude pulmonary embolism.
2. A combination of multiple and segmentary perfusion defects and normal ventilation in these areas almost certainly indicates pulmonary embolism. A rare disease called congenital stenosis of the pulmonary artery branches is the only entity which, despite its different clinical features, can simulate the features of pulmonary embolism.

When the scintigraphic pattern reveals only a single, although segmentary, perfusion defect, the accuracy of

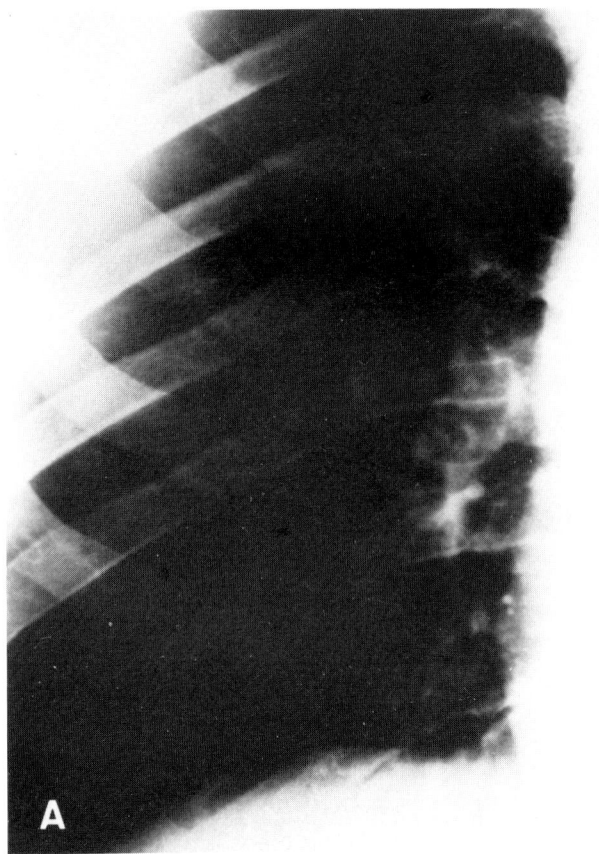
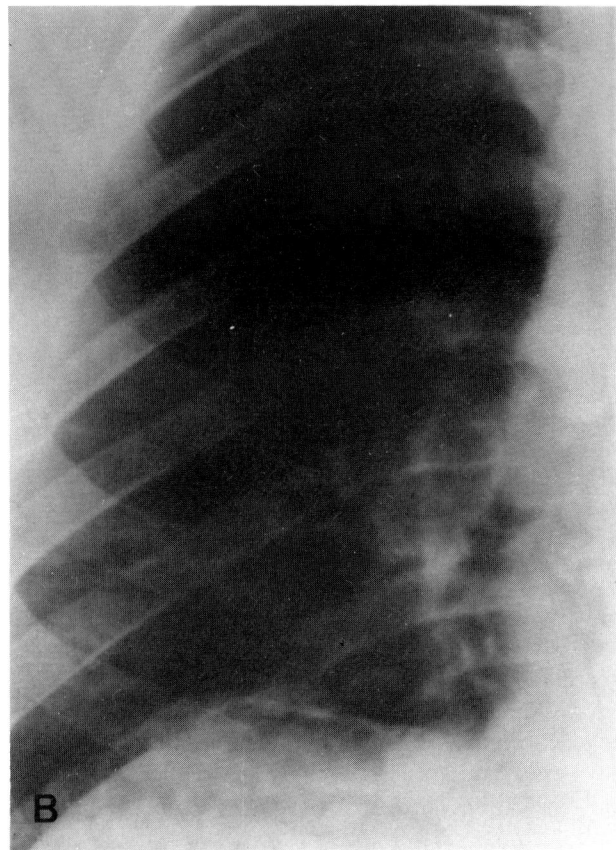
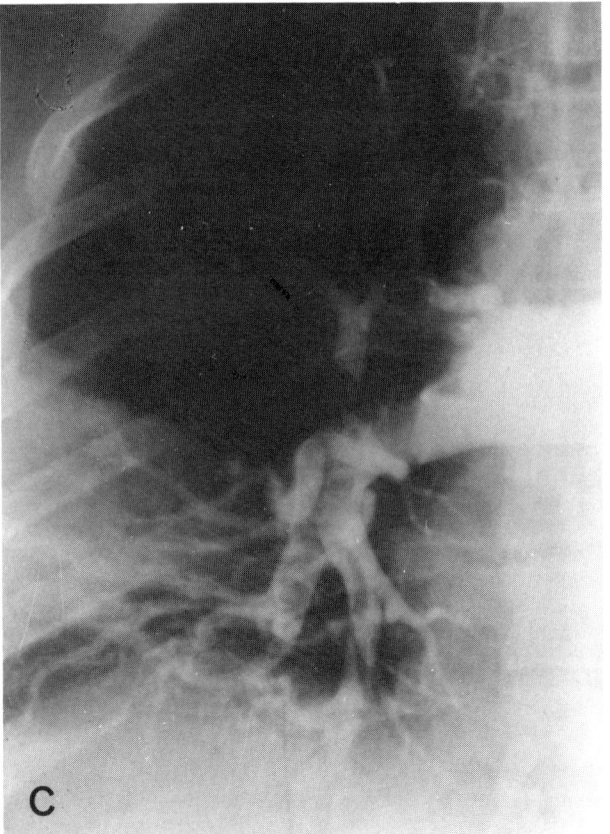

Figure 9.1 A 49-year-old patient who presented with sudden chest pain after prostate surgery.
(A) Preoperative chest x-ray showing a normal-diameter pulmonary artery. (B) Chest x-ray after an episode of chest pain and dyspnea. The main findings were elevation of the right phrenic cupula, reduction of the peripheral pulmonary circulation, and enlargement of the inferior lobe of the pulmonary artery. (C) Right selective pulmonary arteriography showing a massive pulmonary embolism with amputation of the pulmonary artery and various filling defects in the arterial lumen.

the method decreases significantly and diagnosis becomes more difficult.

Statistical probabilities are rife with inaccuracy; there are no precise quantitative standards that can be applied to the diagnosis and treatment of pulmonary embolism. Some authors require high statistical probabilities to start treating their patients and resort to phlebography of the lower extremities and pulmonary arteriography in patients with abnormal perfusion scintigraphy. Other authors advocate a restricted use of angiography.

PULMONARY ANGIOGRAPHY

Indications for performing pulmonary angiography to detect pulmonary embolism are related to the need to improve the accuracy of diagnosis. These indications include the following:

1. Strong clinical suspicion of pulmonary embolism with low-probability scintigraphy
2. Contraindication for anticoagulation and high-probability scintigraphy
3. A need to confirm the diagnosis of pulmonary embolism before starting a procedure such as embolectomy or introducing a vena cava filter.
4. Indeterminate scintigraphy

If pulmonary angiography is required, many options are available in regard to the approach and the equipment used. The most common approach among vascular radiologists is via the femoral vein, although this pathway is slightly impaired in patients with cardiomegaly. The right antecubital vein approach is easily performed using the Seldinger technique, and is as useful and simple as the femoral vein approach. The antecubital vein approach is essential when iliofemoral thrombosis and occlusion of the inferior vena cava are present.

Pulmonary pressure measurement should be a routine procedure, and an average pulmonary pressure higher than 45 mmHg indicates severe pulmonary hypertension. In this case, the examination must be restricted to selective injections.

Pulmonary arteriography has high sensitivity and specificity in the diagnosis of pulmonary embolism in addition to being the safest and most effective procedure (Figs. 9.2 and 9.3). This procedure can be carried out in

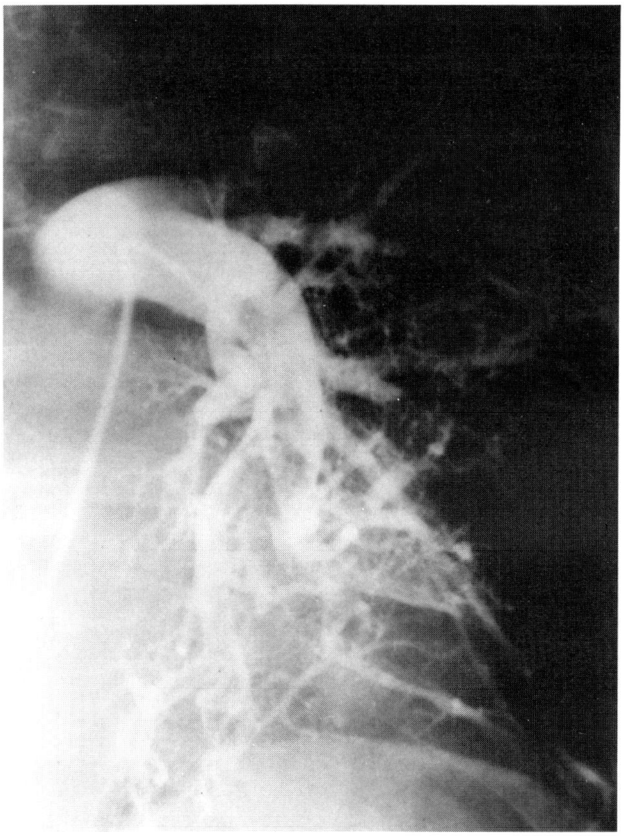

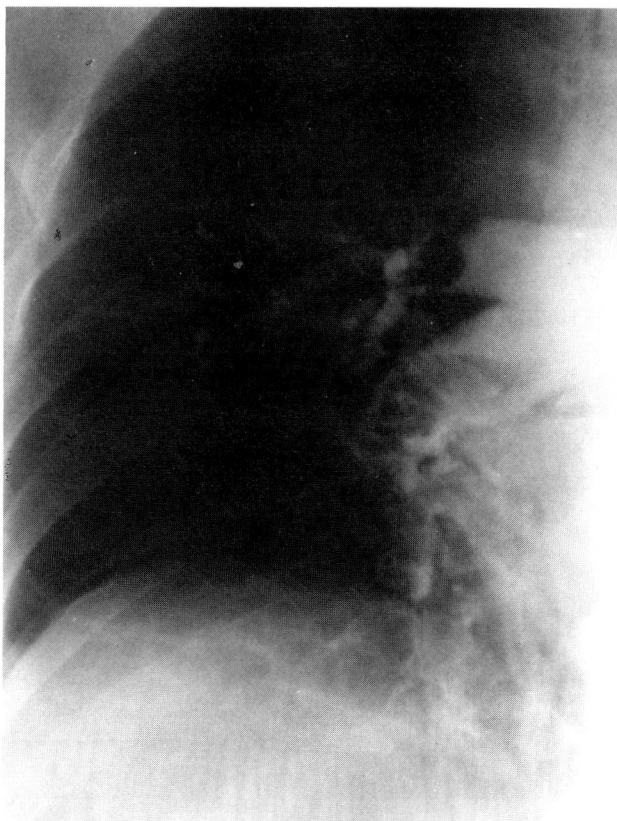

Figure 9.2 Severe pulmonary embolism shown by selective left pulmonary angiography. Note the great number of filling defects in the arterial lumen and the amputation of subsegmental branches.

Figure 9.3 Massive pulmonary embolism 2 weeks after hysterectomy in a 60-year-old female patient. The main finding was amputation of the right pulmonary artery at the level of bifurcation.

Table 9.1 – Classification of pulmonary thromboembolism

Class	Symptoms	Gasometric Values	Pulmonary Occlusion, %	Hemodynamics
I	None	Normal	< 20	Normal
II	Anxiety	Pa_{O_2} < 80 mmHg	20–30	Tachycardia
	Hyperventilation	Pa_{CO_2} < 35 mmHg		
III	Dyspnea	Pa_{O_2} < 65 mmHg	30–50	CVP* high
	Collapse	Pa_{CO_2} < 30 mmHg		APP > 20 mmHg
IV	Shock	Pa_{O_2} < 50 mmHg	> 50	CVP high
	Dyspnea			APP > 25 mmHg
V	Dyspnea	Pa_{O_2} < 50 mmHg	> 50	BP < 100 mmHg
	Syncope	Pa_{CO_2} 30–40 mmHg		APP > 40 mmHg
				CVP high
				CO low, absence of shock

*CVP = Central venous pressure; APP = average pulmonary pressure; BP = blood pressure; CO = cardiac output.

most patients; the few complications basically consist of cardiac arrhythmias during manipulation of the catheter.

However, reactions to the contrast medium can be a serious problem, since the lungs are considered shock organs and therefore are prone to anaphylactic reactions. The use of corticosteroids and H_1 and H_2 blockers may reduce these reactions significantly. Nonionic contrast medium can also help in avoiding severe anaphylactic reactions.

Acute cardiopulmonary failure and cardiac arrest are ominous complications. Alternate selective injections in each pulmonary artery help reduce the risk of cardiac failure during injection. As in other invasive procedures, one should be aware of the risks and benefits of this procedure before resorting to it.

Since the hemodynamic effects of pulmonary embolism are the major consequences in the clinical course of the disease, a physiologic method was developed to classify patients according to cardiorespiratory variables. This method, described by Greenfield in 1982, allows a systematic approach to treatment and a reasonable prognosis while functioning as a pattern of results for treatments in the same patient and among different health centers (Table 9.1).

DEEP VENOUS THROMBOSIS

Venous thromboembolism has aroused interest because it is thought to cause high morbidity and mortality in patients hospitalized for surgical or clinical reasons. Paradoxically, the difficulty of diagnosis of this disease has been a major obstacle in the care of these patients. Frequently, this disease is asymptomatic when it occurs in the lower extremities, and the first symptom is pulmonary embolism.

The use of scintigraphic methods and phlebography in the lower extremities has been the most important means of identifying the origin and cause of an episode of pulmonary embolism related to the venous system of the lower extremities in asymptomatic patients (Fig. 9.4). However, the clinical emphasis has been on the identification of risk groups, the treatment of deep venous thrombosis, and the adoption of prophylactic measures.

The identification of patients with a high probability of developing venous thromboembolism is of the utmost importance in screening this population and determining prophylactic measures which will influence the clinical course of the disease.

The association of venous thromboembolism with heart disease, especially congestive cardiopathy and myocardial infarction, is well established, and these entities are comparable in regard to postoperative risks. In patients with malignant neoplasms, the incidence of venous thrombosis and pulmonary embolism is three times that of patients without these diseases. The incidence of positive tests in postoperative patients is between 30 and 35 percent. The incidence is even higher after surgery of the hip, suprapubic prostatectomy (50 percent), and laparoscopic gynecologic procedures. The incidence of thromboembolism in pregnant patients increases threefold after delivery.

The risk of thromboembolism in women who take oral contraceptives, especially women over 35 years of age, is four times the risk reported among nonusers. Obesity, old age, and a previous history of thromboembolism are also risk elements for the occurrence of venous thrombosis and pulmonary embolism in addition to collagenosis.

Figure 9.4 A 52-year-old male patient who was asymptomatic in the lower limbs developed "pneumonia" with pain, pleural effusion on the left side, and hematic sputum. There was no improvement after therapy with antibiotics. (A) Right lower limb phlebography showing a long thrombus inside the right superficial femoral vein. (B) Digital pulmonary arteriography showing amputation of the branches on the left base with reduction of the perfusion, confirming pulmonary embolism.

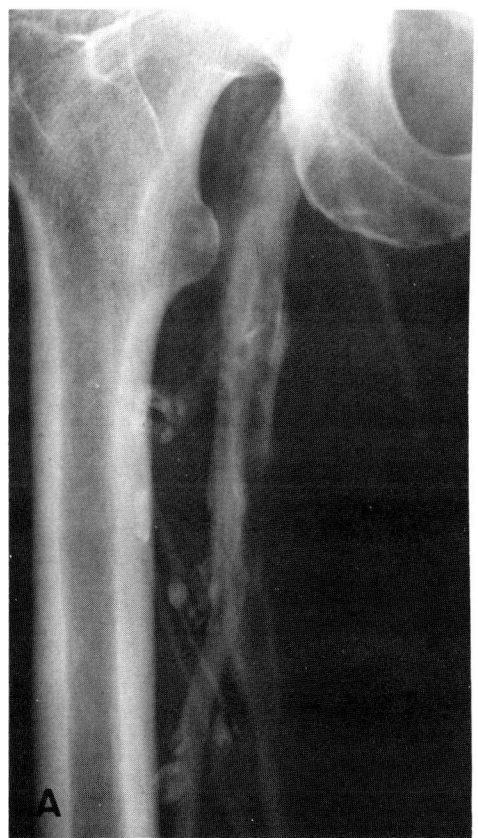
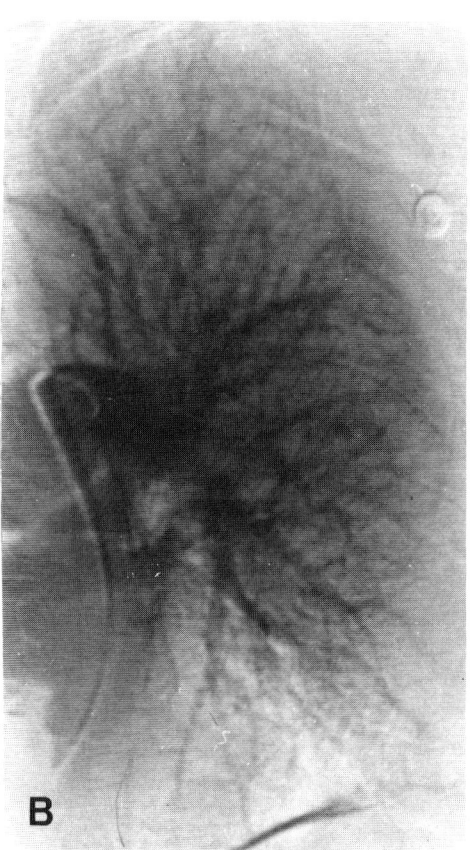

Spontaneous venous thrombosis with pulmonary embolism is not uncommon in patients with no risk factors; in these cases, the thrombosis is called idiopathic. The incidence is high in certain groups, such as paraplegics during the acute phase, and the disease generally follows trauma or any kind of medullary lesion. In these patients, the incidence of thromboembolism decreases with time.

Pathologic studies have indicated that venous thrombosis originates from multiple independent sites within the deep venous system of the lower extremities. Six preferential sites have been identified: iliac veins, common femoral vein, deep femoral vein, popliteal vein, posterior tibial veins, and intramuscular veins of the calf. Thrombosis of the inferior vena cava generally presents as an extension of iliofemoral venous thrombosis.

Phlebography was developed to serve as a standard method in the diagnosis of venous thrombosis in the lower extremities. To obtain radiographs of both the deep and superficial venous systems of the lower extremities, one should inject a large amount of low-osmolality contrast medium. There is no need for a tourniquet, and the patient should be kept in a half-recumbent position.

Scintigraphic techniques, however, are more practical and can be used to follow up patients with repeated examinations. These techniques can also be used to screen a high-risk population.

VENA CAVA FILTERS

The primary therapy for venous thromboembolism is anticoagulation with endovenous heparin in addition to oral administration of coumarin derivatives, whose effectiveness has been documented in both the treatment of venous thrombosis and the prevention of recurrent pulmonary embolism. However, contraindications to anticoagulants sometimes are present. It is sometimes necessary to discontinue drug administration because of hemorrhagic complications and the putative inefficacy of drugs in the treatment of venous thromboembolic disease. In these cases, surgery may be needed to save the patient's life. Venous ligation has been indicated since the last century as an effective measure to forestall pulmonary embolism in patients with venous thrombosis of the lower extremities. Since venous ligature has been carried out proximally to the inferior vena cava, interruption of the vena cava has become the most popular way to avoid repeated pulmonary embolism. With increasing knowledge and improved techniques, it became evident that mere ligature of the inferior vena cava entails morbidity, high recurrence rates of embolism, and mortality beyond acceptable standards. Up to 36 percent of patients with vena cava ligation showed recurrent pulmonary embolism with venous stasis in the extremities and postphlebitic syndrome. For these reasons and because of the advantages of using vena cava filtration instead of occlusion, surgeons adopted partial caval interruption with plication procedures; this entailed fixing clamps which could intermittently obstruct the lumen of the vena cava. Consequently, caval permeability up to 65 percent could be achieved.

Since these techniques required highly technical surgical procedures, research on intraluminal procedures was carried out in the 1960s. This study resulted in the methods of inferior vena cava filtration by the transvenous and percutaneous approach that is used at present. Only local anesthesia or minor surgical procedures are needed to achieve successful results with these techniques.

INDICATIONS

The most common indications for vena cava interruption by means of a system of filters are the same as those for vena cava ligation or plication. Only high-risk patients were treated with these methods initially; nevertheless, their indication has increased progressively because filters are less invasive and more tolerable than are surgical ligations.

Vena cava filters are used in accordance with the following indications:

1. Contraindication to anticoagulation (peptic ulcer, recent trauma, hemorrhagic diathesis, severe systemic hypertension, hemoptysis, and digestive hemorrhage)
2. Complications of anticoagulation, such as gastrointestinal and retroperitoneal bleeding, or after recent surgeries as well as thrombocytopenia
3. Systemic anticoagulation that did not prevent recurrent pulmonary embolism
4. Septic pulmonary embolism
5. Chronic pulmonary embolism with pulmonary hypertension and cor pulmonale (class V patients)
6. Percutaneous pulmonary embolectomy due to massive embolism, using a Greenfield catheter
7. Prophylactic use of an inferior vena cava filter (relative indication):
    a. Class III and class IV patients who present with more than 50 percent of the vascular bed occluded and cannot tolerate subsequent episodes of embolism
    b. Patients with a propagating iliofemoral thrombus in whom treatment with anticoagulation proves to be of no value
    c. Patients who present with a large fluctuating iliofemoral thrombus on phlebography

TYPES OF TRANSVENOUS DEVICES

There are basically two methods for performing inferior vena cava interruption: occlusion and filtering.

The Hunter balloon was designed to occlude the vena cava acutely and keep it closed even after progressive deflation of the balloon within the next few months. The occlusive balloon is preferred because this procedure causes no perforation of the vena cava and achieves complete obstruction of the vena cava as a result of the perfect adaptation of the device to the vascular diameter. Another advantage is the lack of formation of new thrombi in the site of vascular occlusion. At present, this device is considered obsolete and is used in only a few health centers.

The design and functioning of the filtering elements are basically aimed at maintaining flow in the vena cava, keeping the cava permeable, and retaining only specific migratory particles above a certain diameter.

The oldest system of inferior vena cava filtration is the Mobin-Uddin umbrella, which consists of six flattened stems with pointed tips which are radially arranged around the central axis. These stems are covered and united by a Silastic membrane impregnated with heparin. The filter ranges in diameter from 23 to 28 mm and can be adapted to the patient's anatomic characteristics.

The Mobin-Uddin umbrella filter was designed to be introduced by venotomy of the right jugular vein under fluoroscopic guidance, using local anesthesia. It should always be positioned below the renal veins. The filter is inserted into the vena cava inside a 7-mm-wide and 32-mm-long capsule up to the desired level and then released from the capsule; slight traction is applied to the catheter to fix its extremities to the wall of the vena cava. Once the system has been introduced and fixed to the vena cava, the catheter is unscrewed from the central axis of the filter and then withdrawn.

This type of filter occludes the inferior vena cava in 60 to 75 percent of patients; 51 percent of these patients have edema formation, and 1.5 percent have phlebitis. Filters with a diameter smaller than 23 mm are no longer used because they are more subject to displacement and migration. A 0.5 percent incidence of recurrent pulmonary embolism was detected in many patients using the Mobin-Uddin filter.

As a result of the high incidence of caval occlusions

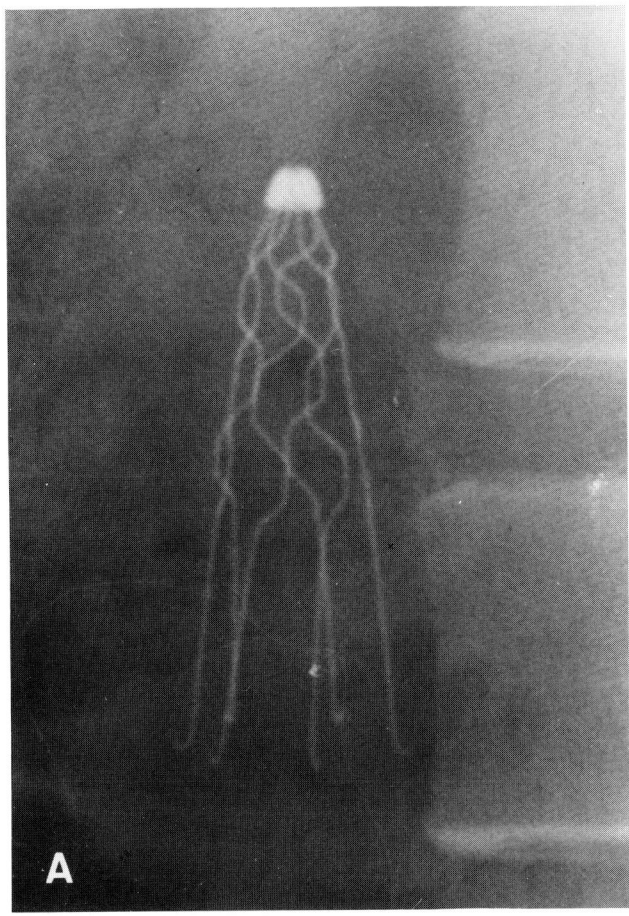
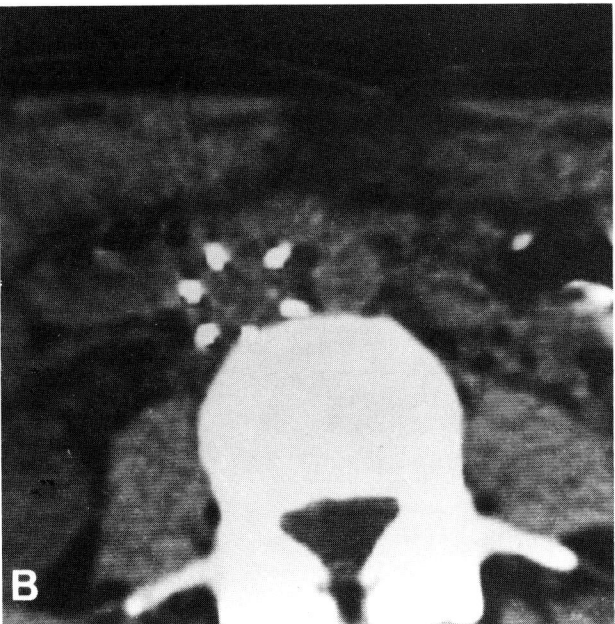

Figure 9.5 (A) A Greenfield vena cava filter. It has the shape of a conal segment with six stainless steel legs which are curved proximally and are straight distally, with a diameter of 3 cm at the base. Note the sharp hooks in contact with the wall of the vena cava. (B) Computed tomography shows the circular aspect of the filter base and the close contact of the legs with the vena cava as well as the relation of the filter to adjacent structures.

and the high risk of migration, there has been a marked reduction in the use of this kind of filter. In fact, production of this device has been discontinued.

Another type of inferior vena cava filter called the Kinray-Greenfield (K-G) filter was developed by Greenfield to avoid caval occlusion by thrombi and proximal displacement of the device to the heart. This device can be inserted by means of venotomy through either the jugular vein or the femoral vein. The 6-cm-long filter consists of six stainless steel legs symmetrically arranged around a small central capsule. The legs are ondulated in their proximal portion and have small sharp pointed "hooks" at the extremities to fix them to the wall of the vena cava (Fig. 9.5). At present, this is the most popular system for filtration of the inferior vena cava.

The first step consists of reverting the patient's heparinization or discontinuing anticoagulation for at least 3 days. The K-G filter may be introduced via the jugular vein or the femoral vein by percutaneous puncture without the need of a venotomy. However, this technique is a recently developed improvement which requires additional equipment such as a system of dilators and Amplatz sheaths (percutaneous nephrostomy tract dilator). These devices are used to dilate the site of the puncture to allow placement of a No. 24 French sheath, which then receives the capsule with the filter inside. The K-G filter has two specific catheters: the first for the jugular approach and the second for the femoral approach (Fig. 9.6).

The method used to introduce the filter by means of percutaneous femoral puncture is as follows:

1. Insert the filter in the capsule of the catheter that will be introduced; the "hooks" are disposed proximally.
2. Check the filter to make sure the hooks are not overlapping.
3. Fill the catheter that will be introduced with heparinized saline.
4. Under local anesthesia puncture both femoral veins, or only one if occlusion is observed, and introduce a straight catheter to perform cavography. Locate the confluence of the iliac veins and that of the renal veins.
5. Dilate the right venous puncture with the dilator system or a balloon after making a 1-cm cut in the

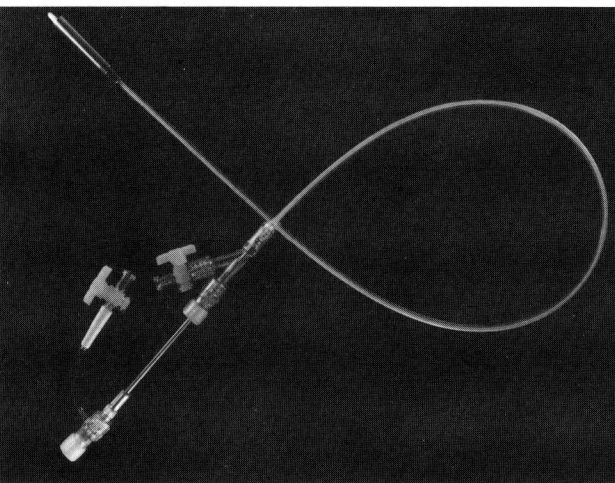

Figure 9.6 The Greenfield femoral introducing catheter. Note the coaxial system and the 8-mm-diameter steel capsule at the distal end (No. 24 French).

skin with a No. 11 scalpel. Exchange progressively the Amplatz dilator and its sheath carefully until it reaches No. 24 French (Fig. 9.7).
6. Insert the catheter with the delivery system through the sheath after assembling the filter on the carrying capsule. Only the guidewire and the sheath are kept partially inside the vein. During this procedure, abundant bleeding may take place and can be controlled manually with either the finger or a soft rubber tube (Fig. 9.8).
7. Fluoroscopically, direct the whole system to the previously determined site, keeping the tip of the filter just below the renal veins.
8. With the filter in position, carefully withdraw the external capsule while keeping the system's central catheter, which holds the filter, stable and stationary. When the hooks of the filter are released, the filter expands and is anchored to the caval wall (Fig. 9.9).
9. Remove the guidewire and the introducing system through the No. 24 French sheath; after this, withdraw the sheath immediately. A 10- to 15-min compression is sufficient to control the bleeding at the puncture site. Close the small incision in the skin with sutures.
10. Perform a cavography through the catheter, in the left femoral vein, to control the filter's position.

If there is occlusion in both femoral veins, the same procedure can be carried out in reverse through the right jugular vein by either puncture or venotomy. In this case a special introductory system is used for the jugular vein.

In patients who receive prolonged follow-up, the Greenfield vena cava filter has revealed approximately 95 percent permeability of blood flow in the inferior vena cava. After its insertion, the filter prevents the displacement of emboli with diameters ranging from 3 mm to several centimeters. Recurrent pulmonary embolism may occur in about 2 to 4 percent of patients who receive this type of filter. A controlled study of some patients revealed that the filter may forestall the displacement of large thrombi without occluding the inferior vena cava (Fig. 9.10).

It is possible to introduce the filter through the femoral vein using a percutaneous technique, even in the presence of a large fluctuating thrombus in the iliac veins. Computed tomography shows how the filter and adjacent structures are positioned (Figs. 9.11 and 9.12).

COMPLICATIONS

Recurrent pulmonary embolism after the insertion of a filter has already been mentioned. The most frequent problem with currently available vena cava filters results from the difficulty of inserting the large-bore introductory system through the venous vessels and positioning the filter adequately. Occasionally, the filter may be prematurely released and inadequately placed—either above the renal veins or inside an iliac vein—as a result of difficulties in manipulation or abrupt movements by the operator.

Migration of the filtering devices has become infrequent with the use of the Greenfield filter and has been markedly reduced with the use of the Mobin-Uddin filter, which has a larger diameter (28 mm). Surgical retrieval of embolized filters near the heart, however, is associated with high mortality.

Owing to its structure, the Greenfield filter does not migrate, although a case of displacement toward the right ventricle has been reported. Nevertheless, its hooks and legs can penetrate into and perforate the wall of the vena cava and thus cause perforation in adjacent organs such as the duodenum and right ureter.

It is not possible to perform percutaneous retrieval of a Greenfield filter after 3 or 4 weeks, because the proliferation of the intimal layer of the vena cava will cover the legs and hooks adjacent to the vascular wall.

The snare technique is a percutaneous alternative for retrieval of the Greenfield filter within the first few days of placement (Chap. 7). A large-caliber catheter with a wire loop is introduced percutaneously. This loop encircles the filter downward and is then carefully closed by means of external traction of its tips. The loops must encircle the filter legs and trap the hooks. As the filter is

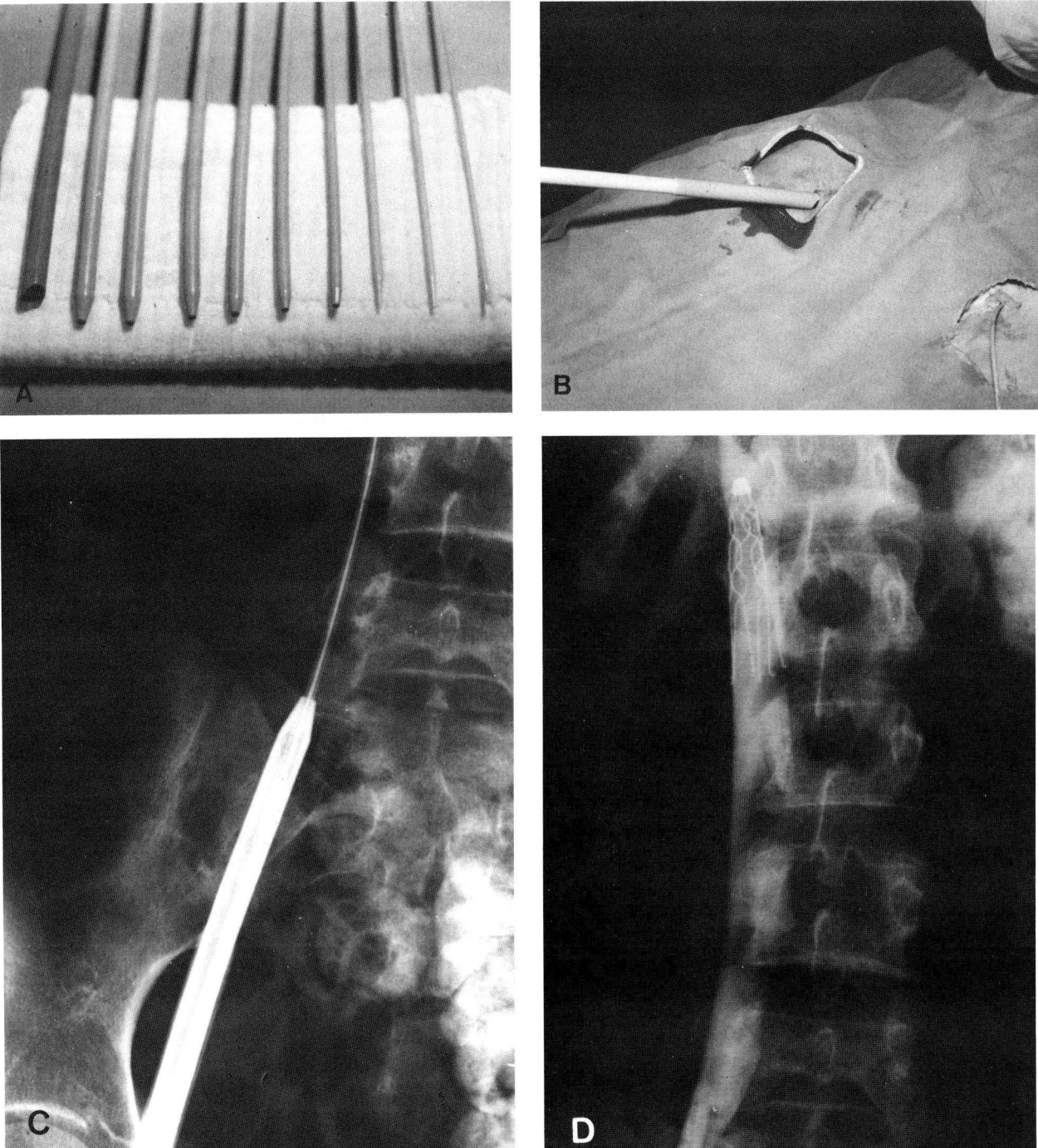

Figure 9.7 A 19-year-old female patient, tetraplegic after a traumatic lesion of the medulla, who developed partial caval thrombosis, pulmonary embolism, and hemorrhagic complications in the intracath with hematoma and hemothorax while taking heparin.

(A) An Amplatz dilator system with a No. 24 French sheath on the left. (B) A No. 24 French dilator system with a sheath positioned for placement of the filter by the percutaneous approach. The catheter is positioned to perform cavography of the left femoral vein. (C) A guidewire, a No. 8 French catheter, a No. 24 French dilator, and a No. 24 French sheath positioned inside the right femoral vein and right iliac vein. (D) A vena cava filter positioned in the inferior vena cava above the thrombus. Note the spasm of the right femoral vein and right iliac vein after retrieval of the sheath.

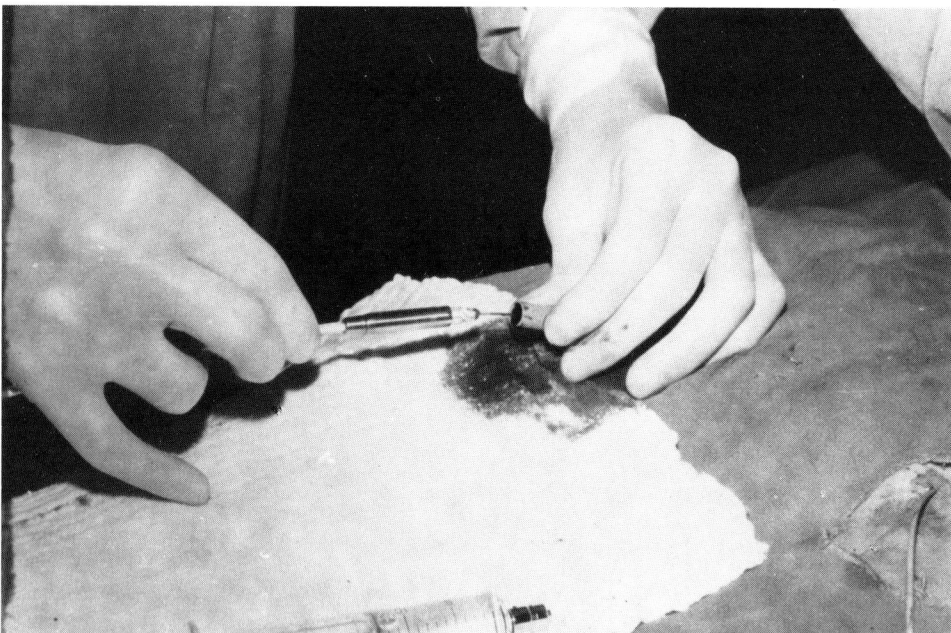

Figure 9.8 The precise moment for the introduction of a Greenfield filter in its capsule through a No. 24 French sheath. Note the guidewire passing through the introducing catheter and inside the sheath as far as the inferior vena cava. No significant bleeding was detected.

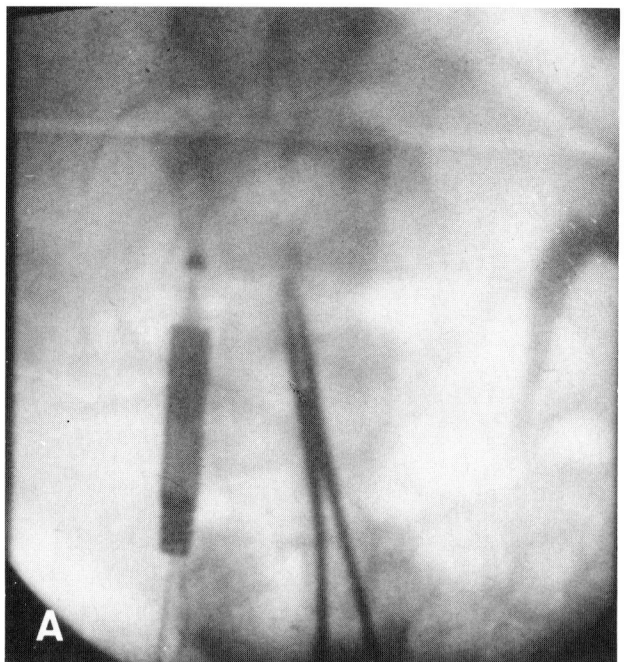
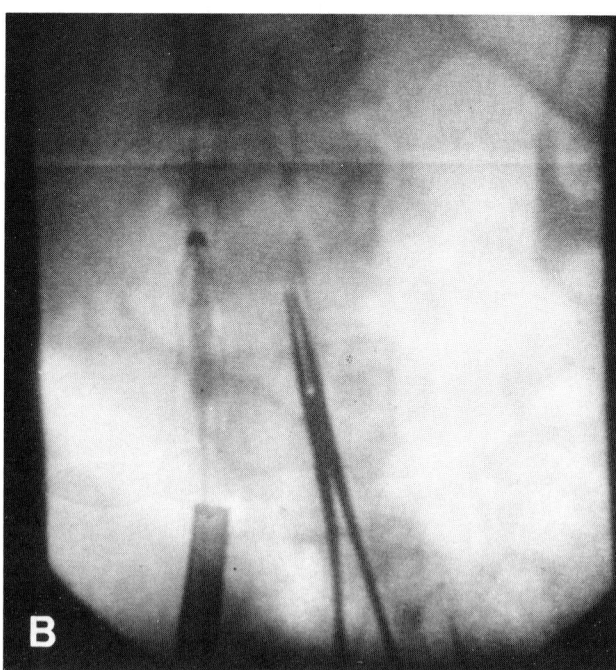

Figure 9.9 (A) A Greenfield filter still inside the capsule and in position to be released. (B) Filter positioning soon after capsule retrieval, with the filter kept stationary. (Photos were obtained from TV screen images.)

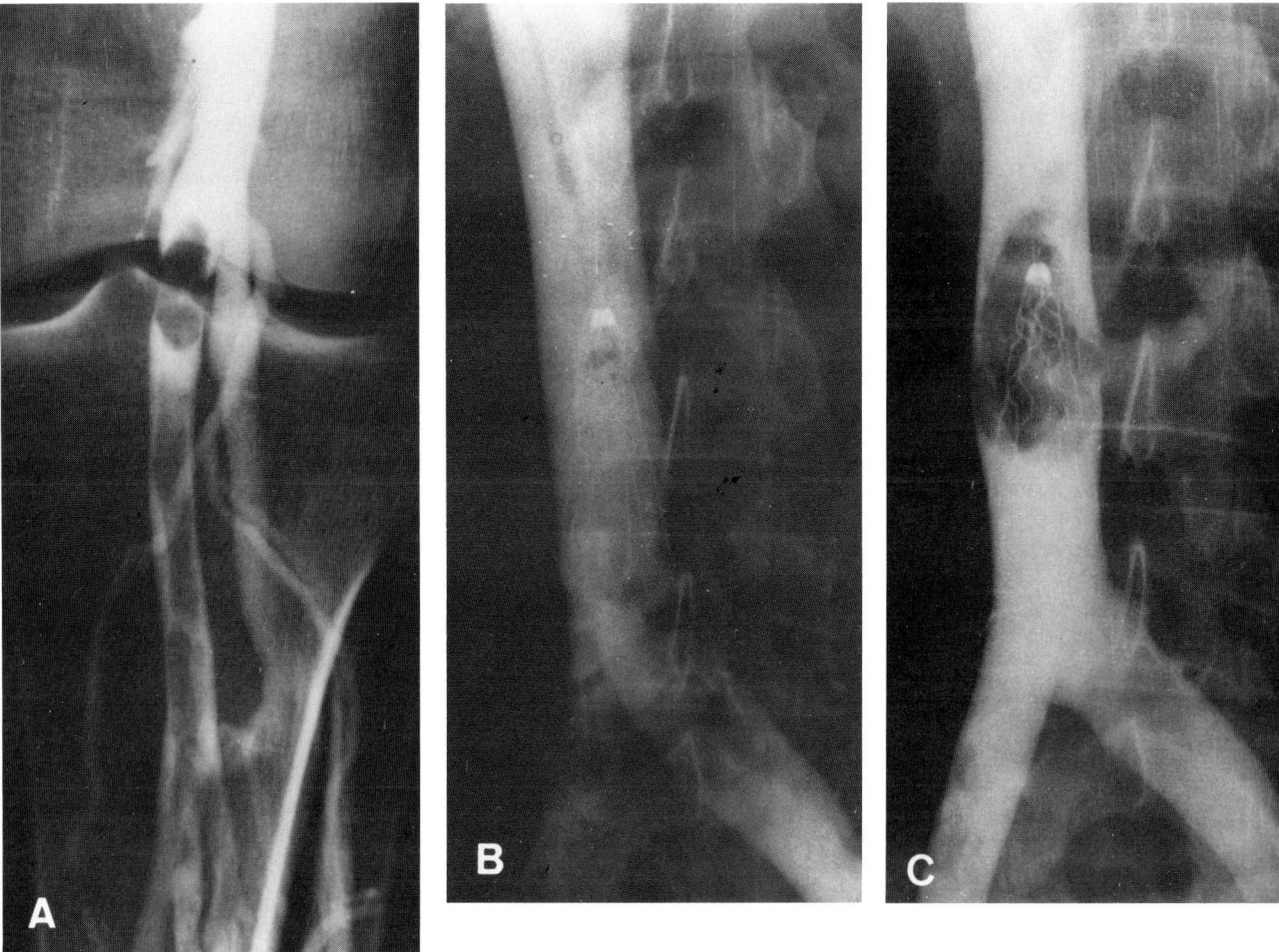

Figure 9.10 A 36-year-old male patient who presented with myocardiopathy, chronic heart failure, recurrent thrombophlebitis in the lower limbs, and various episodes of pulmonary embolism resulting in cor pulmonale.
(A) Left lower limb phlebography showing multiple thrombi inside the left tibial and popliteal veins. (B) Cavography immediately after placement of the vena cava filter shows an embolus captured by the filter. (C) Control cavography 2 months after placement of the filter shows a great number of thrombi inside and around the filter without occlusion of the vena cava. If the whole filter had not been placed, this thromboembolic material would have migrated to the pulmonary circulation.

knotted, it can be tractioned and displaced or even retrieved through a sheath in the right femoral vein.

NEW DEVELOPMENTS IN FILTERS

Other types of percutaneously inserted vena cava filters have been developed recently. However, they have not been employed worldwide.

Bird's Nest Filter

The bird's nest filter is made of stainless steel wire mesh and has distal and proximal tips for fixation. It is introduced through a No. 10 French catheter, using a percutaneous puncture via the femoral vein. Its filtrating capacity is lower than that of the other available filters.

Amplatz Filter (Spider)

This umbrella-shaped metal filter is highly flexible and stable and is capable of filtering small particles. It is percutaneously introduced through a No. 14 French catheter and has a proximal hook that is withdrawn with a simple wire loop. Its circular shape with a sequence of bearing points keeps the filter's axis oblique to the vena cava.

Günther Filter

This stainless steel filter is made of 12 stainless steel wires that form a helical basket similar to the Dormia

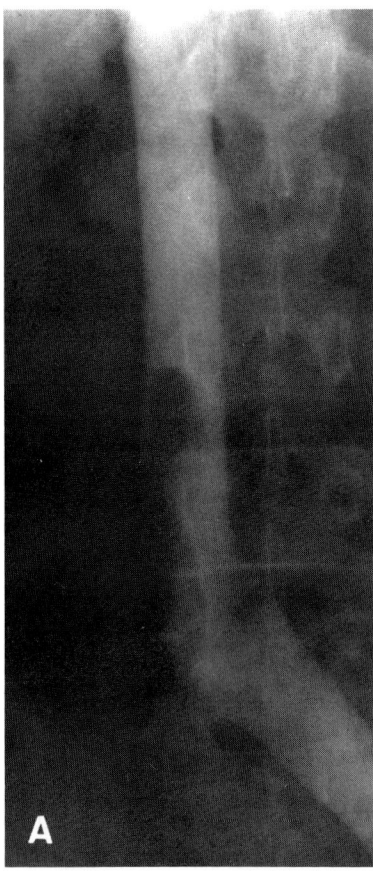
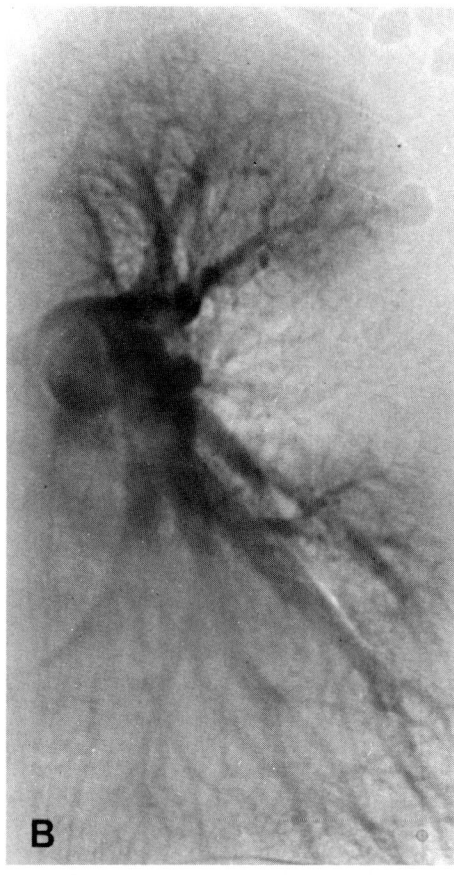

Figure 9.11 A 31-year-old male patient who presented with recurrent thrombophlebitis for 12 years. Phlebography of the lower limbs showed deep venous thrombosis of the entire right lower limb.

(A) Cavography and phlebography of the iliac veins showing occlusion of the right iliac vein and a large thrombus inside the vena cava, originating in the right iliac vein. (B) Pulmonary arteriography performed through puncture of the basilic vein of the right upper limb showing signs of pulmonary embolism in the right hemithorax (defect of perfusion). Signs of embolism were also present on the right side (not shown). (C) Cavography after placement of the filter in the inferior vena cava above the thrombus, via the left femoral vein. Note thrombi inside the filter. (D) Computed tomography showing the filter in the vena cava and the close relation between one of its legs and the end hook and the right ureter.

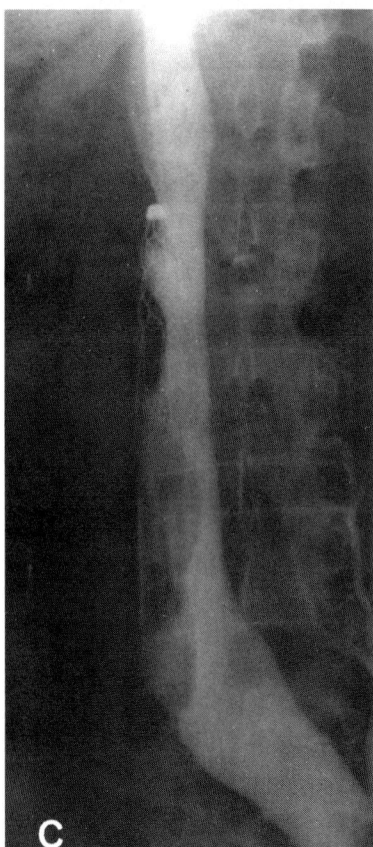
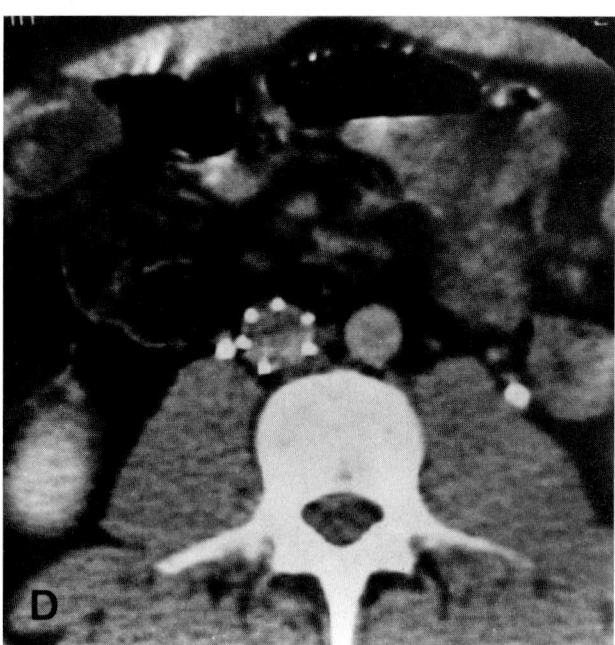

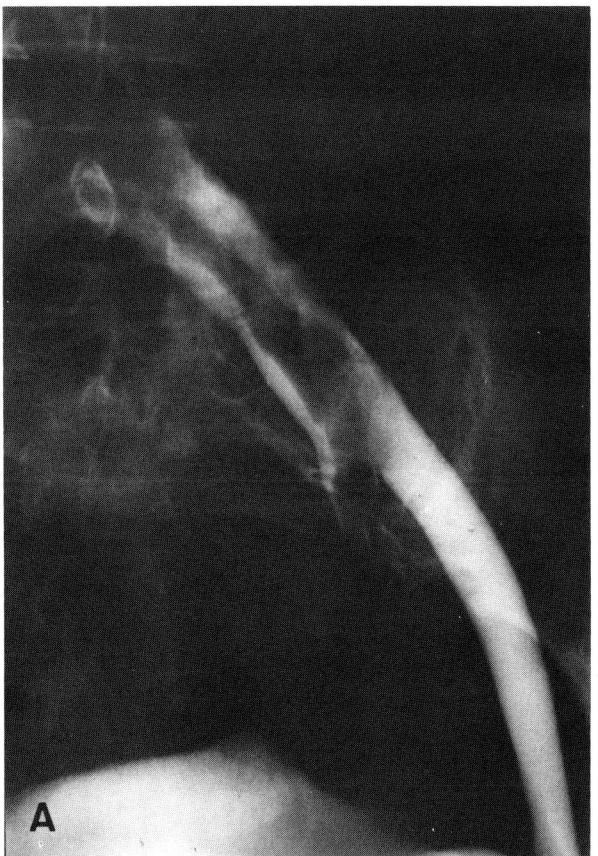
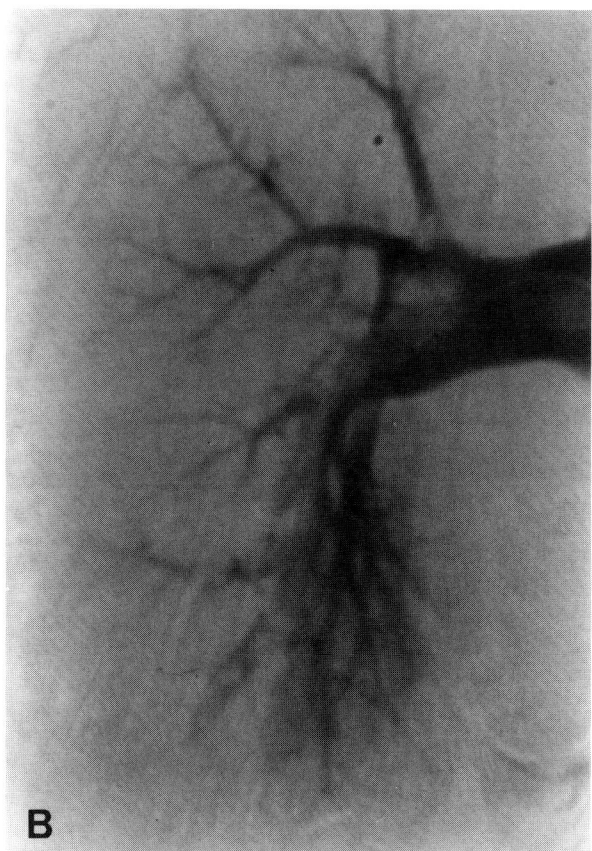
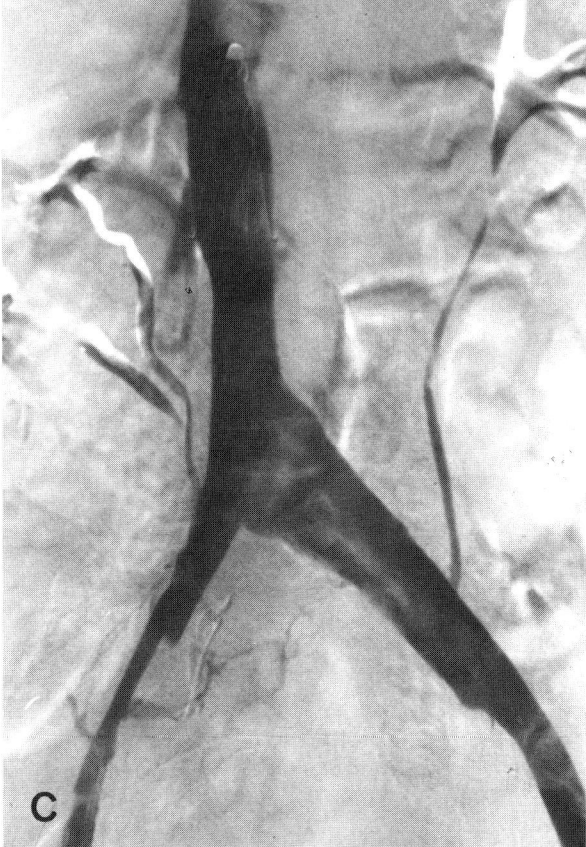

Figure 9.12 A postoperative 4-year-old patient who underwent a hysterectomy because of myomatosis and bleeding. This patient developed a vesicovaginal fistula and a right-sided pulmonary embolism.
(A) Phlebography showing a thrombus coming out of the left hypogastric vein and floating in the left iliac vein. (B) A right digital pulmonary angiogram showing severe pulmonary embolism with filling defects in the main artery and devascularization of the peripheral circulation. (C) Follow-up cavography after insertion of the vena cava filter by a percutaneous technique. Note the spasm in the right iliac vein.

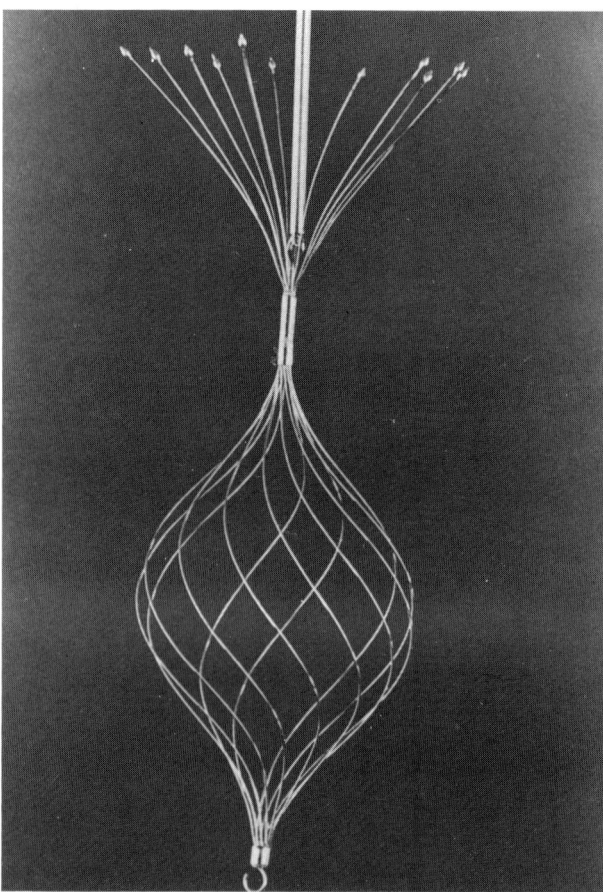

Figure 9.13 The Günther filter is made of 12 steel wires that form a basket-like configuration. There is an upper crown with prongs for fixation. Note the proximal and distal hooks for retrieval.

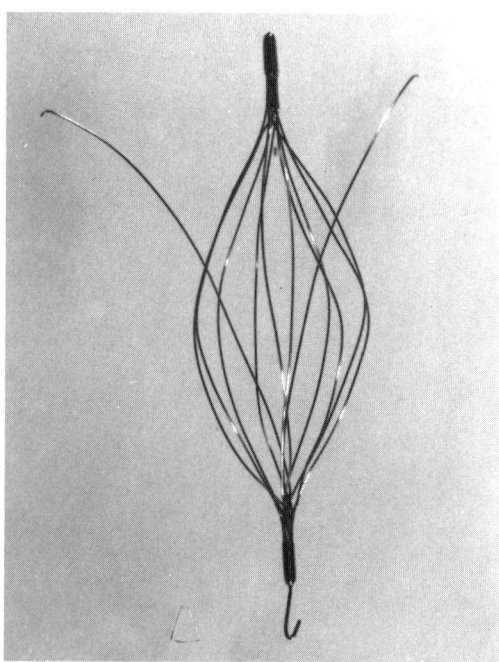

Figure 9.14 An Uflacker vena cava filter. It is similar to a Dormia basket and is connected to three stainless steel legs that fix the filter to the walls of the vena cava. The legs are shown open; in the axial position, the structure has a radiate aspect and shows the legs medially gathered (in the center) and fixed to the caval walls.

basket. It is connected to a crown with legs for fixation that are used for placement of the filter along the axis of the vena cava. The filter is percutaneously introduced through a No. 10 French catheter. It is percutaneously retrieved by its proximal hook and wire loop (Fig. 9.13).

Uflacker Filter

This zeppelin-shaped stainless steel filter consists of 9 to 12 stainless steel wires and has only three legs for fixation. The legs emerge from the proximal center and, together with the filter's body, establish two bearing points in the vena cava.

Because of the filter's stability, the axis always lies parallel to the caval axis. The filter is percutaneously introduced through a No. 10 to 12 French catheter. It can be percutaneously withdrawn with a wire loop, since it has a hook in the proximal tip (Fig. 9.14).

Simon Nitinol Filter

The Simon nitinol filter is made from a set of seven 0.015-in-diameter nitinol wires that are fused together at two points. The termal-shape memory of nitinol permits the device to have two functional forms. The first is a set of straight and pliable wires that are suitable for delivery through a standard angiographic catheter; the second is a complex and rigid filter shape for filtering emboli from the bloodstream. The filter form has two sections: the filter mesh and the anchoring limbs (Fig. 9.15). The filter mesh consists of a set of seven overlapping loops and has an overall outside diameter of 25 mm. The anchoring limbs can spread to a 32-mm diameter and have small termal hooks that engage the caval wall to hold the filter in place.

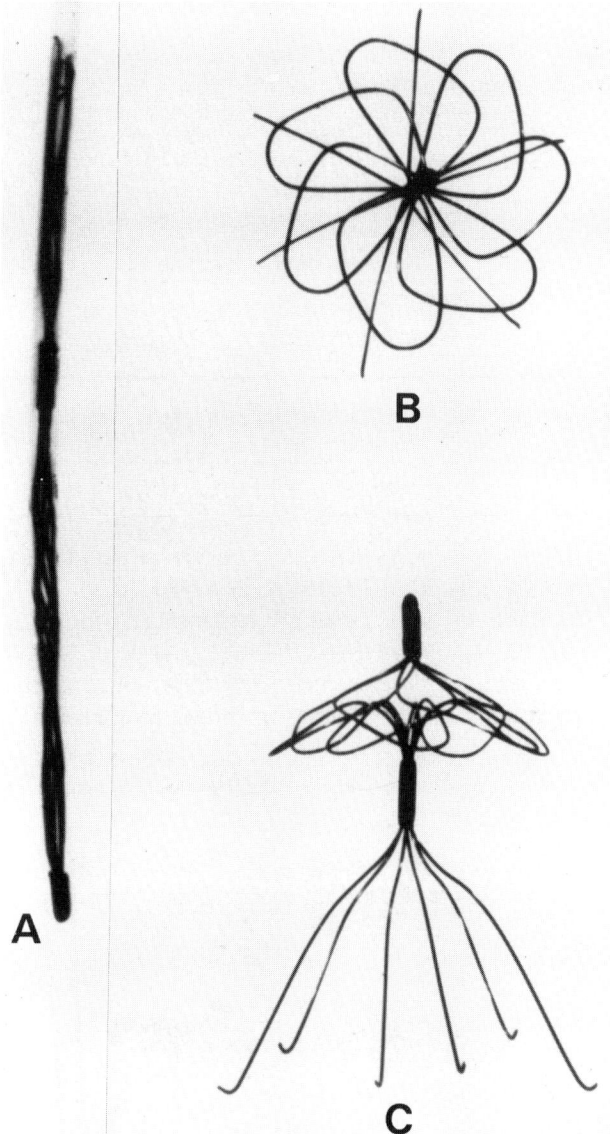

Figure 9.15 A Simon nitinol inferior vena cava filter. (A) Straight wires loaded into a standard angiographic No. 10 French catheter at room temperature. (B,C) Filter configuration at body temperature after delivery. Note the radial configuration of the filter mesh and the six anchoring limbs.

Vena Tech Filter

The vena tech filter consists of six stainless steel wires in a pyramid configuration with six additional lateral stabilizing wires. The stabilizing wires allow central positioning without angulation after insertion within the cava. The filter can be placed percutaneously through a No. 12 French sheath from either common femoral vein or a transjugular approach. Occasionally, positioning the filter from a left-sided percutaneous femoral vein approach may require gentle manipulation of the sheath as the filter passes this particular angulated segment. In our series of approximately 60 percutaneous vena tech filter placements, there have been no major untoward complications. No instances of retroperitoneal bleeding and no filter migration or inadequate expansion have been incurred in this series. There have been occasional reports of incomplete expansion when the filter has been positioned from a jugular approach. The filter is ordinarily positioned at the completion of a pulmonary arteriogram. Evaluation of the inferior vena cava and assuming the caval dimensions are 28 mm or less, the vena tech filter can be positioned with the apex of the cone just beneath the level of the renal veins. The entire procedure takes less than 5 min operator time. The filter itself is loaded within a 5-ml syringe and compressed to No. 10 French dimensions within the syringe. After connecting the syringe to the distal aspect of the No. 12 French introducer, the filter is then injected into the introducer via the syringe. A blunt-tipped cannula is then positioned within the introducer and the filter is pushed down the lumen until the desired position within the inferior vena cava is reached. The entire procedure is monitored fluoroscopically.

SUMMARY OF IN VITRO STUDIES OF THE RESULTS OF DIFFERENT FILTERING DEVICES

The optimal filter should exhibit most of the following characteristics: It traps all emboli, large and small; does not impede blood flow and is not thrombogenic; and can be percutaneously inserted through a small-caliber catheter. Its extrusion mechanism is simple and controlled; fixation to the wall of the inferior vena cava is secure enough to prevent migration; and although the point is debatable, retrievability is desirable.

It is difficult to find all these characteristics in a single type of filter, although some filters come close. However, no currently available vena cava device will never thrombose or migrate, and these filters cannot be 100 percent effective in preventing recurrent pulmonary thromboembolism. The filters discussed in this chapter are described in Table 9.2.

OVERVIEW

Intravascular filters are not intended to resolve thrombi already present in the lungs; their use is considered a prophylactic procedure to protect against thrombi which have not yet migrated to the lungs. There are no known contraindications for the use of inferior vena cava filters, and no concomitant drug therapy is contraindicated by the presence of the filter.

Table 9.2 – Comparison of clot-trapping capacity and flow dynamics

Filter	Small Clots, %	Large Clots, %	Blood Flow Dynamics	Filter Rating
Mobin-Uddin	80–100	100	Marked turbulence	Poor
Amplatz spider	80–100	100	Marked turbulence	Poor
Günther basket	80–100	100	Moderate turbulence	Superior
Simon nitinol	80–100	100	Least turbulent	Superior
Bird's nest	80–100	100	Least turbulent	Superior
Kimray-Greenfield	0–100	60–100	Moderate turbulence	Acceptable

Source: Katsamouris et al., 1988.

For each of the available devices, clinical trials have already been conducted and have shown the effectiveness of these filters in preventing recurrent pulmonary emboli. There are still some problems concerning migration of the device (Mobin-Uddin and bird's nest), insertion failure (bird's nest), misplacement (Mobin-Uddin and Kimray-Greenfield), caval wall penetration (Kimray-Greenfield), occlusion of the inferior vena cava (Mobin-Uddin, Kimray-Greenfield, and bird's nest), and recurrent pulmonary thromboembolism (Mobin-Uddin and bird's nest).

On the basis of the currently available data, the most effective and safe devices are the Kimray-Greenfield and Günther filters. Studies of new devices are in progress. Improvements in the Kimray-Greenfield filter that will allow percutaneous introduction through a smaller-caliber catheter will soon be available.

Percutaneous Transluminal Pulmonary Embolectomy

Surgical pulmonary embolectomy can cause extremely high mortality. In the first significant series of studies, only 16 percent of patients who received surgical pulmonary embolectomy survived. At present, the mortality from surgical pulmonary embolectomy is 57 percent.

More recently, Greenfield advocated percutaneous transvenous pulmonary embolectomy followed by the introduction of a vena cava filter (Greenfield filter) in patients with massive pulmonary embolism. This procedure was successful in Greenfield's patients and caused immediate reduction of pulmonary hypertension and excessive right-sided heart congestion.

Patients with massive pulmonary embolism whose hemodynamic features place them in class III and IV (Greenfield's classification) are the most likely candidates for percutaneous pulmonary embolectomy.

A 1-m-long No. 10 French catheter with a wide diameter is used for this technique. The catheter has a steerable tip with a screwed cupula which is used to aspirate the thrombotic mass. The available cupulas can be of two sizes: 5 mm and 7 mm in diameter (Fig. 9.16).

By resorting to the four control wires embedded in the walls of this type of catheter, one can adapt the catheter to a Medi-Tech control handle and steer its tip (Fig. 9.16). The system containing the cupula is introduced via the femoral vein by surgical venotomy or percutaneous insertion through a No. 22 or 24 French Amplatz sheath. Under fluoroscopy and with the help of the control handle, the steerable catheter connected to the cupula is directed to the pulmonary artery and to the position predetermined by angiographic diagnosis. Injection of contrast medium and subsequent impregnation of the thrombotic mass will determine the precise position of the thrombus. The embolus is kept trapped in the cupula by means of continuous aspiration, and the catheter is withdrawn by means of venotomy or through the sheath in the femoral vein.

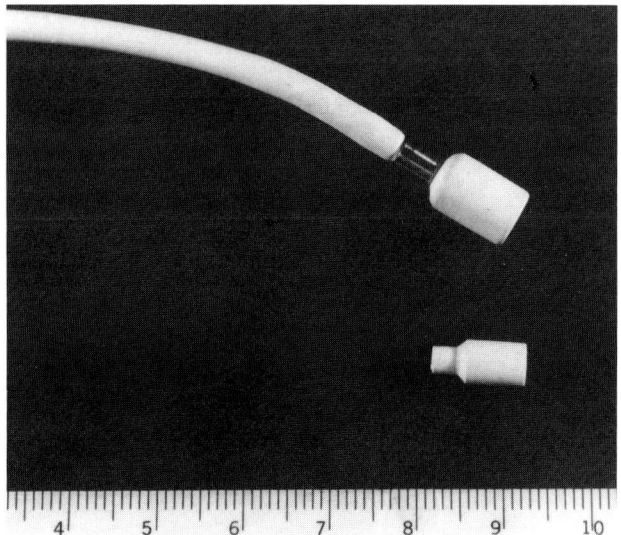

Figure 9.16 A catheter with a cupula for the performance of percutaneous transvenous embolectomy. This is a No. 10 French catheter with a steerable tip and a 5- to 7-mm-diameter cupula screwed into its tip. The cupula is attached to the pulmonary embolus through continuous aspiration; this allows transvenous retrieval.

The catheter should be introduced several times until pulmonary pressure is reduced to almost normal levels (about 20 mmHg) and large thrombotic masses can no longer be observed in the pulmonary arteries. After embolectomy, a vena cava filter should be inserted.

If this procedure does not retrieve a significant number of emboli within an hour, it should be abandoned and surgery should be considered.

REFERENCES

Brewster DC. Introduction to symposium on transvenous vena cava interruption. *J Vasc Surg* 1984;1:487–490.

Castaneda F, Herrera M, Cragg AH, Salamonowitz E, Lund G, Castaneda-Zuniga WR, Amplatz K. Migration of a Kimray-Greenfield filter to the right ventricle. *Radiology* 1983;149:690.

Cimochowski GE, Evans RH, Zarins CK, Lu CT, De Meester TR. Greenfield filter versus Mobin-Uddin umbrella. *J Thorac Cardiovasc Surg* 1980;358–365.

Coon WW. Epidemiology of venous thromboembolism. *Ann Surg* 1977;186:149–164.

Dunnick NR, Ravin CE, Sullivan DC. Pulmonary embolism. Course No. 301, 71st Scientific Assembly and Annual Meeting. Radiological Society of North America. Chicago, November 17–22, 1985.

Greenfield LJ. Current indications for and results of Greenfield filter placement. *J Vasc Surg* 1984;1:502–504.

Greenfield LJ, Peyton MD, Brown DP, Elkins RC. Transvenous management of pulmonary embolic disease. *Ann Surg* 1974;461–468.

Greenfield LJ, Perton R, Crute S, Barnes R. Greenfield vena caval filter experience: Late results in 156 patients. *Arch Surg* 1981;116:1451–1456.

Greenfield LJ, Stewart JR, Crute S. Improved technique for insertion of Greenfield vena caval filter. *Surg Gynecol Obstet* 1983;156:217–219.

Günther RW, Schild H, Fries A, Storkel S. Vena caval filter to prevent pulmonary embolism: Experimental study, work in progress. *Radiology* 1985;156:315–320.

Hunter JA, Delaria GA. Hunter vena cava balloon: Rationale and results. *J Vasc Surg* 1984;1:491–497.

Katsamouris AA, Waltman AC, Delichatrios MA, Athanasoulis CA. Inferior vena cava filters: In vitro comparison of clot trapping and flow dynamics. *Radiology* 1988;166:361–366.

Mobin-Uddin K, McLean R, Jude JR. A new catheter technique of interruption of inferior vena cava for prevention of pulmonary embolism. *Ann Surg* 1969;35:889–893.

Palestrant AM, Prince M, Simon M. Comparative in vitro evaluation of the nitinol inferior vena cava filter. *Radiology* 1982;145:351–355.

Prince MR, Novelline RA, Athanasoulis CA, Simon M. Diameter of the inferior vena cava and its implications for the use of vena cava filters. *Radiology* 1983;149:687–689.

Roehm JOF. The bird's nest filter: A new percutaneous transcatheter inferior vena cava filter. *J Vasc Surg* 1984;1:498–501.

Schneider PA, Bednarkiewica M. Percutaneous retrieval of Kimray-Greenfield vena caval filter. *Radiology* 1985;156:547.

Simon M, Palestrant AM. Tranvenous devices for the management of pulmonary embolism. *Cardiovasc Intervent Radiol* 1980;3:308–318.

Steward JR, Greenfield LJ. Tranvenous vena cava filtration and pulmonary embolectomy. *Surg Clin North Am* 1982;62:411–430.

Tadavarthy SM, Castaneda-Zuniga WR, Salomonowitz E, Lund G, Gragg AH, Hunter D, Coleman C, Amplatz K. Kimray-Greenfield vena cava filter: Percutaneous introduction. *Radiology* 1984;151:525–526.

Chapter Ten

Percutaneous Drainage of Abdominal Fluid Collections

RENAN UFLACKER

INTRODUCTION

Abdominal abscesses have traditionally been treated surgically with large incisions and extensive drainage through large tubes; this has generally been uncomfortable for patients. Until recently exploratory surgery was also an analytic method for diagnosing and locating abdominal abscesses when a strongly suggestive clinical picture was present. However, this type of procedure may lead to a mortality rate of 28 percent for hepatic abscesses and 43 percent for subphrenic and subhepatic abscesses, including a 49 percent recurrence rate for subphrenic and subhepatic abscesses.

Conventional x-rays and nuclear medicine did not supply accurate diagnostic data but provided only non-specific findings. The use of gallium in nuclear medicine made it possible to visualize abscesses. Abdominal abscesses became directly visible only with the advent of modern imaging methods which made visualization of the abdomen in different planes possible. Since the development of imaging and percutaneous treatment, exploratory surgery and drainage were replaced almost completely by percutaneous drainage.

Actually, both ultrasonography (US) and computed tomography (CT) can be used to diagnose abdominal collections. The choice of one method over the other depends on local availability, the cost of examination, and professional expertise.

Location in relation to adjacent structures and identification of a safe access route are the most significant aspects of the image diagnosis of abscesses; this information also helps in planning a percutaneous approach. A few criteria should be followed to identify a safe access window, for instance, the shortest distance between the collection and the skin and the possibility of bypassing interposing structures or intestinal loops. Image-guided puncture is the next step. Once the lesion type has been defined, an appropriate catheter is introduced and the abscess is evacuated.

Percutaneous drainage of abdominal fluid collections and abscesses was described as "one of the decade's greatest advances" by Welch and Malt in 1983 in a review of abdominal surgery.

It is currently accepted that this procedure is here to stay and will have a reasonably rapid growth of its applications. This is in contrast to other interventional techniques, which have proved to be merely transitional, such as transhepatic embolization of esophageal varices and percutaneous renal lithotripsy. The first technique is being replaced by endoscopic sclerosis, and the second will soon be replaced by shock wave lithotripsy.

Although US is more than adequate for diagnosing and locating abdominal collections, the literature and our experience suggest that CT is more appropriate for planning a percutaneous approach to a lesion. With CT one can more easily find the right window and identify and distinguish intestinal loops.

There are five different signs of abscess on CT scan:

1. A low-attenuation soft tissue mass [0 to 25 Hounsfield units (HU)]. Irregular or well-defined contours may be seen, depending on the maturity and arrangement of the abscess.
2. A peripheral rim of enhancement after contrast injection has distinguished the lesion from adjacent normal structures.
3. Abnormal presence of gas in the form of small bubbles or air-fluid levels.
4. Edema of tissue planes next to the lesion.
5. Displacement of surrounding structures.

When these signs are present, CT has been shown to be the most accurate and effective method for diagnosing abdominal abscesses, especially compared with US, in which the signs vary according to the homogeneity of the collection content and the type of device used.

Most abscesses appear as hypoechoic masses, which have good transmission of US waves as a result of their fluid content. Air fluid levels are occasionally identified when debris layers are formed. Air fluid levels also may hinder visualization of deep layers, causing the abscess to appear to be similar to an intestinal loop. Gas bubbles seen inside an abscess may produce an image indistinguishable from that of surrounding structures, particularly intestinal loops.

Although 80 to 90 percent of intraabdominal abscesses can be drained, a considerable number of attempts fail. The main cause of failure in percutaneous and surgical drainage of intraabdominal abscesses is inadequate diagnosis of the magnitude, extension, complexity, location, and response of the abscess.

The mortality rate in drainage of abdominal abscesses is frequently related to a low physiologic score, and even rapid and precise drainage may not be beneficial. Technical errors in approaching and choosing the drainage method are significant causes of failure. These errors can be divided into two groups: inadequate diagnosis and inappropriate technique.

Inadequate diagnosis is usually related to nonrecognition of enteric or biliary fistulas. Identification of a phlegmonous process when one is draining a poorly developed abscess, i.e., one without a complete capsule, frequently results in hemorrhage. Another example of inadequate diagnosis is failure to identify loculation or residual abscesses. The most common technical errors are related to premature removal of the drainage catheter and the use of an inadequate access window which fails to locate the puncture site on the dependent portion of the cavity.

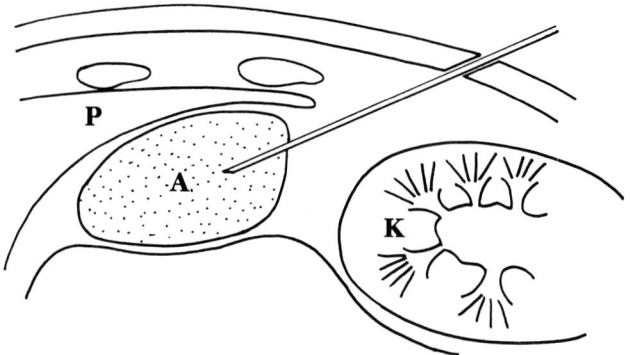

Figure 10.1 Schematic drawing of the posterior approach by triangulation to subphrenic abscesses. This technique prevents violation of the pleural space, with the needle penetrating through a small interspace between the kidney and the pleura. P = pleural space; A = abscess; R = kidney.

process based on the Pythagorean theorem (Fig. 10.1). This access route is useful in cases of SA posterior to the liver, the spleen, or the gastric body or fundus (Fig. 10.2). Transpleural vertical posterior puncture violates this space and can lead to extraabdominal contamination (Fig. 10.3).

SUBPHRENIC COLLECTIONS

Subphrenic abscesses (SAs) are defined as collections of sometimes purulent material in the immediate space between the lower surface of the diaphragm and the organs at the supramesocolic level. These abscesses can occupy the locus of any of these organs which have been surgically removed.

A range of diseases may cause spontaneous formation of an SA with gastrointestinal perforation, biliary disease, or sepsis. The most common cause, however, is contamination of the peritoneal cavity during surgery, especially surgery for intestinal inflammatory disease, gastrectomy, incidental splenectomy, and partial hepatectomy.

Surgeries infected by inflammatory intestinal disease tend to produce abscesses in subphrenic or subhepatic positions, while the presence of subphrenic empty spaces as a result of organ ablation favors the collection of purulent fluid in the area previously occupied by the organ on both the right and left sides.

Approach routes to subphrenic abscesses vary depending on size and location. In a patient with a posterior SA, special care should be taken in regard to pleural reflection which reaches the 11th and 12th ribs posteriorly. The approach used is puncture in the cephalic, subcostal, and extraperitoneal direction, following a course dorsal to the kidney and ventral to the diaphragm. The angular approach is obtained through a triangulation

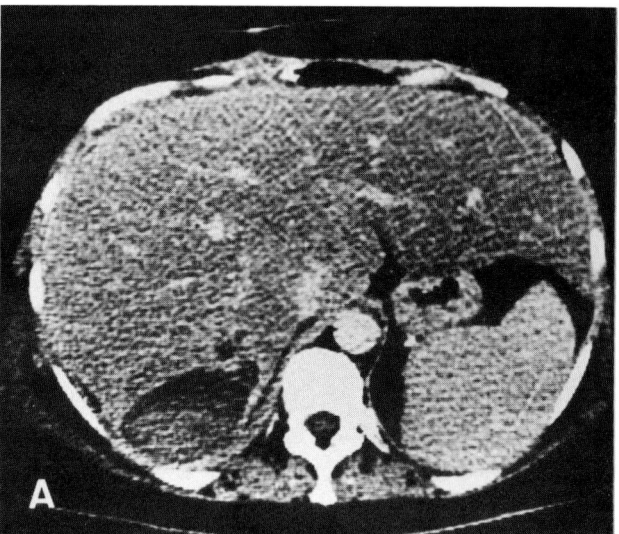

Figure 10.2 (A) A 63-year-old patient on the thirtieth postoperative day after a cholecystectomy with a biliary fistula and a retrohepatic subphrenic abscess. (B) A cholangiogram performed through the drain shows a biliary fistula. (C) Puncture of the lesion by the posterior approach performed cranially with triangulation. Opacification of the right subphrenic cavity. (D) A sump-type (No. 12 French) catheter for irrigation inside the lesion. (E) Control CT scan a few hours after drainage shows contrast in the interior and some reduction in cavity volume. Total drainage time was 12 days.

Figure 10.2 *Continued*

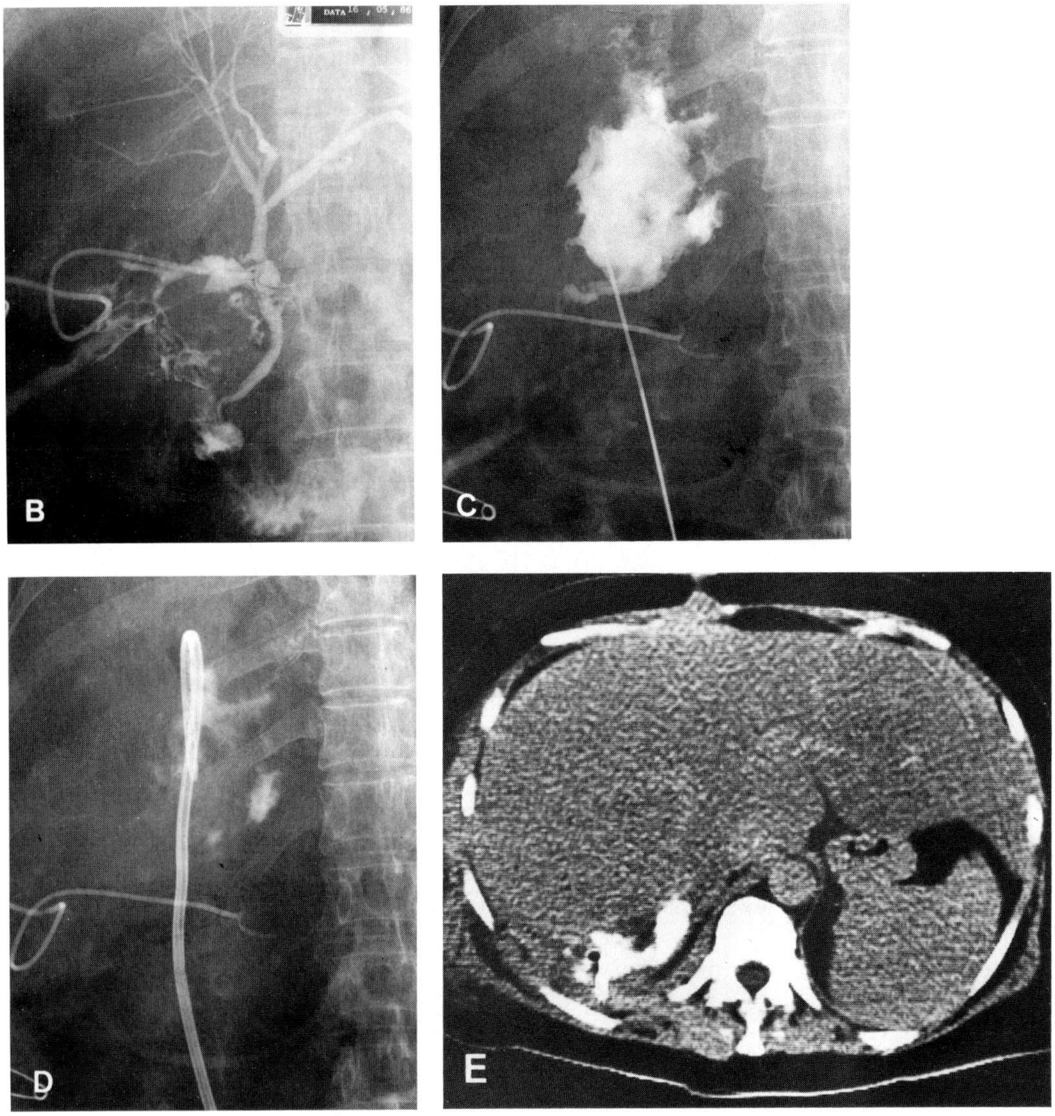

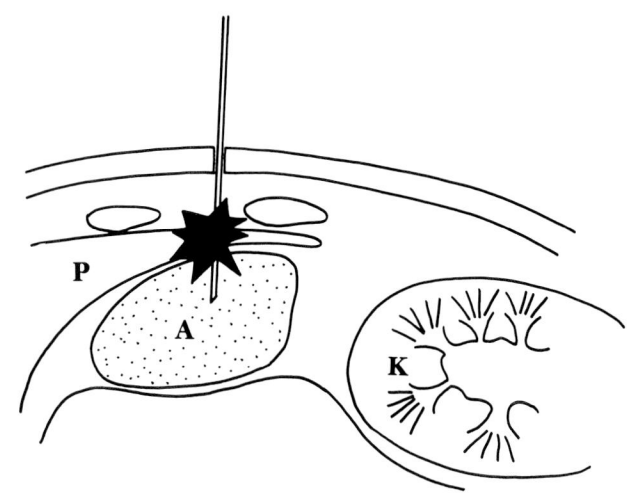

Figure 10.3 Schematic drawing illustrates violation of the pleural space (P) when a high vertical posterior puncture is performed toward the abscess (A). The relation of the kidney (R) to the pleura was not observed, and there was a risk of dissemination of the infection to the thorax.

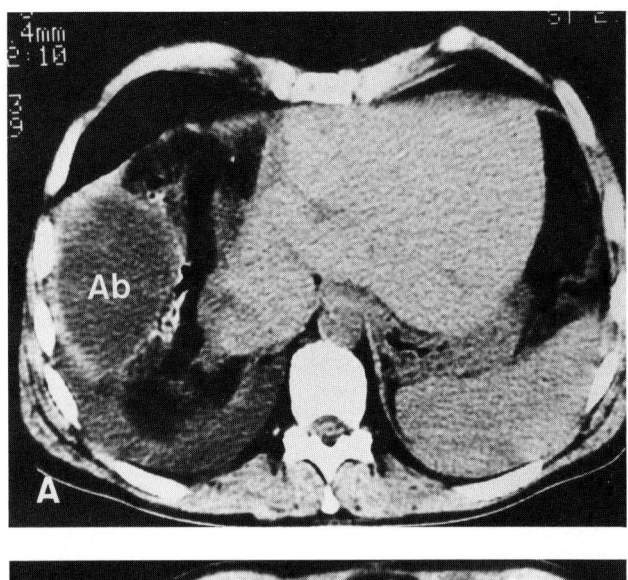
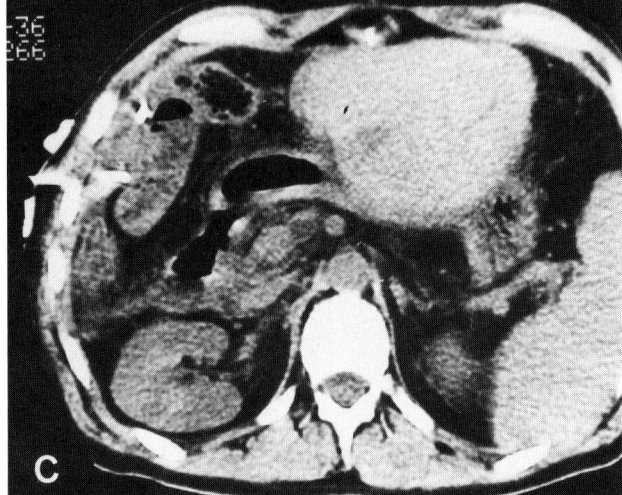
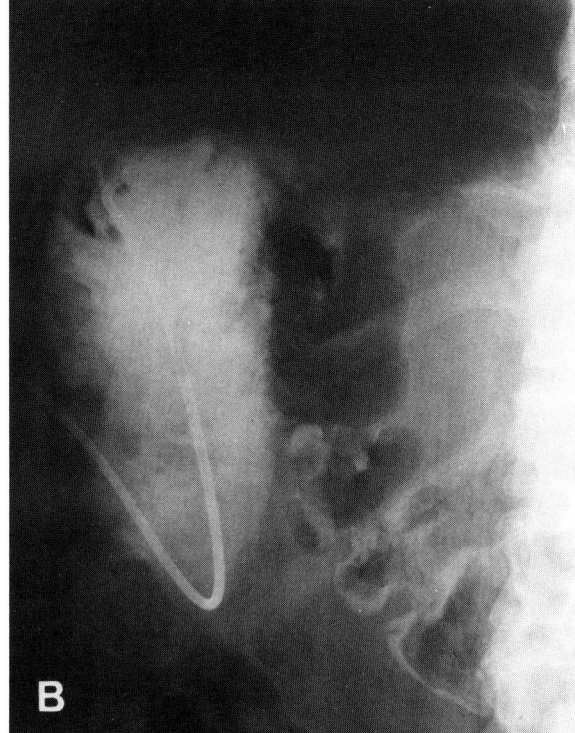
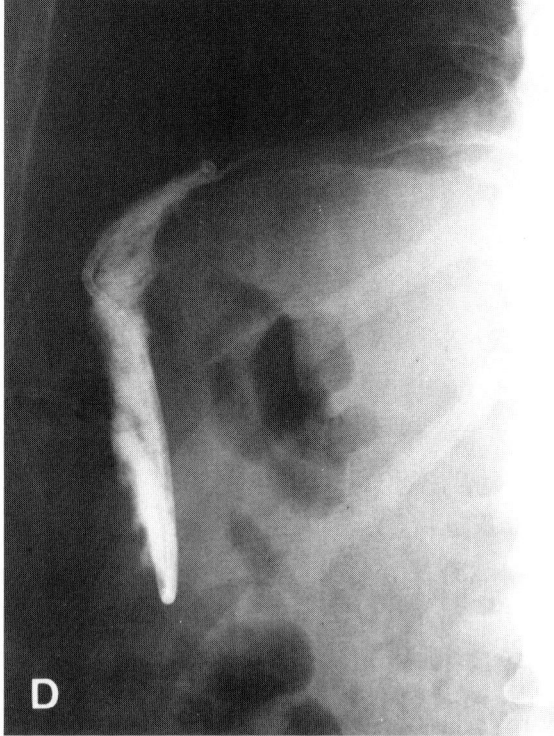

Figure 10.4 (A) A 47-year-old patient with fever and jaundice 15 days after right hepatectomy (trisegmentectomy) for a hepatic metastasis of a previously operated colonic carcinoma. Note the right subphrenic abscess (Ab) with the colon displaced medially. (B) After puncture, the purulent material assumed the aspect of bile. A pigtail catheter with multiple lateral holes was used to drain the cavity. (C) Control CT about 10 days after puncture shows considerable reduction in lesion volume. (D) A sinogram showing the virtual cavity which remained. The catheter was kept in place for 20 additional days until biliary secretion disappeared; it was then removed.

Laterally or anteriorly located SAs can be drained through lateral (Fig. 10.4) or anterior windows (Fig. 10.5), provided that one can prove the absence of intestinal loops that are in the way. Window demarcation on the skin with radiopaque material by CT makes it possible for the abscess to be drained in the CT room or the angiography laboratory under fluoroscopic guidance after a reference point has been obtained.

Occasionally, without CT references, it is possible to drain a subphrenic locus under fluoroscopic guidance

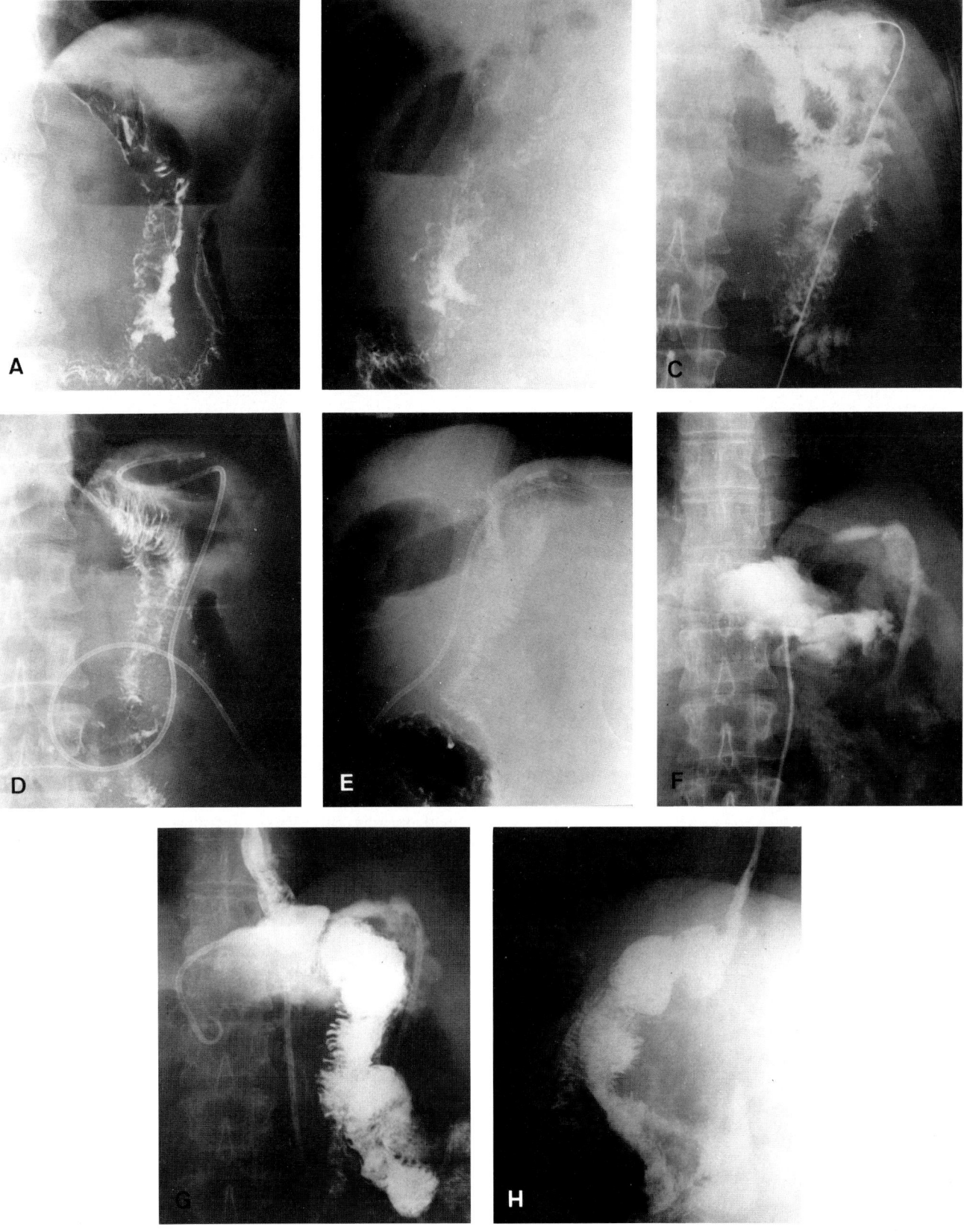

Figure 10.5 (A,B) A 40-year-old patient with a subphrenic abscess after a gastrectomy for carcinoma. Barium contrast outlines the esophagoenteric anastomosis. Frontal (A) and profile (B) images of air fluid levels in the abscess. (C) Cavity puncture and catheterization; intestinal loops on the left extending below the phrenic dome. Note that the spleen is present and should be preserved. (D,E) Drainage catheter (biliary Ring type) in the left subphrenic space. In the lateral view (E), reduction of the posterior-superior cavity is seen, with a persistent anterior cavity. (F,G) A new puncture of the anterior cavity performed by the anterior route shows no communication between the two cavities. The posterior-superior cavity is almost totally collapsed. (H) Final control after removal of the posterior catheter and effective drainage of the anterior cavity. Fever disappeared. Total drainage time was 13 days: 6 days for the first drainage and 7 for the second.

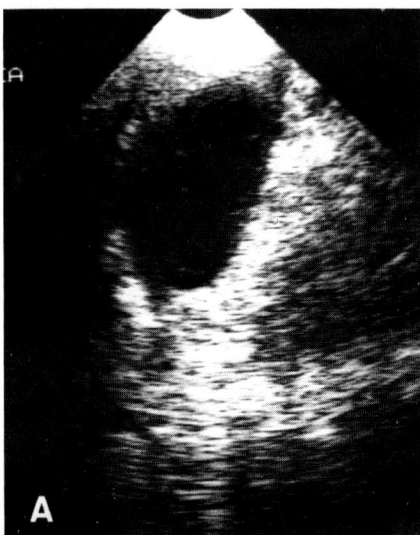 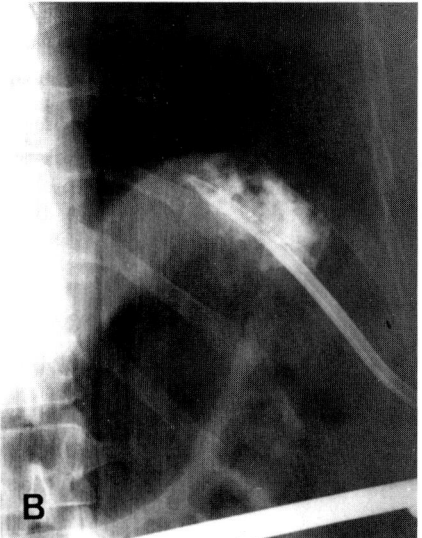 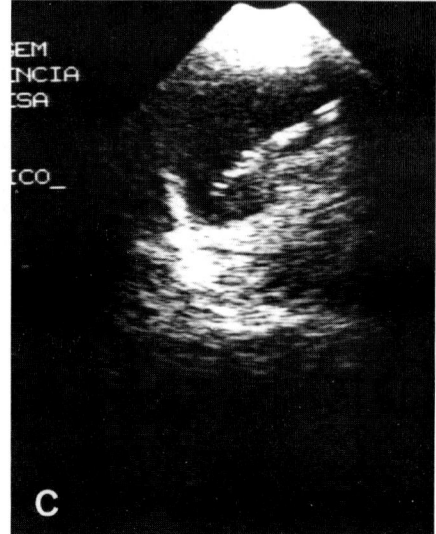

Figure 10.6 (A) A 34-year-old patient who was involved in an automobile accident, with spleen rupture and fracture of the pelvis. Ultrasonography (US) shows a left subphrenic cavity in the splenic bed. The puncture was performed under US guidance. (B) Side x-ray shows the cavity and drainage catheter (sump type). (C) US control showing a partially drained cavity and the catheter in place inside it.

(Fig. 10.5) or by means of ultrasonography alone (Fig. 10.6). When fluoroscopy is used, it is advisable to opacify adjacent intestinal loops (Fig. 10.5).

SA may or may not be related to a biliary fistula or to the intestinal tube. When a fistula is present, the time required for catheter drainage is much longer, varying from 12 to 120 days and averaging 43 days, according to the literature (Fig. 10.4). When there is only one subphrenic cavity and it is not connected to the fistula, the average drainage time is reduced to 18 days (Figs. 10.2 and 10.7). Lesion irrigation and aspiration apparently reduce the drainage time in both cases. More recent findings indicate that when a larger catheter, irrigation, and aspiration are used, drainage time is reduced to 5 to 7 days in patients who have an SA without a fistula (Figs. 10.8 and 10.9).

Abscesses in the liver parenchyma or the perihepatic spaces tend to drain 25 to 50 mL of serous fluid per day, decreasing in volume after 5 to 7 days. Abscesses in potential spaces, i.e., intraperitoneal, pericolic, or pelvic abscesses, can produce larger quantities of fluid for longer periods. When a fistula is present, the drainage time increases to 3 to 4 weeks.

In all these different types of abscesses, however, the most important evaluation parameter is the relative amount of drained fluid, serially measured, not the absolute quantity.

Daily drainage volume is more significant than the presence of infection. Noninfected bilomas and seromas require much longer drainage times, as they produce more fluid than do common abscesses.

In an aseptic collection, needle aspiration or 24-h drainage is appropriate. With this method, the cause of fever is removed and secondary contamination can be prevented (Fig. 10.6).

It is also true, however, that many abscesses of any location can be cured by means of direct aspiration alone, with antibiotic coverage and without prolonged drainage. Breaking the balance of the bacterial ecosystem by means of aspiration or drainage will itself cause definitive involution of the process in most cases.

Subphrenic abscesses belong to the group of abscesses which are more easily treated by percutaneous drainage. Success rates have reached 72 to 94 percent, with just 1 to 4 percent mortality, whereas in recent reports 24 to 84 percent mortality rates have been reported for surgical drainage.

When the abscess is accurately located through CT, it is possible to anticipate the probability of cure with percutaneous drainage. There is an 84 percent chance of curing subphrenic and hepatic abscesses, while for intraabdominal abscesses in other areas, the chances of complete cure are only 47 percent.

LIVER

The incidence of pyogenic abscesses in the liver varies significantly between published series. Before 1933 the incidence at necropsy varied between 0.45 and 1.47 percent. More recently (1975) and compared with the

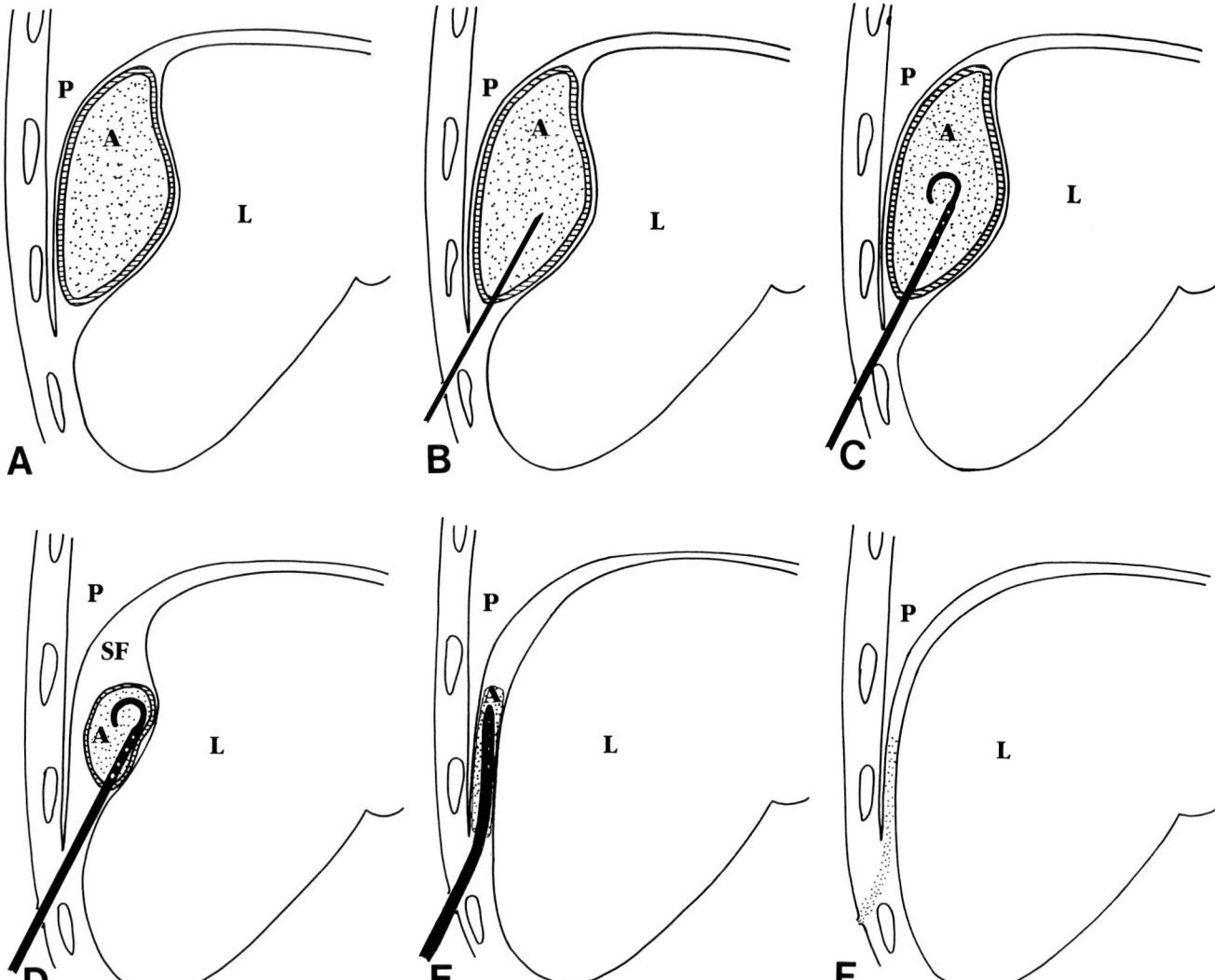

Figure 10.7 (A) Schematic drawing shows a right subphrenic abscess (A) displacing the liver (F) and in contact with the diaphragm and its relationship to the pleural space (P). (B) Abscess puncture by the lateral route with a rigid needle below the pleural reflection. (C) A pigtail drainage catheter is introduced. (D) After the third day of drainage, the cavity was reduced and the subphrenic space (SF) became clearer. (E) On the fifth to seventh day the cavity is only virtually present and the catheter can be removed. (F) After catheter removal, only a track is seen, with granulation tissue and a small scar on the skin.

total number of hospital admissions, it varied from 0.013 to 0.016 percent.

The rate of liver contamination by the portal route was 45 percent before 1938 but has dropped to as low as 18 percent. Patients with diabetes mellitus, polycystic liver disease, hepatic cirrhosis, extensive burns, cancer, biliary obstruction, multiple trauma, or granulomatous disease and those receiving immunosuppressive medication constitute a risk group for hepatic abscess (HA). HA is most prevalent in the sixth and seventh decades of life.

The most frequent location of HA is in the right lobe, distributed by the effect of portal laminar flow (Fig. 10.10). With multiple abscesses in the liver, there is a higher probability of contamination by the arterial route, for instance, by bacterial endocarditis. Obstruction of the biliary tract can also cause multiple abscesses in the liver. Multiple HAs occur in 46.4 to 60 percent of cases, varying between series.

In the liver, it is most common to find a single abscess collection in the right lobe. If the collection is in a lower position, the easiest approach is lateral, intercostal, or subcostal (Fig. 10.11A). A posterior high abscess (close to the diaphragm) can be approached laterally, but a posterior approach is more frequently adopted. The triangulation technique, as previously described, is used to avoid the posterior pleural recess (Fig. 10.11B). When the abscess is in the left hepatic lobe, the puncture

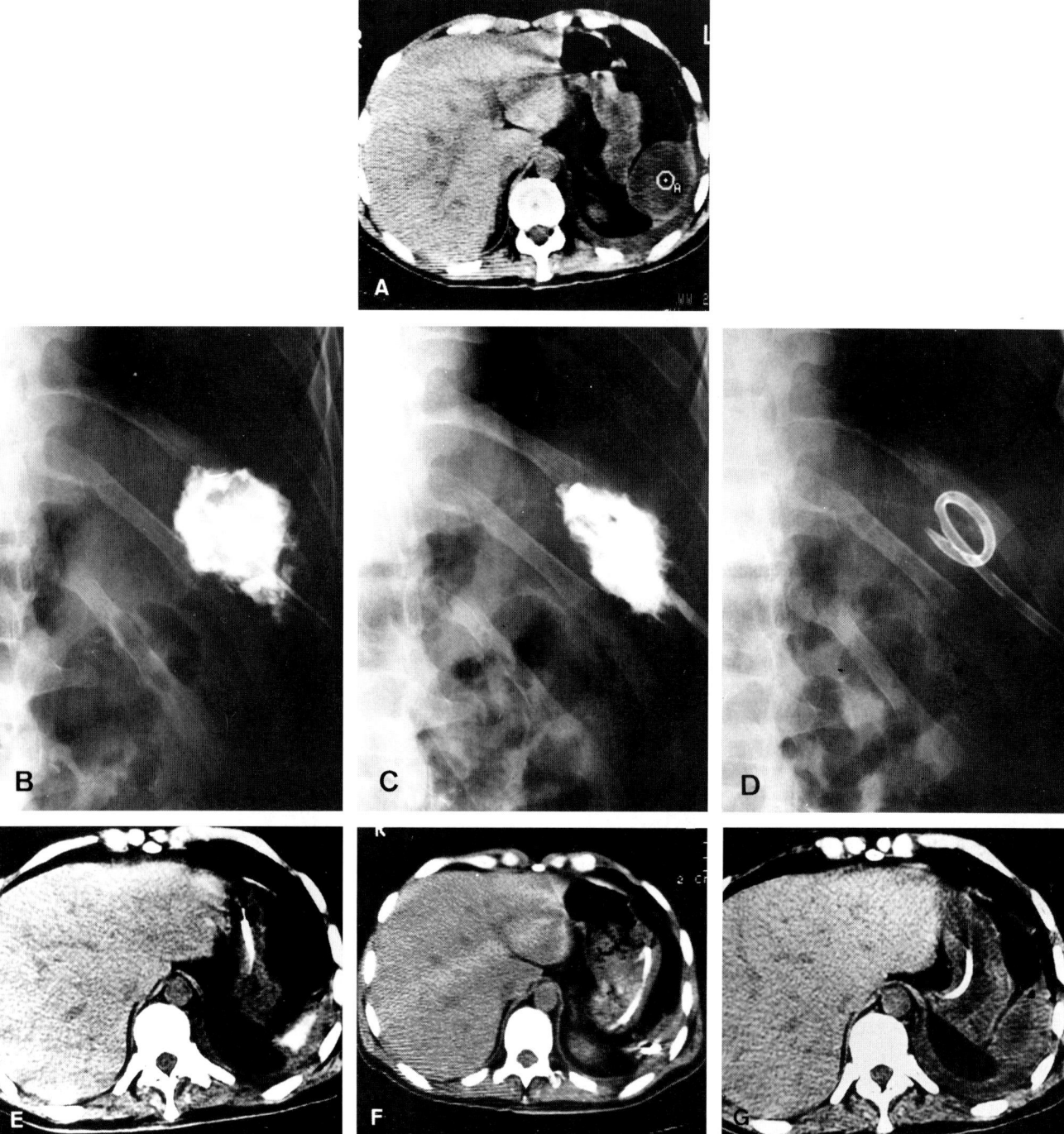

Figure 10.8 (A) Computed tomography (CT) shows the left subphrenic cavity (A) (same patient in Fig. 10.6). (B) Puncture with an 18-gauge needle under CT guidance, followed by contrast injection. (C,D) A pigtail-type drainage catheter inside the cavity. (E,F) Control by CT after drainage shows an emptied cavity. (G) After catheter removal, a small subphrenic collection persisted; it had a good evolution to total cure in 2 weeks.

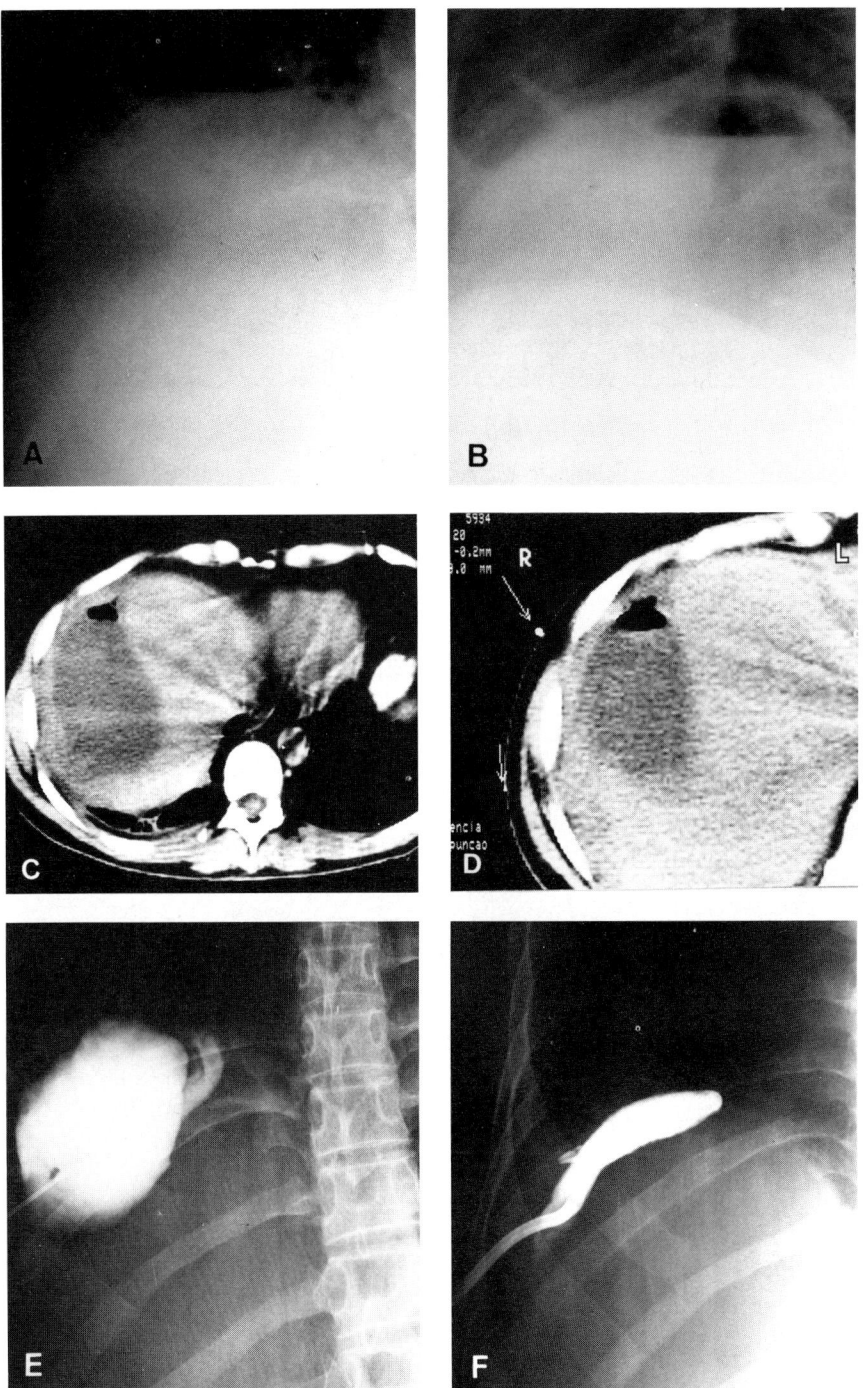

Figure 10.9 (A,B) A 36-year-old patient who developed peritonitis and a subphrenic abscess after appendectomy. Frontal (A) and lateral (B) x-rays showing the right subphrenic air fluid level. (C,D) Computed tomography (CT) showing the subphrenic cavity in close contact with the liver and diaphragm. Note the reference point (arrow) marked on the skin. (E) Subphrenic cavity puncture followed by drainage with a sump-type catheter. (F) A control sinogram 3 days after drainage. The cavity is significantly reduced. Continuous aspiration and irrigation were performed. (G) Control CT showing the catheter inside the cavity. (H,I) Sinogram and control CT on the sixth day showing a practically virtual cavity. (J,K) The catheter was removed on the seventh day, with complete resolution of the abscess. Note, however, the presence of edema and air on the periphery of the liver.

Figure 10.9 *Continued*

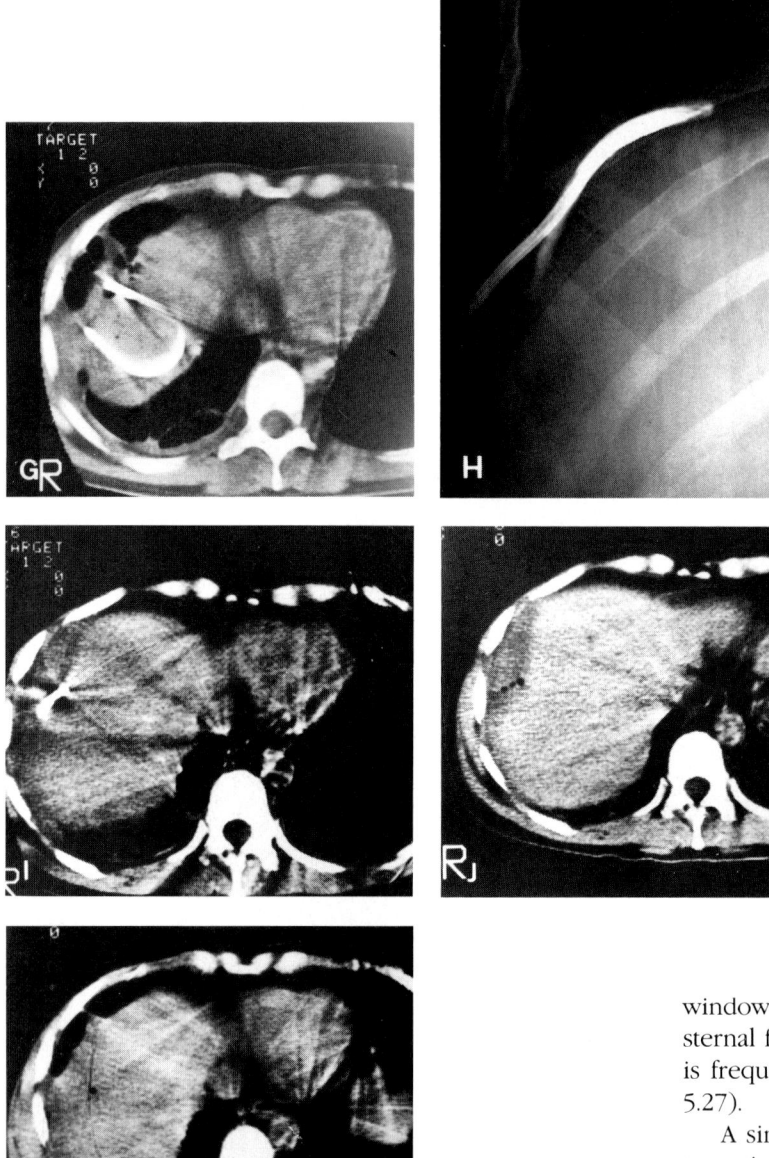

window is anterior, frequently subcostal, and next to the sternal furcula (Fig. 10.11C). Puncture during inhalation is frequently required with the anterior approach (Fig. 5.27).

A single No. 8 or 10 French catheter with a pigtail-type tip and lateral holes is sufficient for draining a solitary small to medium-volume HA. When the collected material is thick, with a volume exceeding 100 mL, a sump-type double-lumen No. 12 to 16 French catheter will be necessary. The approach to multiple HAs must also be multiple, using many different catheters and windows.

US, as previously mentioned, can easily detect multiple HAs, while CT can define the location of HAs more accurately in relation to reference points (Fig. 10.11).

Percutaneous drainage of HAs is successful in 91 percent of cases if infected hematomas and tumors are not included in the statistics. When these two groups of lesions are considered for statistical purposes, the success rate drops to 76 percent.

The puncture methodology adopted is similar to that used for SAs. Once the access window has been defined,

Figure 10.10 (A) A patient with fever, jaundice, dyspnea, and obnubilation resulting from a hepatic abscess. CT shows a collection in the right hepatic lobe. (B) After treatment with antibiotics for 7 days, the limits of the process were better established. Fever persisted, however. (C) A CT-guided percutaneous puncture opacifying the intrahepatic cavity. (D) Drainage with a sump-type No. 16 French catheter, which was maintained with irrigation and aspiration. (E) Sinogram with catheter repositioning. Note the reduction in the size of the collection after 3 days. (F) Control CT on the seventh day after drainage shows absence of the cavity. The catheter was removed because there was no more drainage or fever. (G) Control tomography 13 days after removal of the catheter showing an image that suggests the presence of a residual collection. This was done for observation purposes. (H) Control CT around 45 days after removal of the catheter shows almost complete resolution of the collection. The patient remained asymptomatic. A new drainage of the "lesion" would have been useless, as can be seen in the evolution from (G) to (H).

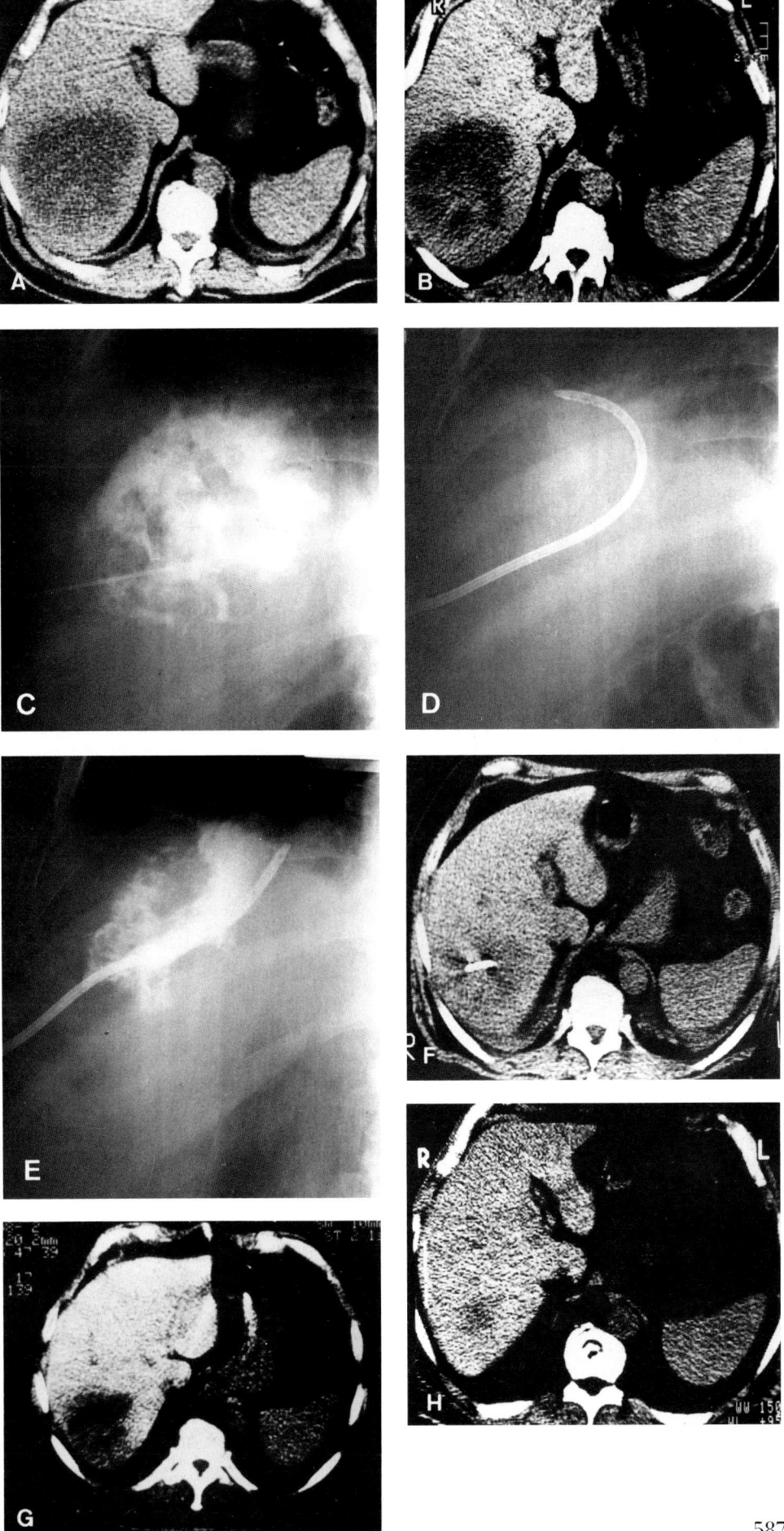

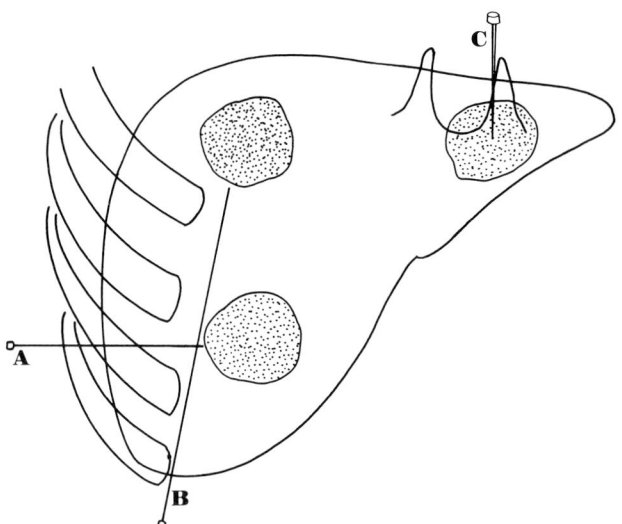

Figure 10.11 Schematic drawing shows a window for approaching intrahepatic lesions according to their location.
(A) A collection in the right hepatic lobe may be approached laterally by the intercostal or subcostal route. (B) A collection in the posterior-superior segment of the right liver lobe should be approached posteriorly by the triangulation technique, as described in Fig. 10.3. (C) Collections in the left hepatic lobe should be approached by anterior puncture near the midline, with the needle in the vertical position.

puncture with a fine needle is performed under fluoroscopy, and material is collected for analysis of contamination. Immediately afterward, the cavity is punctured with an 18-gauge needle; using the Seldinger technique, the access route is dilated and a drainage catheter is introduced, placed in position, and then fixed onto the skin (Fig. 10.12).

A major therapeutic effect occurs almost immediately after puncture and decompression of the collection. This effect is accentuated by careful irrigation and lavage of the cavity with large parceled volumes of simple saline until a clear aspirate is obtained. Maintenance of the catheter with daily intermittent irrigation or continuous irrigation for a few days is a practical measure which permits abscess evacuation and cleaning and keeps the catheter patent for the necessary time period (Figs. 10.13 and 10.14). As with all other types of abdominal collections, drainage times are longer in HAs with connecting fistulas to the biliary tract (Fig. 10.15).

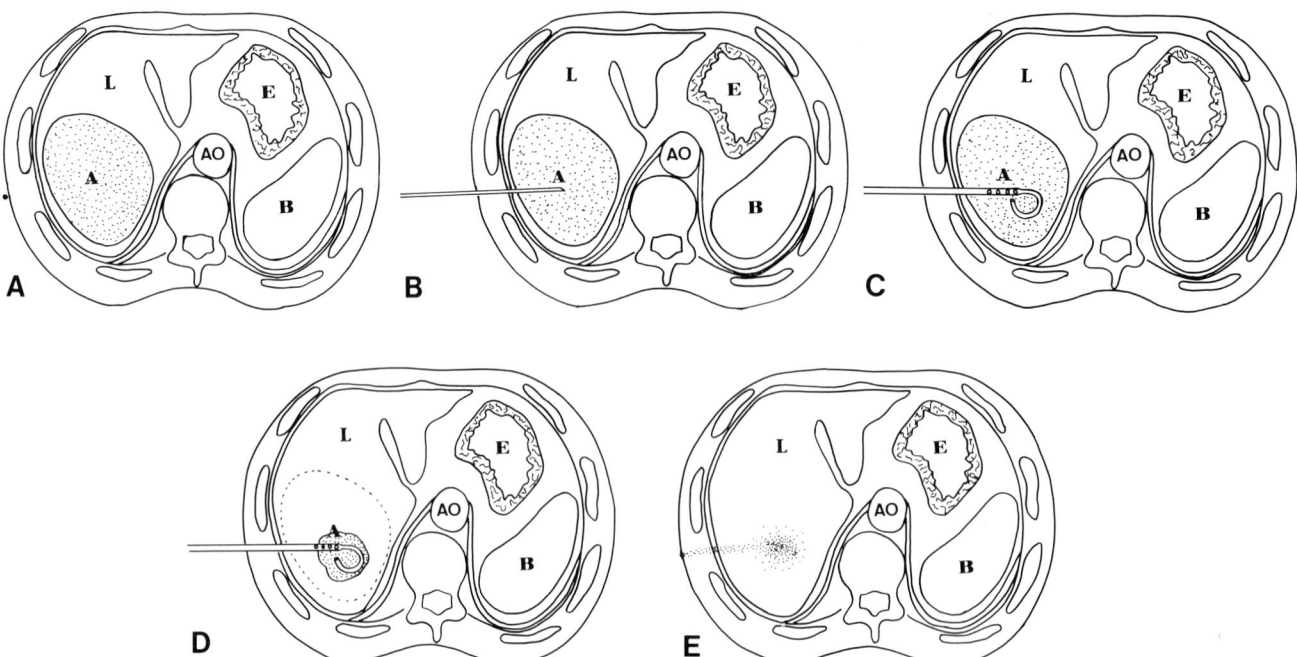

Figure 10.12 Schematic drawing of hepatic abscess drainage.
(A) Tomographic section at the hepatic level (F) showing an intrahepatic abscess (A) and reference marked on the skin (black dot). B = spleen; E = stomach; AO = aorta. (B) Puncture with an 18-gauge rigid needle by the percutaneous route till the needle is inside the abscess. (C) A pigtail-type drainage catheter inside the lesion. (D) After 3 to 5 days the cavity around the catheter becomes smaller. (E) The catheter can be removed in 7 to 9 days, leaving behind only its track with granulation tissue.

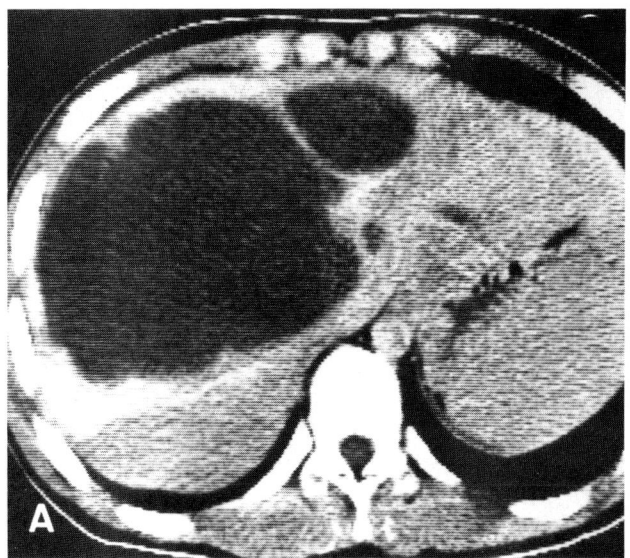

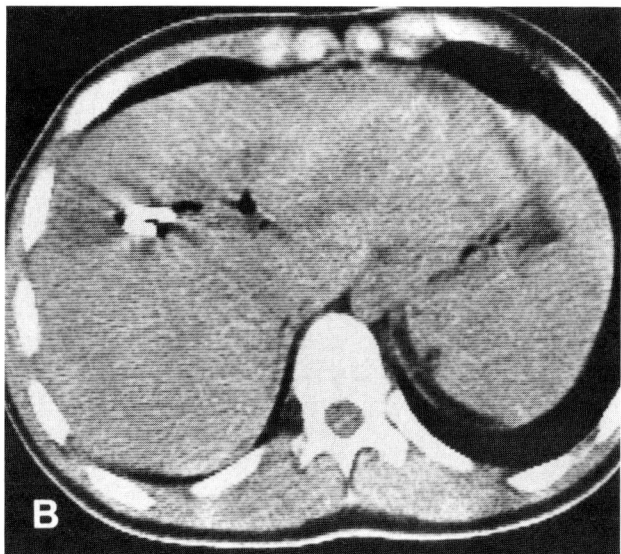

Figure 10.13 (A) A patient with blunt abdominal trauma and a large intrahepatic biloma producing pain and fever. Note the large intrahepatic cavity on computed tomography.

(B) Control after 7 days of drainage showing total regression of the lesion; the catheter was removed immediately after the control examination.

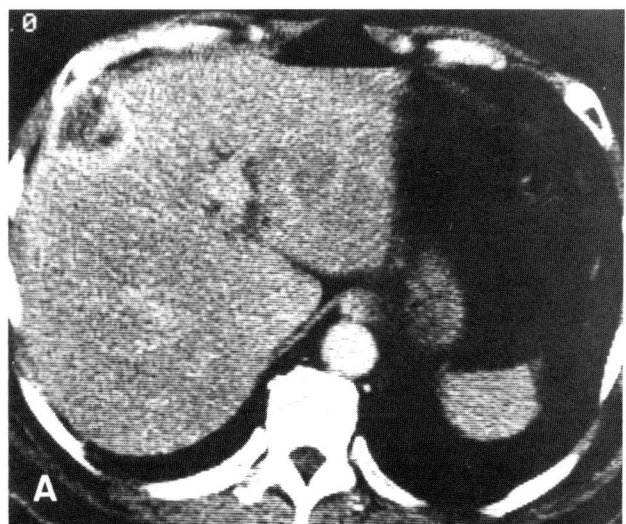

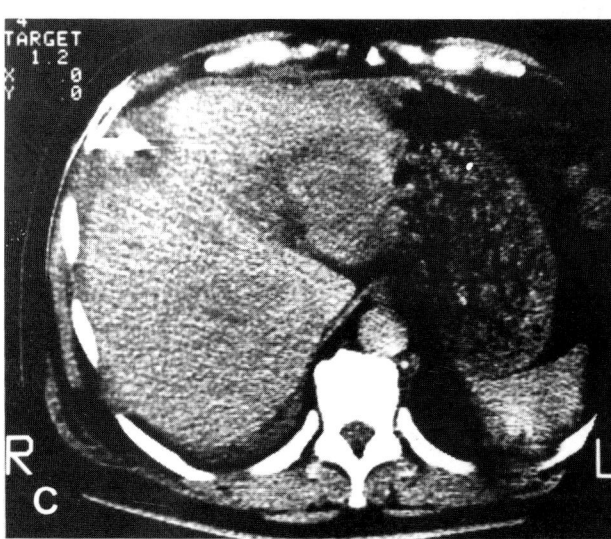

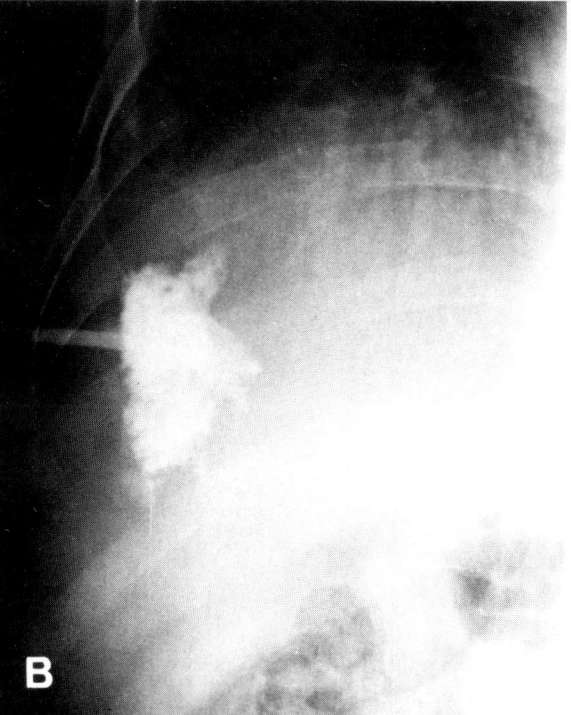

Figure 10.14 (A) A patient with a small spontaneous hepatic abscess on the periphery of the right lobe. (B) Puncture under fluoroscopy, contrast injection, and drainage with a pigtail catheter shows the cavity. (C) Control computed tomography shows cavity reduction. Drainage for 7 days with cure of the lesion.

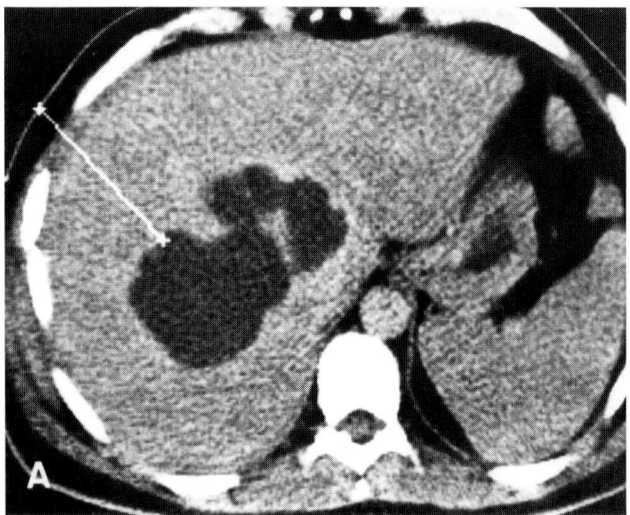
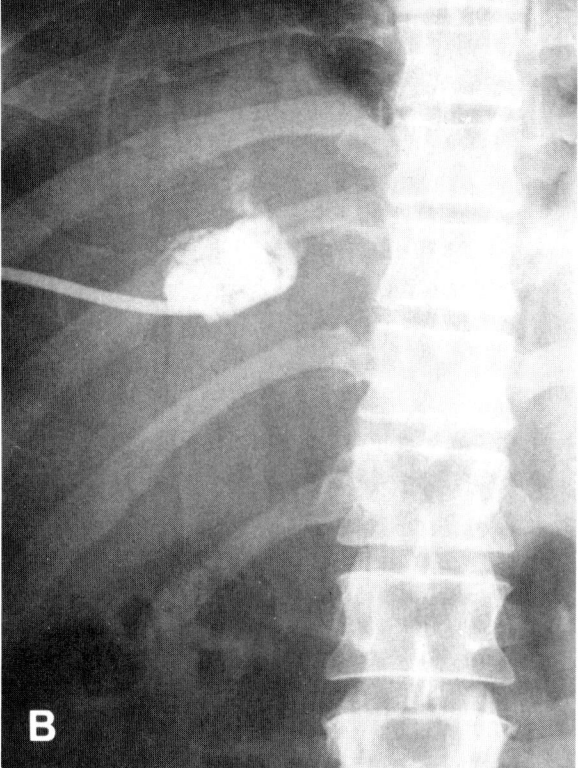
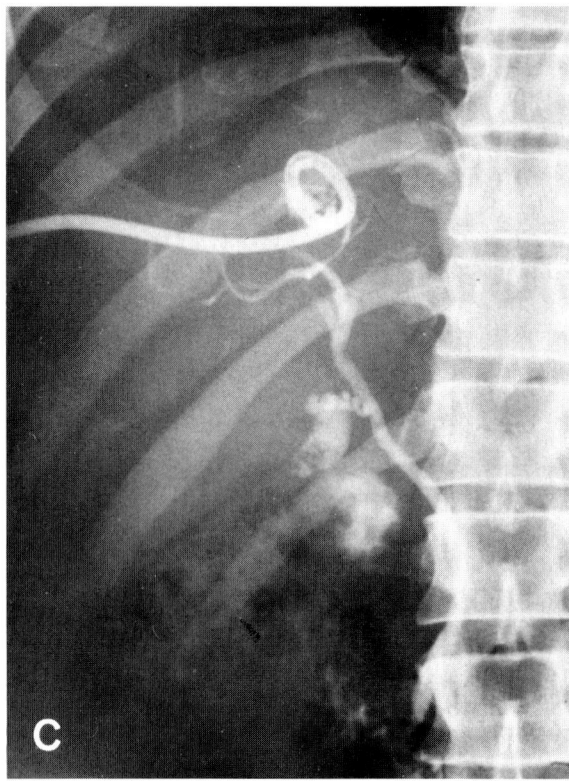
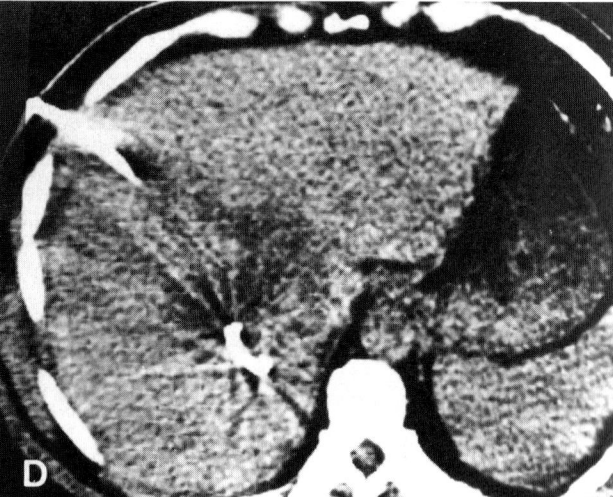

Figure 10.15 (A) A large intrahepatic abscess which appeared spontaneously. Note the marking of the reference point on the skin and the determination of the track to be followd by the needle. (B) Drainage with a catheter for 4 days shows reduction of cavity size. (C,D) The cavity practically disappeared by the seventh day. However, the biliary fistula caused extension of the drainage for 15 days.

Perihepatic abscesses, which are closely related to the liver, behave like HAs, especially when they are found in the subhepatic position. Drainage should be performed by the transhepatic route in most of these cases (Fig. 10.16).

Even though hepatic cysts may become infected and turn into abscesses, this is not a common condition (Fig. 10.17). However, these cysts should be treated as single or multiple HAs, according to each case.

Caroli's disease is included in the differential diagnosis

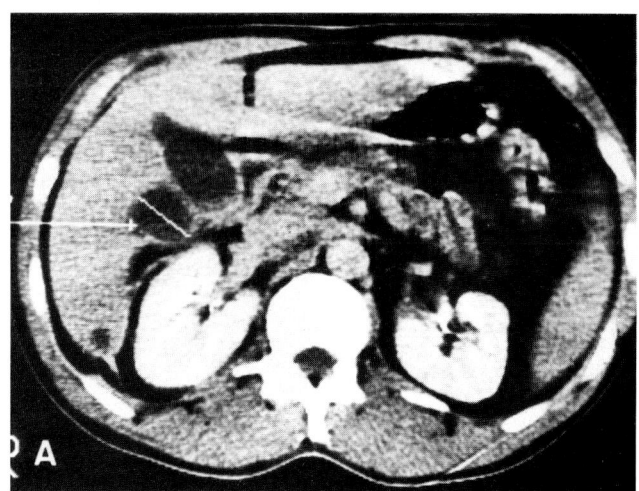
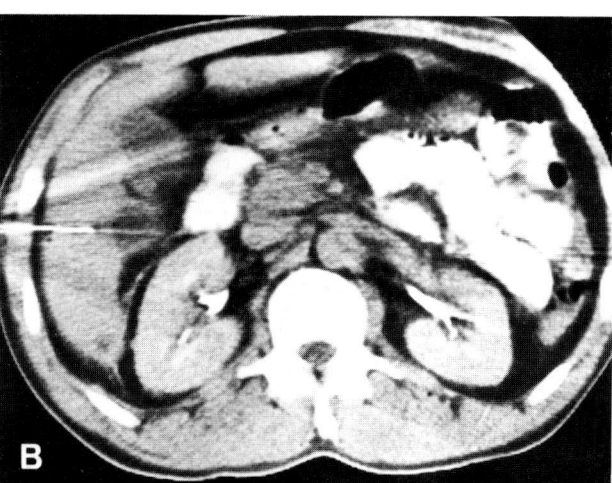
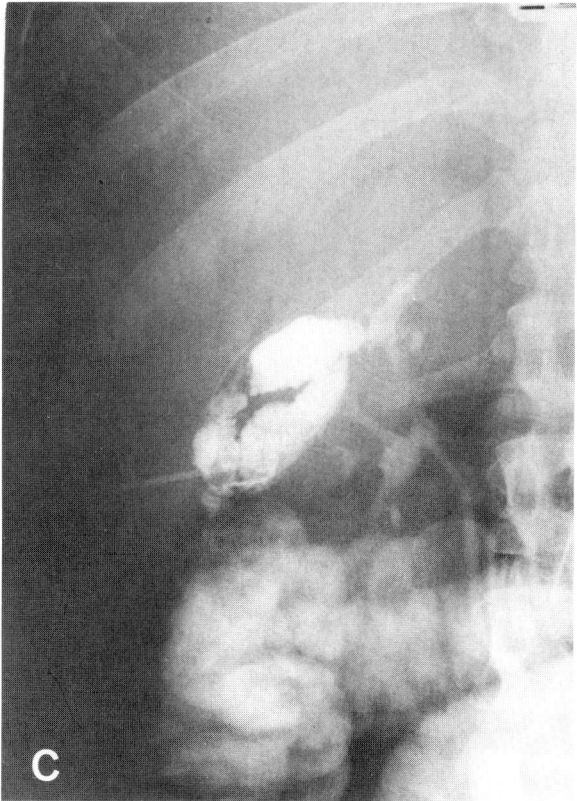
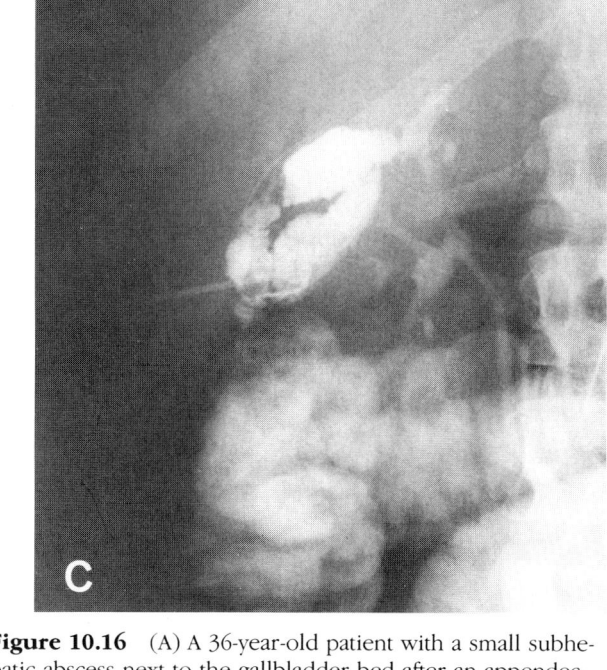

Figure 10.16 (A) A 36-year-old patient with a small subhepatic abscess next to the gallbladder bed after an appendectomy. Note the small right lobe cavity. Skin demarcation suggests a straight-line path. (B) Puncture under computed tomography control directly on the lesion. (C) Contrast injection inside the cavity. (D) Drainage with a pigtail catheter. (E,F) Control tomogram showing the catheter and reduction of the lesion. (G) A minute cavity on the third day. (H) Only the track was visible on the fifth day. The catheter was removed after the symptoms disappeared.

Figure 10.16 *Continued*

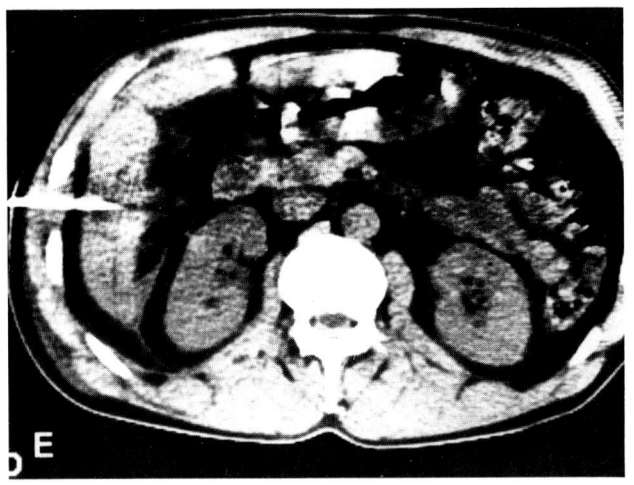
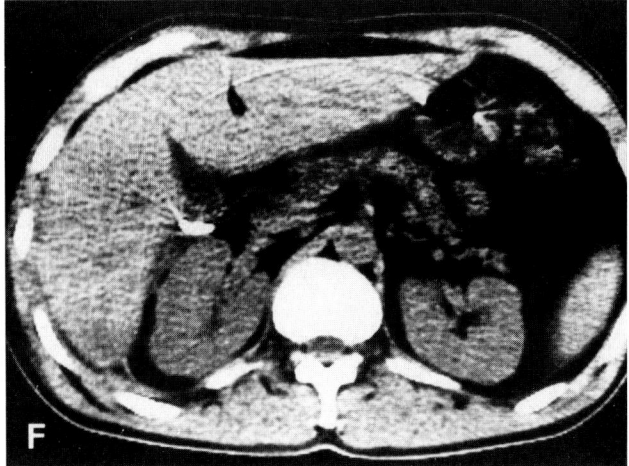
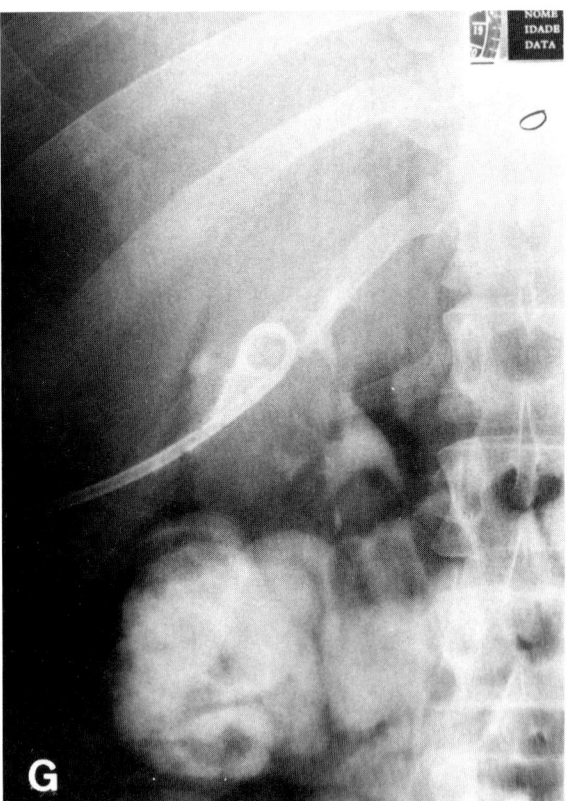
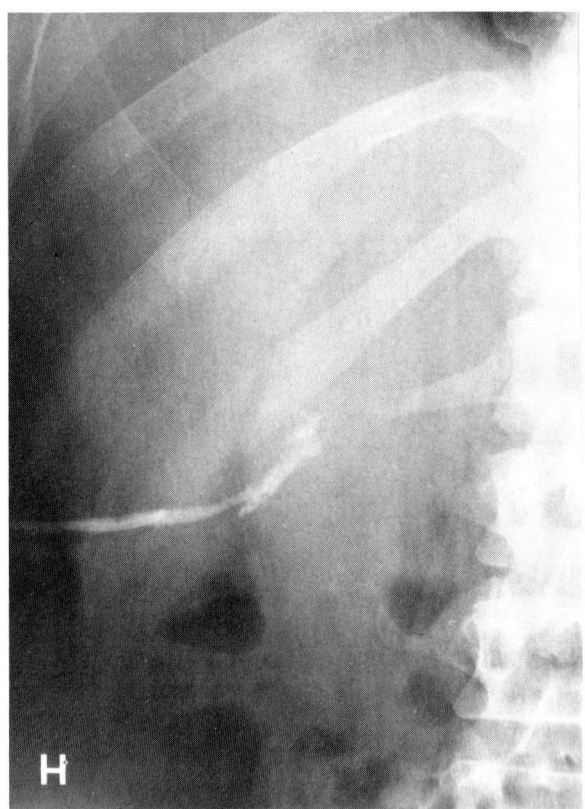

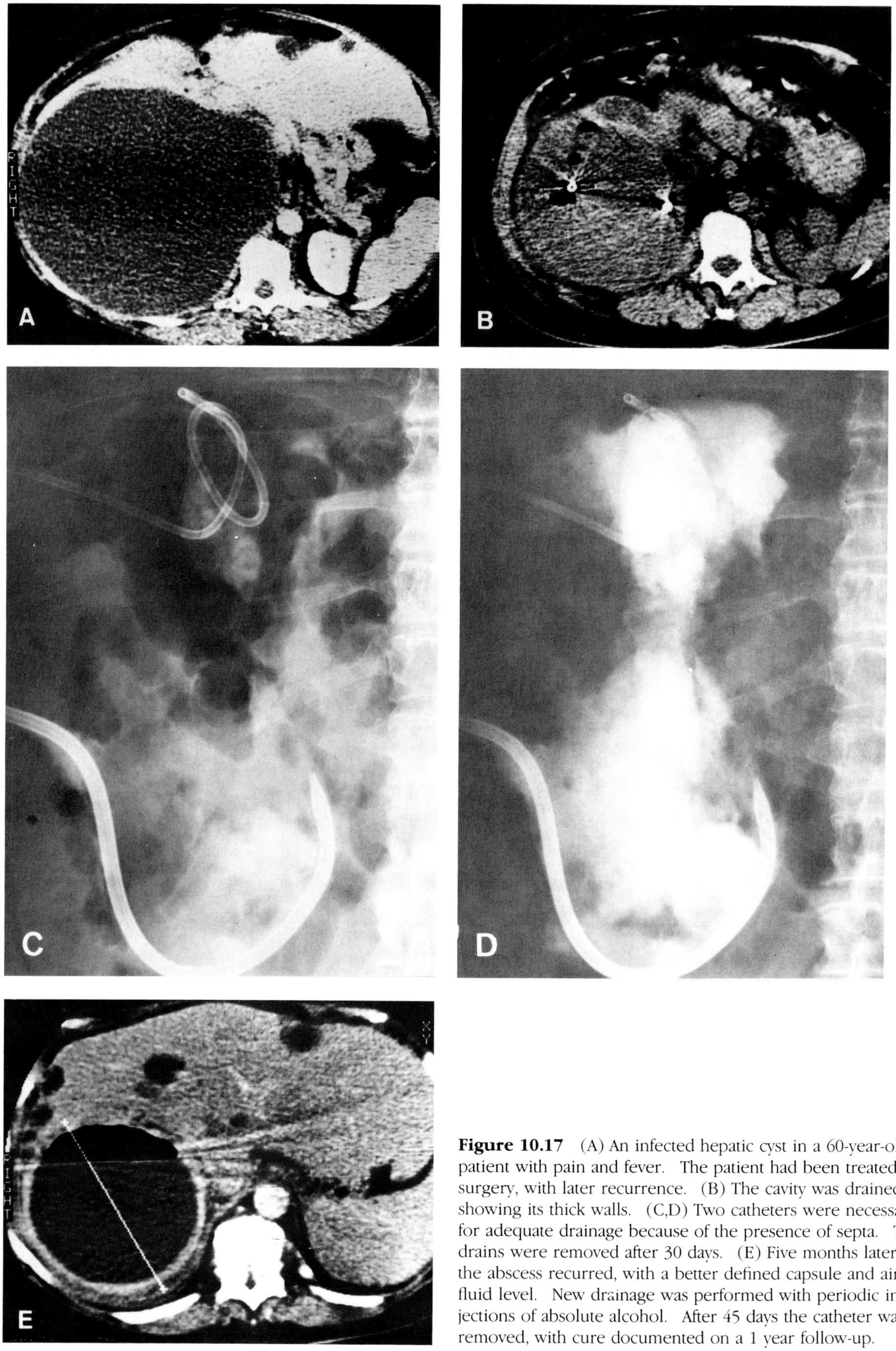

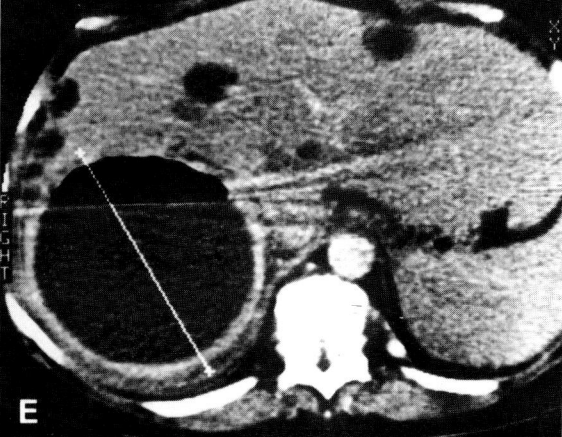

Figure 10.17 (A) An infected hepatic cyst in a 60-year-old patient with pain and fever. The patient had been treated by surgery, with later recurrence. (B) The cavity was drained, showing its thick walls. (C,D) Two catheters were necessary for adequate drainage because of the presence of septa. The drains were removed after 30 days. (E) Five months later the abscess recurred, with a better defined capsule and air fluid level. New drainage was performed with periodic injections of absolute alcohol. After 45 days the catheter was removed, with cure documented on a 1 year follow-up.

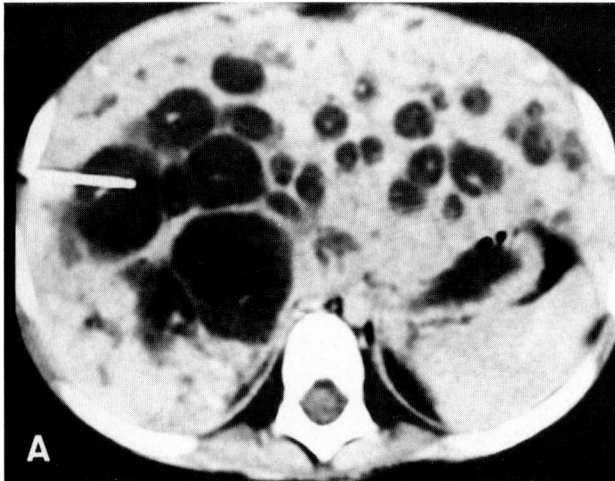
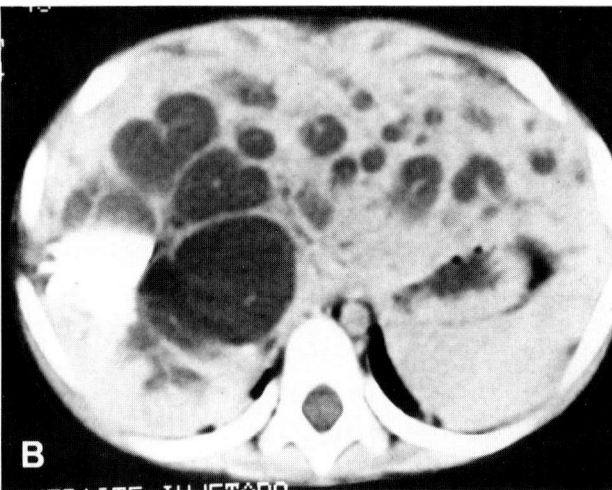
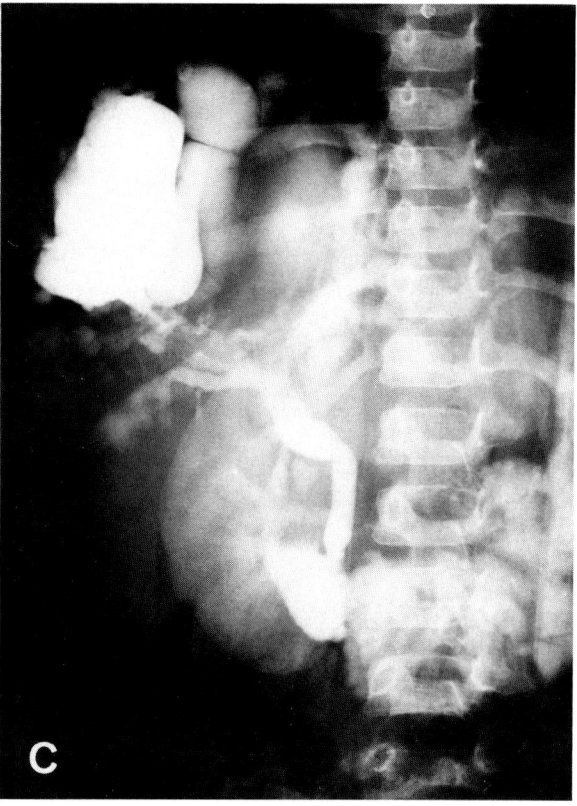

Figure 10.18 (A) A 4-year-old patient with fever for 2 months and hepatomegaly. Previous ultrasonography had shown intrahepatic collections. Puncture was performed, and bile with germ growth was aspirated. (B,C) Contrast injection filled the cavities and opacified the biliary tract. Caroli's disease was diagnosed. Percutaneous drainage was not performed.

of multiple HAs, but the indication for drainage in these cases is not clear, as the cavities are in communication with the biliary tree (Fig. 10.18). However, percutaneous drainage in patients with Caroli's disease has been linked to improvement of the septic condition after drainage.

The presence of a cavitated hepatic tumor or one containing central necrosis and fluid is another source of confusion in regard to the differential diagnosis of HA. In some of these patients drainage may help reduce the lesions and their symptoms (Fig. 10.19).

SPLEEN

Splenic abscess is a rare clinical condition which if not treated can lead to mortality rates varying from 60 to 100 percent. This is such an uncommon condition that a review done at the Mayo Clinic revealed that during a 31-year period, only 19 cases of splenic abscess were found. The estimated incidence at necropsy is 0.14 to 0.70 percent. The incidence of this lesion, however, is expected to increase as newer imaging methods, which can detect earlier and smaller lesions that were previously missed, are introduced.

Splenic abscesses may be related to postoperative sepsis or bacteremia (Fig. 10.20), trauma, blood diseases, and the extension of an adjacent infectious process (pancreatitis, for instance) or may appear spontaneously (Fig. 10.21). The most common symptoms are fever and abdominal pain, which sometimes is accompanied by pleuritic-type thoracic pain.

Splenic abscesses have traditionally been treated with antibiotics and surgical splenectomy. As the present trend

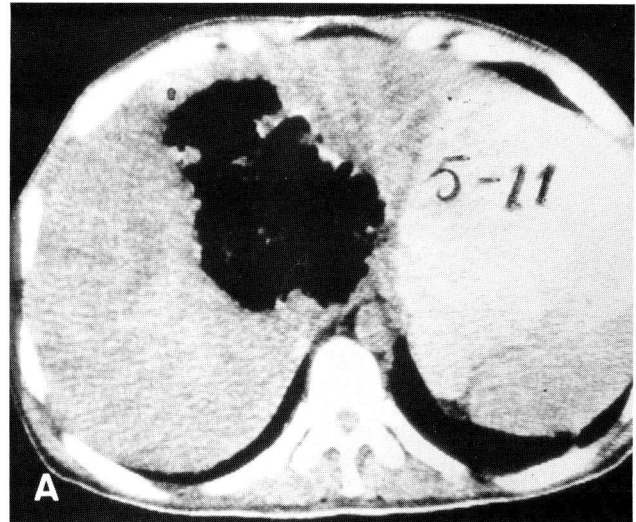
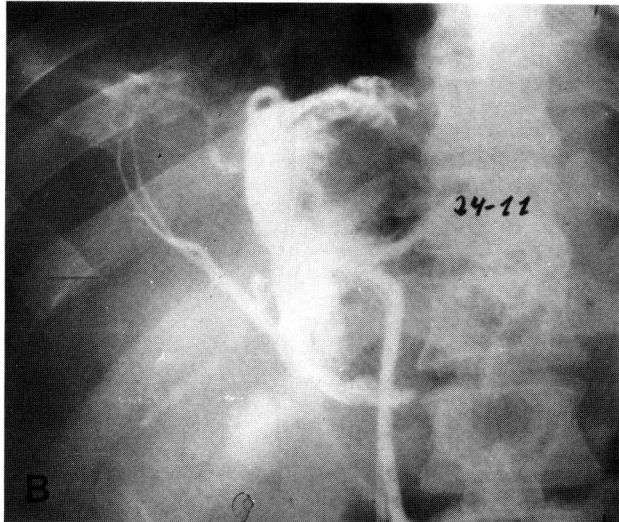
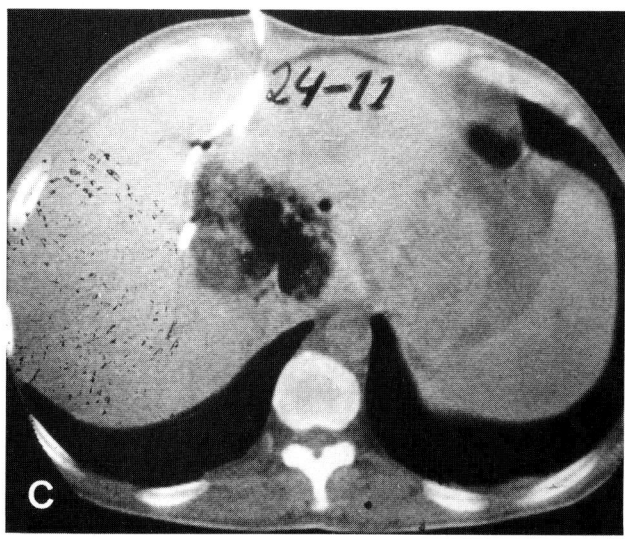

Figure 10.19 (A) A patient with a cavitated colonic carcinoma metastasis simulating an abscess. (B,C) The lesion became smaller after drainage; biliary tract opacification is shown in (B). Drainage is not indicated for this type of lesion. Puncture biopsy should always be performed in case of doubt, with material obtained from the periphery.

is toward preserving the spleen because of the high infection rates in splenectomized patients ("Splenic Embolization," Chap. 4) as well as the reduction in survival rates, percutaneous drainage has come to be considered a valid therapeutic alternative.

Although the spleen may convey the picture of a brittle, hemorrhagic organ which can be easily lacerated by puncture or the introduction of a larger catheter, this is not the case. Percutaneous drainage of a splenic abscess can be performed in all patients in whom access (or a window) is available for percutaneous puncture, using a range of catheter sizes and models (Fig. 10.22).

Puncture of a splenic abscess should be performed with an 18-gauge needle after the puncture site has been located under CT. The pleural space is preserved when this technique is used.

It is advisable to use the Seldinger technique in the spleen, with the introduction of a metallic J-guidewire and with placement of a pigtail-tip No. 8.2 French catheter. In case of a blood collection, a fine catheter may present occlusion problems. However, this problem can be solved by the use of intermittent irrigation. A pigtail-type catheter should be used to prevent the catheter from penetrating the splenic parenchyma when the cavity has collapsed.

Percutaneous drainage in patients with a splenic abscess is effective in practically 100 percent of cases. The incidence of complications is negligible (Figs. 10.20 through 10.22).

KIDNEY

Renal abscesses can be intraparenchymal, subcapsular, or perirenal. These abscesses are not uncommon but can

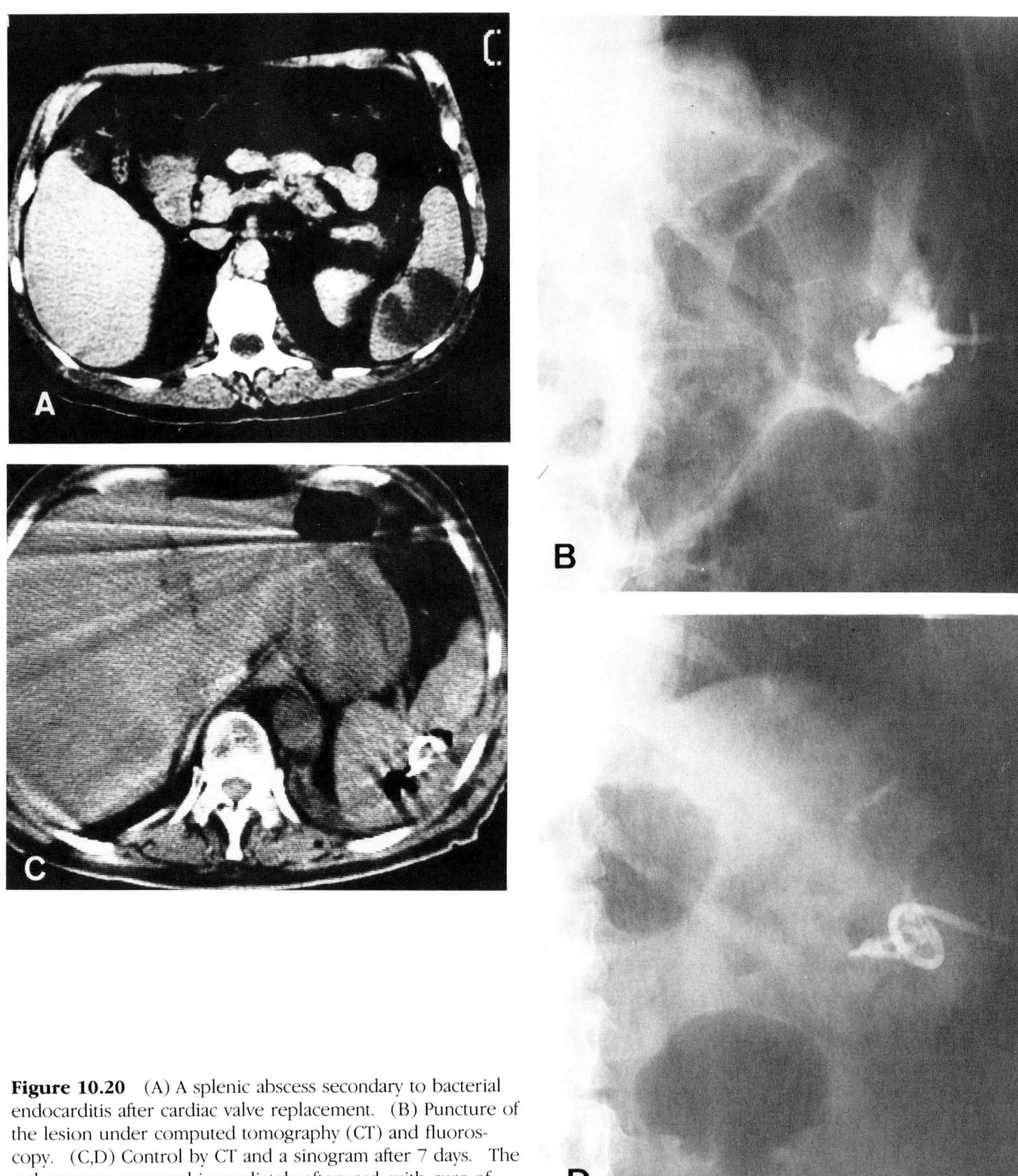

Figure 10.20 (A) A splenic abscess secondary to bacterial endocarditis after cardiac valve replacement. (B) Puncture of the lesion under computed tomography (CT) and fluoroscopy. (C,D) Control by CT and a sinogram after 7 days. The catheter was removed immediately afterward, with cure of the lesion.

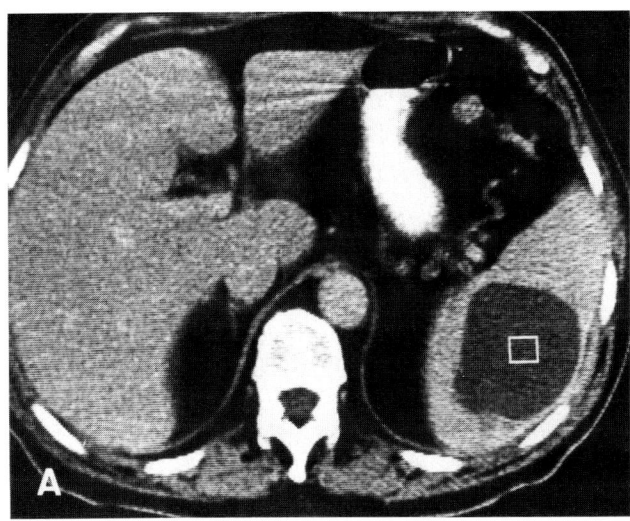
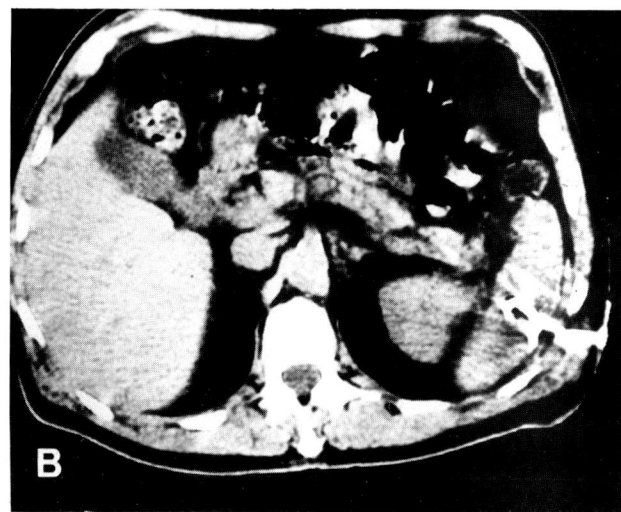

Figure 10.21 (A) An infected cystic lesion of the spleen with fever and septicemia. (B) Control after drainage for 7 days. The catheter was removed a few days later, after fever had disappeared and drain secretion had stopped.

go unnoticed and grow to be very large when they are not detected early enough by US or CT. Percutaneous drainage of these lesions is relatively easy if CT is used as a demarcation method for skin reference points. The risks involved are minimal, since the extraperitoneal route is usually employed. A posterior or lateral posterior puncture is generally performed, and a pigtail-type catheter up to No. 8.2 French should be used (Figs. 8.47 and 8.48).

PANCREAS

Percutaneous drainage of pancreatic abscesses is not easy to perform, since several characteristic features of the pancreas must be considered in the evaluation and in the procedure itself.

The pancreas is clearly a CT domain, although US can be used to identify and locate an increase in parenchymal volume or the presence of a pseudocyst.

Physicians are usually afraid to handle needles and catheters in the pancreas and its vicinity because of the risk of developing pancreatitis. Certain lesions, such as pseudocysts, particularly when they are infected, may be, and in fact should be, drained percutaneously whenever adequate access is available. A pancreatic phlegmon (still not cavitated) should never be punctured and drained.

In these patients drainage is ineffective and involves a high risk of hemorrhage.

The first papers on percutaneous drainage of pancreatic lesions have shown failure rates up to 60 percent because of the presence of unorganized phlegmons which are not drainable. More recent studies, however, have shown a much higher rate of success: 86 percent for noninfected pseudocysts, 78 percent for infected pseudocysts, and 69 percent for pancreatic abscesses. According to these studies, at least 70 percent of patients with infected or noninfected pseudocysts or pancreatic abscesses can be cured with drainage alone, without a need for surgery.

A pseudocyst in a pancreas with adequate percutaneous access can be drained with a catheter. Resolution is usually excellent, although potential spontaneous resolution of an uncomplicated pancreatic pseudocyst should also be considered. As a principle, only symptomatic pseudocysts resulting from volume or infection should be drained with a catheter (Fig. 10.23). An infected pseudocyst is a clear indication for drainage, as its behavior is that of a peripancreatic abscess.

Drainage of extrapancreatic pseudocysts is made easier by distance from the pancreas. A sinogram may show communication between the pseudocyst and the pancreas (Fig. 10.23).

The drainage routine is the same as that used with any other type of lesion. Because of the risk of pancreatitis and bleeding, the pancreas is protected against needle- or catheter-produced trauma.

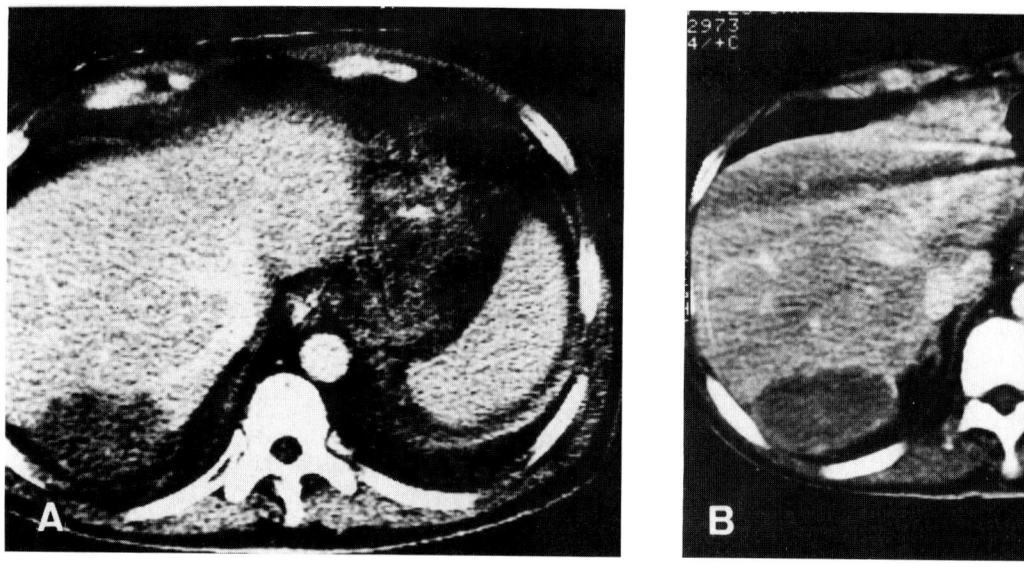
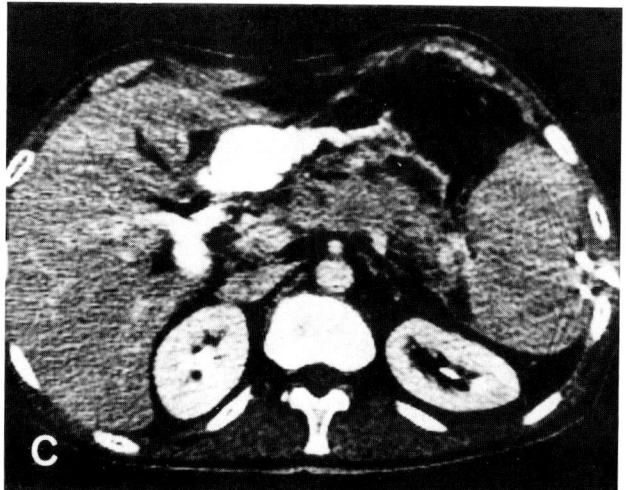
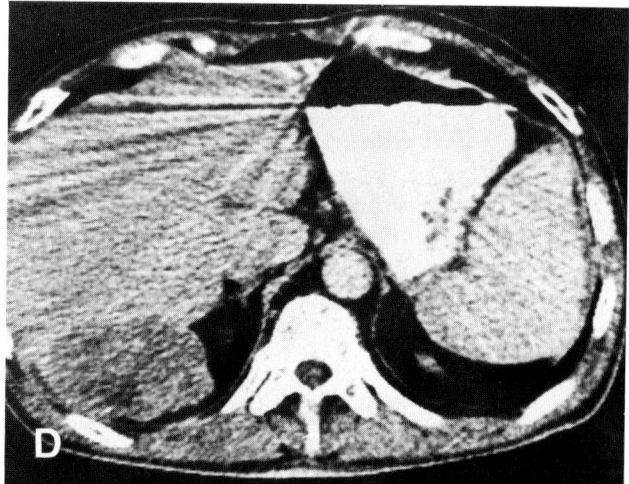

Figure 10.22 An alcoholic 62-year-old patient operated on for a pancreatic pseudocyst.
(A) Preoperative tomography showing a normal spleen and a lesion in the liver. The lesion was a hepatic angioma, as was later established, apart from the pancreatitis. (B) Postoperative control done because of the presence of fever showed a splenic subcapsular collection. (C) CT-guided percutaneous drainage revealed an abscess, which was cured after 10 days. (D) Control tomography about 1 month after drainage shows a normal spleen and an unchanged hepatic angioma. The examination was performed because of a new episode of pancreatitis.

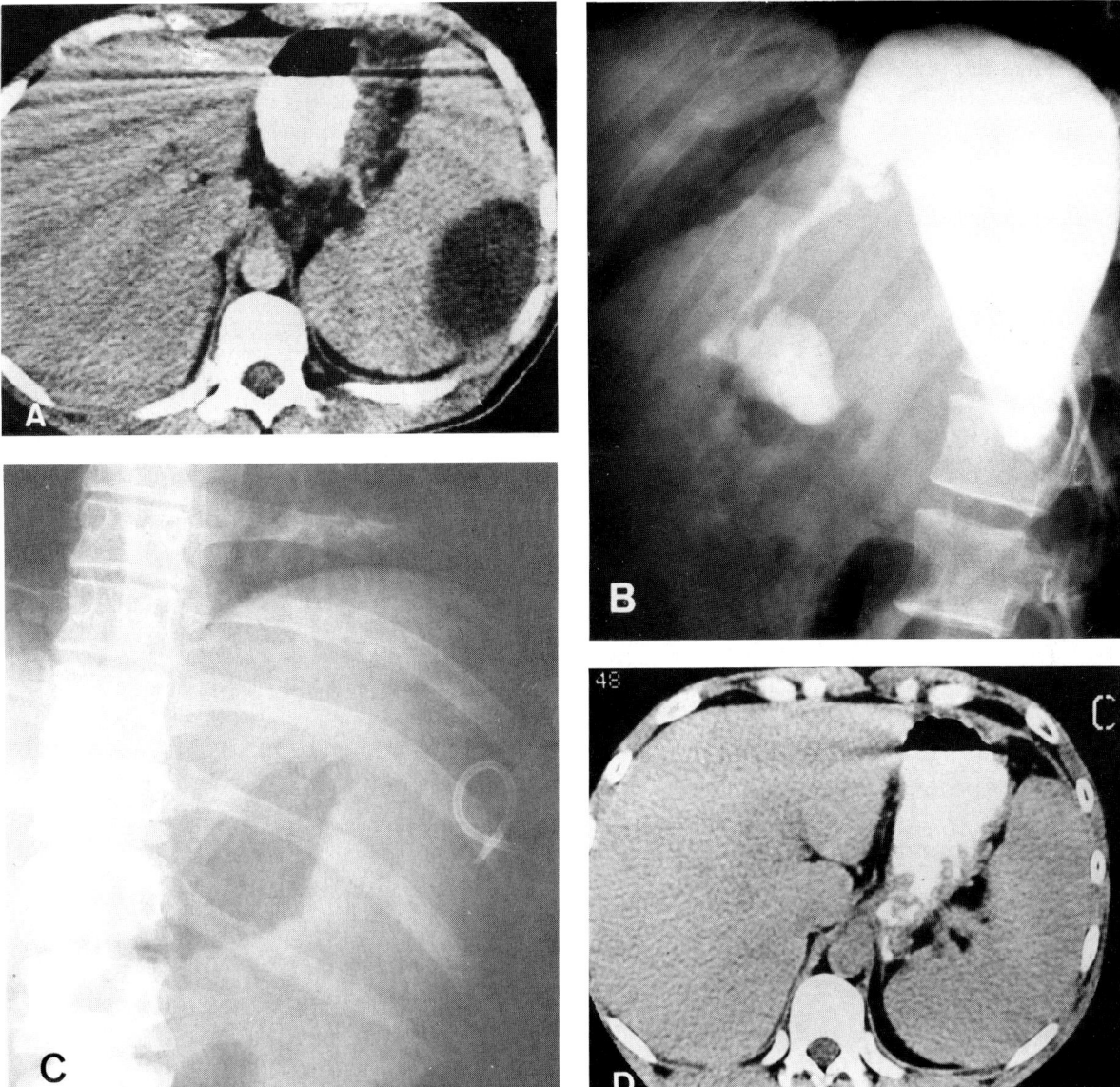

Figure 10.23 (A) A patient with pancreatitis and an infected splenic collection, with bandlike abdominal pain, on November 16, 1984. (B) Percutaneous drainage showing the lesion communicating with another collection in the pancreas on November 16, 1984. (C) A pigtail catheter in place. (D) Control computed tomography performed because of pain in May 1986 shows an enlarged spleen, but with the lesion cured. Changes suggesting inflammatory process were present in the spleen.

INTRAPERITONEAL COLLECTIONS

All abscesses and fluid collections within the limits of the peritoneum, which are not located in the subphrenic or subhepatic space and which are not intraparenchymal lesions, are considered to be intraperitoneal collections. Abscesses and collections in the intestinal loops and the pelvis thus belong in this group.

Abscesses in the midst of intestinal loops are considered the most difficult for drainage by the percutaneous route because of the problems involved in finding an access route and because the results are more precarious. A recent report showed that SAs and HAs can be cured in 84 percent of cases by percutaneous drainage, while for intraabdominal abscesses the chance of a complete cure is only 47 percent.

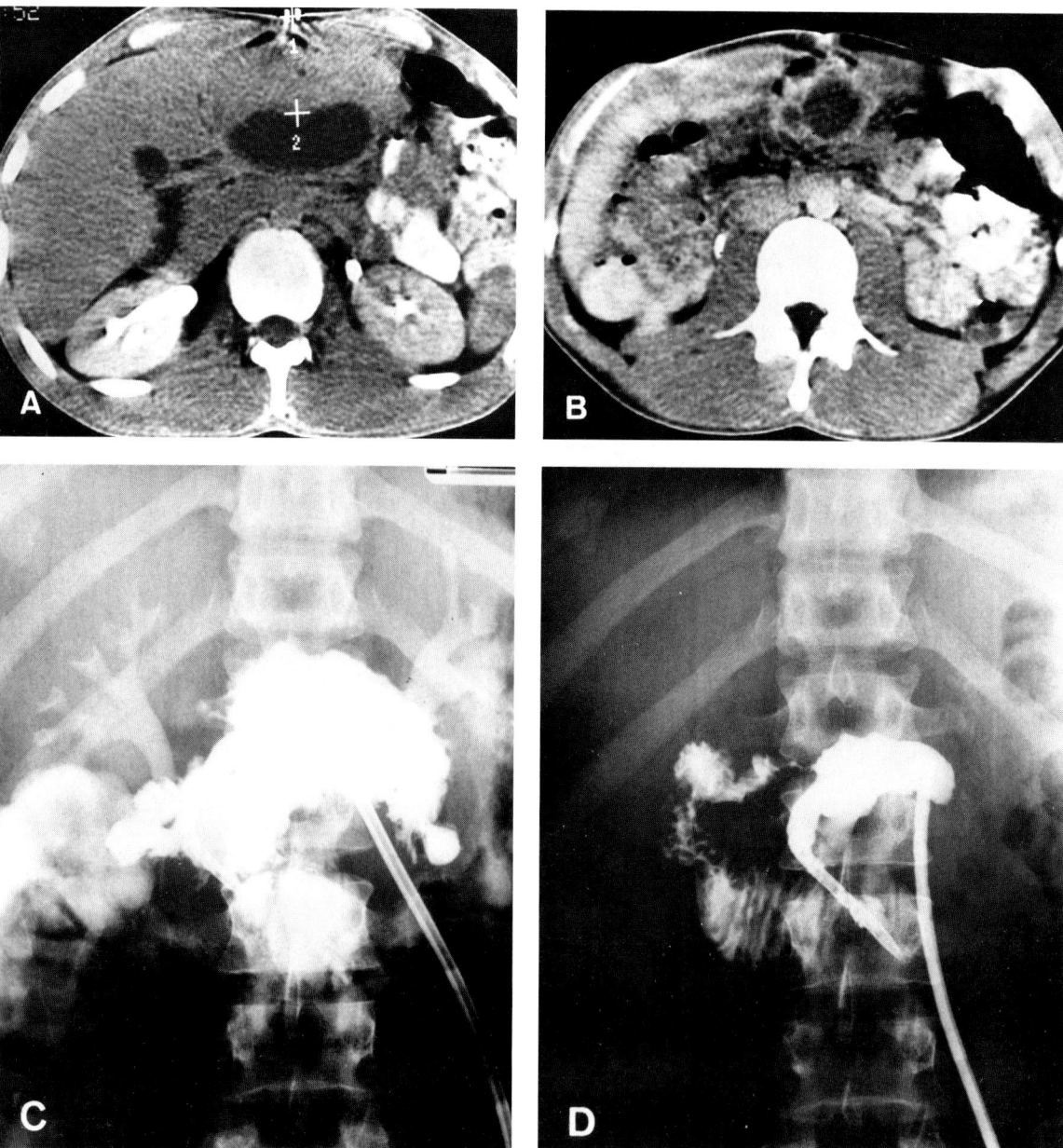

Figure 10.24 (A,B) A 24-year-old patient in the postoperative period of gastrectomy for an ulcer developed an intraperitoneal abscess along the main incision. (C,D) Drainage of a multiloculated cavity with a duodenal stump fistula and bilious content [better seen in D after 1 week of drainage with aspiration and irrigation]. (E) Guidewire and catheter manipulation through the fistula. (F) Embolization of the track was achieved with bucrylate. (G,H) Control after embolization with reduction of the passage through the fistula. (I) Control tomogram shows cavity reduction and cure after catheter removal (H).

Intraperitoneal abscesses that are close to the peritoneal wall are more easily drained. The route used in these patients makes it easy to avoid the intestinal loops.

As in any other type of abscess, the presence of an enteric fistula will hinder resolution and significantly lengthen the duration of drainage (Fig. 10.24). Fistula catheterization and occlusion may be attempted in order to decrease the output. An alternative is nasoenteric intubation simultaneously with drainage, with aspiration of the intestinal content to reduce fistulous output while shortening the draining time. Percutaneous enterostomy is sometimes performed.

Intraperitoneal abscesses usually result from postsurgical contamination of the peritoneal cavity. When the process is initiated by vascular surgery, there is a prognosis of imminent disaster, and percutaneous drainage

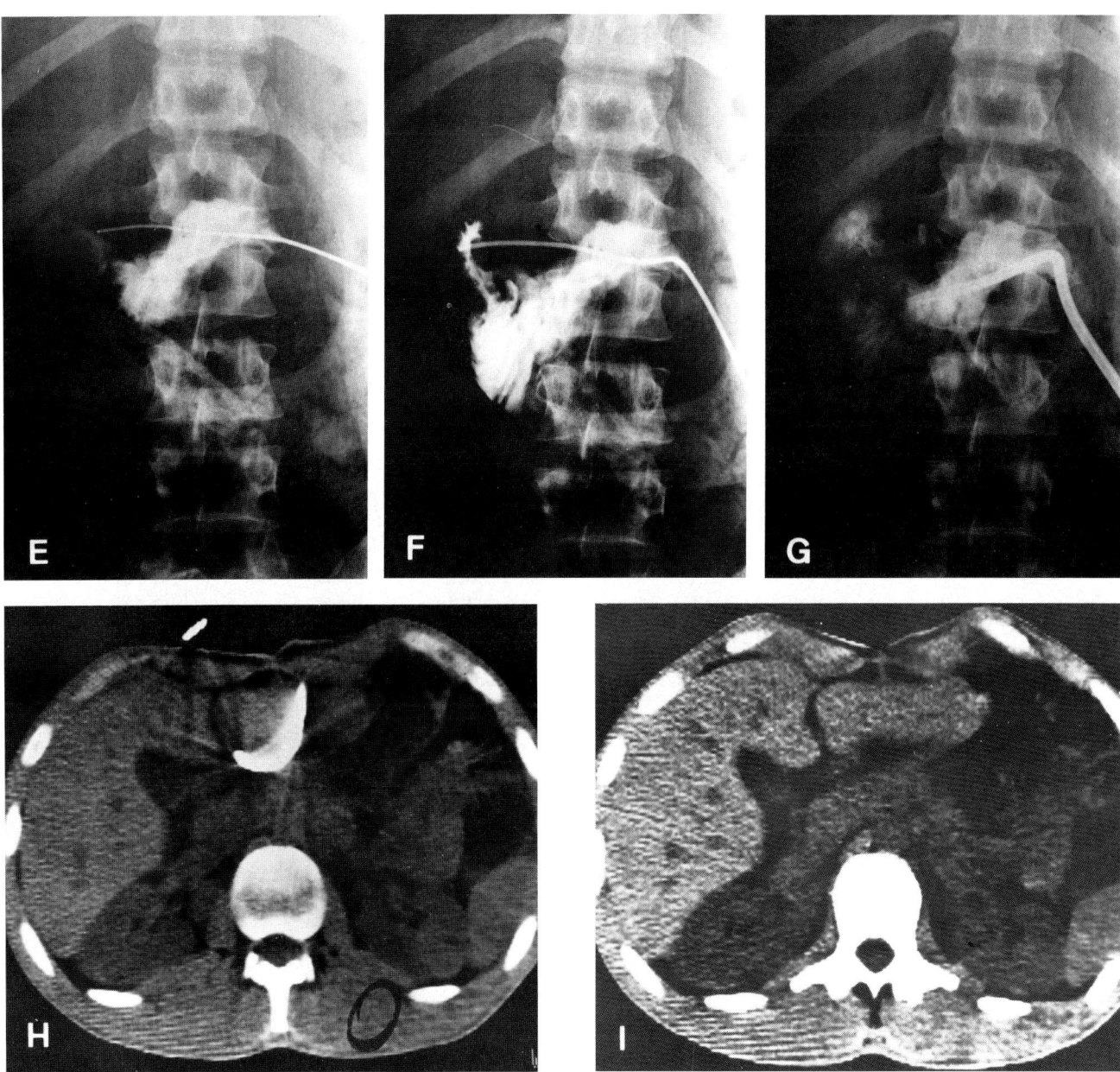

Figure 10.24 *Continued*

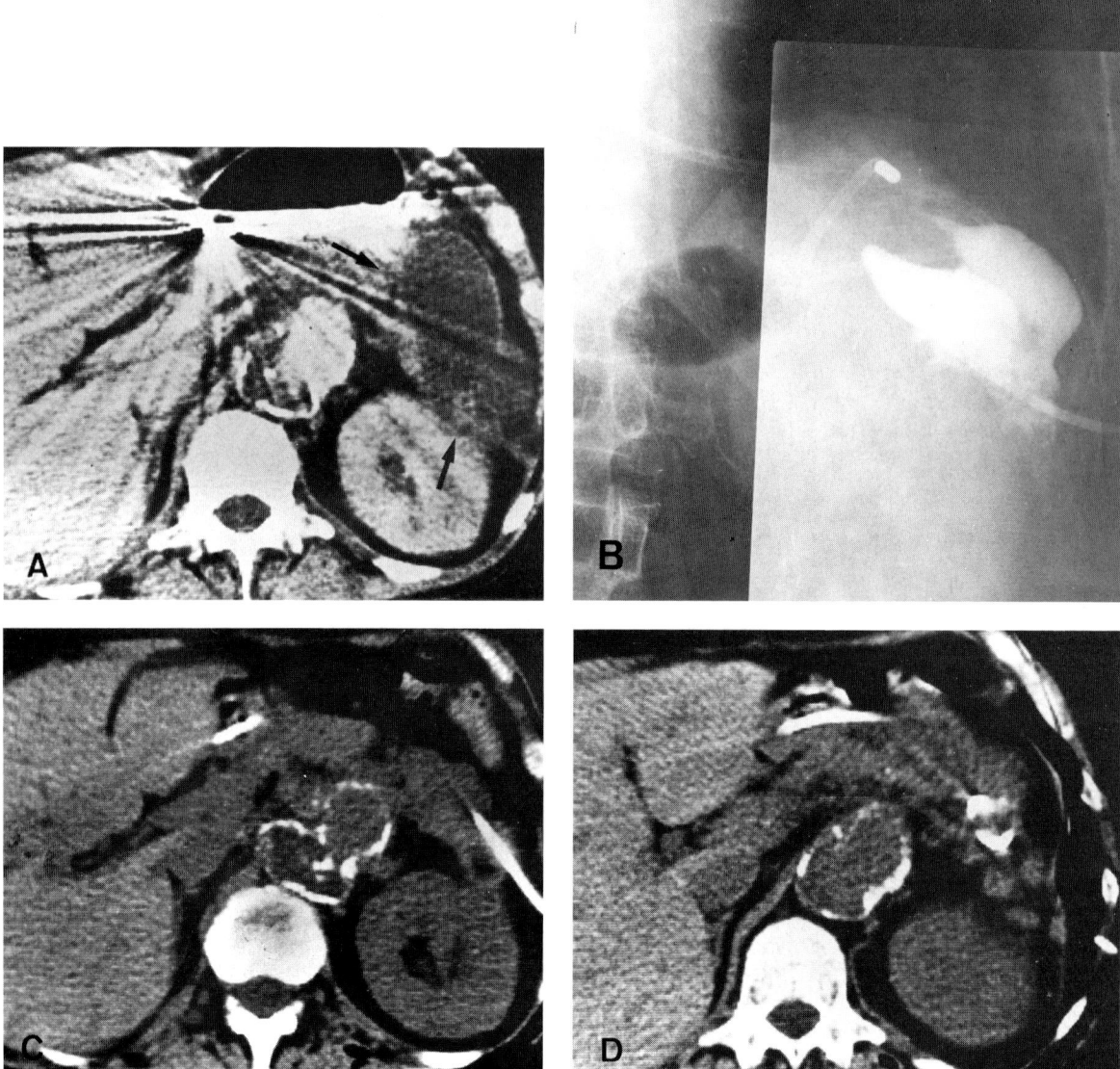

Figure 10.25 A 56-year-old patient on the thirtieth postoperative day of an aortic graft for aneurysm presented with fever and septicemia.
(A) Computed tomography shows a collection in the left hypochondrium and the left flank (arrows). There is an empty space next to the aortic graft, which is normal. (B) Puncture and drainage of the purulent cavity with a Cope-type nephrostomy pigtail catheter. (C,D) Control at 5 and 7 days of drainage showing collection resolution. The risk of graft infection with bleeding leads to high mortality rates in these patients. Surgical correction of this problem is complex and is associated with high morbidity and mortality rates.

should be performed as quickly and carefully as possible (Fig. 10.25). The risk of infection of a vascular graft, possibly resulting in anastomotic dehiscence or massive hemorrhage, is very high. A new surgical intervention is usually contraindicated, and percutaneous drainage plays a special role in these patients. Obviously, the risk of percutaneous drainage is also higher in these patients, since a catheter is introduced close to fragile vessels and contaminated vascular grafts. Bleeding is the most serious risk in these patients.

Multiple intraperitoneal abscesses present a mechanical obstacle to successful drainage because of inaccessibility, the presence of multiple foci in spaces between the intestinal loops, and the association with inflammatory changes in the peritoneum and intestinal wall.

Pelvic abscesses usually collect in the pouch of Douglas in women and in the prerectal space in men. However, collections may be located anteriorly, adjacent to the urinary bladder, and in the sigmoid region or even the retrorectal space.

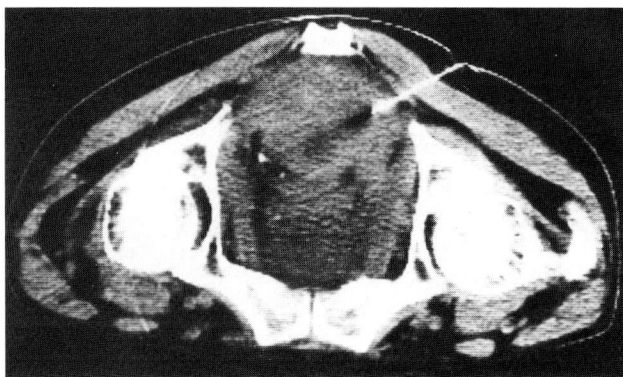

Figure 10.26 A patient with an irradiated rectal carcinoma followed by resection and a fistula with a pelvic abscess.
The posterior approach was adopted, with puncture with a rigid needle through the great sciatic foramen. Puncture is performed in the gluteal region, just below the sacroiliac joint.

Pelvic abscesses can be approached through the anterior route if an adequate puncture window and pathway are identified and there are no intestinal loops in the chosen route. Two other approaches have been described recently: the transrectal (or transvaginal) route in lesions posterior to the uterus (pouch of Douglas) in women and the prerectal space in men and through the large sciatic foramen by puncture of the gluteal region just below the sacroiliac joint (Fig. 10.26). In multiloculated lesions that extend from the anterior to the posterior pelvic regions, simultaneous posterior and anterior catheters may be necessary.

DETERMINING THE ACCESS ROUTE

As has been stressed, CT supplies fast and accurate data as well as the diagnosis for intraperitoneal and intraparenchymal abdominal collections.

There are abscesses which, as a result of their significant growth, may displace intestinal loops, pushing them aside and reaching the parietal peritoneum. These processes are easy to diagnose, and any imaging method can be used to establish safe drainage. The contact point with the peritoneum provides a safe window for drainage (Fig. 10.24). In the case of an abscess between intestinal loops, the importance of CT increases significantly, since it can be employed to differentiate between the cavity and the intestinal loops (Fig. 10.25).

Primary fluoroscopic guidance is usually limited to lesions in which the access route is parallel to the x-ray and the central beam can be positioned perpendicularly to the collection. However, fluoroscopy is also extremely useful during guidewire and catheter handling.

Four different factors should be considered in planning a percutaneous access route: (1) skin entry point, (2) entry angle, (3) depth, and (4) anatomy.

After the skin has been marked with radiopaque material (small parallel segments of angiographic catheters), the location is checked with a new CT section and the angle of abscess puncture can be measured with the device. The depth from the skin to the abscess surface should be measured, and the puncture needle should be introduced as deeply as necessary to pierce the abscess capsule.

The extraperitoneal route is preferred. However, there is no reason not to go beyond the peritoneum.

DRAINAGE TECHNIQUE

A drainage procedure should begin with diagnostic aspiration with a fine needle such as a Chiba-type needle (22-gauge) or a slightly thicker needle (20- or 18-gauge). A finer needle will cause more difficulties when one is aspirating a more viscous collection. However, when one is not sure of the approach route, it is preferable to begin with a fine needle.

The skin is prepared by antisepsis to avoid contamination of sterile collections during the puncture. After local infiltration with 2% lidocaine (Xylocaine) or 0.5% bupivacaine (Marcaine) (which lasts longer), a small incision of 3 to 4 mm is made with a No. 11 blade knife. A fine-tip hemostat can be used for divulsion of subcutaneous and muscle tissue. After puncture with the drainage needle, with the desired length marked as previously measured with CT, the mandrel is removed and about 5 to 8 mL of material is aspirated and sent for bacteriologic examination. A rigid 18-gauge needle is preferred, as it goes directly into the collection with only one pass. After the mandrel is removed, a large J-guidewire (0.038 in.) is introduced and winds itself inside the cavity. The path is dilated progressively with rigid Teflon dilators up to the size of the catheter that has been selected.

If only nonpurulent fluid is aspirated, the cavity should be emptied and the needle should be removed without drainage being performed. If purulent material is aspirated, one should proceed with dilation, and the drainage catheter should be introduced using the Seldinger technique. The J-guidewire is then introduced into the cavity, and after dilation, the drainage catheter is introduced. With a small abscess (less than 80 to 100 mL), a pigtail No. 8.2 French catheter with 12 side holes is indicated. Soon after the catheter has been positioned and the guidewire has been removed, the tube reshapes itself, adopting a spiral configuration; this prevents perforation of the cavity wall. The abscess is manually evacuated with a syringe, and the catheter is fixed onto the skin with stitches and connected to a gravitational or negative-pressure drainage system.

If a trocar catheter technique is used with a No. 12 to 16 French Silastic catheter and a self-contained stylet with a cutting edge, the catheter is introduced through the route used for diagnostic puncture. The central stylet provides the system with rigidity, and the catheter has a beveled shape for penetrating and dilating the entry route. This system requires considerable linear force during its introduction, and great care should be taken to prevent penetration with rupture of the wall opposite to the collection. A needle stop should be used. When the central portion of the collection is reached, the stylet is held firmly in the stationary mode and the catheter is slowly advanced into the lesion. These catheters usually have curve memory in the distal extremity and tend to curve as they are introduced. The stylet is removed, and the abscess is aspirated and rinsed. The catheter is sutured to the skin and then connected to a drainage system.

A coaxial needle system became available recently. This system uses a 22-gauge needle with a removable hub for puncture, and then another 18-gauge needle is introduced over the first one. This makes it possible to introduce the guidewire, dilators, and catheters.

SELECTION OF MATERIALS AND TECHNIQUE

The technique chosen should be the easiest possible for the person doing the procedure. Currently, the most commonly used method is the modified Seldinger technique. However, there is no significant difference between these techniques in terms of the effects produced.

A No. 8 or 9 French pigtail catheter should be used for small, deep lesions and those found in parenchymal organs and for abscesses in the vicinity of vital structures (blood vessels, intestinal loops). The trocar technique can be used for larger, more superficial cavities and retroperitoneal collections. Larger catheters, such as the sump Ring-McLean and VanSonnenberg types, can generally be used as "angiographic" catheters, employing a modified Seldinger technique.

MAINTENANCE OF DRAINAGE

After aspiration has been completed, drainage should be followed with US or CT in order to document all accessory cavities, loculated sacs, and residual septations. X-rays are always useful in evaluating catheter position. The catheter is sutured onto the skin with cotton or 0 silk thread, using tension stitches. It is advisable to apply a sterile dressing. Adhesive tape should be used to hold the catheter in place to prevent the drain from being displaced by stronger pulling.

Purulent abscesses usually do not coagulate or obstruct the drainage catheter. Continuous or intermittent irrigation with simple saline thus is not necessary. However, in our experience, continuous irrigation during the first 3 days of drainage helps keep the cavity clean. A sump-type double-lumen catheter should be used for this type of irrigation. When single-lumen catheters are used, intermittent irrigation can be performed once or twice a day with a small volume of simple saline (5 to 10 mL). The volume can be reduced progressively.

Drainage can be only gravitational, aided by breathing movements and external pressures over the abscess "capsule." Continuous aspiration with low negative pressure can be particularly useful as an alternative to continuous irrigation and when one is dealing with voluminous cavities which produce residua and fluids or hematomas. In our experience, continuous aspiration can reduce drainage and hospitalization times to a few days.

The decision to remove the percutaneous catheter is perhaps the most difficult aspect of treatment. The radiologist's fear of leaving the catheter in place for an insufficient period is counterbalanced by the patient's anxiety about having the abscess drained in the shortest time possible.

However, the radiologist's decision to remove the catheter should be based on the patient's clinical evolution. If temperature is lowered and the leukocyte count returns to normal, the volume of material drained will drop considerably (to less than 5 mL/d). If follow-up or CT does not show residual cavities or a pus residue, the catheter can be removed, usually within 7 to 14 days. However, in most patients all these criteria may be met by the fifth day.

Contrast injection through the catheter (sinogram) used as a control usually shows significant cavity reduction around the fifth day (Fig. 10.9). A sinogram is generally indicated for lesions which continue to drain significant fluid volumes after 5 to 7 days of drainage, because an enteric or biliary fistula may be present. In these cases, the drainage time will be extended, even though other maneuvers may be tried for occluding the fistulous pathway with bucrylate.

Catheter removal should not be done too early or too late. If it is performed too early, CT may show an area of edema which should not be mistaken for abscess recurrence. This is especially true in patients with parenchymal lesions (Fig. 10.10).

CONCLUSIONS

Percutaneous access to abscesses is determined through the most advanced imaging methods (US and CT).

Most lesions offer an adequate window and pathway for percutaneous puncture. The function of the radiologist is to find them.

Computed tomography is more effective than US in determining the precise location of an abscess and its relationship to adjacent structures, particularly intestinal loops.

The great majority of intraabdominal abscesses are of the simple type, without loculations, and are ideal for the use of the percutaneous approach.

Percutaneous drainage of abscesses is a radiologic procedure, and every radiologist who has experience with US, CT, and intervention should be able to perform it.

From a strictly radiologic point of view, percutaneous drainage of an abscess may seem too invasive; however, from a surgical point of view, this is a rather conservative but effective procedure that is applicable even to patients who are considered poor candidates for surgery.

REFERENCES

Berger L, Osborne DR. Treatment of pyogenic liver abscesses by percutaneous needle aspiration. *Lancet* 1982;1:132–136.

Butch RJ, Mueller PR, Ferrucci JT, Wittenberg J, Simeone JF, White EM, Brown AS. Drainage of pelvic abscesses through the greater sciatic foramen. *Radiology* 1986;158:487–491.

Chulay JD, Lanherani MR. Splenic abscess: Report of 10 cases and review of the literature. *Am J Med* 1976;61:513–522.

Chun CH, Roff MJ, Contreras L, Varghese R, Waterman N, Daffner R, Melo JC. Splenic abscess. *Medicine* 1980;59:50–63.

Dawson SL, Mueller PR, Ferrucci JT. Mucomyst for abscesses: A clinical comment. *Radiology* 1984;151:342.

Gerzof SG, Robbins AH, Biskett DH, Johnson WC, Pugatch RD, Vincent ME. Percutaneous catheter drainage of abdominal abscesses guided by ultrasound and computed tomography. *AJR* 1979;133:1–8.

Gerzof SG, Robbins AH, Johnson WC, Birket DH, Nabseth DC. Percutaneous catheter drainage of abdominal abscesses: A five-year experience. *N Engl J Med* 1981;305:653–657.

Greenwood LH, Collins TL, Yrizary JM. Percutaneous management of multiple liver abscesses. *AJR* 1982;139:390–392.

Haaga JR, Alfidi RJ, Havrilla TR, Cooperman AM, Seidelman FE, Reich NE, Weinstein AJ, Meaney TF. CT detection and aspiration of abdominal abscesses. *AJR* 1977;128:465–474.

Haaga JR, Weinstein AJ. CT-guided percutaneous aspiration and drainage of abscesses. *AJR* 1980;135:1187–1194.

Herbert DA, Rothman J, Simmons F, Fogel DA, Wilson S, Ruskin J. Pyogenic liver abscesses: Successful non-surgical therapy. *Lancet* 1982;1:134–136.

Jaques P, Mauro M, Safrit H, Vankarkas B, Piggott B. CT features of intraabdominal abscesses: Prediction of successful percutaneous drainage. *AJR* 1986;146:1041–1045.

Johnson RJ, Mueller PR, Ferrucci JT, Dawson SL, Butch RJ, Papanicolau N, VanSonnenberg E, Simeone JF, Wittenberg J. Percutaneous drainage of pyogenic liver abscesses. *AJR* 1985;144:463–467.

Johnson WC, Gerzof SG, Robbins AH, Nabseth DC. Comparative evaluation of operative drainage versus percutaneous catheter drainage guided by computed tomography or ultrasound. *Ann Surg* 1981;194:510–520.

Lang EK, Springer RM, Glorioso LW, Cammarata CA. Abdominal abscess drainage under radiologic guidance: Causes of failure. *Radiology* 1986;159:329–336.

Linos DA, Nagorney DM, McIbrath DC. Splenic abscess: The importance of early diagnosis. *Mayo Clin Proc* 1983;58:261–264.

Mauro MA, Jaques PF, Mandell LVS, Mandel SR. Pelvic abscess drainage by the transrectal catheter approach in men. *AJR* 1985;144:477–479.

Mueller PF, VanSonnenberg E, Ferrucci JT. Percutaneous drainage of 250 abdominal abscesses and fluid collection: II. *Radiology* 1984;151:343–347.

Papanicolau N, Mueller PRE, Ferrucci JT, Dawson SL, Johnson RD, Simeone J, Butch RJ, Wittenberg J. Abscess fistula association: Radiologic recognition and percutaneous management. *AJR* 1984;143:811–815.

Percutaneous drainage of the abdominal abscess (editorial). *Lancet* 1982;889–890.

Quinn SF, VanSonnenberg E, Casola G, et al. Interventional radiology in the spleen. *Radiology* 1986;161:289–291.

Torres WE, Evert MB, Baumgartner BR, Bernardino ME. Percutaneous aspiration and drainage of pancreatic pseudocysts. *AJR* 1986;147:1007–1009.

VanSonnenberg E, Verrucci JT, Mueller PR, Wittenberg J, Simeone JF, Malt RA. Percutaneous radiographically guided catheter drainage of abdominal abscesses. *JAMA* 1982;247:190–192.

VanSonnenberg E, Mueller PR, Ferrucci JT. Percutaneous drainage of 250 abdominal abscesses and fluid collections: I. *Radiology* 1984;151:337–341.

VanSonnenberg E, Wittich GR, Casola G, Stauffer AE, Polansky AD, Coons HG, Cabrera OA, Gerver PS. Complicated pancreatic inflammatory disease: Diagnostic and therapeutic role of interventional radiology. *Radiology* 1985;155:335–340.

VanWaes PFGM, Feldberg MAM, Mali WPTM, Ruijs SH, Eenhoorn PC, Buijs PHO, Kruis FJ, Ramos LRM. Management of loculated abscesses that are difficult to drain: A new approach. *Radiology* 1983;147:57–63.

Index

Abdominal collections, percutaneous drainage of (*see* Percutaneous drainage)
Abdominal organs:
  traumatic lesions of, 221–222
  (*See also specific organs*)
Abscess(es):
  abdominal, 577
    computed tomographic signs of, 577
    inadequate diagnosis of, 578
  hepatic, percutaneous drainage of, 582–583, 586, *587–595*, 588, 591, 594
  intraperitoneal, percutaneous drainage of, 600–603, *600–603*
  pancreatic, percutaneous drainage of, 597, *599*
  pericolic, 96
  perihepatic, percutaneous drainage of, 591, *591–593*
  perirenal, 533, *534*, 535
  renal
    cortical, 531
    percutaneous drainage of, 595, 597
  splenic, percutaneous drainage of, 594–595, *596–598*
  subphrenic, percutaneous drainage of, 578, *578–586*, 580, 582
  (*See also specific sites*)
Absolute alcohol, 17, 27–28, *28*
  gallbladder ablation and cystic duct occlusion and, 374, 376
  hemangiomas and arteriovenous malformations and, 248
  hepatic tumors and, 155–156
  postembolization pain and, 32
  precautions with, 34, 35, 39
  renal tumors and, 177, 178
  tumoral lesions in soft tissue and bones and, 227
Age:
  axillary approach to abdominal aorta and, 4–5, *5*
  immune system and, splenectomy and, 170
  as risk factor for renal hypertension, 411
Alcohol:
  portal hypertension and, 102
  as risk factor for renal hypertension, 412
ε-Aminocaproic acid, 18
Amplatz filter, 569
Amplatz guidewire, ureteral obstructions and, 544
Anastomoses:
  arterial, in renal transplants, 416–417
  enteric loop, 95–96, *97*
  between iliolumbar and sacral lateral arteries, 217
  postgastrectomy, gastrojejunal, 84
Anastomotic stenosis, of arterial grafts, angioplasty and, 384

and Vasopressin, in lower gastrointestinal bleeding, 68–70, *69*
Anesthesia, general, percutaneous lithotripsy and, 557
Aneurysm(s), 222–223, *224–225*
  Charcot–Bouchard, renal hypertension and, 412
  embolization and, 31
  hepatic, 64, *64*
  of hepatic artery, embolization and, 138, *140–144*, 141
  mycotic, 64, *64*
  Rasmussen, 205, *206*
  of renal artery, spontaneous rupture of, 185, *187–189*
  of splenic artery, 172, *172*
Angina, abdominal, angioplasty and, 446
Angiodysplasia, 86, *88*, 88–89
  cecal, 86, 88
  pathology of, 89, *89*
  treatment of, 89, *90*
Angiofibroma(s), nasopharyngeal, 290, 292
  angiographic protocol and, 292
  embolization of, 292, *292–293*
Angiography:
  angiodysplasia and, 88, *88*
  bleeding from gastric mucosa and, 50
  carotid cavernous fistulas and, 252–253
  colonic diverticula and, 86
  colonic neoplastic bleeding and, 91, *91*
  digital, hemoptysis and, 200, 202, *202–204*
  epistaxis and, 296, 300, *300–301*
  hemorrhage secondary to pancreatitis and, *174*, 174–175
  lower gastrointestinal bleeding and, 68
  nasopharyngeal angiofibromas and, 292
  paragangliomas and, 293–294
  pelvic lesions and, 222
  portal hypertension and, 103
    Budd-Chiari syndrome and, 128
    hepatic cirrhosis and, 115, *115*
    portal vein obstruction and, 105–107, *106*
    schistosomiasis and, 110
  pulmonary embolism and, *561*, 561–562, 562t
  splenic, 167–168
  tumors of small intestine and, 75, 77, 79, *79–80*
  upper gastrointestinal bleeding and, 45, *47–49*, 48
Angioma(s):
  arteriovenous, intracerebral, 260, *264–266*
  vertebral, embolization of, 17
Angiomatoses, 246, 284, *284*
Angiomatous lesions, 260–287
  intracerebral arteriovenous angiomas and, 260
  embolization in, 260, *264–266*

Angioplasty, *383*, 383–485, *384*
  of aorta and aortic bifurcation, 419–420, *419–421*
  axillary versus femoral approach to, 390
  basic techniques of, 385–386, *385–391*, 388, 390
  of carotid and vertebral arteries, 446, *447*
  complications of, 455t, 455–460
    associated with arterial puncture, 455, *455*
    local reactions as, 456–457, *456–460*, 460
  coronary, 384
  dilatation and, 390–392, *391–392*, 484
  femoral, 433, *434–439*, 435, 437
  fibrinolytic therapy and (*see* Fibrinolytic therapy)
  flow dynamics and, 399, *399*
  of hypogastric arteries, 448–449, *450*
  of iliac arteries, 423–429
    iliac occlusion and, 427–428, *428–429*
    iliac stenosis and, 423, *424–427*, 426–427
    simultaneous treatment of iliac and distal arteries and, 429, *430–431*
  indications and contraindications for, 383–385
  intravascular stents and (*see* Intravascular stents)
  mechanics and hemodynamics of, 395, *398*, 398–399, *399*
  mechanism of, 392, *392–393*, 394
  of mesenteric vessels, 446–448, *448–449*
  percutaneous mechanical recanalization techniques and (*see* Percutaneous mechanical recanalization techniques)
  of popliteal and distal branch arteries, 437, 439, *440–441*, 442
  renal artery percutaneous transluminal angioplasty and (*see* Renal artery percutaneous transluminal angioplasty)
  of subclavian and brachial arteries, 443, *443–445*, 445–446
  transluminal
    Budd-Chiari syndrome and, 128
    (*See also* Renal artery percutaneous transluminal angioplasty)
  venous, 452, *452–453*, 454
Antibiotics:
  gallbladder ablation and cystic duct occlusion and, 374
  percutaneous lithotripsy and, 553
  percutaneous nephrostomy and, 511
  postembolization sepsis and, 32, 34
  prophylactic
    biliary drainage and, 306
    hepatic metastatic endocrine tumors and, 152
    splenic embolization and, 169

Note: Pages in italics refer to pages of illustrations.

Anticoagulation therapy:
   venous thromboembolism and, 563
   (*See also* Heparinization; *specific drugs*)
Anuria, obstructive, from tumors, 519, *520–523*, 523
Aorta:
   abdominal, axillary approach to, 4–5, *5*
   angioplasty of, 419–420, *419–421*, 443–445, *443–446*, *447*
   reflux of embolization material into, *33*, 34
   thoracic, angioplasty of, 443–445, *443–446*, *447*
Aortic bifurcation, angioplasty of, 419–420, *419–421*
Aortic coarctation, angioplasty of, 384
Apudoma(s), 175
Arterial stenosis, hypertension of renal origin and, 190, *190*
Arteriography, renal artery stenosis and, caused by arteritis, 409, *411–412*
Arterioportal fistulas, intrahepatic, congenital, 104, *104*
Arteriotomy, for removal of intravascular foreign bodies, 492
Arteriovenous fistulas, 233–234, 238, 242, *244–246*, 249, *249–250*
   bleeding due to, 340
   cavernous, carotid, *251–259*, 251–260
   as complication of percutaneous nephrostomy, 535
   congenital, 242, *244*
   for dialysis, 452, *452–453*
   of face, neck, and scalp, 260, *261–263*
   hepatic, 144–145, *144–147*
      congenital, 144
      traumatic, 144, *144–145*
      tumoral, 144–145, *146–147*
   lesions of extremities and, 222
   in portal hypertension, hyperkinetic, 104, *104–105*
   pulmonary, 192, *192–194*, 194–195
      embolization in, 31
   renal, 181
   traumatic, of head and neck, *251–259*, 251–260, *261–263*
   visceral, embolization in, 31
Arteriovenous malformations:
   angiomatosis and, 246
   colonic, 92, *93–95*
   dural, 284–285, *285–286*, 287, 287t, *288*
   embolization in, 31
   renal, detachable balloons in, 39, *41–42*
   of skin, 233, 233t, 236, *237–243*
   of small intestine, 75, *77–78*, 79–80, 82, *83*
Arteritis:
   caused by radium therapy, in supraaortic vessels, 445
   colonic, 90
   renal artery stenosis caused by, 409, *411–412*
   Takayasu's, in supraaortic vessels, 445
Aspiration biopsy, in pancreatic carcinoma, 334
Atherolytic reperfusion wires, 469, 471, *471–473*
Atheromatosis, mesenteric arterial stenosis and, 446–447, *449*

Atheromatous lesions:
   angioplasty of carotid and vertebral arteries and, 446, *447*
   angioplasty of renal arteries and, 395
Atherosclerosis:
   guidewire introduction and, 3, *3–4*
   iliac stenosis and, angioplasty and, 423, *424*
   percutaneous transluminal treatment of, 383
   renal artery stenosis caused by, 402, *403*
   in supraaortic vessels, 445
Autologous clot, 17–18
Axillary approach, 1
   to abdominal aorta, 4–5, *5*
   for angioplasty, 386
      femoral approach versus, 390
      of mesenteric vessels, 447–448, *449*
      of subclavian artery, 446
   intraarterial infusion of chemotherapeutic agents and, 153

Bacteremia:
   as complication of percutaneous nephrostomy, 535
   pyonephrosis and, 516
Balloon(s):
   detachable (*see* Detachable balloons)
   latex, in intracerebral arteriovenous angiomas, 260, *264–266*
   occlusion
      catheters with, 28, *29*
      diagnostic, prevention of reflux and, 34
      hepatic artery aneurysms and, 141, *143–144*
   pulmonary arteriovenous fistulas and, 195
   renal hematuria of nontumoral origin and, 182, *184–185*
Balloon abnormalities, 460, *460*
Balloon angioplasty, of carotid and vertebral arteries, 446
Balloon catheters:
   for angioplasty, 383, 385, 390–392, *391–392*
   for biliary drainage, 306
   dilatation of benign biliary stenoses and, 357, *359*
   double-lumen, angioplasty and, 383
   extraction of renal calculi with, 540
   occlusion, in hepatic artery aneurysms, 141, *143–144*
   for removal of intravascular foreign bodies, 496
   splenic artery aneurysm embolization and, 172, *172*
   ureteral stenoses and, 526–527, *527*
Balloon dilatation:
   of biliary stenoses, *364*, 365
   percutaneous lithotripsy and, 557
   ureteral obstruction and, 543–544, *545–547*
   congenital, 551, *553*
Barium studies, contraindication in acute upper gastrointestinal bleeding, 46
Benign biliary stenoses, dilatation of, 357–359, *358*
   results with, 357, 359
   technique for, 357, *359*

Bentson-type guidewire, angioplasty of renal arteries and, 395, *396*
Bile:
   aspiration of, 308–309
   cytopathologic study of, 322
Bile ducts, 308
   common (*see* Common bile duct)
   cystic, occlusion of, 374, 376
   reconstruction of, 362–366, *363*
      technique for, 362, *364–367*, 365–366
   traumatic lesions of, reconstruction and, 365–366, *365–367*
Bile salts, oral, 370
Biliary decompression, in pancreatic carcinoma, 334
Biliary drainage, 362
   in association with brachytherapy, 361, *361*
   complications of, 336t, 336–344
      catheter displacement and, 341–342, *343*
      catheter occlusion and, 336, *337–340*, 339
      caused by technique, 344
      hemorrhage and, 339–340, *341–342*
      perforation of hollow viscera and, 341
      sepsis as, 344, *345*
      thoracic, 342, 344, *344*
   external, 305, 309, *309*, 310, *310*
      technique for, 310, *313*
   indications and contraindications for, 305t, 305–306
   internal, 305
      technique for, 322–323, *322–325*, 326
      types of endoprostheses and, 322–323, *324–325*
   internal-external
      in cholangiocarcinoma, 334
      failure of, 321
      percutaneous biopsy and, *321*, 321–322
      postoperative fistulas and, 365
      technique for, 310, 314–316, *314–320*, 318–322
      temporary, 320–321
   materials for, 306–307, *307*
   patient preparation for, 306
   results with, 344–345
   technique for, *307–312*, 307–344
      anterior approach and, *326*, 326–327, *327*
      cholangiocarcinoma and, 334, *335*
      gallbladder carcinoma and, 334
      metastatic disease of porta hepatis and, 333–334
      pancreatic carcinoma and, 334
      placing endoprostheses or multiple catheters and, 327–328, *328–333*, 332
Biliary fistulas, subphrenic abscesses and, 582, *583–586*
Biliary obstruction:
   as indication for drainage, 306
   malignant, internal drainage and, 323
Biliary stenoses, benign, dilatation of, 357–359, *358*
   results with, 357, 359
   technique for, 357, 359
Biliary stones, 368
   extraction of (*see* Common bile duct, extraction of residual stones from)
   percutaneous lithotripsy and, 373, *375*

Biliary tract:
  drainage and (see Biliary drainage)
  percutaneous cholangiography and (see Percutaneous transhepatic cholangiography)
Bilirubin stones, 370
Biopsy:
  aspiration, in pancreatic carcinoma, 334
  percutaneous, biliary, *321*, 321–322
Bird's nest filter, 569, *572–573*
Bleeding:
  acute, advantage of embolization for, 17
  adventitial laceration and, 456–457, *457–459*
  as complication of biliary drainage, 339–340, *341–342*
  as complication of fibrinolytic therapy, 485, *488–489*
  gastrointestinal (see Gastrointestinal bleeding; Lower gastrointestinal bleeding; Upper gastrointestinal bleeding)
  embolization in, 30
  hemangiomas and, 234
  from hepatic tumors, 149, *151*
  intraabdominal, extraluminal, embolization in, 30
  intraperitoneal, 222
  neoplastic, embolization in, 30
  from pelvic organs, 216–217
    anatomic considerations and, 216
    complications of embolization in, 217, *217–219*
    embolization technique in, *216*, 216–217
    portosystemic encephalopathy created by shunts and, 129, *130*
  secondary to pancreatitis, *174*, 174–175
  secondary to trauma, embolization in, 30
  thoracic, postsurgical, 195, *196*
  vascular tumors and, 267, *269–270*
Blood pressure (see Hypertension; Hypotension; Portal hypertension; Renovascular hypertension)
Boijsen catheter, *6*, 8
Bovine collagen, 19
Brachial approach, 1
Brachial artery, angioplasty of, 443, *443–445*, 445–446
Brachytherapy:
  in cholangiocarcinoma, 334
  with iridium-192 wire, 360–361
  with iridium-192 wire, in cholangiocarcinoma, technique for, *360*, 360–361, *361*
Brescia-Cimino fistula, 452
Bristle brushes, 26
Brödel's avascular plane, 508, *509*
Brödel's white line, 508, *510*
Bronchial artery(ies):
  embolization of, risks associated with, 205, 208
  postsurgical bleeding from, 195
Bronchiectasis, 200
Brown-Séquard's paralysis, 217
Bucrylate, 24–26, *25*
  bleeding secondary to trauma and, 30
  carotid cavernous fistulas and, 253, 260
  duodenal ulcer and, 58–59, *60*
  epistaxis and, 300

hemangiomas and arteriovenous malformations and, 248–249
hemoptysis and, 31
hemorrhage secondary to pancreatitis and, 175
intraabdominal extraluminal hemorrhage and, 30
pulmonary sequestration and, *208*, 209
upper gastrointestinal bleeding and, 66
vascular malformations of head and neck and, 271
visceral arteriovenous fistulas and, 30
Budd-Chiari syndrome, 103, 121–122, *123–127*, 125, 128
  venous angioplasty and, 452
Bupivacaine (Marcaine):
  for percutaneous drainage, 603
  for percutaneous nephrostomy, 511

Calcium renal stones, 540
Capsular arteries, perforating, 409
Captopryl test, renal hypertension and, 413
Carcinoid syndrome, 152
Cardiac arrest, pulmonary angiography and, 562
Cardiopathy, congenital, angioplasty and, 384
Cardiopulmonary failure, pulmonary angiography and, 562
Cardiovascular system, percutaneous retrieval of foreign bodies from (see Intravascular foreign bodies, percutaneous retrieval of)
Caroli's disease, 591, 594
Carotid artery:
  angioplasty of, 446, *447*
  arteriovenous fistulas of, *251–259*, 251–260
  external
    arteriovenous fistulas of, 260, *261–262*
    embolization of extracranial vessels of, 39
  internal, protrusion of embolization material into, 39, *40*
Catalyzer(s), for silicon rubber, 27
Catalyzer M, 27
Catheter(s):
  balloon (see Balloon catheters)
  Boijsen, *6*, 8
  for chemotherapy, 13, *13*
  coaxial, 11–13, *12–14*, 15
  Cobra, 6, 7, 12, *12–13*
    for percutaneous nephrostomy, 515, *515*
    varicocele and, 212, *214*
  complications of biliary drainage caused by, 336–344
    catheter displacement as, 341–342, *343*
    hemorrhage as, 339–340, *341–342*
    occlusion as, 336, *337–340*, 339
    perforation of hollow viscera as, 341
    thoracic, 342, 344, *344*
  dilatation with, ureteral obstruction and, 544, *548–551*, 550
  displacement of, as complication of percutaneous nephrostomy, 535
  Dormia-type, percutaneous nephrostomy and, 531
  French, 13, *14*, 15
    subselective, 17

hook-tip, for removal of intravascular foreign bodies, 493
intravascular foreign bodies and, 491–492
irritating cystitis and trigonitis and, 523
Judkins-type left coronary, for removal of intravascular foreign bodies, 493, 496, *497*
Kensey, 467–469, *468–470*
  complications with, 469, *470*
  percutaneous lithotripsy and, 374
Mikaelsson type, *6*, 7
  reshaping, 7, *8*
obstruction of, as complication of percutaneous nephrostomy, 535
with occlusion balloons, 28, *29*
open-curve, 8, *10*
for percutaneous drainage, 604
pigtail, *6*, 6–7
  for percutaneous drainage, 604
  for removal of intravascular foreign bodies, 493
with reversed curve, *6*, 7
right coronary, for percutaneous nephrostomy, 515, *515*
Ring, for internal-external biliary drainage, 319
Ring-McLean, for percutaneous drainage, 604
for selective and superselective catheterization, curves most used in, *6*, 6–7
shepherd hook, 7, *8*
Simmons, *6*, 7
  angioplasty of renal arteries and, 395
  reshaping, 7–8, *8–9*
straight-type, 7
Tracker, 12
translumimal extraction, 472, *474–477*, 478
Van Sonnenberg, for percutaneous drainage, 604
visceral, selective, *6*, 7
Waltman's cobra loop, 8
Catheterization, *1*, 1–15, *5–10*
  guidewire introduction and, *3*, 3–4, *4*
  puncture and, 1–3, *2*
  Seldinger technique for (see Seldinger technique)
  superselective, *10*, 10–15
    coaxial catheters and, 11–13, *12–14*, 15
    exchange catheter technique for, 10, *11*
    steerable devices and, 10, *11*
Caval stenosis, secondary to neoplasm and radiotherapy, 452–453
Cavernous fistulas, carotid, *251–253*, 251–260
  angiographic protocol and, 252–253
  arterial access and, 256–257
  treatment of, 253, *254–257*, 256
  venous access and, 258, *258–259*, 260
CDDP (see Cisplatin)
Cecal angiodysplasia, 86, 88
Cefoxitin:
  for percutaneous nephrostomy, 511
  prophylactic, for biliary drainage, 306
Celiac axis:
  in lower gastrointestinal bleeding, 68
  vasopressin infusion into, 64
Cellulose, oxidized, 19, *19*
Cerebral arteries, Charcot-Bouchard aneurysms in, renal hypertension and, 412

Charcot-Bouchard aneurysms, renal hypertension and, 412
Chemoembolization, 29–30
    of hepatic neoplasms, 156, *157–165*
Chemotherapy:
    catheters for, 13, *13*
    intraarterial infusion and, 153
    tumoral lesions in soft tissue and bones and, 227, *228–230*
Chenodeoxycholate, 370
Chiba needle, for percutaneous transhepatic cholangiography, 305, 307
Children, hemangiomas in, 233–234, 247
Chloroform, 371
p-Chlorophenylalanine, in hepatic metastatic endocrine tumors, 152
Cholangiocarcinoma, 334, *335*
    brachytherapy with iridium-192 wire in, 360–361
    technique for, *360*, 360–361, *361*
Cholangitis:
    acute, as complication of biliary drainage, 344
    sclerosing, bile duct reconstruction and, 362
Cholecystectomy, 368
Cholecystitis, acute, 368
Cholecystostomy, percutaneous, *368*, 368–369, *369*
Cholelithiasis (*see* Common bile duct, extraction of residual stones from)
Cholesterol stones, 370
    oral bile salts and, 370
Chondrosarcoma(s), 227
Circumferential stress, dilatation force and, 398–399, *399*
Cirrhosis, hepatic, portal hypertension and, 112–113, *113–122*, 115–116, 118–119, 121
Cisplatin (CDDP), tumoral lesions in soft tissue and bones and, 227
Claudication, intermittent, 384
    Kensey catheter and, 468
Clot:
    autologous, 17–18
    heating, 18
Coagulopathy, vascular tumors and, 267
Coaxial catheters, 11–13, *12–14*, 15
Coaxial needle system, for percutaneous drainage, 604
Coaxial technique, for removal of intravascular foreign bodies, 496, *497–498*
Cobra catheter, 6, 7, 12, *12–13*
    for percutaneous nephrostomy, 515, *515*
    varicocele and, 212, *214*
Coil(s):
    in gastric ulcer, 54
    giant, 21
    Gianturco (*see* Gianturco coils)
    Gianturco-Anderson-Wallace, 19–22, *20–22*
    "microcoils" and, 20–21
    minicoils and, 17, 20, *20*
Coil baffle, 29
Coiled silk threads, 29
Colectomy, 68
Colic, nephretic, 516
Colic artery, middle, embolization of, 70, *73*
Collagen:
    bovine, 19

in hepatic metastatic endocrine tumors, 152
Collateral vessels:
    guidewire entering, 4, *4*
    hepatofugal, hepatic cirrhosis and, 113, *114*
    intrahepatic, 138
    in portal hypertension, 102
    renal vascular disease and, 409
    spleen and, 167
Collecting system:
    opacifying, 511–512, *512*
    pus in, diagnostic pyelography and, 516
    pyonephrosis and, 516, *517–519*
Colon:
    carcinoma of, 153
    lower gastrointestinal bleeding related to (*see* Lower gastrointestinal bleeding, related to colon)
    in posterolateral position, 504, *505*
    puncture of, as complication of percutaneous nephrostomy, 535
Colonoscopy, diverticula and, 85
Common bile duct:
    extraction of residual stones from, 348–356
    complications of, 354, 356, *356*
    indications for, 349, 351, *352*
    methodology for, 348–349, *348–351*
    results with, 354
    stone impaction and, 352, *353–355*, 354
    stone size and, 351–352
    obstruction of, as indication for drainage, 306
    perforation by catheter, 341
Common bile duct diaphragm, as indication for drainage, 306
Compression treatment, in hemangiomas and arteriovenous malformations, 247–248
Computed tomography (CT):
    percutaneous drainage of subphrenic abscesses and, 580
    signs of abdominal abscesses on, 577
Congestive cardiopathy, venous thromboembolism and, 562
Contralateral approach:
    antegrade, angioplasty of renal arteries and, 426–427
    for fibrinolytic therapy, 483–484, *485*
Contralateral puncture, for angioplasty, 386, *387*, 388
Contrast injection, dissection of intima by, 456, *456*
Contrast medium:
    extravasation of
        bleeding from gastric mucosa and, 50
        hemoptysis and, 200, *201*
    reaction to, 460, 562
Controllable-tip guidewire, for removal of intravascular foreign bodies, 493
Cook deflecting handle, 10
Coronary angioplasty, 384
Coronary catheter, right, for percutaneous nephrostomy, 515, *515*
Coronary ischemia, vasopressin infusion and, 70
Corticosteroids:
    hemangiomas and, 247
    vascular tumors and, 267

Coumarin derivatives, venous thromboembolism and, 563
Crohn's disease:
    colonic, 93
    in small intestine, 70
Curling's ulcer, 50
Cyproheptadine, in hepatic metastatic endocrine tumors, 152
Cystine renal stones, 540
Cystitis, irritating, catheters and, 523

DAVMs (*see* Dural arteriovenous malformations)
Deep venous thrombosis, 562–563, *563*
    treatment of (*see* Vena cava filters)
Dehydration, as complication of angioplasty, 460
Desilet-Hoffman-type angiographic sheath, for removal of intravascular foreign bodies, 492, *493–494*
Detachable balloons, 23, *23–24*, *24*
    arteriovenous fistulas and, 249, *249*
    bleeding secondary to trauma and, 30
    carotid cavernous fistulas and, 253, *256*, 256–257, *257*
    hemorrhage secondary to pancreatitis and, 175
    hepatic artery aneurysms and, 141, *143–144*
    hepatic hemangiomas and, 149
    introduction of, 23–24
    latex, in carotid cavernous fistulas, *256*, 256–257, *257*
    portal hypertension and, portosystemic encephalopathy created by shunts and, 129
    pseudoaneurysms and, 222–223
    pulmonary arteriovenous fistulas and, 31
    renal arteriovenous malformations and, 39, *41–42*
    splenic artery aneurysm embolization and, 172, *172*
    visceral arteriovenous fistulas and, 31
Diabetes, as risk factor for renal hypertension, 412
Dialysis, arteriovenous fistulas for, 452, *452–453*
Diazepam:
    for biliary drainage, 306
    for percutaneous nephrostomy, 511
Digital angiography, hemoptysis and, 200, *202*, *202–204*
Digital ischemia, subclavian arterial stenosis and occlusion and, 443, *444*, 445, *445*
Dilatation, of growing vessels, 464
Dilatation balloons:
    for angioplasty, 390–392, *391–392*
    (*See also* Balloon dilatation)
Dilatation force, circumferential stress and, 398–399, *399*
Dipyrone, postembolization pain and, splenic embolization and, 169
Distal branch artery, angioplasty of, 437, 439, *440–441*, 442
Disulfiram silicon coagulant, 27
Diuresis, pyonephrosis and, 516, *519*
Diverticula, colonic, 84–86, *86–87*
Diverticulitis, 68

Dormia basket:
  for extraction of ureteral calculi, 541, *542–543*
  percutaneous lithotripsy and, 373
  for removal of intravascular foreign bodies, 493
Dormia stone basket, 348, *348–350*, 349, 351
Dormia-type catheter, percutaneous nephrostomy and, 531
Dotter's coaxial system, 383, *383*
Drainage, percutaneous, of abdominal collections (*see* Percutaneous drainage)
Duodenal ulcer(s), 55, 57–59, *57–60*
  diagnosis of, 51, 53
Duodenum, perforation by catheter, 341
Dura mater, 22–23
  in hepatic metastatic endocrine tumors, 152
Dural arteriovenous malformations (DAVMs), 284–285, *285–286*, 287, 287t, *288*

Electrocardiography, renal hypertension and, 413
Electrocoagulation, transarterial, 28
Electrohydraulic lithotripsy, 373
Embolectomy, percutaneous transluminal pulmonary, 574, *574*
Embolism:
  cerebral, during angioplasty of internal carotid arteries, 446
  peripheral, during angioplasty, 445
  pulmonary (*see* Pulmonary embolism)
Embolization, 17–39, 137–300
  angiomatosis and, 246
  arteriovenous fistulas and, 238, 242, *244–246*
    therapeutic approach to, 246–247
    treatment and, 247–250, *249*
  arteriovenous malformations and, 236, *237–243*
    therapeutic approach to, 246–247
    treatment and, 247–250, *249*
  with bleeding from pelvic organs, 216–217
    anatomic considerations and, 216
    complications of, 217, *217–219*
    technique for, *216*, 216–217
  bronchial (*see* Embolization, thoracic, hemoptysis and)
  chemoembolization and, 29–30
  complications of, 31–32, *32–42*, 34, 37, 39
    bleeding from pelvic organs and, 217, *217–219*
    gastroesophageal varices and, 133–134, *134*
    pulmonary arteriovenous fistulas and, 195
  ferromagnetic, 29
  of gastroesophageal varices, complications from, 133–134, *134*
  of head and neck lesions, 251–300
    angiomatous lesions and, 260–287, *264–266*, 267t, *268–286*, 287t, *288*
    traumatic arteriovenous fistulas and, *251–259*, 251–260, *261–263*
    tumors and, 289–300, *289–301*
  in hemangiomas, 234, 234t, *235–236*
    therapeutic approach to, 246–247
    treatment and, 247–250, *249*

hemobilia and, 340
  due to pseudoaneurysm, 339, *342*
hepatic
  complications of, 152–153
  contraindications for, 152
inadvertent, *38–40*, 39
in liver, 138–156, *139*
  bleeding from hepatic tumors and, 149, *151*
  chemoembolization of hepatic neoplasms and, 156, *157–165*
  hemangiomas and, 147, *148–150*, 149
  hepatic arterial embolization and, 153, 155–156, *156*
  hepatic artery aneurysms and hemobilia and, 138, *140–144*, 141
  hepatic neoplasms and, 153
  intraarterial infusion of chemotherapeutic agents and, 153
  metastatic endocrine tumors and, 152–153, *154–155*
  traumatic, congenital, and tumoral arteriovenous fistulas and, 144–145, *144–147*
lower gastrointestinal bleeding and, 70, *71–73*, 92
  abscesses and, 96
  complications of, 86, *87*
  diverticula and, 86, *87*
  neoplastic, 91, *91–92*
  postoperative, 95–96
  stress ulcers and, 93, *96*
  superselective, 70, *71*, 80, 82, *83*, 89, *90*
materials for, 17–30, 18t
  bleeding from pelvic organs and, 217
  chemoembolization and, 29–30
  coil baffle and modified guidewire and, 29
  coiled silk threads and, 29
  in dural arteriovenous malformations, 287
  ferromagnetic embolization and, 29
  in hepatic metastatic endocrine tumors, 152
  intermediate-term, 18–19, *19*
  iodinated contrast material and, 29
  long-term, 19–28, *20–29*
  protrusion into internal carotid artery, 39, *40*
  reflux into vessels, *33*, 34
  short-term, 17–18
  splenic embolization and, 169
  Terbal and, 29, *30*
in pancreas, 174–176
  functional pancreatic tumors and, *175*, 175–176
  hemorrhage secondary to pancreatitis and, *174*, 174–175
portal hypertension and, 102, 104
  hepatic cirrhosis and, 113, 116, *118, 119*, 119–120, 121
  portal vein obstruction and, 110
  portosystemic encephalopathy created by shunts and, 129
renal, 177–190
  hypertension of renal origin and, 190, *190*
  renal hematuria of nontumoral origin and, 181–182, *181–189*, 185
  renal tumors and, 177, *178–179*

selective
  bleeding from gastric mucosa and, 49, *50*
  colonic diverticula and, 86, *87*
  colonic ulcerations and, 93, *96*
  hepatic arteriovenous fistulas and, 145, *147*
  hepatic hemangiomas and, 147, *148–150*, 149
splenic, 167–172
  partial, in hypersplenism, 167–169
  portal hypertension and, 131, *132*, 133, *133*
  splenic artery aneurysms and, 172, *172*
  in trauma cases, 169–172, *171*
superselective
  angiodysplasia and, 89, *90*
  dural arteriovenous malformations and, 287
  functional pancreatic tumors and, *175*, 175–176
  hemangiomas and arteriovenous malformations and, 248–250, *249*
  hepatic artery aneurysms and, 141
  intracerebral arteriovenous angiomas and, 260
  lower gastrointestinal bleeding and, 80, 82, *83*
  splenic, 168
  in upper gastrointestinal bleeding, 64, *65*
techniques for, selection of, 137–300
therapeutic uses of, 30–31
  aneurysms and, 31
  arteriovenous malformations and, 31
  bleeding secondary to trauma and, 30
  gastrointestinal bleeding and, 30
  hemoptysis and, 30–31
  intraabdominal extraluminal hemorrhage and, 30
  neoplastic bleeding and, 30
  pulmonary arteriovenous fistulas and, 31
  visceral arteriovenous fistulas and, 31
thoracic, 192–209
  hemoptysis and, 195–196, *197–207*, 198, 198t, 200, 202, 205, *208–209*
  postsurgical thoracic bleeding and, 195, *196*
  pulmonary arteriovenous fistulas and, 192, *192–194*, 194–195
  pulmonary sequestration and, *208*, 209
traumatic and aneurysmal lesions and, 221–223, *224–225*
  abdominal organs and, 221–222
  of extremities, 222, *223–224*
  pelvic, 222
tumoral lesions in soft tissues and bones and, 227
  technique of, 227, *228–232*
upper gastrointestinal bleeding and, 59, 60–65, *61–62*, *64–66*
  duodenal ulcer and, 57–59, *57–60*
  from gastric mucosa, 51, *52*
  gastric ulcer and, 53–54, *53–56*
  selective, 49, *50*
  superselective, 64, *65*
varicocele and, 211–215
  anatomic considerations and, 211–212, *211–213*

Embolization (*Cont.*):
  results with, 215
  technique for, 212, *214*, 215
  (*See also* Percutaneous transhepatic embolization)
Encephalopathy, portosystemic, created by shunts, 128–129, *129–133*, 131, 133
Endoprostheses, 305, 322–323, *322–325*, 326
  in metastatic disease of porta hepatis, 334
  occlusion of, 323, 336, *337–340*, 339
  placement of, 326–328, *328–333*, 332
  types of, 322–323, *324–325*
Endoscopic sclerosis:
  in esophageal varicose bleeding, 101
  in portal hypertension, hepatic cirrhosis and, 115
Endoscopic sphincterotomy, 373
Endoscopy:
  differential diagnosis of gastric and duodenal ulcers and, 51, 53
  gastrointestinal bleeding and, portal hypertension and, 101
  upper gastrointestinal bleeding and, 46, 48
Endourology, 501
Enteric fistulas, intraperitoneal abscesses and, *600–601*, 601
Enterostomy, percutaneous, 601
Epistaxis, 296–300
  angiographic protocol and embolization of, 296, 300, *300–301*
Ethanolamine oleate (Ethanolin), 27–28, *28*
  hemangiomas and arteriovenous malformations and, 248
  varicocele and, 215
Ethibloc gel, 19
Exchange catheter technique, 10, *11*
Exophthalmos, 234, 251
Extracorporeal shock wave lithotripsy (ESWL), 376–379, 377t
  patient selection for, 376–378, 378t
  principles of, 376
  results with, 378–379, *380*
  technique for, 378, *379*
Extravasation:
  angiographic identification of, 48–49, *49*
  of contrast medium
    bleeding from gastric mucosa and, 50
    hemoptysis and, 200, *201*
Eyelid, tumors of, 234, 267, *268*

Fascia lata, as embolization material, 27
Fascia of Gerota, 502, *503*
Fascia of Zuckerchandl, 502
Femoral approach, 1, 5
  for angioplasty, 385–386, *385–389*
    axillary approach versus, 390
    of brachial artery, 446
    of mesenteric vessels, 447
    of renal arteries, 394
    of subclavian artery, 445
  carotid cavernous fistulas and, 256–257
  intraarterial infusion of chemotherapeutic agents and, 153
  for removal of intravascular foreign bodies, 492
  splenic embolization and, 168
  varicocele and, 212, *214*

Femoral artery:
  angioplasty of, 433, *434–439*, 435, 437
  antegrade puncture of, 2, *2*
  recanalization of, 384
  retrograde puncture of, 2, *2*
Fentanyl:
  control of pain during embolization by, 32
  for percutaneous nephrostomy, 511
Ferromagnetic embolization, 29
Fever, embolization and, 32
  splenic, 169
Fibrinolytic agents:
  reaction to, 460
  types of, 479
Fibrinolytic therapy, *486–489*
  angioplasty and, 437
  clinical indications for, 479–480, *480–483*
  contraindications for, 480
  fibrinolytic agents and, 479
  for peripheral vascular disease, 479–485
  regional, 485
  treatment with, 481, 483–484, *484–485*
Fibromuscular disease, supraaortic vessels and, 445
Fibromuscular dysplasia:
  angioplasty of renal arteries and, 395
  mesenteric arterial stenosis and, 446–447, 449
  renal artery stenosis caused by, 402, 403t, *404–408*, 405–406, 409, *410*
    adventitial periarterial fibroplasia and, 406, 409, *410*
    branch involvement and, 409
    focal fibromuscular dysplasia and, 405–406
    intimal fibromuscular dysplasia and, 402, *405*
    multifocal medial fibromuscular dysplasia and, 402, 405, *407*
    subadventitial (perimedial) fibroplasia and, 406, *408*
Fibroplasia, medial, angioplasty of renal arteries and, 395
Flow artifacts, upper gastrointestinal bleeding and, 59, *60–65*, 61–62
Fluids and electrolytes, splenic embolization and, 169
Fluoroscopy:
  identification of catheter position by, 5
  percutaneous drainage guided by, 603
Forceps technique, for removal of intravascular foreign bodies, 493
Foreign bodies, intravascular, percutaneous retrieval of (*see* Intravascular foreign bodies, percutaneous retrieval of)
Fractures, pelvic, 222
Fungus ball, in lung cavity, 209

Gallbladder:
  ablation of, 373, 376
  carcinoma of, 334
  necrosis of, hepatic embolization and, 152–153
Gallbladder sclerotherapy, 376
Gallstones, stone dissolution agents and, 370–374

oral bile salts as, 370
  topical, 370–374
Gangrene, occlusive diseases and, 385
Garamycin (*see* Gentamicin)
Gastric artery:
  left
    embolization of, 54
    vasopressin infusion into, 64
  vasopressin infusion into, 53, 64
Gastric mucosa, bleeding from, 49–51, *51–52*
  treatment of, 49, 50
Gastric ulcer, 51, 53, *53–56*, 54
  diagnosis of, 51, 53
Gastroduodenal artery:
  embolization of, 57, *57*, *60–62*, 61
  vasopressin infusion into, 64
Gastroepiploic artery, embolization of, 54
Gastrointestinal bleeding:
  occult, fibrinolytic therapy and, 484
  portal hypertension and, 101–134
    complications from percutaneous transhepatic portography and embolization of gastroesophageal varices and, 133–134, *134*
    extrahepatic presinusoidal, 105–110, *105–110*
    hyperkinetic, 103–104, *104–105*
    intrahepatic, 112–121, *113–122*
    intrahepatic presinusoidal, 110–112, *111–112*
    portosystemic encephalopathy caused by shunts and, 128–129, *129–133*, 131, 133
    postsinusoidal, 121–128, *123–127*
  (*See also* Lower gastrointestinal bleeding; Upper gastrointestinal bleeding)
Gastrointestinal malfunction, arteriovenous fistulas and, 242, *246*
Gel, Ethibloc, 19
Gelfoam, 17–19, *19*
  bleeding from pelvic organs and, 217
  duodenal ulcer and, 57, *57*, 58
  epistaxis and, 300, *301*
  gastric ulcer and, 54
  gastrointestinal bleeding and, 30
  hemangiomas and arteriovenous malformations and, 248
  hemoptysis and, 200
  hemorrhage secondary to pancreatitis and, 174–175
  hepatic hemangiomas and, 147, 149
  hepatic metastatic endocrine tumors and, 152
  lower gastrointestinal bleeding and, 70, 72, 92
    postoperative, 96
  meningiomas and, 289
  nasopharyngeal angiofibromas and, 292
  paragangliomas and, 295
  postembolization fever and, 32
  postembolization pain and, 32
  pseudoaneurysms and, 222
  reflux into aorta, 34
  renal tumors and, 177
  splenic embolization and, 169, 172
  traumatic lesions of abdominal lesions and, 221–222

Gelfoam (*Cont.*):
  tumoral lesions in soft tissue and bones and, 227
  upper gastrointestinal bleeding and, 66
General anesthesia, percutaneous lithotripsy and, 557
Genetic factors, as risk factors for renal hypertension, 411
Gentamicin (Garamycin):
  for percutaneous nephrostomy, 511
  prophylactic, for biliary drainage, 306
Giant-cell malignant tumors, 227
Giant coils, 21, 29
Gianturco-Anderson-Wallace coils, 19–22, *20–22*
Gianturco coils, 17, 21–22
  aneurysms and, 31
  arteriovenous fistulas and, 249, *249*
  bleeding from pelvic organs and, 217
  duodenal ulcer and, 58, *59*
  epistaxis and, 300, *301*
  giant, 29
  hemorrhage secondary to pancreatitis and, 175
  hepatic artery aneurysms and, 141
  hepatic hemangiomas and, 149
  hepatic tumors and, 155, *156*
  intraabdominal extraluminal hemorrhage and, 30
  intraarterial infusion of chemotherapeutic agents and, 153
  percutaneous removal of, 34
  portal hypertension, portosystemic encephalopathy created by shunts and, 129, *130*
  pseudoaneurysms and, 222–223
  pulmonary arteriovenous fistulas and, 195
  pulmonary sequestration and, *208*, 209
  reflux into aorta, *33*, 34
  renal hematuria of nontumoral origin and, 182, *184*, 185, *185*, *187–189*
  splenic artery aneurysm embolization and, 172, *172*
  splenic embolization and, 172
  traumatic lesions of abdominal lesions and, 221–222
  tumoral lesions in soft tissue and bones and, 227
  visceral arteriovenous fistulas and, 31
Gianturco Z-stent:
  bile duct reconstruction and, 362, *363*
  self-expandable, dilatation of benign biliary stenoses and, 359
Glucose (50%), 27–28, *28*
Granuloma(s), lethal midline, of small intestine, 80, *82*
Granulomatosis:
  lymphomatoid, of small intestine, 80, *82*
  Wegener's, 99
    simulation by ischemic ulcerations, 80
    vasculitis and, 74
Granulomatous hyperproliferative disease, colonic, 90
Greenfield filter, 566, 574
  retrieval of, 566, 569
Guidewire(s):
  Amplatz, ureteral obstructions and, 544
  arterial perforation by, 456

Bentson-type, angioplasty or renal arteries and, 395, *396*
controllable-tip, for removal of intravascular foreign bodies, 493
deflecting, 10, *11*
dissection of intima by, 456, *456*
for internal-external biliary drainage, *319*, 314–318
introducing, *3*, 3–4, *4*
Lunderquist
  for percutaneous nephrostomy, 515, *515*
  ureteral obstructions and, 543–544
modified, 29
resistance to, 3
Sos, 11–12
Terumo, ureteral obstructions and, 543
Günther filter, 569, 572–573, *572*

HA (*see* Hepatic abscesses)
Heart, renal hypertension and, 412
Heart failure, due to high output, arteriovenous fistulas and, 242, *245*
Hemangioendothelioma(s), hepatic, in children, 149
Hemangioma(s), 234, 234t, *235–236*
  angiomatosis and, 246
  capillary, 233–234
  cavernous, 234, 267
  in children, 247
  hepatic, 147, *148–150*, 149
  terminology for, 233, 233t
Hemangiopericytoma(s), 296, *299*
Hematochezia, upper gastrointestinal bleeding and, 45
Hematoma, as complication of angioplasty, 455, *455*
Hematoma(s), axillary punctures and, 1
Hematuria:
  as complication of percutaneous nephrostomy, 535
  fibrinolytic therapy and, 484
  renal, of nontumoral origin, 181–182, *181–189*, 185
Hemicolectomy, right, in angiodysplasia, 89, *90*
Hemobilia, 62, 64
  as complication of biliary drainage, 339
  hepatic artery aneurysms and, embolization and, 138, *140–144*, 141
Hemodynamics:
  angioplasty and, 460
  pulmonary angiography and, 562
  renal artery stenosis and, 402
Hemolymphangioma(s), 281
Hemoptysis, 195–196, *197–207*, 198, 198t, 200, 202, 205, 208–209
  embolization in, 30–31
  pulmonary sequestration and, *208*, 209
  recurrence of, 208–209
Hemorrhage (*see* Bleeding)
Hemorrhoidal arteries, superior, embolization of, 91, *91–92*
Hemostatic gelatin (*see* Gelfoam)
Heparin:
  reaction to, 460
  stone dissolution and, 371
  venous thromboembolism and, 563

Heparinization:
  catheterization and, 1
  fibrinolytic therapy and, 483, 485
  intraarterial infusion of chemotherapeutic agents and, 153
Hepatic abscesses (HA), percutaneous drainage of, 582–583, 586, *587–595*, 588, 591, 594
Hepatic artery(ies), 138, 307
  accidental puncture of, 134, *134*
  aneurysms of, embolization and, 138, *140–144*, 141
  common, vasopressin infusion into, 64
  embolization of, 153, 155–156, *156*
  intraarterial infusion of chemotherapeutic agents and, 153
  ligation of, in bleeding from hepatic tumors, 149
  vasopressin infusion into, 64
Hepatic cirrhosis, portal hypertension and, 112–113, *113–122*, 115–116, 118–119, 121
Hepatic fibrosis, congenital, 112, *112*
Hepatic veins, 308
Hepatic venography, with manometry, 103
Hepatitis, portal hypertension and, 102
Hepatitis B virus, hepatocarcinomas and, 153
Hepatocarcinoma(s):
  hepatitis B virus and, 153
  infusion and embolization of, 153
Hepatoma(s), infusion and embolization of, 153
Hereditary hemorrhagic telangiectasis (HHT), 92, *94–95*, 192, 195, 246, 284
High-dose routine, for fibrinolytic therapy, 483, *484*
Hook-tip catheter, for removal of intravascular foreign bodies, 493
Hunter balloon, 564
Hydration, for biliary drainage, 306
Hyperlipidemia, as risk factor for renal hypertension, 412
Hypernephroma(s), 177
Hyperplastic polyps, 98, *98–99*
Hypersplenism:
  partial splenic embolization in, 167–169
  portal hypertension and, 129, 131, *132*, 133, *133*
Hypertension:
  portal (*see* Portal hypertension)
  of renal origin, 190, *190*
  renovascular (*see* Renovascular hypertension)
Hyperuricemia, as risk factor for renal hypertension, 412
Hypogastric artery(ies):
  anastomosis with, in renal transplants, 416–417
  angioplasty of, 448–449, *450*
  embolization of, 216, 222
  posterior branch of, occlusion of, 217
Hypotension, as complication of angioplasty, 460

IBC (*see* Bucrylate)
Iliac artery(ies):
  angioplasty of, 384

Iliac artery(ies): (Cont.):
  simultaneous angioplasty of distal arteries and, 429, 430–431
  stents in, 464, 464
Iliac occlusion, angioplasty and, 427–428, 428–429
Iliac stenosis, angioplasty and, 423, 424–427, 426–427
Immune system, splenectomy and, 170
Immunosuppressive states, hypersplenism related to, 167
Impotence, radicular artery occlusion and, 217, 217
Infantile capillary hemangiomas, 233
Infection:
  hemangiomas and, 234
  resistance to, spleen and, 169–170
Inferior vena cava, thrombosis of, 563
Inflammatory diseases:
  colonic, 93, 95
  of small intestine, 70
Insulinoma(s), control of hormone secretion by, 175, 175–176
Intercostal arteries, embolization of, 208
Intestinal loops, abscesses in, 600, 603
Intestinal varices, 82, 84
Intima:
  dissection of perforation of, by guidewire or contrast injection, 456, 456
  dissection or perforation of, 2, 3
  rupture of, 456
Intimal fibrosis:
  renal artery stenosis caused by, 402, 405
  venous angioplasty and, 452, 452
Intraperitoneal abscesses, percutaneous drainage of, 600–603, 600–603
Intrarenal abscesses, 531
Intravascular foreign bodies:
  causes of, 491–492
  percutaneous retrieval of, 491–499, 499
    coaxial technique for, 496, 497–498
    contraindications for, 497
    difficulties with, 496, 498
    Dormia basket for, 493
    forceps technique for, 493
    materials and results with, 492, 492
    modified snare technique for, 493, 496, 497
    snare technique for, 492–493, 493–496, 497, 499
Intravascular stents, 462–465
  current use and clinical application of, 464, 464–465, 465
  stent types and, 462–463, 463
Intravenous pyelography (IVP), renal hypertension and, 413
Intravenous urography, intrarenal and extrarenal collections and, 531
Iodinated contrast medium, 29
Ipsilateral antegrade approach, for fibrinolytic therapy, 481
Iridium-192 wire, brachytherapy in cholangiocarcinoma with, 360–361
  technique for, 360, 360–361, 361
Irrigation, extraction of ureteral calculi and, 540
Ischemia:
  coronary, vasopressin infusion and, 70

digital, subclavian arterial stenosis and occlusion and, 443, 444, 445, 445
myocardial, renal hypertension and, 412
rest, Kensey catheter and, 468
ulcerations and
  colonic, 89–90
  of small intestine, 80, 81–82
Isobutyl-2-cyanoacrylate (see Bucrylate)
Isodose calculation, for brachytherapy with iridium-192 wire, 360, 360
Isotope renography, renal hypertension and, 413
Ivalon, 22, 22
  carotid cavernous fistulas and, 260
  hemangiomas and arteriovenous malformations and, 248
  hemoptysis and, 30–31, 200
  hepatic hemangiomas and, 147
  hepatic metastatic endocrine tumors and, 152
  lower gastrointestinal bleeding and, 70, 72, 92
  nasopharyngeal angiofibromas and, 292
  neoplastic bleeding and, 30
  renal tumors and, 177
  tumoral lesions in soft tissue and bones and, 227
  vascular malformations of head and neck and, 271
IVP (see Intravenous pyelography)

Judkins-type left coronary catheter, for removal of intravascular foreign bodies, 493, 496, 497
Jugular approach, in varicocele, 215

K-G filter, 565–566, 565–571
Kasabach-Merritt syndrome, 234, 236, 248
  vascular tumors and, 267
Kensey catheter, percutaneous lithotripsy and, 373
Kensey dynamic angioplasty catheter, 467–469, 468–470
  complications with, 469, 470
Kensey-Nash device, percutaneous lithotripsy and, 373
Kidney, embolization of (see Embolization, renal)
Kidney(s):
  anatomy of, 502–508
    position and location of kidneys and, 502, 502
    renal beds, fasciae, and renal spaces and, 502–504, 503–504
    topographic relationships of kidney and, 504, 504–505
    vascular supply and, 507–508, 508–510
  (See also headings beginning with term Renal)
Kidney transplantation, renal artery percutaneous transluminal angioplasty and, 415–417, 416–417
  technique for, 416–417
Kimray-Greenfield (K-G) filter, 565–566, 565–571, 573
"Kissing balloons" technique, 419–420, 420–421

Klatzkin's tumor, biliary drainage and, 328, 332, 332–333, 334, 335
Klippel-Trenaunay syndrome, 246

Laser lithotripsy, 374
Latex detachable balloons, 23, 23, 24, 24
Leiomyoma(s), of small intestine, 74–75
Leiomyosarcoma(s), of small intestine, 75, 77–78, 79
Lethal midline granuloma, of small intestine, 80, 82
Leukosis, chronic myeloid, 99
Lidocaine (Xylocaine), for percutaneous drainage, 603
Lipiodol, 25
  arteriovenous fistulas of face, neck, and scalp and, 260, 263
  meningiomas and, 289
Lithiasis:
  residual stones and (see Common bile duct, extraction of residual stones from)
  urinary (see Ureteral stones)
Lithotripsy:
  electrohydraulic, 373
  extracorporeal shock wave lithotripsy and (see Extracorporeal shock wave lithotripsy)
  laser, 373
  mechanical, 373
  nephrolithotripsy and, 512
  percutaneous (see Percutaneous lithotripsy)
  ultrasonic, 374
Liver:
  embolization in (see Embolization, in liver)
  (See also headings beginning with term Hepatic)
Lower gastrointestinal bleeding, 68–98
  acute, massive, 68
  chronic
    massive intermittent, 68
    small-volume, 68
  embolization in, 70, 71–73
  related to colon, 84–99
    abscesses and, 96
    adenomatous, villous, and hyperplastic polyps and, 96, 98, 98–99
    angiodysplasia and, 86, 88–89, 88–90
    arteriovenous malformations and, 92, 93–95
    diverticula and, 84–86, 86–87
    inflammatory diseases and, 93, 95
    ischemic ulcers and, 89–90
    postoperative, 95–96, 97
    stress ulcers and, 93, 96
    tumors and, 90–91, 91–92
  related to small intestine, 70–84
    arteriovenous malformations and, 80, 82, 83
    inflammatory disease and, 70
    intestinal varices and, 82, 84
    ischemic ulcerations and, 80, 81–82
    nonspecific ulcerations and, 70, 74, 74–75
    postoperative, 84, 85

Lower gastrointestinal bleeding,
  related to small intestine, (Cont.):
    tumors and, 74–75, 77–80, 79
    vasculitis and, 74, 76
    vasoconstrictor infusion in, 68–70, 69
Lunderquist guidewire:
  internal-external biliary drainage and, 314
  for percutaneous nephrostomy, 515, *515*
  ureteral obstructions and, 543
Lung cavity, fungus ball in, 209
Lymphangioma(s), 281
Lymphomatoid granulomatosis, of small intestine, 80, *82*
Lymphoproliferative disorders, vasculitis and, 74
Lyodura:
  in carotid cavernous fistulas, 260
  nasopharyngeal angiofibromas and, 292

Malignant fibrous histiocytoma(s), 227
Mallory-Weiss tears, upper gastrointestinal bleeding from, 49, *50*
Marcaine (*see* Bupivacaine)
Medi-Tech instrument, 10
Medullary lesions, embolization of intercostal arteries and, 208
Melena, upper gastrointestinal bleeding and, 45
Meningioma(s), 289, *289–290*
  embolization of, 289, *291*
Meperidine:
  control of pain during embolization by, 32
  for percutaneous nephrostomy, 511
  postembolization pain and, splenic embolization and, 169
Mesenteric artery(ies):
  inferior, in lower gastrointestinal bleeding, 68
  stenosis of, 446–447, *449*
  superior
    fistulas of, 104, *105*
    in lower gastrointestinal bleeding, 68
Mesenteric vein, superior, fistulas of, 104, *105*
Mesenteric vessels, angioplasty of, 446–448, *448–449*
Metastatic disease, of porta hepatis, 333–334
Metastatic polyps, 98, *98–99*
Methacrylate, in gallbladder ablation and cystic duct occlusion, 374
Methyl tert-butyl ether (MTBE), *371*, 371–373
  patient selection for, 371, *372*
  results with, 372, *373*
  technique for, 371–372, *374*
Methylcellulose, hepatic neoplasms and, 156, *157–165*
Meticortelone (*see* Prednisolone)
Meticorten (*see* Prednisone)
"Microcoils," 20–21
Microfistulas, 238
Mikaelsson catheter, 6, *7*
  reshaping, *7, 8*
Minicoils, 17, 20, *20*
Mitomycin C:
  chemoembolization and, 29–30
  hepatic neoplasms and, 156, *157–165*
Mitral valvuloplasty, angioplasty and, 384

Mobin-Uddin umbrella, 564–566, *572–573*
Mono-octanoin, 371
Morphine, control of pain during embolization by, 32
MTBE (*see* Methyl tert-butyl ether)
Muscle, as embolization material, 27
Myeloid leukosis, chronic, 99
Myocardial infarction:
  as complication of angioplasty, 460
  venous thromboembolism and, 562
Myocardial ischemia, renal hypertension and, 412
Myoma(s):
  colonic, 91
  of small intestine, 75

Nasopharynx, hypervascular lesions in, embolization of, 39, *39*
Needle(s):
  catheterization and, 1–2, *2*
  for percutaneous drainage, 603–604
  for percutaneous transhepatic cholangiography, 305, *307*
Neoplasm(s), 289–300
  angiographic protocol and, 289
  biliary, internal biliary drainage and, 323
  caval stenosis secondary to, 452–453
  cholangiocarcinoma and (*see* Cholangiocarcinoma)
  colonic, 90–91, *91, 92*
  embolization for control of, 17
  of gallbladder, 334
  glandular, polypoid, 96, 98
  hepatic
    bleeding from, 149, *151*
    endocrine, metastatic, 152–153, *154–155*
    hepatic abscesses differentiated from, 594, *595*
    infusion and embolization of, 153, 155–156, *156–165*
    hepatic arteriovenous fistulas and, 144–145, *146–147*
    as indication for drainage, 306
    lower gastrointestinal bleeding and, small intestine and, 74–75, 77–80, 79
    malignant, venous thromboembolism and, 562
    obstructive anuria and, 519, *520–523*, 523
    pancreatic, 334
      functional, *175*, 175–176
      renal, 177, *178–179*
    in soft tissue and bones, 227
      embolization technique for, 227, *228–232*
    vascular, 267, *268–270*
Neoplastic bleeding, embolization in, 30
  gastric bleeding and, 62, *63*
Nephretic colic, 516
Nephrolithotomy, percutaneous, 540
Nephrolithotripsy, 512
  percutaneous, 553
Nephrosclerosis, benign, renal hypertension and, 412
Nephroscopy, percutaneous nephrostomy and, 531, 535, *536–537*

Nephrostomy:
  neoplastic obstructions and, 519, *522*
  percutaneous (*see* Percutaneous nephrostomy)
  percutaneous lithotripsy and, 557
  ureteral obstruction and, 543, 551
Neuroblastoma(s), 296, *298*
Nuclear imaging, in upper gastrointestinal bleeding, 45–46
Nylon brushes, 26

Obesity, as risk factor for renal hypertension, 412
Occlusion balloons:
  catheters with, 28, *29*
  diagnostic, prevention of reflux and, 34
  renal tumors and, 177
Occlusive diseases, Fontaine's classification of, 384–385
Oliguria, vasopressin infusion and, 70
Open-curve catheter, 8, *10*
Opiate analgesics, for biliary drainage, 306
Optic nerve compression, 234
Oral bile salts, 370
Oral contraceptives, venous thromboembolism and, 562
Orbit, hemangioma in, 234
Osteosarcoma, 227
Oxidized cellulose, 19, *19*
Oxylate renal stones, 540

Pain:
  control of, during embolization, 32
  occlusive diseases and, 384–385
  postembolization, 31–32
    splenic embolization and, 169
  renal tumor occlusion and, 177
  vasopressin infusion and, 69
Palmaz stent, bile duct reconstruction and, 362
Pancreas:
  abscesses of, percutaneous drainage of, 597, *599*
  carcinoma of, 334
  embolization in (*see* Embolization, in pancreas)
Pancreatic artery:
  dorsal, 167
  transverse, 167
Pancreatic caudal artery, 167
Pancreatic phlegmon, 597
Pancreatica magna, 167
Pancreatitis:
  as complication of removal of stones from common bile duct, 354, 356
  hemorrhage secondary to, *174*, 174–175
Paraganglioma(s), 292–296
  angiographic protocol and, 293–294
  embolization of, *294–295*, 295–296
Paraplegia, venous thrombosis and, 563
Pararenal space, posterior, 504
Parkes-Weber syndrome, 246
Partial splenic embolization (PSE), 167–169
  embolization technique and, 168–169, *170*
  postembolization treatment and, 169, *171*
  preembolization treatment and, 168

Pass-over technique, for removal of intravascular foreign bodies, 496, *497–498*
PAVF (*see* Pulmonary arteriovenous fistulas)
PTCA (*see* Percutaneous transluminal coronary angioplasty)
Pelvic lesions, 222
Percutaneous biopsy, biliary, *321*, 321–322
Percutaneous cholecystostomy, *368*, 368–369, *369*
Percutaneous drainage, 577–605
  determining access route for, 603
  of hepatic abscesses, 582–583, 586, *587– 595*, 588, 591, 594
  of intraperitoneal collections, 600–603, *600–603*
  maintenance of, 604
  of pancreatic abscesses, 597, *599*
  of renal abscesses, 595, 597
  selection of materials and technique for, 604
  of splenic abscesses, 594–595, *596–598*
  of subphrenic collections, 578, *578–586*, 580, 582
  technique for, 603–604
Percutaneous enterostomy, 601
Percutaneous lithotripsy, 374, *375*, 553–557
  access and, 553, 556
  complications of, 557
  indications for, 553, *554–555*
  nephrostomy and stone extraction and, 557
  previous examinations and, 553
  track dilatation and, 556, 556–557
Percutaneous mechanical recanalization techniques, 467–478
  atherolytic reperfusion wires and, 469, 471, *471–473*
  Kensey dynamic angioplasty catheter and, 467–469, *468–470*
  transluminal extraction catheters and, 472, *474–477*, 478
Percutaneous nephrolithotomy, 540
Percutaneous nephrolithotripsy, 553
Percutaneous nephrostomy, 501–535
  complications of, 535, *538*
  indications and contraindications for, 535
  percutaneous lithotripsy and, 553
  renal anatomy and, 502–508
    position and location of kidneys and, 502, *502*
    renal beds, fasciae, and renal spaces and, 502–504, *503–504*
    renal calices and, 504–507, *506–507*
    renal vascular supply and, 507–508, *508–510*
    topographic relationships of kidney and, 504, *504–505*
  technical procedure for, 508–509, *511*, 511–535
    correction of fistulas and stenoses and, 523–524, *524–530*, 526–527
    diagnostic pyelography and, 516
    general considerations and, 508–509, *510*, 511, *511*
    intrarenal and extrarenal collections and, 531, 533, *533–534*, 535
    neoplastic obstructions and, 519, *520– 523*, 523
    nephroscopy and, 535, *536–537*
    opacifying collection system and, 511–512, *512*
    pyonephrosis and, 516, *517–519*
    renal puncture and, 512, *513–515*, 514–515
    urinary lithiasis and, 531, *532*
  technique for, translumbar, 531, *533*
Percutaneous transcatheter embolization, pulmonary arteriovenous fistulas and, *193–194*, 195
Percutaneous transhepatic cholangiography, 305, 307, *307*
Percutaneous transhepatic embolization, intestinal varices and, 82
Percutaneous transhepatic portography:
  complications from, 133–134, *134*
  in portal hypertension
    hepatic cirrhosis and, 119, *120*, 121, *121*
    portal vein obstruction and, 106, *106*
Percutaneous transluminal coronary angioplasty (PTCA), 462
Percutaneous transluminal pulmonary embolectomy, 574, *574*
Periarterial fibrosis, as complication of angioplasty, 457, *459–460*
Pericolic abscesses, 96
Perihepatic abscesses, percutaneous drainage of, 582, 591, *591–593*
Perirenal abscesses, 533, *534*, 535
Perirenal fat, 502, *503*
Peritoneum, posterior reflection of, anatomic relationships of, 503–504, *504*
PH (*see* Portal hypertension)
Phlebography:
  portal, 115–116, *115–117*
  in varicocele, 215
  venous thrombosis and, 563
Phlegmon, pancreatic, 597
Phosphate renal stones, 540
Phrenic artery, vasopressin infusion into, 64–65
Pigment stones, 370
Pigtail catheters, 6, *6–7*
  for percutaneous drainage, 604
  for removal of intravascular foreign bodies, 493
Pitressin infusion, in portal hypertension, 102
Plaque, in atrial ostium, angioplasty of renal arteries and, 395, *398*
Plasma renin, renal hypertension and, 413
Plastic-deformation stents, 463, *463*
Pleural effusion, as complication of percutaneous nephrostomy, 535
Pleural puncture, as complication of percutaneous nephrostomy, 535
Pneumothorax, as complication of percutaneous nephrostomy, 535
Poiseuille's law, flow dynamics and, 399, *399*
Polyarteritis nodosa, 99
  vasculitis and, 74
Polymorphous reticulosis, of small intestine, 80, 82
Polyp(s):
  colonic, adenomatous, villous, and hyperplastic, 96, 98, *98–99*
  of small intestine, 79
Polystyrene spheres, 26
Polyvinyl alcohol (*see* Ivalon)
Popliteal artery:
  angioplasty of, 437, 439, *440–441*, 442
  recanalization of, 384
Port wine syndrome, 246
Porta hepatis, metastatic disease of, 333–334
Portal hypertension (PH), 101–134
  complications from percutaneous transhepatic portography and embolization of gastroesophageal varices and, 133–134, *134*
  extrahepatic, presinusoidal, 105–110, *105–110*
  gastrointestinal bleeding and (see Gastrointestinal bleeding, portal hypertension and)
  hyperkinetic, 103–104, *104–105*
  hypersplenism and, 129, 131, *132*, 133, *133*, 167
  intestinal varices and, 82
  intrahepatic, 112–121, *113–122*
    postsinusoidal, 121–128, *123–127*
    presinusoidal, 110–112, *111–112*
  portosystemic encephalopathy and, caused by shunts, 128–129, *129–133*, 131, 133
  presinusoidal
    extrahepatic, 102
    intrahepatic, 102–103
    schistosomiasis and, 110
Portal radicles, 307–308
Portal vein, 138
  dilatation of, portal vein obstruction and, 108, *109–110*
  obstruction of, 105–108, *105–110*, 110
  venous angioplasty and, 452, 454
Portography:
  arterial, in portal hypertension, 103
  transhepatic
    percutaneous (*see* Percutaneous transhepatic portography)
    in portal hypertension, 110, 112, *112*, 116, 118
    portal vein obstruction and, 107, *108*
  (*See also* Splenoportography)
Portosystemic encephalopathy, created by shunts, 128–129, *129–133*, 131, 133
Portosystemic shunts, angiography and, 103
Postembolization syndrome, 31, 169
Postoperative bleeding:
  colonic, 95–96, *97*
  in small intestine, 84, *85*
Postoperative fibrosis, venous angioplasty and, 452, *453*
Postoperative fistulas, bile duct reconstruction and, 362, *364*, 365
Postoperative stenosis, as indication for drainage, 306
Prednisolone (Meticortelone), hemangiomas and, 247
Prednisone (Meticorten), hemangiomas and, 247
Proctitis, hemorrhagic, colonic ulcerations and, 93, *96*
PSE (*see* Partial splenic embolization)
Pseudoaneurysm(s), 62, 64, 222–223, *224– 225*
  adventitial laceration and, 456
  as complication of biliary drainage, 339–340, *341–342*

Pseudoaneurysm(s) (*Cont.*):
  as complication of percutaneous nephrostomy, 535
  of hepatic artery, 138, 141, *142–143*
  pancreatic, 174
  radiation-induced, 223, *225*
  renal, 181
Pseudocysts, pancreatic, percutaneous drainage of, 597, *599*
"Pseudovein," in upper gastrointestinal bleeding, 48
Pulmonary angiography:
  complications of, 562
    pulmonary embolism and, *561*, 561–562, 562t
Pulmonary arteriovenous fistulas (PAVF), 192, *192–194*, 194–195
  embolization in, 31
Pulmonary artery, dilatation of, 559, *560*
Pulmonary embolism, 559–562
  angiography and, *561*, 561–562, 562t
  percutaneous transluminal pulmonary embolectomy and, 574
  radiology of thorax and, 559, *560*
  scintigraphy and, 559, 561
  venous thrombosis with, 563
Pulmonary scintigraphy, pulmonary embolism and, 559, 561
Pulmonary sequestration, *208*, 209
Pulmonary stenosis, peripheral, angioplasty and, 384
Pulmonary system shunts, 205, *207*
Pulmonary valvuloplasty, angioplasty and, 384
Pus, in collecting system, diagnostic pyelography and, 516
PVA (*see* Ivalon)
Pyelography:
  diagnostic, 516
    urine in retroperitoneum and, 524, *535*
Pyelonephritis, chronic, hypertension of renal origin and, 190, *190*
Pyloroduodenal bleeding, vasopressin infusion and, 64
Pyonephrosis, 516, *517–519*

Race, as risk factor for renal hypertension, 411
Radiation, pseudoaneurysm induced by, 223, *225*
Radiation exposure, to operator, in percutaneous nephrostomy, 512
Radicular arteries, occlusion of, 217, *217*
Radiofrequency electrocoagulation technique (RFE), 376
Radiology, pulmonary embolism and, 559, *560*
Radiotherapy, caval stenosis secondary to, 452–453
RAPTA (*see* Renal artery percutaneous transluminal angioplasty)
Rasmussen aneurysm, 205, *206*
Recanalization (*see* Percutaneous mechanical recanalization techniques)
Rectocolitis, ulcerative, 93
Reflux, of embolization material, *33*, 34
Renal abscesses:
  cortical, 531
  percutaneous drainage of, 595, 597

Renal artery(ies):
  aneurysm of, spontaneous rupture of, 185, *187–189*
  anterior, 507, *508*
  first branch of, 507, *509*
  posterior, 507, *508*
  transluminal angioplasty of, technique for, 394–395, *394–398*
Renal artery percutaneous transluminal angioplasty, technique for, 394–395, *394–398*
Renal artery percutaneous transluminal angioplasty (RAPTA), 414–417
  basic technique of, *414*, 414–415, 415t
  indications and contraindications for, 414
  in kidney transplant recipients, 415–417, *416–417*
  technique for, 416–417
Renal artery stenosis:
  caused by arteritis, 409, *411–412*
  caused by atherosclerosis, 402, *403*
  caused by fibromuscular dysplasia, 402, 403t, *404–408*, 405–406, 409, *410*
  branch involvement and, 409
  hemodynamic effects of, 402
  measurement of, 409
Renal calices, 504–507, *506–507*
Renal capsule, 502, *503*
Renal carcinoma:
  bone metastases of, 227, *230*
  hypervascular metastases of, 296, *296–297*
Renal hypertension:
  primary, 409
  secondary, 409
Renal pelvis, anatomic relationships of, 503–504, *504*
Renal puncture, 512, *513–515*, 514–515
Renal stones, 540
  intracaliceal, 556
  percutaneous lithotripsy and (*see* Percutaneous lithotripsy)
  pyonephrosis and, 516, *517*
Rendu-Osler-Weber disease (*see* Hereditary hemorrhagic telangiectasis)
Renography, isotope, renal hypertension and, 413
Renovascular hypertension, 401–413
  clinical and laboratory evaluation of, 409–413
  clinical approach and, 412–413
  collateral circulation and, 409
  etiology of, 409
  frequency of, 402
  laboratory tests and, 413
  pathophysiology of, *401*, 401–402
  renal artery stenosis and
    caused by arteritis, 409, *411–412*
    caused by atherosclerosis, 402, *403*
    caused by fibromuscular dysplasia, 402, 403t, *404–408*, 405–406, 409, *410*
    hemodynamic effects of, 402
    measurement of, 409
  risk factors for, 409, 411–412
  target-organ involvement and, 412
  two-kidney versus one-kidney model of, *401*, 401–402
Reperfusion wires, atherolytic, 469, 471, *471–473*

Reticulosis, polymorphous, of small intestine, 80, *82*
Retrograde approach, angioplasty of renal arteries and, 423, *425*, 426, *426*
RFE (*see* Radiofrequency electrocoagulation technique)
Ring catheter, for internal-external biliary drainage, 319
Ring-McLean catheters, for percutaneous drainage, 604

Saline solutions, stone dissolution and, 371
Sarcoma(s), 227
SAs (*see* Subphrenic abscesses)
Schistosomiasis, portal hypertension and, 102–103, 110, *111*, 112, *112*
Scintigraphy:
  colonic diverticula and, 85
  pulmonary embolism and, 559, 561
Sclerosing agents, 17, 18t, 27–28, *28*
Sclerotherapy:
  of gallbladder, 376
  in hemangiomas and arteriovenous malformations, 248
Screw syringes, for angioplasty, 390, *391–392*
Sedation:
  for percutaneous lithotripsy, 557
  for percutaneous nephrostomy, 511
Seldinger technique, 1, *1*
  angioplasty and, 385
  modified, for percutaneous drainage, 604
  for removal of intravascular foreign bodies, 492
  splenic embolization and, 168
Selective embolization (*see* Embolization, selective)
Selective visceral catheter, 6, *7*
Sepsis:
  as complication of biliary drainage, 344, *345*
  embolization and, 32, 34
  ischemic ulcerations of small intestine and, 80
Septic shock, pyonephrosis and, 516
Serum creatinine, renal hypertension and, 413
Serum potassium, renal hypertension and, 413
Sex, as risk factor for renal hypertension, 411
Sexual impotence, angioplasty of hypogastric arteries and, 448–449, *450*
Shepherd hook catheter, 7, *8*
Shock, septic, pyonephrosis and, 516
Shunt(s):
  portosystemic encephalopathy created by, 128–129, *129–133*, 131, 133
  pulmonary systemic, 205, *207*
Silicon detachable balloons, 23–24
Silicon rubber, 27
Silicon spheres, 26
Silk threads, coiled, 29
Simmons catheter, 6, *7*
  angioplasty of renal arteries and, 395
  reshaping, 7–8, *8–9*
  retrograde catheterization of left duct with, 328, 330, *331*
Simon nitinol filter, 572, *573*

Sinogram, for percutaneous drainage, 604
Small intestine, lower gastrointestinal bleeding related to (see Lower gastrointestinal bleeding, related to small intestine)
Smoking, as risk factor for renal hypertension, 412
Snare technique:
  modified, for removal of intravascular foreign bodies, 493, 496, *497*
  for removal of intravascular foreign bodies, 492–493, *493–496*, 497, *499*
Sodium intake, as risk factor for renal hypertension, 412
Sodium tetradecyl sulfate, in gallbladder ablation and cystic duct occlusion, 376
Sos guidewire, 11–12
Spermatic vein, left, selective catheterization of, 212, *214*
Sphincterotomy, endoscopic, 373
Spider(s), stainless steel, 26, *26–27, 27*
Spider filter, 569
"Spiderlon," 26
"Spiderweb," in portal hypertension, Budd-Chiari syndrome and, 128
Spleen:
  abscesses of, percutaneous drainage of, 594–595, *596–598*
  embolization of (see Embolization, splenic)
  puncture of, as complication of percutaneous nephrostomy, 535
Splenectomy, 167, 169
  immune system and, 170
Splenic artery, 167
  aneurysms of, 172, *172*, 174
  embolization of, 54, *55*
  vasopressin infusion into, 64
Splenic manometry, in portal hypertension, 102
Splenic vein, increase in flow in, in portal hypertension, 103
Splenomegaly, 168, 504, *505*
Splenoportography, in portal hypertension, 102
  portal vein obstruction and, 107
  schistosomiasis and, 110, 112, *112*
Spring-loaded stents, 462–463, *463*
Stainless steel spiders, 26, *26–27, 27*
Steerable devices, 10, *11*
Stent(s):
  Gianturco Z-stent
    bile duct reconstruction and, 362, *363*
    dilatation of benign biliary stenoses and, 359
  intravascular (see Intravascular stents)
  Palmaz, bile duct reconstruction and, 362
  plastic-deformation, 463, *463*
  spring-loaded, 462–463, *463*
  thermal-memory, 462
  ureteral, ureteral obstruction and, 544, 550, *551*
Stone basket:
  Dormia-type, 348, *348–350*, 349, 351
  percutaneous lithotripsy and, 374
  modified, for extraction of ureteral calculi, 541

Stone dissolution agents, 370–373
  oral bile salts as, 370
  topical, 370–373
Stortz system, percutaneous lithotripsy and, 557
Straight-type catheter, 7
Streptokinase, 479, 484
  reaction to, 460
Stress, as risk factor for renal hypertension, 412
Stress ulcers, 50
  colonic, 93, *96*
  in small intestine, 70, 74, *74–75*
Struvite renal stones, 540
Sturge-Weber's syndrome, 246
Subclavian artery:
  angioplasty of, 443, *443–445*, 445–446
  lesions in, 222
Subphrenic abscesses (SAs), percutaneous drainage of, 578, *578–586*, 580, 582
Sulfuric ether, 370–371
Superficial segmental fistulas, 260, *263*
Superior vena cava stenosis, stents and, 464
Superior vena cava syndrome, venous angioplasty and, 452
Superselective embolization, in upper gastrointestinal bleeding, 64, *65*
Suprahepatic vein, angioplasty of, Budd-Chiari syndrome and, 128
Surgery:
  angioplasty and, 384
  bleeding from gastric mucosa and, 50–51, *51*
  colonic arteriovenous malformations and, 92
  contamination of peritoneal cavity during, subphrenic abscesses and, 578
  venous thromboembolism and, 562
Surgical exploration, in upper gastrointestinal bleeding, 46
Symmers' fibrosis, 110, 112, *112*
Syringes, angioplasty of renal arteries and, 398
Systemic artery, embolization of, *208*, 209

t-PA (see Tissue plasminogen activator)
Takayasu's arteritis, in supraaortic vessels, 445
Tantalum, 24
TEC (see Transluminal extraction catheter)
10 percent rule, 5
Terbal, 29, *30*
Terumo guidewire, ureteral obstructions and, 543
Tetracycline, in gallbladder ablation and cystic duct occlusion, 373, 376
Thermal-memory stents, 462
Thoracic embolization (see Embolization, thoracic)
Thoracotomy, hemoptysis and, 195
Thrombocytopenia, 234, *236*, 248
Thrombocytopenic purpura, 234, *236*
Thrombosis:
  deep venous, 562–563, *563*
  of portal vein, portal hypertension and, 121, *122*
Thyroid tumors, 296, *298*

TIA (see Transient ischemic vascular attacks)
Tibiofibular truncus, dilatation of, 439, *441*, 442
Tissue plasminogen activator (t-PA), 479
Tissue sclerosing agents, 27–28, *28*
Toldt's fascia, 502
Track dilatation, percutaneous lithotripsy and, *556*, 556–557
Tracker catheter, 12
Transarterial electrocoagulation, 28
Transhepatic needle puncture, 369
Transhepatic percutaneous portography, with manometry, 102
Transient ischemic vascular attacks (TIA), 446
Transjejunal percutaneous biliary dilatation, 357, 359
Transluminal extraction catheter (TEC), 472, *474–477*, 478
Transplanted patients:
  renal hematuria of nontumoral origin and, 185
  ulcers in
    colonic, 93, *96*
    in small intestine, 70, 74, *74–75*
Trauma, 221–222
  of abdominal organs, 221–222
  bleeding secondary to, embolization in, 30
  of extremities, 222, *223–224*
  pelvic, 222
  splenic embolization in, 169–172, *171*
Trifluoroacetic acid, in gallbladder ablation and cystic duct occlusion, 373, 376
Trigonitis, irritating, 523
Trocar catheter technique, for percutaneous drainage, 604
Trypsin, pancreatic pseudoaneurysms and, 174
Tuberculosis:
  hemoptysis and, 195
  inflammatory colonic disease and, 93
Tumoral necrosis, biliary drainage and, 339, *341*
Tunica media, rupture of, 456
Typhoid fever, inflammatory colonic disease and, 93

Uflacker filter, 572, *572*
Ulcer(s):
  Curling's, 50
  duodenal, 55, 57–59, *57–60*
    diagnosis of, 51, 53
  gastric, 51, 53, *53–56*, 54
    diagnosis of, 51, 53
  hemangiomas and, 234
  ischemic
    colonic, 89–90
    of small intestine, 80, *81–82*
  stress, 50
    colonic, 93, *96*
    in small intestine, 70, 74, *74–75*
  uremic
    colonic, 93, *96*
    in small intestine, 70, 74, *74–75*
Ultrasonic lithotripsy, 373
Upper gastrointestinal bleeding, 45–66, *46–47*, 47
  anatomy and, 47, *47*

Upper gastrointestinal bleeding (*Cont.*):
  aneurysms and, hepatic and mycotic, 64, *64*
  angiography and, 47–49, *48*
    difficulties of interpretation and treatment and, 48–49, *49*
  duodenal ulcer and, 55, 57–59, *57–60*
  embolization in, 30
  flow artifacts and, 59, *60–65*, 61–62
  gastric mucosal, 49–51, *51–52*
  gastric ulcer and, 51, 53, *53–56*, 54
  hemobilia and, 62, 64
  from Mallory-Weiss tears, 49, *50*
  neoplastic, gastric, 62, *63*
  percutaneous embolization and, 66
  superselective embolization and, 64, *65*
  vasopressin infusion and, 64–66
Uremic ulcers:
  colonic, 93, *96*
  in small intestine, 70, 74, *74–75*
Ureteral fistulas, 523–524, *524–530*, 526–527
Ureteral obstruction, 540–551
  congenital, 551, *552*
  dilation and
    with balloon, 543–544, *545–547*
    with catheter, 544, *548–551*, 550
    congenital obstructions and, 551, *552*
    extraction of ureteral calculi and, 540–541, *541–543*
  urolithiasis and, 540
Ureteral stenoses, 523–524, *524–530*, 526–527
Ureteral stents, ureteral obstruction and, 544, 550, *551*
Ureteral stones, 526–527, *527*, 531, *532*, 540
  extraction of, 540–541, *541–543*
  pyonephrosis and, 516, *517*
Ureterolithotomy, urinary fistulas and, 523, *524*
Ureterorenoscopy, 540
Uric acid renal stones, 540
Urine:
  outside collecting system, 524, *525*, 526
  (*See also* Anuria; Hematuria; Oliguria)
Urinoma(s), 524, 526, 533–534
Urography, intravenous, intrarenal and extrarenal collections and, 531
Urokinase, 479, 483–484
  reaction to, 460
Urolithiasis, 540
Ursodeoxycholate, 370

Valvuloplasty:
  mitral, angioplasty, and, 384
  pulmonary, angioplasty, and, 384
Van Sonnenberg catheters, for percutaneous drainage, 604
Varices:
  cirrhosis and, transhepatic occlusion of, 113, *113*
  embolization of, complications from, 133–134, *134*
  secondary to noncirrhotic portal obstruction, bleeding from, 108, 110
  of small intestine, 82, *84*
Varicocele, 211–215
  anatomic considerations and, 211–212, *211–213*
  embolization technique in, 212, *214*, 215
Vas rectus, colonic diverticula and, 85–86
Vascular arcade, 61
Vascular dilatation, objectives of, 395, 398
Vascular lesions:
  of face and neck, 264, 267, 267t
  of head and neck
    malformations and, 267, 271–281, *271–281*, 281
    tumoral, 267, *268–270*
Vascular resistance, increased, portal hypertension and, 102
Vasculitis:
  colonic, 99, *99*
  of small intestine, 74, *76*
Vasoconstrictors:
  intraarterial infusion of, 17
  in portal hypertension, hepatic cirrhosis and, 113
Vasopressin:
  bleeding from gastric mucosa and, 49, *50*, 51
  colonic abscesses and, 96
  colonic diverticula and, 86
  colonic ulcerations and, 93, *96*
  duodenal ulcer and, 57, *57*, 59
  gastric ulcer and, 53
  gastrojejunal postgastrectomy anastomoses and, 84
  ischemic colonic ulcers, 90
  portal hypertension, hepatic cirrhosis and and, 113
  upper gastrointestinal bleeding and, 61–62, 64–66
  complications of, 66

  routine for, 65–66
  solution for, 65
  vasculitis and, of small intestine, 74, 76
Vena cava:
  inferior, thrombosis of, 563
  superior
    stenosis of, stents and, 464
    superior vena cava syndrome and, venous angioplasty and, 452
Vena cava filters, 563–573
  Amplatz, 569
  bird's nest, 569
  complications with, 566, 569
  Günther, 569, 572
  indications for, 564
  overview of, 572–573
  percutaneous transluminal pulmonary embolectomy and, 574
  results with, 572, 573t
  Simon nitinol, 572, *573*
  types of, 564–566, *565–571*
  Uflacker, 572, *572*
Vena tech, 573
Venotomy, for removal of intravascular foreign bodies, 492, *495*
Venous angioplasty, 452, *452–453*, 454
Venous ligation, venous thromboembolism and, 563–564
Venous thromboembolism, 562–563, *563*
  treatment of (*see* Vena cava filters)
Vertebral artery, angioplasty of, 446
Vertebrojugular fistulas, 260
Vertebrovertebral fistulas, 260
Visceral arteriovenous fistulas, embolization in, 31

Wall hyperemia, in inflammatory disease of small intestine, 70
Waltman's cobra loop, 8
Wedged sinusoidal pressure, 103
Wegener's granulomatosis, 99
  simulation by ischemic ulcerations, 80
  vasculitis and, 74
Wolf system, percutaneous lithotripsy and, 557

Xylocaine (lidocaine), for percutaneous drainage, 603